Histopathology
of the
Skin

6
TH EDITION

**445 Light Microscopic Illustrations
with 8 in Color, and
50 Electron Microscopic Plates**

Histopathology of the Skin

Walter F. Lever, M.D.

Professor Emeritus of Dermatology
Tufts University School of Medicine;
Associate in Dermatology
New England Medical Center;
Honorary Dermatologist
Massachusetts General Hospital
Boston, Massachusetts

Gundula Schaumburg-Lever, M.D.

Assistant Professor of Dermatology
Tufts University School of Medicine;
Associate in Dermatology
New England Medical Center;
Associate in Dermatology
St. Elizabeth Hospital
Boston, Massachusetts

J. B. Lippincott Company
PHILADELPHIA
London · Mexico City · New York ·
St. Louis · São Paulo · Sydney

Sponsoring Editor: Darlene D. Pedersen
Manuscript Editor: Martha Hicks-Courant
Indexer: Ruth Elwell
Art Director: Maria S. Karkucinski
Designer: Patrick Turner
Production Supervisor: N. Carol Kerr
Production Assistant: J. Corey Gray
Compositor: Monotype Composition Company, Inc.
Printer/Binder: Halliday Lithograph

The authors and publisher have exerted every effort to ensure that drug selection and dosage set forth in this text are in accord with current recommendations and practice at the time of publication. However, in view of ongoing research, changes in government regulations, and the constant flow of information relating to drug therapy and drug reactions, the reader is urged to check the package insert for each drug for any change in indications and dosage and for added warnings and precautions. This is particularly important when the recommended agent is a new or infrequently employed drug.

6th Edition

3 5 6 4

Library of Congress Cataloging in Publication Data

Lever, Walter F.
  Histopathology of the skin.

  Bibliography: p.
  Includes index.
  1. Skin—Diseases.   2. Histology, Pathological.
I. Schaumburg-Lever, Gundula.
II. Title. [DNLM: 1. Skin diseases—Pathology.
WR 105 L659h]
RL95.L48   1983   616.5'07   82-13994
ISBN 0-397-52095-6

Preface

With each new edition, the size of this book has increased. This is understandable, because, in the years since 1949, when the first edition was published, the amount of knowledge in dermatopathology has greatly increased. This increase has also been quite impressive during the 8 years that have passed since publication of the previous edition.

The primary purpose in writing this new edition has been to bring up to date the histologic findings and the histogenesis of each dermatosis. Even though the histogenesis, like the clinical introduction, is printed in small print, the information contained in it concerning electron microscopy, histochemistry, and immunology is regarded as important for an adequate understanding of the histologic findings in most dermatoses.

The following are examples of recent progress made in the field of diagnostic histopathology: (1) the recognition of the existence of two types of parapsoriasis en plaques, a small plaque and a large plaque type; (2) the description of the dysplastic nevus syndrome, providing new evidence of the capability of melanocytic nevi to transform into malignant melanoma and thus illustrating the difficulty that may arise in deciding whether a melanocytic lesion is benign or malignant, particularly when the clinical data are inadequate; (3) the Breslow measurement of the thickness of melanomas, which has proved valuable, particularly in combination with Clark's levels, in determining the prognosis of stage I melanoma; and (4) the continued usefulness of the Rappaport classification of lymphoma when correlated with the terms and concepts of the more "modern" classifications of Lukes and Collins and of Lennert.

Examples of advances based on the correlation of histologic and laboratory findings are (1) the subdivision of cryoglobulinemia into a monoclonal and a mixed type with different histologic manifestations; (2) the identification of linear IgA bullous dermatosis as an entity; (3) the recognition of the different origins of the amyloid in the three types of amyloidosis: immunoglobulin light chains in primary systemic amyloidosis, serum amyloid A in secondary systemic amyloidosis, and tonofilaments in lichenoid and macular amyloidosis; and (4) recognition of the important role played by Langerhans cells in the histogenesis of allergic contact dermatitis and mycosis fungoides.

In addition to bringing the book up to date on the dermatoses that were already described in the fifth edition, we have included about 100 dermatoses that were not previously described. About half of them are "new" dermatoses that were either unknown or not fully established as entities when the fifth edition was written. The other half are dermatoses that were already known but were regarded as too rare to be included. However, in order to make this edition not only a textbook but also a book of reference, it was decided to include them. A list of these "new" and "newly included" dermatoses follows.

The bibliography following each chapter has been brought up to date with deletion of some of the older references. As in previous editions, references in English have been given preference, since they will be understood by all readers of the book, but references in French or German regarded as important have also been included.

Because of a significant increase in the volume of the text, it was decided, with regret, to add only a few light microscopic illustrations and not to increase the number of electron microscopic plates.

Walter F. Lever, M.D.
Gundula Schaumburg-Lever, M.D.

"New" Diseases

(listed in order of discussion)

Transient neonatal pustular melanosis
Acropustulosis of infancy
Graft-versus-host disease
Mucocutaneous lymph node syndrome
  (Kawasaki's disease)
Keratosis lichenoides chronica
Pustulosis acuta generalisata
Lymphomatoid granulomatosis
Angioimmunoblastic lymphadenopathy
Sinus histiocytosis with massive lymph-
  adenopathy
Glucagonoma syndrome
Intestinal bypass syndrome
Hypereosinophilic syndrome
Histiocytic cytophagic panniculitis
Eosinophilic pustular folliculitis
Eosinophilic cellulitis (Wells' syndrome)
Minocycline pigmentation
Penicillamine-induced elastosis
  perforans serpiginosa
Perforating calcific elastosis (periumbilical
  perforating pseudoxanthoma elasticum)
Annular elastolytic granuloma
Bowenoid papulosis of the genitalia
Oral focal epithelial hyperplasia
Verruciform xanthoma
Necrobiotic xanthogranuloma with
  paraproteinemia
Congenital self-healing reticulohistiocytosis
Progressive nodular histiocytoma

Eosinophilic fasciitis
Eruptive vellus hair cysts
Necrotizing sialometaplasia
Eosinophilic ulcer of the tongue
Sebaceous trichofolliculoma
Pilar sheath acanthoma
Multiple fibrofolliculomas
Multiple trichodiscomas
Desmoplastic trichoepithelioma
Multiple trichilemmomas in Cowden's disease
Trichilemmocarcinoma
Torre's syndrome of multiple sebaceous
  tumors
Tubular apocrine adenoma
Mucinous syringometaplasia
Malignant eccrine spiradenoma
Trabecular carcinoma (Merkel cell carcinoma)
Cranial fasciitis of childhood
Arteriovenous (venous) hemangioma
Intravascular papillary endothelial hyper-
  plasia (Masson's pseudoangiosarcoma)
Folded skin with lipomatous nevus (Michelin-
  tire baby)
Spindle cell lipoma
Pleomorphic lipoma
Cutaneous cartilaginous tumor
Acral lentiginous melanoma, in situ or invasive
Dysplastic nevus syndrome (B-K mole
  syndrome)
Cutaneous extramedullary hematopoiesis

"Newly Included" Diseases

(listed in order of discussion)

Acrokeratoelastoidosis
Linear melorheostotic scleroderma
Winchester syndrome
Cutaneous cholesterol embolism
Sclerosing lymphangitis of the penis
Actinic prurigo
Subcutaneous fibrosis after megavoltage
    radiotherapy
Subcutaneous dirofilariasis
Schistosomiasis
Subcutaneous cysticercosis
Erythema chronicum migrans
Acanthoma fissuratum
Blastomycosislike pyoderma (pyoderma
    vegetans)
Malakoplakia
Rocky Mountain spotted fever
Cutaneous protothecosis
Cutaneous alternariosis
Lobomycosis
African histoplasmosis
Botryomycosis
Plaquelike mucinosis (reticular erythematous
    mucinosis)
Oculocutaneous tyrosinosis
Reticulated pigmented dermatosis of the
    flexures
Mixed connective tissue disease
Leser–Trélat sign
Bronchogenic and thyroglossal duct cysts

Cutaneous ciliated cyst
Median raphe cyst of the penis
Verrucous carcinoma
Dilated pore
Trichoadenoma
Erosive adenomatosis of the nipple
Carcinoma of the inframammary crease
Bazex syndrome with multiple basal cell
    epitheliomas
Multiple perifollicular fibromas
Giant cell tumor of tendon sheath
Congenital generalized fibromatosis
Fibrous hamartoma of infancy
Juvenile hyalin fibromatosis
Malignant fibrous histiocytoma
Unilateral nevoid telangiectasia
Smooth muscle hamartoma
Cutaneous endosalpingiosis
Umbilical omphalomesenteric duct polyp
Storiform neurofibroma
Pacinian neurofibroma
Pseudomelanomatous changes in
    melanocytic nevi (after incomplete
    removal)
Melanonychia striata
Dermal melanocyte hamartoma
Generalized melanosis in metastatic melanoma
Lennert's lymphoma
Woringer–Kolopp disease
Macroglobulinemia of Waldenström

Preface to the First Edition

This book is based on the courses of dermatopathology which I have been giving in recent years to graduate students of dermatology enrolled at Harvard Medical School and Massachusetts General Hospital. The book is written primarily for dermatologists; I hope, however, that it may be useful also to pathologists, since dermatopathology is given little consideration in most textbooks of pathology.

I have attempted to keep this book short. Emphasis has been placed on the essential histologic features. Minor details and rare aberrations from the typical histologic picture have been omitted. I have allotted more space to the cutaneous diseases in which histologic examination is of diagnostic value than to those in which the histologic picture is not characteristic. In spite of my striving for brevity I have discussed the histogenesis of several dermatoses, because knowledge of the histogenesis often is of great value for the understanding of the pathologic process.

Primarily for the benefit of pathologists who usually are not too familiar with dermatologic diseases, I have preceded the histologic discussion of each disease with a short description of the clinical features.

A fairly extensive bibliography has been supplied for readers who are interested in obtaining additional information. In the selection of articles for the bibliography preference has been given, whenever possible, to those written in English.

I wish to express my deep gratitude to Dr. Tracy B. Mallory and Dr. Benjamin Castleman of the Pathology Laboratory at the Massachusetts General Hospital for the training in pathology they have given me. It has been invaluable to me. Their teaching is reflected in this book. Furthermore, I wish to thank Mr. Richard W. St. Clair, who with great skill and patience produced all the photomicrographs in this book.

Walter F. Lever
1949

Contents

5

Morphology of the Cells in the Dermal Infiltrate   47

6

Congenital Diseases (Genodermatoses)   57

7

Noninfectious Vesicular and Bullous Diseases   92

8

Noninfectious Erythematous, Papular, and Squamous Diseases   136

9

Vascular Diseases   164

Systemic Diseases with Cutaneous Manifestations   190

10

Inflammatory Diseases of the Epidermal Appendages and of Cartilage   198

11

Inflammatory Diseases Due to Physical Agents and Foreign Substances   211

12

13

Noninfectious Granulomas   229

14

Inflammatory Diseases of the Subcutaneous Fat   245

15

Eruptions Due to Drugs   259

16

Degenerative Diseases   271

17

Bacterial Diseases   290

18

Treponemal Diseases   320

19

Fungal Diseases   328

20

Diseases Caused by Protozoa   356

21

Diseases Caused by Viruses   360

25

Connective Tissue Diseases 445

26

Tumors and Cysts of the Epidermis 472

27

Tumors of the Epidermal Appendages 522

28

Metastatic Carcinoma and Carcinoid   590

29

Tumors of Fibrous Tissue   597

30

Tumors of Vascular Tissue   623

31

Tumors of Fatty, Muscular, and Osseous Tissue   652

32

Tumors of Neural Tissue   667

33

Melanocytic Nevi and Malignant Melanoma   681

34

Lymphoma and Leukemia   726

COLOR PLATES

Histopathology
of the
Skin

Introduction

1

TECHNIC FOR BIOPSY

Four technics can be used for obtaining a specimen for biopsy: scalpel, punch, shave biopsy, and curettage. Aside from excising lesions, scalpel biopsies often are advisable for the study of subcutaneous lesions, since it usually is not possible to obtain adequate amounts of subcutaneous tissue by punch biopsy.

Punch biopsies represent the standard procedure for obtaining specimens of skin for histologic examination. It is important to select a proper site for biopsy. In most instances, histologic examination of a fully developed lesion will give more information than examination of an early or involuting lesion. Vesicular, bullous, and pustular lesions represent exceptions to this rule. For their histologic examination, a very early lesion is required; otherwise, secondary changes (such as regeneration, degeneration, or secondary infection) may obscure essential features and make recognition of their mode of formation impossible. Generally, it is inadvisable to include normal tissue in the biopsy specimen unless a large specimen is taken or the physician personally supervises the processing of the specimen, because improper sectioning by the technician may result in only normal skin being seen in the section. If the submitted specimen is supposed to contain tumor tissue but the sections do not show it, it is advisable that deeper sections into the tissue block be carried out in the laboratory before a final report of absence of tumor tissue is rendered; if the laboratory fails to do this, the physician who submitted the specimen should request it.

The biopsy specimen should include subcutaneous fat, because, in many dermatoses, characteristic histologic features are found in the lower dermis or in the subcutaneous fat. If several lesions are present and the diagnosis hinges on the histologic findings, much time may be saved by taking specimens for biopsy from more than one lesion.

In most instances, a specimen obtained with a 4-mm biopsy punch is adequate for histologic study. Often, a specimen obtained with even a 3-mm punch is adequate. After the biopsy specimen has been loosened with the biopsy punch, it should be handled very gently and, above all, not be grasped with a forceps. It should either be squeezed manually out of its socket or be "speared" with the syringe needle that was used for injection of the local anesthetic (Ackerman, 1975). Scissors may then be used to cut through the subcutaneous fat at the base of the specimen. After use of the 3-mm punch, no suturing is required except on the face; application of a "butterfly tape" to approximate the wound edges and over it a "Band-Aid" type of tape is sufficient. Whenever sutures are used, insertion of two sutures is preferable, since one suture may become loose.

Shave biopsies should be employed only for lesions in which characteristic histologic changes are expected to be present in the epidermis or the upper dermis. This includes seborrheic keratoses,

1

solar keratoses, verrucae, benign nevi, and basal cell epitheliomas. Shave biopsies obviously are inadequate for differentiating between squamous cell carcinoma and keratoacanthoma, and they are contraindicated if there is even the slightest suspicion of malignant melanoma because determination of the depth of penetration is of great importance. To carry out a shave biopsy, one raises the skin as a fold and cuts with the scalpel parallel to the skin surface. This method has the advantage of leaving the lower portion of the dermis intact so that, immediately afterwards, lesions such as nevi and basal cell epitheliomas can be fully removed by curettage with or without electrodesiccation. (It is not recommended that a curettage be performed immediately after a punch biopsy, because this will result in a deep scar at the site of the biopsy. Rather, one should wait to perform curettage for about 2 months.)

Curettage is the least satisfactory method for obtaining material for histologic examination, because the submitted material usually is scanty and superficial in location and has lost its architecture. If this method is used, the most satisfactory specimen obtainable by curet is one taken by a single, firm stroke; however, even so, fragmentation and distortion cannot be avoided (Bart and Kopf, 1979).

As fixative, 10% formalin in aqueous solution can be used in nearly all instances (see p. 42). However, if the specimen is to be mailed in winter, 10% aqueous formalin, which freezes at $-11°$ C, may allow the formation of ice crystals in the specimen. This causes damage and distortion in the specimen, particularly in epithelial cells, and thus makes adequate histologic evaluation impossible. Freezing can be prevented by the addition to the formalin of 95% ethyl alcohol, 10% by volume (Ackerman, 1978).

If any special stains are desired, this should be indicated on the requisition sheet that is being sent to the laboratory with the specimen. If, for instance, a stain for lipids is to be carried out, the specimen must not be processed in the Autotechnicon (see Table 4-1, p. 44).

LIMITATIONS OF HISTOLOGIC DIAGNOSIS

Although histologic study is one of the most valuable means of diagnosis in dermatology, it has its limitations. Often, no definitive diagnosis can be made. Few inflammatory dermatoses are associated regularly with a diagnostic histologic picture. Instead, the histologic features may be merely suggestive of a diagnosis or may be entirely nonspecific. In cases of infectious granulomas, such as tuberculosis, leprosy, and the deep mycoses, a specific diagnosis often cannot be made unless the causative organism can be demonstrated. In some diseases of the large group of noninfectious inflammatory dermatoses, such as lichen planus and lupus erythematosus, the histologic picture, although diagnostic in most instances, may be merely suggestive, especially in cases in which the clinical picture is not typical. In other noninfectious inflammatory dermatoses, such as psoriasis, the histologic picture is rarely diagnostic. Similarly, in subacute and chronic dermatitis, the histologic findings generally are nonspecific and resemble those seen also in other dermatoses, such as pityriasis rosea, prurigo simplex, and the small plaque type of parapsoriasis en plaques. Nevertheless, when the histologic picture is not diagnostic, correlation of the histologic with the clinical findings frequently makes a diagnosis possible.

In the case of tumors, difficulties in diagnosis may also arise. For instance, distinction of squamous cell carcinoma from pseudocarcinomatous hyperplasia or from keratoacanthoma is not always possible. Similarly, distinction between malignant melanoma and a Spitz nevus (formerly called benign juvenile melanoma or spindle and epithelial cell nevus), or between lymphoma and pseudolymphomas, such as lymphocytoma cutis or lymphomatoid papulosis, may be exceedingly difficult and is occasionally impossible.

It is obvious that the histopathologist can give the clinician a maximum amount of information only if every specimen submitted for histologic diagnosis is accompanied by detailed clinical information, including a differential diagnosis.

BIBLIOGRAPHY
ACKERMAN AB: Biopsy: Why, where, when, how. J Dermatol Surg 1:21–23, 1975
ACKERMAN AB: Histologic Diagnosis of Inflammatory Skin Diseases, pp 149–155. Philadelphia, Lea & Febiger, 1978
BART RS, KOPF AW: Techniques of biopsy of cutaneous neoplasms. J Dermatol Surg Oncol 5:979–987, 1979

Embryology of the Skin

2

THE EPIDERMIS

Keratinocytes. The youngest human embryos in whom the skin has been examined histologically were 5 to 6 weeks old, with a crown-to-rump length of 14 mm (Breathnach and Robins; Holbrook and Odland). At this stage, the epidermis in a few areas still consists of only a single layer of ectodermal cells. However, in most areas, there already are two layers, the basal cell layer, or stratum germinativum, and, above it, the periderm layer.

When the fetus reaches the age of 10 weeks (crown-to-rump length, 5 cm), another row of cells, the stratum intermedium, forms between the two layers through upward movement of cells of the basal cell layer. The cells of the periderm are large and protrude into the amniotic cavity. Because of the large size of its cells, the periderm layer accounts for approximately one half of the epidermal thickness. At 19 weeks (length, 17 cm), there are two to three layers of intermediate cells, and the cells of the periderm begin to flatten (Fig. 2-1). At

Fig. 2-1. The skin of an embryo 5 months old
The epidermis consists of three layers: the stratum germinativum (*S.G.*), the stratum intermedium (*S.I.*), and the periderm (*P*). Two primary epithelial germs (*P.E.G.*) are shown. The fetal dermis shows many more fibroblasts than the adult dermis. (×400)

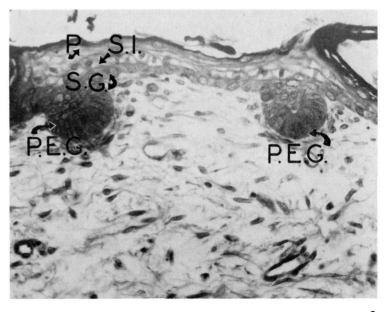

23 weeks (length, 19 cm), keratinization has taken place in the upper cell layer of the stratum intermedium, and small keratohyaline granules are apparent in the subjacent cells. The cells of the periderm have largely been shed, leaving only fragments of degenerated periderm cells above the keratinized cells of the newly formed stratum corneum (Holbrook and Odland).

Histogenesis. On *electron microscopic examination,* embryos 6 to 7 weeks of age show immature desmosomes between the epidermal cells but no tonofilaments as yet; and, although a distinct basement membrane is seen, half-desmosomes either are absent or are just beginning to appear (Hashimoto et al; Matsunaka and Mishima). The surface of the cells of the periderm shows indentations and numerous microvilli, providing a large area of exposure to the amniotic fluid. This, together with the presence of numerous cytoplasmic vesicles within the periderm cells, suggests an active exchange between the periderm cells and the amniotic fluid (Breathnach). When the fetus is 14 weeks old, numerous desmosomes connect the cells of the epidermis, but few tonofilaments are apparent. At 16 weeks, however, dense accumulations of tonofilaments are present in the cells of the intermediate layer as evidence of beginning keratinization (Holbrook and Odland).

Melanocytes.   The appearance of melanocytes in the epidermis takes place in a craniocaudal direction, in accordance with the development of the neural crest, from which the melanocytes are derived. By use of light microscopy on sections that have been either treated with impregnation by Masson's ammoniated silver nitrate technic or exposed to the dopa reaction, melanocytes can be identified in the epidermis of the head region during the latter part of the third fetal month,

Neural Crest [handwritten margin note]

whereas, in the more caudal body regions, the earliest formed melanin can be observed only in the latter part of the fourth month. Since melanocytes are functionally immature during their migration through the fetal dermis, they cannot be identified by histochemical methods until they have reached the epidermis (Becker and Zimmermann).

Histogenesis. *Electron microscopy* has led to an earlier recognition of melanocytes in the epidermis than is possible by light microscopy. At 6 weeks, the first obvious nonkeratinocytes are present in the epidermis (Breathnach and Robins). Such cells are distinguishable from keratinocytes by the absence of desmosomal attachments and a greater cytoplasmic density. However, since the characteristic cytoplasmic organelles are still absent, a decision as to whether these cells are "primordial" melanocytes or Langerhans cells is not possible. Melanocytes with recognizable melanosomes may be seen in the epidermis of feti at a gestational age of 8 to 10 weeks (Sagebiel and Odland). Synthesis of melanin within the melanosomes occurs on the head in the latter part of the third month and elsewhere in the fourth month (Holbrook). Langerhans cells that contain the characteristic cytoplasmic granules are present at 14 weeks (Breathnach and Wyllie).

THE EPIDERMAL APPENDAGES

The embryonal stratum germinativum, or basal cell layer, differentiates not only into basal cells, which give rise to the keratinizing epidermis, but also into hair germs, also called primary epithelial germs, which give rise to the hair, sebaceous glands, and apocrine glands, and into eccrine gland germs, which give rise to the eccrine glands (Chart 2-1).

Chart 1. Embryology of the Epidermis

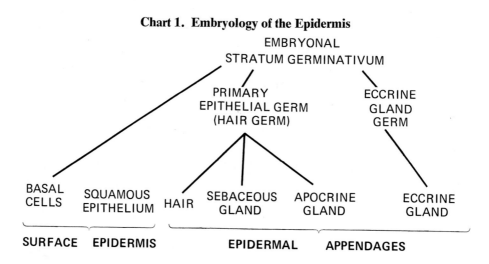

EMBRYONAL STRATUM GERMINATIVUM

PRIMARY EPITHELIAL GERM (HAIR GERM)

ECCRINE GLAND GERM

BASAL CELLS   SQUAMOUS EPITHELIUM   HAIR   SEBACEOUS GLAND   APOCRINE GLAND   ECCRINE GLAND

SURFACE EPIDERMIS   **EPIDERMAL   APPENDAGES**

Hair. Hair germs, or primary epithelial germs, are first observed in embryos in the eyebrow region and the scalp during the third month of gestation (Hashimoto, 1970a). The general development of hair begins in the fourth fetal month in the face and scalp and gradually extends in a cephalocaudal direction. Thus, during the fourth month, while some hair follicles on the head are already well matured and are producing hair, most of those on the trunk are barely differentiated (Serri et al). In addition, new primary epithelial germs keep developing between earlier ones so that, in any section obtained from the beginning of the fifth month up to birth, hair structures in different stages of development are found (Mishima and Widlan).

Hair germs, or primary epithelial germs, in their earliest stage of development consist of an area of crowding of deeply basophilic cells in the basal cell layer of the epidermis. Subsequently, the areas of crowding develop into buds that protrude into the dermis (Fig. 2-1). Beneath each bud lies a group of mesenchymal cells from which the dermal hair papilla is later formed. As the primary epithelial germ grows deeper into the dermis under induction by the underlying mesenchymal cells, it forms first the hair peg and then, as the hair matrix cells and the dermal hair papilla develop, the bulbous hair peg (Pinkus).

As the bulbous peg stage is reached, differentiation occurs in the lower and upper portions of the hair follicle as well as in the overlying epidermis. Differentiation in the lower portion of the follicle leads to the formation of the hair cone and subsequently to the formation of the hair, the cuticle, and the two inner root sheaths. The hair canal in the upper portion of the hair follicle, located at the level of the upper dermis, is formed by the premature death of the central core cells before they have become keratinized. In contrast, the intraepidermal portion of the hair canal is produced by means of premature keratinization and subsequent dissolution of the matrix cells of the cordlike hair canal extending obliquely through the epidermis. By the time the hair cone has reached the upper portion of the hair follicle, the hair canal is already open within the dermis and epidermis (Hashimoto, 1970c).

The hair follicles grow at a slant and, in the late hair peg or early bulbous stage, develop two or three bulges on their undersurface. The lowest of the three bulges develops into the attachment for the arrector pili muscle, whereas the middle bulge differentiates into the sebaceous gland. The up-permost bulge develops into the apocrine gland; however, the apocrine bud does not develop on all hair follicles but only on those located in certain regions (see p. 22) (Hashimoto, 1970b).

In sections treated with the dopa reaction or stained with ammoniated silver nitrate, melanocytes are distributed at random in primary epithelial germs and in hair pegs. During the bulbous peg stage, the melanocytes concentrate in the so-called pigment matrix region, that is, in the basal cell layer lying on top of the dermal hair papilla, and, to a lesser degree, in the lower hair bulb located lateral to the dermal hair papilla (Mishima and Widlan).

Histogenesis. *Electron microscopic examination* of hair germ buds and hair pegs of the embryo has revealed that relatively large cytoplasmic processes extend like pseudopodia from their basal cells through breaks in the basement membrane into the dermal mesenchyme. The mesenchymal cells that are concentrated beneath the hair germs are in contact with the basement membrane of the hair germs either directly, or indirectly through various types of fibrils. Also, the mesenchymal cells are connected to each other through desmosomelike cell-to-cell contacts (Hashimoto, 1970a). These morphologic findings suggest that the "hair germ mesenchymal cells" provide a force pulling down the hair germ as they move deeper in the dermal mesenchyme.

Formation of the intraepidermal portion of the hair canal through cellular destruction is found on electron microscopy to be associated with the presence of lysosomelike dense bodies. Thus, the intraepidermal portion of the hair canal seems to form by lysosomal digestion of cellular cytoplasm analogous to the formation of the intraepidermal eccrine duct and of the intrafollicular apocrine duct (see below) (Hashimoto, 1970c).

Sebaceous Glands. The development of sebaceous glands from the middle bulge of hair follicles begins on the scalp and face in the fourth month of fetal life. Their development, like that of the hairs, spreads caudad. By the time of birth, the sebaceous glands are considerably larger than they are in infancy and contribute their secretion to the vernix caseosa (Serri et al).

Apocrine Glands. Apocrine glands develop only in certain areas (see p. 22). Wherever they form, they develop from the upper bulge of hair follicles that are in the early bulbous peg stage and show a hair cone. The formation of apocrine glands thus begins late in the fourth month and continues until late in embryonic life as long as new hair follicles develop. In the earliest stage, a solid epithelial cord projects into the perifollicular mesenchyme at a right angle to the long axis of the hair follicle and then grows downward past the developing sebaceous gland and arrector pili bulge. By the time the tip of the epithelial cord has reached the level of the sebaceous gland, the intradermal ductal lumen begins to form, as does the intrafollicular lumen (Hashimoto, 1970b). At the time of birth, there is as yet no recognizable myoepithelial layer of cells around the secretory portion of the apocrine glands (Serri et al).

Histogenesis. *Electron microscopic examination* shows that the apocrine dermal duct forms through separation of apposing luminal cells. In contrast, the intrafollicular lumen forms through lysosomal formation of intracytoplasmic vacuoles in neighboring cells and subsequent extracytoplasmic coalescence of these vacuoles (Hashimoto, 1970b). The formation of the intrafollicular portion of the apocrine duct is analogous to the formation of the intraepidermal portion of the eccrine duct. (See below for a more detailed description.)

Eccrine Glands.   Eccrine glands are present in mammals, with the exception of anthropoid apes, only on the soles. Their presence in other parts of the skin in humans thus is a late development from the phylogenetic point of view. Accordingly, the eccrine glands develop in humans earlier on the palms and soles than elsewhere. On the palms and soles, eccrine gland germs are first seen in 12- to 13-week-old embryos (Hashimoto et al, 1965). In the early part of the fifth fetal month, they develop in the axillae, and, near the end of the fifth month, they begin to appear over the remainder of the body (Serri et al). The eccrine gland germs begin as areas of crowding of deeply basophilic cells in the basal layer of the epidermis. They differ from primary epithelial germs only slightly by being narrrower and by showing fewer mesenchymal cells at their base. Like hair follicles, eccrine glands may be seen at one time in different stages of development. Thus, in embryos 16 weeks old, some eccrine glands are already beginning to form coils on the palms and soles, while new eccrine gland germs are still forming in the epidermis (Hashimoto et al, 1966). At 16 weeks, both intraepidermal and intradermal lumina begin to form on the palms and soles.

At the time of lumen formation, the intradermal duct as well as the secretory segment show a wall composed of two layers of cells, an inner layer of luminal cells and an outer layer of basal cells. Whereas the dermal duct continues to consist of these two layers of cells throughout life, the two layers in the secretory segment undergo differen-

tiation: the luminal cells differentiate into tall, columnar secretory cells extending from the basement membrane to the luminal border, while the basal cells differentiate either into secretory cells or into myoepithelial cells, which appear as pyramidal, relatively small cells wedged at the base between secretory cells (Hashimoto et al, 1966). The differentiation into secretory and myoepithelial cells in the secretory segment is well advanced on the palms and soles of embryos 22 weeks old. At the time of birth, the appearance of the eccrine glands resembles that of adult eccrine glands.

Histogenesis. On *electron microscopic examination,* the embryonic lumen formation occurring in the eccrine dermal duct and in the secretory segment differs from the lumen formation occurring in the intraepidermal portion of the eccrine duct. (This difference exists also in the apocrine gland, in regard to which it is discussed briefly in the first column on this page.)

In the eccrine dermal duct, lumen formation results from a separation of desmosomes between apposing luminal cells and the subsequent formation of microvilli at the luminal surfaces. In the secretory portion, lumen formation also begins with the separation of luminal cells from one another and is followed by the appearance of numerous small secretory vesicles and dense secretory granules in the secretory cells (Hashimoto et al, 1966).

In the intraepidermal portion of the eccrine duct, intracytoplasmic vacuoles form through lysosomal action within the inner cells of the intraepidermal eccrine duct units. These vacuoles enlarge, coalesce, and break through the plasma membrane. Through coalescence with similarly produced vacuoles from adjoining inner cells, a patent extracellular lumen is formed. After formation of the lumen, the intraepidermal eccrine duct unit undergoes keratinization, the outer cells at the level of the midsquamous layer and the inner cells at the level of the stratum granulosum (Hashimoto et al, 1965).

THE DERMIS

The dermis of a 2-month-old embryo consists of loosely arranged mesenchymal cells that are embedded in ground substance. During the third month, argyrophilic reticulum fibers appear. As these fibers increase in number and in thickness, they arrange themselves in bundles that no longer can be impregnated with silver and, instead, stain with the methods for collagen (Montagna). Simultaneously, the mesenchymal cells develop into fibroblasts. The skin of the human fetus contains a large percentage of type III collagen, in contrast to the skin of the adult, which contains a large proportion of type I collagen (Stenn) (p. 31).

Elastic fibers appear in the dermis at 22 weeks, much later than the collagenous fibers. At this time, acid orcein stains show elastic tissue in the reticular dermis either as granular material interspersed with occasional short fibers or as a delicate network of branching fibers. As gestation progresses, elastic fibers increase in quantity. At 32 weeks, a well-developed network of elastic fibers indistinguishable from that seen in term infants is present in both the papillary and the reticular dermis (Deutsch and Esterly).

Fat cells begin to develop in the subcutaneous tissue toward the end of the fifth month. Histologic examination at that time shows (1) spindle-shaped, lipid-free mesenchymal cells as precursor cells; (2) young-type fat cells containing two or more small lipid droplets; and (3) mature fat cells possessing one large central lipid droplet and a peripherally located nucleus, so-called signet-ring cells (Fujita et al). Although some of the cells containing multiple small lipid droplets resemble the multivacuolated mulberry cells present in brown fat and in hibernoma, they are but few in number in embryonic white fat. Brown and white fat are two separate entities incapable of interconversion (Seemayer et al) (see p. 655).

Histogenesis. *Electron microscopic examination* of the fetal dermis from week 6 to week 14 reveals, apart from Schwann cells identified by their association with neuraxons, three main types of cells: (1) stellate mesenchymal cells with long processes; (2) phagocytic macrophages of probable yolk-sac origin; and (3) cells containing granules, which could be either melanoblasts or mast stem cells. From week 14 on, fibroblasts become numerous (Breathnach).

Young elastic fibers, as seen in a 22-week-old fetal dermis, show masses of peripheral microfibrils surrounding a small amorphous electron-lucent core representing elastin, with only a few internal microfibrils. As the embryo matures, the amount of elastin and the number of microfibrils within the elastin increase while the number of peripheral microfibrils decreases (Varadi).

BIBLIOGRAPHY

The Epidermis
BECKER SW, JR., ZIMMERMANN AA: Further studies on melanocytes and melanogenesis in the human fetus and newborn. J Invest Dermatol 25:103–112, 1955

BREATHNACH AS: Embryology of human skin. J Invest Dermatol 57:133–143, 1971

BREATHNACH AS, ROBINS J: Ultrastructural features of epidermis of a 14-mm (6 weeks) human embryo. Br J Dermatol 81:504–516, 1969

BREATHNACH AS, WYLLIE LM: Electron microscopy of melanocytes and Langerhans cells in human fetal epidermis at fourteen weeks. J Invest Dermatol 44:51–60, 1965

HASHIMOTO K, GROSS BG, DIBELLA RJ et al: The ultrastructure of the skin of human embryos. IV. The epidermis. J Invest Dermatol 47:317–335, 1966

HOLBROOK KA: Human epidermal embryogenesis. (Review) Int J Dermatol 18:329–356, 1979

HOLBROOK KA, ODLAND GF: The fine structure of developing human epidermis: Light, scanning, and transmission electron microscopy of the periderm. J Invest Dermatol 65:16–38, 1975

MATSUNAKA M, MISHIMA Y: Electron microscopy of embryonic human epidermis at seven and ten weeks. Acta Derm Venereol (Stockh) 49:241–250, 1969

SAGEBIEL RW, ODLAND GF: Ultrastructural identification of melanocytes in early human embryos. (Abstr) J Invest Dermatol 54:96, 1970

The Epidermal Appendages
HASHIMOTO K: The ultrastructure of the skin of human embryos. V. The hair germs and perifollicular mesenchymal cells. Br J Dermatol 83:167–176, 1970a

HASHIMOTO K: The ultrastructure of the skin of human embryos. VII. Formation of the apocrine gland. Acta Derm Venereol (Stockh), 50:241–251, 1970b

HASHIMOTO K: The ultrastructure of the skin of human embryos. IX. Formation of the hair cone and intraepidermal hair canal. Arch Klin Exp Dermatol 238:333–345, 1970c

HASHIMOTO K, GROSS BG, LEVER WF: The ultrastructure of the skin of human embryos. I. The intraepidermal eccrine sweat duct. J Invest Dermatol 45:139–151, 1965

HASHIMOTO K, GROSS BG, LEVER WF: The ultrastructure of human embryo skin. II. The formation of intradermal portion of the eccrine sweat duct and of the secretory segment during the first half of embryonic life. J Invest Dermatol 46:513–529, 1966

MISHIMA Y, WIDLAN S: Embryonic development of melanocytes in human hair and epidermis. J Invest Dermatol 46:263–277, 1966

PINKUS H: Embryology of hair. In Montagna W, Ellis RA (eds): The Biology of Hair Growth, pp. 1–23. New York, Academic Press, 1958

SERRI F, MONTAGNA W, MESCON H: Studies of the skin of the fetus and the child. J Invest Dermatol 39:199–217, 1962

The Dermis
BREATHNACH AS: Development and differentiation of dermal cells in man. J Invest Dermatol 71:2–8, 1978

DEUTSCH TA, ESTERLY NB: Elastic fibers in fetal dermis. J Invest Dermatol 65:320–323, 1975

FUJITA H, ASAGAMI C, ODA Y et al: Electron microscopic studies of the differentiation of fat cells in human fetal skin. J Invest Dermatol 53:122–139, 1969

MONTAGNA W: The Structure and Function of Skin, 2nd ed, pp 122–173. New York, Academic Press, 1962

SEEMAYER TA, KNAACK J, WANG NS et al: On the ultrastructure of hibernoma. Cancer 36:1785–1793, 1975

STENN KS: Collagen heterogeneity of skin. Am J Dermatopathol 1:87–88, 1979

VARADI DP: Study on the chemistry and fine structure of elastic fibers from normal adult skin. J Invest Dermatol 59:238–246, 1972

Histology
of the Skin

3

In histologic sections of normal skin, the border between the epidermis and the dermis is irregular because numerous cone-shaped dermal papillae extend upward into the epidermis. Even though they appear as pegs in histologic sections, the ridges of epidermis separating the papillae should be called rete ridges, not rete pegs.

KERATINOCYTES OF THE EPIDERMIS

Two types of cells constitute the epidermis: keratinocytes and dendritic cells. The keratinocytes differ from the dendritic cells, or clear cells, by possessing intercellular bridges and ample amounts of stainable cytoplasm. As they differentiate into horny cells, the keratinocytes are arranged in four layers: (1) the basal cell layer, (2) the squamous cell layer, (3) the granular layer, and (4) the horny layer (Fig. 3-1). The terms *stratum malpighii* and *rete malpighii* are often applied to the three lower layers, which contain the basal, squamous, and granular cells and comprise the nucleated, viable epidermis. An additional layer, the stratum lucidum, can be recognized in areas having a thick stratum granulosum and corneum as forming the lowest portion of the horny layer, especially on the palms and soles.

Basal Cell Layer. The basal cells form a single layer, are columnar in shape, and lie with their long axis perpendicular to the dividing line between the epidermis and the dermis. They have a deeply basophilic cytoplasm and a dark-staining oval or elongated nucleus. They are connected with each other and with the overlying squamous cells by intercellular bridges or desmosomes. These desmosomes are less distinct than those in the squamous cell layer. At their base, the basal cells are attached to the subepidermal basement membrane zone, which, however, can be demonstrated only with special stains, such as the periodic acid-Schiff (PAS) stain (see below). The amount of melanin present in the basal cells parallels skin color. In light-skinned Caucasoids, the basal cells contain only a few small melanin granules that are hardly visible with a routine hematoxylin-eosin stain, whereas, in Caucasoids with sun-tanned skin or dark complexions and in Mongoloids and Negroids, numerous distinct melanin granules are present, often with a predominant localization as supranuclear caps. (For a discussion of the transfer of melanin from melanocytes to basal cells and the autophagocytosis of melanin in basal cells, see p. 17.)

Mitotic Activity. Mitoses denoting nuclear and cellular division are found in the normal human epidermis largely in the basal cell layer. Even mitoses that appear to be located at a level above the basal cell layer often are found on serial sectioning to be in juxtaposition with a dermal papilla and thus to represent basal cells (Van Scott and Ekel). A more efficient method of determining the location of proliferating cells in the human epidermis consists of either the intradermal injection of tritiated thymidine in vivo or the incubation of skin slices with tritiated thymidine in vitro. This method labels all cells

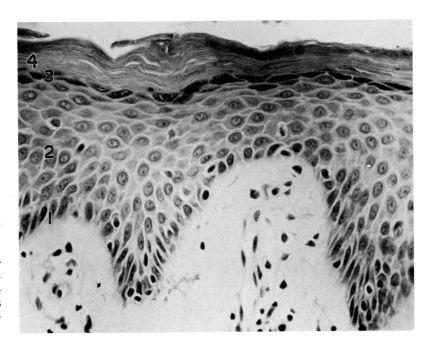

Fig. 3-1.   Normal epidermis, dorsum of hand
Four layers can be recognized: (1) basal layer, (2) squamous cell layer, (3) granular layer, and (4) horny layer. Note the presence of intercellular bridges between the basal cells. Several clear cells (melanocytes) are present in the basal layer. They possess a small, dark nucleus and clear cytoplasm. (×400)

in the S phase of DNA synthesis, which is approximately 7 times longer than the mitotic or M phase. Thus, many more tritiated-thymidine-labeled cells can be visualized than mitoses. With the labeling method, 45% of the labeled cells in normal human epidermis were found in one study to be suprabasal in location; however, after the examination of tracings of serial sections, the corrected value was 32% (Penneys et al). Accordingly, the germinative cell population in normal human epidermis can be considered to consist of 1½ cell layers.

Reproduction of Cells and Transit Through the Epidermis. The average normal epidermal germinative cell has a DNA synthesis time of 16 hr and divides approximately every 19 days (Weinstein and Frost). If it is assumed that the germinative layer is 1½ cell layers thick, it can be concluded that, once a cell has been formed, the time required for it to travel from the basal cell layer to the surface of the granular layer is probably between 26 and 42 days in normal human skin (Halprin). The passage of the horny cells through the normal horny layer has been calculated to require about 14 days, both on the basis of autoradiographs with radioactive glycine (Frost et al) and on the basis of disappearance of fluorescence from the stratum corneum after it has been permeated by a fluorescent dye (Baker and Kligman). Thus, the total epidermal renewal time is 59 to 75 days, if the reproduction time of germinal cells is presumed to be 19 days, the transit time through the stratum malpighii 26 to 42 days, and the transit time through the stratum corneum 14 days (Halprin).

The transit time of epidermal cells through the stratum malpighii varies greatly for individual cells. When the nuclei of the normal epidermis were labeled by the intradermal injection of tritiated thymidine, it was found that the labeled nuclei migrate at differing speeds, so that some of them reach the granular layer within 1 week whereas others require 6 weeks (Epstein and Maibach). This indicates that the intercellular bridges can open up and form anew, a characteristic that allows the epidermal cells to alter their size, shape, and movement. In contrast to the situation in the viable epidermis, where cells are released to pass upward in a random fashion, once they get to the stratum corneum they are tightly attached to one another and travel in unison, so that autoradiographs taken at intervals show a horizontal band of labeled protein moving upward through the stratum corneum (Weinstein; Frost et al).

Subepidermal Basement Membrane Zone. A subepidermal basement membrane zone not visible in sections stained with hematoxylin-eosin is seen on staining with the PAS stain (see p. 43). It appears as a homogeneous band, 0.5 μm to 1 μm thick, at the epidermal-dermal junction (Fig. 3-2) (Bourlond and Vandooren-Deflorenne). Its positive PAS reaction indicates the presence of a relatively large number of neutral mucopolysaccharides in this zone (Stoughton and Wells). Furthermore, impregnation with silver nitrate reveals in the uppermost dermis a meshwork of reticulum fibers (Fig. 3-2). Staining with alcian blue, which stains the band of polysaccharides as well as the reticulum meshwork, reveals that the band of polysaccharides is located above the reticulum layer (Cooper).

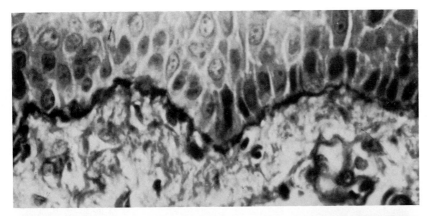

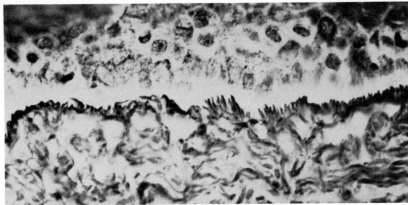

Fig. 3-2.   Subepidermal basement membrane zone
(*Top*) Periodic acid-Schiff stain shows a homogeneous band. (×400) (*Bottom*) Impregnation with silver nitrate shows a meshwork of reticulum fibers in the uppermost dermis. (×400)

The light microscopic PAS-positive subepidermal basement membrane zone appears heterogeneous on electron microscopy (see Electron Microscopy of Keratinocytes, p. 13). It must be differentiated from the electron microscopic basement membrane, or basal lamina, which is a true membrane and, being only 35 nm to 45 nm thick, is submicroscopic. Thus, the light microscopic PAS-positive basement membrane zone is on the average 20 times thicker than the electron microscopic basement membrane, or basal lamina (Bourlond and Vandooren-Deflorenne). (The factors causing the firm attachment of the epidermis to the dermis are discussed under Electron Microscopy of Keratinocytes; see p. 12.) A basement membrane zone similar to that seen at the epidermal-dermal border is present also around the cutaneous appendages.

Squamous Cell Layer.   The cells of the squamous cell layer are polygonal and form a mosaic of cells usually five to ten layers thick. They become flattened toward the surface, with their long axis arranged parallel to the skin surface (see Fig. 3-1). The cells are separated by spaces that are traversed by intercellular bridges. These intercellular spaces stain slightly with the PAS stain and with alcian blue and colloidal iron, suggesting that they contain neutral mucopolysaccharides as well as acid mucopolysaccharides (glycosaminoglycans). Pretreatment with hyaluronidase largely prevents staining with colloidal iron, indicating that hyaluronic acid (hyaluronate) is an important component of the glycosaminoglycans (Cerimele et al).

X Chromatin.   The so-called X chromatin, also called sex chromatin or Barr body, can be found in the nuclei of epidermal cells. However, as a rule, buccal scrapings are used for X-chromatin determinations. The X chromatin can be seen in sections stained with hematoxylin-eosin, although the Feulgen stain is preferable (Goldman and Goldman). The X chromatin appears as a basophilic, Feulgen-positive, planoconvex body about 1 μm in diameter flattened against the nuclear membrane. It is found in the epidermal nuclei of skin biopsy specimens in 25% to 54% of the cells in females and in 0% to 9% of the cells in males (Emery and McMillan). The observation of an X chromatin in the cells of normal males is based on artifacts resembling the X chromatin, and the observation of the X chromatin in less than 100% of the cells of normal females is explained by its location on the nuclear border at points other than the plane of sectioning (Platt and Kailin). The presence of the X chromatin is due to the fact that female cells possess two X chromosomes, in contrast to male cells, which have only one. Since only one X chromosome is utilized during mitosis, the other is inactivated and is deposited as the X chromatin during the interphase.

Granular Cell Layer. The cells of the granular layer are diamond-shaped or flattened. Their cytoplasm is filled with keratohyaline granules that are deeply basophilic and irregular in size and shape (see Fig. 3-1). The thickness of the granular layer in normal skin is proportional to the thickness of the horny layer: it is only one to three cell layers thick in areas in which the horny layer is thin but measures up to ten layers in thickness in areas with a thick horny layer, such as the palms and soles.

In the process of keratinization, the keratohyaline granules form two structures: (1) the interfibrillary matrix, which cements the keratin fibrils, or tonofibrils, together and (2) the inner lining of the horny cells, the so-called marginal band. Whereas the tonofibrils contain only small amounts of sulfur as sulfhydryl groups, the interfibrillary matrix and the marginal band contain about 10 times the amount of sulfur that is present in the tonofibrils, predominantly as disulfide bonds of cystine (Matoltsy, 1975, 1976). Consequently, the tonofibrils are soft and flexible, while the matrix and marginal band provide necessary strength and stability (Matoltsy, 1976) (for more details, see p. 13). Thus, the keratin of the epidermis represents "soft" keratin, in contrast to the "hard" keratin of the hair and nails, in which keratohyaline granules are lacking and the tonofibrils themselves harden through the incorporation of disulfide bonds (Schwarz). Whereas "soft" keratin desquamates as the result of enzymatic action (see p. 14), the "hard" keratin of the hair and nails does not, thus requiring periodic cutting.

The granular cell layer represents the keratogenous zone of the epidermis, in which the dissolution of the nucleus and other cell organelles is prepared. In contrast to the basal and squamous cell layers, in which lysosomal enzymes, such as acid phosphatase and aryl sulfatase, are present as only a few granular aggregates, there is diffuse staining for lysosomal enzymes in the granular cell layer. These diffusely staining lysosomal enzymes probably play an important role in the autolytic changes occurring in the granular layer (Lazarus

et al) (see also Electron Microscopy of the Epidermis).

Horny Layer. As a result of their abrupt keratinization, the cells of the horny layer are anuclear. The horny layer stains eosinophilic, in contrast to the underlying stratum malpighii. The thickness of the horny layer is often difficult to ascertain in formalin-fixed specimens, because some of the outer cell layers frequently detach themselves. Most of the horny layer is apt to show a basket-weave pattern in formalin-fixed specimens because of the presence of large intracellular spaces. These spaces are the result of inadequate fixation of soluble constituents within the horny cells by the formalin and the subsequent removal of these constituents by water, ethanol, and xylene during histologic processing. Thus, the portion of the cytoplasm that contains disulfide bonds of cystine has shrunk to form a shell along the cell membrane (Spearman). In contrast, glutaraldehyde fixation as used for electron microscopy causes precipitation of the formalin-soluble substances within the horny cells and allows staining of the contents of the horny cells with stains such as uranyl acetate and lead citrate. With a fluorescent staining technic, it can be shown that the cells of the horny layer are arranged in orderly vertical stacks and do not overlie each other in a random manner (Christophers).

Stratum Lucidum. In many sections fixed with formalin, the lowest portion of the horny layer appears after processing and staining as a thin homogeneous eosinophilic zone, referred to as the stratum lucidum. This zone is most pronounced in areas in which the horny layer is thick, especially on the palms and soles. The stratum lucidum differs histochemically from the rest of the horny layer by being rich in protein-bound phospholipids contained in the Odland bodies (see p. 14). It has been referred to also as the stratum conjunctum, in contrast to the overlying stratum disjunctum with its basketweave pattern (Spearman).

Oral Mucosa. With the exception of the dorsum of the tongue and the hard palate, the mucous membrane of the mouth possesses neither a granular nor a horny layer. Where these layers are absent, the epithelial cells in their migration from the basal layer to the surface first appear vacuolated, largely as a result of their glycogen content, then shrink, and finally desquamate (Fig. 3-3).

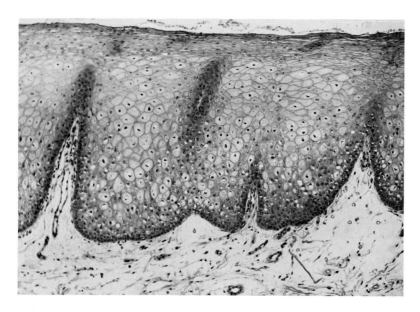

Fig. 3-3.   Epithelium of the oral mucosa
No horny layer is formed. The epithelial cells in their migration from the basal layer to the surface become vacuolated, then shrink, and finally desquamate. (×200)

Electron Microscopy of Keratinocytes. A characteristic electron microscopic feature of keratinocytes, in contrast to the dendritic cells in the epidermis, is the presence of desmosome–tonofilament complexes (EM 1).

DESMOSOME–TONOFILAMENT COMPLEXES. The tonofilaments within the cytoplasm of the keratinocytes of the stratum malpighii are loose bundles of electron-dense filaments (EM 2), each filament measuring 7 nm to 8 nm in diameter. The tonofilaments at one end are attached to the attachment plaque of a desmosome, while the other end lies free in the cytoplasm near the nucleus. The desmosomes represent the intercellular bridges (EM 3). Each desmosome possesses two electron-dense attachment plaques, one at either end, that are located in the cytoplasm of the two keratinocytes that the desmosome connects (EM 3, inset). Next to each attachment plaque lies the trilaminar plasma membrane of the two keratinocytes. Each trilaminar plasma membrane is 8 nm thick and consists of two electron-dense lines, called the inner and the outer leaflets, enclosing an electron-lucent line (EM 3, inset). In the center of the desmosome lies the intercellular cement substance (EM 3, inset), which shows greatest electron density in the portion directly adjoining the outer leaflet of the trilaminar plasma membrane representing the so-called cell surface coat (Hashimoto and Lever, 1970b). The *cell surface coat* often cannot be separated visually from the outer leaflet, and the two components have therefore been referred to also as the intermediate dense layer (Odland). The remaining central portion of the intercellular cement appears electron-lucent, except for a thin electron-dense line exactly in the center of the intercellular cement and thus also of the desmosome called the intercellular contact layer (Odland) (EM 3, inset). The irregular location of the desmosomes shows that the plasma membrane of keratinocytes is remarkably convoluted.

INTERCELLULAR CEMENT SUBSTANCE. The intercellular cement substance between adjoining keratinocytes, referred to also as glycocalyx, contains glycoproteins, which are stainable in vivo as well as in vitro with ruthenium red and with lanthanum. Staining with either of these agents often results in greater electron density along the cell surface than in the center of the intercellular space because of a higher concentration of cement substance there as cell surface coat (Wolff and Schreiner, 1968). The fact that the intercellular cement substance has a gel-like consistency explains why it on the one hand provides cohesion between the epidermal cells and on the other hand allows the rapid passage of water-soluble substances such as ruthenium red through the intercellular spaces and, furthermore, allows the opening up of desmosomes and individual cell movement (Wolff and Wolff-Schreiner).

ATTACHMENT OF BASAL CELLS TO THE DERMIS. The plasma membrane at the undersurface of basal cells shows half-desmosomes possessing only one intracytoplasmic attachment plaque to which tonofilaments from the interior of the basal cell are attached (EM 2, inset). Beneath the plasma membrane of the basal cells, a rather electron-lucent zone called the lamina lucida, 35 nm to 40 nm wide, separates the trilaminar plasma membrane, about 8 nm wide, from the medium electron-dense basement membrane, or basal lamina, 35 nm to 45 nm wide (Bourlond and Vandooren-Deflorenne). Within the electron-lucent zone, one observes beneath each half-desmosome attachment plaque and extending parallel to it a plaque 7 nm to 9 nm thick, the sub-basal cell dense plaque (EM 2, inset), which lies about 10 nm from the outer leaflet of the basal cell plasma membrane (Hashimoto and Lever, 1970a; Tarnowski). Filaments, 5 nm to 7 nm thick, called anchoring filaments, extend from the basal cell plasma membrane to the basement membrane (EM 2, inset). Filaments arising from the plasma membrane beneath the attachment plaque of a half-desmosome extend vertically to the underlying sub-basal cell dense plaque and from there to the basement membrane, whereas filaments not attached to sub-basal cell dense plaques show an irregular "criss-crossing" course from the basal cell plasma membrane to the basement membrane.

The basement membrane, or basal lamina, is 35 nm to 45 nm thick and consists of very fine filaments (EM 2, inset). Basement membranes are extracellular matrices synthesized by a variety of cells, including the basal cells of the epidermis, the capillary endothelium, and the epithelial cells of the glomerulus. They contain a procollagenlike molecule, that is, a triple-helical collagen molecule to which the nonhelical extensions at either end are still attached (see Biosynthesis and Electron Microscopy of Collagen, p. 31). The procollagenlike molecule, instead of undergoing conversion to a true collagen molecule, interacts with glycoprotein (Kefalides). The basement membrane collagen is classified as type IV collagen (Yaoita et al).

Two types of fibrous structures are found attached to the undersurface of the basement membrane: anchoring fibrils and microfibrils. Anchoring fibrils are collagen fibrils varying in thickness from 20 nm to 60 nm (EM 2, inset). They thus approach the thickness of collagen fibrils but differ from them by showing nonperiodic striation rather than a regular periodicity of 68 nm (see p. 31). The dermal end of the anchoring fibrils is difficult to determine. They seem to form an interlocking meshwork at a depth of 150 nm to 200 nm beneath the basement membrane (Briggaman and Wheeler, 1975a). Collagen fibrils are sometimes caught up in this meshwork or are surrounded by loops of anchoring fibrils (Briggaman). Besides anchoring fibrils, microfibril bundles and individual microfibrils approximately 10 nm in diameter are attached to the undersurface of the basement membrane. These microfibrils may course relatively long distances into the deeper dermis. They resemble the microfibrils that are found at the periphery of elastic fibers and thus may represent an extension of the dermal elastic tissue system (Briggaman and Wheeler, 1975b; Kobayasi, 1977). However, effective anchoring of the epidermis to the dermis is a function largely of the anchoring fibrils; elastic microfibril anchoring of the basement membrane is quite sparse (Kobayasi, 1978). As a third component, solitary collagen fibrils are present in the zone immediately beneath the basement membrane. They are randomly oriented and not attached to the basement membrane.

The PAS-positive basement membrane zone, which is 0.5 μm to 1 μm thick and thus about 20 times thicker than the basement membrane, comprises the fibrous zone immediately beneath the basement membrane. This zone stains with PAS because of its high content of neutral mucopolysaccharides (Briggaman and Wheeler, 1975a).

KERATINIZATION OF KERATINOCYTES. The number of tonofilaments increases in the upper portion of the squamous layer. The decisive change initiating keratinization occurs in the granular cells and is characterized by the appearance of keratohyaline granules (EM 4).

The earliest formation of keratohyaline granules consists of the aggregation of electron-dense ribonucleoprotein particles largely along tonofilaments. The keratohyaline granules increase in size through further peripheral aggregation of ribonucleoprotein particles, and, as they do so, surround more and more tonofilaments (Bell and Kellum). By extending along numerous tonofilaments, the keratohyaline granules assume an irregular, often star-shaped outline (EM 4) and may reach a size of 1 μm or 2 μm. After ultimately ensheathing all tonofilaments, they form in the horny cells the electron-dense interfilamentous protein matrix of mature epidermal keratin.

Keratohyaline granules are quite heterogeneous in their composition, and different methods used for their isolation have given different results. Thus, whereas some authors (Ugel; Tezuka and Freedberg) have isolated a protein component rich in histidine and low in sulfur, Matoltsy (1975, 1976) obtained a protein component rich in sulfur and with a high content of cystine. Quantitative autoradiography after injection of cystine-3H and histidine-3H provided evidence that keratohyaline granules contain both types of protein (Fukuyama and Epstein). It may be concluded that keratohyaline granules are sulfur-rich but are coated by a protein that is rich in histidine (Matoltsy, 1975). It seems well established that the tonofilaments, which constitute about 50% of horny cells, are composed of sulfur-poor alpha-keratin, whereas the matrix and the marginal band, which constitute about 45% and 5%, respectively, of horny cells, are derived from keratohyaline granules and are rich in sulfur, particularly cystine, the disulfide bonds of which give stability to horny cells.

HORNY CELLS. The transformation of granular cells into horny cells usually is abrupt. Fixation with glutaraldehyde and osmium tetroxide as used for electron microscopy preserves the internal structure of horny cells (EM 5), in contrast to formalin fixation for light microscopy (see p. 11). By electron microscopy, the cytoplasm of the cells in the lower portion of the horny layer shows relatively electron-lucent tonofilaments, about 8 nm thick, embedded in an interfilamentous substance having the same high degree of electron density as the keratohyaline granules (Brody). In the upper portions of the horny layer, however, the cells lose their filamentous structure. Together with the sudden keratinization of the horny cells, an electron-dense, homogeneous marginal band forms in their peripheral cytoplasm in close approximation to the trilaminar plasma membrane. Fully developed, the marginal band measures 16 nm in thickness, as compared with 8 nm for the trilaminar plasma membrane. Whereas in the lowermost horny layer the trilaminar plasma membrane is still preserved outside the marginal band, in the midportion of the horny layer it becomes discontinuous and then desquamates so that the marginal band serves as the real cell membrane (Hashimoto). In the uppermost portion of the horny layer, even the marginal band often disappears concomitant with the degeneration and desquamation of the horny cells. Desmosomal contacts are at first still present in the horny layer but disappear prior to desquamation of the horny cells.

ODLAND BODIES. Odland bodies, also called membrane-coating granules and keratinosomes, are small organelles that are discharged from the granular cells into the intercellular space and have two important functions: they establish a barrier to water loss, and they mediate stratum corneum cell cohesion. Odland bodies appear first in the perinuclear cytoplasm in the squamous cell layer. Higher up in the epidermis, they rapidly increase in number and size (Wolff-Schreiner). Both within and outside the granular cells, Odland bodies are round or oval, measure approximately 300 nm by 500 nm in diameter, and possess a trilaminar membrane and a laminated interior (EM 4, insets). They contain acid phosphatase, just as do lysosomes, as well as phospholipids and cholesterol sulfate. As they are extruded from the granular cells into the intercellular space (EM 4, right inset), they form densely packed lamellar masses. The lipids within Odland bodies are responsible for the appearance of a stratum lucidum in epidermis having a thickened stratum granulosum and stratum corneum (see p. 11).

An indication that the Odland bodies contribute to the physiologic water barrier was the following observation, made by Schreiner and Wolff in 1969. When these investigators injected intradermally in vivo a solution of horseradish peroxidase as an electron microscopic tracer protein, they found that it penetrated the basement membrane and the intercellular spaces of the epidermis up to the upper portion of the granular layer, where Odland bodies block the intercellular spaces. Conclusive evidence was provided by Elias and colleagues, who showed by freeze fracture techniques that the Odland bodies fuse and completely fill the intercellular spaces at the level of the granular layer. They concluded that the phospholipids formed in the Odland bodies act as hydrophobic material, which is important to the barrier function. A similar permeability barrier as seen in the epidermis exists also in the oral mucosa (Squier and Hopps).

The second function, that of providing cohesion between the cells of the lower stratum corneum, is brought about by the lipids of the Odland bodies. The action of enzymes, such as steroid sulfatase, removes the lipids from the upper stratum corneum and brings about desquamation of the cells there (Epstein et al). (For a discussion of the role of steroid sulfatase deficiency in X-linked ichthyosis, see p. 58.)

LYSOSOMES IN KERATINOCYTES. Primary lysosomes that are membrane-bound and contain a variety of hydrolytic enzymes, such as acid phosphatase, aryl sulfatase, and beta-galactosidase, are seen in small numbers within keratinocytes, largely but not exclusively in the basal cell layer and lower squamous cell layer (Wolff and Schreiner, 1970). These primary lysosomes are seen in the Golgi area, where they arise, and elsewhere in the cytoplasm. A great number of lysosomal enzymes is demonstrable also in the granular layer and in the lowermost horny layer, as already mentioned in the light microscopic description (see p. 11). However, on electron microscopic examination, only a very small proportion of these lysosomal enzymes is seen inside of primary lysosomes; most of the lysosomal enzymes are found free in the cytoplasm as irregularly shaped aggregates that are not membrane-bound (Braun-Falco and Rupec). As already discussed, lysosomal enzymes are found also in the Odland bodies, not only while they are within granular cells but also after they have been discharged into the intercellular space (Wolff and Schreiner, 1970).

In addition to primary lysosomes, some secondary lysosomes, also called phagolysosomes, are present in the lower epidermis, especially in the basal cells. They digest phagocytized melanosomes, usually as melanosome complexes. (For a detailed description, see p. 18.) In cases of epidermal injury, such as sunburn or contact dermatitis, numerous phagosomes containing cellular organelles are present in the keratinocytes, which, as the result of the influx of lysosomal enzymes from primary lysosomes, become phagolysosomes (Wolff and Schreiner, 1970).

ORAL MUCOSA. In the epithelial cells of the oral mucosa, in contrast to those of the epidermis, electron microscopic examination reveals poor development of tonofilaments. Instead of increasing, the tonofilaments diminish in number in the upper layers and become dispersed. Large aggregates of glycogen are present in the cells. The epithelial cells of the oral mucosa show only few well-developed desmosomes. Instead, they show numerous microvilli at their borders. They are held together by an amorphous, moderately electron-dense intercellular cement substance, the resolution of which causes the detachment of the uppermost cells (Hashimoto et al).

DENDRITIC CELLS OF THE EPIDERMIS

Of the three types of dendritic cells present in the epidermis, only one type, the melanocyte, can easily be identified in histologic sections stained with hematoxylin-eosin. The second type, the Langerhans cell, can be identified with certainty only with histochemical methods or by electron microscopy. The third type, the indeterminate dendritic cell, can be identified only with the electron microscope.

Melanocytes. In sections stained with hematoxylin-eosin, melanocytes appear as clear cells having a small, dark-staining nucleus and, largely as the result of shrinkage, a clear cytoplasm. They are found wedged between the basal cells of the epidermis. Although the number of melanocytes in relation to basal cells varies with the body region and increases with repeated exposure to ultraviolet light (see p. 16), the average number of clear cells in hematoxylin-eosin-stained vertical sections is 1 of 10 cells in the basal layer (Cochran). However, not all clear cells seen in routine sections necessarily are melanocytes; occasionally, basal keratinocytes show the same shrinkage artifact and then are indistinguishable from melanocytes (Clark et al). As a rule, melanocytes stain with Bloch's dopa reaction because they possess the ability to form melanin, and they stain with silver stains because they contain melanin (for details, see p. 16). The dendritic processes of melanocytes can be recognized with the dopa reaction; usually, they can also be seen on staining with silver, provided that they contain a sufficient amount of melanin (Fig. 3-4). Melanin is transferred by means of the dendritic processes from the melanocytes to the basal keratinocytes, where it is first stored and later degraded. As a rule, a greater amount of melanin is present in the basal keratinocytes than in the melanocytes. Since only about 10% of the cells in the basal layer are melanocytes, each melanocyte supplies several keratinocytes with melanin, forming with them an epidermal melanin unit (Fitzpatrick et al).

In persons with a light skin color, staining with hematoxylin-eosin may reveal only few or even no melanin granules. On staining with silver nitrate

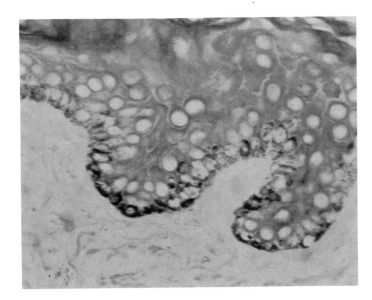

Fig. 3-4.   Moderately pigmented epidermis of Caucasoid skin
Masson–Fontana stain. Melanin is present in melanocytes as well as basal keratinocytes. In melanocytes, it extends into the dentritis processes. (×400)

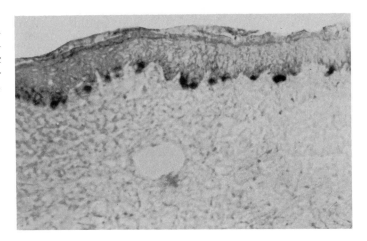

Fig. 3-5.   Melanocytes stained with dopa
On incubation in a solution of 3,4-dihydroxyphenylalanine, called dopa for short, melanocytes stain blackish, because the melanogenic enzyme they contain oxidizes dopa to dopa-melanin. (×300) (Courtesy of Milton R. Okun, M.D.)

or with the Fontana-Masson stain, however, melanin granules are seen in the basal layer. In persons with a dark skin color, especially Negroids, melanin granules, even though present predominantly in the basal layer, are found throughout the epidermis, including the horny layer, and in some instances also in the upper dermis within macrophages, called melanophages.

Staining Reactions.   The dopa reaction, originated by Bloch in 1917, requires that fresh unfixed tissue be submitted to the laboratory. Sections of the skin are then incubated in a 0.01% solution of 3,4-dihydroxyphenylalanine (called *dopa* for short) (Gilchrest et al). Melanocytes stain blackish, because the melanogenic enzyme they contain (see p. 17) changes the colorless dopa of the staining solution through oxidation into *dopa-melanin* at sites at which the enzyme is located (Fig. 3-5). Dopa-melanin generally is easily distinguished from naturally formed melanin by light microscopy, since dopa-melanin appears black and homogeneous rather than brown and granular (Okun). The dopa reaction imitates physiologic melanin formation, which begins with the enzymatic hydroxylation of tyrosine to dopa and the oxidation of dopa to dopa-quinone. Through nonenzymatic oxidation, the latter is polymerized into melanin, and melanin then combines with protein to form melanoprotein (Fitzpatrick et al). (For more details about enzymatic melanogenesis, see p. 17.)

Silver stains indicate the presence of melanin, which is both argyrophilic and argentaffin. Because melanin is argyrophilic, it can be impregnated with silver nitrate solutions and, through reducing the silver nitrate with hydroquinone to silver, it stains black. Because melanin is argentaffin, the Fontana-Masson stain with ammoniated silver nitrate may be used. With this staining method, the phenolic groups present in melanin reduce the silver salt to free black silver. Impregnation with silver nitrate is not specific for melanin but also demonstrates nerve fibers and reticulum fibers. Bleaching of melanin by strong oxidizing agents, such as hydrogen peroxide or potassium permanganate, is of value as a specific identifying measure (Pearse).

Density of Distribution of Melanocytes. The density of melanocytes is determined on biopsy specimens 4 mm in diameter. The epidermis is separated from the dermis by incubation of the specimen in a 2N solution of sodium bromide. The epidermal sheet is treated with a 1:1000 solution of dopa for 2 hr to 4 hr and then is fixed in formalin, cleared, and mounted (Staricco and Pinkus; Gilchrest et al). It has thus been determined

that the concentration of melanocytes in such epidermal sheets varies in different areas but is quite constant for any particular region. The highest concentration of melanocytes has been found on the face and the male genitals, about 2000/mm^2 melanocytes, and the lowest on the trunk, about 800/mm^2 melanocytes (Staricco and Pinkus; Fitzpatrick and Szabo). No significant difference in the density of distribution of melanocytes for any given area of the skin exists between Negroid and Caucasoid skin. However, whereas in Negroid skin the melanocytes are uniformly highly reactive, the melanocytes of Caucasoids, when not exposed to sunlight, are highly variable in dopa-reactivity (Quevedo et al). In addition, Negroid skin contains larger and more highly dendritic melanocytes than Caucasoid skin (Staricco and Pinkus; Fitzpatrick and Szabo) (see also Electron Microscopy of Melanocytes).

Exposure to Ultraviolet Light. After a single exposure to ultraviolet light in vivo, the skin of Caucasoids, when examined with the dopa reaction, shows no increase in the density of the melanocyte population but does show an increase in the size and functional activity of the existing melanocytes (Pathak et al). Repeated exposure to ultraviolet light, however, causes an increase in the concentration of dopa-positive melanocytes, as well as an increase in their size and functional activity (Quevedo et al; Mishima and Tanay). Thus, examination of habitually exposed and of unexposed skin from adjacent anatomic sites, such as the lateral and medial aspects of the upper arm, has shown a twofold higher concentration of melanocytes in the habitually exposed skin (Gilchrest et al).

Because mitotic melanocytes are seen only rarely in nonstimulated unexposed skin and only occasionally in skin repeatedly exposed to the sun, it was previously thought that at least some of the increase in melanocytes seen after repeated exposure was from previously dormant or marginally active melanocytes (Quevedo et al). However, in experiments in which mice were repeatedly exposed to the sun and vincristine was then administered to them to arrest all dividing cells in metaphase, the mitotic rate was of such a magnitude as to account for the increase in the concentration of melanocytes (Rosdahl).

Enzymatic Melanogenesis in Melanocytes. The traditional view of enzymatic melanogenesis, expressed by Lerner and Fitzpatrick in 1950 and subsequently by Fitzpatrick and Szabo in 1959 and by Lerner in 1971, holds that tyrosinase is the melanogenic enzyme. According to this view, tyrosinase, a copper-containing enzyme, catalyzes the hydroxylation of tyrosine to dihydroxyphenylalanine (dopa) and the oxidation of dopa to dopa-quinone. However, before tyrosinase can act on tyrosine, two cupric atoms present in tyrosinase must be reduced to cuprous atoms. It is believed that, in addition to being a substrate, dopa activates this reduction, thereby acting as a cofactor in the reaction. The conversion of tyrosine to melanin by tyrosinase is characterized by a variable lag period. When tyrosinase is present in low concentrations, as in epidermal melanocytes of nonirradiated skin, this lag period is markedly prolonged, and no utilization of tyrosine by tyrosinase is detectable. In contrast, in skin exposed in vivo to ultraviolet light (Fitzpatrick), as well as in epidermal sheets (Szabo) and in hair bulbs (Fitzpatrick and Szabo), tyrosinase activity is detectable with tyrosine as substrate. Since there is no lag period with dopa as substrate, tyrosinase in epidermal melanocytes can be readily demonstrated even in nonirradiated skin when skin sections are incubated in dopa rather than in tyrosine. The enzyme acting on dopa is therefore thought to be tyrosinase, rather than dopa-oxidase, as Bloch originally assumed in 1917.

The role of tyrosinase as the enzyme causing the hydroxylation of tyrosine to dopa has been questioned by Okun and his associates (Okun et al; Edelstein et al; Shapiro et al). They believe that peroxidase, rather than copper-dependent tyrosinase, mediates the conversion of tyrosine to melanin in the presence of dopa as cofactor. They have found no conclusive evidence that tyrosinase is capable of oxidizing tyrosine to melanin. However, because tyrosinase oxidizes dopa to melanin, they assume that tyrosinase functions as a dopa-oxidase as conceived by Bloch. Objections to the view of Okun and his associates include the findings that peroxidase from mouse melanoma does not significantly catalyze the hydroxylation of tyrosine whereas soluble tyrosinase does (White and Hu) and that tyrosinase retains the ability to convert tyrosine and dopa to melanin when catalase is present in sufficient quantities to block peroxidase (Holstein et al).

Electron Microscopy of Melanocytes. Melanocytes differ from keratinocytes by possessing no tonofilaments or desmosomes (EM 6). However, at their base, where they lie in close apposition to the basement membrane, melanocytes show structures resembling the half-desmosomes of basal keratinocytes (Tarnowski). Each of these structures consists of a cytoplasmic dense plate attached to the inner leaflet of the trilaminar plasma membrane and, except for being slightly smaller, has the same appearance as the attachment plaque of a half-desmosome. Anchoring filaments extend from the outer leaflet of the plasma membrane to the basement membrane. However, there is no sub-basal cell dense plaque as in the case of basal keratinocytes.

The melanogenic enzyme, usually referred to as tyrosinase (but thought to be peroxidase by Okun and his associates; see above), is synthesized in the so-called Golgi-associated endoplasmic reticulum, where tyrosinase condenses in membrane-limited vesicles. This process has been observed by electron microscopy in epidermal melanocytes after in vivo ultraviolet irradiation with either dopa or tyrosine as substrate (Hunter et al). Subsequently, these tyrosinase units are transferred to dilated tubules of the smooth endoplasmic reticulum.

There, tyrosinase is incorporated into a structural protein matrix containing filaments that have a distinctive periodicity. This then represents a stage I melanosome (Jimbow et al; Frenk).

Melanosomes in their development from stage I to stage IV (EM 6, insets) gradually move from the cytoplasm of the melanocyte into the dendritic processes. However, even in the dendritic processes, stage II melanosomes may be seen. As melanosomes mature, their content of melanin increases, while their concentration of melanogenic enzyme as measured by the electron microscopic dopa reaction decreases (Fitzpatrick et al; Toda et al, 1969).

Stage I melanosomes are round, measure about $0.3 \mu m$ in size, and possess very intense enzyme activity concentrated along filaments. They contain no melanin (Toshima et al).

Stage II melanosomes are ellipsoid and measure approximately $0.5 \mu m$ in length, as do the melanosomes of stages III and IV. They contain longitudinal filaments that are cross-linked with one another (EM 6, upper inset). Enzyme activity is present both on the enveloping membrane and on the filaments. Melanin deposition on the cross-linked filaments begins at this stage.

Stage III melanosomes have very little enzyme activity but show continued melanin deposition (EM 6, middle inset), partially through nonenzymatic polymerization.

Stage IV melanosomes no longer possess enzyme activity. Melanin, which now is formed entirely by nonenzymatic polymerization, fills the entire organelle and obscures its internal structure (EM 6, lower inset).

Transfer of Melanosomes to Keratinocytes. The transfer of melanosomes from melanocytes to epidermal keratinocytes and to hair cortex cells is the result of active phagocytosis of the tips of melanocytic dendrites by keratinocytes and hair cortex cells as demonstrated in tissue cultures (Cruickshank and Harcourt). With electron microscopy, one can observe that pseudopodlike cytoplasmic projections of keratinocytes or hair cortex cells are wrapped around the tips of dendrites. After such a projection has completely enveloped the tip of a dendrite, it is pinched off. At first, the melanosomes in the pinched-off dendrite are separated from the cytoplasm of the keratinocyte by the plasma membranes of the dendrite and of the keratinocyte (Mottaz and Zelickson). After the breakdown of these two plasma membranes, the melanosomes are dispersed throughout the cytoplasm of the keratinocyte.

Melanosomes in Keratinocytes. In the nonexposed skin of Caucasoids, especially those with light skin, melanosomes are found almost exclusively in the basal cell layer and, to a slight degree, in the layer of keratinocytes above the basal cell layer. However, in Negroids, in whom melanosomes are also principally seen in the basal cell layer, moderate quantities of melanosomes are found throughout the epidermis, including the stratum corneum (Olson et al).

In addition to this difference in the distribution of melanosomes, already known through light microscopy, the following important difference exists: in Caucasoids and Mongoloids, the melanosomes present in keratinocytes lie largely aggregated within membrane-bound melanosome complexes containing two or three melanosomes, and only a small proportion of melanosomes are seen to be singly dispersed. The melanosomes present within complexes often show signs of degeneration (Olson et al; Szabo et al). In contrast, in Negroids and Australian Aborigines, the great majority of melanosomes lie singly dispersed, and relatively few melanosome complexes are found (Olson et al; Szabo et al; Mitchell).

The reason for the lack of aggregation of melanosomes in Negroids seems to be their larger size. Whereas in Caucasoids individual melanosomes range in length from 0.3 μm to 0.5 μm, in Negroids they range in length from 0.5 μm to 0.8 μm (Flaxman et al). Since the membrane-bound melanosome complexes show considerable acid phosphatase activity, it is clear that they represent phagolysosomes in which the melanosomes are being degraded (Wolff and Schreiner, 1971). Thus, melanosomes are removed more rapidly in Caucasoids than in Negroids. It may be concluded that the difference in skin color between Caucasoids and Negroids is due to the following: in Negroid skin, (1) there is greater production of melanosomes in melanocytes, (2) individual melanosomes show a higher degree of melanization, and (3) melanosomes are larger, as a consequence of which, (4) there is a higher degree of dispersion in the keratinocytes, and (5) there is a slower rate of degradation (Flaxman et al). However, the predominant size of the melanosomes does not depend only on racial factors. Thus, topical treatment of the skin with trimethylpsoralen followed by irradiation with ultraviolet A light leads to an increase in the size of melanosomes in Caucasoids (Toda et al, 1972).

Langerhans Cells. Langerhans cells, the second type of dendritic cell in the epidermis, are seen in histologic sections stained with hematoxylin-eosin as high-level clear cells in the suprabasal epidermis. Even though in hematoxylin-eosin-stained sections they resemble basal layer clear cells or melanocytes, being completely surrounded by keratinocytes they are more difficult to distinguish from keratinocytes than basal layer clear cells.

Staining Reactions. Langerhans cells appear as dendritic cells in sections impregnated with gold chloride, a stain that is specific for Langerhans cells (Zelickson and Mottaz). Fixation with osmium zinc iodide, in contrast, demonstrates both melanocytes and Langerhans cells as dendritic cells (Niebauer et al, 1969).

Several enzyme histochemical stains may be used for identifying Langerhans cells and differentiating them from melanocytes. Among them are adenosine triphosphatase and aminopeptidase (Wolff and Winkelmann). In addition, Langerhans cells can be demonstrated with the monoclonal antibody OKT6 when the antibody is labeled with either peroxidase or fluorescein (Chu et al).

Langerhans cells are present in the epidermis in a concentration similar to that of melanocytes, between 460/mm^2 and 1000/mm^2 (Baer). In contrast to melanocytes, their number does not increase with repeated exposure to ultraviolet light (Wolff and Winkelmann). Their number does increase, however, in contact allergic reactions (Baer). This is due to the fact that they are involved in the processing of antigen and its conveyance to lymphocytes (Silberberg) (see below). Their number in the epidermis is increased also in mycosis fungoides, where they are seen in contact with T helper lymphocytes (MacKie and Turbitt). (For details, see Mycosis Fungoides, p. 745.) Langerhans cells are present not only in the skin but also in the oral mucosa, the vagina, lymph nodes, and the thymus; occasionally, they are seen in the dermis as well (Hashimoto and Tarnowski; Kiistala and Mustakallio).

Electron Microscopy of Langerhans Cells. On electron microscopic examination, Langerhans cells show a markedly folded nucleus and no tonofilaments or desmosomes (EM 7). Melanosomes are only rarely found in them and, if they are, they always are located within lysosomes (EM 7), indicating that they have been phagocytized (Breathnach and Wyllie).

Of great interest is the regular presence of an organelle, referred to as the Langerhans granule, in the cytoplasm of all Langerhans cells (EM 7). The size of these granules varies considerably, from 100 nm to 1 μm (Niebauer et al, 1970). The granule has the shape of a disk or a flat bowl and often shows a vesicle at one end and occasionally at both ends. A cross section of the central portion has the appearance of a rod, and, if a vesicle is attached to the rod at one end, the Langerhans granule has the highly characteristic appearance of a tennis racquet (EM 7, inset). Viewed in rod-shaped cross sections, the central portion has a central lamella showing cross striation with a periodicity of 6 nm (Niebauer et al, 1969; 1970). On fixation with osmium zinc iodide, the cross striations of the central lamella and the vesicles of the "tennis racquets" stain deeply, whereas the limiting membrane of the organelle does not stain. The nuclear membrane and the Golgi complex of the Langerhans cells are also stained, but the plasma membrane is not.

There is no full agreement as to whether the Langerhans granules arise in the Golgi area and migrate to the plasma membrane (Niebauer et al, 1969; Wolff and Schreiner, 1970) or arise from the plasma membrane by endocytosis and migrate to the Golgi region (Hashimoto, 1971). Niebauer and co-workers (1969) point out that the failure of the plasma membrane to stain with osmium zinc iodide, in contrast to the Langerhans granules and the Golgi region, makes the Golgi region a more likely origin of the Langerhans granules than the plasma membrane. In addition, these authors have observed a discharge of the osmium zinc iodide-positive contents of the granules into the intercellular space. Furthermore, Wolff and Schreiner (1970) and Sagebiel, after an intradermal injection in vivo of peroxidase or ferritin as electron microscopic tracer, observed no tracer substance in intracytoplasmic Langerhans granules, even though the Langerhans cells phagocytized the tracer substance by endocytosis and stored it in phagolysosomes. In contrast, Hashimoto observed the ingestion of peroxidase by Langerhans granules at the cell periphery and the migration of such labeled granules into the interior of Langerhans cells.

Origin and Functions of Langerhans Cells. It is generally accepted that Langerhans cells originate in the bone marrow and that they are functionally and immunologically related to the monocyte–macrophage–histiocyte series (Tamaki et al).

The presence of Langerhans cells in the normal dermis, especially in the dermal papillae and in the subpapillary region, has been described in several electron microscopic studies (Hashimoto and Tarnowski; Kiistala and Mustakallio). Furthermore, Langerhans cells have been seen in electron micrographs to cross the basal lamina, presumably from the dermis into the epidermis (Hashimoto and Tarnowski) and to undergo mitosis in the epidermis (Konrad and Hönigsmann). In addition, Langerhans cells have been found in the dermis by electron microscopy in various dermatoses, such as pityriasis rosea (Hashimoto and Tarnowski), Ehlers–Danlos disease (Ebner), and necrobiosis lipoidica and granuloma annulare (Carrington and Winkelmann). A significant number of Langerhans cells is also seen by electron microscopy in the dermis in mycosis fungoides. Here, the Langerhans cells lie in close apposition to the cells of the lymphoid infiltrate (Jimbow et al). (For details, see Mycosis Fungoides, p. 745.)

The histiocytes present in the cutaneous and visceral lesions of histiocytosis X contain Langerhans granules (see p. 396). These granules are indistinguishable in their electron microscopic appearance from those seen in epidermal Langerhans cells (Wolff; Nezelof et al).

The Langerhans cells in the epidermis, like the cells of the monocyte–macrophage–histiocyte series, bear surface receptors for the Fc portion of immunoglobulin G (IgG) and for the third component of complement (C3), and they synthesize and express immune response gene-associated (Ia) antigens on their cell membranes (Katz). Both types of cells are capable of presenting immunologically relevant antigen to T lymphocytes and of causing proliferation of T lymphocytes (Stingl et al). Although epidermal Langerhans cells have a poor uptake

of lipids and of enzyme proteins, they have a special selective uptake of small molecules, ions, and dyes (Hunziker and Winkelmann). They thus represent a special population of macrophages that function as the initial receptors for the cutaneous response to external antigens, many of which are of rather small molecular size. Like macrophages, epidermal Langerhans cells are derived from cells originating in bone marrow (Katz).

Epidermal Langerhans cells, analogous to macrophages, present contact allergens, which they carry on the cell surface, to specifically sensitized T lymphocytes. The T lymphocytes interact with the allergen or antigen and release lymphokines. Furthermore, some epidermal Langerhans cells carry antigen by way of the dermal lymphatics to regional lymph nodes where, in the paracortical region, they participate in immunoproliferative processes (Silberberg; Silberberg et al). (For a more detailed description of the role of Langerhans cells in contact dermatitis, see p. 97.)

Indeterminate Cells. Indeterminate dendritic cells are identifiable only by electron microscopy and are characterized by the absence of both melanosomes and Langerhans granules. Whereas it used to be thought that such cells could differentiate into either melanocytes or Langerhans cells, it has now been established that they are related to Langerhans cells, since, like Langerhans cells, they react specifically with the monoclonal antibody OKT6 (Chu et al).

NERVES OF THE EPIDERMIS

Intraepidermal nerve endings are present as Merkel cell–neurite complexes (see below). It is doubtful whether, in addition, free nerve endings exist in the human epidermis. Light microscopic examinations are not decisive, because the staining methods used for the demonstration of nerves are not sufficiently specific. Thus, in sections impregnated with silver nitrate (Montagna and Ford) or stained with methylene blue (Arthur and Shelley), not only nerves but also melanocytes and their dendrites are stained (Fitzpatrick et al), and in thick sections stained for cholinesterase (Montagna), it is impossible to decide whether a nerve is located within a papilla or intraepidermally. In any case, electron microscopic examinations have failed so far to prove conclusively the presence of free nerve endings in normal human epidermis (Orfanos and Mahrle).

Merkel Cells. Merkel cells are present at the undersurface of the epidermis and oral mucosa. They are quite scarce, are irregularly distributed, and are occasionally arranged in groups (Hashimoto). It is assumed that the Merkel cell is a touch receptor (Kidd et al). The Merkel cell as such cannot be recognized in light microscopic sections; however, in silver-impregnated sections, the meniscoid neural terminal that covers the basal portion of each Merkel cell can be seen as a Merkel disk (Smith). A sensory nerve fiber terminates at the disk.

Histogenesis. On *electron microscopic examination,* Merkel cells usually are located directly above the basement membrane (EM 8). They are quite easily recognized by electron microscopy, since they possess electron-dense granules, strands of filaments, and occasional desmosomes on their cell membranes connecting them with neighboring keratinocytes (EM 8) (Kidd et al). The electron-dense granules vary in size between 80 nm and 200 nm and are membrane-bound (EM 8, inset). The filaments resemble tonofilaments and, like tonofilaments, are seen in some areas to converge upon desmosomes. In some sections, the Merkel disk can be seen above the basement membrane as a cushion on which the Merkel cell rests. It consists of a mitochondria-rich, nonmyelinated axon terminal (Hashimoto).

The electron-dense granules in Merkel cells appear identical to the norepinephrine-containing granules of the adrenal medulla and to the granules in other chromaffin cells, including the cells of carcinoid tumors (see p. 595). These granules are characteristic of the neurosecretory system of cells capable of elaborating a variety of amine and polypeptide hormones. They are referred to as *APUD cells,* an acronym for *a*mino *p*recursor *up*take and *d*ecarboxylation. Because of their granules, it is likely that Merkel cells belong to the APUD cell system (Winkelmann).

ECCRINE GLANDS

Eccrine glands are present everywhere in the human skin; however, they are absent in areas of modified skin that lack all cutaneous appendages, that is, the vermilion border of the lips, the nail beds, the labia minora, the glans penis, and the inner aspect of the prepuce. They are found in greatest abundance on the palms and soles and in the axillae. They are tubular glands the secretory cells of which can produce large amounts of sweat under appropriate stimulation, especially heat. During secretion, the secretory cells do not change their size and shape. Eccrine sweat is not visible in the lumen on staining with hematoxylin-eosin. Schiefferdecker called the sweat glands eccrine glands because, as merocrine glands, their secretory cells simply excrete.

Eccrine glands possess a basal coil from which a duct leads through the dermis directly into the epidermis (Fig. 3-6). They are composed of three

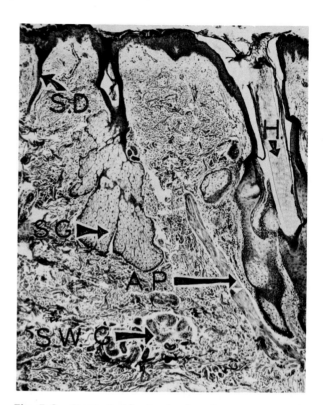

Fig. 3-6. Normal skin, back of neck
On the left side, an eccrine sweat duct (*S.D.*) enters the epidermis. In the center, a large sebaceous gland (*S.G.*) leads into a follicle containing a vellus hair. On the right rise, a large hair (*H.*) lies within a follicle surrounded by sebaceous lobules. An arrector pili muscle (*A.P.*) is situated in the obtuse angle of the hair. Beneath the large sebaceous gland, the basal coil of an eccrine sweat gland (*S.W.G.*) is seen. (×50)

segments: the secretory portion, the intradermal duct, and the intraepidermal duct. The secretory portion makes up about one half of the basal coil, the other half being composed of duct. The basal coil lies either at the border between the dermis and the subcutaneous fat or in the lower third of the dermis (Fig. 3-6). When located in the lower dermis, it is surrounded by fatty tissue that connects with the subcutaneous fat.

The *secretory portion* of the eccrine gland shows only one distinct layer composed of secretory cells (Fig. 3-7). The presence of only one distinct layer is due to the fact that the cells of the outer layer have become differentiated either into secretory or into myoepithelial cells during the sixth to eighth months of embryonic life (see p. 6). The secretory cells lining the lumen consist of two types, clear cells and dark cells, which are present in about

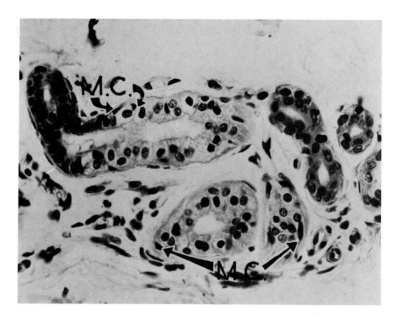

Fig. 3-7. Eccrine gland
A basal coil is shown. In the center, three secretory tubules are visible, and on the right side, three ductal tubules are seen. On the left side, the secretory portion changes into the duct. The wall of the secretory portion is composed of only one layer of secretory cells. Here and there, small myoepithelial cells are wedged in at their bases (M.C.). The wall of the duct is composed of two layers of small, cuboidal, dark-staining cells. The lumen of the duct is lined with a homogeneous cuticle. (×400)

equal numbers. The clear cells generally are broader at the base than they are near the lumen, appear somewhat larger than the dark cells, and contain very faint, small granules. The dark cells, in contrast, are broadest near the lumen and contain numerous basophilic granules (Montagna et al). The clear cells contain PAS-positive, diastase-labile glycogen, and the dark cells contain PAS-positive, diastase-resistant mucopolysaccharides. The clear cells secrete abundant amounts of aqueous material together with glycogen, whereas the dark cells secrete sialomucin (Headington). This substance contains both neutral and nonsulfated acid mucopolysaccharides, is positive for PAS and for alcian blue at pH 2.4, and is resistant to diastase and hyaluronidase. Prolonged sweating leads to a depletion of glycogen in the clear cells (Dobson et al). The myoepithelial cells possess a small spindle-shaped nucleus and long contractile fibrils. The fibrils run in a spiral, their long axes aligned obliquely to the direction of the secretory tubule. Delivery of sweat to the skin surface is greatly aided by myoepithelial contraction (Hurley and Witkowski). Peripheral to the myoepithelial cells lies a hyaline basement membrane zone containing collagen fibers. The transition from the secretory to the ductal epithelium is abrupt (Fig. 3-7).

The *intradermal eccrine duct* is composed of two layers of small, cuboidal, deeply basophilic epithelial cells. Unlike the secretory portion of the eccrine gland, the eccrine duct has no peripheral hyaline basement membrane zone, but the lumen of the duct is lined with a deeply eosinophilic, homogeneous cuticle that is PAS-positive and diastase-resistant.

The *intraepidermal eccrine duct* extends from the base of a rete ridge to the surface and follows a spiral course (Fig. 3-8). The cells composing the duct are different from the cells of the surrounding epidermis in that they are derived from dermal duct cells through mitosis and upward migration (Christophers and Plewig). For this reason, the intraepidermal eccrine duct has been referred to as acrosyringium or the epidermal sweat duct unit. The intraepidermal eccrine duct consists of a single layer of inner or luminal cells and two or three rows of outer cells. The ductal cells begin to keratinize, as evidenced by the presence of kera-tohyaline granules, at a lower level than the cells of the surrounding epidermis, that is, in the middle squamous layer, and are fully keratinized at the level of the stratum granulosum of the surrounding epidermis (Hashimoto et al). Prior to keratinization, the intraepidermal lumen is lined by an eosinophilic cuticle.

The lumen of the secretory portion of the eccrine gland, measuring approximately 20 μm in diameter, is small in comparison with that of the apocrine gland (see p. 23). The lumen of the eccrine duct measures about 15 μm across.

Histogenesis. By *electron microscopy,* the clear cells in the secretory portion are seen to contain numerous small aggregates of electron-dense glycogen granules (EM 9). The most striking feature is the presence of numerous

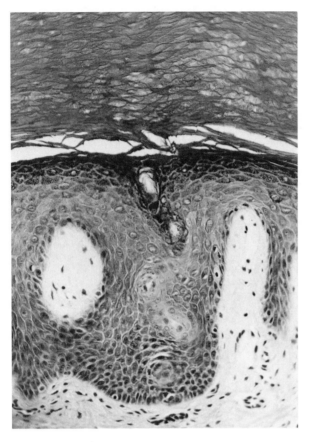

Fig. 3-8.   Eccrine gland
An intraepidermal eccrine duct follows a spiral course. The ductal cells keratinize at a lower level than the cells of the surrounding epidermis. (× 200)

The luminal cells show a periluminal filamentous zone composed of tonofilaments, which give a certain rigidity to the periluminal region and thus assure patency of the ductal lumen. Their luminal border possesses numerous tortuous microvilli covered with amorphous material, which together form the eosinophilic cuticle seen by light microscopy (Hashimoto et al). It is likely that the PAS-positive, diastase-resistant granules of the dark cells contribute to the PAS-positive, diastase-resistant cuticle.

The intraepidermal duct has luminal cells that, until they keratinize, also have tortuous microvilli coated with amorphous material, resulting in the eosinophilic cuticle seen by light microscopy.

APOCRINE GLANDS

The apocrine glands differ from eccrine glands in origin, distribution, size, and mode of secretion. Whereas the eccrine glands primarily serve in the regulation of heat, the apocrine glands represent scent glands.

Apocrine glands, together with hair and sebaceous glands, originate from the hair germ, or primary epithelial germ (see p. 4). Accordingly, the duct of an apocrine gland usually leads to a pilosebaceous follicle, entering it in the infundibulum, above the entrance of the sebaceous duct. An occasional apocrine duct, however, opens directly on the skin surface close to a pilosebaceous follicle.

Apocrine glands are encountered in only a few areas: in the axillae, in the anogenital region, and as modified glands in the external ear canal (ceruminous glands), in the eyelid (Moll's glands), and in the breast (mammary glands). Occasionally, a few apocrine glands are found on the face, in the scalp, and on the abdomen; they usually are small and nonfunctional (Hurley and Shelley). Apocrine glands develop their secretory portion and thus become functional only at puberty (Pinkus).

The 12 to 20 protuberances present in the areola of the female breast and referred to as *Montgomery's areolar tubercles* each contain a lactiferous duct and several superficially located sebaceous lobules whose ducts lead into the lactiferous duct (Montagna and Yun; Smith et al).

Apocrine glands are tubular glands the secretory cells of which pass through various stages. Schiefferdecker, who in 1917 first described these glands, observed that, during secretion, part of the cell was pinched off and released into the lumen. He referred to this process as *decapitation secretion*. He chose the name apocrine for these glands to indi-

villous folds wherever two clear cells lie side by side. The villous folds of adjacent clear cells interdigitate with one another (Ellis). In addition, intercellular canaliculi are present between adjoining clear cells, showing many tortuous microvilli protruding into their central opening (EM 9). The luminal surface of clear cells is generally small, since dark cells occupy most of the luminal border. Only a few short microvilli are seen at the luminal surface of the clear cells. Nearly all their aqueous secretion reaches the secretory lumen by way of the intercellular canaliculi (Dobson and Sato). The dark cells contain, particularly in their luminal portion, large electron-dense granules (EM 9) containing a mucoid substance (Ellis). After the granules have dissolved in the apical cytoplasm, the mucoid material is excreted into the lumen. The luminal surface of the dark cells, like that of the clear cells, shows only short microvilli.

The intradermal duct shows an outer layer of basal cells and an inner layer of luminal cells. The cells of both layers show pronounced folding of their lateral borders and, in addition, well-developed desmosomes.

cate that part of the cytoplasm of the secretory cells was pinched off (apo = off).

Apocrine glands, like eccrine glands, are composed of three segments: the secretory portion, the intradermal duct, and the intraepidermal duct. In contrast to eccrine glands, the basal coil of apocrine glands, which is located in the subcutaneous fat, is composed entirely of secretory cells and contains no ductal cells.

The *secretory portion* of the apocrine gland shows a single layer of secretory cells, since the outer layer of cells consists, just as in the eccrine gland, of myoepithelial cells. The secretory cells vary greatly in height, depending on the stage of secretion. Variation in height may be seen even in the cross section of the same secretory tubule (Schaumburg-Lever and Lever). The secretory cells possess an eosinophilic cytoplasm. Except in the apical portion, they contain in their cytoplasm fairly large, PAS-positive, diastase-resistant granules, which appear much larger than similar granules seen in the dark secretory cells of eccrine glands. In addition, the apocrine granules frequently contain iron (Soltermann). The lumen of the secretory portion of apocrine glands is large, measuring up to 200 μm in diameter, 10 times the average diameter of the lumen of eccrine glands (Fig. 3-9). The myoepithelial cells contain numerous contractile fibers extending in a spiral fashion around the secretory tubules (Pinkus). A hyaline basement membrane zone containing collagen is seen peripheral to the myoepithelium.

The type of secretion occurring in apocrine glands, referred to as decapitation secretion by Schiefferdecker, consists of the release of portions of cytoplasm into the lumen (Fig. 3-10). Because of the presence of portions of cytoplasm in the secretion, apocrine secretion, in contrast to eccrine secretion, is visible in histologic sections stained with hematoxylin-eosin. (For details of the process of apocrine secretion, see Histogenesis.) The apocrine secretion contains amorphous, PAS-positive, diastase-resistant material originating from the granules that have dissolved in the apical portion of the secretory cells (Montes et al). This PAS-positive material, like the secretion of the dark cells in eccrine glands, consists of sialomucin (Headington) (see p. 21).

Mucinous metaplasia in some of the axillary apocrine glands is fairly common. The secretory portion of the involved glands shows considerable cystic dilatation with flattening of the secretory cells and the presence of mucinous material in the lumen, which is PAS-positive and diastase-resistant and stains orthochromatically with toluidine blue. Since these changes can be found in persons of all ages, they cannot be regarded as abnormal (Winkelmann and Hultin).

The *ductal portion* of the apocrine glands has the same histologic appearance as the eccrine duct, showing a double layer of basophilic cells and a periluminal eosinophilic cuticle. The intrafollicular or intraepidermal portion of the apocrine duct is straight and not spiral in appearance, as is the intraepidermal eccrine duct (Hurley and Shelley).

Fig. 3-9. Apocrine glands and eccrine glands in the axilla
Note the great difference in the size of the lumina of the apocrine glands on the left and the eccrine glands on the right. (× 100)

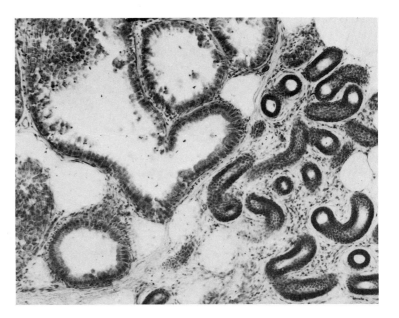

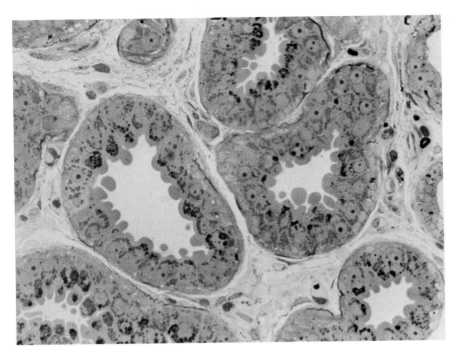

Fig. 3-10. Apocrine glands
On fixation in Karnowsky's solution, semi-thin sections, ½ μm thick, show decapitation secretion of the apocrine secretory cells. The secretory granules are deeply stained with methylene blue. (×120)

Histogenesis. *Electron microscopic examination* reveals an abundant amount of large granules surrounding the nucleus of the secretory cells. Two types of large granules are readily distinguished: dark and light (EM 10, insets) (Hashimoto et al). The dark granules initially consist of a dense protein substance within a small membrane-bound vesicle. By growth and coalescence, large dark granules form up to 5 μm in diameter. They contain, in addition to the dense protein substance, lipid globules (EM 10, left inset), ferritin particles, and myelin figures. Their strong reaction for acid phosphatase and beta-glucuronidase indicates that the dark granules are lysosomes. The second type of granules, the light granules, are derived from mitochondria, since, like mitochondria, they possess cristae and a double-layered membrane (EM 10, right inset).

Maturation of the secretory cells is indicated by the formation of a dome-shaped apical cap. Most of the apical cap is nearly free of large granules, but it contains numerous small, smooth vesicles about 50 nm in diameter. Beneath the apical cap, numerous large granules, both of the dark and of the light type, are seen. The luminal plasma membrane shows a moderate number of microvilli.

No agreement has been reached among electron microscopists about the mode of secretion in apocrine secretory cells. Several authors have denied the existence of an apocrine type of secretion, since they have found no cellular debris in the secretory lumen. They have concluded that secretion takes place as merocrine secretion, as in eccrine glands, through the excretion of small, smooth vesicles present in the apical cap (Biempica and Montes; Ellis). Other authors have observed, in addition

to merocrine secretion, the discharge of cellular contents into the lumen through small discontinuities in the luminal plasma membrane of secretory cells (Hibbs; Hashimoto et al). In addition, in a few instances, dissolution of entire secretory cells suggestive of holocrine secretion has been observed (Braun-Falco and Rupec).

Decapitation secretion comparable to that seen by light microscopy has been found on electron microscopic examination by Kurosumi and associates and by Schaumburg-Lever and Lever. Although Kurosumi and co-workers did not actually observe decapitation, they found detached apical caps.

Schaumburg-Lever and Lever found three types of secretion: merocrine, apocrine, and holocrine. In the apocrine type of secretion, three stages were observed: (1) formation of an apical cap; (2) formation of a dividing membrane at the base of the apical cap; and (3) formation of tubules above and parallel to the dividing membrane, supplying a new plasma membrane for both the under-surface of the apical cap and the top of the residual cell, thus bringing about detachment of the apical cap (EM 10).

Decapitation secretion with formation of an apical cap and a dividing membrane has since been found to occur also in the secretory cells of an apocrine cystadenoma (Hassan et al). Convincing proof of the detachment of entire apical caps in apocrine glands has been provided through scanning microscopy by Inoue, who observed on each secretory cell a cytoplasmic luminal protuberance about 2 μm in diameter. In the early stage of secretion, the protuberance was hemispheric, but, at a later stage, it increased in height to form a linguiform process.

SEBACEOUS GLANDS

Sebaceous glands are present everywhere on the skin except on the palms and soles. On the skin, they are found in association with hair structures. In addition, free sebaceous glands that are not associated with hair structures occur in some areas of modified skin, such as the nipple and areola of both the male and female breasts. There, they occur over the entire surface of the nipple and in Montgomery's areolar tubercles, each of which contains several sebaceous lobules in association with a lactiferous duct (see p. 22). Free sebaceous glands are found also on the labia minora and the inner aspect of the prepuce. However, sebaceous glands occur only very rarely on the glans of the penis (Hyman and Brownstein). The not infrequent presence of free sebaceous glands on the vermilion border of the lips and on the buccal mucosa is known as Fordyce's condition (see p. 539). The meibomian glands of the eyelids are modified sebaceous glands.

The sebaceous glands are well developed at the time of birth, most likely owing to the effect of maternal hormones. After a few months, they undergo considerable atrophy. At puberty, as a result of increased androgen output, the sebaceous glands become greatly enlarged (Strauss and Pochi). (See also Nevus Sebaceus, p. 536.)

A sebaceous gland may consist of only one lobule but often has several lobules leading into a common excretory duct composed of stratified squamous epithelium (see Fig. 3-6). Sebaceous glands, being holocrine glands, form their secretion by decomposition of their cells. In sebaceous glands of the skin, the pilosebaceous follicle into which the sebaceous duct leads may possess a large hair or a vellus hair that may be too small to reach the skin surface. There is no relationship between the size of the sebaceous gland and the size of the associated hair. For example, in the center of the face and on the forehead, where the sebaceous glands are very large, the associated hairs are of the vellus type.

Each sebaceous lobule possesses a peripheral layer of cuboidal, deeply basophilic cells that usually contain no lipid droplets. The more centrally located cells contain lipid droplets if lipid stains are used on formalin-fixed frozen sections; but in routinely processed sections in which the lipid has been extracted, the cytoplasm of these cells appears as a delicate network. The nucleus is centrally located. In the portion of the lobule located closest to the duct, the cells disintegrate. One sees coa-lesced lipid droplets in the excretory duct in lipid stains and amorphous material in routine stains.

Histogenesis. The composition of lipids in the sebaceous glands is not uniform. Thus, under polarized light, doubly refractile lipids may be present in small to moderate amounts or may be absent (Suskind). Histochemical examination reveals the presence of triglycerides and small amounts of phospholipids. Esterified cholesterol is present, but there is no free cholesterol. Waxes are also present, but they are not identifiable by histochemical means (Suskind).

Electron microscopic studies have confirmed that the cells of the peripheral layer usually contain no lipid vacuoles (EM 11). Analogous to the basal cells of the epidermis, they are attached to a basement membrane by half-desmosomes (Cashion et al). In the cells located farther inside, one can observe a marked increase in the volume of cytoplasm and, at the same time, the appearance of smooth endoplasmic reticulum and the formation of fine lipid material within its cisterns (EM 11). This indicates that the smooth endoplasmic reticulum synthesizes the lipid (Cashion et al; Rupec). In the Golgi region, the synthesized lipid material aggregates as lipid droplets. Toward the center of the sebaceous lobules, the cells, as a result of continued lipid synthesis, are almost completely filled with lipid droplets. Although a true limiting membrane is clearly present around the lipid droplets in the incipient stages, none is detectable in mature droplets (Niizuma).

Lysosomal enzymes bring about the physiologic autolysis that occurs in the holocrine secretion. Histochemical staining of electron microscopic sections for lysosomal enzymes, such as acid phosphatase and aryl sulfatase, reveals an increasing number of lysosomes as the sebaceous cells become more lipidized. In the disintegrating cells located in the preductal region, the acid phosphatase and aryl sulfatase activity is most pronounced, but this activity is now present largely outside of lysosomes, since the lysosomes have released their contents in their function as "suicide bags" (Rowden; Rupec and Braun-Falco).

HAIR

The hair follicle, with its hair in longitudinal sections, consists of three parts: (1) the lower portion, extending from the base of the follicle to the insertion of the arrector pili muscle; (2) the middle portion, or isthmus, a rather short section, extending from the insertion of the arrector pili to the entrance of the sebaceous duct; and (3) the upper portion, or infundibulum, extending from the entrance of the sebaceous duct to the follicular orifice.

The lower portion of the hair follicle is composed of five major portions: (1) the dermal hair papilla, (2) the hair matrix, (3) the hair, consisting inward to outward of medulla, cortex, and hair cuticle, (4) the inner root sheath, consisting inward to outward of inner root sheath cuticle, Huxley layer, and Henle layer, and (5) the outer root sheath.

The histologic appearance of the hair follicle changes considerably during the hair cycle, which causes the hair to turn from an anagen hair into a catagen hair, then into a telogen hair, and finally into a new anagen hair (see Histogenesis below). Since the anagen phase persists for years, in contrast to the catagen phase, which lasts for two to three weeks, and to the telogen phase, which lasts a few months, anagen hairs comprise more than 80% of the hair present in the normal scalp (Van Scott et al).

During its active growth, or anagen stage, the hair follicle shows at its lower pole a knoblike expansion, the hair bulb, composed of matrix cells and melanocytes. A small, egg-shaped dermal structure, the *dermal hair papilla,* protrudes into the hair bulb (Fig. 3-11). The papilla induces and

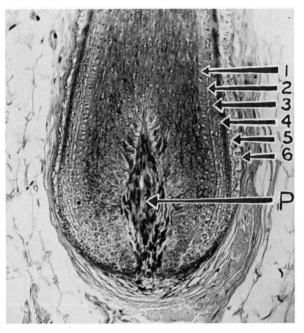

Fig. 3-11.   Lower part of an anagen hair follicle
The dermal hair papilla (*P*), composed of connective tissue, protrudes into the hair bulb. The various linings of the hair can be recognized. They are, from the inside to the outside: (*1*) the hair cuticle, (*2*) the inner root sheath cuticle, (*3*) the Huxley layer, (*4*) the Henle layer (which stains dark because of the presence of trichohyaline granules), (*5*) the outer root sheath, and (*6*) the glassy or vitreous layer. (× 200)

maintains the growth of the hair follicle (Kollar). Because of the presence of large amounts of acid mucopolysaccharides in its ground substance, the dermal hair papilla stains positively with alcian blue and metachromatically with toluidine blue. Since positive staining with alcian blue takes place not only at pH 2.5 but also at pH 0.5, it can be concluded that the ground substance of the hair papilla contains not only nonsulfated acid mucopolysaccharides, such as hyaluronic acid, but also sulfated acid mucopolysaccharides, such as chondroitin sulfate (Johnson and Helwig). In addition, there is considerable alkaline phosphatase activity in the hair papilla during the anagen stage as a result of the presence of large numbers of capillary loops (Kopf and Orentreich; Cormia). In persons with dark hair, large amounts of melanin can be seen in the dermal hair papilla situated within melanophages.

The pluripotential cells of the *hair matrix* present in the hair bulb give rise to the hair and to the inner root sheath. In contrast, the outer root sheath represents a downward extension of the epidermis. The cells of the hair matrix have large vesicular nuclei and a deeply basophilic cytoplasm. Dopapositive melanocytes are interspersed mainly between the basal cells of the hair matrix lying on top of the dermal hair papilla and, to a lesser degree, between the basal cells of the hair matrix located lateral to the hair papilla (Mishima and Widlan). Melanin, varying in quantity in accordance with the color of the hair, is produced in these melanocytes and is incorporated into the future cells of the hair through phagocytosis of the distal portion of dendritic processes by future hair cells. This transfer of melanin is analogous to that observed from epidermal melanocytes to keratinocytes (see p. 17).

As they move upward, the cells arising from the hair matrix differentiate into six different types of cells, each of which keratinizes at a different level. The outermost layer of the inner root sheath, the Henle layer, keratinizes first, thus establishing a firm coat around the soft central parts. The two apposed cuticles covering the inside of the inner root sheath and the outside of the hair keratinize next, followed by Huxley's layer. The hair cortex then follows, and the medulla is last (Pinkus, 1972). (For a discussion of keratinization of the outer root sheath as the seventh follicular structure to keratinize, see below.)

The *hair medulla* of human hair is often difficult to find by routine light microscopy, since it may be discontinuous or even absent (Zaun). It is more readily recognizable by polariscopic examination, since, unlike the cortex, the only partially keratinized medulla contains hardly any doubly refractile structures (Garn). If the medulla is seen by light microscopy in human hairs, it appears amorphous because of only partial keratinization.

The *hair cortex* consists of cells that, during their upward growth from the hair matrix, keratinize gradually by losing their nuclei and becoming filled with keratin fibrils. The process of keratinization takes place without the formation of keratohyaline granules, as seen in the keratinizing epidermis, or of trichohyaline granules, as seen in the inner root sheath. Thus, the keratin of the hair cortex represents hard keratin, in contrast to the keratin of the inner root sheath, which, like that of the epidermis, represents soft keratin (Leppard et al) (see also p. 13).

The *hair cuticle* (1 in Fig. 3-11), located peripheral to the hair cortex, consists of overlapping cells arranged like shingles and pointing upward with their peripheral portion. The cells of the hair cuticle are tightly interlocked with the cells of the inner root sheath cuticle (see below), resulting in the firm attachment of the hair to its inner root sheath. The hair and the inner root sheath thus move upward in unison.

The *inner root sheath* is composed of three concentric layers; from the inside to the outside, these are the inner root sheath cuticle (2 in Fig. 3-11), the Huxley layer (3 in Fig. 3-11), and the Henle layer (4 in Fig. 3-11). None of these three layers contains melanin. All three layers keratinize, unlike the cells of the hair cortex and of the hair cuticle, by means of trichohyaline granules. These granules in many respects resemble the keratohyaline granules of the epidermis, although they stain eosinophilic, in contrast to the basophilic-staining keratohyaline granules of the epidermis. Closest to the hair is the single-layered inner root sheath cuticle, consisting of flattened overlapping cells that point downward in the direction of the hair bulb. Since the cells of the hair cuticle point upward, these two types of cells interlock tightly. Trichohyaline granules are few in the inner root sheath cuticle cells. The Huxley layer, which usually consists of two rows of cells, develops numerous trichohyaline granules at the level of the keratogenous zone of the hair. The Henle layer, only one cell layer thick and the first layer to undergo keratinization, already shows numerous trichohyaline granules at its emergence from the hair matrix (Montagna). After having become fully keratinized, the cells of all three layers composing the inner root sheath disintegrate when they reach the isthmus of the hair follicle, which extends from the area of attachment of the arrector pili muscle to the entrance of the sebaceous duct. The cells of the inner root sheath thus do not contribute to the emerging hair (Parakkal and Matoltsy).

The *outer root sheath* (5 in Fig. 3-11) extends upward from the matrix cells at the lower end of the hair bulb to the entrance of the sebaceous duct, where it changes into surface epidermis, which lines the upper portion, or infundibulum, of the hair follicle. The outer root sheath is thinnest at the level of the hair bulb, gradually increases in thickness, and is thickest in the middle portion of the hair follicle, the isthmus. In its lower portion, below the isthmus, the outer root sheath is covered by the inner root sheath and does not undergo keratinization. The outer root sheath cells have a clear, vacuolated cytoplasm because of the presence of considerable amounts of glycogen. In contrast to the surface epidermis lining the infundibulum, which contains active, melanin-producing melanocytes in its basal layer, the basal layer of the outer root sheath contains only inactive, amelanotic melanocytes demonstrable with toluidine blue. However, these inactive melanocytes can become melanin-producing cells after skin injuries, such as dermabrasion, when they increase in number and migrate upward into the regenerating upper portion of the outer root sheath and into the regenerating epidermis (Staricco).

In the middle portion of the hair follicle, the so-called isthmus, which extends upward from the attachment of the arrector pili muscle to the entrance of the sebaceous duct, the outer root sheath is no longer covered by the inner root sheath, which by then has keratinized and disintegrated. The outer root sheath therefore undergoes keratinization. This type of keratinization, referred to as *trichilemmal keratinization* (Pinkus, 1969), produces large, homogeneous keratinized cells without the formation of keratohyaline granules. Trichilemmal keratinization is found also in catagen and telogen hairs and in trichilemmal cysts and trichilemmal tumors (see pp. 485 and 533).

The upper portion of the hair follicle above the entrance of the sebaceous duct, the infundibulum, is lined by surface epidermis, which, like the sebaceous duct, undergoes keratinization with the formation of keratohyaline granules.

The *glassy* or *vitreous layer* (6 in Fig. 3-11) forms a homogeneous, eosinophilic zone peripheral to the outer root sheath. Like the subepidermal basement membrane zone, it is PAS-positive and diastase-resistant, but it differs from the subepidermal basement membrane zone by being thicker and visible with routine stains. It is thickest around the lower third of the hair follicle. Peripheral to the vitreous layer lies the fibrous root sheath, which is composed of thick collagen bundles.

Histogenesis. The *hair cycle* consists of the involutionary stage (catagen) and the end stage (telogen) of the old hair and its replacement by a young, new hair (early anagen). At the onset of the catagen stage, mitotic activity and melanin production in the hair bulb cease. Next, the bulb shrinks, setting the dermal hair papilla free (Montagna). As the hair moves upward, the lower portion of the follicle involutes. The reduction in follicle size results from cell deletion by apoptosis (Weedon and Strutton). (For a definition of apoptosis, see Lichen Planus and the Glossary.) The lower follicle thus becomes a thin cord of epithelial cells surrounded by the fibrous root sheath, which is wrinkled in thick folds. Also, as the hair moves upward, growth of the inner root sheath

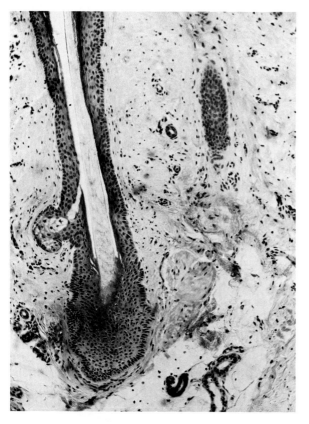

Fig. 3-12.   Telogen stage of a hair follicle
The lower portion of the hair is encased in trichilemmal keratin and is completely surrounded by the outer root sheath. (×50)

ceases, so that the lower end of the hair shaft becomes surrounded by dense keratin, referred to as trichilemmal keratin, that is formed by the outer root sheath without the interposition of keratohyaline granules (Pinkus, 1969). This then represents the club hair of the *catagen stage.*

Next, the thin cord of epithelial cells retracts upward, faithfully followed by the underlying dermal hair papilla, which thus also moves upward. The cord of epithelial cells shortens until it forms only a small nipplelike downward protrusion from the club hair, called the secondary hair germ. Under it lies the dermal hair papilla. With the hair follicle decreased to about one third of its former length, the lowest portion of the hair follicle lies at the level of the attachment of the arrector pili. The lower portion of the hair is encased in trichilemmal keratin and completely surrounded by the outer root sheath (Fig. 3-12). Folds of the fibrous root sheath extend downward from the hair follicle. At this point, the hair has reached the *telogen stage* (Kligman).

When regrowth of the hair begins, the secondary hair germ begins to elongate by cell division and grows down as an epithelial column together with the dermal hair papilla inside of the old, collapsed fibrous root sheath of the previous hair. As it is growing down, the lower end of the epithelial column becomes invaginated by the dermal hair papilla. A new hair bulb is thus formed, representing the *early anagen stage.* By subsequent differentiation, a new hair arises. Thus, the formation of an active hair follicle from the secondary germ recapitulates the embryonic pattern of development of the hair from the primary hair germ (Kligman).

Electron microscopic examination of a hair follicle in its anagen stage shows the *hair medulla* to be composed of an irregular network of immature keratin containing in its spaces large, irregular vacuoles and a homogeneous electron-dense material. The latter is analogous to the interfibrillary material of the hair cortex but is present in much greater amounts than in the hair cortex. Melanosomes are present in both the immature keratin and the interfibrillary material of the hair medulla (Mahrle and Orfanos, 1971). The *hair cortex* consists of closely packed keratinized spindle cells. The keratin within these cells consists of filaments arranged in fibrils that are separated by small amounts of electron-dense interfibrillary material. The melanosomes of the hair cortex are larger than those of the epidermis. They lie singly or in groups but not within lysosomes. They are located usually in the interfibrillary matrix within the cells and only rarely in the intercellular space (Orfanos and Ruska).

Three types of melanosomes are present in hair. Erythromelanin granules, seen in red hair, are polymorphous and have an irregular internal structure. The other two types of granules, homogeneous eumelanin granules and lamellated pheomelanin granules, are found in varying proportions in blond and dark hair and are round to oval. Dark hair contains more melanosomes than light hair, and the melanosomes are largely of the homogeneous eumelanin type; in light hair, lamellated pheomelanin melanosomes predominate (Mahrle and Orfanos, 1973).

In grey and white hair, the melanocytes in the basal layer of the hair matrix are greatly reduced in number or are absent. The melanocytes that are present show degenerative changes, especially of their melanosomes (Herzberg and Gusek). The hair shafts contain only detritus of melanin or none at all (Mahrle and Orfanos, 1973).

NAILS

The nail plate is composed of keratinized cells. They originate in the thick epidermis of the nail matrix, formerly referred to as the ventral nail matrix, and keratinize without the formation of keratohyaline granules (Zaias). The proximal nail fold, formerly referred to as the dorsal nail matrix, merely forms the nail cuticle, which keratinizes with the formation of keratohyaline granules. Neither the proximal nail fold nor the nail bed contributes to the nail plate (Zaias and Alvarez). The rete ridges of the nail bed are oriented not as a network of anastomosing ridges, as elsewhere in the skin, but as parallel longitudinal ridges, so that the boundary between the epidermis and the dermis of the nail bed is serrated in transverse sections but flat in longitudinal sections (Lewin).

Histogenesis. The conclusion reached by Zaias and Alvarez that only the nail matrix is responsible for the formation of the nail plate was based on their in vivo experiments on monkeys with tritiated glycine. An additional observation made by Norton on human volunteers with tritiated thymidine and glycine was that, even though the main stream of labeled cells is from the nail matrix into the nail plate, there is some cellular progression distally from the nail plate into the nail bed, indicating that some nail bed cells have their origin in the nail matrix. Norton assumes that the migration of nail matrix cells into the nail bed allows for distal movement of the nail bed together with the attached nail plate. He points out that, in the experiments conducted by Zaias and Alvarez, labeling of the nail bed was obscured by an abundance of melanin in the primate nail bed.

Electron microscopic examination has confirmed that keratinization in nail cells, analogous to the formation of "hard" keratin in hair cortex cells, takes place by accretion of tonofilaments without the formation of keratohyaline granules. The cellular envelope of the horny cells of the nail, similar to the horny cells of the epidermis, becomes thickened through the cytoplasmic formation of a marginal band (Hashimoto) (see p. 13).

CONNECTIVE TISSUE OF THE DERMIS

The connective tissue of the dermis consists of collagenous and elastic fibers embedded into ground substance. All three components are formed by fibroblasts.

Collagenous Fibers. Collagen represents by far the most abundant constituent of the connective tissue of the dermis. On light microscopy, collagen consists of fibers. The diameter of collagen fibers is quite variable, ranging from 2 μm to 15 μm. The collagen fibers are present either as a finely woven network or as thick bundles. Collagen as a finely woven meshwork of collagen fibers is found in the papillary layer of the dermis, which includes not only the subepidermal papillae situated between the rete ridges but also the subpapillary layer forming a narrow ribbon between the rete ridges and the subpapillary blood vessels. This is referred to as the *papillary dermis.* In addition, the pilosebaceous units and the eccrine and apocrine glands are encircled by a thin meshwork of collagen fibers similar to that present in the papillary dermis. Therefore, the papillary and the periadnexal dermis is regarded as an anatomical unit, the *adventitial dermis* (Reed and Ackerman). The blood vessels of the dermis are also surrounded by a thin layer of fine collagen fibers. The rest of the dermis, constituting by far the largest portion of the dermis and referred to as the *reticular dermis,* shows the collagen fibers united into thick bundles. These collagen bundles are arranged nearly parallel to the surface of the skin and interlace. Nevertheless, they extend in various directions horizontally, and thus some are cut lengthwise and others across in histologic sections. As a rule, collagen bundles that are cut lengthwise appear slightly wavy. A small number of fibroblasts are interspersed between the collagen bundles. Their nuclei are rather palestaining and, when cut lengthwise, appear spindle-shaped. The cytoplasmic border of the fibroblasts cannot be recognized with routine stains. The only other cell type present in the normal dermis is the mast cell, seen generally in small numbers in perivascular arrangement. Usually, mast cells can be recognized only with special stains such as the Giemsa stain, which stains the mast cell granules metachromatically purple (see p. 53 and 81).

Reticulum Fibers. Reticulum fibers are not recognizable with routine stains; but, being argyrophilic, they can be impregnated with silver nitrate, which, by being subsequently reduced to silver, stains black. Reticulum fibers represent a special type of thin collagen fiber that measures from 0.2 µm to 1 µm in diameter, in contrast to collagen fibers, which measure 2 µm to 15 µm in diameter (Schmidt). The argyrophilia shown by reticulum fibers, in contrast to collagen fibers, probably is related to the fact that reticulum fibers represent type III collagen rather than type I collagen. (For details, see Histogenesis.)

Reticulum fibers are the first-formed fibers during embryonic life (see p. 6) and in various pathologic conditions associated with increased fibroblastic activity (see below).

In normal skin, even though collagen is being continuously replaced, the formation of new collagen is not preceded by an argyrophilic phase. Rather, all newly formed collagen consists of large fibers. However, there are a few areas in which normally small collagen fibers are present as reticulum fibers without transforming into larger, nonargyrophilic collagen fibers. This occurs above all in the basement membrane zone, that is, the region of the adventitial dermis that lies closest to the epidermis and its appendages (see Fig. 3-3). In addition, reticulum fibers are present normally around blood vessels and as a basketlike capsule around each fat cell.

In contrast to the sparsity of reticulum fibers in normal skin is the abundance of reticulum fibers in pathologic conditions in which active fibroblasts form new collagen. Thus, large numbers of reticulum fibers are present in granulomas, such a tuberculosis and sarcoidosis, in fibroblastic tumors, such as dermatofibroma and fibrosarcoma, and in healing wounds. In all these conditions, histologic sections impregnated with silver nitrate show an extensive network of reticulum fibers (Rehtijärvi). As healing of granulomas or wounds takes place, the reticulum fibers are gradually replaced by nonargyrophilic collagen fibers (see Fig. 13-3).

Ground Substance.   The ground substance, an amorphous substance that fills the spaces between collagen fibers and collagen bundles, contains glycosaminoglycans, or acid mucopolysaccharides. These glycosaminoglycans are covalently linked to peptide chains to form high-molecular-weight complexes called proteoglycans (Winand).

Glycosaminoglycans are present in normal skin in such small amounts that they cannot be demonstrated with either routine or special histologic staining methods except in the hair papilla of anagen hair, which contains both nonsulfated and sulfated acid mucopolysaccharides (see p. 26).

However, through the study of tissues with an active growth of fibroblasts, as seen in the papillary dermis in dermatofibroma and in the connective tissue around the tumor islands of basal cell epithelioma, it is known that the dermal ground substance consists largely of nonsulfated acid mucopolysaccharides such as hyaluronic acid (Johnson and Helwig). In healing wounds, however, in which new collagen is laid down, the ground substance contains sulfated as well as nonsulfated acid mucopolysaccharides (Jacques and Cameron).

The *nonsulfated acid* mucopolysaccharides consist largely of hyaluronic acid, are stainable with alcian blue at pH 3.0 but not at pH 0.5, and show metachromasia with toluidine blue at pH 3.0 but not at pH 1.5. The *sulfated acid* mucopolysaccharides consist largely of chondroitin sulfate, are stainable with alcian blue at pH 0.5 as well as at pH 3.0, and show metachromasia with toluidine blue at pH 1.5 as well as at pH 3.0. Both nonsulfated and sulfated acid mucopolysaccharides stain with colloidal iron. Testicular hyaluronidase hydrolyzes hyaluronic acid but not the sulfated acid mucopolysaccharides (Johnson and Helwig).

Elastic Fibers.   In light microscopic sections that are routinely stained, elastic fibers are not visible. With special elastic tissue stains, such as orcein or resorcin–fuchsin, they are found entwined among the collagen bundles. Since elastic fibers are thin in comparison with collagen bundles, measuring from 1 µm to 3 µm in diameter, and are wavy, only a small portion of any fiber is seen in histologic sections, giving even normal elastic fibers a fragmented appearance. The elastic fibers are thickest in the lower portion of the dermis, where they are arranged, like collagen bundles, chiefly parallel to the surface of the skin. In the lower papillary dermis, thin elastic fibers form a dense network, and, from there, still thinner elastic fibers ascend almost vertically toward the epidermis and end free just below the dermal-epidermal border (Pinkus).

Histogenesis.   With regard to the *function of the collagenous and elastic fibers,* it is generally agreed that collagen is not extensible, although its wavy arrangement in the dermis allows for the skin to stretch somewhat. In contrast, the elastic fibers are extensible like rubber and return to their original shape after stretching (Jansen; Smith). Thus, the bovine ligamentum nuchae is very extensible, and its elastic fibers, though coarser, are of the same type as the elastic fibers of human skin (Jansen). It appears likely that the papillary dermis, because of the vertical arrangement of the elastic fibers in it, serves as an elastic interface between the epidermis and the less pliable reticular dermis (Reed and Ackerman).

ELECTRON MICROSCOPY OF FIBROBLASTS. Fibroblasts that actively synthesize collagen have a prominent rough endoplasmic reticulum composed of many membrane-lined cisternae with large numbers of attached ribosomes (EM 12). The dilated cisternae are filled with an amorphous material produced by the ribosomes lining the cisternae (Scarpelli and Goodman). This apparently amorphous material consists of triple helical procollagen molecules, each molecule being composed of three pro-alpha polypeptide chains (see below). The procollagen molecules pass from the cisternae of the rough endoplasmic reticulum to the Golgi area, whence they are excreted into the extracellular space by means of secretory vesicles (Ross and Benditt; Uitto and Lichtenstein). Conversion of procollagen molecules into collagen molecules composed of three alpha chains then occurs outside the cell (Nigra et al).

BIOSYNTHESIS AND ELECTRON MICROSCOPY OF COLLAGEN. The biosynthesis of collagen begins within the fibroblast by the assembly of three pro-alpha polypeptide chains into a triple helical procollagen molecule (Nigra et al). After excretion into the extracellular space, the three pro-alpha chains of each procollagen molecule are shortened by 30% to 40% through removal of the carboxy-terminal and amino-terminal peptide extensions brought about by the action of two enzymes produced by the fibroblast: carboxy-terminal peptidase and amino-terminal peptidase (Uitto and Lictenstein). This then results in conversion of the procollagen molecule into the collagen molecule. Whereas the additional peptides present in procollagen keep it soluble and prevent its intracellular polymerization, collagen molecules polymerize readily. The collagen molecule is a rigid rod in which each of the three coiled alpha-chains consists of about 1000 amino acids (Nigra et al). The collagen molecule is about 300 nm long and 1.5 nm wide (Lazarus; Grant and Prockop). Collagen fibrils form by both lateral and longitudinal association of collagen molecules. However, the collagen fibrils vary in diameter as a result of varying degrees of polymerization of collagen molecules, with younger collagen fibrils being thinner than older fibrils. In the normal dermis, the thickness of collagen fibrils ranges from 70 nm to 140 nm, most of the fibrils being around 100 nm thick (EM 2,6,8,13) (Hayes and Rodnan).

Collagen fibrils possess characteristic cross striations with a periodicity of 68 nm. The periodicity of the cross striations in the collagen fibrils can be explained as follows. Each collagen molecule possesses along its length of 300 nm five charged regions 68 nm apart, and, although neighboring collagen molecules overlap each other, they always have their charged regions lying side by side. This parallel alignment of the charged regions produces the cross striations (Grant and Prockop).

Reticulum fibrils possess the same 68-nm periodicity of their cross striations as collagen fibrils but have a smaller diameter than collagen fibrils, varying between 40 nm and 65 nm rather than between 70 nm and 140 nm (Schmidt). Furthermore, reticulum and collagen differ in the number of fibrils present in the cross section of each fiber and in the amount of ground substance present within and around each fiber. The amount of ground substance around the fibrils and on the surface of the fiber may explain the presence of argyrophilia in reticulum fibers and its absence in collagen fibers (Schmidt).

HETEROGENEITY OF COLLAGEN. Five different types of collagen have been recognized that differ in composition and antigenicity. Type I collagen, the predominant collagen in postfetal skin, is found in the large fiber bundles of the reticular dermis. Reticulum fibers are composed of type III collagen. Although type III collagen is the prevalent type of collagen in early fetal life, in postfetal life it is limited to the subepidermal and periappendageal regions, that is, the basement membrane zones and the perivascular regions (Meigel et al) (see p. 30). Basement membrane collagen (basal lamina collagen) is type IV, and the collagen of cartilage is type II. A fifth type of collagen has been recognized in the epidermis (Stenn). It is a somewhat heterogeneous type referred to also as cell-surface-related collagens (Byers et al). The various types of collagen can be identified by indirect immunofluorescent techniques using purified antibodies from rabbits or similar animals that have been immunized with the various types of collagen (Meigel et al; Yaoita et al).

Among the differences in composition are the following. In type I collagen, the three alpha chains in the collagen molecule consist of two different kinds: two identical alpha chains designated as alpha-1(I), and a third chain called alpha-2. In type II collagen, the collagen molecules are composed of three identical, genetically distinct alpha chains, alpha-1(II). Type III collagen is also composed of three identical, distinct alpha chains (Uitto and Lichtenstein). Type IV collagen consists of procollagen composed of three identical pro-alpha chains that have retained their nonhelical extensions (Kefalides). Type V collagen has not been clearly characterized.

ELECTRON MICROSCOPY OF ELASTIC FIBERS. The elastic fiber of the dermis consists of two components: the microfibrils and the matrix elastin. The microfibrils are electron-dense and measure 10 nm to 12 nm in diameter. They are aggregated at the periphery of the elastic fiber, giving the fiber its characteristic frayed appearance (EM 13) (Breathnach). In addition, microfibrils are present within the elastin as strands 15 nm to 80 nm in diameter, extending in a longitudinal direction (Hashimoto and DiBella). The microfibril component amounts to only 15% of the elastic fiber, whereas the amorphous electron-lucid elastin makes up 85% of the fiber (Varadi). It is the elastin that stains with elastic tissue stains, is removable by elastase, and is markedly extensible, whereas the microfibrils are the elastic resilient component of the elastic fiber (Hashimoto and DiBella).

Elastic fibers undergo significant changes during life. One change, representing aging, is best studied in nonexposed skin. The other change, elastotic degeneration, is the result of chronic sun exposure and will be described elsewhere (see Solar Degeneration, p. 27).

In young children up to the age of 10 years, the elastic fibers may not be fully matured, so that microfibrils predominate (Stadler and Orfanos). Physiologic aging is a gradual process and usually becomes quite apparent by ages 30 to 50. There is a gradual decrease in the number of peripheral microfibrils, so that ultimately there may be none and, instead, the surface of the elastic fiber appears irregular and granular (Stadler and Orfanos). The microfibrils within the elastin matrix become thicker and show electron-lucent holes of varying sizes (Marsch et al). In very old persons, fragmentation and disintegration of some of the elastic fibers may be observed (Stadler and Orfanos).

NERVES AND NERVE END-ORGANS OF THE DERMIS

In sections stained with routine methods, one can recognize only the large nerve bundles and the Meissner and Vater–Pacini end organs. The finer nerves require special staining. Among the staining methods used are impregnation with silver salts (Winkelmann, 1955), vital staining with methylene blue (Woollard et al), and in vitro staining of thick sections with methylene blue (Arthur and Shelley).

Nerves are composed of neuraxons, a cytoplasmic process that conducts neural impulses, and Schwann cells (sheath cells or neurilemmal cells) enveloping the neuraxons. Such a primary functioning unit may or may not be myelinated and is surrounded by an endoneurium, a mucinous or fibrous matrix containing fibroblasts, which supports the primary functioning unit. A perineurium composed of elongated, flattened cells surrounds several primary functioning units and their endoneurial matrix (Reed).

The skin is supplied with sensory nerves as well as autonomic nerves, both of which permeate the entire dermis with nerve fibers showing frequent branching. Sensory and autonomic nerves differ in that sensory nerves possess a myelin sheath up to their terminal ramifications, whereas autonomic nerves do not. The autonomic nerves, derived from the sympathetic nervous system, supply the blood vessels, the arrectores pilorum, and the eccrine and apocrine glands. The sebaceous glands possess no autonomic innervation, and their functioning depends on endocrine stimuli.

All autonomic nerves end in fine arborizations. So do the sensory nerves, except in a few areas in which there are, in addition to fine arborizations, special nerve end-organs (see below). Hair follicles, especially large hair follicles, are also surrounded below the entry of the sebaceous duct by a network of sensory nerves that lose their myelin sheaths a short distance from the outer root sheath and end in numerous arborizations of fine nonmyelinated fibers.

Histogenesis. On *electron microscopic examination*, myelinated nerves are seen to possess myelin sheaths composed of regular, concentric layers of plasmalemma of Schwann cells, each only 3 nm thick and separated by intervals of 10 nm (Sian and Ryan). After losing their myelin sheaths, cutaneous nerves terminate either as free nerve endings just beneath the basement membrane of the epidermis or in association with specialized receptor organs, such as the Merkel cells in the epidermal basal layer (see p. 19) or the special nerve end-organs (see below). However, the free nerve endings are not naked axons, but axons surrounded by small Schwann cell processes and by a basement membrane (Breathnach). In some instances, instead of terminating just beneath the epidermal basement membrane, the nerves show direct continuity between their basement membranes and the basement membrane of the epidermis (Orfanos and Mahrle).

Special Nerve End-Organs. In the areas of hairless skin on the palms and the soles and in the areas of modified hairless skin at the mucocutaneous junctions, some of the sensory nerves end in special nerve end-organs. They are of three types: mucocutaneous end-organs, Meissner corpuscles, and Vater–Pacini corpuscles. Although it is customary to speak of them as end organs, they actually represent starting organs in a functional sense, since nerve impulses start there and are transmitted to the sensory cells of the spinal cord (Orfanos and Mahrle).

Mucocutaneous End-Organs. The mucocutaneous end-organs, on the average 50 μm in diameter, are found in the modified hairless skin at the mucocutaneous junctions, namely, the glans, the prepuce, the clitoris, the labia minora, the perianal region, and the vermilion border of the lip. They are in the papillary dermis. They cannot be recognized in routinely stained sections, in contrast to the Meissner corpuscles in the dermal papillae. Impregnation with silver nitrate reveals that from two to six myelinated nerve fibers enter each mucocutaneous end-organ and, after losing their myelin sheaths, form many loops of nerve fibers resembling an irregularly wound ball of yarn (Winkelmann, 1960).

Histogenesis. The *electron microscopic* features of mucocutaneous end-organs are similar to those of Meissner corpuscles (MacDonald and Schmitt) (see below), despite minor differences in their light microscopic appearance. They show a subdivision into lobules, each containing a complex arrangement of axon terminals. These axon terminals are surrounded by concentric lamellar processes derived from so-called laminar cells, the nuclei of which are situated toward the periphery of the lobules. It is assumed that the laminar cells represent modified Schwann cells. The mucocutaneous end-organs are always separated from the basal layer of the epidermis by a band of papillary dermal collagen.

Meissner Corpuscles.   Meissner corpuscles are located in dermal papillae (Fig. 3-13) and mediate a sense of touch. They occur exclusively on the ventral aspects of the hands and feet, their number increasing distally. There are more Meissner corpuscles on the hands than on the feet. At the site of their greatest concentration, the fingertips, approximately every fourth papilla contains a Meissner corpuscle (Winkelmann, 1960). The size of the Meissner corpuscles averages 30 μm by 80 μm in diameter. Owing to their size and their elongated shape, resembling that of a pine cone, they occupy the greater part of the papilla in which they are located. They possess a capsule composed of several layers of flattened Schwann cells that are arranged transverse to the long axis of the corpuscle. Impregnation with silver salts reveals that several myelinated nerves, as they approach the base or the side of the corpuscle, lose their myelin sheaths and then enter it. Within the corpuscle, the nerves take a meandering course upward.

Histogenesis. *Electron microscopic studies* reveal that the principal part of the Meissner corpuscle is made up of irregular layers of flattened, greatly elongated laminar cells. The nuclei of the laminar cells are located largely at the periphery of the corpuscle. The axons terminating within the Meissner corpuscle are surrounded by slender processes of the laminar cells. This enveloping of axons by laminar cells or their lamellar processes is analogous to the enveloping of axons by infolding of the plasma membrane of Schwann cells and indicates that the laminar cells are modified Schwann cells (Cauna and Ross).

The axon terminals and laminar cells are in direct contact with the epidermal basal cells at the upper end of the Meissner corpuscle without interposition of a basement membrane (Hashimoto).

Vater–Pacini Corpuscles.   Vater–Pacini corpuscles are large nerve end-organs that are located

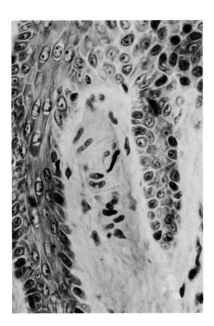

Fig. 3-13.   Meissner tactile corpuscle located in the papilla of a fingertip
It is composed of several layers of flattened Schwann cells that are arranged transversely to the long axis of the corpuscle. Since this is a hematoxylin-eosin stain, the nerve fibers cannot be visualized. (×400)

in the subcutis and mediate a sense of pressure. They measure up to 1 mm in diameter and thus are detected easily by light microscopy (Fig. 3-14). They are found most commonly below the skin of the volar aspects of the palms and soles, showing their greatest concentration at the tips of the fingers and toes. In addition, a few Vater–Pacini corpuscles occur in the subcutis of the nipple and of the anogenital region (Winkelmann, 1960). Vater–Pacini corpuscles vary in shape. Some are ovoid, others have the appearance of a flattened sphere, and still others have an irregular shape (Winkelmann and Osment). They consist of a stalk and of the body proper, the latter having a small core and a thick capsule. In the stalk, the single thick nerve supplying the Vater–Pacini corpuscle makes several turns and, just after entering the stalk, loses its myelin sheath. The core shows a granular substance surrounding the ascending meandering nerve. The thick capsule consists of 30 or more concentric, loosely arranged lamellae.

Histogenesis. On *electron microscopic examination*, the single nerve fiber present in the inner portion of the core retains its Schwann cell cytoplasmic covering for a short distance. The outer portion of the core shows

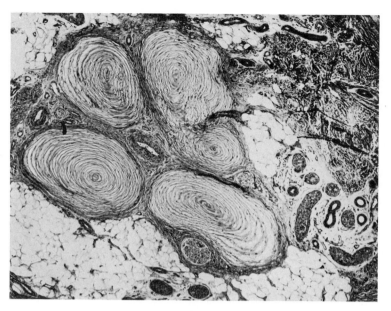

Fig. 3-14. Vater–Pacini corpuscles in the subcutaneous fat of a fingertip
Their large size becomes apparent if one compares it with the size of the eccrine sweat glands and their ducts, which are located on the right side of the field. (×50)

closely packed, greatly elongated laminar cells. The thick capsule consists of at least 30 layers of flattened laminar cells separated from one another by fluid-filled spaces (Pease and Quilliam). The laminar cells of the Vater–Pacini corpuscle, analogous to those of the Meissner corpuscle, are modified Schwann cells.

BLOOD VESSELS AND LYMPH VESSELS

Dermal Blood Vessels. The arrangement of the cutaneous blood vessels consists of a subcutaneous plexus of small arteries from which arterioles ascend into the dermis and are interconnected. The arterioles and venules form three important plexuses in the dermis: a subpapillary plexus and plexuses around hair follicles and eccrine glands (Yen and Braverman). Each of the three plexuses gives rise to numerous capillaries located largely in the adventitial portion of the dermis (see p. 29). From the subpapillary plexus, one capillary loop supplies each subepidermal dermal papilla. Each loop consists of an ascending arterial limb and a descending venous limb. The venous portion empties into the subpapillary plexus of postcapillary venules and further through larger venules into the subcutaneous plexus of small veins.

Histologically, the small arteries of the subcutaneous plexus and the arterioles of the dermis possess three layers: (1) an intima, composed of endothelial cells and an internal elastic lamina; (2) a media, which contains two or more layers of muscle cells in the small arteries, but only a single layer of muscle cells in the arterioles of the lower dermis, and a discontinuous layer of muscle cells in the arterioles of the upper dermis; and (3) an adventitia of connective tissue (Moretti). The capillaries that are present throughout the dermis but especially in the adventitial dermis are composed of a layer of endothelial cells surrounded by an incomplete layer of pericytes. A basement membrane, composed of reticulum fibers, is present peripheral to the endothelial cells and surrounds the pericytes. There is alkaline phosphatase activity in the endothelial cells of all capillaries (Kopf; Klingmüller). Staining for alkaline phosphatase thus demonstrates well the capillary loop in each subepidermal dermal papilla, with the ascending, arterial limb of the loop staining more heavily than the descending, venous limb (Klingmüller). The abundant capillaries present in the hair papilla of anagen hairs also stain heavily (Kopf and Orentreich).

The walls of veins generally are thinner than those of arteries and less clearly divided into the three classic layers. The postcapillary venules resemble capillaries, since they consist of endothelial cells, pericytes, and a basement membrane. In medium-sized venules, muscle cells as well as elastic fibers appear, but the latter are diffusely arranged and do not form an internal elastic lamina. In contrast, large venules and veins show an internal elastic lamina but differ from arteries in that they possess valves (Moretti).

Histogenesis. On *electron microscopy*, the endothelial cells of capillaries show a well-developed endoplasmic

34

reticulum, bundles of fairly thick cytoplasmic filaments with a diameter of 5 nm to 10 nm, and many pinocytotic vesicles at their luminal surface (EM 14). Peripheral to the endothelium lies a basement membrane. The peripheral row of cells, the pericytes (EM 14), have long cytoplasmic processes and form a discontinuous layer. They are completely surrounded by the capillary basement membrane. Pericytes are poorly differentiated mesenchymal cells that are capable of forming basement membranelike material (Eimoto) and may develop phagocytic properties (Meade et al). They also may serve as precursors of other vascular cells such as smooth muscle cells, endothelial cells, and fibroblasts (Eimoto). In larger capillaries, more than one layer of pericytes may be present, and transitional forms between pericytes and smooth muscle cells (see p. 36) may be seen (Weber and Braun-Falco).

Seen on electron microscopic examination, the subpapillary horizontal plexus is composed of terminal arterioles, arterial and venous capillaries, and postcapillary venules. The arteriolar and venous segments can be distinguished from each other on the basis of the basement membrane, which has a homogeneous appearance in the former and is multilaminated in the latter. Furthermore terminal arterioles have elastin and smooth muscle cells in their walls, whereas postcapillary venules have only pericytes in their walls (Yen and Braverman). The capillary loops leading from the subpapillary plexus to the dermal papillae and back can be divided into an intrapapillary portion and an extrapapillary portion. The extrapapillary ascending limb and the intrapapillary portion have the characteristics of an arterial capillary, that is, a homogeneous basement membrane, whereas the extrapapillary descending limb has venous characteristics, that is, a multilayered basement membrane (Braverman and Yen). Although some investigators have observed areas of fenestration at the tips of the capillary loops between the endothelial cells (Seifert and Klingmüller), others have failed to find them (Braverman and Yen).

Glomus.

A special vascular structure, the glomus, is located within the reticular dermis in certain areas. Glomus formations occur most abundantly in the pads and nailbeds of the fingers and toes but also elsewhere on the volar aspect of the hands and feet, in the skin of the ears, and in the center of the face. The glomus is concerned with temperature regulation and represents a special arteriovenous shunt that, without the interposition of capillaries, connects an arteriole with a venule. When open, these shunts cause a great increase in blood flow in the area. Each glomus consists of an arterial and a venous segment. The arterial segment, called the Sucquet–Hoyer canal, branches from an arteriole and has a narrow lumen and a thick wall measuring 20 μm to 40 μm in diameter. The wall shows a single layer of endothelium,

surrounded by a PAS-positive, diastase-resistant basement membrane zone, and a media that is densely packed with four to six layers of glomus cells. These are large cells with a clear cytoplasm resembling epithelioid cells. Although myofibrils cannot be recognized within glomus cells with light microscopic staining methods, these cells have generally been regarded as smooth muscle cells (Mescon et al). Peripheral to the glomus cells is a zone of loose connective tissue. Staining with silver salts shows many nerve fibers extending to the glomus cells within this zone. The venous segment of the glomus is thin-walled and has a wide lumen. This wide collecting venule functions as a reservoir and drains into a dermal venule. As many as four Sucquet–Hoyer canals may be found in a single glomus body, which is encapsulated (Pepper et al).

Histogenesis. *Electron microscopic study* of the Sucquet–Hoyer canal reveals the glomus cells to be vascular smooth muscle cells. As such, each glomus cell is surrounded by a basement membrane. The cytoplasm of the glomus cells is filled with filaments with a diameter of about 5 nm. Cytoplasmic as well as peripheral dense bodies, 300 nm to 400 nm in diameter, are present in the glomus cells as a result of condensations of the myofilaments. Numerous nonmyelinated nerves ensheathed by Schwann cells are present peripheral to the glomus cells (Goodman).

Lymph Vessels.

Lymph vessels are difficult to recognize in histologic sections because of their resemblance to blood vessels. They can be divided into lymph capillaries, postcapillary lymph vessels, and deep lymph vessels (Pfleger).

Lymph capillaries are not recognizable in histologic sections of normal skin, not even by means of lymphangiography. However, in areas of lymph stasis, they can be recognized in the subpapillary and deeper dermis as lumina lined only by a few endothelial cells. In contrast to blood capillaries, they lack pericytes and do not possess a basement membrane (Seifert and Klingmüller). The lumina are surrounded by loosely arranged collagen fibers and elastic fibers.

The postcapillary lymph vessels located in the deep layers of the dermis, at the border between the dermis and the subcutis, and in the subcutaneous septa are as a rule stained by lymphangiography (Pfleger). They have a wider lumen and a thicker connective tissue wall than lymph capillaries. Also, a few smooth muscle cells are present in the wall. The postcapillary lymph vessels possess valves lined by endothelium.

The deep lymph vessels located at the border between the dermis and subcutis and in the subcutaneous septa possess three layers and valves, similar to veins. An internal elastic lamina between the intima and media is regularly present (Pfleger).

MUSCLES OF THE SKIN

Smooth Muscle.   Smooth or involuntary muscle of the skin occurs as arrectores pilorum, as tunica dartos of the external genitals, and in the areola of the nipples. The muscle fibers of the arrectores pilorum arise in the connective tissue of the upper dermis and are attached to the hair follicle below the sebaceous glands. They are situated in the obtuse angle of the hair follicle (see Fig. 3-6). Thus, when contracted, they pull the hair follicle into a vertical position and produce the perifollicular elevations of "gooseflesh."

Histopathology.   Smooth muscle is characterized by the absence of striation and by the location of the nucleus in the center of the muscle cell. Argyrophilic reticulum fibers surround each muscle cell.

Histogenesis.   *Electron microscopic examination* reveals that smooth muscle cells possess a basement membrane peripheral to the plasma membrane. The cytoplasm of the cells is filled with myofilaments, 5 nm in diameter, that form cytoplasmic and peripheral dense bodies as a result of condensations, just as the myofilaments do in myoepithelial cells, in vascular smooth muscle cells, and in glomus cells (Breathnach) (see p. 35). The rather narrow spaces between the muscle cells are occupied by collagen fibrils and by Schwann cells with associated nonmyelinated axons (Orfanos).

Striated Muscle.   Striated or voluntary muscle is found in the skin of the neck as platysma and in the skin of the face as muscles of expression.

Histopathology.   The striated muscle bundles take their origin either from a fascia or from the periosteum, or they form a closed ring, as in the musculus sphincter oris. They extend through the subcutaneous tissue into the lower dermis (Schmidt). The muscle fibers, like skeletal muscle, show cross striation. Their nuclei are located at the periphery of the fibers immediately beneath the sarcolemma, the limiting membrane of the fibers.

BIBLIOGRAPHY

Keratinocytes of the Epidermis

BAKER H, KLIGMAN AM: Technique for estimating turnover time of human stratum corneum. Arch Dermatol 95:408–411, 1967

BELL RF, KELLUM RE: Early formation of keratohyalin granules in rat epidermis. Acta Derm Venereol (Stockh) 47:350–353, 1967

BOURLOND A, VANDOOREN-DEFLORENNE R: La membrane basale sous-épidermique: Sa structure et son ultrastructure. Arch Belg Derm Syph 24:119–135, 1968

BRAUN-FALCO O, RUPEC M: Die Verteilung der sauren Phosphatase bei normaler und psoriatischer Verhornung. Dermatologica 134:225–242, 1967

BRIGGAMAN RA: Biochemical composition of the epidermal-dermal junction and other basement membranes. J Invest Dermatol 78:1–6, 1982

BRIGGAMAN RA, WHEELER CE, JR.: The epidermal–dermal junction. J Invest Dermatol 65:71–84, 1975a

BRIGGAMAN RA, WHEELER CE, JR.: Epidermolysis bullosa dystrophica—recessive: A possible role of anchoring fibrils in the pathogenesis. J Invest Dermatol 65:203–211, 1975b

BRODY I: An electron microscopic study of the fibrillar density in the normal human stratum corneum. J Ultrastruct Res 30:209–217, 1970

CERIMELE D, DEL FORNO C, SERRI F: Histochemistry of the intercellular substance of the normal and psoriatic human epidermis. Arch Dermatol Res 262:27–36, 1978

CHRISTOPHERS E: Cellular architecture of the stratum corneum. J Invest Dermatol 56:165–169, 1971

COOPER JH: Microanatomical and histochemical observations on the dermal–epidermal junction. Arch Dermatol 77:18–22, 1958

ELIAS PM, GOERKE J, FRIEND DS: Mammalian epidermal barrier layer lipids: Composition and influence on structure. J Invest Dermatol 69:535–546, 1977

EMERY JL, MCMILLAN M: Observations on the female sex chromatin in human epidermis and on the value of skin biopsy in determining sex. J Pathol Bacteriol 68:17–22, 1954

EPSTEIN EH, JR, WILLIAMS ML, ELIAS PM: Editorial: Steroid sulfatase, X-linked ichthyosis, and stratum corneum cell cohesion. Arch Dermatol 117:761–763, 1981

EPSTEIN WL, MAIBACH HI: Cell renewal in human epidermis. Arch Dermatol 92:462–468, 1965

FROST P, WEINSTEIN GD, VAN SCOTT EJ: The ichthyosiform dermatoses. II. Autoradiographic studies of epidermal proliferation. J Invest Dermatol 47:561–567, 1966

FUKUYAMA K, EPSTEIN WL: Heterogenous protein in keratohyaline granules studied by quantitative autoradiography. J Invest Dermatol 65:113–117, 1975

GOLDMAN L, GOLDMAN J: Some studies of sex chromatin in dermatology. Dermatologica 127:445–456, 1963

HALPRIN KM: Epidermal "turnover time": A reexamination. Br J Dermatol 86:14–19, 1972

HASHIMOTO K: Cellular envelopes of keratinized cells of the human epidermis. Arch Klin Exp Dermatol 235:374–385, 1969

HASHIMOTO K, DIBELLA RJ, SHKLAR A: Electron microscopic studies of the normal human buccal mucosa. J Invest Dermatol 47:512–525, 1966

HASHIMOTO K, LEVER WF: An ultrastructural study of cell junctions in pemphigus vulgaris. Arch Dermatol 101:287–298, 1970

HASHIMOTO K, LEVER WF: The cell surface coat of normal keratinocytes and of acantholytic keratinocytes in pemphigus. Br J Dermatol 83:282–290, 1970

KEFALIDES NA: Basement membranes: Structural and biosynthetic considerations. J Invest Dermatol 65:85–92, 1975

KOBAYASI T: Anchoring of basal lamina to elastic fibers by elastic fibrils. J Invest Dermatol 68:389–390, 1977

KOBAYASI T: Dermoepidermal junction of normal skin. J Dermatol (Tokyo) 5:157–165, 1978

LAZARUS GS, HATCHER VB, LEVINE N: Lysosomes and the skin. J Invest Dermatol 65:259–271, 1975

MATOLTSY AG: Desmosomes, filaments, and keratohyaline granules: Their role in stabilization and keratinization of the epidermis. J Invest Dermatol 65:127–142, 1975

MATOLTSY AG: Keratinization. J Invest Dermatol 67:20–25, 1976

ODLAND GF: The fine structure of the interrelationship of cells in the human epidermis. J Biophys Biochem Cytol 4:529–538, 1958

PENNEYS NS, FULTON JE, JR., WEINSTEIN GD et al: Location of proliferating cells in human epidermis. Arch Dermatol 101:323–327, 1970

PLATT LI, KAILIN EW: Sex chromatin frequency. JAMA 187:182–186, 1964

SCHREINER E, WOLFF K: Die Permeabilität des epidermalen Intercellularraums für kleinmolekulares Protein. Arch Klin Exp Dermatol 235:78–88, 1969

SCHWARZ E: Biochemie der epidermalen Keratinisation. In: Marchionini A (ed): Handbuch der Haut- und Geschlechtskrankheiten, Vol. 1, Part 4A, pp 1–115. Berlin, Springer-Verlag, 1979

SPEARMAN RIC: Some light microscopical observations on the stratum corneum of the guinea pig, man and common seal. Br J Dermatol 83:582–590, 1970

SQUIER CA, HOPPS RM: A study of the permeability barrier in epidermis and oral epithelium using horseradish peroxidase as a tracer in vitro. Br J Dermatol 95:123–129, 1976

STOUGHTON R, WELLS G: A histochemical study on polysaccharides in normal and diseased skin. J Invest Dermatol 14:37–51, 1950

TARNOWSKI WM: Ultrastructure of the epidermal melanocyte-dense plate. J Invest Dermatol 55:265–268, 1970

TEZUKA T, FREEDBERG IM: Epidermal structural proteins. III. Isolation and purification of histidine-rich protein of the newborn rat. J Invest Dermatol 63:402–406, 1974

UGEL AR: Bovine keratohyalin: Anatomical, histochemical, ultrastructural, immunologic, and biochemical studies. J Invest Dermatol 65:118–126, 1975

VAN SCOTT EJ, EKEL TM: Kinetics of hyperplasia in psoriasis. Arch Dermatol 88:373–381, 1963

WEINSTEIN GD: Autoradiographic studies of turnover time and protein synthesis in pig epidermis. J Invest Dermatol 44:413–419, 1965

WEINSTEIN GD, FROST P: Methotrexate for psoriasis. Arch Dermatol 103:33–38, 1971

WOLFF K, SCHREINER E: An electron microscopic study on the extraneous coat of keratinocytes and the intercellular space of the epidermis. J Invest Dermatol 51:418–430, 1968

WOLFF K, SCHREINER E: Epidermal lysosomes. Electron microscopic cytochemical studies. Arch Dermatol 101:276–286, 1970

WOLFF K, WOLFF-SCHREINER EC: Trends in electron microscopy of skin. J Invest Dermatol 67:39–57, 1976

WOLFF-SCHREINER EC: Ultrastructural cytochemistry of the epidermis. (Review) Int J Dermatol 16:77–102, 1977

YAOITA H, FOIDART JM, KATZ SI: Localization of the collagenous component in the skin basement membrane. J Invest Dermatol 70:191–193, 1978

Dendritic Cells of the Epidermis

BLOCH B: Das Problem der Pigmentbildung in der Haut. Arch Dermatol Syph Berlin 124:129–143, 1917

BREATHNACH AS, WYLLIE LMA: Melanin in Langerhans cells. J Invest Dermatol 45:401–403, 1965

CARRINGTON SG, WINKELMANN R: Ultrastructure of histiocytes in cutaneous pathology. J Invest Dermatol 52:372–373, 1969

CHU A, EISINGER M, LEE JS et al: Immunoelectron microscopic identification of Langerhans cells using a new antigenic marker. J Invest Dermatol 78:177–180, 1982

CLARK WH, JR., WATSON MC, WATSON BEM: Two kinds of "clear" cells in the human epidermis. Am J Pathol 39:333–344, 1961

COCHRAN AJ: The incidence of melanocytes in normal skin. J Invest Dermatol 55:65–70, 1970

CRUICKSHANK CND, HARCOURT SA: Pigment donation in vitro. J Invest Dermatol 42:183–184, 1964

EBNER H: Beitrag zum Ehlers-Danlos Syndrom. Z Hautkr 43:177–182, 1968

EDELSTEIN LM, CARIGLIA N, OKUN MR et al: Inability of murine melanoma melanosomal "tyrosinase" (L-dopa oxidase) to oxidize tyrosine to melanin in polyacrylamide gel systems. J Invest Dermatol 64:364–370, 1975

FITZPATRICK TB: Human melanogenesis. Arch Dermatol Syph 65:379–391, 1952

FITZPATRICK TB, MIYOMATO M, ISHIKAWA K: The evolution of concepts of melanin biology. Arch Dermatol 96:305–323, 1967

FITZPATRICK TB, SZABO G: The melanocytes: Cytology and cytochemistry. J Invest Dermatol 32:197–209, 1959

FLAXMAN BA, SOSIO AC, VAN SCOTT EJ: Changes in melanosome distribution in Caucasoid skin following topical application of N mustard. J Invest Dermatol 60:321–326, 1973

FRENK E: Pigment cell biology and its relation to disorders of melanin pigmentation. (Review) Dermatologica 159:185–194, 1975.

GILCHREST BA, BLOG FB, SZABO G: Effects of aging and chronic sun exposure on melanocytes in human skin. J Invest Dermatol 73:141–143, 1979

HASHIMOTO K: Langerhans' cell granule: An endocytic organelle. Arch Dermatol 104:148–160, 1971

HASHIMOTO K, TARNOWSKI WM: Some new aspects of the Langerhans cell. Arch Dermatol 97:450–464, 1968

HOLSTEIN TJ, STOWELL CP, QUEVEDO WC, JR. et al: Peroxidase "protyrosinase" and the multiple forms of tyrosinase in mice. Yale J Biol Med 46:560–571, 1973

HUNTER JAA, MOTTAZ JH, ZELICKSON AS: Melanogenesis: Ultrastructural histochemical observations on ultraviolet irradiated human melanocytes. J Invest Dermatol 54:213–221, 1970

HUNZIKER N, WINKELMANN RK: Langerhans cells in contact dermatitis of the guinea pig. Arch Dermatol 114:1309–1313, 1978

JIMBOW K, CHIBA M, HORIKOSHI T: Electron microscopic identification of Langerhans cells in the dermal infiltrates of mycosis fungoides. J Invest Dermatol 78:102–107, 1982

JIMBOW K, QUEVEDO WC, JR., FITZPATRICK TB et al: Some aspects of melanin biology. (Review) J Invest Dermatol 67:72–89, 1976

KATZ SI: Editorial: The role of Langerhans cells in immunity. Arch Dermatol 116:1361–1362, 1980

KIISTALA U, MUSTAKALLIO KK: The presence of Langerhans cells in human dermis with special reference to their potential mesenchymal origin. Acta Derm Venereol (Stockh) 48:115–122, 1968

KONRAD K, HÖNIGSMANN H: Elektronenmikroskopischer Nachweis einer mitotischen Langerhans-Zelle in normaler menschlicher Epidermis. Arch Derm Forsch 246:70–76, 1973

LERNER AB: On the etiology of vitiligo and gray hair. Am J Med 51:141–147, 1971

LERNER AB, FITZPATRICK TB: Biochemistry of melanin formation. Physiol Rev 30:91–126, 1950

MACKIE RM, TURBITT ML: The use of a double-label immunoperoxidase monoclonal antibody technique in the investigation of patients with mycosis fungoides. Br J Dermatol 106:379–384, 1982

MISHIMA Y, TANAY A: The effect of alpha-methyldopa and ultraviolet irradiation on melanogenesis. Dermatologica 136:105–114, 1968

MITCHELL RE: Melanocytes in Australian Aboriginal skin. (Abstr) J Invest Dermatol 94:93, 1970

MOTTAZ JH, ZELICKSON AS: Melanin transfer: A possible phagocytic process. J Invest Dermatol 49:605–610, 1967

NEZELOF C, BASSET F, ROUSSEAU MF: Histiocytosis X: Arguments for a Langerhans cell origin. Biomedicine 18:365–371, 1973

NIEBAUER G, KRAWCZYK WS, KIDD RI et al: Osmium zinc iodide reactive sites in the epidermal Langerhans cell. J Cell Biol 43:80–89, 1969

NIEBAUER G, KRAWCZYK WS, WILGRAM GF: Über die Langerhans-Zellorganelle bei Morbus Letterer-Siwe. Arch Klin Exp Dermatol 239:125–137, 1970

OKUN MR: Dermal dopa-positive cells in lichen planus. Arch Dermatol 106:422–423, 1972

OKUN MR, EDELSTEIN LM, OR N et al: The role of peroxidase *vs.* the role of tyrosinase in enzymatic conversion of tyrosine to melanin in melanocytes, mast cells and eosinophils. J Invest Dermatol 55:1–12, 1970

OLSON RL, NORDQUIST J, EVERETT MA: The role of epidermal lysosomes in melanin physiology. Br J Dermatol 83:189–199, 1970

PATHAK MA, SINESI SJ, SZABO G: The effect of a single dose of ultraviolet radiation on epidermal melanocytes. J Invest Dermatol 45:520–528, 1965

PEARSE AGE: Histochemistry: Theoretical and Applied, 3rd ed, p 1056, Edinburgh, Churchill Livingstone, 1972

QUEVEDO WC, JR., SZABO G, VIRKS J et al: Melanocyte populations in UV-radiated human skin. J Invest Dermatol 45:295–298, 1965

ROSDAHL IK: Melanocyte mitosis in UVB-irradiated mouse skin. Acta Derm Venereol (Stockh) 58:217–221, 1978

SAGEBIEL RW: In vivo and in vitro uptake of ferritin by Langerhans cells of the epidermis. J Invest Dermatol 58:47–54, 1972

SHAPIRO HC, EDELSTEIN LM, PATEL RP et al: Inability to demonstrate hydroxylation of tyrosine by murine melanoma "tyrosinase" (L-dopa oxidase), using the tritiated water assay technique. J Invest Dermatol 72:191–193, 1979

SILBERBERG I: Apposition of mononuclear cells to Langerhans cells in contact allergic reactions. Acta Derm Venereol (Stockh) 53:1–12, 1973

SILBERBERG I, BAER RL, ROSENTHAL SA: The role of Langerhans cells in allergic contact hypersensitivity: A review of findings in man and guinea pig. J Invest Dermatol 66:210–217, 1976

STARICCO RJ, PINKUS H: Quantitative and qualitative data on the pigment cells of adult human epidermis. J Invest Dermatol 28:33–45, 1957

STINGL G, KATZ SI, SHEVACH EM et al: Analogous functions of macrophages and Langerhans cells in the initiation of the immune response. J Invest Dermatol 71:59–64, 1978

SZABO G: Tyrosinase in the epidermal melanocytes of white human skin. Arch Dermatol 76:324–329, 1967

SZABO G, GERALD AB, PATHAK MA et al: The ultrastructure of racial color differences in man. (Abstr) J Invest Dermatol 54:98, 1970

TAMAKI K, STINGL G, KATZ SI: The origin of Langerhans cells. J Invest Dermatol 74:309–311, 1980

TARNOWSKI WM: Ultrastructure of the epidermal melanocyte dense plate. J Invest Dermatol 55:265–268, 1970

TODA K, HORI Y, FITZPATRICK TB: The site of tyrosinase activity within the melanosome. (Abstr) J Invest Dermatol 52:380, 1969

TODA K, KATHAK MA, PARRISH JA et al: Alteration of racial differences in melanosome distribution in human epidermis after exposure to ultraviolet light. Nature 236:143–145, 1972

TOSHIMA S, MOORE GE, SANDBERG AA: Ultrastructure of human melanoma in cell culture: Electron microscopic studies. Cancer 21:202–216, 1968

WHITE R, HU F: Characteristics of tyrosinase in B16 melanoma. J Invest Dermatol 68:272–276, 1977

WOLFF K: The Langerhans cell. In Mali JWH (ed): Current Problems in Dermatology, Vol 4, pp 79–145. Basel, S Karger AG, 1972

WOLFF K, SCHREINER E: Uptake, intracellular transport and degradation of exogenous protein by Langerhans cells. J Invest Dermatol 54:37–47, 1970

WOLFF K, SCHREINER E: Melanosomal acid phosphatase. Arch Dermatol Forsch 241:255–272, 1971

WOLFF K, WINKELMANN RK: The influence of ultraviolet light on the Langerhans cell population and its hydrolytic enzymes in guinea pigs. J Invest Dermatol 48:531–539, 1967

ZELICKSON AS, MOTTAZ JH: Epidermal dendritic cells. Arch Dermatol 98:652–659, 1968

Nerves of the Epidermis

ARTHUR RP, SHELLEY WB: The innervation of human epidermis. J Invest Dermatol 32:397–411, 1959

FITZPATRICK TB, SEIJI M, MCGUGAN AD: Melanin pigmentation. N Engl J Med 265:328–332, 1961

HASHIMOTO K: Fine structure of Merkel cell in human oral mucosa. J Invest Dermatol 58:381–387, 1972

KIDD RL, KRAWCZYK WS, WILGRAM GF: The Merkel cell in human epidermis: Its differentiation from other dendritic cells. Arch Dermatol Forsch 241:374–384, 1971

MONTAGNA W: Histology and cytochemistry of human skin. XXXIV. The eyebrows. Arch Dermatol 101:257–263, 1970

MONTAGNA W, FORD DM: Histology and cytochemistry of human skin. XXXIII. The eyelid. Arch Dermatol 100:328–335, 1969.

ORFANOS CE, MAHRLE G: Ultrastructure and cytochemistry of human cutaneous nerve. J Invest Dermatol 61:108–120, 1973

SMITH KR, JR: The ultrastructure of the human Haarscheibe and Merkel cells. J Invest Dermatol 54:150–159, 1970

WINKELMANN RK: The Merkel cell system and a comparison between it and the neurosecretory or APUD cell system. J Invest Dermatol 69:41–46, 1977

Eccrine Glands

CHRISTOPHERS E, PLEWIG G: Formation of the acrosyringium. Arch Dermatol 107:378–382, 1973

DOBSON RL, FORMISANO V, LOBITZ WC, JR. et al: Some histochemical observations on the human eccrine sweat gland. III. The effect of profuse sweating. J Invest Dermatol 31:147–159, 1972

DOBSON RL, SATO K: The secretion of salt and water by the eccrine sweat gland. Arch Dermatol 105:366–370, 1972

ELLIS RA: Eccrine, sebaceous and apocrine glands. In Zelickson AS (ed): Ultrastructure of Normal and Abnormal Skin, pp. 132–162. Philadelphia, Lea & Febiger, 1967

HASHIMOTO K, GROSS BG, LEVER WF: Electron microscopic study of the human adult eccrine gland. I. The duct. J Invest Dermatol 46:172–185, 1966

HEADINGTON JT: Primary mucinous carcinoma of skin: Histochemistry and electron microscopy. Cancer 39:1055–1063, 1977

HURLEY HJ, WITKOWSKI JA: The dynamics of eccrine sweating in man. J Invest Dermatol 39:329–338, 1962

MONTAGNA W, CHASE HB, LOBITZ WC, JR.: Histology and cytochemistry of human skin. IV. The eccrine sweat glands. J Invest Dermatol 20:415–423, 1963

SCHIEFFERDECKER P: Die Hautdrüsen des Menschen und der Säugetiere, ihre biologische und rassenanatomische Bedeutung sowie die Muscularis sexualis. Biol Ztrbl 37:534–562, 1917

Apocrine Glands

BIEMPICA L, MONTES LF: Secretory epithelium of the large axillary sweat glands. Am J Anat 117:47–72, 1965

BRAUN-FALCO O, RUPEC M: Apokrine Schweissdrüsen. In Marchionini A (ed): Handbuch der Haut- und Geschlechtskrankheiten, Ergänzungswerk, Vol 1, Part 1, pp. 267–338. Berlin, Springer-Verlag, 1968

ELLIS RA: Eccrine, sebaceous and apocrine glands. In Zelickson AS (ed): Ultrastructure of Normal and Abnormal Skin, pp. 132–162. Philadelphia, Lea & Febiger, 1967

HASHIMOTO K, GROSS BG, LEVER WF: Electron microscopic study of apocrine secretion. J Invest Dermatol 46:378–390, 1966

HASSAN MO, KHAN MA, KRUSE TV: Apocrine cystadenoma: An ultrastructural study. Arch Dermatol 115:194–200, 1979

HEADINGTON JT: Primary mucinous carcinoma of skin: Histochemistry and electron microscopy. Cancer 39:1055–1063, 1977

HIBBS RG: Electron microscopy of human apocrine sweat glands. J Invest Dermatol 38:77–84, 1962

HURLEY HJ, SHELLEY WB: The Human Apocrine Sweat Gland in Health and Disease. Springfield, IL, Charles C Thomas, 1960

INOUE T: Scanning electron microscope study of the human axillary apocrine glands. J Dermatol (Tokyo) 6:299–308, 1979

KUROSUMI K, YAMAGISHI M, SEKINE M: Mitochondrial deformation and apocrine secretory mechanism in the rabbit submandibular organ as revealed by electron microscopy. Z Zellforsch 55:297–312, 1961

MONTAGNA W, YUN JS: The glands of Montgomery. Br J Dermatol 86:126–133, 1972

MONTES LF, BAKER BL, CURTIS AC: The cytology of the large axillary sweat glands in man. J Invest Dermatol 35:273–291, 1960

PINKUS H: Anatomy and histology of skin. In Graham JH, Johnson WC, Helwig EB (eds): Dermal Pathology, pp. 1–24. Hagerstown, Harper & Row, 1972

SCHAUMBURG-LEVER G, LEVER WF: Secretion from human apocrine glands. J Invest Dermatol 64:38–41, 1975

SCHIEFFERDECKER P: Die Hautdrüsen des Menschen und der Säugetiere, ihre biologische und rassenanatomische Bedeutung, sowie die Muscularis sexualis. Biol Ztrbl 37:534–562, 1917

SMITH DM JR, PETER TG, DONEGAN WL: Montgomery's areolar tubercle. Arch Pathol Lab Med 106:60–63, 1982

SOLTERMANN W: Die Bedeutung des Eisennachweises in der Haut für die Diagnose einer Hämochromatose unter besonderer Berücksichtigung der Axillargegend und der apokrinen Schweissdrüsen. Dermatologica 112:335–356, 1956

WINKELMANN RK, HULTIN JV: Mucinous metaplasia in normal apocrine glands. Arch Dermatol 78:309–313, 1958

Sebaceous Glands

CASHION PD, SKOBE Z, NALBANDIAN J: Ultrastructural observations on sebaceous glands of the human oral mucosa (Fordyce's disease). J Invest Dermatol 53:208–216, 1969

HYMAN AB, BROWNSTEIN MH: Tyson's glands. Arch Dermatol 99:31–36, 1969

NIIZUMA K: Lipid droplets of the sebaceous glands: Some observations from tannic acid fixation. Acta Derm Venereol (Stockh) 59:401–405, 1979

ROWDEN G: Aryl sulfatase in the sebaceous glands of mouse skin. J Invest Dermatol 51:41–50, 1968

RUPEC M: Zur Ultrastruktur der Talgdrüsenzelle. Arch Klin Exp Dermatol 234:273–292, 1969

RUPEC M, BRAUN-FALCO O: Zur Frage lysosomaler Aktivität in normalen menschlichen Talgdrüsen. Arch Klin Exp Dermatol 232:312–324, 1968

STRAUSS JS, POCHI PE: Histology, histochemistry, and electron microscopy of sebaceous glands in man. In Marchionini A (ed): Handbuch der Haut- und Geschlechtskrankheiten, Ergänzungswerk, Vol 1, Part 1, pp 184–223. Berlin, Springer-Verlag, 1968

SUSKIND RK: The chemistry of the human sebaceous gland. I. Histochemical observations. J Invest Dermatol 17:37–54, 1951

Hair

CORMIA F: Vasculature of the normal scalp. Arch Dermatol 88:692–701, 1963

GARN SM: The examination of hair under the polarizing microscope. Ann N Y Acad Sci 53:649–652, 1951

HERZBERG J, GUSEK W: Das Ergrauen des Kopfhaares. Arch Klin Exp Dermatol 236:368–384, 1970

JOHNSON WC, HELWIG EB: Histochemistry of the acid mucopolysaccharides of skin in normal and in certain pathologic conditions. Am J Clin Pathol 40:123–131, 1963

KLIGMAN AM: The human hair cycle. J Invest Dermatol 33:307–316, 1959

KOLLAR EJ: The induction of hair follicles by embryonic dermal papillae. J Invest Dermatol 55:374–378, 1970

KOPF AW, ORENTREICH N: Alkaline phosphatase in alopecia areata. Arch Dermatol 76:288–295, 1957

LEPPARD BJ, SANDERSON KV, WELLS RS: Hereditary trichilemmal cysts. Clin Exp Dermatol 2:23–32, 1976

MAHRLE G, ORFANOS CE: Das spongiöse Keratin und die Marksubstanz des menschlichen Kopfhaares. Arch Dermatol Forsch 241:305–316, 1971

MAHRLE G, ORFANOS CE: Haarfarbe und Haarpigment. Arch Dermatol Forsch 248:109–122, 1973

MISHIMA Y, WIDLAN S: Embryonic development of melanocytes in human hair and epidermis. J Invest Dermatol 46:263–277, 1966

MONTAGNA W: The Structure and Function of Skin, 2nd ed, pp. 174–267. New York, Academic Press, 1962

ORFANOS CE, RUSKA H: Die Feinstruktur des menschlichen Haares. II. Der Haar-Cortex. III. Das Haarpigment. Arch Klin Exp Dermatol 231:264–292, 1968

PARAKKAL PF, MATOLTSY AG: A study of the differentiation products of the hair follicle cells with the electron microscope. J Invest Dermatol 43:23–34, 1964

PINKUS H: "Sebaceous cysts" are trichilemmal cysts. Arch Dermatol 99:544–555, 1969

PINKUS H: Anatomy and histology of skin. In Graham JH, Johnson WC, Helwig EB (eds): Dermal Pathology, pp 1–24. Hagerstown, Haper & Row, 1972

STARICCO RG: The melanocytes and the hair follicle. J Invest Dermatol 35:185–194, 1960

VAN SCOTT EJ, REINERTSON RP, STEINMULLER R: The growing hair roots of the human scalp and morphologic changes therein following amethopterin therapy. J Invest Dermatol 29:197–204, 1957

WEEDON D, STRUTTON G: Apoptosis as the mechanism of the involution of hair follicles in catagen formation. Acta Derm Venereol (Stockh) 61:335–339, 1981

ZAUN H: Histologie, Histochemie und Wachstumsdynamik des Haarfollikels. In Marchionini A (ed): Handbuch der Haut- und Geschlechtskrankheiten. Ergänzungswerk, Vol 1, Part 1, pp 143–183. Berlin, Springer-Verlag, 1968

Nails

HASHIMOTO K: The marginal band: A demonstration of the thickened cellular envelope of the human nail cell with the aid of lanthanum staining. Arch Dermatol 103:387–393, 1971

LEWIN K: The normal finger nail. Br J Dermatol 77:421–430, 1965

NORTON LA: Incorporation of thymidinemethyl-H^3 and glycine-2H^3 in the nail matrix and bed of humans. J Invest Dermatol 56:61–68, 1971

ZAIAS N: The movement of the nail bed. J Invest Dermatol 48:402–403, 1967

ZAIAS N, ALVAREZ J: The formation of the primate nail plate: An autoradiographic study in squirrel monkey. J Invest Dermatol 51:120–136, 1968

Connective Tissue of the Dermis

BREATHNACH AS: An Atlas of the Ultrastructure of Human Skin, pp 174–175. London, J & A Churchill, 1971

BYERS PH, BARSH GS, HOLBROOK KA: Molecular pathology in inherited disorders of collagen metabolism. Hum Pathol 13:89–95, 1982

GRANT ME, PROCKOP DJ: The biosynthesis of collagen. N Engl J Med 286:194–199, 1972

HASHIMOTO K, DIBELLA RJ: Electron microscopic studies of normal and abnormal elastic fibers of the skin. J Invest Dermatol 48:405–423, 1967

HAYES RL, RODNAN GP: The ultrastructure of skin in progressive sclerosis (scleroderma). Am J Pathol 63:433–442, 1971

JACQUES J, CAMERON HCS: Changes in the ground-substance of healing wounds. J Pathol 99:337–340, 1969

JANSEN LH: The structure of the connective tissue: An explanation of the symptoms of the Ehlers-Danlos syndrome. Dermatologica 110:108–120, 1955

JOHNSON WC, HELWIG EB: Histochemistry of the acid mucopolysaccharides of the skin in normal and in certain pathologic conditions. Am J Clin Pathol 40:123–131, 1963

KEFALIDES NA: Basement membranes: Structural and biosynthetic considerations. J Invest Dermatol 65:85–92, 1975

LAZARUS GS: Collagen, collagenase and clinicians. Br J Dermatol 26:193–199, 1972

MARSCH WC, SCHOBER E, NÜRNBERGER F: Zur Ultrastruktur und Morphogenese der elastischen Faser und der aktinischen Elastose. Z Hautkr 54:43–46, 1979

MEIGEL WN, GAY S, WEBER L: Dermal architecture and collagen type distribution. Arch Dermatol Res 259:1–10, 1977

NIGRA TP, FRIEDLAND M, MARTIN GR: Controls of connective tissue synthesis: Collagen metabolism. J Invest Dermatol 59:44–49, 1972

PINKUS H: The direction of growth of human epidermis. Br J Dermatol 83:556–564, 1970

REED RJ, ACKERMAN AB: Pathology of the adventitial dermis. Hum Pathol 4:207–217, 1973

REHTIJÄRVI K: Reticular network and karyometric properties of lymphomas of the skin. Acta Derm Venereol (Stockh) 43, Suppl 53:1–100, 1963

ROSS R, BENDITT EP: Wound healing and collagen formation. V. Quantitative electron microscopic radioautographic observations of proline-H³ utilization by fibroblasts. J Cell Biol 27:83–89, 1965

SCARPELLI DG, GOODMAN RM: Observations on the fine structure of the fibroblast from a case of Ehlers-Danlos syndrome with the Marfan syndrome. J Invest Dermatol 50:214–219, 1968

SCHMIDT W: Die normale Histologie von Corium und Subcutis. In Marchionini A (ed): Handbuch der Haut- und Geschlechtskrankheiten, Ergänzungswerk, Vol 1, Part 1, pp 430–490. Berlin, Springer-Verlag, 1968

SMITH JG, JR.: The dermal elastoses. Arch Dermatol 88:382–392, 1963

STADLER R, ORFANOS CE: Reifung und Alterung der elastischen Fasern. Arch Dermatol Forsch 262:97–111, 1978

STENN K: Collagen heterogeneity of skin. Am J Dermatopathol 1:87–88, 1979

UITTO J, LICHTENSTEIN JR: Defects in the biochemistry of collagen in diseases of connective tissue. J Invest Dermatol 66:59–79, 1976

VARADI DP: Studies on the chemistry and fine structure of elastic fibers from normal adult skin. J Invest Dermatol 59:238–246, 1972

WINAND R: Biosynthesis, organization and degradation of mucopolysaccharides. Arch Belg Derm Syph 28:35–40, 1972

YAOITA H, FOIDART JM, KATZ SI: Localization of the collagenous component in the skin basement membrane. J Invest Dermatol 70:191–193, 1978

Nerves and Nerve End-Organs of the Dermis

ARTHUR RP, SHELLEY WB: The innervation of human epidermis. J Invest Dermatol 32:397–413, 1959

BREATHNACH AS: An Atlas of the Ultrastructure of Human Skin, pp 206–207. London, J & A Churchill, 1971

CAUNA N, ROSS LL: The fine structure of Meissner's touch corpuscles of human fingers. J Biophys Biochem Cytol 8:467–482, 1960

HASHIMOTO K: Fine structure of the Meissner corpuscle of human palmar skin. J Invest Dermatol 60:20–28, 1973

MACDONALD DM, SCHMITT D: Ultrastructure of the human mucocutaneous end organ. J Invest Dermatol 72:181–186, 1979

ORFANOS CE, MAHRLE G: Ultrastructure and cytochemistry of human cutaneous nerves. J Invest Dermatol 61:108–120, 1973

PEASE DC, QUILLIAM TA: Electron microscopy of the Pacinian corpuscle. J Biophys Biochem Cytol 3:331–344, 1957

REED RJ: Cutaneous manifestations of neural crest disorders. Int J Dermatol 16:807–826, 1977

SIAN CS, RYAN SF: The ultrastructure of neurilemoma with emphasis on Antoni B tissue. Hum Pathol 12:145–160, 1981

WINKELMANN RK: Silver impregnation method for peripheral nerve endings. J Invest Dermatol 24:57–64, 1955

WINKELMANN RK: Nerve Endings in Normal and Pathologic Skin, pp 50–80. Springfield, IL, Charles C Thomas, 1960

WINKELMANN RK, OSMENT LS: The Vater–Pacinian corpuscle in the skin of the human finger tip. Arch Dermatol 73:116–122, 1956

WOOLLARD HH, WEDDELL G, HARPMAN JA: Observations on neurohistological basis of cutaneous pain. J Anat 74:413–440, 1940

Blood Vessels and Lymph Vessels

BRAVERMAN IM, YEN A: Ultrastructure of human dermal microcirculation. II. The capillary loop of the dermal papillae. J Invest Dermatol 68:44–52, 1977

EIMOTO T: Ultrastructure of an infantile hemangiopericytoma. Cancer 40:2161–2170, 1977

GOODMAN TF: Fine structure of the cells of the Suquet–Hoyer canal. J Invest Dermatol 59:363–369, 1972

KLINGMÜLLER G: Die Darstellung alkalischer Phosphatase in Capillaren. Hautarzt 9:84–88, 1958

KOPF AW: The distribution of alkaline phosphatase in normal and pathologic human skin. Arch Dermatol 75:1–37, 1957

KOPF AW, ORENTREICH N: Alkaline phosphatase in alopecia areata. Arch Dermatol 76:288–295, 1957

MEADE JB, WHITWELL F, BICKFORD BJ et al: Primary hemangiopericytoma of the lung. Thorax 29:1–15, 1974

MESCON H, HURLEY HJ, MORETTI G: The anatomy and histochemistry of the arteriovenous anastomosis in human digital skin. J Invest Dermatol 27:133–145, 1956

MORETTI G: The blood vessels of the skin. In Marchionini A (ed): Handbuch der Haut- und Geschlechtskrankheiten, Ergänzungswerk, Vol 1, Part 1, pp 491–623. Berlin, Springer-Verlag, 1968

PEPPER M, LAUBENHEIMER R, CRIPPS DJ: Multiple glomus tumors. J Cutan Pathol 4:244–257, 1977

PFLEGER L: Histologie und Histopathologie cutaner Lymphgefässe der unteren Extremitäten. Arch Klin Exp Dermatol 221:1–22, 1964

SEIFERT HW, KLINGMÜLLER G: Elektronenmikroskopische Struktur normaler Kapillaren und das Verhalten alkalischer Phosphatase. Arch Dermatol Forsch 242:97–110, 1972

WEBER K, BRAUN-FALCO O: Ultrastructure of blood vessels in human granulation tissue. Arch Dermatol Forsch 248:29–44, 1973

YEN A, BRAVERMAN IM: Ultrastructure of the human dermal microcirculation: The horizontal plexus of the papillary dermis. J Invest Dermatol 66:131–142, 1976

Muscles of the Skin

BREATHNACH AS: An Atlas of the Ultrastructure of Human Skin, pp 330–333. London, J & A Churchill, 1971

ORFANOS C: Elektronenmikroskopische Untersuchung glatter Hautmuskelfasern und ihrer Innervation. Dermatologica 132:445–459, 1966

SCHMIDT W: Die normale Histologie von Corium und Subcutis. In Marchionini A (ed): Handbuch der Haut- und Geschlechtskrankheiten, Ergänzungswerk, Vol 1, Part 1, pp 430–490, Berlin, Springer-Verlag, 1968

4 Laboratory Methods

PREPARATION OF SPECIMENS

Fixation. As already stated in Chapter 1, the fixative of choice is a 10% aqueous solution of formalin, except during winter, when, in order to prevent freezing of the specimen, it is recommended that 95% ethyl alcohol, 10% by volume, be added to the formalin solution (see p. 2).

It is important that adequate time be allowed for fixation. The minimum period for specimens 4 mm thick is 8 hr; for specimens 6 mm thick, it is 12 hr.

Large specimens, such as excised tumors, should be cut in the laboratory into slices 4 mm to 5 mm thick for further fixation. It is important that such specimens be cut not lengthwise but across so that, after the histologic examination, information can be provided as to whether an adequate margin of normal skin is present between the tumor and the border of the specimen.

Demonstration of Enzyme Activities. With few exceptions (see below), specimens should not be placed in formalin for the demonstration of enzyme activities. Instead, it is recommended that a specimen be delivered to the laboratory wrapped in water-moistened gauze and placed in a plastic bag, since, for enzyme staining, frozen sections cut on a cryostat are usually used. It should be kept in mind that staining for enzyme activities is not routinely done in all pathology laboratories and therefore should not be requested without checking with the laboratory first. Staining for enzymes is necessary only in very rare instances for purposes of diagnosis.

An enzyme stain that is occasionally of value is the stain demonstrating dopa-oxidase activity. Demonstration of dopa-oxidase activity in melanocytes may aid in distinguishing a malignant melanoma from tumors not composed of melanocytes (see pp. 16 and 716). Also, the distinction between eccrine and apocrine differentiation in cutaneous appendage tumors is often possible by means of enzyme stains, since certain enzymes, such as succinic dehydrogenase and phosphorylase, are characteristic of eccrine differentiation (see pp. 552 and 554), whereas others, such as acid phosphatose and beta-glucuronidase, are characteristic of apocrine differentiation (see p. 544).

Enzyme reactions that can be carried out on a formalin-fixed, paraffin-embedded tissue are the following: (1) demonstration of naphthol AS-D chloracetate esterase activity, with naphthol AS-D chloracetate as substrate, present in mature and immature granulocytes, except in myeloblasts (Neiman et al) (see p. 750); (2) demonstration of lysozyme with the antilysozyme immunoperoxidase technic, lysozyme being present in mature and immature granulocytes, even in myeloblasts, as well as in eosinophilic myeloid cells and histiocytes (Neiman et al) (see p. 750); and (3) demonstration of alpha-naphthyl acetate (nonspecific) esterase activity, with alpha-naphthyl acetate as substrate, present in histiocytes (Wohlenberg et al) (see p. 750).

Formalin-fixed, paraffin-embedded specimens of skin can also be used for the immunoperoxidase technic. With this method, various monoclonal antibodies can be demonstrated. Among these antibodies are various OKT mouse monoclonal antisera against T lymphocytes and Langerhans cells (see pp. 49 and 745) and antibodies generated against several tissue proteins, among them carcinoembryogenic antigen, present in eccrine and apocrine glands and tumors, including Paget's disease (Penneys et al, 1982b); myelin, present in nerves and neural tumors, including granular cell tumors (Penneys et al, 1982a); prekeratin, present in the epidermis and epidermal tumors, including even poorly differentiated squamous cell carcinomas (Penneys et al, 1982c); and blood group antigens, present in normal epidermis but largely absent in malignant epidermal tumors (Schaumburg-Lever et al).

In two diseases, scleredema of Buschke and amyloidosis, unfixed frozen sections may show a more conclusive reaction to specific staining methods than is obtainable with formalin-fixed material. It is therefore recommended that, in these two diseases, only part of the tissue be fixed in formalin and the remainder be used for frozen sections. In scleredema, demonstration of hyaluronic acid with toluidine blue at pH 7.0 may be more intense in unfixed, frozen sections than in formalin-fixed sections (see p. 428); in amyloidosis, the reactions of the amyloid with crystal violet or Congo red may be conclusive only in unfixed, frozen sections (see p. 407).

Processing. After having been fixed for a sufficient length of time in formalin, all routine specimens are processed in an automatic processor, such as an Autotechnicon. The only exception is specimens that are to be stained for lipids. Since lipids are extracted by the xylene used in the Autotechnicon for the processing of specimens, formalin-fixed, frozen sections are used for lipid staining.

The Autotechnicon, regulated by clockwork, automatically controls overnight the duration of processing in a succession of beakers. The specimens pass first through increasing concentrations of ethanol for dehydration, then through xylene for lipid extraction, and finally through several changes of hot, melted paraffin or Paraplast. The next morning, the specimens are embedded with the epidermis upward in the still liquid paraffin or Paraplast, which is allowed to harden. The specimens are then cut on a rotary microtome into sections 5 μm to 7 μm thick.

Staining. All routine sections are stained with hematoxylin-eosin, the most widely used routine stain. With this staining method, nuclei stain blue, whereas collagen, muscles, and nerves stain red. Special stains are employed only when needed for the demonstration of particular structures (Table 4-1). (For details, see the *Manual of Histologic Staining Methods of the Armed Forces Institute of Pathology*, Luna LG, ed.)

HISTOCHEMICAL STAINING

Histochemistry, especially enzyme histoc both at the light microscopic and electron scopic level, has gained increasing importar recent years and has been largely responsible the expansion of histopathology from a purely descriptive science to one that is dynamic and functional (Pearse). Most enzyme histochemical methods are used only for research and, as already pointed out, have the limitation of usually requiring fresh tissue in the place of formalin-fixed tissue (see p. 42).

Two histochemical stains that stain chemical substrates rather than enzymes and can be carried out on formalin-fixed, Autotechnicon-processed material have attained considerable diagnostic importance: the periodic acid-Schiff (PAS) reaction (Kligman et al), and the alcian blue reaction (Cawley et al).

The *PAS stain* demonstrates the presence of certain polysaccharides, particularly glycogen and mucoproteins containing neutral mucopolysaccharides, by staining them red. The PAS reaction is of value also in the study of fibrinoid degeneration (see p. 450), since fibrin deposits in areas of fibrinoid degeneration are PAS-positive. Furthermore, since the cell walls of fungi are composed of a mixture of cellulose and chitin and thus contain polysaccharides, all fungi stain bright red with the PAS reaction.

The PAS reaction consists of the oxidation of adjacent hydroxyl groups in 1,2 glycols to aldehydes and the staining of the aldehydes with fuchsin–sulfuric acid (Stoughton and Wells).

For the distinction of neutral mucopolysaccharides and fungi from glycogen deposits, it is necessary to compare two serial sections, one exposed to diastase prior to staining and the other not. Since glycogen is diastase-labile, that is, digested by the diastase, and thus no longer colored red by the PAS reaction, it can be easily distinguished from neutral mucopolysaccharides and fungi that are diastase-resistant. Since glycogen is present in outer root sheath cells and eccrine gland cells, and neutral polysaccharides are found in eccrine and apocrine gland cells, demonstration of the presence of glycogen is of diagnostic value in trichilemmal tumor (see p. 533), in trichilemmoma (see p. 534), in clear cell hidradenoma (see p. 557), and in eccrine poroma (see p. 553). Demonstration of the presence of neutral mucopolysaccharides is of value in Paget's disease of the breast (see p. 510), in extramammary Paget's disease (see p. 512), in clear

elastic fibers dark brown

combines c̄ tyrosine in melanocyte → dopa-melanin —black

Y METHODS

...ft esterase: outlines mast cells or granulocytic myelocytes

mmonly Used Staining Methods

	Purpose of Stain	Results
	Routine	Nuclei: blue; collagen, muscles, nerves: red
	Collagen	Collagen: green; nuclei, muscles, nerves: dark red
	Elastic fibers	Elastic fibers: black; collagen: red; nuclei, muscles, nerves: yellow
	Melanin, reticulum fibers, nerves (argyrophilic)	Melanin, reticulum fibers, nerves: black
Fontana–Masson (ammoniated silver nitrate)	Melanin (argentaffin)	Melanin: black
Methenamine silver	Fungi, Donovan bodies, Frisch bacilli	Fungus walls, Donovan bodies, Frisch bacilli: black
PAS (periodic acid-Schiff) and diastase	Glycogen, neutral MPS, fungi	Glycogen: diastase-labile; neutral MPS, fungus walls: diastase-resistant
Alcian blue	Acid MPS	Acid MPS: blue
Toluidine blue	Acid MPS	Acid MPS: metachromatically purple
Giemsa	Mast cell granules, acid MPS, eosinophils, *Leishmania*	Mast cell granules, acid MPS: metachromatically purple; eosinophil granules, *Leishmania:* red
Fite	Acid-fast bacilli	Acid-fast bacilli: red
Perls' potassium ferrocyanide	Hemosiderin	Hemosiderin: blue
Alkaline Congo red	Amyloid	Amyloid: green birefringence in polarized light
Von Kossa	Calcium	Calcium: black
Scarlet red	Lipids	Lipids: red

Note: All stains, except that for lipids, can be carried out on formalin-fixed specimens that have been processed in the Autotechnicon. The stain for lipids requires formalin-fixed, frozen section. MPS = mucopolysaccharides.

cell hidradenoma (see p. 557), and intraluminally in eccrine spiradenoma (see p. 555) and eccrine poroma (see p. 553).

The *alcian blue reaction* demonstrates the presence of acid mucopolysaccharides by staining them blue. Acid mucopolysaccharides are present in the dermal ground substance, but in amounts too small to be demonstrable in normal skin. However, in the dermal mucinoses, one finds a great increase in nonsulfated acid mucopolysaccharides, mainly hyaluronic acid, so that the mucin stains with alcian blue (see p. 425). In extramammary Paget's

disease of the anus with rectal carcinoma (see p. 513), as well as in cutaneous metastases of carcinoma of the gastrointestinal tract containing goblet cells (see p. 593), tumor cells in the skin, like their parent cells, secrete sialomucin. Sialomucin contains nonsulfated acid mucopolysaccharides staining with alcian blue, as well as PAS-positive neutral mucopolysaccharides. (For details about sialomucin, see p. 593.) Whereas nonsulfated acid mucopolysaccharides stain with alcian blue at *p*H 2.5 but not at *p*H 0.5, strongly acidic sulfated acid mucopolysaccharides, such as heparin in mast cell

Ulex europaeus I } endothelial cells
Factor VIII Ag }

Leu 6 OKT6 – Langerhans Cells

Leu 3a OKT4 CD4 — Helper T
Leu 2a OKT8 CD8   Suppressor T

Keratin
Neurofilaments
Desmin (smooth & striated muscle)
Vimentin (fibroblasts, melanocytes)

Lysozyme
Chymotrypsin } macrophages

IMMUNOFLUORESCENCE TESTING   45

granules and chondroitin sulfate in cartilage, stain with alcian blue both at *pH* 2.5 and at *pH* 0.5 (Johnson and Helwig; Helwig and Graham).

POLARISCOPIC EXAMINATION

Polariscopic examination is the examination of histologic sections under the microscope with polarized light, that is, with light from which all rays except those vibrating in one plane are excluded.

For polariscopic examination, two disks made of polarizing plastics are inserted in the microscope. One disk is placed below the condenser of the microscope and acts as the polarizer. The second disk is placed in the eyepiece of the microscope and acts as the analyzer. When the eyepiece containing the analyzing disk is rotated so that the path of the light through the two disks is broken at a right angle, the field is dark. However, when doubly refractile substances are introduced between the two disks, they break the polarization and are visible as bright white bodies in the dark field.

Polariscopic examination is useful in evaluating lipid deposits, certain foreign bodies, gout, and amyloid.

With regard to lipids, it is not fully known why certain lipids are doubly refractile and others are not. In general, however, cholesterol esters are doubly refractile, whereas free cholesterol, phospholipids, and neutral fat are not. It should be remembered that only formalin-fixed, frozen sections can be used for a polariscopic examination for lipids.

Doubly refractile lipids are present regularly (1) in the tuberous and plane xanthomas and xanthelasmata (but not always in the eruptive xanthomas) of hyperlipoproteinemia (see p. 386), (2) in the cutaneous lesions of diffuse mormolipemic plane xanthoma (see p. 397), and (3) in the vascular walls of angiokertoma corporis diffusum (Fabry's disease) (see p. 390).

Doubly refractile lipids are present, provided that the cutaneous lesions contain a sufficient amount of lipid, (1) in histiocytosis X (Hand–Schüller–Christian type) (see p. 396), (2) in juvenile xanthogranuloma, or nevoxanthoendothelioma (see p. 399), (3) in erythema elevatum diutinum (extracellular cholesterosis) (see p. 176), and (4) in dermatofibroma (lipidized "histiocytoma") (see p. 598).

Doubly refractile lipids are absent in lipid-containing lesions, as a rule, (1) in necrobiosis lipoidica

(see p. 238), (2) in hyalinosis cutis et mucosae, or lipoid proteinosis (see p. 415), and (3) in multicentric reticulohistiocytosis and solitary reticulohistiocytic granuloma (see p. 401).

Among foreign bodies, silica causes granulomas showing doubly refractile spicules. Such granulomas are caused either by particles of soil or glass (silicon dioxide) or by talcum powder (magnesium silicate) (see p. 223). Wooden splinters and suture material also are doubly refractile.

Gout tophi show double refraction of the urate crystals present within them provided that the crystals are sufficiently preserved. This is accomplished by the use of alcohol rather than formalin for fixation (see p. 423).

Amyloid shows a characteristic green birefringence in polarized light after staining with alkaline Congo red (see p. 407).

IMMUNOFLUORESCENCE TESTING

One distinguishes between direct immunofluorescence testing, which uses the patient's own skin or mucous membrane, and indirect immunofluorescence testing, which uses the patient's blood serum. Direct immunofluorescence testing is a valuable diagnostic procedure in three groups of diseases: (1) the chronic "autoimmune" vesiculobullous diseases, (2) all forms of lupus erythematosus, and (3) leukocytoclastic vasculitis. In addition, indirect immunofluorescence testing can be carried out in some of the chronic "autoimmune" vesiculobullous diseases, such as the various forms of pemphigus and pemphigoid, because of the presence of circulating antibodies. The indirect test is less sensitive than the direct test; however, it may be used as a supplementary test when the direct test cannot be relied upon because the specimen is being mailed over long distances or is in danger of freezing. Although, in general, a correlation exists in pemphigus between the level of antibody titers and the degree of disease activity, this correlation is not consistent enough to be used as a guide to therapy or prognosis (Judd and Lever; Fitzpatrick and Newcomer).

Technic of Biopsy. A 3-mm punch biopsy generally is adequate. In the group of chronic "autoimmune" vesiculobullous diseases, lesional skin should not be used for testing, because, in the various forms of pemphigus or pemphigoid, detachment of the top of the blister from the biopsy specimen may result in inadequate material being available for testing and thus cause a falsely negative test. In dermatitis herpetiformis, it has become apparent that the inflammatory infiltrate may phagocytize the immune complexes within the lesions. It is therefore recommended that the biopsy specimen in dermatitis herpetiformis be obtained a good distance from any lesion, preferably from the buttock region (Fry and Seah). In the various forms of pemphigus, it does not seem to matter from which area of uninvolved skin the biopsy is taken (Judd and Lever). In contrast, in the various forms of pemphigoid, the test may be negative when the biopsy specimen is taken from an area far away from active lesions, especially in patients with only a few lesions; therefore, it is recommended that perilesional skin always be used for biopsy. As will be described under the headings of the various vesiculobullous diseases, positive direct tests are obtained in almost 100% of the cases in the various forms of pemphigus, in bullous pemphigoid, and in dermatitis herpetiformis, as well as in a very high percentage of cases in cicatricial pemphigoid and herpes gestationis.

The site of the biopsy for direct immunofluorescence in lupus erythematosus depends on the purpose of the test; if it is to establish the diagnosis, the biopsy is taken from a lesion, whereas, if it is to determine whether the patient has systemic rather than discoid lupus erythematosus, the biopsy is taken from uninvolved skin or even from sun-protected skin (see p. 454).

In cases of vasculitis, the biopsy specimen is taken from a very early lesion, preferably one less than 24 hr old (see p. 169).

Transport of the Biopsy Specimen. It was originally thought necessary to quick-freeze the biopsy specimen and to keep it in a frozen state up to the time of testing. It has since become evident that specimens can be kept in a special "holding solution" for 2 weeks and longer without loss of reactivity (Nisengaard et al); or they can be transported in phosphate-buffered normal saline solution (Judd and Lever). This, of course, has made the direct immunofluorescence technic much more readily applicable.

BIBLIOGRAPHY

CAWLEY EP, LUPTON CH, JR., WHEELER CE et al: Examination of normal and myxedematous skin: Use of Mowry's Alcian blue periodic acid-Schiff technique. Arch Dermatol 76:537–544, 1957

FITZPATRICK RE, NEWCOMER VD: The correlation of disease activity and antibody titers in pemphigus. Arch Dermatol 116:285–290, 1980

FRY L, SEAH PP: Dermatitis herpetiformis: An evaluation of diagnostic criteria. Br J Dermatol 90:137–146, 1974

HELWIG EB, GRAHAM JH: Anogenital (extramammary) Paget's disease. Cancer 16:387–403, 1963

JOHNSON WC, HELWIG EB: Histochemistry of the acid mucopolysaccharides of the skin in normal and in certain pathologic conditions. Am J Clin Pathol 40:123–131, 1963

JUDD KP, LEVER WF: Correlation of antibodies in skin and serum with disease severity in pemphigus. Arch Dermatol 115:428–432, 1979

KLIGMAN AM, MESCON H, DELAMATER ED: The Hotchkiss-McManus stain for the histopathologic diagnosis of fungus diseases. Am J Clin Pathol 21:86–91, 1951

LUNA LG (ed): Manual of Histologic Staining Methods of the Armed Forces Institute of Pathology, 3rd ed. New York, McGraw-Hill, 1968

NEIMAN RS, BARCOS M, BERARD C et al: Granulocytic sarcoma. Cancer 48:1426–1437, 1981

NISENGAARD RJ, BLASZCZYK M, CHORZELSKI T et al: Immunofluorescence of biopsy specimens: Comparison of methods of transportation. Arch Dermatol 114:1329—1332, 1978

PEARSE AGE: Histochemistry, Theoretical and Applied, 3rd ed. Boston, Little, Brown & Co, 1972

PENNEYS NS, ADACHI K, ZIEGELS-WEISSMAN J et al: Granular cell tumors of the skin contain myelin basic protein. Arch Pathol, in press a

PENNEYS NS, NADJI M, MORALES A: Carcinoembryonic antigen in benign sweat gland tumors. Arch Dermatol 118:225–227, 1982b

PENNEYS NS, NADJI M, ZIEGELS-WEISSMAN J et al: Prekeratin in spindle cell tumors of the skin. Arch Dermatol, in press c

SCHAUMBURG-LEVER G, ALROY J, GAVRIS V et al: Cell surface coats in proliferative epidermal lesions. J Invest Dermatol, submitted for publication

STOUGHTON R, WELLS G: A histochemical study on polysaccharides in normal and diseased skin. J Invest Dermatol 14:37–51, 1950

WOHLENBERG H, GRISS P, GOOS M et al: Zur Zytochemie von Hautinfiltraten myelomonocytärer Leukämien. Dtsch Med Wochenschr 95:1439–1443, 1970

Morphology of the Cells in the Dermal Infiltrate

5

Various types of cells, largely derived from the bone marrow, infiltrate the dermis and occasionally also the epidermis in the inflammatory and granulomatous dermatoses. It is important for diagnostic purposes to identify the cell types. Three groups of cells are derived from the bone marrow: (1) the granulocytic group, (2) the lymphocytic group, including plasma cells, and (3) the monocytic or macrophagic group. In addition, two types of cells form in the dermis and may participate in the cellular proliferation occurring in the inflammatory and granulomatous dermatoses: the mast cell and the fibroblast. (For a discussion of the fibroblast and its functions, see p. 31.)

GRANULOCYTIC GROUP

Neutrophilic and eosinophilic granulocytes are found in the skin in various dermatoses. Eosinophils participate in anaphylactic reactions. Basophilic granulocytes, which require special fixation and staining for identification in the skin (see p. 54), participate both in anaphylactic and in delayed hypersensitivity reactions, such as contact dermatitis (Dvorak and Dvorak).

Neutrophilic Granulocytes. The neutrophilic granulocyte, also called a neutrophil or polymorphonuclear leukocyte, is 10 μm to 12 μm in size and has a lobated nucleus consisting of several segments that are connected only by narrow bridges of nucleoplasm. The slightly basophilic cytoplasm contains numerous neutrophilic to slightly eosinophilic granules. On histochemical examination, the granules are seen to contain lysosomal enzymes and thus represent primary lysosomes.

Neutrophilic granulocytes play an important role (1) in the early phase of some inflammatory responses, (2) in the phagocytosis and killing of microorganisms, and (3) in the immobilization and phagocytosis of antigen–antibody complexes in the presence of compliment (Wilkinson). The phagocytosis of microorganisms and of antigen–antibody complexes is accompanied by partial to complete degranulation of the neutrophils, during which the lysosomal granules discharge their contents (Parish).

Examples of the participation of neutrophils in the early phase of inflammation are their presence in primary irritant dermatitis and their occurrence in the early phase of nodular nonsuppurative panniculitis and erythema nodosum. Phagocytosis of microorganisms is seen in the subcorneal pustules of impetigo and candidiasis, in staphylococcal folliculitis, in erysipelas, and in cellulitis. Association of neutrophils with immune complexes occurs in allergic vasculitis (anaphylactoid purpura) and possibly also in its variants, erythema elevatum diutinum and acute febrile neutrophilic dermatosis of Sweet, as well as in the neutrophilic vasculitis and papillary microabscesses of dermatitis herpetiformis. It is unknown why neutrophils are present in the Munro microabscesses and the spongiform pustules of Kogoj observed in psoriasis and its variants, or in the subcorneal pustule of subcorneal pustular dermatosis. In psoriasis, the presence of a leukotactic factor in the psoriatic scales has been postulated (see p. 144).

Histogenesis. Two types of membrane-bound cytoplasmic granules or lysosomes are found to be present in neutrophils on *electron microscopic examination:* azurophilic and specific granules (Weissmann et al). The azurophilic granules, constituting about 20% of all granules, are relatively dense and large, measuring up to 1 μ in diameter. The more numerous specific granules average 300 nm in diameter. Among other substances, *azurophilic* granules contain (1) myeloperoxidase, which mediates the formation of hydrogen peroxide, essential for the killing of many microorganisms; (2) acid hydrolases, such as beta-glucuronidase and acid phosphatase, capable of degrading dead bacteria and other necrotic material; (3) neutral proteases, such as collagenase and elastase, that may break down collagen and elastin; (4) cationic proteins, which cause an increase in vascular permeability; and (5) lysozyme, an enzyme that degrades and lyses bacterial cell walls. The *specific* granules also contain lysozyme and collagenase, as well as lactoferrin, an iron-binding protein with bacteriostatic properties, and alkaline phosphatase.

Neutrophils phagocytize and kill microorganisms by incorporating them into their cytoplasms through endocytosis, resulting in phagocytic vacuoles or phagosomes that are lined by the invaginated plasma membrane. Many cytoplasmic granules discharge their lysosomal enzymes into such a phagosome, making it a phagolysosome. The various lysosomal enzymes then kill the microorganisms. If phagocytosis cannot be accomplished, the neutrophil is capable of extracellular degranulation and extracellular discharge of lysosomal enzymes (Weissmann et al).

Immune complexes, after their activation by complement, may induce the accumulation of neutrophils, possibly by chemotaxis. The immune complexes may be phagocytized by neutrophils, which then discharge lysosomal enzymes into the phagosomes containing the immune complexes; or, if the complexes are attached to a basement membrane located either around a blood vessel or at the epidermal-dermal border, the neutrophils may release their lysosomal constituents by extracellular degranulation (Henson). Since the released enzymes include a collagenase and an elastase, considerable damage can ensue to the basement membrane and even the walls of blood vessels through the exocytosis of neutrophilic granules (Lazarus et al). This destructive event, when it affects blood vessels, represents the so-called Arthus phenomenon or, in a broader sense, an antigen–antibody complex reaction or the type III hypersensitivity reaction in the classification of Gell and Coombs (Gell and Coombs; Patterson et al).

Eosinophilic Granulocytes.   The eosinophil, 12 μm to 17 μm in size, is characterized by the presence in the cytoplasm of eosinophilic granules. They are larger than the granules of neutrophils. Although visible with routine stains, these granules stand out more clearly in brilliant red when a Giemsa stain is used. The nucleus of eosinophils, in contrast to that of neutrophils, is usually bilobed and only occasionally trilobed (Berretty and Cormane, 1978).

Because eosinophils can phagocytize mast cell granules and certain antigen–antibody complexes, tissue eosinophilia in the skin can occur (1) as a result of anaphylactic or atopic hypersensitivity, (2) subsequent to the degranulation of mast cells, and (3) in certain diseases associated with deposits of antigen–antibody complexes in the skin.

The tissue eosinophilia appearing in anaphylactic reactions and other forms of "immediate" allergy such as atopy is based on the presence of antibodies of the IgE type on the surface of mast cells. The anaphylactic reaction, classified as type I hypersensitivity reaction (Gell and Coombs), occurs following the binding of a specific antigen to a specific antibody on the surface of the mast cells. This leads to degranulation of mast cells and to the release of vasoactive substances, especially histamine. Wherever degranulation of mast cells occurs, eosinophils appear and phagocytize the released mast cell granules (Parish, 1970). Eosinophils thus may modify an anaphylactic reaction (Berretty and Cormane, 1981). Degranulation of mast cells as the cause of tissue eosinophilia occurs also in urticaria pigmentosa after stroking of the lesions.

Diseases in which deposition of antigen–antibody complexes is the cause of eosinophilia include pemphigus vulgaris, particularly pemphigus vegetans, pemphigus foliaceus, bullous pemphigoid, and granuloma faciale. The reasons for the occasional presence of tissue eosinophilia in histiocytosis X and in Hodgkin's disease are not fully apparent.

Parasitic infestations often are associated with eosinophilia both in the peripheral blood and in the tissue. It appears likely that eosinophils function as effector cells in parasite destruction (Zucker-Franklin).

Histogenesis. On *electron microscopic examination,* the granules of eosinophils are seen to be oval or boat-shaped. They consist of two components, a central, angular-shaped core, often referred to as the crystalloid, and a surrounding matrix. In electron microscopic sections stained with lead compounds, the crystalloid is more darkly stained than the matrix (Poole). The longer diameter of the granules measures 0.5 μm to 1.5 μm, and the shorter diameter 0.3 μm to 1 μm (Berretty and Cormane, 1978). The granules contain a variety of hydrolytic enzymes, particularly peroxidase and arylsulfatase, and therefore can be classified as lysosomes. The phagocytic potential of eosinophils seems to be limited to immune complexes and mast cell granules. During phagocytosis, which is analogous to that seen in neutrophils, the content of the eosinophilic granules is discharged into phagosomes (Zucker-Franklin).

Eosinophils are attracted in an anaphylactic reaction by sensitized mast cells, which release an eosinophil chemotactic factor of anaphylaxis (ECF-A). Eosinophils thus attracted to the site of an anaphylactic reaction accumulate around degranulating mast cells and phagocytize the free mast cell granules (Goetzl et al). Eosinophils are also attracted by histamine, a fact that was established with the Boyden method of assessing chemotaxis (Zucker-Franklin).

Basophilic Granulocytes. Although basophils and mast cells have similar or identical functions and supplement each other, they are very different cells both in origin and in anatomy (Dvorak and Dvorak). Basophils have their origin in the bone marrow and circulate in the peripheral blood, whereas mast cells develop from undifferentiated perivascular mesenchymal cells.

The demonstration of basophils in light microscopic sections requires the use of electron microscopic fixation and processing techniques; biopsy specimens must be embedded in Epon and sectioned at 1 μm. The sections then are stained with the Giemsa stain. Basophils possess a multilobed nucleus and large, diffusely arranged metachromatic granules, whereas mast cells have a unilobed nucleus and smaller, peripherally located metachromatic granules (Katz). (For a discussion of the function and electron microscopic appearance of the basophil, see Mast Cells, p. 54.)

LYMPHOCYTIC GROUP

Histogenesis. There are two types of peripheral lymphocytes: T and B lymphocytes, both of which arise in the bone marrow. One type migrates to the thymus, where it differentiates to a lymphocyte, and then proceeds to the peripheral lymphoid tissues as a thymus-derived or T lymphocyte. In lymph nodes, T lymphocytes are located predominantly in the interfollicular cortex, also called the paracortical areas. The other type of lymphocyte, the B lymphocyte, matures in the bone marrow (Weissman et al). The term *B lymphocyte*, mean-

ing bursa-derived lymphocyte, originally was given because, in birds, the bursa of Fabricius is held responsible for B cell maturation (Weissman et al). In humans, the term *B lymphocyte* is used to mean bone-marrow-derived lymphocyte (Raff). In lymph nodes, B lymphocytes largely occupy the lymph follicles, including their germinal centers. Whereas the T lymphocyte is the effector cell for cellular immunity, the B lymphocyte mediates humoral immunity. The lymph nodes and other lymphoid organs share three principal functions: (1) to concentrate within them antigens from all parts of the body; (2) to circulate the lymphocyte population through the lymphoid organs so that every antigen is exposed to antigen-specific lymphocytes; and (3) to carry the products of the immune response, that is, humoral antibodies and cells mediating cellular immunity, to the blood and tissues (Weissman et al). T cells can exert important regulating functions on both T cells and B cells as helper T cells and suppressor T cells (Stingl and Knapp).

Although T and B cells are indistinguishable by light microscopy, they can be differentiated by in vitro tests. Human T lymphocytes have receptors for sheep erythrocytes, so that, in the E rosette assay, sheep erythrocytes (E) form rosettes around T lymphocytes. Furthermore, T lymphocytes undergo blastic transformation when exposed to mitogens such as phytohemagglutinin or concanavalin A, and anti-T-lymphocyte antisera have a specific cytotoxic effect on them (Claudy; Luckasen et al). In addition, anti-T-cell sera can be used in vitro as well as in frozen sections for immunofluorescence or immunoperoxidase tests (Stingl and Knapp). Also, T lymphocytes show granular staining with alpha-naphthyl acetate (nonspecific) esterase, in contrast to the diffuse staining of histiocytes (Sterry et al). Unlike T lymphocytes, B lymphocytes, as well as histiocytes, have receptors for the activated third component of complement and are therefore identifiable by their rosette formation both in vitro and in frozen sections with erythrocytes coated with immunoglobulin M antibody and complement (IgM EAC). However, only histiocytes bind erythrocytes coated with IgG antibody (IgG EA) (Edelson). The finding that only B lymphocytes synthesize and carry on their surface either IgD or IgM or both has made detection of these membrane-bound surface immunoglobulins by immunofluorescence the most reliable marker of B lymphocytes in vitro and in frozen sections (Stingl and Knapp). Although both B lymphocytes and monocytes have Fc-IgG receptors, only B cells possess Fc-IgM receptors on their surface. The most reliable marker for T cells in tissue sections is a series of mouse monoclonal antisera against various T-cell antigens. The antigens are identifiable by labeling the antisera with either fluorescein or peroxidase. All peripheral T cells react with OKT3 antiserum. Within this population, cells with helper T-cell function react with OKT4 antiserum, whereas suppressor T cells react with OKT8 antiserum (Holden et al). The percentage of B cells among lymphocytes in normal adult blood is approximately 20%, whereas that of T cells is about 75%. A small percentage of lymphocytes lack surface markers and are referred to as unidentified or null cells (Luckasen et al).

The T lymphocyte is the effector cell of cellular immunity. After "presentation" of the antigen by macrophages to predisposed lymphocytes, which thus become specifically sensitized, the sensitized T lymphocytes migrate to the paracortical area of regional lymph nodes, where they are transformed into T immunoblasts and undergo cell division. After a few days, the T immunoblasts change back into small T lymphocytes, which carry a receptor for the specific antigen on their surface. They leave the lymph nodes as effector cells, also called transformed or activated lymphocytes or memory cells. At sites of antigen localization, the effector cells leave the circulation and discharge lymphokines. (For details, see p. 98.)

The B lymphocyte is the effector cell of humoral immunity. On antigenic stimulation, the primary follicles in lymph nodes, composed of small B lymphocytes, develop into secondary follicles, consisting of a germinal center surrounded by a rim of small B lymphocytes (Weissman et al). In the germinal centers, small B lymphocytes enlarge through an intermediate stage of *centrocytes* with cleaved nuclei into *centroblasts,* which are large cells with noncleaved nuclei (Gerard-Marchant et al). The centroblasts become immunoblasts as a result of antigenic stimulation and produce a clone of activated cells, or memory cells, that mature into immunoglobulin-secreting plasma cells (Wilson Jones; Rywlin). The plasma cells collect in the medullary cords of lymph nodes without circulating in the blood stream but secrete immunoglobulins that circulate as "humoral" antibodies. (For a further discussion of humoral antibodies, see Plasma Cells below.)

Of interest is the role of B lymphocytes and T lymphocytes in the various forms of leukemia and lymphoma, respectively. Most examples of chronic lymphocytic leukemia and most instances of nodular and diffuse lymphoma represent B-cell proliferations (Taylor), whereas mycosis fungoides and Sézary's syndrome represent T-cell proliferations (Schein et al) (see pp. 737 and 744).

Histology of Lymphocytes.   Lymphocytes possess a relatively small, round nucleus that appears deeply basophilic because of the presence of numerous chromatin particles. They have only a very narrow rim of cytoplasm that is hardly recognizable. It is usually impossible by light microscopy to distinguish lymphocytes from monocytes in routinely stained histologic sections; and, in several instances in which it was once assumed that lymphocytes were an important constituent of the dermal infiltrate, such as in contact dermatitis and sarcoidosis, it has been shown through demonstration of the presence of lysosomal enzymes within the cells and through electron microscopy

that many of the cells are monocytes rather than lymphocytes. It is therefore preferable to refer to cells with a histologic appearance of lymphocytes as lymphoid cells.

Lymphocytes in Delayed Hypersensitivity. Delayed hypersensitivity can be evoked by a variety of agents, such as contact allergens, and many microorganisms, such as mycobacteria, viruses, and fungi. In addition, the rejection of tissue homografts represents a delayed hypersensitivity reaction. The number of specifically sensitized, also called activated or transformed lymphocytes, which carry the antibody to the antigen and thus induce the delayed hypersensitivity reaction, generally is small, so that they do not dominate the histologic picture. Thus, in contact dermatitis, monocytes or macrophages predominate, phagocytizing the damaged cells at the site of the antigen–antibody reaction (Macher). The number of macrophages at the reaction site is greatly increased by several lymphokines released by the transformed lymphocytes, such as the chemotactic factor for macrophages, the macrophage migration inhibiting factor (MIF), and the macrophage activation factor. Through these factors, monocytes or macrophages are brought to the cell-mediated immune reaction site, are held there, and are activated to show increased phagocytosis (Krueger). (For further details, see Histogenesis under Contact Dermatitis, p. 97.) In many instances, for example, tuberculosis and many deep fungal infections, such as blastomycosis, the delayed hypersensitivity reaction to microorganisms is granulomatous in nature.

Nonsensitized Lymphocytes.   Lymphocytes are the predominant cells in most chronic inflammations of the skin. They predominate, for instance, in psoriasis, lichen planus, and lupus erythematosus. They also predominate in lymphocytic vasculitis, as seen in pityriasis lichenoides et varioliformis acuta.

Plasma Cells

Plasma cells have an abundant cytoplasm that is deeply basophilic, homogeneous, and sharply defined. The round nucleus is eccentrically placed and shows along its membrane coarse, deeply basophilic, regularly distributed chromatin particles, which give the nucleus a cartwheel appearance. The fact that patients with agammaglobulinemia lack plasma cells was responsible for early recognition of the fact that the plasma cell is the site of formation of all immunoglobulins that circulate as humoral antibodies. The synthesis of immunoglobulins takes place in plasma cells located mainly in the lymph nodes, the spleen, and the bone marrow. Since plasma cells are tissue cells and are not seen in the peripheral circulation, it can be assumed that, if they are present in the dermis, they have developed there from B lymphocytes (see p. 50 and Histogenesis).

Plasma cells are apt to be present in conspicuous numbers in several infectious diseases, such as early syphilis, rhinoscleroma, and granuloma inguinale. It is not clear why, in some instances, the chronic inflammatory infiltrate of mycosis fungoides, solar keratosis, chronic deep folliculitis, or other diseases contains numerous plasma cells, whereas, in most instances, the infiltrate contains few plasma cells or even none. The reason for the presence of plasma cells in balanitis chronica plasmacellularis is also not known.

In the presence of many plasma cells, but especially in rhinoscleroma, round, hyaline, eosinophilic bodies called Russell bodies may be found inside and outside of plasma cells. They form within plasma cells as the result of a very active synthesis of immunoglobulins and may ultimately completely replace the plasma cells in which they have formed (Erlach et al). They may possess a size twice that of normal plasma cells, measuring up to 20 μm in diameter. They contain varying amounts of glycoproteins and are as a rule grampositive as well as PAS-positive and diastase-resistant (Tappeiner et al).

Histogenesis. On *electron microscopy,* plasma cells are characterized by the presence in their cytoplasm of an extensive system of cisternae lined by a rough endoplasmic reticulum. The cisternae usually are flat but may be irregularly dilated. Numerous ribosomes not only line the membranes of the endoplasmic reticulum but are also present in the cytoplasm. The abundant ribosomes and the highly developed endoplasmic reticulum are involved in the synthesis of immunoglobulins. Thus, the cisternae are often filled with a homogeneous to granular substance that is released into the extracellular space.

Russell bodies are also formed within the rough endoplasmic reticulum. When the plasma cell is overloaded with this material, first the nucleus and ultimately the entire cell lyse (Erlach et al). Immunofluorescence staining shows the presence of immunoglobulin within the Russell bodies.

Plasma cells arise from antigenically stimulated B lymphocytes, referred to as centroblasts or immunoblasts, and collect in foci in the medullary cords of lymph nodes or the red pulp of the spleen (Weissman et al). They are the effector cells of humoral immunity. As such, they do not enter the blood stream but discharge the immunoglobulins they produce into the blood. Five different classes of immunoglobulins are recognized: IgG, IgA, IgD, IgE, and IgM. In addition, there are four subclasses of IgG: IgG 1 to 4. Each immunoglobulin is composed of four chains: two identical heavy chains and two identical light chains. The heavy chains determine the class of immunoglobulin. The two identical light chains in each immunoglobulin can be one of two types: kappa or lambda. Two thirds of the immunoglobulins possess kappa light chains, and one third lambda light chains. Each plasma cell produces only one type of immunoglobulin and one type of light chain (Weissman et al).

MONOCYTIC OR MACROPHAGIC GROUP

Macrophages, also called histiocytes, are of bone marrow origin. They circulate in the blood and enter the tissue as monocytes (Spector, 1969). Upon proper stimulation, monocytes develop into macrophages and may develop further into epithelioid cells and foreign body giant cells. Macrophages constitute the "mononuclear phagocytic system," a concept that has replaced that of the reticuloendothelial system. The macrophages of the mononuclear phagocytic system, including the alveolar phagocytes in the lungs and the Kupffer cells in the liver, are the "professional" phagocytes, whereas the reticuloendothial cells, including the fixed reticulum cells in lymph nodes and the endothelial cells of blood vessels, are merely "facultative" phagocytes and are comparatively inadequate (Wells). As "professional" phagocytes, macrophages are capable of ingesting large particles and developing a high concentration of lysosomal enzymes. They can also be stimulated by immunologic factors, having surface receptors for the Fc portion of IgG, for C3, and for Ia antigen. In contrast, the facultative phagocytosis carried out by endothelial cells and fixed reticulum cells consists merely of pinocytosis of small particles without immune stimulation (Wells).

When macrophages aggregate for the purpose of phagocytosis, they form granulomas (Adams). In the skin, four types of granulomas can be recognized: (1) foreign body granulomas, (2) infectious granulomas, (3) immunogenic granulomas, and (4) granulomas associated with tissue injury (Epstein). Most foreign body granulomas are "primary irritant granulomas," and in only a few instances do they form on the basis of a specific sensitization, such as to zirconium, to beryllium, or to metals such as cobalt or cinnabar contained in tattoos. (For a detailed discussion of foreign body granulomas, see pp. 221–226.) Infectious granulomas, which develop without sensitization to the microorganism, show numerous microorganisms within macrophages without the development of epithelioid cells. Such infectious granulomas are seen in rhinoscleroma, granuloma inguinale, acute leishmaniasis, and lepromatous leprosy. Immunogenic granulomas, in which sensitization to the microorganism has taken place and many epithelioid cells but only few microorganisms are usually present, occur in chronic leishmaniasis, tuberculoid leprosy, tertiary syphilis, and the reinfection type of tuberculosis. Sarcoidosis may also be classified as a type of immunogenic granuloma, even though in this disorder, delayed hypersensitivity reactions are depressed (Epstein). Among the granulomas associated with tissue injury are necrobiosis lipoidica and granuloma annulare.

Macrophages may also exert their phagocytic capacity without aggregating to granulomas, as in instances in which they ingest lipids and change into foam cells, ingest melanin and change into melanophages, or ingest hemosiderin.

Besides acting as phagocytes, macrophages play an important role in both cell-mediated and humoral immunity. They operate both in the afferent limb of the immune response in antigen processing and in the efferent limb as effector cells. As such, macrophages can selectively present antigen to immunocompetent T and B lymphocytes. Close contact between macrophages and lymphocytes is important in the transfer of immunologic information and the initiation of the immune response (Cline).

Histopathology. Monocytes are indistinguishable from lymphocytes, since both cells have a small, dark, rounded nucleus and very scanty cytoplasm that cannot be recognized in routine sections. The only means by which monocytes can be differentiated from lymphocytes in histologic sections is through staining for lysosomal enzymes, such as acid phosphatase, which are present in monocytes and absent in lymphocytes. Thus, it has been possible through enzymatic staining and electron microscopy to identify as monocytes most cells with small, dark nuclei present in contact dermatitis and at the periphery of sarcoidal granulomas (see pp. 97 and 232).

Macrophages, or histiocytes, since they are activated monocytes, are larger cells than monocytes and usually have a lightly staining, elongated nucleus with a clearly visible nuclear membrane. Their cytoplasm cannot be recognized in routine stains. It is often impossible in routinely stained sections to distinguish macrophages from fibroblasts or from endothelial cells except through their respective locations or activities, but this is not always a reliable criterion. Histochemical staining for enzymes often is helpful in their distinction, although it must be kept in mind that, in some pathologic conditions, such as dermatofibroma and Kaposi's sarcoma, fibroblasts may also contain many lysosomes and then stain positive for lysosomal enzymes (see pp. 600 and 639).

Epithelioid Cells. Epithelioid cells arise from macrophages (1) after the macrophages have completed phagocytosis of a digestible product such as bacteria; (2) after the macrophages have eliminated by exocytosis an indigestible product, such as certain foreign materials or metabolic by-products; (3) in immunogenic granulomas in which, as the result of delayed hypersensitivity, only few microorganisms are present; and (4) when there is nothing to phagocytize, as in sarcoidosis (Papadimitriou and Spector, 1971). Thus, although epithelioid cells can develop in granulomas without delayed hypersensitivity, it is evident that delayed hypersensitivity greatly augments and accelerates the development of epithelioid cell granulomas (Adams). It seems likely that the majority of epithelioid cells in lesions of reinfection tuberculosis and tuberculoid leprosy are derived from macrophages that have never digested bacilli because more macrophages entered the area than were needed to engulf the organisms present (Papadimitriou and Spector, 1972) (see the discussion of electron microscopic examination below).

Histologically, epithelioid cells, like epithelial cells, lie in groups, either as "naked" epithelioid cell tubercles or intermingled with monocytes, macrophages, and often also foreign body giant cells. (Formerly, the monocytes were misinterpreted as lymphocytes; see p. 233.) Epithelioid cells possess a large, usually oval, pale, vesicular nucleus with a clearly visible nuclear membrane. The nucleus thus does not differ from that of macrophages, except that it is on the average slightly larger. The two cells, however, differ in their cytoplasm. Whereas the cytoplasm of macrophages is difficult to recognize in routine stains, epithelioid cells have abundant, ill-defined, slightly eosinophilic cytoplasm. Pseudopodic elongations of the cytoplasm usually are present, and the cytoplasm of adjoining epithelioid cells often has coalesced.

Foreign Body Giant Cells. As macrophages mature, they show less of a tendency to divide and a greater tendency to fuse into multinucleated giant cells (Carter and Roberts). Thus, foreign body giant cells, like epithelioid cells, no longer are phagocytizing cells. They tend to congregate in areas in which large amounts of indigestible material are located and may even completely surround large particles of such indigestible material. It has been customary to distinguish between multinucleated giant cells of the Langhans type occurring with epithelioid cells in delayed hypersensitivity granulomas and multinucleated giant cells of the foreign body type. Whereas the nuclei of giant cells of the Langhans type are located along the periphery of the giant cell in a semicircular fashion, those of giant cells of the foreign body type lie either irregularly distributed or in clusters. However, transitions between the two forms occur, and they often occur together, both in delayed hypersensitivity granulomas and in foreign body granulomas, so that their morphologic distinction often is impossible. Classic foreign body giant cells are seen (1) in a number of foreign body reactions, as in paraffinomas and suture reactions; (2) in the vicinity of metabolic by-products, as in gout and calcinosis; (3) in areas in which keratin is in direct contact with the dermis, as in calcifying epithelioma of Malherbe, ruptured hair follicles occurring in acne vulgaris and *Trichophyton rubrum* granuloma, and ruptured epidermal cysts or milia; and (4) in areas of tissue necrosis, as in necrobiosis lipoidica.

Histologically, both types of multinucleated giant cells usually show a well-demarcated cytoplasm. The number of nuclei may exceed 100. The occasional presence of asteroid bodies and of Schaumann bodies within them is not specific for any disease. (For discussion of these two bodies, see p. 230.)

Histogenesis. The origin of the tissue monocytes in human skin from blood monocytes has been established in healthy probands through transfusion of tritiated thymidine-labeled monocytes and their observation 3 hr later in skin window exudates (Meuret et al). On the other hand, the dermal infiltrate of monocytes and macrophages in patients with chronic dermatitis is largely self-renewing, since the monocyte recruitment rate from the blood is low in these patients following the autotransfusion of labeled monocytes (Meuret et al).

The derivation of macrophages present in cutaneous granulomas from the circulating blood has also been proved in animals. In rats, fairly persistent cutaneous granulomas can be produced by the intradermal injection of bovine serum albumin, provided that the rats have a high antibody titer against this substance (Spector and Heesom). In rats in which granulomas were thus produced and circulating neutrophils and monocytes were labeled with tritiated thymidine, more labeled neutrophils than monocytes infiltrated the granulomas during the first week. In subsequent weeks, considerably more labeled monocytes than labeled neutrophils emigrated from the capillaries into the granulomas. In the final weeks of the 12-week life span of the granulomas, however, fresh emigration of labeled monocytes made only a minor contribution to the granulomas in comparison with the mitotic division of the macrophages in the granulomas (Spector et al).

Electron microscopic examination reveals in monocytes many primary lysosomes scattered through their cytoplasm as small dense bodies (Papadimitriou and Spector,

1971). Macrophages, which represent stimulated monocytes, differ from monocytes in that they are larger, show longer processes, and contain a greater number of lysosomes (Carr). Many macrophages contain phagocytized material within phagosomes, which, through the influx of the contents of primary lysosomes, have become phagolysosomes. In experimental infections, if the bacteria kill the macrophages, other macrophages take over (Papadimitriou and Spector, 1972). Most epithelioid cells appear to evolve from macrophages that have never ingested any bacteria or antigen–antibody complexes. Only a small percentage of epithelioid cells show some evidence of past phagocytosis in the form of small residual bodies or phagolysosomes. Therefore, it seems that, in general, persistence of active phagolysosomes is an effective deterrent to epithelioid cell formation (Papadimitriou and Spector, 1971). Epithelioid cells possess numerous pseudopods that interlock with those of neighboring epithelioid cells. Their extensive cytoplasm is completely filled with organelles (Adams). The function of epithelioid cells is poorly understood, but the presence of numerous organelles suggests that their function has become diverted from phagocytosis to secretion (Spector, 1976).

Multinucleated foreign body giant cells are formed by the fusion of nonproliferating macrophages. Active phagocytosis by macrophages and giant cell formation are mutually exclusive (Papadimitriou et al). As evidence that the macrophages that form multinucleated giant cells are nondividing cells, the nuclei of macrophages in the vicinity of the giant cells show no DNA synthesis on labeling with tritiated thymidine (Carter and Roberts). Similarly, there is no DNA synthesis in the nuclei of giant cells (Black and Epstein).

MAST CELLS

Mast cells occur in the normal dermis in small numbers as spindle-shaped cells with an oval nucleus. They contain in their cytoplasm numerous granules that do not stain with routine stains such as hematoxylin-eosin. Therefore, mast cells in normal skin usually are indistinguishable from fibroblasts, although one can occasionally recognize in mast cells a small amount of cytoplasm and the cell membrane. The granules stain with methylene blue, which is present in the Giemsa stain, with toluidine blue, and with alcian blue. They also stain metachromatically with methylene blue and toluidine blue, that is, they stain in a color different from that possessed by the dye and appear purplish red rather than blue. The granules measure up to 0.8 μm in diameter (Hashimoto et al).

The normal dermis contains mast cells mainly in the vicinity of capillaries. Since the greatest number of capillaries is present in the subpapillary region and in the vicinity of the cutaneous appendages, most mast cells are observed in these areas (Okonkwo et al). The number of mast cells in the dermis is increased in many inflammatory conditions in which these cells are found intermingled with various "inflammatory" cells, for example, in the granulation tissue of healing wounds and in atopic dermatitis, lichen simplex chronicus, lichen planus, and pemphigus vulgaris (Mikhail and Miller-Milinska). The dermal infiltrate in these conditions is as a rule easily differentiated from that of urticaria pigmentosa, in which the infiltrate, even though it may be fairly slight, consists almost exclusively of mast cells. The exception is the presence of a slight admixture of eosinophils as a result of the degranulation of some of the mast cells (see Histogenesis below and Urticaria Pigmentosa, p. 82). Also, in many tumors, particularly benign tumors, the stroma contains an increased number of mast cells (Cawley and Hoch-Ligeti). The number of mast cells in neurofibromas is particularly large (Crowe et al).

Mast cells and *basophilic granulocytes* (see p. 49) have closely related or even identical functions. This is due to the similarity in the chemistry of their cytoplasmic granules and to the presence of membrane receptors for IgE. Both types of cells are participants in the immediate and the delayed types of hypersensitivity (Dvorak and Dvorak, 1972). Immediate hypersensitivity reactions can be triggered by mast cells and basophils in "anaphylactically" sensitized persons through the presence on their cell surfaces of specific antibodies of the IgE type. When the specific antigen combines with these antibodies, an anaphylactic reaction is elicited through the degranulation of mast cells and basophils and the release of histamine from the granules (Kaliner). Histamine increases the permeability of capillaries and, if released in sufficient amounts, may produce an anaphylactic shock. In delayed hypersensitivity reactions such as allergic contact dermatitis, specifically sensitized lymphocytes exposed to the specific antigen release as one of the lymphokines a "basophil chemotactic factor," which attracts basophils (Katz). Infiltration of the site of contact dermatitis with basophils, which are quickly mobilized from the blood stream, is thus an appropriate initial response to the antigenic challenge. After several days, the basophils gradually decrease in concentration as new mast cells arise at the site of the antigenic challenge (Dvorak and Dvorak, 1972). During the initial basophilic response in allergic contact dermatitis, basophils constitute from 5% to 15% of the infiltrate and are seen to degranulate (Dvorak and Mihm).

Histogenesis. The fact that histamine and heparin are synthesized in mast cells and basophils has been proved with the aid of radioactive compounds. Mast cells and basophils synthesize histamine by means of a specific enzyme, histidine decarboxylase. Thus, when these cells are cultured with ^{3}H-histidine, histamine is newly synthesized (Dvorak and Dvorak, 1979). Similarly, the synthesis of heparin in mast cells has been proved by the incubation of slices of mouse mast cell tumors with radioactive glucose or sulfate and the resulting incorporation of this radioactive material into the heparin extractable from the tumor slices (Korn). The sulfated acid mucopolysaccharides within the granules of mast cells and basophils, which impart metachromatic staining to the granules, consist of a mixture of chondroitin sulfate, dermatan sulfate, and heparin sulfate (Dvorak and Dvorak, 1979).

Electron microscopic examination of mast cells reveals numerous large and long villi at their periphery (see EM 18). The mast cell granules appear as round, oval, or angular-shaped, membrane-bound structures. Mature granules measure up to 0.8 μm in diameter (Hashimoto et al). They contain two components: lamellae and electron-dense, finely granular material (Hashimoto et al; Eady) (EM 18). The lamellae appear in cross sections as thick, curved, parallel filaments forming whorls or scrolls that may resemble fingerprints in their configuration. Each lamella is 7 nm to 12 nm wide, and their spacing is about 12 nm apart. At high magnification, the lamellae show transverse banding with a periodicity of approximately 6 nm. Tangential sectioning of the lamellae reveals paracrystalline lattices as a result of transverse banding. In some granules, distinct lamellae are not identifiable, and the internal appearance instead is finely granular. Other granules contain both lamellae and finely granular material. The granules of basophils are composed largely of electron-dense, finely granular material; only about 5% of the granules show some lamellae with periodic banding (Katz).

Degranulation of human mast cells following stroking of a lesion of urticaria pigmentosa is maximal after 1 min (Kobayasi and Asboe-Hansen). However, in vitro degranulation of peritoneal mast cells of rats induced by the histamine liberator Compound 48/80 requires 4 min, and the in vitro degranulation brought about by the addition of horse serum to the mast cells of sensitized rats is maximal only after an incubation period of 20 min (Mann, 1969b). Degranulation usually consists of the extrusion of entire granules, but some granules may undergo intracellular disintegration (Hashimoto et al; Kobayasi and Asboe-Hansen). Extrusion of granules takes place through extensive membrane fusion between the plasma membrane and perigranular membranes and between adjacent perigranular membranes. This results in extensive labyrinthine channels in the cell through which swollen, less electron-dense granules, all of which have lost their surrounding membranes, are released into the extracellular space (Uvnäs).

Concomitant with their release into the extracellular

space, the granules release histamine and heparin. Many granules are phagocytized by eosinophils through endocytosis in a membrane-lined vacuole. Once within the eosinophil, the phagosomal membrane surrounding the mast cell granule breaks down, and the mast cell granule is digested by the eosinophil not through lysosomal activity but by intracytoplasmic enzymes. In phagocytizing the mast cell granules, the eosinophil reduces the severity of histamine shock (Mann, 1969a).

BIBLIOGRAPHY

Granulocytic Group

BERRETY PJM, CORMANE RH: The eosinophil granulocyte. Int J Dermatol 17:776–784, 1978

BERRETTY PJM, CORMANE RH: Eosinophilic granulocytes and skin disorders. Int J Dermatol 20:531–540,1981

DVORAK HF, DVORAK AM: Basophils, mast cells, and cellular immunity in animal and man. Hum Pathol 3:454–456, 1972

GELL PGH, COOMBS RRA: Classification of hypersensitivity reactions. In Gell PGH, Coombs RRA (eds.): Clinical Aspects of Immunology, 2nd edition. Oxford, Blackwell Scientific Publications, 1968

GOETZL EJ, WASSERMAN SI, AUSTEN KF: Eosinophil polymorphonuclear leukocyte function in immediate hypersensitivity. Arch Pathol 99:1–4, 1975

HENSON PM: Pathological mechanisms in neutrophil-mediated injury. Am J Pathol 68:593–612, 1972

KATZ SI: Recruitment of basophils in delayed hypersensitivity reactions. J Invest Dermatol 71:70–75, 1978

LAZARUS GS, DANIELS JR, LIAN J et al: Role of granulocyte collagenase in collagen degradation. Am J Pathol 68:565–578, 1972

PARISH WE: Effects of neutrophils on tissues. Br J Dermatol 81, Suppl 3:28–35, 1969

PATTERSON R, ZEISS CR, KELLY JF: Classification of hypersensitivity reactions. N Engl J Med 295:277–279, 1976

POOLE JCF: Electron microscopy of polymorphonuclear leukocytes. Br J Dermatol 81, Suppl 3:11–18, 1969

WEISSMANN G, SMOLEN JE, HOFFSTEIN S: Polymorphonuclear leukocytes as secretory organs of inflammation. J Invest Dermatol 71:95–99, 1978

WILKINSON DS: Pustular dermatoses. Br J Dermatol 81, Suppl 3:38–45, 1969

ZUCKER-FRANKLIN D: Eosinophilic function related to cutaneous disorders. J Invest Dermatol 71:100–105, 1978

Lymphocytic Group

CLAUDY AL: The immunological identification of the Sézary cell. Br J Dermatol 91:597–600, 1974

EDELSON RL: Membrane markers of lymphocytes in lymphoma, melanoma and lupus erythematosus. Int J Dermatol 15:577–586, 1976

ERLACH E, GEBHART W, NIEBAUER G: Ultrastructural investigations on the morphogenesis of Russell bodies. (Abstr) J Cutan Pathol 3:145, 1976

GERARD-MARCHANT R, HAMLIN I, LENNERT K et al: Classification of non-Hodgkin's lymphoma. Lancet 2:406–408, 1974

HOLDEN CA, MORGAN EW, MACDONALD DM: The cell population in the cutaneous infiltrate of mycosis fungoides: In situ studies using monoclonal antisera. Br J Dermatol 106:385–392, 1982

KRUEGER GG: Lymphokines in health and disease. Int J Dermatol 16:539–551, 1977

LUCKASEN JR, SABAD A, GOLTZ RW et al: T and B lymphocytes in atopic eczema. Arch Dermatol 110:375–377, 1974

MACHER E: Das entzündliche Hautinfiltrat. In Marchionini A (ed): Handbuch der Haut- und Geschlechtskrankheiten, Ergänzungswerk. Vol 1, Part 2, pp 473–518. Berlin, Springer-Verlag, 1968

RAFF MC: T and B lymphocytes in mice studied by using antisera against surface antigenic markers. Am J Pathol 65:467–478, 1971

RYWLIN AM: Non-Hodgkin's malignant lymphomas. Brief historical review and simple unifying classification. Am J Dermatopathol 2:17–25, 1980

SCHEIN PS, MACDONALD JS, EDELSON R: Cutaneous T-cell lymphoma. Cancer 34:626–633, 1974

STERRY W, STEIGLEDER GK, PULLMAN H: In situ identification and enumeration of T lymphocytes in cutaneous T cell lymphoma by demonstration of granular activity of acid nonspecific esterase. Br J Dermatol 103:67–72, 1980

STINGL G, KNAPP W: Immunological markers for characterization of subpopulations of mononuclear cells. Am J Dermatopathol 3:215–223, 1981

TAPPEINER J, PFLEGER L, WOLFF K: Das Vorkommen und histochemische Verhalten von Russellschen Körperchen bei plasmacellulären Hautinfiltraten. Arch Klin Exp Dermatol 222:71–90, 1965

TAYLOR CR: Classification of lymphoma: New thinking of old thoughts. Arch Pathol 102:549–554, 1978

WEISSMAN IL, WARNKE R, BUTCHER EC et al: The lymphoid system: Its normal architecture and the potential for understanding the system through the study of lymphoproliferative diseases. Hum Pathol 9:25–45, 1978

WILSON JONES E: Prospectives in mycosis fungicides in relation to other lymphomas. Trans St John's Hosp Dermatol Soc 61:16–30, 1975

Monocytic or Macrophagic Group

ADAMS DO: The granulomatous response: A review. Am J Pathol 84:164–191, 1976

BLACK MM, EPSTEIN WL: Formation of multinucleate giant cells in organized epithelioid cell granulomas. Am J Pathol 74:263–274, 1974

CARR I: The cellular basis of reticulo-endothelial stimulation. J Pathol 94:323–330, 1967

CARTER RL, ROBERTS JDB: Macrophages and multinucleate giant cells in nitrosoquinoline-induced granulomata in rats. An autoradiographic study. J Pathol 105:285–288, 1971

CLINE MJ: Monocytes, macrophages, and their diseases in man. J Invest Dermatol 71:56–58, 1978

EPSTEIN WL: Cutaneous granulomas. Int J Dermatol 16:574–579, 1977

MEURET G, MARWENDEL A, BRAND ET: Makrophagenrekrutierung aus Blutmonocyten bei Entzündungsreaktionen der Haut. Arch Dermatol Forsch 245:254–266, 1972

PAPADIMITRIOU JM, SFORSINA D, PAPAELIAS L: Kinetics of multinucleate giant cell formation and their modifications by various agents in foreign body reactions. Am J Pathol 73:349–364, 1973

PAPADIMITRIOU JM, SPECTOR WG: The origin, properties and fate of epithelioid cells. J Pathol 105:187–203, 1971

PAPADIMITRIOU J, SPECTOR WG: The ultrastructure of high- and low-turnover inflammatory granulomata. J Pathol 106:37–43, 1972

SPECTOR WG: Recent advances in the study of leukocyte emigration. Br J Dermatol 81, Suppl 3:19–27, 1969

SPECTOR WG: Epithelioid cells, giant cells, and sarcoidosis. Ann NY Acad Sci 278:3–6, 1976

SPECTOR WG, HEESOM N: The production of granulomata by antigen–antibody complexes. J Pathol 98:31–39, 1969

SPECTOR WG, LYKKE AWJ, WILLOUGHBY DA: A quantitative study of leukocyte emigration in chronic inflammatory granulomata. J Pathol 93:101–107, 1967

WELLS GS: The pathology of adult-type Letterer-Siwe disease. Clin Exp Dermatol 4:407–417, 1979

Mast Cells

CAWLEY EP, HOCH-LIGETI C: Association of tissue mast cells and skin tumors. Arch Dermatol 83:92–96, 1961

CROWE FW, SCHULL WJ, NEEL JV: Multiple neurofibromatosis. Springfield, IL, Charles C Thomas, 1955

DVORAK HF, DVORAK AM: Basophils, mast cells, and cellular immunity in animals and man. Hum Pathol 3:454–456, 1972

DVORAK AM, DVORAK HF: The basophil: Its morphology, biochemistry, motility, release reactions, recovery, and role in inflammatory responses of IgE-mediated and cell-mediated origin. (Review) Arch Pathol 103:551–557, 1979

DVORAK HF, MIHM MC, JR.: Basophilic leukocytes in allergic contact dermatitis. J Exp Med 135:235–254, 1972

EADY RAJ: The mast cells: Distribution and morphology. Clin Exp Dermatol 1:313–329, 1976

HASHIMOTO K, TARNOWSKI WM, LEVER WF: Reifung und Degranulierung der Mastzellen in der menschlichen Haut. Hautarzt 18:318–324, 1967

KALINER MA: Editorial: The mast cell, a fascinating riddle. N Engl J Med 301:498–499, 1979

KATZ SI: Recruitment of basophils in delayed hypersensitivity reactions. J Invest Dermatol 71:70–75, 1978

KOBAYASI T, ASBOE-HANSEN G: Degranulation and regranulation of human mast cells. Acta Derm Venereol (Stockh) 49:369–372, 1969

KORN ED: The synthesis of heparin by slices of mouse mast cell tumor. J Biol Chem 234:1321–1324, 1959

MANN PR: An electron-microscope study of the relations between mast cells and eosinophilic leukocytes. J Pathol 98:183–186, 1969a

MANN PR: An electron-microscope study of the degranulation of rat peritoneal mast cells brought about by four different agents. Br J Dermatol 81:926–936, 1969b

MIKHAIL GR, MILLER-MILINSKA A: Mast cell population in human skin. J Invest Dermatol 43:249–254, 1964

OKONKWO B, RUST S, STEIGLEDER GK: Die Verteilung der Mastzellen in der gesunden menschlichen Haut. Arch Klin Exp Dermatol 223:99–104, 1965

UVNÄS B: Chemistry and storage function of mast cell granules. J Invest Dermatol 71:76–80, 1978

Congenital Diseases (Genodermatoses)

6

ICHTHYOSIS

A classification of ichthyosis includes four major and three minor forms. In addition, there are a number of syndromes that are associated with ichthyosis.

Ichthyosis Vulgaris

Autosomal dominantly inherited ichthyosis vulgaris, a common disorder, develops a few months after birth. The skin shows scales that on the extensor surfaces of the extremities are large and adherent, resembling fish scales, and elsewhere are small. The flexural creases are spared. Keratosis pilaris is often present, and the palms and soles may show hyperkeratosis.

A noninherited form of the disease may appear in patients with lymphoma, particularly Hodgkin's disease (Stevanovic), but this form has been reported also in association with carcinoma (Flint et al) and sarcoidosis (Kauh et al).

Histopathology. The characteristic finding is the association of a moderate degree of hyperkeratosis with a thin or absent granular layer (Fig. 6-1). The hyperkeratosis often extends into the hair follicles, resulting in large keratotic follicular plugs. The dermis is normal.

Histogenesis. Labeling with tritiated thymidine shows a normal rate of epidermal proliferation (Frost et al). The hyperkeratosis is regarded as a retention keratosis resulting from increased adhesiveness of the stratum corneum (Frost and Van Scott). The reason for this, as

seen by *electron microscopy,* is a delay in the dissolution of the desmosomal disks in the horny layer (Anton-Lamprecht, 1973). Keratohyaline granules are regularly seen on electron microscopy, in contrast to light microscopy. The stratum granulosum, however, consists of only a single layer, and the keratohyaline granules appear small and crumbly or spongy, evidence of defective synthesis (Anton-Lamprecht, 1973). In noninherited ichthyosis vulgaris associated with neoplasia, the keratohyaline granules have been described as being small but showing a normal structure, indicating a reduced but not an abnormal synthesis (Perrot et al).

Differential Diagnosis. Although the noninflamed but "dry" skin of patients with atopic dermatitis clinically resembles ichthyosis vulgaris, it does not show on histologic examination the features of ichthyosis vulgaris but rather increased epidermal thickness, patchy parakeratosis, and, in places, slight hypergranulosis as seen in chronic dermatitis (Finley et al).

X-Linked Ichthyosis

X-linked ichthyosis is recessively inherited.* It is only rarely present at birth. Although female heterozygotes

---

* X-chromosomal recessive gene defects also exist in hypohidrotic ectodermal dysplasia (see p. 65), dyskeratosis congenita (see p. 62), Ehlers–Danlos syndrome, type V (see p. 78), Wiskott–Aldrich syndrome (see p. 101), and angiokeratoma corporis diffusum or Fabry's disease (see p. 391). Full expression of these diseases is found only in males who are hemizygotic for the X chromosome, so that they inherit either the healthy or the mutant gene. Women, being heterozygotes, may have a mild form of these diseases.

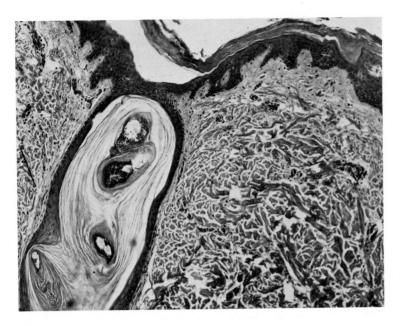

Fig. 6-1. Ichthyosis vulgaris
There is a moderate degree of hyperkeratosis without a granular layer. A large keratotic plug is located within a hair follicle. (× 100)

are frequently affected, males have a more severe form of the disorder. The thickness of the adherent scales increases during childhood (Frost). In contrast to ichthyosis vulgaris, the flexural creases may be involved.

Histopathology.   There is hyperkeratosis. The granular layer is normal or slightly thickened but not thinned as in dominant ichthyosis vulgaris. The epidermis may be slightly thickened (Feinstein et al).

Histogenesis. X-linked ichthyosis, like ichthyosis vulgaris, shows a normal rate of epidermal proliferation. The disorder is a retention hyperkeratosis characterized by delayed dissolution of the desmosomal disks in the horny layer. In contrast to that of ichthyosis vulgaris, the synthesis of keratohyaline granules in X-linked ichthyosis is not defective, and the rate of synthesis is slightly increased (Anton-Lamprecht, 1974). The cause of the retention hyperkeratosis in X-linked ichthyosis is the virtual absence of steroid sulfatase activity. This was first recognized in skin fibroblasts (Shapiro et al) but was found subsequently also in the entire epidermis and in leukocytes (Williams and Elias). Steroid sulfatase normally acts on cholesterol sulfate, a product of the Odland bodies (see p. 14) that is discharged with them from the granular cells into the intercellular space and provides cell cohesion in the lower stratum corneum. Failure of steroid sulfatase to remove cholesterol sulfate results in persistent cell cohesion even in the upper stratum corneum and interferes with the normal process of desquamation (Epstein et al).

Epidermolytic Hyperkeratosis

Epidermolytic hyperkeratosis, an autosomal dominantly inherited disease also known as bullous congenital ichthyosiform erythroderma, shows from the time of birth generalized erythema. Within a few days after birth, there is, in addition to the erythema, thick, brown, verrucous scaling. The flexural surfaces of the extremities show marked involvement often consisting of furrowed hyperkeratosis. Vesicles and bullae are usually encountered only during the first few years.

Histopathology.   A characteristic histologic picture is seen in the epidermis (Fig. 6-2) and is referred to either as epidermolytic hyperkeratosis (Frost and Van Scott) or as granular degeneration (Ishibashi and Klingmüller). It is present in bullous as well as in nonbullous areas. Evident are (1) variously sized clear spaces around the nuclei in the upper stratum spinosum and in the stratum granulosum; (2) peripheral to the clear spaces, indistinct cellular boundaries formed either by lightly staining material or by keratohyaline granules; (3) a markedly thickened granular layer containing an increased number of irregularly shaped keratohyaline granules; and (4) compact hyperkeratosis (Ackerman). When bullae form, they arise intraepidermally through separation of edematous cells from one another (McCurdy and Beare). The upper dermis shows a moderately severe, chronic inflammatory infiltrate. Mitotic figures are 5 times more numerous than in normal epidermis (Frost and Van Scott).

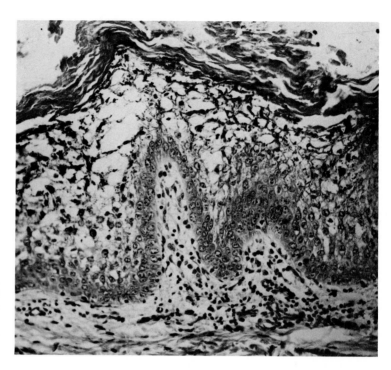

Fig. 6-2.   Epidermolytic hyperkeratosis
There is pronounced vacuolization of the cells in the middle and upper portions of the stratum malpighii. These cells show indistinct cellular boundaries. The keratohyaline granules are large and irregularly shaped. (×400)

Histogenesis. The essential *electron microscopic* features are excessive production of tonofilaments and excessive and premature formation of keratohyaline granules, so that, at the periphery of the cells, numerous keratohyaline granules are embedded in thick shells of irregularly clumped tonofilaments (Ishibashi and Klingmüller; Schnyder). The desmosomes appear normal, but the association of tonofilaments and desmosomes is disturbed, so that many desmosomes are attached to only one keratinocyte instead of connecting two neighboring keratinocytes. Because of this disturbance in desmosomal attachment, blister formation takes place and real acantholysis occurs (Anton-Lamprecht and Schnyder). Labeling with tritiated thymidine reveals greatly increased proliferative activity in the epidermis (Frost et al). It can thus be concluded that keratinization is both excessive and abnormal.

Differential Diagnosis.   Although the histologic picture of epidermolytic hyperkeratosis is diagnostic for the type of ichthyosis referred to as epidermolytic hyperkeratosis, it is not specific for it. It is found also in several other seemingly unrelated conditions (Mehregan; Niizuma): (1) epidermolytic keratosis palmaris et plantaris (see p. 61), (2) linear epidermal nevus, usually of the systematized type (see p. 473), (3) solitary epidermolytic acanthoma (see p. 474), (4) disseminated epidermolytic acanthoma (see p. 474), and (5) epidermolytic hyperkeratosis as an incidental histologic finding in a variety of unrelated conditions (see p. 475).

Lamellar Ichthyosis

Lamellar ichthyosis, inherited as an autosomal recessive trait, is also known as nonbullous congenital ichthyosiform erythroderma. At birth, the infant is encased in a tight, shiny membrane resembling collodion. During the first few days of life, this membrane detaches itself, after which the entire skin, including the flexural surfaces, appears red and scaly. This appearance may persist through life, but, in milder cases, the erythroderma may gradually subside (Bloom and Goodfried).

Histopathology.   The histologic findings are nonspecific, showing moderate hyperkeratosis, a normal or thickened granular layer, moderate acanthosis, and a mild chronic inflammatory infiltrate in the upper dermis (Schnyder and Konrad; Vandersteen and Muller, 1972). After detachment, the "collodion" membrane is seen to be composed of orthokeratotic stratum corneum (Larrèque et al).

Histogenesis. In lamellar ichthyosis, as in epidermolytic hyperkeratosis, labeling with tritiated thymidine reveals greatly increased numbers of labeled cells per unit surface, which is indicative of increased proliferative activity (Frost et al). On *electron microscopy*, a greater than normal amount of intercellular cement in the stratum corneum has been held responsible for increased adherence of the horny cells (Vandersteen and Muller, 1972).

Harlequin Ichthyosis

Harlequin ichthyosis is a rare condition that is invariably fatal. At birth, the child is encased in a thick, horny cuirass with deep fissures. Marked ectropion and eclabium are present.

Histopathology. There usually is a massive hyperkeratosis, the stratum corneum being 20 to 30 times thicker than the stratum malphighii (Luderschmidt et al). The stratum granulosum is either absent or consists of a single layer of flattened cells containing small keratohyaline granules (Buxman et al). A stain for fat has shown small droplets of neutral fat distributed uniformly throughout the cornified cells (Buxman et al). Some cases have shown papillomatosis, in addition to hyperkeratosis or areas of parakeratosis (Baden et al).

Histogenesis. In one case, the stratum corneum showed a cross-beta x-ray diffraction pattern instead of the usual alpha-type (Baden and Goldsmith); however, in other cases, the pattern was completely normal (Buxman et al; Baden et al), suggesting that the disorder may have multiple causes.

Erythrokeratodermia Variabilis

A rare, dominantly inherited disorder, erythrokeratodermia variabilis starts in infancy rather than at birth. It has two morphologic components. First, areas of erythema expand centrifugally and coalesce into circinate figures. These lesions fluctuate, sometimes rapidly, in their configuration and extent and thus are "variable." Second, persistent hyperkeratotic plaques develop both within the areas of erythema and in areas of apparently normal skin (Vandersteen and Muller, 1971). In rare cases, referred to as progressive symmetric erythrokeratodermia, only persistent erythematous hyperkeratotic plaques are present, and they are limited to the extremities (Nir and Tanzer).

Histopathology. The changes are nonspecific. In the hyperkeratotic plaques, they consist of hyperkeratosis with moderate papillomatosis and acanthosis. The granular layer appears normal, being two to three cell layers thick (Vandersteen and Muller, 1971).

Histogenesis. Labeling with tritiated thymidine shows a normal rate of proliferation (Schellander and Fritsch). It is therefore likely that the hyperkeratosis is due to decreased shedding of horny cells and is thus of the retention type (Vandersteen and Muller, 1971).

Ichthyosis Linearis Circumflexa

A recessive disorder that is present at birth or starts shortly thereafter, ichthyosis linearis circumflexa shows extensive migratory polycyclic lesions or erythema and scaling that has at the periphery a distinctive "double-edged" scale. The presence of extensive erythema causes a resemblance to psoriasis. The dermatosis persists through life. In more than half of the reported cases, hair anomalies have been present in the scalp, usually trichorrhexis invaginata, the so-called Netherton syndrome (Mehvorah et al) (see pp. 61 and 202).

Histopathology. The areas of erythema and scaling show nonspecific changes with some resemblance to psoriasis, such as elongation of the rete ridges and hyperkeratosis, as well parakeratosis (Altman and Stroud).

The "double-edged" scale frequently shows in the upper stratum malpighii intracellular edema and irregular spongiosis leading to multilocular vesicles or vesiculopustules within the horny layer (Hersle). In other cases, focal accumulations of periodic acid-Schiff (PAS)-positive, diastase-resistant, homogeneous material representing exuded serum protein are seen within a parakeratotic stratum corneum (Thorne et al). The presence of such exudative changes, however, is not specific or characteristic for ichthyosis linearis circumscripta, as has been claimed (Mevorah and Frenk).

Histogenesis. *Electron microscopic examination* has also shown the presence of multilocular vesicles that are filled with an amorphous substance compatible with serum protein (Zina and Bundino).

Syndromes Associated with Ichthyosis

There is an expanding list of syndromes that combine ichthyosis with neuroectodermal and mesodermal defects (Jorizzo et al). Some of the syndromes described in the literature may be chance associations (Wells). Among the well-established syndromes are the *Sjögren–Larsson syndrome*, which is characterized by lamellar ichthyosis in association with mental retardation and spastic paresis (Heijer and Reed); *Rud's syndrome*, showing generalized ichthyosis with hypogonadism, mental deficiency, and epilepsy (Maldonado et al); *Conradi's syndrome*, in which ichthyosis with a whorled pattern is associated with skeletal and ocular abnormalities (Edidin et al); and *Netherton's syndrome*, which consists of a combination of either ichthyosis linearis circumflexa or, less commonly, lamellar ichthyosis with trichorrhexis invaginata (see p. 202). The only syndrome showing specific histologic changes in the skin is *Refsum's syndrome.*

Refsum's Syndrome. An autosomal recessive disorder, Refsum's syndrome is characterized by generalized ichthyosis, cerebellar ataxia, progressive paresis of the extremities, and retinitis pigmentosa.

Histopathology. The skin shows hyperkeratosis, hypergranulosis, and acanthosis. In the basal and suprabasal cells of the epidermis are variably sized vacuoles that, on staining for lipids, are seen to contain lipid accumulations (Davies et al).

Histogenesis. The primary enzymatic defect in Refsum's disease lies in an inability to convert exogenous phytanic acid to alpha-hydroxophytanic acid, preventing its elimination (Steinberg et al). *Electron microscopy* shows in the basal and suprabasal cells of the epidermis variously sized vacuoles possessing no limiting membrane (Davies et al).

KERATOSIS PALMARIS ET PLANTARIS

Three major autosomal dominant forms and two autosomal recessive forms of keratosis palmaris et plantaris exist. The three dominantly inherited forms are the following:

Keratosis palmaris et plantaris of Unna-Thost, showing either diffuse or localized, occasionally linear hyperkeratosis of the palms and soles. A division into two types as suggested by Greither, a circumscribed type with limitation to the palms and soles and an extending type with gradual progression to the dorsa of the hands and feet, the ankles and wrists, and the elbows and knees, is not tenable because both types may occur in the same family (Kansky and Arzensek).

Epidermolytic keratosis palmaris et plantaris, although clinically indistinguishable from the Unna-Thost type, histologically shows epidermolytic hyperkeratosis.

Keratosis palmo-plantaris punctata (or papulosa), which has multiple keratotic plugs.

The two recessively inherited forms are the following:

Keratosis palmaris et plantaris of the Meleda type, showing diffuse involvement of the palms and soles and a marked tendency toward progression to the dorsa of the hands and feet, the ankles and wrists, and the elbows and knees (Salamon et al).

The *Papillon–Lefèvre syndrome*, which shows the clinical characteristics of the Meleda type in association with periodontosis resulting in the loss first of the deciduous teeth and later of the permanent teeth (Bach and Levan).

In addition, keratosis palmaris et plantaris occurs in three syndromes: pachyonychia congenita (see p. 62), hidrotic ectodermal dysplasia (see p. 65), and the Richner–Hanhart syndrome associated with tyrosinemia (see p. 433). Keratosis palmo-plantaris punctata may occur as part of acrokeratosis verruciformis of Hopf (see p. 74).

Histopathology. In keratosis palmaris et plantaris of the Unna-Thost type and the Meleda type, as well as in the Papillon–Lefèvre syndrome, the histologic picture is nonspecific, consisting of considerable hyperkeratosis, hypergranulosis, acanthosis, and a mild inflammatory infiltrate in the upper dermis (Salamon et al; Callan).

In epidermolytic keratosis palmaris et plantaris, the histologic picture is identical with that seen in epidermolytic hyperkeratosis (see p. 58). Many cells in the middle and upper stratum malpighii appear vacuolated, and scattered cavities are present as a result of ruptured cell walls. Keratohyaline granules are numerous and large (Klaus et al; Moulin and Bouchet; Fritsch et al).

In keratosis palmo-plantaris punctata, there is massive hyperkeratosis over a sharply limited area, with depression of the underlying malpighian layer below the general level of the epidermis. There is an increase in the thickness of the granular layer. The dermis is free of inflammation (Buchanan). In two cases reported as punctate keratoderma, a cornoid lamella was seen in the center of the hyperkeratotic plug; these cases therefore represent punctate porokeratosis with the lesions limited to the palms and soles, rather than keratosis palmo-plantaris punctata (Brown; Herman) (see p. 62).

ACROKERATOELASTOIDOSIS

Acrokeratoelastoidosis is a rare autosomal dominantly inherited condition in which firm, shiny papules are seen at the periphery of the palms and soles with some extension to the dorsa of the fingers and the sides of the feet (Costa; Jung et al).

Histopathology. The essential histologic feature in the papules consists of diminution and fragmentation of the elastic fibers, especially in the deeper portions of the dermis (Costa; Jung et al). Some of the fragmented elastic fibers appear thickened and tortuous (Highet et al). In some instances, the elastic fibers show no obvious damage in histologic sections but only on electron microscopic examination (Johansson et al).

Histogenesis. On *electron microscopic examination,* the elastic fibers in the reticular dermis appear disaggregated, with fragmentation of the microfibrils (Jung et al; Johansson et al).

PACHYONYCHIA CONGENITA

A disorder with autosomal dominant inheritance, pachyonychia congenita is characterized by the following triad: (1) subungual hyperkeratosis, with accumulation of hard, keratinous material beneath the distal portion of the nails, lifting the nails from the nail bed; (2) keratosis palmaris et plantaris with thick callosities, especially on the soles, that are tender and are often associated with blister formation; and (3) thick whitish areas on the oral mucosa that resemble those seen in white sponge nevus and possess no tendency toward malignant degeneration (Kelly and Pinkus). In addition, follicular hyperkeratosis may occur, mainly on the elbows and knees.

Histopathology. The nail bed shows marked hyperkeratosis. As in a normal nail bed, there is no granular layer (Kelly and Pinkus). The blisters that may be seen beneath and around the plantar callosities arise in the upper layers of the stratum malpighii through increasing intracellular edema and vacuolization. Unlike friction blisters, they show no areas of necrosis (Schönfeld) (see p. 128). The oral lesions show thickening of the oral epithelium with extensive intracellular vacuolization, exactly as seen in white sponge nevus (see p. 475), and without evidence of dyskeratosis (Witkop and Gorlin).

DYSKERATOSIS CONGENITA

A rare disorder with an X-linked, recessive inheritance, dyskeratosis congenita is seen mostly in males, occurring only sporadically in women (Sorrow and Hitch). It is characterized by the following triad: (1) dystrophy of the nails, with failure of the nails to form a nail plate, (2) whitish thickening (leukokeratosis) of the oral and occasionally also of the anal mucosa, and (3) extensive areas of netlike pigmentation of the skin suggestive of poikiloderma atrophicans vasculare but with less atrophy and telangiectasia. Carcinoma may develop in the areas of buccal and anal leukokeratosis (Garb). In many cases, a Fanconi type of anemia develops that may begin with leukopenia and thrombocytopenia but terminates in severe pancytopenia (Garb; Gutman et al).

Histopathology. In dyskeratosis congenita, the areas of netlike pigmentation show as their only constant feature melanophages in the upper dermis (Bryan and Nixon). In contrast to poikiloderma

atrophicans vasculare, atrophy of the epidermis, vacuolization of basal cells, and inflammatory infiltration of the upper dermis are either absent (Costello and Buncke) or are mild and thus not diagnostic (Bryan and Nixon). Oral biopsies may show squamous cell carcinoma in situ or invasive squamous cell carcinoma (Garb).

POROKERATOSIS

Porokeratosis has autosomal dominant inheritance and is characterized by one or many atrophic, keratotic patches surrounded by a distinct, raised ridge showing the cornoid lamella as a characteristic histologic finding. Five different forms can be distinguished.

The *plaque type,* as originally described by Mibelli, shows usually a single or only a few lesions several centimeters in diameter. The border often consists of a raised wall having on its top a furrow filled with keratotic material. The lesions have a tendency toward peripheral extension.

The *superficial disseminate form,* often widely distributed, shows lesions especially on the trunk and on the palms and soles. The lesions are small and are surrounded only by a narrow, slightly raised, hyperkeratotic ridge showing no distinct furrow clinically (Guss et al).

Disseminated superficial actinic porokeratosis resembles the last described form, except that the lesions are present in sun-exposed areas, especially on the extensor surfaces of the extremities, and can be elicited by prolonged exposure to the sun (Chernosky and Freeman).

The *linear form* may involve only a segment of the body or may have a generalized distribution. The lesions clinically resemble those of linear verrucous epidermal nevus (Rahbari et al, 1974; Nabai and Mehregan).

The *punctate form* is rare and is limited in distribution, occurring either on the elbows, wrists, and fingers or only on the palms (Rahbari et al, 1977). If located on the palms and soles, the lesions may be clinically indistinguishable from those of keratosis palmo-plantaris punctata (see p. 61).

Development of a squamous cell carcinoma or of Bowen's disease within lesions of porokeratosis has been repeatedly reported in patients with solitary lesions (Oberste-Lehn and Moll) as well as in persons with disseminated lesions (Guss et al) or linear lesions (Coskey and Mehregan).

Histopathology. It is essential that the specimen for biopsy be taken from the peripheral, raised, hyperkeratotic ridge. On histologic examination, the ridge then shows a keratin-filled invagination of the epidermis. In the plaque type, the invagi-

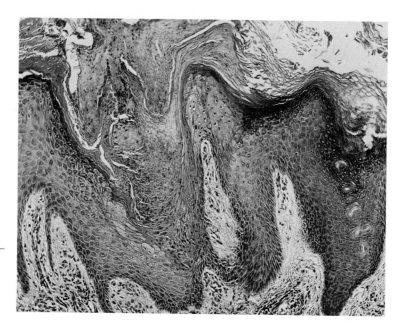

Fig. 6-3. Porokeratosis Mibelli
The section is taken from the peripheral raised ridge showing in its center a keratin-filled furrow or invagination. In the center of the invagination rises a parakerototic column, the so-called cornoid lamella. The parakeratotic column shows at its base epidermal cells that have pyknotic nuclei with perinuclear edema. On the right side is a normal sweat duct. (×100)

nation extends deeply downward at an angle the apex of which points away from the central portion of the lesion. In the center of this keratin-filled invagination rises a parakeratotic column, the so-called cornoid lamella, representing the most characteristic feature of porokeratosis Mibelli (Fig. 6-3). Within the parakeratotic column, the horny cells appear homogeneous and possess deeply basophilic pyknotic nuclei. In the epidermis beneath the parakeratotic column, the keratinocytes are irregularly arranged and have pyknotic nuclei with perinuclear edema. In the upper stratum malpighii, some cells possess an eosinophilic cytoplasm as a result of premature keratinization (Braun-Falco and Balsa). No granular layer is found at the site at which the parakeratotic column arises, whereas, elsewhere, the keratin-filled invagination of the epidermis has a well-developed granular layer.

The histologic changes in the other forms of porokeratosis are similar to those seen in the plaque type but less pronounced, the central invagination being rather shallow, especially in disseminated superficial actinic porokeratosis. The shallow parakeratotic invagination then stands out by showing homogeneous cells rather than the basket-weave pattern seen in the surrounding orthokeratotic stratum corneum (Fig. 6-4).

Since the peripheral raised ridge in porokeratosis slowly moves centrifugally, it stands to reason that the invagination is not bound to a definite structure, such as the sweat pore, as originally assumed by Mibelli. Thus, even though the invagination occasionally may be seen within a sweat pore or a pilosebaceous follicle, most commonly it is found in the epidermis independent of these cutaneous appendages (Reed and Leone).

The epidermis overlying the central portion of a lesion of porokeratosis may be either flattened

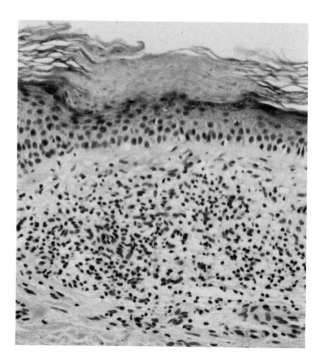

Fig. 6-4. Disseminated superficial actinic porokeratosis
In this type of porokeratosis, the central furrow from which the parakeratotic column arises is quite superficially located and therefore often very shallow. (×100)

or normal in thickness or, rarely, acanthotic. A nonspecific perivascular infiltrate of chronic inflammatory cells is present in the dermis.

Histogenesis. The presence of a clone of abnormal epidermal cells located at the base of the parakeratotic column explains the lesions of porokeratosis. As a result of a gradual centrifugal movement of this clone, the furrow is slanted, its apex pointing away from the center of the lesion (Reed and Leone).

Electron microscopic examination reveals that, in the epidermis beneath the parakeratotic column, many keratinocytes show signs of degeneration. They show a pyknotic nucleus, large perinuclear vacuoles that are separated from one another by cytoplasmic strands, and condensation of tonofilaments at their periphery (Mann et al). At the base of the parakeratotic column, dyskeratotic cells composed of nuclear remnants and aggregated tonofilaments are seen (Sato et al). The parakeratotic column is composed chiefly of cells with a pyknotic nucleus and a cytoplasm possessing high electron density because of the presence of many partially degraded organelles. In addition, a few dyskeratotic cells are present (Sato et al).

Differential Diagnosis. In rare instances, histologic examination of a congenital linear nevus comedonicus located on a palm or sole shows dilated eccrine ducts containing parakeratotic plugs. These plugs resemble cornoid lamellae except for the fact that they are limited to eccrine ducts (p. 474).

XERODERMA PIGMENTOSUM

In xeroderma pigmentosum, an autosomal recessive disorder, excessive solar damage to the skin develops at an early age. Consequently, the lesions occur chiefly in areas of the skin habitually exposed to sunlight. Three stages are recognized (Hadida et al). In the first stage, which usually starts when the child is 1 or 2 years old, one observes slight diffuse erythema associated with scaling and small areas of hyperpigmentation resembling freckles. In the second stage, atrophy of the skin, mottled pigmentation, and telangiectases are present, giving the skin an appearance similar to that of a chronic radiodermatitis. Solar keratoses arise in areas of scaling. In the third stage, which usually starts in adolescence but sometimes much earlier in the patient's life, various types of malignant tumors of the skin appear, often causing death. They include squamous cell carcinoma, basal cell epithelioma, and, rarely, fibrosarcoma (Bell and Rothnem; Hadida et al). In about 3% of the patients with xeroderma pigmentosum, malignant melanomas arise (Lynch et al, 1967). In some patients, they show no tendency to metastasize (Ronchese), but, in others, they metastasize rapidly (McGovern). In addition to the skin, the eyes are affected, showing conjunctivitis and often keratitis with corneal opacities (El-Hefnawi and Mortada).

A very rare variant of xeroderma pigmentosum is the DeSanctis–Cacchione syndrome, which, in addition to severe skin lesions, shows neurologic manifestations, especially microcephaly, retarded growth, and cerebellar ataxia (Reed et al).

Histopathology. In the first stage, the histopathologic appearance is not specific, but the diagnosis is suggested by a combination of changes that normally are not seen in the skin of young persons. They are (1) hyperkeratosis, (2) thinning of the stratum malpighii with atrophy of some of the rete ridges and elongation of others, (3) a chronic inflammatory infiltrate in the upper dermis, and (4) irregular accumulations of melanin in the basal cell layer, either with or without an increase in the number of melanocytes present (Lynch et al, 1967).

In the second stage, the hyperkeratosis and irregular hyperpigmentation already present in the first stage are more pronounced. The epidermis shows atrophy in some areas and acanthosis in others. There may be disorder in the arrangement of the epidermal nuclei, and, in some areas, the epidermis may show atypical downward growth, so that the histologic picture in such areas is identical with that of solar keratosis (see p. 491). The upper dermis shows basophilic degeneration of the collagen and solar elastosis, as also seen in solar degeneration (see p. 271).

In the third, or tumor, stage, histologic evidence of the various malignant tumors mentioned above is found.

Histogenesis. In patients with xeroderma pigmentosum (with the exception of those who have the so-called XP variant; see below), cells of the skin in tissue culture show a decrease in their ability to repair the damage induced by sunlight to their deoxyribonucleic acid (DNA). This repair is brought about by *excision repair*, a system whereby damaged single-strand regions of DNA are excised and replaced with new sequences of bases (Cleaver). The reason for the inadequate excision repair is that the DNA-endonuclease that initiates the excision process is deficient (Lynch et al, 1977). In vitro testing of skin fibroblasts from different patients with xeroderma pigmentosum shows considerable variation in the excision defect, the extent of repair replication varying between 0% and 90% of normal. Affected siblings are usually similar to each other in degree of repair replication (Lynch et al, 1977). However, no correlation exists between the level of repair replication and the severity of clinical symptoms (Akiba et al).

There are at least five patients known in whom excision repair is normal but the cells are defective in a DNA repair mode referred to as postreplication repair. This represents the so-called XP variant form. In cells of this variant form, the rate of conversion from low- to high-molecular-weight DNA is defective (Friedberg).

Electron microscopic examination of the epidermis has revealed in pigmented areas marked pleomorphism and a definite increase in the number of melanosomes (Rasheed et al). In some cases, very large melanosomes, referred to as giant melanosomes, are present in both melanocytes and keratinocytes (Guerrier et al).

ECTODERMAL DYSPLASIA

Two forms of ectodermal dysplasia are recognized: hidrotic and anhidrotic.

The *hidrotic* form, which has an autosomal dominant inheritance, is primarily a disorder of keratinization and is characterized by the triad of hypotrichosis, dystrophic nails, and palmoplantar hyperkeratosis. It is sometimes associated with dental hypoplasia (Pierard et al). The degree of alopecia varies from slight to total (McNaughton et al).

The *anhidrotic* form is an X-linked recessive disorder occurring in its full expression only in males. Females as heterozygotes may be mildly affected, with reduced sweating and faulty dentition. Males affected with anhidrotic ectodermal dysplasia show the tetrad of anhidrosis or hypohidrosis, hypotrichosis, dental hypoplasia, and a characteristic facies. Frequently, there is also dystrophy of the nails (Martin-Pascual et al). The greatly reduced or absent function of the eccrine glands results in intolerance to heat. The face shows prominent frontal bosses and a depressed nasal bridge. In addition, the mucous glands of the mouth and respiratory tract may be absent (Reed et al). The lack of mammary glands and nipples has also been noted (Martin-Pascual et al).

Histopathology. Both the hidrotic and the anhidrotic forms show hypoplasia of the hair and the sebaceous glands, with a decrease in their number, size, and degree of maturation (Pierard et al; Martin-Pascual et al).

In the anhidrotic form, there is, in addition, either a total absence or severe hypoplasia of the eccrine glands. In the case of hypoplasia, eccrine glands are present in only a few areas, especially the axillae and palms; but, even in these areas, they are sparse and poorly developed. Thus, the secretory cells may be small and flat, so that they resemble endothelial rather than epithelial cells, and the excretory ducts may be composed of a single instead of a double layer of epithelial cells (Malagon and Taveras). The apocrine glands of the axillae are present in some patients with the anhidrotic form (Sunderman); in others, these glands are hypoplastic and cannot be distinguished from

hypoplastic eccrine glands (Dominok and Rönisch), and, in still others, both eccrine and apocrine glands are absent (Upshaw and Montgomery).

FOCAL DERMAL HYPOPLASIA SYNDROME

The focal dermal hypoplasia syndrome, or Goltz syndrome, is probably due to an X-linked dominant gene lethal in homozygous males. Therefore, the syndrome occurs largely in females. Its occasional occurrence in males may be the result of a new mutation (Happle and Lenz). The mode of inheritance thus is similar to that of incontinentia pigmenti (see p. 83).

The cutaneous manifestations of the focal dermal hyperplasia syndrome include (1) widely distributed linear areas of hypoplasia of the skin resembling striae distensae; (2) soft yellowish nodules, often in linear arrangement; and (3) large ulcers due to congenital absence of skin that gradually heal with atrophy. Frequent additional abnormalities include (1) lack of a digit, which may be associated with syndactyly and which results in the very characteristic "lobster-claw deformity"; (2) colobomata of the eyes, or microphthalmia, or agenesis of an eye (Gottlieb et al); and (3) hypoplasia of hair, nails, or teeth (Goltz et al). The presence of fine parallel, vertical striations in the metaphysis of long bones on radiography, referred to as osteopathia striata, is a reliable diagnostic marker of the Goltz syndrome (Howell and Reynolds).

Histopathology. The linear areas of hypoplasia of the skin show a marked diminution in the thickness of the dermis, the collagen being present as thin fibers not united into bundles (Howell). The soft yellowish nodules represent accumulations of fat that largely replace the dermis, so that the subcutaneous fat extends upward to the epidermis in some areas (Fig. 6-5) (Howell; Goltz et al; Lever). Thin fibers of collagen and even some bundles of collagen resembling that of normal dermis may be located between the subepidermal adipose tissue and the subcutaneous fat (Howell).

Histogenesis. The question has been debated of whether the subepidermal accumulations of fat represent a herniation of subcutaneous adipose tissue through an underdeveloped dermis or a hamartoma, that is, a nevoid neoplasm. Since herniation of subcutaneous fat does not occur in any other disease with dermal atrophy, the hamartomatous origin of the fat appears more likely (Howell and Reynolds).

Differential Diagnosis. Fat cells are seen in the dermis also in the nevus lipomatosus of Hoffmann and Zurhelle (see p. 652), but the extreme attenuation of the collagen that occurs in some areas of

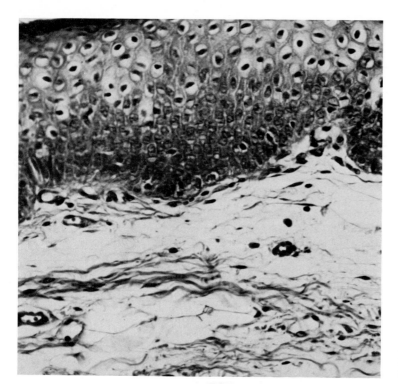

Fig. 6-5. Focal dermal hypoplasia
Adipose tissue is present very near to the epidermis, being separated from it by only a few collagen fibers. ($\times 200$)

the skin in patients with focal dermal hypoplasia syndrome is not seen in nevus lipomatosus.

APLASIA CUTIS CONGENITA

Aplasia cutis congenita consists of a localized absence of skin at the time of birth. Most commonly, one observes a single ulcer or several ulcers on the scalp that measure only 1 cm to 3 cm in diameter and heal uneventfully. In some instances, intrauterine healing has occurred. Occasionally, large defects of the skin are present; but, even then, as a rule, healing takes place within several months (Harari et al; Levin et al).

Histopathology. Ulcers extend through the entire thickness of the dermis, exposing the subcutaneous fat (Deeken and Caplan). Healed areas show, besides a flattened epidermis, fibrosis in the dermis and complete absence of adnexal structures (Harari et al).

POIKILODERMA CONGENITALE (ROTHMUND–THOMSON SYNDROME)

Poikiloderma congenitale is inherited in an autosomal recessive pattern. It begins, a few months after birth, with erythema on the face and subsequently extends to the dorsa of the hands and feet and occasionally also to the arms, legs, and buttocks. Later on, slight atrophy develops with telangiectases and mottled hyper- and hypopigmentation, so that the appearance is that of poikiloderma atrophicans vasculare. Exposure to light aggravates the lesions. Most patients show dwarfism and hypogonadism. In about 40% of the patients, cataracts develop between the ages of 4 and 7 (Rook et al).

Histopathology. During the early phase occurring in infancy and early childhood, one observes hydropic degeneration of the basal layer leading to "pigmentary incontinence" with presence of melanophages in the upper dermis (Tritsch and Lischka). A mild chronic inflammatory infiltrate is intermingled with the melanophages and may show a bandlike arrangement close to the flattened epidermis (Fig. 6-6) (Rook et al). The histologic changes thus may be identical with those seen in the early stage of poikiloderma atrophicans vasculare (see p. 460). In later childhood and adult life, the epidermis is flattened, and dilated capillaries as well as melanophages are present in the upper dermis, but there is no longer any inflammatory infiltrate (Thannhauser).

BLOOM'S SYNDROME (CONGENITAL TELANGIECTATIC ERYTHEMA)

Bloom's syndrome, with autosomal recessive inheritance, resembles poikiloderma congenitale by showing (1) telangiectatic erythema of the face starting in infancy

66

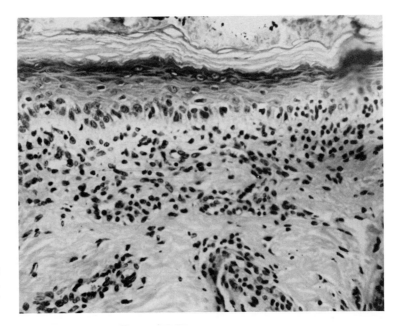

Fig. 6-6. Poikiloderma congenitale (Rothmund–Thomson), early stage
This section, obtained from a young child, shows flattening of the epidermis, hydropic degeneration of the basal layer, and a bandlike inflammatory infiltrate in the upper dermis. (×200)

and often extending to the forearms and dorsa of the hands; (2) sensitivity to sunlight; and (3) growth retardation. It differs from poikiloderma congenitale by (1) the lack of netlike hyper- and hypopigmentation (Braun-Falco and Marghescu); (2) the absence of hypogonadism and cataracts; (3) the occasional presence of immunoglobulin deficiencies, especially of IgA and IgM (Landau et al; Bloom and German); (4) a high incidence of nonspecific chromosomal breakage (Landau et al) and a nine- to tenfold increase in the frequency of another type of chromosome instability, sister chromatid exchanges (Dicken et al); and (5) an increased risk for malignant disease, especially leukemia, lymphoma, and carcinoma of the alimentary tract (Sawitsky et al; Dicken et al).

Histopathology. The epidermis is flattened and may show hydropic degeneration of the basal cell layer (Dicken et al). There is dilatation of the capillaries in the upper dermis, which may be associated with a perivascular mononuclear infiltrate (Katzenellenbogen and Laron; Dicken et al); however, there may be absence of any infiltrate (Braun-Falco and Marghescu).

Histogenesis. Bloom's syndrome shows impairment of both cellular and humoral immunity, although this is not as pronounced as in ataxia–telangiectasia (see below). Evidence of impaired cellular immunity is the occasional absence of delayed hypersensitivity reactions (Bloom and German) and the tendency toward development of malignant disease. Evidence of impaired humoral immunity is the occasional presence of immunoglobulin deficiencies. However, in contrast to ataxia–telangiectasia, susceptibility to infections is not pronounced.

Differential Diagnosis. Pigmentary incontinence is not pronounced in Bloom's syndrome, as it is in poikiloderma congenitale. The presence of hydropic degeneration of the basal cell layer and of a perivascular infiltrate may cause difficulties in differentiation from lupus erythematosus. However, no linear deposits of immunoglobulin are seen at the dermal-epidermal junction in Blooms' syndrome (Dicken et al).

ATAXIA–TELANGIECTASIA

Ataxia–telangiectasia is transmitted in an autosomal recessive mode. The ataxia is evident already in infancy, whereas the telangiectases do not appear until childhood. They usually appear first on the bulbar conjunctivae, with subsequent extension to the cheeks, ears, and neck and often also to other areas, such as the buttocks and extremities. A marked susceptibility to infections, particularly sinopulmonary infections, exists. Death from chronic respiratory infection or lymphoma–leukemia is common in the second or third decade of life (Rosen).

Histopathology. The upper dermis shows numerous markedly dilated vessels that belong to the subpapillary venous plexus (Gschnait et al).

Histogenesis. All patients have severe defects in both humoral and cellular immunity. Thus, in approximately 70% of the patients, IgA, and often also IgE, are absent in the serum, and the antibody response to a variety of bacterial and viral antigens is lower than normal

(McFarlin et al). Autopsies have established maldevelopment of the thymus as an integral part of ataxia–telangiectasia (McFarlin et al). Chromosomal breakage is common, but there is no increased rate of sister chromatid exchanges (Gschnait et al).

PROGERIA OF THE ADULT (WERNER'S SYNDROME)

Werner's syndrome, which has an autosomal recessive mode of inheritance, does not manifest itself until the second or third decade of life. The subcutaneous fat and the musculature of the extremities undergo atrophy, so that the patient exhibits thin arms and legs. The skin of the extremities gradually becomes taut, and ulcers may develop on the legs. As signs of premature senility, patients show graying of the hair, cataracts, and atherosclerosis in early adult life. Diabetes of the late-onset type (Epstein et al) and hypogonadism due to interstitial fibrosis of the testes (Tritsch and Lischka) are common. Death usually occurs in the fifth decade of life because of atherosclerosis.

Histopathology.   On the arms and legs, where the skin is taut, the epidermis is thin and devoid of rete ridges, and the dermis shows fibrosis with or without hyalinization of the collagen, together with disappearance of the pilosebaceous structures and atrophy of the sweat glands. The subcutaneous fat is atrophic (Epstein et al; Tritsch and Lischka).

Differential Diagnosis.   Differentiation from a late lesion of scleroderma may be difficult, because fibrosis and hyalinization of the collagen are seen also in scleroderma (Epstein et al). In its late stage, scleroderma may also show no inflammatory infiltrate, so that differentiation has to be made on the basis of the patient's history and clinical manifestations.

EPIDERMOLYSIS BULLOSA

The following forms of epidermolysis bullosa (EB) exist: two epidermal forms, (1) EB simplex (dominant) and (2) EB of Cockayne of the hands and feet (dominant); two junctional forms, (1) EB letalis (recessive) and (2) generalized atrophic benign EB (recessive); two dermal forms, (1) EB dystrophica-dominant and (2) EB dystrophica-recessive; and EB acquisita, which is not inherited. In all seven forms, the blisters usually form as a result of minor trauma. Distinction of EB letalis, generalized atrophic benign EB, EB dystrophica-dominant, and EB dystrophica-recessive often is impossible on the basis of clinical and histologic data and requires electron microscopic examination.

In EB simplex, the bullae heal without scarring, and the mucous membranes and the nails are rarely affected. In the Cockayne form of EB, the bullae are limited to the hands and feet. In EB letalis, death usually occurs within the first few months of life. The bullae show little tendency to heal; but, when they heal, no scars remain. Oral lesions and dystrophic changes of the nails are present. The other junctional form of EB, generalized atrophic benign EB, has a good prognosis. It shows generalized blister formation, often including oral lesions. The cutaneous lesions result in extensive areas of superficial atrophy together with atrophic alopecia and dystrophic nail changes (Schnyder and Anton-Lamprecht; Hintner et al; Hintner and Wolff). In EB dystrophica-dominant, mild scarring occurs; the oral mucosa is occasionally affected, and the nails are often thickened or lost. In EB dystrophica-recessive, extensive erosions resulting in ulcerations and scarring occur; the oral mucosa is nearly always affected, the nails are rudimentary, and esophageal stenoses can occur (Bergenholtz and Olsson). The ulcers and scars may give rise to squamous cell carcinomas, which tend to metastasize (Reed et al). In especially severe cases of EB dystrophica-recessive, death may occur. In a relatively mild form of EB dystrophica-recessive that has been described under the designation of EB dystrophica inversa, the lesions are located predominantly on the trunk rather than on the extremities, and scarring does not occur until adolescence, thus leading to possible confusion with EB letalis (Gedde-Dahl; Hashimoto et al, 1976; Stevanovic et al). EB acquisita starts in adult life with blisters at sites of trauma resulting in atrophic scars. Dystrophy of the nails is common, and oral lesions are seen occasionally (Roenigk et al).

Histopathology.   Histologic differentiation of the various forms of EB is unsatisfactory even if histologic examination is carried out on very early bullae or on areas that have been exposed to minimal frictional trauma by gentle rubbing with a finger for a few seconds. The location of the bulla or split appears to lie subepidermally in all forms of the disorder. Electron microscopic examination (see below) is much more informative than examination by light microscopy. Nevertheless, the light microscopic features that may be seen in the various forms of EB will be briefly described.

In EB simplex, experimentally produced or early lesions may show vacuolization and degeneration of basal cells. The primary separation occurs either within the basal cell layer (Lowe; Pearson, 1971) or, as the result of complete disintegration of the basal cell layer, subepidermally (Pearson, 1971). In sections stained with the PAS technic, the PAS-positive basement membrane zone is located on the dermal side of the blister (Hintner et al). In bullae of more than one day's duration, the cleavage may be found intraepidermally or subcorneally as a result of epidermal regeneration.

In *EB of the hands and feet*, a cytolytic process associated with necrosis of some of the cells has been assumed to take place in the upper stratum malpighii, as seen in friction blisters (Pearson, 1971) (see p. 128). However, a reinvestigation has shown that the blisters form, just as in EB simplex, in the lowest portion of the basal cells (Haneke and Anton-Lamprecht).

In *EB letalis*, the trauma of having a specimen taken for biopsy generally is sufficient to induce separation. This separation is located between the epidermis and the dermis, with the PAS-positive basement membrane zone usually remaining with the dermis (Pearson et al). Autopsy has in some cases revealed extensive subepithelial separation also in the gastrointestinal, respiratory, and urinary tracts (Pearson et al; Schachner et al).

In *EB dystrophica-dominant* and *EB dystrophica-recessive* as well as in *EB acquisita*, light microscopic examination shows dermal-epidermal separation. A PAS stain usually is of little help in ascertaining the exact level of cleavage, since the PAS-positive basement membrane zone often appears hazy (Pearson, 1971). If recognizable, either it is seen in contact with the detached epidermis (Lowe) or it appears split, being located partially at the base and partially at the top of the bulla (Roenigk et al).

Histogenesis. *Electron microscopic examination* of spontaneously as well as experimentally formed blisters has not only clarified the site of bulla formation in the various forms of EB but has also, in conjunction with biochemical studies and studies by tissue culture and immunofluorescence, greatly clarified the pathogenesis of the various forms of EB. On the basis of the electron microscopic findings, EB simplex and EB of the hands and feet are referred to as epidermolytic forms of EB; EB letalis and generalized atrophic benign EB as junctional forms; and EB dystrophica-dominant, EB dystrophica-recessive, and EB acquisita as dermolytic forms.

In *EB simplex* (Pearson, 1962) and in *EB of the hands and feet* (Haneke and Anton-Lamprecht), cleavage is the result of degenerative, cytolytic changes occurring in the lower portion of the basal cells between the dermal-epidermal junction and the nucleus (EM 15).

In *EB letalis* (Pearson et al; Anton-Lamprecht and Schnyder) and in *generalized atrophic benign EB* (Schnyder and Anton-Lamprecht; Hintner and Wolff), separation takes place between the plasma membrane of the basal cells and the basement membrane, or basal lamina, within the lamina lucida (Pearson et al). The probable cause of the separation is a hypoplasia of the half-desmosomes demonstrable in areas of intact skin. Half-desmosomes are markedly reduced in number, and,

where present, they are small, show a poorly developed attachment plaque, and lack a sub-basal cell dense plaque (Anton-Lamprecht and Schnyder). Thus, a diagnosis of junctional EB can be established with the aid of electron microscopy by examination either of the blister top, which lacks an underlying basement membrane, or of uninvolved skin, which shows poorly developed half-desmosomes.

In both *EB dystrophica-dominant* and *EB dystrophica-recessive*, the bullae form in the uppermost dermis, in the region of the anchoring fibrils. Thus, in both forms of dystrophic EB, the basement membrane, or basal lamina, is seen at the top of the blister, in coherence with the detached epidermis. No agreement exists about the role that the anchoring fibrils play in the production of blisters in the two dystrophic forms of EB. Whereas a defect of the anchoring fibrils in EB dystrophica-dominant is assumed by some authors to be primary (Hashimoto et al, 1975; Anton-Lamprecht), others regard the defect as a secondary event (Briggaman and Wheeler). Similarly, in EB dystrophica-recessive, the defect in the anchoring fibrils is regarded as primary by some (Briggaman and Wheeler) and as secondary by others (Hashimoto et al, 1976). In support of a primary defect in the anchoring fibrils in EB dystrophica-recessive are tissue culture experiments in which anchoring fibrils were not formed by EB dystrophica-recessive dermis when combined with either EB dystrophica-recessive epidermis or normal epidermis (Briggaman and Wheeler). Of interest is the possible role of collagenase in EB dystrophica-recessive: a significant increase in the level of collagenase was found in both involved and normal-appearing skin of patients with EB dystrophica-recessive; in contrast, patients with EB dystrophica-dominant showed no significant increase in collagenase in their normal-appearing skin (Bauer and Uitto).

Attempts have been made to differentiate, even without the use of an electron microscope, junctional forms of EB from the dermolytic or dystrophic forms of EB. For this purpose, fluorescein-labeled antibody-containing bullous pemphigoid serum has been used, but the results have been contradictory: the immunofluorescent staining in junctional EB was found on the floor of the blister by one group (Schachner et al) and mainly on the roof of the blister by another group (Hintner et al). It seems that better differentiation can be obtained by immunofluorescence testing with specific antisera against type IV collagen, localized within the basement membrane, and against laminin, localized in the lamina lucida. In junctional EB, both antisera were found on the floor of the blister, whereas, in dermolytic and dystrophic EB, both antisera were located on the roof of the blister (Hintner et al).

In *EB acquisita*, as in the other dystrophic forms of EB, the blisters arise in the uppermost dermis in the region of the anchoring fibrils, that is, beneath the basement membrane or basal lamina (Gibbs and Minus; Metz et al). The anchoring fibrils are decreased in both normal-appearing and lesional skin (Yaoita et al) and may even be destroyed at the site of blister formation (Richter and McNutt). In most cases of EB acquisita, direct immunofluorescence testing has shown the presence of linear deposits of immunoglobulins and complement components along the dermal-epidermal border in both involved and uninvolved skin (Gibbs and Minus; Livden et al). In some patients, even circulating IgG class anti-basement membrane zone antibodies were found (Nieboer et al; Yaoita et al). These findings have led to the speculation that EB acquisita may be a sign of cicatricial pemphigoid (Dahl). However, with immunoelectron microscopy using peroxidase-labeled antibody, the in vivo deposits of IgG are found to be located beneath the basement membrane, not above the basement membrane as in cicatricial pemphigoid (Nieboer et al; Yaoita et al) (see p. 117). Thus, EB acquisita is a distinct entity in which autoimmune mechanisms seem to play a role.

KERATOSIS FOLLICULARIS (DARIER'S DISEASE)

Darier's disease, although usually transmitted in an autosomal dominant pattern, may occur as a mutation. In typical cases, there is a more or less extensive, persistent, slowly progressive eruption consisting of hyperkeratotic or crusted papules often showing a follicular distribution. By coalescence verrucous, crusted areas may form. Occasionally, hypertrophic lesions are present with elevated, papillomatous formations. In a few cases, the occurrence of vesicles, in addition to papules, has been described (Jablonska and Chorzelski;

Piérard et al). The so-called seborrheic areas are the sites of predilection. In some cases of Darier's disease, there are on the dorsa of the hands and feet keratotic papules that resemble those seen in acrokeratosis verruciformis of Hopf (Panja). The oral mucosa is involved occasionally (Weathers et al). In rare instances, Darier's disease manifests itself without a family history as a unilateral localized linear lesion arising either in late life (Kellum and Haserick; Leeming; Binnick and Fleischmajer; Starink and Woerdeman) or at birth (Demetree et al). The question has been raised as to whether this type of lesion represents a linear epidermal nevus with acantholytic dyskeratosis rather than Darier's disease (Demetree et al), and the designation *acantholytic dyskeratotic epidermal nevus* has been suggested (Starink and Woerdeman) (see p. 473). Although Darier's disease may arise late in life (Gisslén and Mobacken) and may be localized in extent (Delacrétaz and Christeler), it is quite likely that some of the cases with scattered papular lesions of limited extent arising in adult life represent transient acantholytic dermatosis of Grover rather than Darier's disease (Fishman; Gisslén and Mobacken; Carapeto and Armijo) (see p. 127).

Histopathology. The characteristic changes in Darier's disease are (1) a peculiar form of dyskeratosis resulting in the formation of corps ronds and grains, (2) suprabasal acantholysis leading to the formation of suprabasal clefts or lacunae, and (3) irregular upward proliferation into the lacunae of papillae lined with a single layer of basal cells, so-called villi (Fig. 6-7). There are also papilloma-

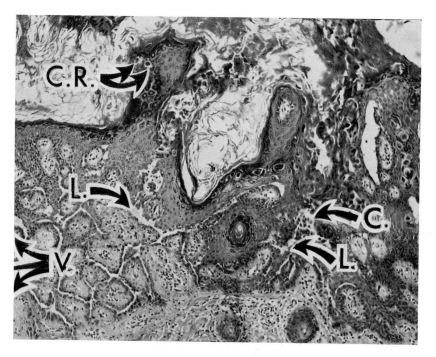

Fig. 6-7. Darier's disease
Low magnification. Hyperkeratosis and papillomatosis are evident. Numerous lacunae (*L.*) are present. On the left are elongated papillae lined by a single layer of cells, so-called villi (*V.*). Corps ronds (*C.R.*) are present in the granular layer, and grains are seen in the horny layer. The lacunae contain desquamated acantholytic cells (*C.*). (×100)

tosis, acanthosis, and hyperkeratosis. The dermis shows a chronic inflammatory infiltrate. In some cases, there is downward proliferation of epidermal cells into the dermis.

The corps ronds occur in the upper stratum malpighii, particularly in the granular and horny layers; grains are found in the horny layer and as acantholytic cells within the lacunae. Corps ronds possess a central homogeneous, basophilic, pyknotic nucleus that is surrounded by a clear halo. By virtue of size and the conspicuous halo, corps ronds stand out clearly (Fig. 6-8). Peripheral to the halo lies basophilic dyskeratotic material as a shell (Sato et al). The nonstaining halo in some instances is partially replaced by homogeneous, eosinophilic dyskeratotic material (Piérard and Kint). In contrast to the corps ronds, the grains are much less conspicuous. They resemble parakeratotic cells but are somewhat larger. The nuclei of grains are elongated and often grain-shaped and are surrounded by homogeneous dyskeratotic material that usually stains basophilic but may stain eosinophilic.

The lacunae represent small, slitlike intraepidermal vesicles most commonly located directly above the basal layer. They contain acantholytic cells that are devoid of intercellular bridges and show premature partial keratinization. Because of shrinkage, some of them are elongated, and these then appear identical with the grains in the horny layer.

The villi projecting into the lacunae may be quite tortuous, so that, on histologic examination, some of them appear in cross section as rounded dermal structures lined by a solitary row of basal cells (see Fig. 6-7).

Hyperkeratosis and papillomatosis may cause the formation of keratotic plugs, which often fill the pilosebaceous follicles but are found also outside of follicles. That Darier's disease is not exclusively a follicular disorder is also proved by the fact that areas devoid of follicles, such as palms, soles, and the oral mucosa, may be affected.

In hypertrophic lesions of Darier's disease, one can occasionally observe considerable downward proliferation of the epidermis, either as proliferations of basal cells or as pseudocarcinomatous hyperplasia. Proliferations of basal cells consist of long, narrow cords composed of two rows of basal cells separated by a narrow lacunar space (Beerman; Krinitz).

The vesicles, which occur in rare instances, differ from lacunae merely in size; they contain numerous

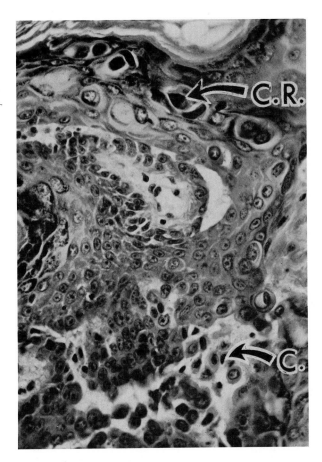

Fig. 6-8.   Darier's disease
High magnification of Figure 6-7. In the upper third of the illustration, within the granular layer, are several corps ronds (*C.R.*) showing a central, large, round, homogeneous, basophilic, dyskeratotic mass surrounded by a clear halo. In the lower third, within a lacuna, are acantholytic cells (*C.*), which, on account of premature partial keratinization, have a shrunken appearance. (× 400)

shrunken cells with the appearance of grains (Jablonska and Chorzelski; Piérard et al).

The keratotic papules that may occur on the dorsa of the hands and feet and that clinically resemble those seen in acrokeratosis verruciformis of Hopf in most instances, especially on serial sectioning, show mild dyskeratotic changes and often suprabasal clefts as well (Panja). They are thus a manifestation of Darier's disease and not of acrokeratosis verruciformis (see p. 74).

The lesions on the oral mucosa are analogous in appearance to those observed on the skin and thus show lacunae and dyskeratosis, although definite well-formed corps ronds generally are absent (Weathers et al).

Histogenesis. The occurrence of suprabasal acantholysis represents a genetic defect. On *electron microscopic examination,* two different mechanisms have been thought to be responsible for the development of acantholysis. Some authors have seen the primary defect in the loss of the intercellular contact layer within desmosomes, which thus pull apart into two halves, after which the tonofilaments become detached from them (Mann and Haye; Biagini et al; Peck et al). Other authors have maintained that the primary event is a separation of tonofilaments from the attachment plaques with subsequent disappearance of the desmosomes (Caulfield and Wilgram; Piérard and Kint). It appears possible that both processes take place (Sato et al). A defect of the tonofilaments would best explain the "dyskeratotic" nature of Darier's disease. In any case, tonofilaments without attachment to desmosomes aggregate around the nuclei of epidermal cells and increase rapidly in number. In association with large keratohyaline granules, the bundles of tonofilaments thus form large aggregates of homogenized dyskeratotic material.

The corps ronds, seen on electron microscopic examination, are characterized by extensive cytoplasmic vacuolization (Gottlieb and Lutzner). They show in their center an irregularly shaped nucleus surrounded by a halo of autolyzed electron-lucid cytoplasm and at their periphery a shell of tonofilaments (EM 16) (Mann and Haye; Sato et al). The grains are seen on electron microscopic examination to consist of nuclear remnants surrounded by dyskeratotic bundles of tonofilaments.

Differential Diagnosis. Although acantholytic dyskeratosis in association with corps ronds is highly characteristic of Darier's disease, it occurs also in several other conditions (Ackerman): (1) in warty dyskeratoma, a solitary lesion with a deep central invagination (see p. 489); (2) in transient or persistent acantholytic dermatosis, in which the lesions consist of discrete papules (see p. 127); (3) in focal acantholytic dyskeratoma, manifesting itself as a solitary papule (see p. 475); and (4) as an incidental small focus in a variety of unrelated lesions (see p. 475). Occasionally, a few corps ronds are seen also in familial benign pemphigus (see below).

FAMILIAL BENIGN PEMPHIGUS (HAILEY–HAILEY DISEASE)

Familial benign pemphigus is inherited as an autosomal dominant trait, with a family history obtainable in about two thirds of the patients (Palmer and Perry). It is characterized by a localized, recurrent eruption of very small vesicles on an erythematous base. By peripheral extension, the lesions may assume a circinate configuration. The sites of predilection are the intertriginous areas, especially the axillae and the groins. Only very few instances of mucosal lesions have been reported, of the mouth (Schneider et al; Botvinick; Heinze), the labia majora (Heinze), and the esophagus (Kahn and Hutchinson).

Histopathology. Although, as in Darier's disease, early lesions may show small suprabasal separations, so-called lacunae, fully developed lesions show large separations, that is, vesicles and even bullae, in a predominantly suprabasal position (Fig. 6-9). Villi, which are elongated papillae lined by a single layer of basal cells, protrude

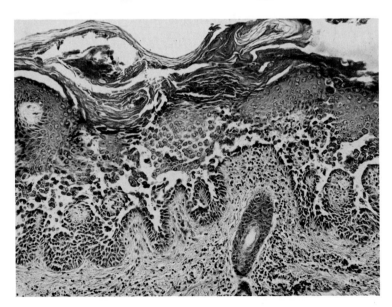

Fig. 6-9. Familial benign pemphigus (Hailey–Hailey disease)
The bulla is largely in a suprabasal position. The extensive loss of intercellular bridges with partial coherence of cells gives the detached epidermis the appearance of a dilapidated brick wall. On the right side, within the granular layer, a corps ronds can be seen. (×200)

upward into the bulla; and, in some cases, narrow strands of epidermal cells proliferate downward into the dermis. Many cells of the detached stratum malpighii show loss of their intercellular bridges, so that acantholysis affects large portions of the epidermis. Individual cells as well as groups of cells usually are seen in large numbers in the bulla cavity. In spite of the extensive loss of intercellular bridges, the cells of the detached epidermis in many places show only slight separation from one another because a few intact intercellular bridges still hold them loosely together. This quite typical feature gives the detached epidermis the appearance of a dilapidated brick wall (Haber and Russell).

Many of the cells of the stratum malpighii that have lost all or most of their intercellular bridges show a fairly normal cytoplasm and a normal nucleus in which mitotic activity has even been observed (Winer and Leeb; Herzberg). Some of the acantholytic cells, however, have a homogenized cytoplasm, suggesting premature partial keratinization. In some instances, such acantholytic cells with premature keratinization resemble the grains of Darier's disease. Occasionally, a few corps ronds are present in the granular layer (Fig. 6-9). (Ellis; Winer and Leeb; Herzberg).

Histogenesis. Based on *electron microscopic* findings, there are two schools of thought about the primary event in the suprabasal acantholysis seen in familial benign pemphigus. One group of authors (Nürnberger and Müller; Thies et al) believes that acantholysis results from an insufficiency of cellular adhesion. This may manifest itself either by primary dissolution of many desmosomes (Thies et al) or by the formation of numerous elongated and branching microvilli at the periphery of the keratinocytes, such as may be seen in early lesions of pemphigus vulgaris (Braun-Falco and Vogell). It is assumed that the microvilli form as a result of faulty synthesis of the intercellular substance (Nürnberger and Müller). The other group of authors (Wilgram et al; Piérard and Kint) believes that the same basic defect in the tonofilament–desmosome complex observed by them in Darier's disease exists also in familial benign pemphigus, resulting in detachment of the tonofilaments from the desmosomes and subsequently leading to the disappearance of desmosomes and thus to acantholysis. Although it seems possible that both processes occur simultaneously and have as a common denominator an abnormal component of the plasma membrane (Gottlieb and Lutzner), recent findings made by the experimental induction of acantholysis on the normal-appearing skin of a patient with familial benign pemphigus favor insufficiency of cellular adhesion as the initial phenomenon: in lesions produced by application of an occlusive dressing, the first alteration, observed after 48 hr of occlusion, was separation of

desmosomes into two halves, each half retaining tonofilaments on its attachment plaque. Separation of tonofilaments from their desmosomes was seen only after 72 hr of occlusion (De Dobbeleer and Achten). It is generally agreed that, after loss of the desmosomes, excessive amounts of tonofilaments form within the keratinocytes and aggregate around the nucleus as thick, electron-dense bundles, often in a whorling configuration; however, even though dyskeratosis is present, it is less pronounced than in Darier's disease, and most of the keratinocytes keratinize normally, only very few becoming grains or corps ronds as the result of dyskeratotic degeneration.

Intradermal injection of tritiated thymidine in vivo into lesions of familial benign pemphigus and of Darier's disease has revealed labeling of many acantholytic epidermal cells in familial benign pemphigus. This suggests that such cells participate in the renewal of the epidermis. No labeling of acantholytic epidermal cells has been seen in Darier's disease, probably because these cells are undergoing keratinization (Lachapelle et al).

Differential Diagnosis. Histologically, familial benign pemphigus shares certain features with both Darier's disease and pemphigus vulgaris. In all three diseases, one finds (1) predominantly suprabasal separation of the epidermis caused by acantholysis and resulting in lacunae or bullae, and (2) upward proliferation of papillae as so-called villi into the lacunae or bullae.

Differentiation of familial benign pemphigus from Darier's disease as a rule is not very difficult, because, in Darier's disease (1) the suprabasal separations usually are smaller, thus appearing as lacunae rather than as bullae; (2) acantholysis is less pronounced, being limited to the lower epidermis, especially the suprabasal region; and (3) dyskeratosis consisting of the formation of corps ronds and grains is much more evident.

Pemphigus vulgaris often resembles familial benign pemphigus to a striking degree, and, in some specimens, histologic differentiation of these two diseases may be impossible. As a rule, however, one observes in pemphigus vulgaris (1) less extensive acantholysis limited largely to the suprabasal region, so that the detached epidermis appears normal and lacks the appearance of a dilapidated brick wall, and (2) more severe degeneration of the acantholytic cells within and near the bulla cavity. The presence of eosinophils in the bulla points toward a diagnosis of pemphigus vulgaris, but their absence does not rule it out.

There used to be much discussion as to whether familial benign pemphigus represents a vesicular variant of Darier's disease. Two points in favor of the basic unity of the two diseases were stressed:

the alleged simultaneous presence of both diseases in the same patient, and the occurrence of corps ronds in both diseases. However, it has become apparent that patients described as having both diseases were either cases of Darier's disease with vesicular lesions (Niordson and Sylvest; Ganor and Sagher) or cases of familial benign pemphigus with the presence of corps ronds (Finnerud and Szymanski; Nicolis et al). Against a relationship is also the fact that, in affected families, always only one of the two diseases occurs (Raaschou-Nielsen and Reymann).

For a discussion of differentiation from transient acantholytic dermatosis, see p. 127.

ACROKERATOSIS VERRUCIFORMIS OF HOPF

In acrokeratosis verruciformis, an autosomal dominant disorder, numerous flat, hyperkeratotic, occasionally verrucous papules are present on the distal part of the extremities, predominantly on the dorsa of the hands and feet (Panja).

Histopathology.   The papules show considerable hyperkeratosis, an increase in thickness of the granular layer, and acanthosis. In addition, there is slight papillomatosis, which is frequently but not always associated with circumscribed elevations of the epidermis resembling church spires (Fig. 6-10) (Waisman; Schueller). The rete ridges are slightly elongated and extend to a uniform level.

Histogenesis. A possible relationship between acrokeratosis verruciformis and Darier's disease has been repeatedly discussed. On the one hand, there is no

question that acrokeratosis verruciformis usually occurs as an independent entity, often in several family members (Panja) and occasionally even in many family members (Niedelman and McKusick) but also as a solitary incidence (Schueller). On the other hand, a relationship to Darier's disease is suggested by the following observations: (1) patients with Darier's disease not infrequently show lesions that are indistinguishable from acrokeratosis verruciformis both clinically and histologically (Waisman; Penrod et al); (2) some of the lesions of presumed acrokeratosis verruciformis occurring in patients with Darier's disease show dyskeratosis and lacunae as seen in Darier's disease, whereas others do not (Waisman); and (3) patients with apparent histologic lesions of acrokeratosis verruciformis may later develop histologic lesions of Darier's disease (Jordan and Spier; Panja). Admittedly, there can be considerable clinical resemblance between the acral lesions of both diseases, but, if multiple specimens for biopsy are taken and serial sections carried out, histologic evidence of Darier's disease is generally obtained only in those patients who have Darier's disease (Beerman; Krause and Ehlers). It seems that there is only one instance in which both diseases were seen in different members of the same family (Herndon and Wilson), and this may well have been coincidence. Thus, it is best to regard acrokeratosis verruciformis as an independent entity (Panja).

Differential Diagnosis.   Although elevations of the epidermis with the configuration of church spires are quite typical of acrokeratosis verruciformis, they may be absent in that disease. Furthermore, they are present in the hyperkeratotic type of seborrheic keratosis (see p. 478). Thus, even though seborrheic keratoses usually are larger than the lesions of acrokeratosis verruciformis, clinical data may be necessary for the differentiation of these two conditions. Also, acrokeratosis verruci-

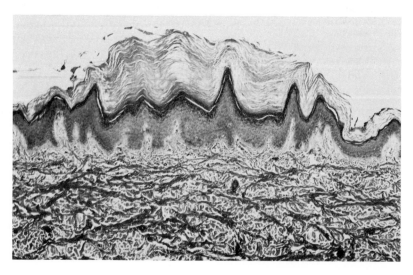

Fig. 6-10.   Acrokeratosis verruciformis of Hopf
A well-circumscribed lesion shows hyperkeratosis and papillomatosis. The latter is associated with elevations of the epidermis resembling church spires. (×100)

formis may resemble verrucae clinically, but it differs from verruca plana by the absence of vacuolization in the cells of the upper epidermis and from verruca vulgaris by the absence of parakeratosis.

PSEUDOXANTHOMA ELASTICUM

In this disorder, genetically abnormal elastic fibers with a tendency toward calcification occur in the skin and frequently also in the retina and within the walls of arteries, particularly the gastric mucosal arteries, coronary arteries, and large peripheral arteries. The inheritance is usually autosomal recessive but occasionally autosomal dominant. It seems that two recessive and two dominant forms exist (Pope, 1975). The classic disorder in this classification is recessive type 1. In the dominant type 1 form, the cutaneous and internal manifestations are more severe than in recessive type 1, whereas, in dominant type 2, they are less severe. The very rare recessive type 2 form shows only cutaneous involvement, which, however, is very extensive (Pope, 1974).

The cutaneous lesions usually appear first in the second or third decade of life and are generally progressive in extent and severity. They consist of soft, yellowish, coalescing papules, and the affected skin appears loose and wrinkled. The sides of the neck, the axillae, and the groin are the most common sites of lesions. In the eyes, so-called angioid streaks of the fundi may cause progressive impairment of vision. Involvement of the arteries of the gastric mucosa may lead to gastric hemorrhage; involvement of coronary arteries may result in attacks of angina pectoris, although

myocardial infarction is rare; and involvement of the large peripheral arteries may cause intermittent claudication (Mendelsohn et al). Radiologic examination in such cases reveals extensive calcification of the affected peripheral arteries (Eddy and Farber).

In rare instances, the coexistence of pseudoxanthoma elasticum with elastosis perforans serpiginosa (see p. 276) has been reported, with perforation and transepidermal elimination present only in the lesions of elastosis perforans serpiginosa (Schutt; Caro et al). Calcific elastosis, which has been referred to also as perforating pseudoxanthoma elasticum or localized acquired pseudoxanthoma elasticum, is not related to pseudoxanthoma elasticum (for a description, see p. 278).

Histopathology.   Histologic examination of the involved skin reveals in the middle and lower thirds of the dermis considerable accumulations of swollen and irregularly clumped fibers staining like elastic fibers; that is, they stain deeply black with orcein or the Verhoeff stain (Figs. 6-11, 6-12). Although normally elastic fibers do not stain with routine stains such as hematoxylin-eosin, the altered elastic fibers in pseudoxanthoma elasticum stain faintly basophilic because of their calcium imbibition. Staining for calcium with the von Kossa method also shows these fibers well. In the vicinity of the altered elastic fibers, one may find accumulations of a slightly basophilic mucoid material, which stains strongly positive with the colloidal iron reaction or with alcian blue (Huang et al). The amount of collagen bundles is reduced in such areas, and numerous reticulum fibers are seen on

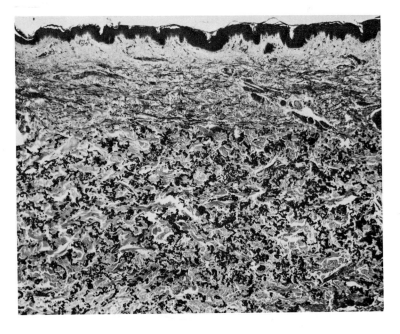

Fig. 6-11.   Pseudoxanthoma elasticum Low magnification, elastic tissue stain. In the middle and lower layers of the dermis, the elastic fibers appear swollen and irregularly clumped. (×50)

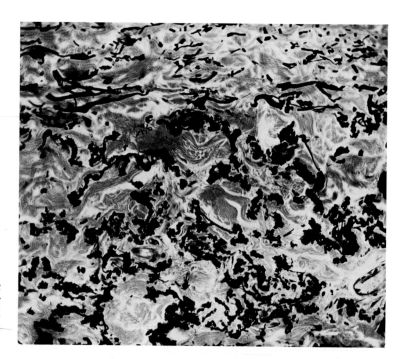

Fig. 6-12. Pseudoxanthoma elasticum
High magnification of Figure 6-11, elastic tissue stain. The elastic fibers in the upper fourth of the illustration have a normal appearance; those in the lower three fourths show marked degeneration. (×200)

impregnation with silver (Danielsen et al). In some cases with pronounced elastic tissue calcification, a macrophage and giant cell reaction may be present (Goodman et al).

The angioid streaks occur in Bruch's membrane, which is located between the retina and the choroid and possesses numerous elastic fibers in its outer portion, the lamina elastica. Calcification of these fibers causes fissures to form in the lamina elastica. These fissures result in repeated hemorrhages and exudates, which in turn cause degenerative changes in the retina consisting of scar formation and pigment shifting (Goodman et al; Kreysel et al).

Gastric bleeding is the result of calcification of elastic fibers in the thin-walled arteries located immediately beneath the gastric mucosa. The internal elastic lamina is particularly affected (Flatley et al). In muscular arteries, such as the coronary arteries and the large peripheral arteries, calcification begins in the internal and external elastic laminae, leading to their fragmentation, and subsequently extends to the media and intima (Mendelsohn et al). Calcification of the elastic fibers in the endocardium is a common occurrence but is clinically silent (Akhtar and Brody).

Histogenesis. *Electron microscopic examination* shows that the calcification occurs in normal-appearing elastic fibers (Hashimoto and DiBella; Danielsen et al; Martinez-Hernandez and Huffer; Akhtar and Brody; McKee et al).

In some patients, especially in young persons, only some of the elastic fibers in the lower dermis are calcified, and the calcification is variable in degree. In adult patients, however, most elastic fibers show considerable calcification and, as a result, degeneration. Early calcification of elastic fibers consists either of diffuse granular deposits throughout the elastic fiber or of dense aggregates that may be located in the center or near the margin of the fiber (EM 17). With progression of the calcification, the elastic fibers ultimately become fully calcified, showing marked swelling and bizarre distortions. In addition, heavy calcium deposits may be seen in the ground substance adjacent to elastic fibers as well as free in the ground substance. The presence of calcified material outside of elastic fibers can be explained by the disintegration of completely calcified elastic fibers (McKee et al).

Besides varying numbers of normal collagen fibrils, irregularly twisted collagen fibrils and granulofilamentous aggregates are present. It appears unlikely that the process of calcification begins in the granulofilamentous material, as maintained by some authors who regard this material as an abnormal precursor of elastic fibers (Huang et al; Saito and Klingmüller). It is probable that this misinterpretation has resulted from the examination of advanced lesions containing disintegrated calcified elastic fibers within the granulofilamentous material (Akhtar and Brody). In favor of a primary location of the calcification within elastic fibers is the important observation that, in decalcified sections of endocardial lesions, the internal structure of the calcified segments of elastic fibers is very similar to that of the adjacent noncalcified segments (Akhtar and Brody).

Differential Diagnosis.   Solar elastosis, like pseudoxanthoma elasticum, shows abnormal elastic tissue. However, in solar elastosis, this material is located in the upper third of the dermis and is present as dense masses rather than as individual curls. Furthermore, these dense masses always show negative staining for calcium. If associated with a perforation, calcific elastosis is easily distinguished from pseudoxanthoma elasticum. In the absence of a perforation the two are indistinguishable, and clinical data are necessary for differentiation. (For a discussion of the differential diagnosis from connective tissue nevus with an increase in elastic tissue, see below.)

CONNECTIVE TISSUE NEVUS

The connective tissue nevus represents a hamartoma in which the amount of collagen is increased whereas the amount of elastic tissue may be decreased, normal, or increased. The lesions consist of slightly elevated, slightly indurated nodules that may be grouped together in one or several plaques or may be widely disseminated. A connective tissue nevus can (1) occur without alterations in other organs and without being genetically determined (Danielsen et al), (2) occur without alterations in other organs, being inherited as an autosomal dominant trait (Uitto et al), or (3) occur with osteopoikilosis, being inherited in an autosomal dominant pattern (Morrison et al). The shagreen patches of tuberous sclerosis do not strictly belong in the category of connective tissue nevi, since they always consist only of excessive amounts of collagen and thus are "collagen nevi" rather than connective tissue nevi (Kobayasi et al) (see p. 603).

In osteopoikilosis, the skin lesions consist of firm, pale papules and plaques in asymmetric distribution with a tendency toward grouping. The extent of involvement may vary from a single lesion to many (Morrison et al). Individual members of affected families may have skin lesions without bone lesions, and vice versa. The bone lesions of osteopoikilosis are asymptomatic and, on x-ray examination, are seen to consist of round or oval densities 2 mm to 10 mm in diameter located in the long bones and in the bones of the hands, feet, and pelvis (Schorr et al).

Histopathology.   The classification of connective tissue nevi into different categories, such as nevus elasticus, nevus anelasticus, and collagenoma, has been generally abandoned since it has become apparent that variations in histologic composition occur not only in different patients but also in different lesions from the same patient (Raque and Wood). Since the lesions are firm, it is obvious that the amount of collagen is always increased, although this may be difficult to ascertain if the collagen

bundles are normal in appearance (Smith and Waisman). In some lesions, however, the collagen bundles are thickened and appear homogeneous (Schorr et al; Uitto et al).

The elastic fibers may appear normal or may be sparse or absent (Schorr et al). In other lesions, they show a marked increase in number and size without signs of degeneration (Fig. 6-13) (Staricco and Mehregan). Broad interlacing bands of elastic fibers may encase the collagen bundles (Morrison et al). Frequently, however, when there is an increase in the amount of elastic tissue, the elastic fibers show coalescence into irregular clusters (Smith and Waisman; Schorr et al; Verbov).

Differential Diagnosis.   In connective tissue nevi with an increase in elastic tissue, the elastic fibers show no breaking up into individual curls and no depositions of calcium, in contrast to pseudoxanthoma elasticum.

LINEAR MELORHEOSTOTIC SCLERODERMA

Melorheostosis is characterized by linear hyperostosis of an extremity. It may be associated with thickening

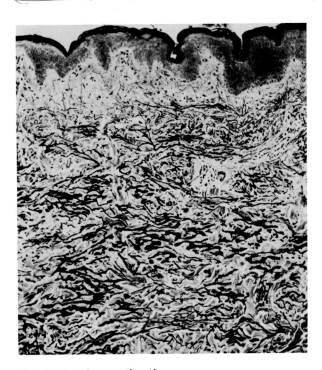

Fig. 6-13.   Connective tissue nevus (nevus elasticus)
The elastic fibers are markedly increased in number and size without showing signs of degeneration. (× 100)

and hypertrichosis of the overlying skin. Although not familial, its start in infancy suggests a congenital disorder (Miyachi et al).

Histopathology.   The skin shows thickening of the dermis caused by the extension of normal-appearing collagen and elastic tissue in strands and lobules into the subcutaneous fat (Wagers et al).

Histogenesis. Hyperplasia of the skin is related to the underlying cortical hyperostosis. The normal appearance of the thickened dermis indicates that the process does not represent localized scleroderma (Wagers et al).

WINCHESTER SYNDROME

A rare inherited disorder described only in the offspring of consanguinous parents, the Winchester syndrome is characterized by dwarfism, small joint destruction, corneal opacities, thickening and hypertrichosis of the skin, and hypertrophic lips and gingivae.

Histopathology.   In the early stage, the skin shows proliferation of fibroblasts in the lower portions of the dermis with extension into the subcutaneous tissue. At a later stage, the collagen appears homogenized and contains only few fibroblasts (Cohen et al). Some areas may show an increase both in the number of fibroblasts and in the density of the collagen bundles (Nabai et al).

Histogenesis. An abnormal function of the fibroblasts is the likely cause for all manifestations. *Electron microscopic examination* has shown dilated and vacuolated mitochondria in the fibroblasts (Cohen et al).

EHLERS–DANLOS SYNDROME

The Ehlers–Danlos syndrome (E–D) has been divided into nine types on the basis of clinical, genetic, and biochemical information. The common clinical features are (1) hyperextensibility of the skin, (2) fragility of the skin with impaired wound healing, resulting in the formation of atrophic scars, and (3) hypermobility of the joints, which may lead to dislocations. Occasionally, one observes at sites of traumatic hematomas raisinlike, or molluscoid, pseudotumors that are raised and soft and have a wrinkled surface. In some cases, firm, spheroid subcutaneous nodules form at sites of traumatic fat necrosis.

E–D types I, II, and III, the most common forms of this syndrome, are inherited in an autosomal dominant pattern and are distinguished by the extent and severity of the symptoms, type I being the gravis type, type II

the mitis form, and type III the benign hypermobile type. No biochemical defect has been detected (Uitto and Lichtenstein).

E–D type IV, the arterial form, is inherited as an autosomal recessive trait. The skin of persons with this disorder is thin and friable. Patients rarely live beyond the second decade of life because of ruptures of large arteries or of the gastrointestinal tract (McFarland and Fuller). This tendency toward rupture is explained by the fact that the fibroblasts in E–D type IV fail to synthesize type III collagen (see p. 31).

E–D type V has an X-linked recessive inheritance pattern and clinical features similar to those of type I. The fibroblasts produce only 15% to 30% of the normal amount of lysyl oxidase. This deficiency results in deficient intramolecular cross-linking in the collagen molecule (Uitto and Lichtenstein).

E–D type VI, the ocular type, with autosomal recessive inheritance, is characterized by severe scoliosis and intraocular bleeding (Pinnell et al). There is a deficiency in lysyl hydroxylase in this form of the disorder.

E–D type VII, the arthrochalasis type, also with autosomal recessive inheritance, shows marked looseness of joints resulting in multiple joint dislocations. The skin and tendons of patients with this form of E–D contain collagen polypeptides with a length intermediate between pro-alpha (procollagen) chains and alpha (collagen) chains. This is due to a structural mutation in the pro-alpha 2 chain that prevents the normal enzymatic removal of the aminopropeptide from it (Prockop et al) (see also p. 31).

E–D type VIII, the periodontal type, inherited as an autosomal dominant trait, is characterized by severe periodontitis and moderate skin fragility. Its biochemical defect is unknown (Nelson and King).

E–D type IX, the fibronectin type, with autosomal recessive inheritance, shows striae, moderate skin extensibility, joint hypermobility, and a platelet aggregation defect caused by a dysfunction of the plasma fibronectin (Arneson et al).

Histopathology.   Aside from areas of the skin that have been altered secondarily by trauma, there are in the great majority of patients no abnormalities either in the thickness of the skin or in the appearance of the collagen or of the elastic fibers. Only an exceptional patient shows thin collagen fibers that are not united to collagen bundles. In such cases, the skin may also be reduced in thickness and show a relative increase in amount of elastic fibers (Sulica et al).

The raisinlike pseudotumors that arise at the site of hematomas show fibrosis and numerous capillaries; they may also show accumulations of foreign body giant cells (Ronchese). The spheroid subcutaneous nodules consist of partially necrotic adipose tissue that may contain areas of dystrophic calcification and that is surrounded by a thick layer of dense collagen (Cullen).

Histogenesis. The enzyme deficiencies observed in the various types of the Ehlers–Danlos syndrome suggest a disturbance in collagen biosynthesis. In several *electron microscopic studies,* no abnormalities were observed in the normal skin of patients with Ehlers–Danlos syndrome (Wechsler and Fisher; Black et al); however, other studies have reported abnormalities. Thus, in a study comparing healing experimental wounds in a patient with Ehlers–Danlos syndrome with those in normal persons, the fibroblasts of the patient with Ehlers–Danlos syndrome showed a paucity of rough-surfaced endoplasmic reticulum, and the bundles of collagen appeared small and sparse (Scarpelli and Goodman). Similar abnormalities were observed also in the normal-appearing skin of five patients with various types of Ehlers–Danlos syndrome: the fibroblasts were smaller than in the skin of normal control persons, the endoplasmic reticulum was underdeveloped, and ribosome content was diminished. In addition, some collagen fibrils possessed an irregular outline, and lateral aggregation of the fibrils into bundles was reduced (Sevenich et al).

Scanning electron microscopic examination in various types of Ehlers–Danlos syndrome has revealed thinner collagen bundles than normal and, within the bundles, gross disorganization of the collagen fibers (Black et al). Thus, scanning electron microscopy has lent support to the previously unsubstantiated proposal by Jansen, made in 1955, that hyperextensibility in the Ehlers–Danlos syndrome is due to defective "wicker work" of the collagen fiber bundles.

CUTIS LAXA (DERMATOCHALASIS)

Cutis laxa, also called dermatochalasis and generalized elastolysis, is characterized by loose, pendulous skin resulting in a prematurely aged appearance. There are two types, congenital and acquired. In the congenital type, the usual mode of inheritance is autosomal recessive (Goltz et al), although autosomal dominant transmission has been described in a few relatively mild cases (Schreiber and Tilley). The acquired type has no genetic background (Reed et al).

In both the congenital and the acquired types, internal organs are frequently involved. There may be pulmonary emphysema causing death in infancy in some of the congenital cases (Goltz et al; Mehregan et al) or later in life in some of the acquired cases (Reed et al). In addition, there may be diverticula in the gastrointestinal tract or in the bladder. Also, rectal prolapse and inguinal, umbilical, and hiatal hernias have been observed (Goltz et al). Some of the cases of acquired cutis laxa are preceded or accompanied by a cutaneous eruption showing urticaria (Scott et al), erythematous plaques (Nanko et al), or a vesicular eruption (Reed et al; Kerl and Burg).

Histopathology. In cases without an inflammatory infiltrate, the changes are limited to the elastic fibers and depend on the stage and the severity of the disease. In the early stage, the elastic fibers are diminished either throughout the dermis or largely in the upper dermis (Reed et al) or the lower dermis (Mehregan et al). Those elastic fibers that are present may be considerably thickened in their midportion and may taper to a point at either end (Goltz et al). Their borders may be indistinct and they may stain unevenly, showing a granular appearance (Fig. 6-14). Ultimately, no intact elastic fibers may be identifiable. Instead, fine, dustlike orceinophilic granules may be scattered in the dermis (Mehregan et al).

In cases in which an inflammatory infiltrate is present, it may consist of a nonspecific chronic inflammatory infiltrate of lymphocytes and histiocytes (Nanko et al). However, it may also contain neutrophils (Jablonska). If vesicles are present, they are subepidermal in location and may show papillary microabscesses composed of neutrophils and eosinophils suggestive of dermatitis herpetiformis (Kerl and Burg).

In patients with involvement of internal organs, the lungs and gastrointestinal tract show the same granular changes in the elastic fibers as seen in the skin (Goltz et al; Reed et al).

Histogenesis. *Electron microscopic examination* shows degenerative changes in the elastic fibers that vary somewhat from case to case. In some instances, the elastic fibers show normal microfibrils but a deficiency of the amorphous, electron-lucent elastin (Hashimoto and Kanzaki; Harris et al), whereas, in other instances, the elastin is preserved and the microfibrils are absent (Sayers et al). In most electron microscopic examinations, the most significant finding is the presence of electron-dense amorphous or granular aggregates in the vicinity of the elastic fibers (Hashimoto and Kanzaki; Sayers et al; Nanko et al). The presence of this electron-dense material outside of elastic fibers suggests that, instead of a primary elastolysis, as generally assumed, a defect in the synthesis of elastic fibers causes the disease (Hashimoto and Kanzaki; Nanko et al).

Another controversy concerns the role of the cutaneous eruption that precedes or accompanies many of the reported cases of acquired cutis laxa. The traditional view has been that the inflammatory infiltrate is in some way responsible for the damage to the elastic fibers (Jablonska; Kerl and Burg; Scott et al; Harris et al). However, sequential biopsies seem to indicate that granular changes in the elastic fibers precede the appearance of the inflammatory infiltrate (Nanko et al), and the possibility therefore exists that the inflammatory infiltrate is a consequence of changes in the fibers.

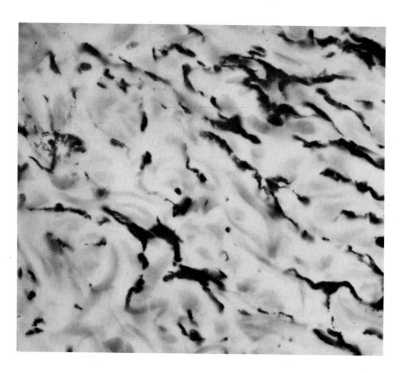

Fig. 6-14. Cutis laxa
Elastic tissue stain. The degenerated elastic fibers stain unevenly, resulting in a granular appearance and indistinct borders. (×400) (Courtesy of Robert W. Goltz, M.D.)

PACHYDERMOPERIOSTOSIS

An idiopathic and an acquired form of pachydermoperiostosis exist, the latter being secondary to carcinoma of the lung. The idiopathic form is transmitted as an autosomal dominant trait, males being more severely affected than females (Rimoin). The manifestations include (1) clubbing of the digits, with periosteal proliferation of the bones of the hands and feet; (2) hyperplasia of the soft parts of the forearms and legs, with periosteal proliferation of the corresponding bones; and (3) thickening and furrowing of the skin of the face and scalp (cutis verticis gyrata). In abortive forms, there may be only clubbing of the fingers with periosteal proliferation of the bones of the hands and forearms (Curth et al).

Histopathology. The skin of the face shows thickening of the dermis, with thick fibrous bands extending into the subcutaneous tissue (Hambrick and Carter). In addition to an increase in the amount and size of the collagen bundles in the dermis, there is an increase in the number of fibroblasts and in the amount of ground substance. The latter stains with colloidal iron, and, because it is composed largely of hyaluronic acid, it stains with alcian blue at pH 2.5 but not at pH 0.45 (Hambrick and Carter).

URTICARIA PIGMENTOSA

Urticaria pigmentosa, although occasionally showing an autosomal dominant mode of transmission (Shaw; Bazex et al), in most instances occurs without a family history. It can be divided into four forms: (1) urticaria pigmentosa arising in infancy or early childhood without significant systemic lesions, (2) urticaria pigmentosa arising in adolescence or adult life without significant systemic lesions, (3) systemic mast cell disease, and (4) mast cell leukemia.

In the first form, the cutaneous lesions often improve or even clear at puberty (Klaus and Winkelmann, 1962). Systemic lesions are absent as a rule and, if present, usually are few in number. Progression into systemic mast cell disease is very rare (see below). In the second form, urticaria pigmentosa arising in adolescence or adult life, systemic lesions are often present but as a rule are rather static in their course (Caplan). However, spontaneous regression has never been documented in adults, in contrast to children (Roberts et al). In only a few patients is there progression to the third form, systemic mast cell disease, which shows extensive and progressive involvement of internal organs (see Systemic Lesions). The rarity of extensive, progressive systemic mast cell disease is attested to by a review of the literature in 1963, which yielded only 29 cases, 5 of which had no cutaneous lesions (Mutter et al). Of the 29 patients, 5 were below 10 years of age, with a fatal outcome in 2 patients (Ellis; Waters and Lacson). In 9 of the 24 adult patients, the disease was fatal, on the average 26 years after the onset of symptoms (Mutter et al). The fourth form, mast cell leukemia, is very rare. It is characterized by the presence of cytologically malignant mast cells in many organs of the body, especially in the bone marrow and the peripheral blood, and is a rapidly fatal disease (Efrati et al; Friedman et al; Brinkmann).

Patients with extensive mast cell infiltration of the skin or the internal organs commonly have attacks of flushing, palpitation, or diarrhea as a result of degranulation of mast cells and the release of histamine.

Five types of cutaneous lesions are seen in urticaria pigmentosa (Klaus and Winkelmann, 1965). Two types can occur in both the infantile and the adult forms: the maculopapular type, consisting usually of dozens or even hundreds of brownish lesions that urticate on stroking, and multiple nodules or plaques also brownish in color and, on stroking, always showing urtication and occasionally also blister formation. The third type, seen almost exclusively in infants, is characterized by a solitary, large cutaneous nodule, which on stroking often shows not only urtication but also large bullae. In rare instances, such solitary nodules have been described as arising in adults without giving rise to bullae (Baraf and Shapiro). The fourth type, the diffuse erythrodermic type, always starts in early infancy and shows generalized brownish red, soft infiltration of the skin, with urtication on stroking and formation of multiple blisters during the first two years of life not only on stroking but also spontaneously (Burgoon et al; Orkin et al). Although visceral lesions are common in the diffuse erythrodermic type, they usually improve (Robinson et al) and only very rarely progress to fatal systemic mast cell disease (Waters and Lacson). On rare occasions, death occurs in early infancy, apparently as a result of histamine shock without or with only insignificant mast cell infiltration of visceral organs (Yasuda and Kukita; Allison). The fifth type of lesion, telangiectasia macularis eruptiva perstans, which usually occurs in adults, consists of an extensive eruption of brownish red macules showing fine telangiectasias, with little or no urtication on stroking (Cramer).

Histopathology. In all five types of lesions, the histologic picture shows an infiltrate composed chiefly of mast cells, which are characterized by the presence of metachromatic granules in their cytoplasm. These granules are not visible with routine stains (see p. 53) but can be seen well after staining with a Giemsa stain or with toluidine blue (Plate 1, facing p. 228).

In the maculopapular type and in telangiectasia macularis eruptiva perstans, the mast cells are limited to the upper third of the dermis and are located especially around capillaries. In some mast cells, the nuclei may be round or oval, but, in most mast cells, they are spindle-shaped (Fig. 6-15). Since the mast cells may be present only in small numbers, and since, in sections stained with hematoxylin-eosin, their nuclei resemble those of fibroblasts or pericytes, the diagnosis may be missed unless special staining is employed (Mihm et al).

In cases with multiple nodules or plaques or with a solitary large nodule, the mast cells lie closely packed in tumorlike aggregates (Figs. 6-16, 6-17). The infiltrate may extend through the entire dermis and even into the subcutaneous fat (Johnson and Helwig). Whenever the mast cells lie in dense aggregates, their nuclei are cuboidal rather than spindle-shaped, and they show ample eosinophilic

Fig. 6-15. Urticaria pigmentosa, maculopapular type
The mast cells are present only in small numbers and are predominantly spindle-shaped and perivascular in location. Since, in routinely stained sections, the mast cells resemble fibroblasts, the diagnosis may be missed. A Giemsa stain will demonstrate the mast cell granules (see Plate 1, facing p. 228). (×100)

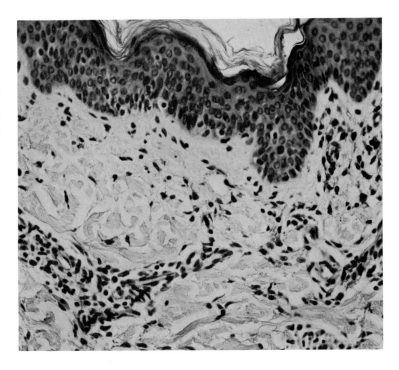

cytoplasm and a well-defined cell border. Because of the shape of their nuclei and ample cytoplasm, they have a rather distinctive appearance, so that the diagnosis usually can be made even before special staining has been carried out.

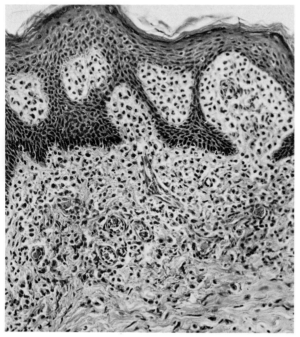

Fig. 6-16. Urticaria pigmentosa, nodular type
Low magnification, hematoxylin-eosin stain. Mast cells, cuboidal in shape, lie closely packed in the upper dermis. Because of staining with hematoxylin-eosin, the granules in the mast cells are not visible. (×200)

In the diffuse, erythrodermic type, one observes in the upper dermis a dense, bandlike infiltrate of mast cells with a rather uniform appearance showing round to oval nuclei and a distinctly outlined cytoplasm (Degos; Braun-Falco and Jung; Robinson et al; Burgoon et al).

Eosinophils may be present in small numbers in all types of urticaria pigmentosa with the exception of telangiectasia macularis eruptiva perstans, in which eosinophils are generally absent because of the small numbers of mast cells within the lesions. If a biopsy is taken shortly after the lesion has been stroked, one observes an increased number of eosinophils and extracellular mast cell granules as an indication that granules have been released by the cells (Drennan).

The bullae that may occur in infants with multiple or solitary nodules or with the diffuse erythrodermic type arise subepidermally (Miller and Shapiro). Because of regeneration of the epidermis at the base of the bulla, older bullae may be located intraepidermally. The bullous cavity often contains mast cells as well as eosinophils (Dewar and Milne). The pigmentation of lesions of urticaria pigmentosa is due to the presence of increased amounts of melanin in the basal cell layer and occasionally also of melanophages in the upper dermis.

Systemic Lesions. It is important to distinguish between asymptomatic systemic involvement of limited degree and true systemic mast cell disease, in which the lesions are symptomatic, widespread, and progressive (see p. 80).

Asymptomatic systemic involvement of a limited degree may occur in urticaria pigmentosa of chil-

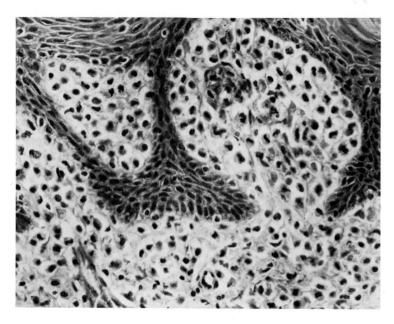

Fig. 6-17. Urticaria pigmentosa, nodular type
High magnification of Fig 6-16, hematoxylin-eosin stain. The mast cells appear as large cuboidal cells. (×400)

dren, but it is not common. It occurs most commonly in the erythrodermic and nodular types and consists of bone and bone marrow involvement or of hepatosplenomegaly (Robinson et al). In urticaria pigmentosa of adults, systemic lesions are more common. For instance, in routinely carried out bone marrow biopsies, as many as 75% of adult patients show mast cell infiltration of bone marrow, in contrast to only 18% of children; and radiologic survey of the skeleton has revealed bone changes in 44% of adult patients but in only 5% of children (Rodermund et al). On radiologic examination, bones with mast cell infiltration may show areas of increased lucency intermingled with areas of increased density owing to the fact that mast cell aggregates in the bone marrow can cause focal bone resorption as well as reactive bone formation (Sostre and Handler).

In true systemic mast cell disease, massive infiltration of the bones may cause collapse of several vertebrae (Mutter et al) or a fracture of long bones (Naveh et al). Myelofibrosis may occur, resulting in anemia, leukopenia, and thrombocytopenia (Monheit et al). Pancytopenia may cause death (Mutter et al). Systemic mastocytosis, besides involving the bone marrow and bones, generally involves the liver and spleen, resulting in hepatosplenomegaly, and various groups of lymph nodes. In some cases, the gastrointestinal tract, lungs, and meninges are also infiltrated with mast cells (Roberts et al). Mature mast cells may be found in the peripheral blood (Burgoon et al; Mutter et al).

Histogenesis. As seen by both light microscopy and *electron microscopy*, the mast cells of urticaria pigmentosa do not differ from normal mast cells either in structure or in mode of degranulation (EM 18) (Freeman; Hashimoto et al). Since mast cells contain histamine and release it during degranulation, chemical analysis of cutaneous lesions of urticaria pigmentosa reveals a considerably higher level of histamine than found in normal skin (Davis et al).

The increased melanin pigmentation in lesions of urticaria pigmentosa is the result of stimulation of epidermal melanocytes by mast cells. Thus, it is not caused by any substance present within the mast cells. In one case of nodular urticaria pigmentosa, however, some mast cells showed dual granulation containing both mast cell granules and melanosomes, as well as granules representing intergrades between mast cell granules and melanosomes (Okun and Bhawan).

Differential Diagnosis.   Even if numerous mast cells are present, an absolutely reliable diagnosis of urticaria pigmentosa requires the demonstration of mast cell granules with the Giemsa stain. On routine staining, the mast cells in macular lesions may resemble fibroblasts or pericytes, whereas those in nodular or erythrodermic lesions may resemble the histiocytes that are seen in Letter–Siwe disease or in eosinophilic granuloma. Differentiation of urticaria pigmentosa from these two diseases on routine staining can be particularly difficult, because, in all three diseases, the infiltrate may contain eosinophils. However, in contrast with Letterer–Siwe disease, the cells of urticaria pigmentosa have no tendency to invade the epidermis. Occasionally, the cuboidal mast cells in nodular urticaria pigmentosa resemble nevus cells, but they show no tendency to nest and no junction activity.

The macular type of urticaria pigmentosa, especially telangiectasia maculosa eruptiva perstans, occasionally may be difficult to diagnose even with the Giemsa stain, because the number of mast cells may be so small that it does not differ significantly from the number normally present (Mihm et al). Some inflammatory dermatoses, such as atopic dermatitis, lichen simplex chronicus, and lichen planus, may contain a high percentage of mast cells in their inflammatory cell infiltrates (Mikhail and Miller-Milinska). In urticaria pigmentosa, however, the infiltrate consists exclusively of mast cells, except for a slight admixture of eosinophils as a result of the degranulation of some of the mast cells.

INCONTINENTIA PIGMENTI

Incontinentia pigmenti is an X-linked dominantly inherited disorder. Females with the abnormal gene on only one of their two X chromosomes are heterozygous for this condition and are not severely affected, whereas males with the abnormal gene on their single X chromosome are hemizygous for this condition and hence are so severely affected that they die in utero. This explains the predominance of female patients with this disorder (Lenz; Gordon and Gordon). Of 609 reported cases, only 16 have been in boys. The fact that these boys were no more severely affected than their female counterparts suggests that the disease in all living male patients is the result of spontaneous mutation (Carney).

The disorder has three stages. The first stage, consisting of erythema and bullae arranged in lines, either is present at birth or starts shortly thereafter. The extremities are predominantly affected. There is also marked blood eosinophilia. In the second stage, which occurs after about two months, the vesicular lesions gradually are superseded by linear, verrucous lesions that persist for several months. As the verrucous lesions subside, widely disseminated areas of irregular, spattered, or whorled pigmentation develop. This pigmentation, representing the third stage, is most pronounced on the trunk. It diminishes gradually after several years and may even clear completely.

In about 80% percent of the cases, incontinentia pigmenti is associated with various congenital abnormalities, particularly of the central nervous system, eyes, and teeth. Partial alopecia at the vertex is also often seen (Carney).

Histopathology. The vesicles seen during the first stage arise within the epidermis and are associated with spongiosis. They are thus of the type seen in dermatitis (Epstein et al; Wodniansky) (see p. 94). However, they differ from the vesicles of dermatitis by the presence of numerous eosinophils within them as well as around them in the epidermis (Fig. 6-18). The epidermis between the vesicles often shows single dyskeratotic cells and whorls of squamous cells with central keratinization (Epstein et al). Like the epidermis, the dermis shows an infiltrate containing many eosinophils and some mononuclear cells.

The alterations in the second stage consist of acanthosis, irregular papillomatosis, and hyperkeratosis. Intraepidermal keratinization, consisting of whorls of keratinocytes and of scattered dyskeratotic cells, is often more pronounced than in the first stage (Epstein et al). The basal cells show vacuolization and a decrease in their melanin content. The dermis shows a mild, chronic inflammatory infiltrate intermingled with melanophages.

This infiltrate extends into the epidermis in many places.

The areas of pigmentation seen in the third stage show extensive deposits of melanin within melanophages located in the upper dermis. Usually, this dermal hyperpigmentation is found in association with a diminution of pigment in the basal layer, the cells of which show vacuolization and degeneration (Sulzberger; Doornink). In some cases, however, the cells of the basal layer contain abundant amounts of melanin (Vilanova and Aguade; Rubin and Becker).

Histogenesis. The fact that the first two stages of incontinentia pigmenti are seen predominantly on the extremities and the third stage mainly on the trunk has led to the assumption by some authors that the pigmentary changes of the third stage occur independently of the bullous and verrucous lesions of the first two stages and represent some sort of nevoid anomaly (Carney). *Electron microscopic studies,* however, have revealed common features, albeit to varying extents, in all three stages of incontinentia pigmenti and thus suggest that the three stages are related to each other (Schaumburg-Lever and Lever; Guerrier and Wong; Caputo et al). Even in the first stage, many keratinocytes and melanocytes show degenerative changes resulting in the migration of macrophages to the epidermis, where they phagocytize dyskeratotic keratinocytes and melanosomes. Subsequently, the macrophages return to the dermis (EM 19). The macrophages seen in the dermis in the second and third stages contain many melanosome

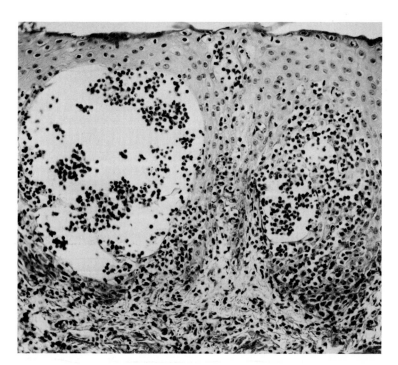

Fig. 6-18.   Incontinentia pigmenti, vesicular stage
The vesicles arise within the epidermis and are associated with spongiosis. Numerous eosinophils and also mononuclear cells are present in the vesicles as well as in the epidermis and the dermis. (×200)

complexes and thus are easily recognizable as melanophages even by light microscopy, whereas the macrophages in the first stage contain only few melanosome complexes and therefore can be identified as melanophages only in the electron microscope (Schaumburg-Lever and Lever). The phagocytosis of melanin by dermal macrophages in the first stage of the disease has been confirmed (Guerrier and Wong), as well as the presence of dyskeratotic keratinocytes in the epidermis during all three stages of the disease (Caputo et al).

HYPOMELANOSIS OF ITO

Hypomelanosis of Ito was originally called incontinentia pigmenti achromians, but, since the disorder shows no pigmentary incontinence, this term has been largely abandoned.

Hypomelanosis of Ito has two forms, cutaneous and neurocutaneous. In the more common cutaneous form, pigmentary loss begins late in childhood and persists until early adulthood, at which time repigmentation takes place. In the neurocutaneous form, pigmentary loss develops in infancy and is accompanied by severe central nervous system dysfunction, including seizures, and by bone abnormalities (Nordlund et al). The inheritance in both forms is autosomal dominant. Although first reported in Japanese patients, hypomelanosis of Ito has since been observed in many races. The pattern and distribution of the hypopigmentation in hypomelanosis of Ito is similar to the pattern of the hyperpigmentation seen in incontinentia pigmenti.

Histopathology.   In the hypopigmented areas, a Fontana–Masson stain shows a decrease in the amount of melanin granules in the basal cell layer, with a complete absence of melanin in some areas (Grosshans et al). With the dopa reaction, the hypopigmented areas are seen to contain fewer and smaller melanocytes than normal, with sparse, short dendrites (Nordlund et al).

Histogenesis. The *electron microscopic findings* show a significant decrease in the number of melanosomes within melanocytes and keratinocytes (Nordlund et al). In addition, some melanocytes show degenerative changes and an absence of melanosomes (Morohashi et al.)

BIBLIOGRAPHY

Ichthyosis

ACKERMAN AB: Histopathologic concept of epidermolytic hyperkeratosis. Arch Dermatol 102:253–259, 1970

ALTMAN J, STROUD J: Netherton's syndrome and ichthyosis linearis circumflexa: Psoriasiform ichthyosis. Arch Dermatol 100:550–558, 1969

ANTON-LAMPRECHT I: Zur Ultrastruktur hereditärer Verhornungsstörungen. III. Autosomal-dominante Ichthyosis vulgaris. Arch Dermatol Forsch 248:149–172, 1973

ANTON-LAMPRECHT I: Zur Ultrastruktur hereditärer Verhornungsstörungen. IV. X-chromosomal-recessive Ichthyosis. Arch Dermatol Forsch 248:361–378, 1974

ANTON-LAMPRECHT I, SCHNYDER UW: Ultrastructure in inborn errors of keratinization. Arch Dermatol Forsch 250:207–227, 1974

BADEN HP, GOLDSMITH LA: The structural proteins of the harlequin fetus: Stratum corneum. J Invest Dermatol 61:25–26, 1973

BADEN HP, KUBILUS J, ROSENBAUM K et al: Keratinization in the harlequin fetus. Arch Dermatol 118:14–18, 1982

BLOOM D, GOODFRIED MS: Lamellar ichthyosis of the newborn. Arch Dermatol 86:336–342, 1962

BUXMAN MM, GOODKIN PE, FAHRENBACH WH et al: Harlequin ichthyosis with epidermal lipid abnormality. Arch Dermatol 115:189–193, 1979

DAVIES MG, MARKS R, DYKES PJ et al: Epidermal abnormalities in Refsum's disease. Br J Dermatol 97:401–406, 1977

EDIDIN DV, ESTERLY NB, BAMZAI AK et al: Chondrodysplasia punctata: Conradi-Hünermann syndrome. Arch Dermatol 113:1431–1434, 1977

EPSTEIN EH, JR., WILLIAMS ML, ELIAS PM: Editorial: Steroid sulfatase, X-linked ichthyosis, and stratum corneum cohesion. Arch Dermatol 117:761–763, 1981

FEINSTEIN A, ACKERMAN AB, ZIPRKOWSKI L: Histology of autosomal dominant ichthyosis vulgaris and X-linked ichthyosis. Arch Dermatol 101:524–527, 1970

FINLEY AY, NICHOLLS S, KING CS et al: The "dry" non-eczematous skin associated with atopic eczema. Br J Dermatol 103:249–256, 1980

FLINT GL, FLAM M, SOTER NA: Acquired ichthyosis: A sign of nonlymphoproliferative malignant disorder. Arch Dermatol 111:1446–1447, 1975

FROST P: Ichthyosiform dermatoses. J Invest Dermatol 60:541–552, 1973

FROST P, VAN SCOTT EJ: Ichthyosiform dermatoses. Arch Dermatol 94:113–126, 1966

FROST P, WEINSTEIN GD, VAN SCOTT EJ: The ichthyosiform dermatoses. II. Autoradiographic studies of epidermal proliferation. J Invest Dermatol 47:561–567, 1966

HEIJER A, REED WB: Sjögren-Larsson syndrome. Arch Dermatol 92:545–552, 1965

HERSLE K: Netherton's disease and ichthyosis linearis circumflexa. Acta Derm Venereol (Stockh) 52:298–302, 1972

ISHIBASHI Y, KLINGMÜLLER G: Erythrodermia ichthyosiformis congenita bullosa Brocq. Arch Klin Exp Dermatol 232:205–224, 1968

JORIZZO JL, CROUNSE RG, WHEELER CE, JR.: Lamellar ichthyosis, dwarfism, mental retardation, and hair shaft anomalies. J Am Acad Dermatol 2:309–317, 1980

KAUH YC, GOODY HE, LUSCOMBE HA: Ichthyosiform sarcoidosis. Arch Dermatol 114:100–101, 1978

LARRÈQUE M, GHARBI R, DANIEL J et al: Le bébé collodion. Ann Dermatol Venereol 103:31–56, 1976

LUDERSCHMIDT C, DORN M, BASSERMANN R et al: Kollodiumbaby und Harlekinfetus. Hautarzt 31:154–158, 1980

MALDONADO RR, TAMAYO L, CARNEVALE A: Neuroichthyosis with hypogonadism (Rud's syndrome). Int J Dermatol 14:347–352, 1975

MCCURDY J, BEARE JM: Congenital bullous ichthyosiform erythroderma. Br J Dermatol 79:294–297, 1967

MEHREGAN AH: Epidermolytic hyperkeratosis. J Cutan Pathol 5:76–80, 1978

MEHVORAH B, FRENK E: Ichthyosis linearis circumflexa Comèl with trichorrhexis invaginata (Netherton's syndrome). Dermatologica 149:193–200, 1974

MEHVORAH B, FRENK E, BROOKE EM: Ichthyosis linearis circumflexa Comèl. Dermatologica 149:201–209, 1974

NIIZUMA K: Isolated epidermolytic acanthoma. Dermatologica 159:30–36, 1979

NIR M, TANZER F: Progressive symmetric erythrokeratodermia. Dermatologica 156:268–273, 1978

PERROT H, SCHMITT D, THIVOLET J: Ichtyose paranéoplasique: Etude ultrastructurale. Ann Dermatol Syph 103:413–421, 1976

SCHELLANDER FG, FRITSCH PO: Variable erythrokeratoderma. Arch Dermatol 100:744–748, 1969

SCHNYDER UW: Inherited ichthyosis. Arch Dermatol 102:240–259, 1970

SCHNYDER UW, KONRAD B: Zur Histogenetik der Ichthyosen. Hautarzt 18:445–450, 1967

SHAPIRO LJ, WEISS R, WEBSTER D et al: X-linked ichthyosis due to steroid-sulphatase deficiency. Lancet 1:70–72, 1978

STEINBERG D, MIZE CE, HERNDON JH, JR.: Phytanic acid in patients with Refsum's syndrome and response to dietary treatment. Arch Intern Med 125:75–87, 1970

STEVANOVIC DV: Hodgkin's disease of the skin. Arch Dermatol 82:96–99, 1960

THORNE EG, ZELICKSON AS, MOTTAZ JH et al: Netherton's syndrome: An electron microscopic study. Arch Dermatol Res 253:177–183, 1975

VANDERSTEEN PR, MULLER SA: Erythrokeratodermia variabilis. Arch Dermatol 103:362–370, 1971

VANDERSTEEN PR, MULLER SA: Lamellar ichthyosis. Arch Dermatol 106:694–701, 1972

WELLS RS: Some genetic aspects of dermatology: A review. Clin Exp Dermatol 5:1–11, 1980

WILLIAMS ML, ELIAS PM: X-linked ichthyosis: Elevated cholesterol sulfate in pathological stratum corneum. (Abstr) J Invest Dermatol 76:312, 1981

ZINA AM, BUNDINO S: Ichthyosis linearis circumflexa Comèl and Netherton's syndrome: An ultrastructural study. Dermatologica 158:404–412, 1979

Keratosis Palmaris et Plantaris

BACH JN, LEVAN NE: Papillon-Lefèvre syndrome. Arch Dermatol 97:154–158, 1968

BROWN FC: Punctate keratoderma. Arch Dermatol 104:682–683, 1971

BUCHANAN RN, JR.: Keratosis punctata palmaris et plantaris. Arch Dermatol 88:644–650, 1963

CALLAN NJ: Circumscribed palmoplantar keratoderma. Aust J Dermatol 11:76–81, 1970

FRITSCH P, HÖNIGSMANN H, JASCHKE E: Epidermolytic hereditary palmoplantar keratoderma. Br J Dermatol 99:561–568, 1978

GREITHER A: Keratosis extremitatum hereditaria progrediens mit dominantem Erbgang. Hautarzt 3:198–203, 1952

HERMAN PS: Punctate porokeratotic keratoderma. Dermatologica 147:206–213, 1973

KANSKY A, ARZENSEK J: Is palmoplantar keratoderma of Greither's type a separate nosologic entity? Dermatologica 158:244–248, 1979

KLAUS S, WEINSTEIN GD, FROST P: Localized epidermolytic hyperkeratosis: A form of keratoderma of the palms and soles. Arch Dermatol 101:272–275, 1970

MOULIN G, BOUCHET B: La kératodermie palmo-plantaire familiale avec hyperkératose épidermolytique. Ann Dermatol Venereol 104:38–44, 1977

SALAMON T, BOGDANOVIC B, LAZOVIC-TEPAVAC O: Die Krankheit von Mljet. Dermatologica 138:433–443, 1969

Acrokeratoelastoidosis

COSTA OG: Acrokeratoelastoidosis. Arch Dermatol 70:228–231, 1954

HIGHET AS, ROOK A, ANDERSON JR: Acrokeratoelastoidosis. Br J Dermatol 106:337–344, 1982

JOHANSSON EA, KARINIEMI AL, NIEMI KM: Palmoplantar keratoderma of punctate type: Acrokeratoelastoidosis Costa. Acta Derm Venereol (Stockh) 60:149–153, 1980

JUNG EG, BEIL FU, ANTON-LAMPRECHT I et al: Akrokeratoelastoidosis. Hautarzt 25:127–133, 1974

Pachyonychia Congenita

KELLY EW, JR., PINKUS H: Report of a case of pachyonychia congenita. Arch Dermatol 77:724–726, 1958

SCHÖNFELD PHIR: The pachyonychia congenita syndrome. Acta Derm Venereol (Stockh) 60:45–49, 1980

WITKOP CJ, GORLIN RJ: Four hereditary mucosal syndromes. Arch Dermatol 84:762–771, 1961

Dyskeratosis Congenita

BRYAN HG, NIXON RK: Dyskeratosis congenita and familial pancytopenia. JAMA 192:203–208, 1965

COSTELLO MJ, BUNCKE CM: Dyskeratosis congenita. Arch Dermatol 73:123–132, 1956

GARB J: Dyskeratosis congenita with pigmentation, dystrophia ungium, and leukokeratosis oris. Arch Dermatol 77:704–712, 1958

GUTMAN A, FRUMKIN A, ADAM A et al: X-linked dyskeratosis congenita with pancytopenia. Arch Dermatol 114:1667–1671, 1978

SORROW JM, JR., HITCH JM: Dyskeratosis congenita. Arch Dermatol 88:340–347, 1963

Porokeratosis

BRAUN-FALCO O, BALSA RE: Zur Histochemie der cornoiden Lamelle. Hautarzt 28:543–550, 1969

CHERNOSKY ME, FREEMAN RG: Disseminated superficial actinic porokeratosis (DSAP). Arch Dermatol 96:611–624, 1967

COSKEY RJ, MEHREGAN A: Bowen disease associated with porokeratosis of Mibelli. Arch Dermatol 111:1480–1481, 1975

GUSS SB, OSBOURN RA, LUTZNER MA: Porokeratosis plantaris, palmaris et disseminata. Arch Dermatol 104:366–373, 1971

MANN PR, CORT DF, FAIRBURN EA et al: Ultrastructural studies on two cases of porokeratosis of Mibelli. Br J Dermatol 90:607–617, 1974

MIBELLI V: Contributo allo studio della ipercheratosi dei canali sudoriferi. G Ital Mal Ven 28:313–355, 1893

NABAI H, MEHREGAN AH: Porokeratosis of Mibelli: A report of two unusual cases. Dermatologica 159:325–331, 1979

OBERSTE-LEHN H, MOLL B: Porokeratosis Mibelli und Stachelzellcarcinom. Hautarzt 19:399–403, 1968

RAHBARI H, CORDERO AA, MEHREGAN AH: Linear porokeratosis. Arch Dermatol 109:526–528, 1974

RAHBARI H, CORDERO AA, MEHREGAN AH: Punctate porokeratosis: A clinical variant of porokeratosis of Mibelli. J Cutan Pathol 4:338–341, 1977

REED RJ, LEONE P: Porokeratosis: A mutant clonal keratosis of the epidermis. Arch Dermatol 101:340–347, 1970

SATO A, ANTON-LAMPRECHT I, SCHNYDER UW: Ultrastructure of inborn errors of keratinization. VII. Porokeratosis Mibelli and disseminated superficial actinic porokeratosis. Arch Dermatol Res 255:271–284, 1976

Xeroderma Pigmentosum

AKIBA H, KATO T, SEIJI M: Enzyme defects in xeroderma pigmentosum. J Dermatol (Tokyo), 3:163–170, 1976

BELL ET, ROTHNEM TP: Xeroderma pigmentosum with carcinoma of the lower lip in two brothers aged 16 and 13 years. Am J Cancer 30:574–579, 1937

CLEAVER JF: Xeroderma pigmentosum: Genetic and environmental influences in skin carcinogenesis. Int J Dermatol 17:435–444, 1978

FRIEDBERG EC: Recent studies on the DNA repair defects. Arch Pathol 102:3–7, 1978

GUERRIER CJ, LUTZNER MA, DEVICO V et al: An electron microscopical study of the skin in 18 cases of xeroderma pigmentosum. Dermatologica 146:211–221, 1973

HADIDA E, MARILL FG, SAYAG J: Xeroderma pigmentosum. Ann Dermatol Syph 90:467–496, 1963

EL-HEFNAWI H, MORTADA A: Ocular manifestations of xeroderma pigmentosum. Br J Dermatol 77:261–276, 1965

LYNCH HT, ANDERSON DE, SMITH JL, JR. et al: Xeroderma pigmentosum, malignant melanoma and congenital ichthyosis. Arch Dermatol 96:625–635, 1967

LYNCH HT, FRICHOT BC, III, LYNCH JF: Cancer control in xeroderma pigmentosum. Arch Dermatol 113:193–195, 1977

MCGOVERN VJ: Melanoblastoma, with particular reference to its incidence in childhood. Aust J Dermatol 6:190–192, 1962

RASHEED A, EL-HEFNAWI H, NAGY G et al: Elektronenmikroskopische Untersuchungen bei Xeroderma pigmentosum. Arch Klin Exp Dermatol 234:321–344, 1969

REED WB, SUGARMAN GI, MATHIS RA: DeSanctis-Cacchione syndrome. Arch Dermatol 113:1561–1563, 1977

RONCHESE F: Melanomata: Pathologically malignant, clinically nonmalignant, in a case of xeroderma pigmentosum. Arch Dermatol Syph 68:355–358, 1953

Ectodermal Dysplasia

DOMINOK GW, RÖNISCH P: Histologische Hautbefunde bei ektodermaler Dysplasie vom anhidrotischen Typ. Dermatol Wochenschr 154:774–778, 1968

MALAGON V, TAVERAS JE: Congenital anhidrotic ectodermal and mesodermal dysplasia. Arch Dermatol 74:253–258, 1956

MARTIN-PASCUAL A, DE UNAMUNO P, APARICIO M et al: Anhidrotic (or hypohidrotic) ectodermal dysplasia. Dermatologica 154:235–243, 1977

MCNAUGHTON PZ, PIERSON DL, RODMAN RG: Hidrotic ectodermal dysplasia in a black mother and daughter. Arch Dermatol 112:1448–1450, 1976

PIERARD GE, VAN NESTE D, LETOT B: Hidrotic ectodermal dysplasia. Dermatologica 158:168–174, 1979

REED WB, LOPEX DA, LANDING B: Clinical spectrum of anhidrotic ectodermal dysplasia. Arch Dermatol 102:134–143, 1970

SUNDERMAN FW: Persons lacking sweat glands. Arch Intern Med 67:846–854, 1941

UPSHAW BY, MONTGOMERY H: Hereditary anhidrotic ectodermal dysplasia. Arch Dermatol Syph 60:1170–1183, 1949

Focal Dermal Hypoplasia Syndrome

GOLTZ RW, HENDERSON RR, HITCH JM et al: Focal dermal hypoplasia syndrome. Arch Dermatol 101:1–11, 1970

GOTTLIEB SK, FISHER BK, VIOLIN GA: Focal dermal hypoplasia. Arch Dermatol 108:551–553, 1973

HAPPLE R, LENZ W: Striation of bone in focal dermal hypoplasia: Manifestation of functional mosaicism. Br J Dermatol 96:133–138, 1977

HOWELL JB: Nevus angiolipomatosus versus focal dermal hypoplasia. Arch Dermatol 92:238–248, 1965

HOWELL JB, REYNOLDS J: Osteopathia striata. Trans St John's Hosp Dermatol Soc 60:178–182, 1974

LEVER WF: Hypoplasia cutis congenita. (Case presentation) Arch Dermatol 90:340, 1964

Aplasia Cutis Congenita

DEEKEN JH, CAPLAN RM: Aplasia cutis congenita. Arch Dermatol 102:386–389, 1970

HARARI Z, PUSMANIK A, DVORETSKY I et al: Aplasia cutis congenita with dystrophic nail changes. Dermatologica 153:363–368, 1976

LEVIN DL, NOLAN KS, ESTERLY NB: Congenital absence of skin. J Am Acad Dermatol 2:203–206, 1980

Poikiloderma Congenitale
(Rothmund–Thomson Syndrome)

ROOK A, DAVIS R, STEVANOVIC D: Poikiloderma congenitale: Rothmund-Thomson syndrome. (Review) Acta Derm Venereol (Stockh) 39:392–420, 1959

THANNHAUSER SJ: Werner's syndrome (progeria of the adult) and Rothmund's syndrome: Two types of closely related heredofamilial atrophic dermatoses with juvenile cataracts and endocrine features. Ann Intern Med 23:559–626, 1945

TRITSCH H, LISCHKA G: Zur Histopathologie der kongenitalen Poikilodermie Thomson. Z Hautkr 43:(155–166), 1968

Bloom's Syndrome (Congenital Telangiectatic Erythema)

BLOOM D, GERMAN J: The syndrome of congenital telangiectatic erythema and stunted growth. Arch Dermatol 103:545–546, 1971

BRAUN-FALCO O, MARGHESCU S: Kongenitales telangiektatisches Erythem (Bloom-Syndrom) mit Diabetes insipidus. Hautarzt 17:155–161, 1966

DICKEN CH, DEWALD G, GORDON H: Sister chromatid exchanges in Bloom's syndrome. Arch Dermatol 114:755–760, 1978

KATZENELLENBOGEN I, LARON Z: A contribution to Bloom's syndrome. Arch Dermatol 82:609–616, 1960

LANDAU IW, SASAKI MS, NEWCOMER VD et al: Bloom's syndrome. Arch Dermatol 94:687–694, 1966

SAWITSKY A, BLOOM D, GERMAN J: Chromosomal breakage and acute leukemia in congenital telangiectatic erythema and stunted growth. Ann Intern Med 65:487–495, 1966

Ataxia–Telangiectasia

GSCHNAIT F, GRABNER G, BRENNER W et al: Ataxia teleangiectatica (Louis-Bar-Syndrom). Hautarzt 30:527–531, 1979

MCFARLIN DE, STROBER W, WALDMANN TA: Ataxia–telangiectasia. (Review) Medicine (Baltimore) 51:281–314, 1972

ROSEN FS: The primary immunodeficiencies: Dermatologic manifestations. J Invest Dermatol 67:402–411, 1976

Progeria of the Adult (Werner's Syndrome)

EPSTEIN CJ, MARTIN GM, SCHULTZ AL et al: Werner's syndrome. (Review) Medicine (Baltimore) 45:177–221, 1966

TRITSCH H, LISCHKA, G: Werner Syndrom, kombiniert mit Pseudo-Klinefelter-Syndrom. Hautarzt 19:547–551, 1968

Epidermolysis Bullosa

ANTON-LAMPRECHT I: Electron microscopy in the early diagnosis of genetic disorders of the skin. Dermatologica 157:65–85, 1978

ANTON-LAMPRECHT I, SCHNYDER UW: Zur Ultrastruktur der Epidermolysen mit junktionaler Blasenbildung. Dermatologica 159:377–382, 1979

BAUER EA, UITTO J: Collagen in cutaneous diseases. Int J Dermatol 18:251–270, 1979

BERGENHOLTZ A, OLSSON O: Die Epidermolysis bullosa hereditaria dystrophica mit Oesophagusveränderungen. Arch Klin Exp Dermatol 217:518–533, 1963

BRIGGAMAN RA, WHEELER CE, JR.: Epidermolysis bullosa dystrophica-recessive: A possible role of anchoring fibrils in the pathogenesis. J Invest Dermatol 65:203–211, 1975

DAHL MGC: Epidermolysis bullosa acquisita: A sign of cicatricial pemphigoid. Br J Dermatol 101:475–484, 1979

GEDDE-DAHL T, JR.: Epidermolysis Bullosa: A Clinical, Genetic and Epidemiological Study. Baltimore, Johns Hopkins Press, 1971

GIBBS RB, MINUS HR: Epidermolysis bullosa acquisita with electron microscopic studies. Arch Dermatol 111:215–220, 1975

HANEKE E, ANTON-LAMPRECHT I: Ultrastructure of blister formation in epidermolysis bullosa hereditaria. V. Epidermolysis bullosa simplex localisata Type Weber-Cockayne. J Invest Dermatol 78:219–223, 1982

HASHIMOTO I, ANTON-LAMPRECHT I, GEDDE-DAHL T, JR. et al: Ultrastructural studies in epidermolysis bullosa hereditaria. I. Dominant-dystrophic type of Pasini. Arch Dermatol Forsch 252:167–178, 1975

HASHIMOTO I, SCHNYDER UW, ANTON-LAMPRECHT I et al: Ultrastructural studies in epidermolysis bullosa hereditaria. III. Recessive dystrophic types with dermolytic blisters (Hallopeau-Siemens types and inverse type). Arch Dermatol Res 256:137–150, 1976

HINTNER H, STINGL G, SCHULER G et al: Immunofluorescence mapping of antigen determinants within the dermal–epidermal junction in mechanobullous diseases. J Invest Dermatol 76:113–118, 1981

HINTNER H, WOLFF K: Generalized atrophic benign epidermolysis bullosa. Arch Dermatol 118:375–384, 1982

LIVDEN JK, NILSEN R, THUNOLD S et al: Epidermolysis bullosa acquisita with Crohn's disease. Acta Derm Venereol (Stockh) 58:241–244, 1978

LOWE LB: Hereditary epidermolysis bullosa. Arch Dermatol 95:587–595, 1967

METZ J, FRANK H, METZ G: Zur Pathogenese der Blasenbildung bei Epidermolysis bullosa acquisita und Epidermolysis bullosa dystrophica. Arch Dermatol Forsch 254:103–112, 1975

NIEBOER C, BOORSMA DM, WOERDEMAN MJ et al: Epidermolysis bullosa acquisita. Br J Dermatol 102:383–392, 1980

PEARSON RW: Studies on the pathogenesis of epidermolysis bullosa. J Invest Dermatol 39:551–575, 1962

PEARSON RW: The mechanobullous diseases. In Fitzpatrick TB, Arndt KA, Clark WH Jr et al (eds): Dermatology in General Medicine, pp 621–643. New York, McGraw-Hill, 1971

PEARSON RW, POTTER B, STRAUSS F: Epidermolysis bullosa hereditaria letalis. Arch Dermatol 109:349–355, 1974

REED WB, COLLEGE, J, JR., FRANCIS MJO et al: Epidermolysis bullosa dystrophica with epidermal neoplasms. Arch Dermatol 110:894–902, 1974

RICHTER BJ, MCNUTT NS: The spectrum of epidermolysis bullosa acquisita. Arch Dermatol 115:1325–1328, 1979

ROENIGK HM, JR., RYAN JG, BERGFELD WF: Epidermolysis bullosa acquisita. Arch Dermatol 103:1–10, 1971

SCHACHNER L, LAZARUS GS, DEMBITZER H: Epidermolysis bullosa hereditaria letalis. Br J Dermatol 96:51–58, 1977

SCHNYDER UW, ANTON-LAMPRECHT I: Zur Klinik der Epidermolysen mit junktionaler Blasenbildung. Dermatologica 159:402–406, 1979

STEVANOVIC P, LALEVIC B, JOVOVIC D et al: La forme inverse de l'épidermolyse bulleuse polydysplasique (Gedde-Dahl). Ann Dermatol Venereol 106:65–67, 1979

TURNER TW: Two cases of junctional epidermolysis bullosa (Herlitz-Pearson). Br J Dermatol 102:97–107, 1980

YAOITA H, BRIGGAMAN RA, LAWLEY TJ et al: Epidermolysis bullosa acquisita: Ultrastructural and immunological studies. J Invest Dermatol 76:288–292, 1981

Keratosis Follicularis (Darier's Disease)

ACKERMAN AB: Focal acantholytic dyskeratosis. Arch Dermatol 106:702–706, 1972

BEERMAN H: Hypertrophic Darier's disease and nevus syringocystadenomatosus papilliferus. Arch Dermatol Syph 60:500–527, 1949

BIAGINI G, COSTA AM, LASCHI R: An electron microscope study of Darier's disease. J Cutan Pathol 2:47–49, 1975

BINNICK SA, FLEISCHMAJER R: Unilateral keratosis follicularis. Arch Dermatol 113:1459–1460, 1977

CARAPETO FJ, ARMIJO M: Maladie de Darier à minimes lésions ou variété Darier-like de la maladie de Grover. Ann Dermatol Venereol 106:279–282, 1979

CAULFIELD JB, WILGRAM GF: An electronmicroscope study of dyskeratosis and acantholysis in Darier's disease. J Invest Dermatol 41:57–65, 1963

DELACRÉTAZ J, CHRISTELER A: Dyskératose acantholytique régionale. Dermatologica 163:113–116, 1981

DEMETREE JW, LANG PG, ST CLAIR JT: Unilateral, linear, zosteriform epidermal nevus with acantholytic dyskeratosis. Arch Dermatol 115:875–877, 1979

FISHMAN HC: Acute, eruptive Darier disease (keratosis follicularis). Arch Dermatol 111:221–222, 1975

GISSLÉN H, MOBACKEN H: Acute adult-onset Darier-like dermatosis. Br J Dermatol 98:217–220, 1978

GOTTLIEB SK, LUTZNER MA: Darier's disease. Arch Dermatol 107:225–230, 1973

JABLONSKA S, CHORZELSKI T: Zur Klassifikation des Pemphigus Hailey-Hailey. Dermatologica 117:24–38, 1958

KELLUM RE, HASERICK JR: Localized linear keratosis follicularis. Arch Dermatol 86:450–454, 1962

KRINITZ K: Tumoröse Veränderungen bei Morbus Darier. Hautarzt 17:445–450, 1966

LEEMING JAL: Acquired linear naevus showing histological features of keratosis follicularis. Br J Dermatol 81:128–131, 1969

MANN PR, HAYE KR: An electron microscope study on the acantholytic and dyskeratotic processes in Darier's disease. Br J Dermatol 82:561–566, 1970

PANJA RK: Acrokeratosis verruciformis (Hopf): A clinical entity? Br J Dermatol 96:643–652, 1977

PECK GL, KRAEMER KH, WETZEL B et al: Cornifying Darier disease: A unique variant. Arch Dermatol 112:495–503, 1976

PIÉRARD J, GEERTS ML, VANDEPUTTE H et al: A propos de quelques cas de dyskératose folliculaire. Arch Belges Dermatol 24:381–397, 1968

PIÉRARD J, KINT A: Die Dariersche Krankheit. Arch Klin Exp Dermatol 231:382–397, 1968

SATO A, ANTON-LAMPRECHT J, SCHNYDER UW: Ultrastructure of dyskeratosis in Morbus Darier. J Cutan Pathol 4:173–184, 1977

STARINK TM, WOERDEMAN MJ: Unilateral systematized keratosis follicularis: A variant of Darier's disease or an epidermal nevus (acantholytic dyskeratotic epidermal nevus)? Br J Dermatol 105:207–214, 1981

WEATHERS DR, OLANSKY S, SHARPE LO: Darier's disease with mucous membrane involvement. Arch Dermatol 100:50–53, 1969

Familial Benign Pemphigus (Hailey–Hailey Disease)

BOTVINICK I: Familial benign pemphigus with oral mucous membrane lesions. Cutis 12:371–373, 1973

BRAUN-FALCO O, VOGELL W: Elektronenmikroskopische Untersuchungen zur Dynamik der Acantholyse bei Pemphigus vulgaris. Arch Klin Exp Dermatol 223:328–346, 1965

DE DOBBELEER G, ACHTEN G: Disrupted desmosomes in induced lesions of familial benign chronic pemphigus. J Cutan Pathol 6:418–424, 1979

ELLIS FA: Vesicular Darier's disease (so-called benign familial pemphigus). Arch Dermatol Syph 61:715–736, 1950

FINNERUD CW, SZYMANSKI FJ: Chronic benign familial pemphigus: A possible vesicular variant of keratosis follicularis. Arch Dermatol Syph 61:737–749, 1950

GANOR S, SAGHER F: Keratosis follicularis (Darier) and familial benign chronic pemphigus (Hailey–Hailey) in the same patient. Br J Dermatol 77:24–29, 1965

GOTTLIEB SK, LUTZNER MA: Hailey–Hailey disease: An electron microscopic study. J Invest Dermatol 54:368–376, 1970

HABER H, RUSSELL B: Sisters with familial benign chronic pemphigus (Gougerot, Hailey and Hailey). Br J Dermatol 62:458–460, 1950

HEINZE R: Pemphigus chronicus benignus familiaris (Gougerot-Hailey-Hailey) mit Schleimhautbeteiligung bei einer Diabetikerin. Dermatol Monatsschr 165:862–867, 1979

HERZBERG JJ: Pemphigus Gougerot/Hailey–Hailey. Arch Klin Exp Dermatol, 202:21–44, 1971

KAHN D, HUTCHINSON E: Esophageal involvement in familial benign chronic pemphigus. Arch Dermatol 109:718–719, 1974

LACHAPELLE JM, DE LA BRASSINNE M, GEERTS ML: Maladies de Darier et de Hailey–Hailey: Etude comparative de l'incorporation de thymidine tritiée dans les cellules épidermiques. Arch Belges Dermatol 29:241–245, 1973

NICOLIS G, TOSCA A, MAROULI O et al: Keratosis follicularis and familial benign chronic pemphigus in the same patient. Dermatologica 159:346–351, 1979

NIORDSON AM, SYLVEST B: Bullous dyskeratosis follicularis and acrokeratosis verruciformis. Arch Dermatol 92:166–168, 1965

NÜRNBERGER F, MÜLLER G: Elektronenmikroskopische Untersuchungen über die Akantholyse bei Pemphigus familiaris benignus. Arch Klin Exp Dermatol 228:208–219, 1967

PALMER DD, PERRY HO: Benign familial chronic pemphigus. Arch Dermatol 86:493–502, 1962

PIÉRARD J, KINT A: Pemphigus familial bénin chronique (maladie de Hailey–Hailey). Dermatologica 139:1–17, 1969

RAASCHOU-NIELSEN W, REYMANN F: Familial benign chronic pemphigus. Acta Derm Venereol (Stockh) 39:280–291, 1959

SCHNEIDER W, FISCHER H, WIEHL R: Zur Frage der Schleimhautbeteiligung beim Pemphigus benignus familiaris chronicus. Arch Klin Exp Dermatol 225:74–81, 1966

THIES W, MERKER HJ, FASSBINDER K: Zur Kasuistik des Pemphigus chronicus benignus (Hailey–Hailey) unter Berücksichtigung elektronenmikroskopischer Befunde. Hautarzt 23:244–251, 1972

WILGRAM GF, CAULFIELD JB, LEVER WF: An electron microscopic study of acantholysis and dyskeratosis in Hailey and Hailey's disease. J Invest Dermatol 39:373–381, 1962

WINER LH, LEEB AJ: Benign familial pemphigus. Arch Dermatol 67:77–83, 1953

Acrokeratosis Verruciformis of Hopf

BEERMAN H: in discussion of Waisman M: Verruciform manifestations of keratosis follicularis. Arch Dermatol 81:1–14, 1960

HERNDON JH, JR., WILSON JD: Acrokeratosis verruciformis (Hopf) and Darier's disease. Arch Dermatol 93:305–310, 1966

JORDAN P, SPIER HW: Morbus Darier-Veränderungen als Späterscheinungen bei Akrokeratosis verruciformis. Arch Dermatol Syph (Berlin) 189:441–442, 1949

KRAUSE W, EHLERS G: Uber die Beziehung zwischen Akrokera-tosis verruciformis Hopf und Dyskeratosis follicularis vegetans Darier. Hautarzt 20:297–403, 1949

NIEDELMAN ML, MCKUSICK VA: Acrokeratosis verruciformis (Hopf). Arch Dermatol 86:779–782, 1962

PANJA RK: Acrokeratosis verruciformis (Hopf): A clinical entity? Br J Dermatol 96:643–652, 1977

PENROD JN, EVERETT MA, MCCREIGHT WG: Observations on keratosis follicularis. Arch Dermatol 82:367–370, 1960

SCHUELLER WA: Acrokeratosis verruciformis of Hopf. Arch Dermatol 106:81–83, 1972

WAISMAN M: Verruciform manifestations of keratosis follicularis. Arch Dermatol 81:1–14, 1960

Pseudoxanthoma Elasticum

AKHTAR M, BRODY H: Elastic tissue in pseudoxanthoma elasticum: Ultrastructural study of endocardial lesions. Arch Pathol 99:667–671, 1975

CARO I, SHER A, RIPPEY JJ: Pseudoxanthoma elasticum and elastosis perforans serpiginosum. Dermatologica 150:36–42, 1975

DANIELSEN L, KOBAYASI T, LARSEN HW et al: Pseudoxanthoma elasticum. Acta Derm Venereol (Stockh) 50:355–373, 1970

EDDY DD, FARBER EM: Pseudoxanthoma elasticum. Arch Dermatol 86:729–740, 1962

FLATLEY FJ, ATWELL ME, MCEVOY RK: Pseudoxanthoma elasticum with gastric hemorrhage. Arch Intern Med 112:352–356, 1963

GOODMAN RM, SMITH EW, PATON D et al: Pseudoxanthoma elasticum: A clinical and histopathological study. (Review) Medicine (Baltimore) 42:297–334, 1963

HASHIMOTO K, DIBELLA RJ: Electron microscopic studies of normal and abnormal elastic fibers of the skin. J Invest Dermatol 48:405–423, 1967

HUANG SN, STEELE HD, KUMAR G et al: Ultrastructural changes of elastic fibers in pseudoxanthoma elasticum. Arch Pathol 83:108–113, 1967

KREYSEL HW, LERCHE W, JÄNNER M: Beobachtungen zum Grönblad-Strandberg-Syndrom (Angioid streaks, Pseudoxanthoma elasticum). Hautarzt 18:24–28, 1967

MARTINEZ-HERNANDEZ A, HUFFER WE: Pseudoxanthoma elasticum: Dermal polyanions and the mineralization of elastic fibers. Lab Invest 31:181–186, 1974

MCKEE PH, CAMERON CHS, ARCHER DB et al: A study of four cases of pseudoxanthoma elasticum. J Cutan Pathol 4:146–153, 1977

MENDELSOHN G, BULKLEY BH, HUTCHINS GM: Cardiovascular manifestations of pseudoxanthoma elasticum. Arch Pathol 102:298–302, 1978

POPE FM: Two types of autosomal recessive pseudoxanthoma elasticum. Arch Dermatol 110:209–212, 1974

POPE FM: Historical evidence for the genetic heterogeneity of pseudoxanthoma elasticum. Br J Dermatol 92:493–509, 1975

SAITO Y, KLINGMÜLLER G: Elektronenmikroskopische Untersuchungen zur Morphogenese elastischer Fasern bei der senilen Elastose und dem Pseudoxanthoma elasticum. Arch Dermatol Res 260:179–191, 1977

SCHUTT D: Pseudoxanthoma elasticum and elastosis perforans serpiginosa. Arch Dermatol 91:151–152, 1965

Connective Tissue Nevus

DANIELSEN L, KOBAYASI T, JACOBSEN GK: Ultrastructural changes in disseminated connective tissue nevi. Acta Derm Venereol (Stockh) 57:93–101, 1977

KOBAYASI T, WOLF-JÜRGENSEN P, DANIELSEN L: Ultrastructure of shagreen patch. Acta Derm Venereol (Stockh) 53:275–278, 1973

MORRISON JGL, WILSON JONES E, MACDONALD DM: Juvenile elastoma (the Buschke-Ollendorff syndrome). Br J Dermatol 97:417–422, 1977

RAQUE CJ, WOOD MG: Connective-tissue nevus. Arch Dermatol 102:390–396, 1970

SCHORR WF, OPITZ JM, REYES CN: The connective tissue nevus–osteopoikilosis syndrome. Arch Dermatol 106:208–214, 1972

SMITH AD, WAISMAN M: Connective tissue nevi. Arch Dermatol 81:249–252, 1960

STARICCO RG, MEHREGAN AH: Nevus elasticus and nevus elasticus vascularis. Arch Dermatol 84:943–947, 1961

UITTO J, SANTA-CRUZ J, EISEN AZ: Famial cutaneous collagenoma: Genetic studies on a family. Br J Dermatol 101:185–195, 1979

VERBOV J: Buschke-Ollendorff syndrome (disseminated dermatofibrosis with osteopoikilosis). Br J Dermatol 96:87–90, 1977

Linear Melorheostotic Scleroderma

MIYACHI Y, HORIO T, YAMADA A et al: Linear melorheostotic scleroderma with hypertrichosis. Arch Dermatol 115:1233–1234, 1979

WAGERS LT, YOUNG AW, JR., RYAN SF: Linear melorheostotic scleroderma. Br J Dermatol 86:297–301, 1972

Winchester Syndrome

COHEN AH, HOLLISTER DW, REED WB: The skin in the Winchester syndrome. Arch Dermatol 111:230–236, 1975

NABAI H, MEHREGAN AH, MORTEZAI A et al: Winchester syndrome: Report of a case from Iran. J Cutan Pathol 4:281–285, 1977

Ehlers–Danlos Syndrome

ARNESON MA, HAMMERSCHMIDT DE, FURCHT LT et al: A new form of Ehlers–Danlos syndrome. JAMA 244:144–147, 1980

BLACK CM, GATHERCOLE LJ, BAILEY AJ et al: The Ehlers–Danlos syndrome: An analysis of the structure of the collagen fibres of the skin. Br J Dermatol 102:85–96, 1980

CULLIN SI: Localized Ehlers–Danlos syndrome. Arch Dermatol 115:332–333, 1979

JANSEN LH: The structure of the connective tissue: An explanation of the symptoms of the Ehlers–Danlos syndrome. Dermatologica 110:108–120, 1955

MCFARLAND W, FULLER DE: Mortality in Ehlers–Danlos syndrome due to spontaneous rupture of large arteries. N Engl J Med 271:1309–1310, 1964

NELSON DL, KING RA: Ehlers–Danlos syndrome type VIII. J Am Acad Dermatol 5:297–303, 1981

PINNELL SR, KRANE SM, KENZORA JE et al: A heritable disorder of connective tissue. N Engl J Med 286:1013–1020, 1972

PROCKOP DJ, KIVIRIKKO KI, TUDERMAN L et al: The biosynthesis of collagen and its disorders. N Engl J Med 301:77–85, 1979

RONCHESE F: Dermatorrhexis. Am J Dis Child 51:1403–1412, 1936.

SCARPELLI DG, GOODMAN RM: Observations on the fine structure of the fibroblast from a case of Ehlers–Danlos syndrome with the Marfan syndrome. J Invest Dermatol 50:214–219, 1968

SEVENICH M, SCHULTZ-EHRENBURG U, ORFANOS CE: Ehlers–Danlos Syndrom: Eine Fibroblasten- und Kollagenkrankheit. Arch Dermatol Res 267:237–251, 1980

SULICA VI, COOPER PH, POPE FM et al: Cutaneous histologic features in Ehlers–Danlos syndrome. Arch Dermatol 115:40–42, 1979

UITTO J, LICHTENSTEIN JR: Defects in the biochemistry of collagen in diseases of connective tissue. (Review) J Invest Dermatol 66:59–79, 1976

WECHSLER HL, FISHER ER: Ehlers–Danlos syndrome. Arch Pathol 77:613–619, 1964

Cutis Laxa (Dermatochalasis)

GOLTZ RW, HULT AM, GOLDFARB M et al: Cutis laxa. Arch Dermatol 92:373–387, 1965

HARRIS RB, HEAPY MR, PERRY HO: Generalized elastolysis (cutis laxa). Am J Med 65:815–822, 1979

HASHIMOTO K, KANZAKI T: Cutis laxa. Arch Dermatol 111:861–873, 1975

JABLONSKA S: Inflammatorische Hautveränderungen, die einer erworbenen Cutis laxa vorausgehen. Hautarzt 17:341–346, 1966

KERL H, BURG G: Erworbene (postinflammatorische) Dermatochalasis. Hautarzt 26:191–196, 1975

MEHREGAN AH, LEE SC, NABAI H: Cutis laxa (generalized elastolysis). J Cutan Pathol 5:116–126, 1978

NANKO H, JEPSEN LV, ZACHARIAE H et al: Acquired cutis laxa (generalized elastolysis). Acta Derm Venereol (Stockh) 59:315–324, 1979

REED WB, HOROWITZ RE, BEIGHTON P: Acquired cutis laxa. Arch Dermatol 103:661–669, 1971

SAYERS CP, GOLTZ RW, MOTTAZ J: Pulmonary elastic tissue in generalized elastolysis (cutis laxa) and Marfan's syndrome. J Invest Dermatol 65:451–457, 1975

SCOTT MA, KAUH YC, LUSCOMBE HA: Acquired cutis laxa associated with multiple myeloma. Arch Dermatol 112:853–855, 1976

SCHREIBER MM, TILLEY JC: Cutis laxa. Arch Dermatol 84:266–272, 1961

Pachydermoperiostosis

CURTH HO, FIRSCHEIN IL, ALPERT M: Familial clubbed fingers. Arch Dermatol 83:828–836, 1961

HAMBRICK GW, CARTER DM: Pachydermoperiostosis. Arch Dermatol 94:594–608, 1966

RIMOIN DL: Pachydermoperiostosis (idiopathic clubbing and periostosis). N Engl J Med 272:923–931, 1965

Urticaria Pigmentosa

ALLISON J: Skin mastocytosis presenting as a neonatal bullous eruption. Aust J Dermatol 9:83–85, 1967

BARAF CS, SHAPIRO L: Solitary mastocytoma. Arch Dermatol 99:589–590, 1969

BAZEX A, DUPRÉ A, CHRISTOL B et al: Les mastocytoses familiales. Ann Dermatol Syph 98:241–260, 1971

BRAUN-FALCO O, JUNG J: Über klinische und experimentelle Beobachtungen bei einem Fall von diffuser Haut-Mastocytose. Arch Klin Exp Dermatol 213:639–650, 1961

BRINKMANN E: Mastzellenreticulose (Gewebsbasophiliom) mit histaminbedingtem Flush und Übergang in Gewebsbasophilen-Leukämie. Schweiz Med Wochenschr 89:1046–1048, 1959

BURGOON CF, GRAHAM JH, MCCAFFREE DL: Mast cell disease. Arch Dermatol 98:590–605, 1968

CAPLAN RM: The natural course of urticaria pigmentosa. Arch Dermatol 87:146–157, 1963

CRAMER HJ: Telangiectasia macularis eruptiva perstans, eine Sonderform der Urticaria pigmentosa. Hautarzt 15:370–374, 1964

DAVIS MJ, LAWLER JC, HIGDON RS: Studies on an adult with urticaria pigmentosa. Arch Dermatol 77:224–226, 1958

DEGOS R: Mastocytoses en dehors de l'urticaire pigmentaire, reticuloses mastocytaires diffuses. Arch Belg Derm Syph 11:10–22, 1955

DEWAR WA, MILNE JA: Bullous urticaria pigmentosa. Arch Dermatol 71:717–721, 1955

DRENNAN JM: The mast cells in urticaria pigmentosa. J Pathol Bacteriol 63:513–520, 1951

EFRATI P, KLAJMAN A, SPITZ H: Mast cell leukemia? Malignant mastocytosis with leukemia-like manifestations. Blood 12:869–888, 1957

ELLIS JM: Urticaria pigmentosa. Arch Pathol 48:426–435, 1949

FREEMAN RG: Diffuse urticaria pigmentosa. Am J Clin Pathol 48:187–199, 1967

FRIEDMAN BI, WILL JJ, FREIMAN DG et al: Tissue mast cell leukemia. Blood 13:70–75, 1958

HASHIMOTO K, GROSS BG, LEVER WF: An electron microscopic study of the degranulation of mast cell granules in urticaria pigmentosa. J Invest Dermatol 46:139–149, 1966

JOHNSON WC, HELWIG EB: Solitary mastocytosis (urticaria pigmentosa). Arch Dermatol 84:806–815, 1961

KLAUS SN, WINKELMANN RK: Course of urticaria pigmentosa in children. Arch Dermatol 86:68–71, 1962

KLAUS SN, WINKELMANN RK: The clinical spectrum of urticaria pigmentosa. Mayo Clin Proc 40:923–931, 1965

MIHM MC, CLARK WH, REED RJ et al: Mast cell infiltrates of the skin and the mastocytosis syndrome. Hum Pathol 4:231–239, 1973

MIKHAIL GR, MILLER-MILINSKA A: Mast cell population in human skin. J Invest Dermatol 43:249–254, 1964

MILLER RO, SHAPIRO L: Bullous urticaria pigmentosa in infancy. Arch Dermatol 91:595–598, 1965

MONHEIT GD, MURAD T, CONRAD M: Systemic mastocytosis and the mastocytosis syndrome. J Cutan Pathol 6:42–52, 1979

MUTTER RD, TANNENBAUM M, ULTMAN JE: Systemic mast cell disease. (Review) Ann Intern Med 57:887–904, 1963

NAVEH Y, LUDATSCHER R, GELLEI B et al: Ultrastructural features of mast cells in systemic mastocytosis. Acta Derm Venereol (Stockh) 55:443–450, 1970

OKUN MR, BHAWAN J: Combined melanocytoma-mastocytoma in a case of nodular mastocytosis. J Am Acad Dermatol 1:338–347, 1979

ORKIN M, GOOD RA, CLAWSON CC et al: Bullous mastocytosis. Arch Dermatol 101:547–564, 1970

ROBERTS PL, MCDONALD HB, WELLS RF: Systemic mast cell disease in a patient with unusual gastrointestinal and pulmonary abnormalities. Am J Med 45:638–644, 1968

ROBINSON HM, JR., KILE RL, HITCH JM et al: Bullous urticaria pigmentosa. Arch Dermatol 85:346–357, 1962

RODERMUND OR, KLINGMÜLLER G, ROHNER HG: Interne Befunde bei Mastozytose. Hautarzt 31:175–178, 1980

SHAW JM: Genetic aspects of urticaria pigmentosa. Arch Dermatol 97:137–138, 1968

SOSTRE S, HANDLER HL: Bony lesions in systemic mastocytosis. Arch Dermatol 113:1245–1247, 1977

WATERS WJ, LACSON PS: Mast cell leukemia presenting as urticaria pigmentosa. Pediatrics 19:1033–1042, 1957

YASUDA T, KUKITA A: A fatal case of purely cutaneous form of diffuse mastocytosis. Proc XII Int Cong Dermatol, Vol 2:1558–1561. Washington, DC, 1962

Incontinentia Pigmenti

CAPUTO R, GIANOTTI F, INNOCENTI M: Ultrastructural findings in incontinentia pigmenti. Int J Dermatol 14:46–55, 1975

CARNEY RG, JR.: Incontinentia pigmenti: A world statistical analysis. Arch Dermatol 112:535–542, 1976

DOORNINK FJ: Über Incontinentia pigmenti und über die Siemens-Bloch'sche Pigmentdermatose. Dermatologica 102:63–72, 1951

EPSTEIN S, VEDDER JS, PINKUS H: Bullous variety of incontinentia pigmenti (Bloch-Sulzberger). Arch Dermatol Syph 65:557–567, 1952

GORDON H, GORDON W: Incontinentia pigmenti: Clinical and genetical studies of two familial cases. Dermatologica 140:150–168, 1961

GUERRIER LJW, WONG CK: Ultrastructural evolution of the skin in incontinentia pigmenti (Bloch-Sulzberger). Dermatologica 149:10–22, 1974

LENZ W: Zur Genetik der Incontinentia pigmenti. Ann Paediatr 196:149–165, 1961

RUBIN L, BECKER SW, JR.: Pigmentation in the Bloch-Sulzberger syndrome (incontinentia pigmenti). Arch Dermatol 74:263–268, 1956

SCHAUMBURG-LEVER G, LEVER WF: Electron microscopy of incontinentia pigmenti. J Invest Dermatol 61:151–158, 1973

SULZBERGER MB: Incontinentia pigmenti (Bloch-Sulzberger). Arch Dermatol Syph 38:57–69, 1938

VILANOVA X, AGUADE JP: Incontinentia pigmenti. Ann Dermatol Syph 86:247–258, 1959

WODNIANSKY P: Das Syndrom der Incontinentia pigmenti. Arch Klin Exp Dermatol 201:49–72, 1955

Hypomelanosis of Ito

GROSSHANS EM, STOEBNER P, BERGOEND H et al: Incontinentia pigmenti achromians (Ito). Dermatologica 142:65–78, 1971

MOROHASHI M, HASHIMOTO K, GOODMAN TF, JR. et al: Ultrastructural studies of vitiligo, Vogt-Koyanagi syndrome, and incontinentia pigmenti achromians. Arch Dermatol 113:755–766, 1977

NORDLUND JJ, KLAUS SN, GINO J: Hypomelanosis of Ito. Acta Derm Venereol (Stockh) 57:261–264, 1977

Noninfectious Vesicular and Bullous Diseases

CLASSIFICATION OF BLISTERS

Before discussing individual vesicular and bullous diseases, it seems appropriate to present a classification of the different types of vesicles and bullae and to outline briefly their mode of formation. (Since, from a histologic or histogenetic point of view, it is immaterial whether a lesion is a vesicle or a bulla, only the term *blister* will be used in the classification.)

Seven types of blisters can be recognized (Table 7-1):

Subcorneal blister, in which detachment of the horny layer occurs (for a detailed description, see p. 126).

Blister due to intracellular degeneration, in which pronounced intracellular degeneration leads to intraepidermal bulla formation below the granular layer (for detailed descriptions, see pp. 58 and 128).

Spongiotic blister. Intercellular edema (spongiosis), an early and characteristic feature of this type of bulla, is accompanied by intracellular edema and a mononuclear cell infiltrate extending from the upper dermis into the epidermis (exocytosis). Pronounced intercellular edema stretches the intercellular bridges (desmosomes) until they disappear, and pronounced intracellular edema leads to reticular degeneration of the epidermis. (For a detailed description, see p. 94.)

Acantholytic blister. As a result of dissolution of the intercellular cement substance, including the intradesmosomal substance, epidermal cells lose their coherence, leading to rifts between them that can enlarge into bullae. Detached (acantholytic) cells are present in the bulla cavity. Acantholysis takes place predominantly in the suprabasal region in some diseases and predominantly in the subcorneal region in others (see Table 7-1). (For detailed descriptions, see pp. 72 and 105–112.)

Viral blister. Invasion of epidermal cells by certain viruses causes two types of degenerative changes in epidermal cells: ballooning and reticular degeneration. Ballooning degeneration leads to extensive secondary acantholysis affecting even the basal layer. (For a detailed description, see p. 362.)

Blister due to degeneration of basal cells. Degenerative changes in basal cells lead to the formation of subepidermal bullae in several diseases (see Table 7-1). (For a detailed description, see pp. 153 and 448.)

Blister due to degeneration of the basement membrane zone. Degenerative changes in one or several of the structures causing coherence of the basal cells with the dermis lead to the formation of subepidermal bullae. On light microscopic examination, splitting, thinning, or absence of the periodic acid-Schiff (PAS)-positive basement membrane zone may be seen. (For detailed descriptions, see pp. 113 and 119.)

On *electron microscopic examination,* the primary damage in blisters, due to degeneration of the basement membrane zone, is seen in some diseases primarily on the half-desmosomes and in the lamina lucida, as in epi-

Table 7-1. Classification of Blisters

Type of Blister	Mode of Formation	Site of Formation	Disease
Subcorneal blister	Detachment of horny layer	Subcorneal	Miliaria crystallina Erythema toxicum neonatorum Subcorneal pustular dermatosis Impetigo
Blister due to intracellular degeneration	Separation of cells from one another	Upper epidermis	Epidermolytic hyperkeratosis Erythema multiforme, epidermal type Friction blisters
Spongiotic blister	Intercellular edema	Intraepidermal	Dermatitis (eczema) Incontinentia pigmenti Miliaria rubra
Acantholytic blister	Dissolution of intercellular cement substance	Intraepidermal (1) Suprabasal (2) Subcorneal	 Pemphigus vulgaris Familial benign pemphigus Darier's disease Transient acantholytic dermatosis Pemphigus foliaceus
Viral blister	Ballooning degeneration leading to acantholysis	Intraepidermal	Variola Herpes simplex Varicella–herpes zoster
Blister due to degeneration of basal cells	Damaged basal cells lose contact with dermis	Subepidermal	Epidermolysis bullosa, epidermal types Lichen planus Lichen sclerosus et atrophicus Lupus erythematosus
Blister due to degeneration of basement membrane zone	Damage in the structures causing coherence of basal cells with dermis	Subepidermal	Epidermolysis bullosa, junctional and dystrophic types Urticaria pigmentosa Bullous pemphigoid Cicatricial pemphigoid Herpes gestationis Dermatitis herpetiformis Erythema multiforme, dermal type Porphyria cutanea tarda

dermolysis bullosa letalis, bullous pemphigoid, cicatricial pemphigoid, herpes gestationis, and exceptional cases of dermatitis herpetiformis. In other diseases, the primary damage occurs beneath the basement membrane (or basal lamina), such as in the dystrophic types of epidermolysis bullosa, the great majority of cases of dermatitis herpetiformis, and the dermal type of erythema multiforme.

DERMATITIS (ECZEMA)

The terms *dermatitis* and *eczema* are used by many dermatologists as synonyms. They refer to an inflammation of the skin that often represents an allergic response to a variety of agents such as chemicals, proteins, bacteria, and fungi. They may act on the skin from either the outside or the inside. In many types of dermatitis, however, the cause is obscure.

Dermatitis may be acute, subacute, or chronic. The clinical picture is characterized by polymorphism of the eruption. Among the primary lesions that may be observed are macules, papules, and vesicles. If macules coalesce, they form patches of erythema that may be edematous; if papules coalesce, they form plaques. Among the secondary lesions are oozing, crusting, scaling, lichenification, and fissuring. Usually, the lesions of dermatitis are not sharply demarcated but merge gradually into the surrounding normal skin. Itching is common in all types of dermatitis.

Even though, literally translated, *dermatitis* means *inflammation of the dermis*, the diagnostic term *dermatitis* refers to a reasonably well defined group of diseases that clinically show the features just mentioned and histologically represent an "epidermodermatitis," with changes in both the epidermis and the dermis.

No generally accepted classification of dermatitis exists, and some cases defy assignment to any definite type. In this section, the following types of dermatitis will be discussed: contact dermatitis, nummular dermatitis, atopic dermatitis, lichen simplex chronicus, seborrheic dermatitis, stasis dermatitis, and generalized exfoliative dermatitis. In addition, lesions of dermatitis may occur in superficial fungal infections as drug eruptions, and in lymphoma. The last three types will be discussed when the respective diseases are described.

Contact dermatitis is caused by contact of the skin with either a substance to which the patient has become specifically sensitized (allergic contact dermatitis) or a substance that acts as a primary irritant (primary irritant contact dermatitis). Contact dermatitis may be acute, subacute, or chronic. In the acute and subacute forms, diffuse erythema, edema, oozing, and crusting predominate; in addition, vesicles and bullae are often present, particularly in allergic contact dermatitis. In the chronic form, erythema, scaling, and lichenification prevail.

Nummular dermatitis presents as the most characteristic lesion fairly sharply demarcated patches of erythema studded with "pinpoint vesicles" or "pinpoint erosions." In addition, there are scattered papulovesicles with a tendency to coalescence. In cases with exclusive or predominant involvement of the palms and soles, where vesicles often predominate, the term *chronic vesicular dermatitis of the palms and soles* is often used. However, the terms *dyshidrotic eruption* or *pompholyx* are best avoided (Calnan).

Atopic dermatitis, a genetically determined disorder that may occur in association with asthma and hay fever in the same patient or family, shows erythematous, scaling, and lichenified areas, which, when active, also show oozing and crusting but no vesicles.

Lichen simplex chronicus shows one or several areas of erythema, scaling, and lichenification. Oozing may be present, but vesiculation is absent. The designation *neurodermatitis* for this eruption is misleading and should be avoided.

Seborrheic dermatitis shows fairly sharply demarcated, brownish red areas that exhibit only slight infiltration and often have on their surface fine scaling, causing some resemblance to psoriasis. Oozing may be present, but there are no vesicles. Generalized seborrheic dermatitis may occur in infants as a self-limited disorder and is often referred to as Leiner's disease. (For a discussion of familial Leiner's disease, see p. 101.)

Stasis dermatitis occurs as a result of venous stasis on the lower portions of the legs. It presents erythema, edema, scaling, and, occasionally, oozing and crusting. It differs from other forms of dermatitis, first, by showing brownish pigmentation and, second, by resulting in some instances in ulceration and atrophic scarring.

Generalized exfoliative dermatitis or generalized erythroderma shows involvement of the entire skin with erythema, scaling, and, in severe cases, oozing. It represents a peak reaction to which several types of dermatitis may lead; these are contact dermatitis, atopic dermatitis, seborrheic dermatitis, stasis dermatitis, and drug dermatitis. In addition, it may occur as a chronic idiopathic disease. When occurring as an apparently idiopathic disease, especially in elderly persons, and in association with peripheral lymphadenopathy, mainly of inguinal and axillary lymph nodes, it often represents Sézary's syndrome, a form of mycosis fungoides (see p. 746). A generalized erythroderma may also be seen in psoriasis, pemphigus foliaceus, and lamellar ichthyosis. However, in psoriasis, the erythroderma has a more uniform appearance because of the absence of oozing; in pemphigus foliaceus, the Nikolsky sign is positive, and, on histologic examination, acantholysis is found to be present; and, in lamellar ichthyosis, the eruption has been present since birth.

Histopathology.   In all clinical types of dermatitis, there are both epidermal and dermal changes. The various types of dermatitis rarely present a histologic picture sufficiently diagnostic to allow their differentiation, because similar histologic reactions occur in all forms of dermatitis: spongiotic microvesicles or macrovesicles with oozing in acute dermatitis; acanthosis with parakeratosis in chronic dermatitis; and a combination of these two reaction patterns in subacute dermatitis. Since, as a rule, no diagnosis more specific than acute, subacute, or chronic dermatitis can be made, the histologic pictures as presented by an acute, a subacute, and a chronic dermatitis will be described first. Thereafter, the more or less distinctive features occasionally presented by the various types of dermatitis will be listed.

In *acute dermatitis*, intraepidermally located vesicles or bullae dominate the histologic picture. Considerable intercellular edema (spongiosis) and intracellular edema may be present in the epidermis surrounding the vesicles. If the number of vesicles is great and the intracellular edema is pronounced, the histologic picture of reticular degeneration of the epidermis results. The vesicles then are separated from one another only by thin septa formed by the resisting walls of edematous epidermal cells and thus form a multilocular bulla (Fig. 7-1). The vesicles and bullae as well as the edematous portions of the epidermis may be permeated by an inflammatory infiltrate composed mainly of mononuclear cells. Lesions more than a few days old may also contain neutrophils, particularly in the stratum corneum. The stratum corneum may be parakeratotic and contain aggregates of coagulated plasma, the substrate of crusts. The upper dermis shows vascular dilatation, edema, and a mononuclear cellular infiltrate around the superficial capillaries extending from there into the epidermis (exocytosis).

In subacute dermatitis one observes spongiosis, intracellular edema, and, usually, vesicles. The vesicles, although smaller in size, arise, like those of acute dermatitis, at sites of spongiosis and intracellular edema and enlarge through reticular degeneration of epidermal cells (Fig. 7-2). The

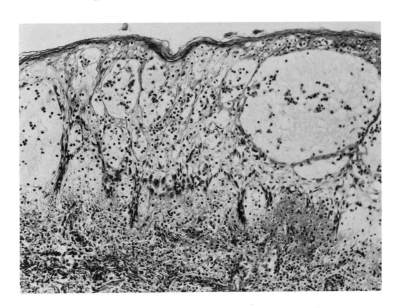

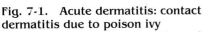
Fig. 7-1.   Acute dermatitis: contact dermatitis due to poison ivy
Numerous intraepidermal vesicles and pronounced intracellular edema are present, resulting in the histologic picture of reticular degeneration of the epidermis. The vesicles are separated from one another only by thin septa formed by the resisting walls of edematous epidermal cells and thus form a multilocular bulla. (×100)

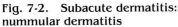
Fig. 7-2.   Subacute dermatitis: nummular dermatitis
The vesicles arise at sites of spongiosis and intracellular edema and enlarge through reticular degeneration of epidermal cells. The epidermis shows moderate acanthosis. The dermis contains a perivascular infiltrate. (×100)

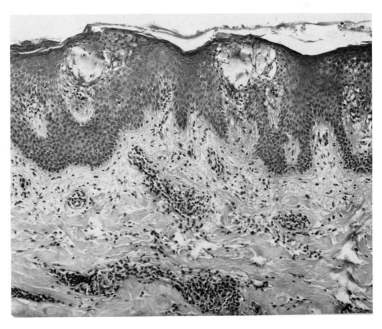

vesicles are seen at various levels of the epidermis. Even though they probably form in the lower epidermis, the rapid proliferation of the epidermis causes vesicles that are only a few days old and are still increasing in size to be located in the upper stratum malpighii. One finds moderate acanthosis and, in the stratum corneum, varying degrees of parakeratosis and crusting. The inflammatory infiltrate is similar to that seen in acute dermatitis.

In *chronic dermatitis* one encounters moderate to marked acanthosis with elongation of the rete ridges. There is also hyperkeratosis with areas of parakeratosis (Fig. 7-3). Slight spongiosis may be present, but vesicles are absent. Intracellular vacuolization, if present, may be the result not of edema but of glycogen accumulation (Neumann and Winter). The inflammatory infiltrate generally has a perivascular distribution in the upper dermis. Exocytosis, that is, extension of the infiltrate into the epidermis, as a rule is absent. The number of capillaries is increased, and their walls may be thickened. There also may be some increase of collagen, manifesting itself as fibrosis, in the upper dermis, including the papillae.

A few words about the histologic aspects of the various types of dermatitis are now in order.

Contact Dermatitis. Contact dermatitis may be acute, subacute, or chronic. The histologic descriptions given above for acute, subacute, and chronic dermatitis apply in general to contact dermatitis. Usually, it is not possible to distinguish histologically between an allergic contact dermatitis and a primary irritant contact dermatitis. This is due to the fact that a biopsy usually is carried out days or weeks after the appearance of the dermatitis. By that time, secondary changes brought on by regeneration, traumatization through scratching, or secondary infection have altered the original picture of the dermatitis, and the findings are those of a nonspecific subacute or chronic dermatitis. However, the patch testing of a sensitized person with the specific sensitizing substance and of a nonsensitized person with a primary irritant results in different histologic responses. Similarly, it often is not possible to distinguish histologically between a photoallergic and a phototoxic contact dermatitis, although such distinction may be important, since some drugs such as chlorpromazine are capable of producing either. However, differentiation of a photoallergic from a phototoxic reaction usually is possible through the histologic examination of photopatch tests, since the histologic responses differ in a manner similar to that of the patch test results in allergic and primary irritant contact dermatitis (see below) (Epstein, 1968).

Experimental Induction. The histologic evolution of allergic contact dermatitis has been studied both in humans and in guinea pigs mainly by the local application of a 0.1% to 0.3% solution of dinitrochlorobenzine (DNCB) after previous sensitization to this substance (Baer et al; Medenica and Rostenberg). The earliest changes are seen 3 hr to 6 hr after the application of the DNCB solution. They consist of vasodilatation and extravasation of mononuclear cells in the uppermost portion of the dermis (Miescher; Baer et al). Subsequently,

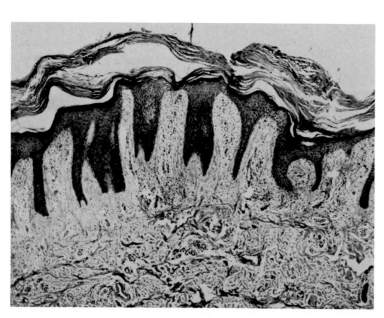

Fig. 7-3. Chronic dermatitis: lichen simplex chronicus
There are hyperkeratosis, acanthosis, elongation of the rete ridges, and elongation and broadening of the papillae. The dermis shows a chronic inflammatory infiltrate and fibrosis. (× 50)

about 8 hr after application of the test solution, the mononuclear cells are seen also in the lower epidermis, where spongiosis is present. By 72 hr, as the spongiosis increases, intraepidermal vesicles form. The reaction reaches maximal intensity after 3 to 6 days (Dvorak et al). Whereas, during the first 24 hr, most mononuclear cells are lymphocytes, a large proportion of the cells can subsequently be identified as monocytes or macrophages by means of staining for enzymes, such as peroxidase (Bandmann). The presence of so many monocytes and macrophages, necessary for the lysosomal removal of damaged keratinocytes, is induced by lymphokines such as the macrophage migration inhibitory factor (MIF) (see p. 98).

A prominent role is played in allergic contact dermatitis by basophilic leukocytes and mast cells. For adequate visualization of basophilic leukocytes, Epon-embedded semithick sections stained with the Giemsa stain are required. Basophils become evident at 24 hr and reach a peak concentration on day 3, when they constitute from 5% to 15% of the cellular infiltrate (Dvorak et al). In reactions 3 days old and older, mast cell mitoses are observed, and mast cells increase in number. Thus, basophils and mast cells, with their similar or identical functions, are supplementary to one another. Basophils, because they can be quickly mobilized from the blood, are important early in the course of the inflammatory reaction. By contrast, new mast cells arise by a process of replication, which requires several days. Whereas, in anaphylactic reactions, basophils and mast cells degranulate rapidly, the degranulation of these cells in allergic contact dermatitis proceeds gradually and incompletely (Dvorak et al).

The histologic evolution of primary irritant contact dermatitis proceeds at a much more rapid pace than that of allergic contact dermatitis. Primary irritants induce damage to the epidermis usually within a few hours, although the speed with which the damage occurs and the degree of damage depend on the type and concentration of the primary irritant (Hall et al). With moderately strong primary irritants, such as a 10% solution of DNCB, both intracellular and intercellular edema throughout the epidermis is evident after 3 hr to 6 hr. Within 24 hr, epidermal necrosis characterized by cellular vacuolation and nuclear pyknosis occurs (Epstein, 1968). This may result in subepidermal blister formation (Kerl et al). There is less of a dermal infiltrate and less exocytosis than on patch testing with allergens, and neutrophils, usually absent in patch tests with allergens, make up a significant proportion of the infiltrate (Epstein, 1968).

Histogenesis. Contact dermatitis represents a delayed hypersensitivity reaction in which Langerhans cells are the antigen-processing and antigen-presenting cells while primed (or specifically sensitized, committed) T lymphocytes are the reacting cells, as first established in 1973 (Silberberg). If, in a previously sensitized human or guinea pig, the agent that produced the sensitization is applied to the skin, epidermal Langerhans cells con-

jugate the agent, called a hapten, with constituents on their surface to form an immunogenic complex or complete antigen. The complete antigen then attracts primed or specifically sensitized T lymphocytes from the circulation to the Langerhans cells (Baer, 1978). Langerhans cells act as macrophages (see p. 19), and, like macrophages, they bear on their cell surface receptors for the Fc portion of the immunoglobulin G (IgG) molecule and for the third component of complement (C3). In addition, they carry so-called immune response-associated antigens (Ia antigens). It seems that such Ia antigens not only form the immunogenic complexes with the hapten but also are responsible for the presentation of these complexes to primed T lymphocytes having the identical Ia antigens as the Langerhans cells (Baer, 1978). The importance of the Langerhans cell in converting haptens into an immunogenic form has been established by the finding that cutaneous surfaces of mice or hamsters that are temporarily deprived of adenosine triphosphatase (ATPase)-positive Langerhans cells by means of ultraviolet radiation fail to become sensitized to dinitrofluorobenzene (DNFB) and, when previously sensitized, fail to react to DNFB (Streilein and Bergstresser).

Electron microscopic studies have revealed that, in sensitized guinea pigs, as in humans, application of a 0.3% solution of DNCB leads to apposition of lymphocytes to Langerhans cells within 3 hr to 5 hr (Silberberg et al, 1974). This is associated with an increase in the number of Langerhans cells present in the epidermis (Baer, 1976), and this increase takes place through the transformation of indeterminate dendritic cells in the epidermis into mature Langerhans cells (see p. 19). Contact with the antigen-presenting Langerhans cells causes stimulation of the primed, or specifically sensitized, T lymphocytes, which thereupon discharge a variety of lymphokines (see below). These lymphokines damage the Langerhans cells, and this possibly results in their discharging inflammation-producing substances (Baer, 1976).

Of great importance is the fact that, in biopsy specimens taken 2 hr to 3 hr after the application of the DNCB solution, Langerhans cells are seen in the lymph vessels of the dermis, before any damage has occurred to them; after 4 hr, they are seen also in regional lymph nodes (Silberberg-Sinakin, 1977). The migration of Langerhans cells to the regional lymph nodes has been well demonstrated in guinea pigs passively sensitized to ferritin (Silberberg-Sinakin et al, 1976, 1978). Upon challenge with ferritin, ferritin-containing Langerhans cells were observed not only in the ferritin-challenged skin sites but also in the draining dermal lymphatics and the regional lymph nodes. In the regional lymph nodes, Langerhans cells are found mainly in the paracortical region, that is, in the region in which T lymphocytes predominate. There, the antigen-carrying Langerhans cells encounter additional specifically sensitized T lymphocytes, react with them, and induce an immunoproliferative reaction resulting in a significant increase in circulating specifically sensitized T lymphocytes, which gradually accumulate at the site of challenge and release various lymphokines.

A considerable number of lymphokines are released by specifically sensitized lymphocytes at the site of challenge. They are responsible for most of the clinical and histologic manifestations of allergic contact dermatitis. Lymphokines recruit other cells into the area and exert an effect on them. The recruited cells include lymphocytes, macrophages, neutrophils, and basophils, which greatly influence the process of inflammation through phagocytosis and the release of various enzymes (Krueger). Among the lymphokines affecting macrophages is the migration inhibiting factor (MIF), which not only inhibits the migration of macrophages but also causes their aggregation and activation. There are lymphokines with chemotactic factors for neutrophils, basophils, and eosinophils, as well as a lymphokine acting as a mitogenic factor for lymphocytes (Krueger). In addition, there are lymphokines, such as lymphotoxin, that damage their target cells (Cohen).

The role of the regional lymph nodes in the re-exposure, or eliciting, phase of contact dermatitis is well understood. A similar mechanism can be postulated for the primary immune response, or sensitization phase, of allergic contact dermatitis, particularly since Langerhans cells exhibit a selective uptake of small molecules and dyes (Hunziker and Winkelmann), and the migration of Langerhans cells from the skin to regional lymph nodes occurs not only in immunologically challenged skin but also in normal skin (Silberberg-Sinakin et al, 1978). It can therefore be assumed that Langerhans cells conjugate potential allergens, carry them to the regional lymph nodes, and present them there to uncommitted T lymphocytes (Epstein, 1975). If sensitization takes place, these uncommitted T lymphocytes develop the ability to recognize the antigen. During the process of specific sensitization, or "programming," which requires 5 to 7 days, T lymphocytes acquire on their surface receptors capable of reacting with the specific antigen (Weston, 1975). The population of specifically sensitized, or committed, T lymphocytes proliferates during the "programming" period in the paracortical area of the regional lymph nodes. Contact sensitization can be prevented by the removal of these nodes during that time but not afterward, because the process becomes generalized as specifically sensitized T lymphocytes are released into the circulation (Epstein et al). When the epidermis is then challenged with the antigen in a certain area, the specifically sensitized T lymphocytes migrate there. At the site of challenge, Langerhans cells have processed the antigen and are ready to present it to the specifically sensitized T lymphocytes.

ELECTRON MICROSCOPY. Sequential electron microscopic examination of biopsy specimens taken after the application of an allergen to the skin of sensitized humans has shown in specimens taken 3 hr to 4 hr after the application intercellular edema in the lower epidermis without the presence of an epidermal cellular infiltrate (Carr et al; Metz; Komura and Ofuji). This edema is thought to be an extension of the edema present in the uppermost dermis (Komura and Ofuji). A cellular infiltrate extending from the dermis into the epidermis and containing both lymphocytes and monocytes is observed usually after 6 hr to 12 hr. As the intercellular edema increases in severity, alterations occur on the desmosomes, leading ultimately to the absence of most desmosomes. Initially, there are two different processes that cause damage to the desmosomes: either the desmosomal unit holds firmly, and there is severe stretching of the cytoplasmic extensions leading from each of the two keratinocytes to the desmosomal unit until one of the cytoplasmic extensions breaks (Carr et al; Komura and Ofuji), or there is dissolution of the intradesmosomal cement substance, resulting in separation of the desmosomal unit in the middle. Because of its resemblance to the acantholysis occurring in pemphigus (see p. 107), this intradesmosomal separation has been referred to as microacantholysis (Metz). The nearly complete absence of desmosomes, seen as early as 12 hr after testing but especially after 24 hr to 48 hr, can best be explained by a failure of new desmosomes to form (Braun-Falco and Wolff).

Compared with the severe intercellular changes, the intracellular alterations within keratinocytes during the first two days are mild. As the result of their loss of coherence with the desmosomal attachment plaques, tonofilaments aggregate in the middle of the cytoplasm (Komura and Ofuji), and there may be mild intracellular edema (Metz) and aggregation of glycogen granula (Braun-Falco and Wolff). After several days, however, the keratinocytes in untreated acute contact dermatitis demonstrate striking cellular breakdown, with large vacuoles in the cytoplasm and pyknotic nuclei (Frichot and Zelickson).

Nummular Dermatitis. Characterized clinically by "pinpoint vesicles," nummular dermatitis usually shows the histologic picture of a subacute dermatitis (Fig. 7-2). In a moderately acanthotic epidermis, one finds scattered intraepidermal vesicles at various levels surrounded by spongiosis. In addition, there is lymphocytic exocytosis in the areas of spongiosis and extensive parakeratosis (Braun-Falco and Petry).

Histogenesis. The *electron microscopic* changes observed in nummular dermatitis resemble those seen in allergic contact dermatitis. Intercellular edema is the most outstanding finding (Braun-Falco and Petry). In the basal cell layer, the number of desmosomes is greatly reduced as a result of microacantholysis (see Contact Dermatitis above). Instead, the keratinocytes may show many cytoplasmic processes. In the stratum spinosum, however, the desmosomes are largely preserved, and thick tonofilament bundles extend through greatly elongated cytoplasmic processes to the desmosomes. When, ultimately, tearing occurs, it is seen in one of the two cytoplasmic processes rather than in the central intradesmosomal area.

Atopic Dermatitis. The histologic picture is that of a chronic dermatitis showing acanthosis with varying degrees of spongiosis (Prose and Sedlis). In areas of spongiosis, exocytosis of mononuclear cells as well as parakeratosis may be seen. In cases of long standing, the rete ridges usually show regular elongation. On the basis of enzyme determinations, the dermal infiltrate is seen to consist mainly of lymphocytes, but it also contains fairly numerous monocytes. Mast cells are present in increased number, but eosinophils are found only rarely (Braun-Falco and Burg).

Histogenesis. A T-cell regulatory defect has been shown to exist in atopic dermatitis (Cooper et al). There is also evidence of impaired suppressor activity of suppressor T cells (Stingl et al). This would account for aberrations in humoral immunity such as elevated IgE and for depressed cell-mediated immunity. However, a direct correlation between serum level of IgE and disease activity does not always exist. Some authors have observed a correlation (Ogawa et al; Byrom et al); however, others have observed a correlation with the extent but not with the severity of the dermatitis (Stone et al), and still others have found consistently elevated levels of IgE only in patients who also have respiratory atopy (MacKie et al, 1979). It seems that, although the mean serum level of IgE is elevated, there are considerable differences in individual patients' IgE levels (Jones et al, 1975). With regard to the depression of cellular immunity in atopic dermatitis, cutaneous anergy is found in the great majority of patients, with as many as 96% of the patients not responding to candidin and 84% not responding to streptokinase–streptodornase (Elliott and Hanifin). Also, on patch testing with rhus oleoresin, fewer atopics (15%) show a positive test than normal controls (61%) (Jones et al, 1973). Only patients with severe atopic dermatitis show depressed responses to the in vitro lymphocyte transformation by mitogens such as phytohemagglutinin (Elliott and Hanifin).

Electron microscopic examination has revealed in atopic dermatitis, particularly in areas of parakeratosis, the presence of rather numerous lysosomes in the keratinocytes of the upper portions of the epidermis (Prose et al). It can be assumed that the lysosomes form as a response to cellular damage.

Lichen Simplex Chronicus. The histologic appearance of lichen simplex chronicus is essentially that of a chronic dermatitis (Fig. 7-3). One observes hyperkeratosis interspersed with small areas of parakeratosis, acanthosis with rather regular elongation of the rete ridges, and elongation and broadening of the papillae. There may be some spongiosis, but vesiculation does not occur. In addition to a chronic inflammatory infiltrate, the dermis often shows a fair number of fibroblasts and some fibrosis even in the papillae.

Seborrheic Dermatitis. The histologic picture of seborrheic dermatitis is not diagnostic. It may be said to be halfway between psoriasis and chronic dermatitis. The horny layer shows focal areas of parakeratosis occasionally containing a few pyknotic neutrophils similar to those seen in the Munro microabscesses of psoriasis (Pinkus and Mehregan). The epidermis shows slight to moderate acanthosis, with some elongation of the rete ridges, and slight to moderate spongiosis. Exocytosis of mononuclear cells may be seen in the areas of spongiosis (Metz and Metz). The dermis shows a mild chronic inflammatory infiltrate. Thus, the only major difference between psoriasis and seborrheic dermatitis is the presence of spongiosis in the latter.

Histogenesis. Seborrheic dermatitis and psoriasis appear to have a similar histogenesis; in both diseases, the papillary capillaries intermittently release neutrophils, which then migrate through the epidermis and accumulate in the parakeratotic horny layer (Pinkus and Mehregan) (see p. 140).

Stasis Dermatitis. Histologic examination shows either a subacute or a chronic dermatitis. Quite frequently, considerable amounts of hemosiderin are scattered through the dermis. Old lesions show numerous dilated capillaries embedded in a fibrotic dermis.

Histogenesis. Inadequate venous circulation in the legs is caused usually by thrombophlebitis or varicose veins. Occasionally, it is a result of congenital arteriovenous fistulae of the legs associated with a portwine nevus, the so-called Klippel–Trenaunay syndrome (see p. 623) (Bluefarb and Adams). Any of these factors can cause venous and capillary stasis on the medial portions of the legs just above the ankles. The stasis leads to hypoxia and poor nutrition of the tissue and thus results in dermatitis. Changes in the arterioles and venules consisting of intimal proliferation and medial hyperplasia are secondary, but arteriolar obstruction may be an important factor in the development of the ulcers in stasis dermatitis (Wiedmann).

Generalized Exfoliative Dermatitis or Generalized Erythroderma. The histologic picture shows either a subacute or a chronic dermatitis. If the dermatitis is subacute, one observes parakeratosis, marked intercellular and intracellular edema, acanthosis with elongation of the rete ridges, and migration of inflammatory cells through the epidermis, so-called exocytosis. The upper dermis shows edema and a considerable chronic inflammatory infiltrate (Fig. 7-4). If the edema in the upper stratum malpighii is pronounced, as seen

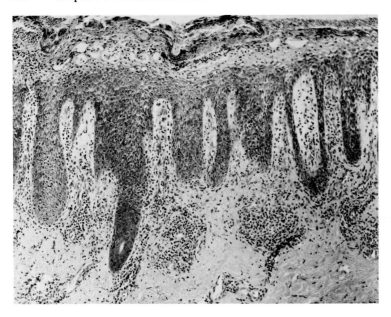

Fig. 7-4. Generalized exfoliative dermatitis due to drug allergy, subacute
There are parakeratosis, marked intercellular and intracellular edema, acanthosis with elongation of the rete ridges, and migration of inflammatory cells through the epidermis. The upper dermis shows edema and a considerable amount of the inflammatory infiltrate. (×100)

especially in drug-induced generalized exfoliative dermatitis, marked oozing is apt to be present in addition to the exfoliation of the parakeratotic horny cells.

In the chronic type of generalized exfoliative dermatitis, the histologic picture is that of a chronic dermatitis. Although the epidermis may have a psoriasiform appearance owing to the regular elongation of the rete ridges, the common presence of spongiosis and eosinophils, and occasionally also of plasma cells, excludes psoriasis (Nicolis and Helwig). Each case of undetermined origin requires thorough histologic examination through multiple skin biopsies and a lymph node biopsy to rule out lymphoma. From 15% to 25% of the cases of undetermined origin occur in association with Sézary's syndrome (Nicolis and Helwig; Edelson et al). Furthermore, generalized erythroderma may precede the fully developed Sézary's syndrome by several years (Winkelmann et al). Even if the histologic examination at first shows no evidence of lymphoma, it is advisable to perform further biopsies as well as hematologic studies at intervals (see Differential Diagnosis below and p. 746).

Differential Diagnosis. Histologic differentiation of acute dermatitis, particularly of a vesicular or bullous contact dermatitis, from erythema multiforme, especially the mixed dermal-epidermal type, may be difficult on a histologic basis and may require clinical information, since erythema multiforme may show invasion of the epidermis by mononuclear cells associated with spongiosis

and formation of intraepidermal vesicles. However, in most cases of erythema multiforme with blisters, there also are subepidermal vesicles or bullae. Furthermore, in instances of erythema multiforme with epidermal changes, one often finds scattered necrotic keratinocytes as a characteristic feature (see p. 122).

It should be stressed that many diseases not belonging to the dermatitis–eczema group either regularly or occasionally show a histologic picture allowing no more specific a diagnosis than chronic dermatitis.* Diseases that regularly show the nonspecific histologic picture of chronic dermatitis include pityriasis rosea, the small plaque type of parapsoriasis en plaques, and pellagra. Many other diseases, especially psoriasis but also lichen planus and pityriasis rubra pilaris, to name but a few, present a diagnostic histologic picture in clinically typical cases but may show a nonspecific histologic picture, that of a chronic dermatitis, in clinically less typical cases. In contrast, a chronic dermatitis may simulate the histologic picture of psoriasis through the presence of evenly elongated rete ridges. However, at least in typical cases, psoriasis shows more pronounced parakeratosis, as well as thinning of the suprapapillary epidermis, edema of the papillae with dilatation of the papillary capillaries, and, usually, Munro microabscesses (see p. 141).

---

* The term *chronic dermatitis* is used if there are both epidermal and nonspecific dermal changes; the term *chronic inflammation* is used if only dermal changes are present.

Early mycosis fungoides must always be kept in mind as a possible diagnosis when a section showing chronic dermatitis is examined, particularly if it shows a fairly marked dermal infiltrate. Often, it is very difficult to establish or to rule out early mycosis fungoides in such instances. One should search for atypical mononuclear cells (so-called mycosis cells). A patchy infiltrate, mitotic figures, and Pautrier microabscesses are also points in favor of mycosis fungoides. However, now and then, a patchy infiltrate, some atypicality ("pleomorphism") in some of the mononuclear cells, and occasional mitotic figures are seen also in chronic dermatitis. This leaves Pautrier microabscesses as a most valuable differential diagnostic feature (see p. 741). Unfortunately, not all cases of mycosis fungoides show them even on "step sectioning." Furthermore, microvesicles of dermatitis may simulate Pautrier microabscesses, although they differ from them by showing spongiosis in their vicinity (Ackerman et al). Similarly, the exocytosis seen in dermatitis differs from the epidermotropism of mycosis fungoides by being associated with spongiosis. If the diagnosis is in doubt, it is advisable to request additional specimens for histologic examination.

Dermatitis Associated with Systemic Diseases

Four systemic diseases characterized by severe immune deficiencies are frequently or regularly associated with a dermatitis.

Familial Leiner's Disease. In familial Leiner's disease, a frequently fatal disorder of infancy, a generalized seborrheic dermatitis indistinguishable from that of ordinary Leiner's disease (see p. 94) is combined with severe diarrhea, recurrent local and systemic infections, and marked wasting. Death usually is due to septicemia. A dysfunction of C5 exists (Jacobs and Miller), but there are also other immune defects, such as severely reduced cellular and humoral chemotaxis (Weston and Humbert).

Hyperimmunoglobulin E Syndrome. Recurrent pyogenic skin infections are associated with extreme elevations of serum IgE and with defective neutrophil chemotaxis (Stanley et al). In addition, most patients have atopic dermatitis (Hill and Quie).

Wiscott–Aldrich Syndrome. A disease with X-linked recessive inheritance, the Wiscott–Aldrich syndrome occurs only in males. It is characterized by recurrent, severe systemic bacterial and viral infections due to defects in both the humoral and the cellular immune

systems and purpura due to thrombocytopenia. Frequently, there also is an eruption resembling atopic dermatitis (MacKie et al, 1978). Because of progressive deterioration of the cellular immunity, death from severe infection or lymphoma occurs during the first decade of life (Rosen).

Chronic Granulomatous Disease. An X-linked recessively inherited disorder affecting only boys, chronic granulomatous disease starts in infancy with a dermatitis particularly around the mouth. The dermatitis often progresses to granulomatous lesions accompanied by cervical adenitis (Weston, 1976). Infections of the lungs, bones, and liver develop with granulomas at the sites of infection. With rare exceptions, death occurs in adolescence. The defect lies in the neutrophils, which are unable to consume oxygen and to produce hydrogen peroxide. Thus, bacteria containing peroxide are killed normally by the neutrophils of patients with this disorder, whereas bacteria not containing peroxide are not killed (Dilworth and Mandell). The inability of the neutrophils to reduce nitroblue tetrazolium dye demonstrates the defect in vitro.

Histopathology. The seborrheic dermatitis in familial Leiner's disease and the eczema or atopic dermatitis in the other three diseases show the histologic features described previously for seborrheic dermatitis (see p. 99) and atopic dermatitis (see p. 99), respectively.

Dermatopathic Lymphadenopathy

Any extensive dermatitis, but particularly generalized exfoliative dermatitis, may cause asymptomatic enlargement of the subcutaneous lymph nodes, especially of the inguinal, axillary, and cervical nodes. The presence of palpably enlarged lymph nodes is common in mycosis fungoides. It is found in about one fourth of early cases, in 70% to 75% of advanced cases, and in 90% of patients with generalized erythroderma, that is, with Sézary's syndrome (Fuks et al).

Histopathology. The architecture of the lymph node is well preserved in dermatopathic lymphadenopathy. However, the lymph follicles may be increased in size and may possess fairly large germinal centers (Laipply). The most conspicuous feature is the presence of enlarged paracortical areas, often reaching the capsule of the lymph node. They stand out as pale patches because of the presence of many histiocytes, or macrophages, with abundant pale cytoplasms and large, pale nuclei (Hurwitt). Some of the histiocytes contain lipid material, whereas others contain melanin or hemosiderin. Intermingled among the histiocytes are varying amounts of lymphoid cells, some of which have hyperchromatic, irregularly shaped "cerebriform" nuclei (Scheffer et al). Eosinophils may also be present.

Histogenesis. It has been postulated that melanin present in the lymph nodes is responsible for the development of dermatopathic lymphadenopathy, since an identical histologic picture can be produced in the lymph nodes of guinea pigs by the parenteral injection of melanin obtained from the choroid of cattle (Hohenadl and de Paola).

The enlargement of the lymph nodes concerns the thymus-dependent area. *Electron microscopic studies* have shown that a great number of the pale-staining macrophages can be identified as interdigitating reticulum cells or as Langerhans cells. The presence of Langerhans cells also in the sinuses suggests that these cells are carried from the skin to the lymph node parenchyma by way of afferent lymphatics (Rausch et al).

Differential Diagnosis. The histologic differentiation of dermatopathic lymphadenopathy from Hodgkin's disease and from non-Hodgkin's lymphoma usually is not difficult, since, in dermatopathic lymphadenopathy, the capsule of the lymph node is not invaded, the lymph node architecture is preserved, and there is evidence of phagocytic activity in the histiocytes.

Considerable difficulty can arise, however, in the distinction of dermatopathic lymphadenopathy from the lymph node changes seen in the early stages of mycosis fungoides and Sézary's syndrome. Indeed, there is evidence of a gradual transition of dermatopathic lymphadenopathy into true mycosis fungoides. Four categories have thus been distinguished in the histopathology of lymph nodes in mycosis fungoides: category I represents dermatopathic lymphadenopathy, category II shows preserved lymph node architecture but atypical nuclei, category III shows focal obliteration of lymph node structure, and category IV shows complete obliteration (Scheffer et al). (For details concerning the lymph nodes in mycosis fungoides, see p. 743.) On performing sequential lymph node biopsies on patients with mycosis fungoides, several authors have found dermatopathic lymphadenopathy initially and specific involvement with mycosis fungoides subsequently (Block et al; Epstein et al; Fuks et al). Thus, it seems that early involvement of lymph nodes with mycosis fungoides may present the nonspecific histologic picture of dermatopathic lymphadenopathy (Constantine). This probably is analogous to the nonspecific appearance that early mycosis fungoides may present in the skin.

MILIARIA

Miliaria occurs when sweating is associated with obstruction of the intraepidermal sweat duct. There are two types: miliaria crystallina and miliaria rubra.

Miliaria crystallina occurs when the sweat duct is obstructed within the stratum corneum. It is seen generally in sunburned areas or after sudden profuse sweating as may occur during a febrile illness. It shows asymptomatic, small, superficial, clear, noninflammatory vesicles resembling dewdrops. The vesicles rapidly subside when sweating ceases or the horny layer overlying the vesicles exfoliates.

Miliaria rubra occurs when the sweat duct is obstructed within the deeper layers of the epidermis. It is seen generally following excessive sweating in parts of the skin covered by clothing. It may also occur following prolonged covering of the skin by occlusive polyethylene wraps. The lesions consist of pruritic small papulovesicles surrounded by erythema. In severe cases, some of the lesions may be pustular (Lyons et al).

Histopathology. In *miliaria crystallina*, one observes intracorneal or subcorneal vesicles. On serial sectioning, the vesicles are found to be in direct communication with an underlying sweat duct (Shelley and Horvath).

In *miliaria rubra*, spongiotic vesicles similar in appearance to those seen in dermatitis are found in the stratum malpighii. Serial sectioning shows these vesicles to be in continuity with a sweat duct. A chronic inflammatory infiltrate is seen around and within the vesicles as well as in the subjacent dermis (Sulzberger and Zimmerman; Loewenthal). In many instances, the intraepidermal sweat duct is filled with an amorphous substance that is PAS-positive and diastase-resistant (Dobson and Lobitz; Hölzle and Kligman).

Histogenesis. In *miliaria crystallina*, the obstruction of the sweat duct within the stratum corneum is caused either by mild damage to the epidermis from a preceding sunburn or by excessive hydration of the stratum corneum.

In *miliaria rubra*, aerobic bacteria, notably staphylococci, are thought to play a decisive role, inducing the obstruction of the acrosyringium. In favor of this view is not only the frequent presence of gram-positive cocci, identifiable as *Staphylococcus aureus*, within the sweat ducts in miliaria rubra (O'Brien; Lyons et al), but also the fact that the development of miliaria rubra under an occlusive polyethylene film can be prevented by the topical application of antibacterial solutions (Singh; Hölzle and Kligman).

The PAS-positive, diastase-resistant, amorphous plug within the acrosyringium was at one time regarded as a secretory product of the dark eccrine secretory cells (see p. 21) and as the sole cause of miliaria rubra (Dobson and Lobitz). However, because of the inhibitory effect of antibiotics on the development of miliaria rubra, it is more likely that cocci secrete a toxin that causes not only inflammation and ductal as well as periductal spongiosis but also precipitation of the intraluminal cast secondary to injury to the luminal cells (Hölzle and Kligman).

ERYTHEMA TOXICUM NEONATORUM

A benign, asymptomatic eruption, erythema toxicum neonatorum affects the skin of about 40% of all infants, usually within 12 hr but in any case within the first 48 hr after birth. Very rarely, the eruption is present at birth (Pohlandt et al). Lasting only two to three days, the eruption usually consists of macules, papules, and large, irregular areas of erythema. Pustules occur in about 10% of the cases. The eruption is associated with eosinophilia of the blood. The cause is unknown.

Histopathology. The macules and areas of erythema show only a few eosinophils in the upper dermis, largely in a perivascular location.

The papules show an accumulation of numerous eosinophils and some neutrophils among the cells of the outer root sheath of the hair from the entry of the sebaceous duct upward to the surface epidermis. In addition, eosinophils are present in the upper dermis.

The pustules form as a result of the upward migration of eosinophils to the surface epidermis around the hair follicles (Freeman et al). Mature pustules usually have an intrafollicular subcorneal location (Fig. 7-5).

Differential Diagnosis. The subcorneal pustules of staphylococcal impetigo of the newborn (see p. 291) contain neutrophils rather than eosinophils and do not have a follicular distribution. Although many eosinophils are present also in the vesicles of incontinentia pigmenti, the intraepidermal rather than subcorneal location of the vesicles and the presence of spongiosis in incontinentia pigmenti help in the differentiation.

TRANSIENT NEONATAL PUSTULAR MELANOSIS

Transient neonatal pustular melanosis, affecting about 2% of all newborn, is invariably present at birth. There are flaccid vesicopustules that rupture after one or two days and develop into hyperpigmented macules. The

Fig. 7-5. Erythema toxicum neonatorum
The pustule has a follicular location and is filled with eosinophils. The outer root sheath beneath the pustule is infiltrated with eosinophils. (×100) (Courtesy of Dieter Lüders, M.D.)

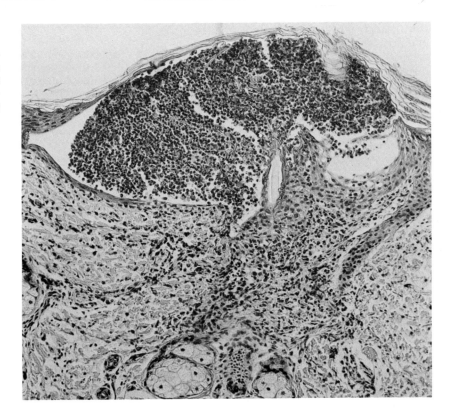

latter persist for several weeks or months and often are the only clinical manifestation present (Ramamurthy et al). The coincidental presence of the melanotic macules with lesions of erythema toxicum neonatorum has been observed (Barr et al). This coexistence is understandable on the basis of the frequent occurrence of the latter.

Histopathology.   The vesicopustules show intracorneal or subcorneal aggregates of neutrophils with a small admixture of eosinophils. The dermis either shows an inflammatory infiltrate with some neutrophils and eosinophils or appears uninvolved. The macules merely show focal basilar hyperpigmentation (Ramamurthy et al).

Differential Diagnosis.   A smear of pustular content shows neutrophils and sparse eosinophils in transient neonatal pustular melanosis and numerous eosinophils in erythema toxicum neonatorum.

ACROPUSTULOSIS OF INFANCY

Recurrent crops of vesicopustules or pustules 1 mm to 3 mm in size are seen predominantly on the distal portions of the extremities, beginning either at birth or during the first year of life. Spontaneous clearing occurs after about two years (Jarratt and Ramsdell).

Histopathology.   Well-circumscribed subcorneal aggregates of neutrophils are seen. The underlying dermis shows a mononuclear infiltrate intermingled with a few neutrophils (Kahn and Rywlin).

Differential Diagnosis.   The histologic picture of impetigo and subcorneal pustular dermatosis is identical with that of acropustulosis of infancy, so that clinical data are necessary for differentiation.

PEMPHIGUS

There are two types of pemphigus, each of which has a variant: pemphigus vulgaris with pemphigus vegetans, and pemphigus foliaceus with pemphigus erythematosus. As first demonstrated in 1943 (Civatte), the bullae of pemphigus show acantholysis as a characteristic feature (see Table 7-1 and Glossary). Acantholysis is absent in the two types of pemphigoid, bullous pemphigoid and cicatricial pemphigoid (see pp. 113 and 117); however, acantholysis occurs not only in pemphigus but also in Darier's disease, focal acantholytic dyskeratosis, familial benign pemphigus, and transient acantholytic dermatosis.

Pemphigus Vulgaris

Pemphigus vulgaris shows flaccid bullae. They break easily and leave denuded areas that tend to increase in size by progressive peripheral detachment of the epidermis. By the increase of lesions in size as well as in number, large areas of the skin can become involved. Oral lesions are almost invariably present and are often the first manifestation of the disease. Before corticosteroids became available, the mortality rate of this disease was very high.

Both pemphigus vulgaris and pemphigus foliaceus are regarded as autoimmune diseases because of the presence of specific antibodies, first demonstrated in 1964 (Beutner and Jordon). In vivo bound antibodies are almost invariably present in the epidermis and demonstrable by direct immunofluorescence testing, and circulating antibodies are usually present in the blood serum and demonstrable by indirect immunofluorescence testing. (For details about the technic of biopsy and transport of the specimen, see p. 45.)

In rare instances, both pemphigus vulgaris and pem-

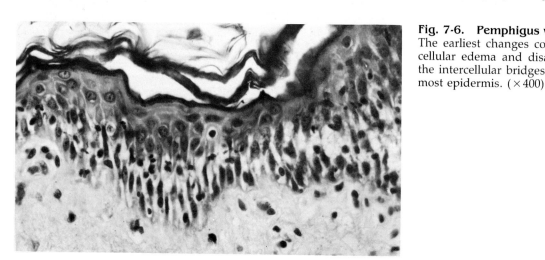

Fig. 7-6.   Pemphigus vulgaris
The earliest changes consist of intercellular edema and disappearance of the intercellular bridges in the lowermost epidermis. (×400)

phigus foliaceus are induced by the prolonged intake of penicillamine (see p. 262).

Histopathology. It is important that early bullae be selected for biopsy, preferably small ones that can be removed in their entirety with a skin punch. If there is reduced cohesion between the epidermal cells, as shown by a positive Nikolsky sign, it is advisable either to use a refrigerant spray before excising the blister with a punch or to excise it widely with a scalpel. If no recent blister is available, an old one may be moved into the neighboring skin by gentle vertical pressure with a finger (Asboe-Hansen). Such a newly created cleavage will reveal quite early histologic changes.

The earliest changes consist of intercellular edema and disappearance of the intercellular bridges in the lowermost epidermis (Fig. 7-6). The resulting loss of coherence between the epidermal cells (acantholysis) leads to the formation first of clefts and then of bullae in a predominantly suprabasal location (Fig. 7-7, top) (Civatte; Lever, 1965; Tappeiner and Pfleger). The basal cells, although separated from one another through the loss of inter-

Fig. 7-7. Pemphigus vulgaris
(*Top*) The bulla lies in a predominantly suprabasal position and leads at its periphery into suprabasal clefts. (× 100) (*Bottom*) The floor of a bulla shows the basal layer adherent to the dermis. The cavity contains single acantholytic epidermal cells, as well as clusters. (× 400)

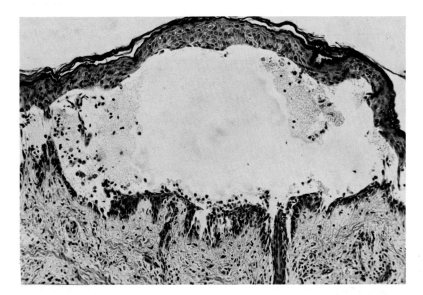

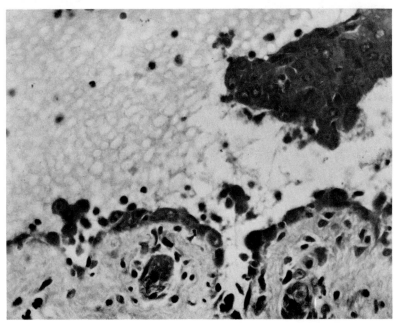

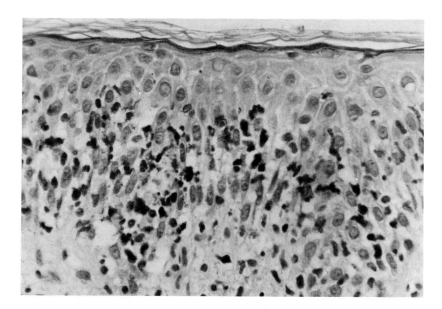

Fig. 7-8. Pemphigus vulgaris
In rare instances, the earliest manifestation consists of "eosinophilic
spongiosis," in which eosinophils
invade a spongiotic epidermis with
little or no evidence of acantholysis.
($\times 400$)

cellular bridges, remain attached to the dermis like
a row of tombstones. As a rule, there is little
evidence of inflammation in pemphigus vulgaris
during the early phase of blister formation. In rare
instances, however, eosinophils invade the epidermis before acantholysis has become evident,
and this has been referred to as eosinophilic spongiosis (Emmerson and Wilson Jones) (Fig. 7-8).
Evidence of acantholysis may or may not be present
within or adjoining the areas of eosinophilic spongiosis. The phenomenon of eosinophilic spongiosis
occurs occasionally also in pemphigus vegetans
and pemphigus foliaceus and even in bullous
eruptions other than pemphigus (Knight et al).

The bullae in pemphigus vulgaris contain single
as well as clusters of epidermal cells that, because
of the loss of coherence with their neighboring
cells, have drifted into the bulla cavity. These
acantholytic cells appear rounded, with a large
hyperchromatic nucleus and homogeneous cytoplasm (Fig. 7-7, bottom). Frequently, one observes
at the floor of the bullae, even of early bullae,
irregular upward growth of papillae that are lined
by a single row of basal cells, so-called villi, as well
as downward proliferation of strands of epidermal
cells into the spaces between the papillae. Acantholysis may also affect the epithelium of the outer
root sheath of the hair. As in the surface epidermis,
clefts form predominantly right above the basal
layer (Fig. 7-9).

Owing to regeneration, the base of an old bulla
may consist of more than one layer of cells
(Fig. 7-9). Denuded areas usually show the basal

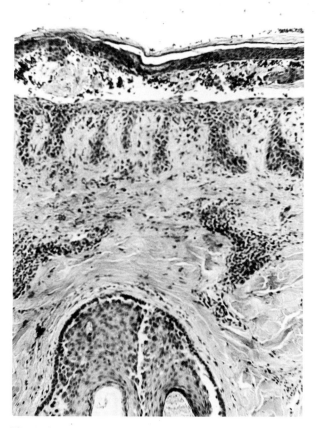

Fig. 7-9. Pemphigus vulgaris
Suprabasal acantholysis may also be seen in the outer
root sheath of hairs. In the epidermis, an old bulla shows
a base consisting of more than one layer of cells. ($\times 200$)

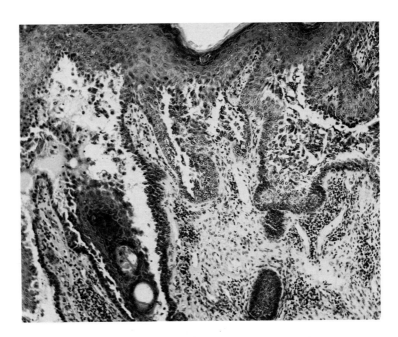

Fig. 7-10.   Pemphigus vulgaris
An intraepidermal, predominantly supra-basal bulla is visible. The bulla cavity contains many acantholytic cells. In addition, there is irregular upward growth of papillae lined predominantly by a single layer of epidermal cells, so-called villi. (×200)

cell layer still adherent to the dermis. During the stage of healing, there may be considerable irregular upward proliferation of villi and downward growth of epidermal strands (Fig. 7-10). The histologic picture then approaches that of pemphigus vegetans.

The dermis beneath early bullae usually shows only slight inflammation, although a few eosinophils generally are present beneath and within the bullae. In old lesions, the number of inflammatory cells, including eosinophils and plasma cells, may be considerable.

In patients with only oral lesions, intact blisters are rarely encountered, and specimens for biopsy are thus best taken from the active border of a denuded area by means of a biopsy punch.

Cytologic examination (Tzanck) is useful for the rapid demonstration of acantholytic epidermal cells in the bullae of pemphigus vulgaris. For this purpose, a smear is taken from the base of an early, freshly opened bulla. The smear is fixed in absolute alcohol for 10 min and then stained with a Giemsa or Papanicolaou stain. However, since acantholytic epidermal cells are occasionally seen also in various nonacantholytic vesiculobullous or pustular diseases as a result of secondary acantholysis, cytologic examination represents merely a preliminary test and should not supplant the histologic examination (Graham et al).

Histogenesis. *Electron microscopic examination* of very early lesions shows that, wherever there is beginning acantholysis, the intercellular cement substance, or glycocalyx, is partially or entirely dissolved (Hashimoto and Lever, 1967a). This phenomenon is best observed in the oral mucosa, where the epithelial cells have only few desmosomes and are held together largely by the intercellular cement substance. Concomitant with the dissolution of the intercellular substance, one observes widening of intercellular spaces while intact desmosomes are still present. Similarly, in the epidermis, where the cells have many more and better developed desmosomes than in the oral mucosa, one observes dissolution of the intercellular cement substance when the desmosomes are still intact. On widening of the intercellular spaces, separation of the two opposing attachment plaques of a desmosome may occur, so that single attachment plaques are seen at the periphery of a cell, the tonofilaments still adherent to them (Hashimoto and Lever, 1967b). As acantholysis progresses, the desmosomes gradually disappear, and the epidermal cells develop numerous cytoplasmic processes that often interdigitate with one another (EM 20). That dissolution of the intercellular cement substance is the primary event in acantholysis is particularly well demonstrated by staining of the intercellular substance with ruthenium red. Adjoining epidermal or oral epithelial cells then are often seen to be still partially attached to one another by the intercellular cement substance which is stained. Wherever two adjoining cells are separated from one another, one merely sees small particles of the stained intercellular substance attached to the plasma membrane of the cells as granular, amorphous material (Hashimoto and Lever, 1970). Immunoelectron microscopy, for which peroxidase rather than fluorescein is coupled to antihuman IgG, shows the reaction product, indicative of the location of the pemphigus antibodies, in the intercellular space in a pattern very similar to that obtained with ruthenium red (Hönigsmann et al).

All the early changes in pemphigus vulgaris are extracellular. Only subsequent to the dissolution of the desmosomes does one find retraction of the tonofilaments to the perinuclear area (EM 20) and, ultimately, degeneration of the acantholytic cells. As a rule, no dyskeratosis occurs because of this degeneration.

The reason the cohesion of the basal cells with the dermis is not affected in pemphigus vulgaris (EM 21) lies in the preservation of the structures connecting the basal cells with the dermis. These structures include the half-desmosomes, the anchoring filaments traversing the lamina lucida and attaching themselves to the basement membrane, or basal lamina, and the anchoring fibrils extending from the basement membrane into the dermis (see p. 12). The connection between basal cells and dermis thus contains no intercellular cement substance and therefore remains intact even at a stage at which the basal cells show severe damage.

IMMUNOFLUORESCENCE TESTING. For direct immunofluorescence testing of the skin of patients with pemphigus vulgaris, unfixed, frozen sections of perilesional or normal skin are used. Fluorescein-labeled antihuman IgG, IgA, IgM, and C3 are applied to various sections. In a positive test, there is fluorescence of the intercellular spaces of the epidermis. The antibodies thus are seen at exactly the site at which blister formation takes place. In a positive direct test, IgG is almost invariably present, and, in about half of the patients, there are deposits also of IgA, IgM, and/or C3. The direct immunofluorescence test is a very reliable diagnostic test for pemphigus vulgaris, since it is positive in close to 100% of the patients, including even those who are in the very early stage of the disease and show only a few lesions. It remains positive often for many years after the disease has subsided (Judd and Lever).

For indirect immunofluorescence testing, unfixed frozen sections of either guinea pig or monkey esophagus are used as substrate. First the patient's serum and then fluorescein-labeled antihuman IgG are applied at various dilutions to these sections. (Only IgG is applied, since the circulating pemphigus antibodies are always of the IgG class.) In a positive test, there is fluorescence of the intercellular spaces of the esophagus mucosa (Fig. 7-11). The highest dilution of the serum that still shows fluorescence indicates the antibody titer. Fluorescence at dilutions of 1:20 or 1:40 indicates a low titer, at dilutions of 1:80 or 1:160 a medium high titer, and at dilutions of 1:320 or more a high titer. In many instances, the titer of antibodies in the sera of patients with pemphigus vulgaris is proportional to the severity of the disease; however, there are too many exceptions to this for the titer to be regarded as a reliable indicator of disease severity (Judd and Lever; Fitzpatrick and Newcomer; Creswell et al; Barrière). Also, considerable discrepancies in the titer may be seen with different substrates (Judd and Mescon). In addition, the indirect test is less sensitive than the direct test, so that it is sometimes negative in patients with early, localized disease (Tuffanelli; Judd and Lever).

PATHOGENICITY OF PEMPHIGUS ANTIBODY. Convincing experiments about the role of pemphigus antibodies in the production of acantholysis have been carried out in vitro. In these experiments, normal human skin was maintained in organ cultures to which serum of patients with pemphigus vulgaris was added. Direct immunofluorescence staining of the explants with fluorescein-labeled goat antihuman IgG showed that, after an incubation of 6 hr, binding of the pemphigus IgG had occurred in the intercellular spaces of the epidermis. After 24 hr, suprabasal acantholysis was seen (Michel and Ko). Partially purified IgG fraction from the pooled serum of patients with pemphigus vulgaris had the same in vitro effect as

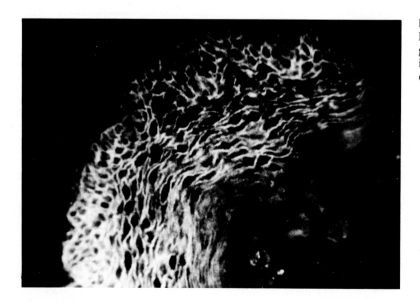

Fig. 7-11. Pemphigus vulgaris
Indirect immunofluorescence testing with guinea pig esophagus as substrate. There is fluorescence of the intercellular spaces of the esophageal mucosa.

whole serum, proving that it is the IgG fraction of pemphigus serum that is responsible for the acantholysis (Schiltz and Michel).

Differential Diagnosis.
In early bullae that are free of secondary changes such as degeneration or regeneration of epidermal cells, the histologic picture of pemphigus vulgaris is highly diagnostic. There are only three conditions that may have the same histologic appearance: pemphigus vegetans, familial benign pemphigus, and transient acantholytic dermatosis. Since pemphigus vegetans is merely a variant of pemphigus vulgaris, they quite naturally resemble each other. However, the histologic resemblance of the other two diseases to pemphigus vulgaris is curious, since they have little in common clinically. If difficulties arise in differentiation, direct immunofluorescence testing is advisable, since only pemphigus vulgaris has intercellular antibodies. (For differentiation of pemphigus vulgaris from familial benign pemphigus, see p. 73; for differentiation from transient acantholytic dermatosis, see p. 127.)

Pemphigus Vegetans

There are two types of pemphigus vegetans, the Neumann type and the Hallopeau type. In the Neumann type, the disease begins and ends as pemphigus vulgaris, differing from that disorder only by having many of the denuded areas heal not with normal skin but instead with verrucous vegetations that, in their early stage, sometimes are studded with small pustules.

The Hallopeau type of pemphigus vegetans, also referred to as pyodermite végétante, is relatively benign. Instead of bullae, pustules are the primary lesions. Their occurrence is followed by the formation of gradually extending verrucous vegetations, especially in the intertriginous areas. Oral lesions are present almost invariably in both types of pemphigus vegetans.

Histopathology.
In the usual type of pemphigus vegetans, the *Neumann type*, the early lesions, consisting of bullae and denuded areas, show essentially the same histologic picture as that seen in pemphigus vulgaris. However, the formation of villi and the downward proliferation of epithelial strands are much more pronounced than in pemphigus vulgaris (see Fig. 7-10). The verrucous vegetations that develop subsequently are characterized by considerable papillomatosis and acanthosis. Although acantholysis often is no longer apparent, one not infrequently observes intraepidermal abscesses composed almost entirely of eosinophils (Fig. 7-12). These abscesses are highly diagnostic of pemphigus vegetans (Lever, 1965). Old vegetations merely show considerable papillomatosis and hyperkeratosis with few or no eosinophils, so that the histologic picture is no longer diagnostic.

Fig. 7-12. Pemphigus vegetans
The section, obtained from a verrucous vegetation, shows considerable acanthosis and intraepidermal abscesses composed almost entirely of eosinophils. (×100)

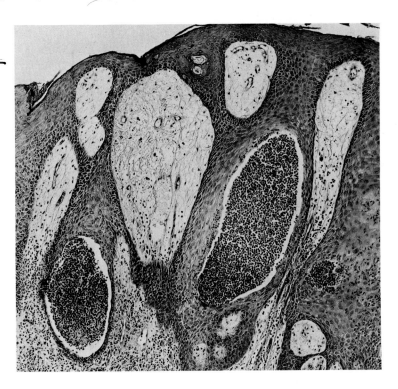

In the *Hallopeau type* of pemphigus vegetans, the early lesions, consisting of pustules arising on normal skin, show acantholysis with formation of small clefts and cavities, many in a suprabasal location. These cavities are filled with numerous eosinophils and degenerated, acantholytic epidermal cells (Röckl). A pronounced inflammatory infiltrate composed largely of eosinophils is present both in the epidermis, where it may present the histologic picture of eosinophilic spongiosis (Pearson et al), and in the dermis. The late verrucous vegetations, including the intraepidermal eosinophilic abscesses, show the same histologic picture as those of the Neumann type of pemphigus vegetans.

Histogenesis. Pemphigus vegetans is a variant of pemphigus vulgaris occurring in patients who have an increased resistance to their disease. This increased resistance finds its expression in the presence of numerous eosinophils. Specific intercellular antibodies are demonstrable by immunofluorescence in the epidermis and usually also in the blood serum (Nelson et al; Neumann and Faber).

Differential Diagnosis. There has been some controversy as to whether pemphigus vegetans of Hallopeau and pyodermite végétante (pyoderma vegetans) are separate diseases. The literature contains cases described with the designation *pyodermite végétante of Hallopeau* (pyoderma vegetans) that clearly are not pemphigus vegetans; they show no oral lesions, no acantholysis, and no positive immunofluorescence (Forman; Ruzicka and Goetz). It is advisable, therefore, to avoid the ambiguous term *pyodermite végétante* entirely and to distinguish between pemphigus vegetans of Hallopeau, in which immunofluorescence studies are positive, and pyoderma vegetans, also referred to as blastomycosislike pyoderma, in which they are negative (see p. 294). Clearly, immunofluorescence studies are the key in this controversy (Nelson; Lever, 1979).

Pemphigus Foliaceus

Pemphigus foliaceus begins with flaccid bullae that usually arise on an erythematous base. Erythema, oozing, and crusting are present from the beginning, not only around the bullae but also in other areas. The bullae break easily and, because of their superficial location, leave shallow erosions, rather than denuded areas as in pemphigus vulgaris. Gradual extension of the lesions may lead to involvement of most of if not the entire body surface. In the advanced stage, bullae are few and

may even be absent, so that the resemblance to generalized exfoliative dermatitis is great. However, pemphigus foliaceus has a positive Nikolsky sign, in contrast to generalized exfoliative dermatitis. Also, the presence of thick hyperkeratotic scales in some areas of erythema is common. In contrast with pemphigus vulgaris, oral lesions do not occur. Even before corticosteroids became available, the prognosis of pemphigus foliaceus was better than that of pemphigus vulgaris.

In some instances, pemphigus foliaceus in its initial stage presents a clinical picture suggestive of dermatitis herpetiformis, showing grouped papules, vesicles, and bullae as well as erythematous patches with vesicles at their periphery (Winkelmann and Roth; Osteen et al). Some of the patients with this clinical picture respond well to the administration of sulfonamides or sulfones. The histologic picture, however, is that of pemphigus foliaceus. The term *pemphigus herpetiformis* is used for this variant (Jablonska et al, 1975; Haensch; Lagerholm et al).

Fogo selvagem, a disease endemic in some parts of Brazil, is clinically, histologically, and immunologically indistinguishable from pemphigus foliaceus (Beutner et al) and can be regarded as identical with it (Furtado).

Histopathology. The earliest change in pemphigus foliaceus consists of the appearance of areas of acantholysis in the upper epidermis, usually in the granular layer or right beneath it, leading to the formation of a cleft in a superficial, often subcorneal, location (Lever, 1965; Perry and Brunsting).

This cleft may develop into a bulla, with acantholysis present at its floor as well as at its roof (Fig. 7-13). Usually, however, enlargement of the cleft leads to detachment of the uppermost epidermis without formation of a bulla (Fig. 7-14). The cells bordering the cleft show an absence of intercellular bridges and a tendency to break off into the space formed by the cleft. It should be emphasized that the number of acantholytic cells bordering the bullae and clefts in pemphigus foliaceus is often small, requiring a careful search for them. Occasionally, secondary clefts develop, resulting in detachment within the middle section of the epidermis. Detachment immediately above the basal layer, as seen typically in pemphigus vulgaris, occurs only very rarely and then over limited areas (Perry).

Old lesions show acanthosis, a mild degree of papillomatosis, and, in addition, hyperkeratosis and parakeratosis. The hyperkeratosis may be associated with keratotic plugging of the follicles. In areas of hyperkeratosis, the thickness of the granular layer is increased. A striking change frequently observed in old lesions of pemphigus foliaceus and

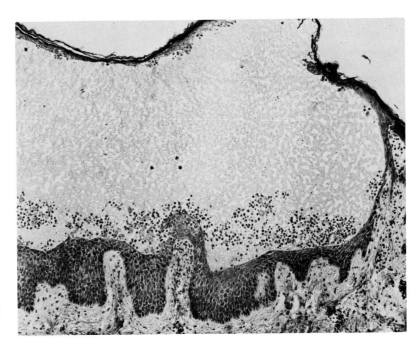

Fig. 7-13. Pemphigus foliaceus
An intact bulla is in a superficial, partly subcorneal position. Acantholysis is present at the base, as well as at the top, of the bulla. (×100)

Fig. 7-14. Pemphigus foliaceus
An early lesion shows detachment of the horny layer and part of the granular layer without bulla formation. The epidermal cells at the base of the cleft show a loss of intercellular bridges resulting in acantholysis. (×200)

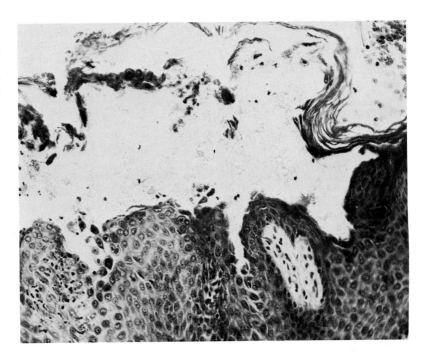

diagnostic for this disease is the presence of dyskeratotic changes in cells of the granular layer (Fig. 7-15). The granular cells show acantholysis and appear deeply basophilic and shrunken, thus resembling the grains of Darier's disease.

The dermis shows a moderate number of inflammatory cells, among which eosinophils are often present.

Eosinophilic spongiosis, already mentioned in the descriptions of pemphigus vulgaris and pemphigus vegetans, can be seen also in pemphigus foliaceus, particularly in the variant referred to as pemphigus herpetiformis. Permeation of the epidermis with eosinophils and intraepidermal eosinophilic pustules are seen together with acantholysis. The latter may be quite inconspicuous initially

111

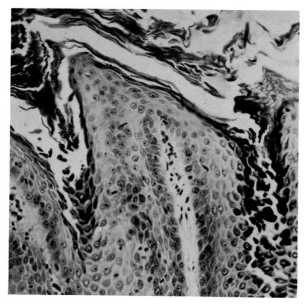

Fig. 7-15.   Pemphigus foliaceus
This represents a late lesion showing considerable acanthosis and hyperkeratosis with cleft formation and acantholysis in the granular layer. The granular cells appear shrunken and hyperchromatic; thus, they resemble the grains of Darier's disease. (× 200)

(Emmerson and Wilson Jones; Jablonska et al, 1975; Lagerholm et al). Direct immunofluorescence, however, shows intercellular immunofluorescence.

Histogenesis. *Electron microscopic examination* reveals some early loss of intercellular cement substance in the lower epidermis associated with a decrease in the number of desmosomes and replacement by tortuous microvilli. However, acantholysis is most pronounced in the upper layers of the epidermis (EM 22) (Lever and Hashimoto). In the midepidermis, many cells show perinuclear arrangement of the tonofilaments and homogenization of the perinuclear tonofilament bundles as evidence of dyskeratosis. The presence of marked dyskeratosis distinguishes pemphigus foliaceus from pemphigus vulgaris (Wilgram et al).
Immunofluorescence testing shows the autoantibodies encountered in pemphigus foliaceus to be identical with those found in pemphigus vulgaris. They are IgG antibodies and are present regularly in the intercellular spaces of the epidermis and usually also in the blood serum.

Differential Diagnosis.   The location of the bullae in pemphigus foliaceus is the same as in subcorneal pustular dermatosis and in impetigo. For their differentiation, see Subcorneal Pustular Dermatosis, p. 126.

Pemphigus Erythematosus

Pemphigus erythematosus (Senear–Usher syndrome) represents either an abortive form or an initial stage of pemphigus foliaceus. In the former case, the eruption remains localized; in the latter case, it advances gradually into pemphigus foliaceus. Clinically, the lesions are the same as in pemphigus foliaceus. There is some clinical resemblance to lupus erythematosus and seborrheic dermatitis both in localization and in appearance. Thus, facial lesions may show follicular hyperkeratosis, although atrophy as in lupus erythematosus does not occur.

Histopathology.   The histopathologic picture is identical with that of pemphigus foliaceus (Lever, 1965; Perry and Brunsting). In old lesions, follicular hyperkeratosis with acantholysis and dyskeratosis of the granular layer often is pronounced.

Histogenesis. Pemphigus erythematosus is identical with pemphigus foliaceus in its *electron microscopic* and *immunologic* manifestations. Although pemphigus erythematosus is the mildest form of pemphigus, it is the one most commonly found in clinical association with other autoimmune diseases, especially myasthenia gravis and thymoma (Tagami et al). There also are a few instances of clinical coexistence with lupus erythematosus (Orfanos et al; Jablonska et al, 1977). Much more common than the clinical association is the immunologic association of pemphigus erythematosus with lupus erythematosus. The presence of a "lupus erythematosus band" in the uppermost dermis, in addition to the presence of intercellular pemphigus antibodies in the epidermis, is surprisingly common. Thus, in a large series of 48 patients with pemphigus erythematosus, a "lupus band" was found not only in 81% of the skin specimens taken from exposed lesions but also in 23% of the skin specimens taken from unexposed lesions (Jablonska et al, 1977). This finding is best regarded as a "serologic stigma" (Thivolet et al) rather than as evidence of the coexistence of pemphigus erythematosus and lupus erythematosus (Chorzelski et al).

Differential Diagnosis.   The lesions of pemphigus erythematosus may clinically resemble those of lupus erythematosus, but they differ sufficiently in their histologic appearance to make differentiation possible. Even though both diseases may show follicular hyperkeratosis, one observes acantholytic and dyskeratotic changes in the granular layer only in pemphigus erythematosus, and hydropic degeneration in the basal cell layer and a patchy inflammatory infiltrate in the dermis only in lupus erythematosus. If bullae are present in pemphigus erythematosus, they are located in the upper layers of the epidermis; in contrast, in lupus erythematosus, they have a subepidermal location, since they form secondary to the hydropic degeneration of the basal layer.

BULLOUS PEMPHIGOID

Bullous pemphigoid, first described in 1953 (Lever), usually shows large, tense bullae over wide areas. Commonly, the groins, the axillae, and the flexor surfaces of the forearms show the largest number of bullae. When the bullae break, the resulting denuded areas in most cases do not materially increase in size as they do in pemphigus vulgaris; rather, they show a tendency to heal. In addition to bullae, there also are areas of erythema with an irregular outline and central clearing. Bullae arise not only on noninflamed skin but also within the areas of erythema. Involvement of the oral mucosa is found in about one third of the cases and is usually mild. Bullous pemphigoid most commonly occurs in elderly persons but occasionally is seen in young adults and even in children. (For a discussion of the occurrence of bullous pemphigoid in children, see Chronic Bullous Dermatosis of Childhood, p. 121.) Although in aged, debilitated people, the disease may result in death, the prognosis in well-preserved individuals usually was good even prior to the availability of corticosteroids, the disease usually subsiding after several months or years. Occasionally, there are recurrences.

Three variants of bullous pemphigoid exist: localized, vesicular, and vegetating. The localized variant most commonly occurs on the lower extremities (Person et al). In vesicular pemphigoid, the blisters are small, tense, and occasionally grouped (Bean et al). In vegetating pemphigoid, verrucous vegetations are found mainly in the axillae and groins (Winkelmann and Su; Kuokkanen and Helin). An association with malignant neoplasms has often been described in individual cases of bullous pemphigoid, but evaluation of large series of cases has not borne out such an association (Ahmed et al, 1977a; Stone and Schroeter). It has been suggested that concurrent malignant disease is prevalent only in patients without circulating antibodies, occurring in 23% of these cases (Hodge et al).

On rare occasions, bullous pemphigoid has been induced by the treatment of renal failure with furosemide (see p. 420).

Histopathology.   The dermal changes in bullous pemphigoid differ, depending on whether the bulla selected for biopsy is located on normal-appearing or on erythematous skin. Since the histologic findings in erythematous skin are often of diagnostic value, it is recommended that specimens for biopsy be taken from early bullae arising on an erythematous base.

The epidermal changes are the same in both inflamed and noninflamed skin and consist of bullae arising through detachment of the epidermis from the dermis (Fig. 7-16) (Lever, 1953; Rook and Waddington). Early bullae are found fully beneath the epidermis, but, after two days, one can already observe regeneration of the epidermis at the floor of the bullae, beginning at the periphery and extending gradually over the entire floor (Fig. 7-17). This regeneration results in an intraepidermal location of the bullae. The epidermis at the roof of the bullae is intact at first but, in older bullae, may become necrotic and then, with the exception of the horny layer, disintegrate. In this way, the bullae that form subepidermally may ultimately become subcorneal in location.

Fig. 7-16.   Bullous pemphigoid
A large subepidermal bulla is shown. The bulla contains a net of fibrin but only few inflammatory cells. (×100)

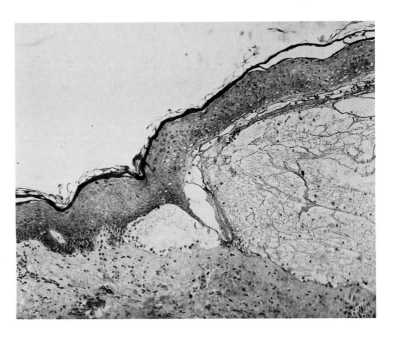

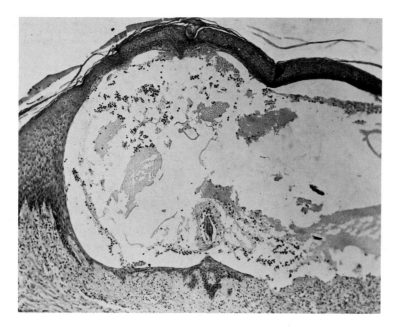

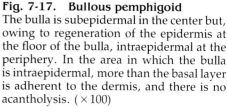

Fig. 7-17. Bullous pemphigoid
The bulla is subepidermal in the center but, owing to regeneration of the epidermis at the floor of the bulla, intraepidermal at the periphery. In the area in which the bulla is intraepidermal, more than the basal layer is adherent to the dermis, and there is no acantholysis. (×100)

Fig. 7-18. Bullous pemphigoid
Bulla arising on erythematous skin. In the dermis and the cavity of the bulla is an inflammatory infiltrate containing many eosinophils. (×200)

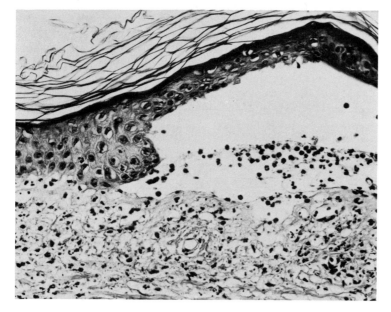

The dermal changes in noninflammatory bullae generally are slight. Beneath the bullae, the dermis shows a rather sparse perivascular infiltrate consisting mainly of mononuclear cells with an admixture of a few eosinophils. The bulla cavity may also contain a few eosinophils within a net of fibrin (see Fig. 7-16) (Kresbach and Hartwagner; van der Meer; Eng and Moncada).

In contrast, the dermal changes in inflammatory bullae consist of extensive accumulations of usually numerous eosinophils intermingled with mononuclear cells and some neutrophils. This infiltrate is seen around the upper dermal blood vessels, in the upper dermis, often in close approximation to the epidermis, and in the bulla cavity. The infiltrate extends beyond the bullae in the upper dermis (Fig. 7-18). At the periphery of some bullae, one may see microabscesses at the tips of papillae that are composed largely of eosinophils (Fig. 7-19) (Jablonska and Chorzelski; van der Meer). They are similar to the papillary microabscesses seen in dermatitis herpetiformis, in which, however, the predominant cells are neutrophils.

In pemphigoid vegetans, one observes pseudocarcinomatous hyperplasia of the epidermis, in addition to subepidermal bulla formation and accumulations of eosinophils and mononuclear cells (Winkelmann and Su; Kuokkanen and Helin).

Histogenesis. Most *electron microscopic examinations* in bullous pemphigoid have been carried out on noninflammatory bullae and have shown formation of the bullae between the plasma membrane of basal cells and the electron-dense basement membrane, that is, within the lamina lucida (EM 23) (Braun-Falco and Rupec). Separation of the basal cells from the basement membrane takes place as a result of the tearing and subsequent disappearance of the anchoring filaments (Kobayasi; Lever and Hashimoto). As the blister forms, one observes not only the disappearance of the half-desmosomes and damage to the plasma membrane of the basal cells but also degenerative alterations within the cytoplasm of the basal cells and intercellular edema between the basal cells (Jakubowicz et al).

In contrast, in inflammatory lesions of bullous pemphigoid, the earliest finding is a pronounced cellular infiltrate of eosinophils and histiocytes in the dermis (Schaumburg-Lever et al, 1972). Subsequently, the basement membrane develops small discontinuities that progress to fragmentation and disappearance of large portions of the basement membrane even before a bulla has formed. When eosinophils migrate into the epidermis and degranulate, a blister forms. In a fully developed blister, the basement membrane is usually destroyed (EM 24), as it is in dermatitis herpetiformis. Also, again as in dermatitis herpetiformis, precipitates of fibrin and amorphous protein are seen in the uppermost dermis.

The sequence of events in bullous pemphigoid is thought to be antibody deposition at the cutaneous dermal-epidermal junction followed by mast cell degranulation resulting in a release of chemotactic factors for eosinophils (Dvorak et al). Accumulation of eosinophils is followed by their degranulation. The release of proteolytic enzymes present in their granules is thought to cause damage to the lamina lucida and thus to initiate the blister formation in bullous pemphigoid (Dubertret et al).

IMMUNOFLUORESCENCE TESTING. For direct immunofluorescence testing, unfixed frozen sections of perilesional skin are used. In a positive test, linear immunofluorescence is seen along the basement membrane zone (Fig. 7-20). Thus, in bullous pemphigoid, as in pemphigus, the in vivo bound antibodies are seen at exactly the site at which blister formation takes place. Whenever immunoglobulins are present, IgG is found (Jordon et al, 1971). Occasionally, IgG is absent, especially in early disease, and only C3 is found. However, IgG then may be found a few weeks later (Ahmed et al, 1977b). IgA

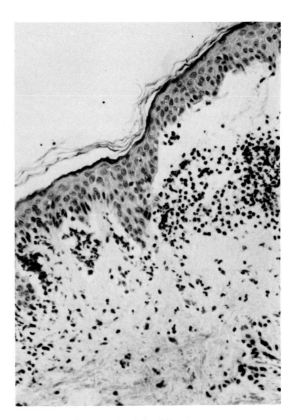

Fig. 7-19. Bullous pemphigoid
At its periphery, an inflammatory bulla arising on erythematous skin shows microabscesses at the tips of papillae that are similar to those seen in dermatitis herpetiformis. The predominant cell type, however, is eosinophils, in contrast with dermatitis herpetiformis, in which neutrophils usually predominate. ($\times 100$)

and IgM are each present in about 25% of the cases. The direct immunofluorescence test is a very reliable diagnostic assay for bullous pemphigoid, since it is positive in close to 100% of the patients.

Indirect immunofluorescence testing, for which either guinea pig or monkey esophagus is used as substrate, is much less sensitive than direct testing, since circulating antibodies are encountered in only about 70% of the cases (Person and Rogers; Ahmed et al, 1977b). If antibodies are present, they always are of the IgG class. No correlation exists between the titer and the clinical condition of the patient (Sams and Jordon; Person and Rogers).

The electron microscopic localization of the in vivo bound IgG has been investigated by the coupling of peroxidase to antihuman gamma-globulin. This has shown that the IgG is located above the basement membrane within the lamina lucida (Schaumburg-Lever et al, 1975; Holubar et al). Thus, the localization differs from the "lupus band" in lupus erythematosus, in which immunoglobulins are found mainly below the basement

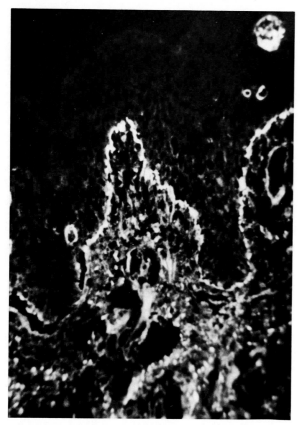

Fig. 7-20.   Bullous pemphigoid
Direct immunofluorescence test. Linear immunofluorescence is seen along the basement membrane zone.

membrane (Ueki et al). Analogous to the electron microscopic findings, immunofluorescence testing has shown that antibodies against type IV collagen, that is, against basement membrane collagen, are located on the floor of the blister (Weber et al).

PATHOGENICITY OF BULLOUS PEMPHIGOID ANTIBODIES. In cultures of normal human skin, separation of the epidermis from the dermis takes place on incubation with antibody containing blister fluid from patients with bullous pemphigoid but not on incubation with blood serum from such patients. The reason for this discrepancy is not known. In contrast to pemphigus, in which in vitro acantholysis occurs even in the absence of complement, complement must be present in bullous pemphigoid for the in vitro dermal-epidermal separation to occur (Naito et al).

Differential Diagnosis. Histologic differentiation of bullous pemphigoid from *pemphigus vulgaris* is not difficult, because, even though the bullae in bullous pemphigoid may be located within the epidermis as a result of regeneration, they are never found above a "tombstone" row of basal cells (see p. 106), and acantholytic cells are not present in the bulla cavity. However, differentiation from other diseases associated with subepidermal bullae often is impossible. Bullae removed from areas without inflammation may not show any eosinophils and then are indistinguishable from bullae of epidermolysis bullosa or porphyria cutanea tarda. In contrast, bullae removed from areas of inflammation and showing an inflammatory infiltrate may be very difficult to differentiate from bullae occurring in cicatricial pemphigoid and dermatitis herpetiformis.

Differentiation of *cicatricial pemphigoid* from bullous pemphigoid may be impossible, since the bullae in both conditions may contain eosinophils in their infiltrate. The immunofluorescence findings are also essentially the same.

Differentiation of *dermatitis herpetiformis* from bullous pemphigoid lies in the degree rather than the type of changes, since (1) in dermatitis herpetiformis, papillary microabscesses are present in great number, extending over several neighboring papillae and resulting in a multilocular blister, whereas, in bullous pemphigoid, microabscesses are seen only rarely and then at the periphery of a blister; and (2) in dermatitis herpetiformis, especially in early lesions, neutrophils predominate over eosinophils. However, differentiation can be impossible, since, in dermatitis herpetiformis, eosinophils and neutrophils occasionally are present in about equal proportions, and, in some cases, eosinophils even predominate (Connor et al); and, conversely, the papillary microabscesses in bullous pemphigoid at times are composed largely of neutrophils (Person and Rogers).

In cases in which a reliable differentiation cannot be made on the basis of the clinical and histologic findings, indirect and direct immunofluorescence testing can be of great value (Lever, 1979), because (1) on indirect testing, dermatitis herpetiformis only rarely shows circulating IgA antibodies, whereas bullous pemphigoid has circulating IgG in 70% of the cases; (2) on direct testing, dermatitis herpetiformis in 80% of the cases shows granular deposits of IgA and only in 20% shows linear deposits like those seen in bullous pemphigoid; and (3) the linear deposits in dermatitis herpetiformis usually are composed only of IgA, and those in bullous pemphigoid only of IgG. However, in rare instances, both dermatitis herpetiformis and bullous pemphigoid may show linear deposits of IgA as well as IgG in the absence of circulating antibodies (Jablonska et al). In such a situation, immunoelectron microscopy may be carried out, because, in some instances, the linear deposits in dermatitis herpetiformis are not above the basement membrane, as in bullous pemphigoid, but rather below it (see p. 121).

Differentiation of *erythema multiforme* from bullous pemphigoid is usually possible, since, in spite of the variability of the histologic picture from case to case, one finds in erythema multiforme that (1) eosinophils, if present at all, are located largely perivascularly and not near the epidermis; (2) if cells are seen near the dermal-epidermal junction, they are mononuclear cells rather than eosinophils; and (3) epidermal changes often are prominent even in early lesions, in which they consist sometimes of exocytosis, spongiosis, and intracellular edema and sometimes of necrotic changes affecting either individual keratinocytes or the entire epidermis.

CICATRICIAL PEMPHIGOID

Cicatricial pemphigoid is characterized by its chronic course, its scarring nature, and its predilection for the mucosal surfaces. Small blisters resulting in erosions are found most commonly on the oral mucosa but occasionally also on the mucous membranes of the larynx, esophagus, nose, vulva, and anus. Scarring occurs occasionally on these mucous membranes. The conjunctivae are frequently but not invariably inflamed without, however, showing blisters. Scarring to the point of near blindness commonly results. Cutaneous lesions are present in about one fourth of the patients and may be of two types: (1) a more or less extensive eruption of bullae that heal without scarring (Lever, 1953); Behlen and Mackay; Brauner and Jimbow), and (2) areas of erythema, mainly on the face and scalp, in which bullae erupt intermittently, ultimately followed by atrophic scarring (Lever, 1942, 1944; Hardy et al). Both types of eruption may be present in the same patient (Kleine-Natrop and Haustein; Tagami and Imamura).

In the variant referred to as the Brunsting-Perry type, there are no mucosal lesions but instead one or several circumscribed erythematous patches on which recurrent crops of blisters appear. Ultimately, atrophic scarring results. The patches are generally confined to the head and neck (Brunsting and Perry; Michel et al). Two variants of the Brunsting-Perry type of cicatricial pemphigoid have been described. In one, there is a widespread, nonscarring bullous eruption in addition to scarring lesions on the head (Hanno et al). In the other, there are widespread bullous lesions that heal with atrophic scars (Provost et al; Braun-Falco et al).

Histopathology.   The bullae on the skin and mucous membranes form subepidermally. In cases with a more or less extensive eruption of bullae in which the bullae heal without scarring, the dermis usually shows only a slight to moderate perivascular infiltrate in which eosinophils may be present (Kleine-Natrop and Haustein) or absent (Behlen and Mackay). The bullae in areas of scarring often show a considerable chronic inflammatory infiltrate and, in late stages, fibrosis.

Histogenesis. *Electron microscopic studies* have revealed in some instances that the oral lesions (Susi and Shklar) and the cutaneous lesions (Brauner and Jimbow) possess an intact basement membrane at the base of the blister. In another study, however, the basement membrane of both the cutaneous and oral lesions was found to be largely destroyed (Caputo et al). The findings are analogous to those made in bullous pemphigoid, in which the basement membrane too may be preserved or destroyed (see p. 115).

IMMUNOFLUORESCENCE TESTING. Direct immunofluorescence testing of lesional or perilesional skin has shown in the majority of the patients in vivo fixed immunoglobulins and/or complement in the basement membrane zone. In the three largest series, a total of 35 of 46 patients showed linear deposits (Bean; Griffith et al; Rogers et al). In most of the tested patients, both IgG and C3 were present, occasionally in association with IgA and/or IgM. However, there were cases in which only C3 was present and others in which IgA was the only immunoglobulin (Rogers et al).

Of the eight patients with the Brunsting-Perry type of cicatricial pemphigoid in whom direct immunofluorescence was carried out, seven showed the presence of IgG. Two of them also showed the presence of C3 (Michel et al; Jacoby et al).

Circulating basement membrane zone antibodies can be demonstrated only rarely. Thus, in one series, IgG was found in only 3 of 12 patients at low titers of 1:20 or less (Bean), and, in another series, IgG was demonstrated in 2 of 23 patients, but only temporarily (Rogers et al). However, in individual patients with unusually widespread involvement, circulating IgG antibodies have been demonstrated at titers of 1:40 and 1:80 (Dantzig; Tagami and Imamura).

The frequent presence of in vivo fixed deposits along the basement membrane zone in cicatricial pemphigoid and the occasional presence of circulating anti-basement membrane zone antibodies has suggested to some authors that cicatricial pemphigoid and bullous pemphigoid are variants of the same disease process (Bean; Rogers et al). However, the clinical manifestations of the two diseases are quite different and distinct. The situation thus is analogous to that of pemphigus vulgaris and pemphigus foliaceus, which clinically are also different and distinct diseases, even though the immunologic findings are the same for both.

HERPES GESTATIONIS

Herpes gestationis, a rare eruption occurring during pregnancy and puerperium, shows vesicles and bullae associated with areas of erythema and edema. Oral lesions are uncommon. Itching is severe. The clinical resemblance to bullous pemphigoid is often great.

The disease carries with it a significantly higher than normal fetal mortality rate (Lawley et al). In some instances, the baby is born with a mild vesicular or bullous eruption (Chorzelski et al; Katz et al).

Histopathology. In areas of erythema and edema, the dermis shows a perivascular infiltrate composed of mononuclear cells and many eosinophils. There is marked papillary edema. The epidermis shows spongiosis and intracellular edema (Piérard et al). There is focal necrosis of the basal cells, some of which have the appearance of colloid bodies as seen in lichen planus (Hertz et al). Eosinophils can be seen within the epidermis.

In bullous lesions, basal cell necrosis leads to the formation of subepidermal bullae (Hertz et al). A pronounced inflammatory infiltrate is present within and around the bullae. It consists mainly of eosinophils, many of which show fragmentation of their nuclei ("nuclear dust") (Schaumburg-Lever et al).

Histogenesis. *Electron microscopic examination* of the epidermis at the periphery of bullae shows significant damage, most pronounced in basal cells but present also in squamous cells and resulting in partial or complete necrosis of epidermal cells, with disappearance of their organelles but partial preservation of their desmosomes (Schaumburg-Lever et al). Although the basal cells show severe damage internally, the basal cell plasma membrane and the basement membrane usually are well preserved and are found at the floor of the bulla (EM 27). Even the half-desmosomes may still be found intact in some areas (Yaoita et al). Epidermal damage thus can be regarded as an important factor in bulla formation, just as it is in the epidermal type of erythema multiforme (Schaumburg-Lever et al).

IMMUNOFLUORESCENCE TESTING. Direct immunofluorescence testing of perilesional skin invariably shows linear deposition of C3 along the basement membrane zone. In addition, other complement factors, such as C1q, C4, and properdin may be present (Chorzelski et al). However, immunoglobulins are absent in approximately half of the cases. If present, IgG is always found, whereas IgA and IgM are only rarely encountered (Kocsis et al; Carruthers et al). Immunoelectron microscopy with peroxidase labeling reveals the localization of C3 and, if it is present, of IgG above the basement membrane within the lamina lucida (Hönigsmann et al; Yaoita et al). The localization thus is the same as in bullous pemphigoid.

Indirect immunofluorescence studies have identified circulating anti-basement membrane IgG antibodies in only a few instances (Reunala et al). Of interest is the presence in the blood serum of most patients with herpes gestationis of the so-called HG factor, first described in 1973 (Provost and Tomasi). This factor, a thermostable IgG, is capable of fixing in vitro C3 obtained from fresh, normal human serum along the basement membrane zone of normal human skin (Katz et al).

In several instances, even in the absence of lesions in the infant, testing of the cord blood or blood of an infant born to a mother with herpes gestationis has shown the presence of complement factors (Chorzelski et al), of the HG factor (Carruthers et al), and, when present in the mother's blood, of IgG (Reunala et al).

Differential Diagnosis. If may be difficult to differentiate herpes gestationis from inflammatory, cell-rich lesions of bullous pemphigoid, particularly since both have an infiltrate rich in eosinophils. However, the presence of necrotic basal cells is a feature that is not observed in bullous pemphigoid. Although the dermal-epidermal type of erythema multiforme shows epidermal necrosis and a dermal infiltrate, the infiltrate in this disorder shows hardly any eosinophils.

DERMATITIS HERPETIFORMIS

Dermatitis herpetiformis is a pruritic, very chronic disease displaying in symmetric distribution groups of papules and vesicles surrounded by erythema. In rare instances, a few bullae are present. The extensor surfaces of the extremities, the shoulders, and the buttocks are affected predominantly. Lesions of the oral mucosa are absent (Tolman et al). The eruption is well suppressed by sulfapyridine or the sulfones. Dermatitis herpetiformis most commonly starts in early adult life, although it may have its onset at any time, including childhood. (For a discussion of dermatitis herpetiformis in childhood, see Chronic Bullous Dermatosis of Childhood, p. 121.)

Linear IgA dermatosis differs from "classic" dermatitis herpetiformis by showing linear rather than granular deposits of IgA, as well as by the absence of a gluten-sensitive enteropathy and by differences in HLA-typing (see Histogenesis). Some authors believe that the clinical features seen in the linear type of the disorder are similar or identical to those seen in granular dermatitis herpetiformis and prefer *linear IgA dermatitis herpetiformis* as the designation (Lawley et al; Seah and Fry; Pehamberger et al, 1977). Other authors, however, believe that, in the linear type, bullae predominate in herpetiform clusters rather than papulovesicles, and they regard this form as a disease separate from dermatitis herpetiformis (Jablonska and Chorzelski, 1979; Dabrowski et al; Honeyman et al). Some authors who have proposed the term *linear IgA bullous dermatosis,* regard the disease as closely related to, if not identical with, chronic bullous dermatosis of childhood with linear IgA (see p. 121), even though, in the adult form, some cases show vesicles rather than bullae. Both the adult and the childhood forms of linear IgA bullous dermatosis differ from dermatitis herpetiformis by the absence of a gluten-sensitive enteropathy (Jablonska and Chorzelski, 1979, 1981; Dabrowski et al).

Histopathology. The typical histologic features of dermatitis herpetiformis are best seen in erythematous, not yet blistering areas located in the vicinity of early blisters. In these areas, one observes at the tips of adjoining papillae accumulations of neutrophils and usually also some eosinophils (Piérard). Early accumulations often consist entirely of neutrophils, whereas, with an increase

in size to microabscesses, they may have a significant admixture of eosinophils. As the microabscesses form, separations appear between the tips of adjoining papillae and the epidermis, so that early blisters are multilocular (Fig. 7-21) (van der Meer). The presence of fibrin in the papillae gives them a necrotic appearance. At first, the interpapillary ridges of the epidermis remain attached to the dermis, so that the blisters of dermatitis herpetiformis are multilocular when they are still too small to be clinically apparent. However, within one to two days, the rete ridges lose their coherence with the dermis, and the blisters then become unilocular and clinically apparent (Fig. 7-22) (MacVicar et al). At that time, one may often still see at the periphery of such unilocular blisters the characteristic papillary microabscesses. For this

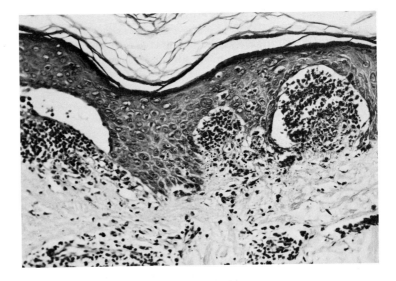

Fig. 7-21. Dermatitis herpetiformis
On the left side, part of an early blister is seen. On the right, two papillae show papillary microabscesses composed of neutrophils. The microabscesses cause separations between the tips of papillae and the epidermis, so that early blisters are multilocular. The presence of fibrin in the papillae gives them a necrotic appearance. (×200)

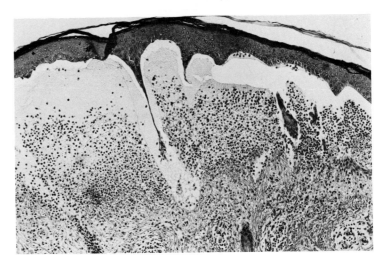

Fig. 7-22. Dermatitis herpetiformis
A fully developed blister is no longer multilocular. Some of the rete ridges that originally subdivided the blister can still be recognized. Most of the cells in the blister and around the dermal vessels are neutrophils. (×50)

reason, the inclusion of perivesicular skin in the biopsy specimen is of considerable value.

The subpapillary dermis usually shows a moderately severe inflammatory infiltrate of neutrophils and some eosinophils. Many neutrophils show disintegration of their nuclei to "nuclear dust." In addition, the underlying subpapillary vessels show a perivascular infiltrate composed of mononuclear cells as well as neutrophils and eosinophils (Kresbach and Hartwagner; Eng and Moncada).

The frequency with which papillary microabscesses have been found in various reported series of patients varies considerably. In one series, papillary microabscesses were present in all 14 patients examined (Kint et al). In another, larger, series of 105 biopsy specimens, papillary microabscesses were seen in only 52% of the cases (Connor et al). It can be assumed that, in the latter series, not all the reviewed specimens were from typical areas, that is, from erythematous, not yet blistering lesions in the vicinity of early blisters, because, in such locations, papillary microabscesses usually are present in dermatitis herpetiformis.

Histogenesis. The *electron microscopic* findings in dermatitis herpetiformis resemble the changes seen during development of the "inflammatory bullae" in bullous pemphigoid (Schaumburg-Lever et al). The only differences are the prevalence in the former of neutrophils over eosinophils, especially in early lesions, and the earlier appearance and greater amount of fibrin present (EM 25), particularly in dermal papillae, where it often is attached to the dermal side of the basement membrane

(EM 25, inset). In more advanced blisters, the basal lamina has disappeared in many areas (Piérard and Kint; Jakubowicz et al), as has been noted in the "inflammatory bullae" of bullous pemphigoid (EM 25, inset).

IMMUNOFLUORESCENCE TESTING. *Direct immunofluorescence testing* almost invariably shows deposits of IgA at the dermal-epidermal junction, provided that uninvolved skin is used for testing. In areas of vesicular lesions, no immunofluorescence is found, as a rule; even areas adjacent to lesions sometimes fail to reveal deposits (Chorzelski et al, 1971). It is likely that, in involved skin, the IgA deposits are destroyed through phagocytosis. In over 80% of the cases, the deposits found in uninvolved skin are granular; in 12% to 18% of the cases, they are linear (Seah and Fry; Katz and Strober). The concurrent presence of both the granular and linear patterns has been observed in only two cases (Seah and Fry). The granular deposits are often located only at the tips of the papillae (Fig. 7-23). In some instances, however, granular deposits are present also beneath the epidermal rete ridges and throughout the dermal papillae. Both granular and linear deposits of IgA are frequently associated with deposits of C3. Immunoglobulins other than IgA are found in about half of the patients with either granular or linear deposits of IgA (Katz and Strober). However, the association of IgA and IgG in the linear pattern is rare, having been observed in only a few cases of dermatitis herpetiformis (Seah et al; Jablonska et al, 1976); it is observed more often in bullous pemphigoid than in dermatitis herpetiformis (see p. 115).

On *immunoelectron microscopy* using staining with peroxidase, granular deposits appear as densely stained clumps and yarnlike fibrils in the dermis (Yaoita and Katz, 1976). They are localized beneath the basement

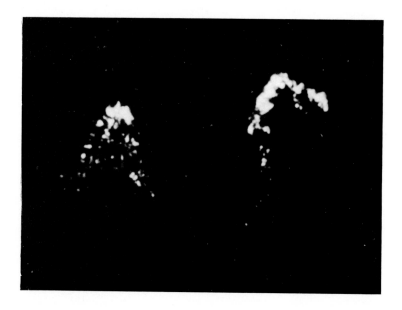

Fig. 7-23. Dermatitis herpetiformis
Direct immunofluorescence test. Granular deposits are seen at the tips of two subepidermal papillae.

membrane and the area of the anchoring fibrils and in some instances appear to be closely associated with bundles of microfibrils of the elastic fibers (Pehamberger et al, 1979). Linear deposits are seen in one of two locations: either in the lamina lucida, in a location identical with that seen in bullous pemphigoid, or beneath the basement membrane, limited to the area in which the anchoring fibrils are located (Yaoita and Katz, 1976; Pehamberger et al, 1977). In some instances, deposits have been seen in both locations (Dabrowski et al).

On *indirect immunofluorescence testing*, circulating anti-basement membrane zone antibodies of the IgA class are encountered only in about 2% of the cases of dermatitis herpetiformis with granular deposits (Yaoita and Katz, 1977). In contrast, in linear dermatitis herpetiformis, circulating IgA antibodies are present in about one third of the cases (Yaoita and Katz, 1977; Honeyman et al). They have been found in patients with either type of linear IgA deposit (Yaoita and Katz, 1977).

A *gluten-sensitive enteropathy* can be demonstrated in nearly all patients with the granular type of dermatitis herpetiformis, whereas patients with the linear type are free from it (Jablonska and Chorzelski, 1979; Lawley et al). The steatorrhea in patients with the granular type of dermatitis herpetiformis usually is mild and asymptomatic, but, when multiple jejunal suction biopsies are taken, evidence of celiac disease, consisting of villous atrophy and a raised intraepithelial lymphocyte count, can be found (Marks; Thune et al). In every patient on a gluten-free diet, the jejunal lesions improve greatly (Reunala). The cutaneous lesions are less responsive: although most patients improve somewhat, only one quarter to one half become asymptomatic (Heading et al; Reunala et al; Frödin et al). In asymptomatic patients, however, the granular IgA deposits do not disappear, suggesting that IgA is not the main factor inducing the symptoms of dermatitis herpetiformis but rather a secondary phenomenon (Frödin et al).

Differences in *HLA typing* between the granular and the linear types of dermatitis herpetiformis suggest that the two forms are pathophysiologically different diseases. Only 30% to 35% of patients with linear deposits have HLA-B8, a prevalence not significantly different from that of the normal population (24%). In contrast, 85% to 88% of patients with granular deposits have HLA-B8 (Lawley et al; Chorzelski and Jablonska, 1981).

Differential Diagnosis.   The presence of an early multilocular vesicle with a microabscess at the tip of each papilla can be regarded as diagnostic for dermatitis herpetiformis. However, microabscesses may be seen also in papillae adjoining the inflammatory bullae of bullous pemphigoid (Jablonska and Chorzelski, 1963; van der Meer). Therefore, in patients suspected of having dermatitis herpetiformis, it is best to select for biopsy

an erythematous area without clinically visible vesicles (Piérard). In the case of dermatitis herpetiformis, such an area is most apt to show a diagnostic multilocular vesicle still too small to be clinically visible. The prevalence of neutrophils in microabscesses certainly speaks in favor of a diagnosis of dermatitis herpetiformis, but a prevalence of eosinophils does not necessarily rule out dermatitis herpetiformis in favor of bullous pemphigoid.

Chronic Bullous Dermatosis of Childhood (Linear IgA Bullous Dermatosis)

Aside from typical papulovesicular dermatitis herpetiformis showing granular deposits of IgA (van der Meer; Pehamberger et al, 1979; Marsden et al), which occurs rarely in children, there are two types of bullous eruption that may be seen in children, usually those of preschool age: bullous pemphigoid and linear IgA bullous dermatosis of childhood. Their clinical distinction may be impossible, although a fairly typical feature in many cases of linear IgA bullous dermatosis of childhood is the presence of annular and serpiginous erythematous patches with bullae arranged at the periphery of the patches like a string of pearls (Chorzelski and Jablonska, 1979; van der Meer et al; Marsden et al). Oral lesions can occur in both diseases (Marsden et al). The response of children with linear IgA bullous dermatosis to sulfones or sulfapyridine is generally good (Lever). In contrast to dermatitis herpetiformis, no gluten-sensitive enteropathy exists, and the incidence of HLA-B8 is very high (Marsden et al).

Histopathology.   In some cases of linear IgA bullous dermatosis of childhood, neutrophilic microabscesses have been observed at the tips of dermal papillae (van der Meer et al; McGuire and Nordlund). However, in other cases, the histologic findings either are inconclusive because of the absence of microabscesses (Chorzelski and Jablonska) or are suggestive of bullous pemphigoid because of the prevalence of eosinophils (Esterly et al; Marsden et al). The differentiation from bullous pemphigoid thus often requires immunofluorescence studies (see below).

Histogenesis.   *Immunofluorescence testing* in linear IgA bullous dermatosis of childhood almost invariably shows the presence of linear deposits of IgA in the basement membrane zone (McGuire and Nordlund; Esterly et al) and often shows the presence of circulating IgA as well (van der Meer et al; Chorzelski and Jablonska, 1979; Marsden et al). Circulating IgA antibodies have been found in as many as two thirds of the cases (Marsden et al). In some cases, there are linear deposits of IgG in addition to linear deposits of IgA, making differentiation from bullous pemphigoid difficult (Faber and van Joost; Chorzelski and Jablonska, 1979) (see also p. 120). In rare instances, no deposits are found (Esterly et al; Marsden et al). As already stated (see p. 119), it is likely that linear IgA dermatitis herpetiformis of adults and linear IgA bullous dermatosis of childhood represent one and the same disease (Jablonska and Chorzelski, 1979, 1981; Dabrowski et al).

ERYTHEMA MULTIFORME

Erythema multiforme is an acute, self-limited dermatosis showing in some patients a tendency toward periodic recurrence. Acute attacks usually resolve within 3 to 6 weeks, and patients with recurrent erythema multiforme in most instances are free of lesions for long periods between episodes. Occasionally, however, attacks occur with such frequency that lesions persist from one episode to the next (Russell Jones). As the name implies, the lesions may be multiform. They include macules, papules, vesicles, and bullae. Quite commonly, one observes so-called iris lesions, or target lesions, representing macules or papules with a central vesicle. Not infrequently, some of the lesions are hemorrhagic. Erythema multiforme may be idiopathic, but it may occur also as a drug reaction. Several infections can induce erythema multiforme, for instance, infection with herpes simplex virus (Shelley) or with *Mycoplasma pneumoniae*, a cause of primary atypical pneumonia (Sontheimer et al). In erythema multiforme associated with herpes simplex, the herpes infection precedes the erythema multiforme by a mean interval of 9 days. Herpes simplex-associated erythema multiforme tends to be recurrent (Huff and Weston).

There are two forms of severe erythema multiforme that start abruptly with high fever, prostration, and a very extensive eruption. They are Stevens–Johnson disease and the "subepidermal" type of Lyell's toxic epidermal necrolysis. Both have a high mortality, between 30% and 40%, unless corticosteroids are given in large doses as soon as possible. Not infrequently, these disorders are caused by allergy to drugs.

In *Stevens–Johnson disease,* one observes, in addition to extensive inflammatory skin lesions, severe involvement of the mucous surfaces of the mouth and nose and the conjunctivae. In rare instances, conjunctival scarring with synechiae and symblepharon ensues (Kopf et al).

In the "subepidermal" type of Lyell's *toxic epidermal necrolysis,* the eruption begins with a widespread blotchy erythema. This is soon followed by large, flaccid bullae and detachment of the epidermis in large sheets, leaving the dermis exposed and giving the skin a scalded appearance. Involvement of the mucous membranes usually is less severe than in Stevens–Johnson disease. The "subepidermal" type of this disease usually occurs in adults and only rarely in small children.

It is important to recognize that toxic epidermal necrolysis, as originally described in 1956 (Lyell), comprised two entirely different diseases (Lyell, 1979): a "subcorneal" staphylococcal type and a "subepidermal" type. The "subcorneal" type is now generally called *staphylococcal scalded skin syndrome* or *Ritter's disease,* its original designation (see p. 291). The "subepidermal" type is now the only type to which the designation *toxic epidermal necrolysis* is still applied. This type is widely regarded as a variant of severe erythema multiforme because of its acute course, its frequent occurrence as a drug allergy, its frequent overlap with Stevens–Johnson disease (according to Lyell [1967], in 22 of 97 cases), and, especially, its histologic identity with the epidermal type of erythema multiforme (see below).

Histopathology.   Erythema multiforme presents a varied histologic picture analogous to its clinical multiformity. It represents a tissue reaction with spectral expression varying from very mild to very severe changes (Bedi and Pinkus). Review of many cases of erythema multiforme with multiple biopsies has revealed in some biopsies predominantly dermal changes, in others predominantly epidermal changes, and in still others both types of changes to nearly equal degrees. Thus, it seems best to distinguish histologically among three types of lesions in erythema multiforme: the dermal type, the mixed dermal-epidermal type, and the epidermal type (Orfanos et al).

Dermal Type.   The dermal type of erythema multiforme is seen in the macular lesions and also in most papular lesions. In macular lesions, only a rather slight perivascular infiltrate composed of mononuclear cells is present. In papular lesions, one finds a fairly pronounced perivascular infiltrate of cells, largely mononuclear but often also containing eosinophils (Bedi and Pinkus). There may be pronounced edema of the papillary dermis. In cases in which the edema has led to the formation of a bulla, the epidermis together with part or all of the PAS-positive basement membrane zone forms the top of the bulla (Fig. 7-24) (MacVicar et al). In some instances, instead of causing a subepidermal bulla, the edema in the upper dermis leads to epidermal edema and multiple intraepidermal vesicles associated with exocytosis (Bedi and Pinkus). Extravasated red blood cells are seen occasionally, but signs of vasculitis are absent.

Mixed Dermal-Epidermal Type.   The mixed type of erythema multiforme is seen in association with papular, plaquelike, and target lesions. A mononuclear infiltrate is present around the superficial blood vessels and along the dermal-epidermal border, with the basal cells showing hydropic degeneration (Ackerman et al). The epidermis contains numerous scattered individually necrotic keratinocytes showing a strongly eosinophilic, homogeneous cytoplasm and pyknotic or absent nuclei. In some lesions, the dermal mononuclear infiltrate extends into the epidermis, and mild spongiosis and intracellular edema may be seen in the epidermis. The hydropic degeneration of the basal cells in association with the focal necrosis of the epidermis may lead to the formation of subepidermal vesicles and bullae showing extensive necrosis of the overlying epidermis. Extravasated erythrocytes often are present in the upper dermis.

Epidermal Type. The epidermal type of erythema multiforme is seen in some target lesions and in the severe forms of erythema multiforme, that is, in Stevens–Johnson disease and in toxic epidermal necrolysis. Whereas the dermal changes in the epidermal type of erythema multiforme consist of only a mild mononuclear infiltrate around the superficial blood vessels, the epidermis in early lesions contains groups of keratinocytes showing eosinophilic necrosis (Fig. 7-25). Mononuclear cells and neutrophils may invade such areas of necrosis, and the necrotic cells subsequently lose their nuclei and coalesce. In severely affected areas, hydropic degeneration of the basal cells may result in subepidermal separation, and all keratinocytes appear necrotic, only the horny layer remaining preserved. In other areas, however, there may be severe damage to the upper epidermal layers and less

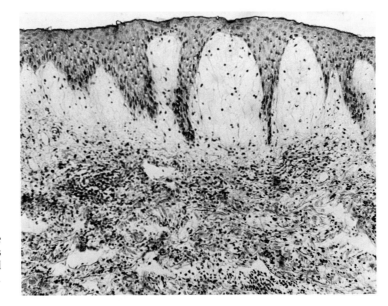

Fig. 7-24. Erythema multiforme, dermal type
A fairly pronounced perivascular infiltrate composed largely of mononuclear cells is present. The upper dermis shows marked edema resulting in subepidermal blisters. (×100)

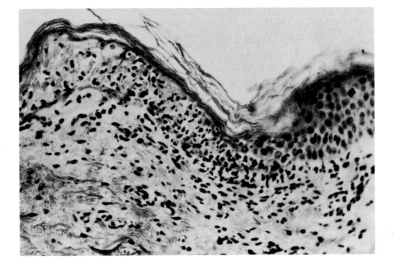

Fig. 7-25. Erythema multiforme, epidermal type
On the left side, the epidermis consists largely of keratinocytes showing eosinophilic necrosis. (×200)

severe damage to the lower epidermal layers, resulting in intraepidermal cleavage (Orfanos et al). These changes are identical with those described for toxic epidermal necrosis (Braun-Falco; Tritsch).

Histogenesis. *Electron microscopic examination* of bullae of the dermal type have shown that the basement membrane is located on top of the blister and that there are no significant alterations within the detached epidermis (Orfanos et al). In contrast, in blisters of the dermal–epidermal or epidermal type, the basal lamina is in some instances destroyed; if present, it is located at the floor of the bulla. The basal cells show marked intracytoplasmic damage with a loss of organelles. Neutrophils and macrophages rich in lysosomes are seen in the lower epidermis phagocytizing the damaged keratinocytes (EM 26). In the midepidermis, large, electron-dense, dyskeratotic bodies may be located, corresponding to the cells with eosinophilic necrosis seen by light microscopy (Orfanos et al; Prutkin and Fellner). In the necrotic epidermis of the epidermal type of erythema multiforme, the damaged epidermal cells often contain few or no organelles (Orfanos et al). The epidermal changes thus are the same as those described in the "subepidermal" type of Lyell's toxic epidermal necrolysis (Braun-Falco and Wolff).

Immunologic studies have shown in many patients with erythema multiforme deposits of IgM and C3 in the walls of the superficial dermal vessels (Imamura et al; Bushkell et al). It has been noted that such deposits are generally found only in biopsy specimens taken from lesions less than 24 hr old (Kazmierowski and Wuepper). In addition, circulating immune complexes have been demonstrated with both a monoclonal rheumatoid factor inhibition assay (Bushkell et al) and a C1q binding radioassay (Imamura et al). These findings suggest that immune complex formation and subsequent deposition in the cutaneous microvasculature play a role in the pathogenesis of erythema multiforme.

GRAFT-VERSUS-HOST DISEASE

Two types of graft-versus-host disease exist: the iatrogenic form, in which immunodeficient patients receive transplants of immunocompetent lymphocytes, and the rare congenital form, in which, owing to an immunologic abnormality of the fetus, maternal lymphocytes normally present in the fetal circulation establish themselves in the fetus and react against their host (Morhenn and Maibach).

The iatrogenic form of graft-versus-host disease may follow bone marrow transplantation to patients with aplastic anemia, acute leukemia, or genetic immunodeficiency states. Graft-versus-host reactions occur in approximately 70% of recipients of bone marrow transplantation, and over 50% of the patients with a graft-

versus-host reaction die of infectious complications (Glucksberg et al).

The disease can be divided into an acute and a chronic phase. The acute phase begins between 7 and 21 days after the transplantation, and the chronic phase between several months to a year after the transplantation. Either phase may occur alone, but many patients have both phases either merging with one another or separated by an asymptomatic period (Shulman et al).

In the *acute phase*, besides the cutaneous lesions, diarrhea, vomiting, and hepatic dysfunction may occur. The skin shows an extensive macular, erythematous eruption. In severe cases, there are extensive erythematous to violaceous scaling lesions and even bullae (De Dobbeleer et al). In one reported case, there was detachment of large sheets of epidermis as seen in toxic epidermal necrolysis (Peck et al). Oral lesions may be present.

In the *chronic phase*, an early lichenoid stage and a late sclerotic stage can be distinguished. Although usually generalized, the involvement is in rare instances localized to a few areas (Shulman et al). In the lichenoid stage, both the cutaneous and oral lesions may show a clinical resemblance to lesions seen in lichen planus (Saurat et al). In addition, the skin may show extensive erythema and irregular hyperpigmentation. In the late sclerotic stage, dermal sclerosis and poikiloderma develop. The skin becomes firm and inelastic and shows atrophy and reticulate pigmentation. There is cicatricial alopecia, and chronic ulcerations may develop (Shulman et al).

Histopathology. In the *acute phase*, one usually finds a sparse, diffuse lymphocytic infiltrate in the upper dermis with extensive exocytosis. Scattered throughout the epidermis are many degenerate keratinocytes, some with a pyknotic nucleus and eosinophilic, hyalinized cytoplasm (Fig. 7-26). These necrotic keratinocytes are often associated with one or more satellite lymphocytes, an association referred to as satellite cell necrosis (Grogan et al; Mascaro et al). In some cases, there is also vacuolar degeneration of basal cells (Hood et al), which may lead to the formation of bullae (Peck et al; De Dobbeleer et al).

In the *chronic phase*, the early lichenoid stage may still show evidence of satellite cell necrosis within the epidermis (Janin-Mercier et al). The overall histologic picture greatly resembles that of lichen planus; one observes acanthosis, eosinophilic keratinocytes in the epidermis resembling colloid or Civatte bodies, cell necrosis in the basal cell layer, and a mononuclear cell infiltrate immediately below the epidermis with pigmentary deposits (Saurat et al; Spielvogel et al). As in lichen planus, colloid bodies may also be seen in the upper dermis as a result of apoptosis (Janin-Mercier et al). There may be areas of separation of the basal cell layer from

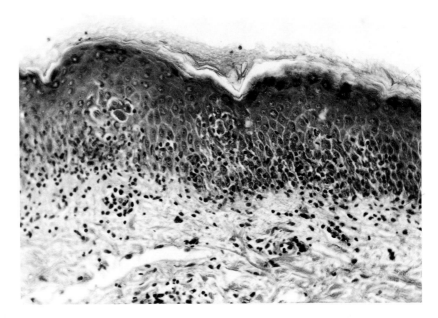

Fig. 7-26. Graft-versus-host reaction, acute phase
Eosinophilic necrotic keratinocytes are scattered through the epidermis. Some of them show an associated lymphocyte, a process referred to as satellite cell necrosis. (×200)

the dermal papillae resembling the clefts seen in severe lichen planus (Shulman et al).

In the late sclerotic stage, the epidermis has changed from an acanthotic to an atrophic state, the keratinocytes being small, flattened, and hyperpigmented. Basal layer vacuolar degeneration, inflammation, and eosinophilic body formation are rare or absent (Shulman et al). The dermis shows thickened and hyalinized collagen bundles extending into the subcutaneous tissue together with destruction of the adnexal structures (Spielvogel et al).

Histogenesis. Graft-versus-host disease is composed of two distinct clinical entities that have a different pathogenesis. Acute graft-versus-host disease is produced by the attack of donor immunocompetent T or null lymphocytes against recipient histocompatibility antigens, whereas chronic graft-versus-host disease is produced by immunocompetent lymphocytes that differentiate in the recipient (Parkman et al). The lymphocytes that are seen as satellites to necrotic keratinocytes are immunocompetent suppressor ("killer") T cells, and the keratinocytes the target cells (Schmitt and Thivolet).

Immunofluorescence studies have revealed basement membrane zone IgM deposition in 39% of the patients with the acute form and 86% of the patients with the chronic form of graft-versus-host disease (Tsoi et al). In addition, IgM and C3 have been found in the walls of dermal vessels (Ullman; Spielvogel et al). These deposits suggest a possible role for humoral immunity in the pathogenesis of graft-versus-host disease in addition to the well-established role of cellular immunity.

On *electron microscopic examination,* the necrotic or dyskeratotic keratinocytes show that the entire cytoplasm is filled with numerous aggregated tonofilaments (De Dobbeleer et al).

Differential Diagnosis. The acute phase of graft-versus-host disease shares with the epidermal type of erythema multiforme the presence of scattered necrotic keratinocytes and the formation of subepidermal bullae through hydropic degeneration of basal cells. However, the presence of satellite lymphocytes adjoining the necrotic keratinocytes has not been described in erythema multiforme (see p. 123).

Distinction of the lichenoid lesions from lichen planus is often impossible. However, late sclerotic lesions can be differentiated from scleroderma by the marked atrophy of the epidermis and by the fact that active synthesis of collagen takes place largely in the upper third of the dermis; in scleroderma, collagen is synthesized mainly in the lower dermis and in the subcutaneous tissue (Janin-Mercier et al).

SUBCORNEAL PUSTULAR DERMATOSIS

A chronic disorder first described in 1956 (Sneddon and Wilkinson), subcorneal pustular dermatosis shows pustules, especially on the abdomen and in the axillary and inguinal folds. Often, the pustules are seen in an annular or serpiginous arrangement. Pus characteristically accumulates in the lower half of large pustules (Sneddon and Wilkinson, 1979). Oral lesions do not occur. The pustules are sterile. In some instances, the eruption responds well to sulfapyridine and the sulfones.

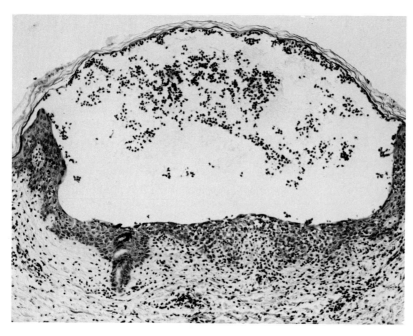

Fig. 7-27.   Subcorneal pustular dermatosis
The pustule has formed beneath the horny layer. No acantholysis is present. (×100)

Histopathology. The pustules are located directly beneath the stratum corneum (Fig. 7-27). Their content consists almost entirely of neutrophils, with only an occasional eosinophil. The stratum malpighii beneath the pustules contains a fairly small number of neutrophils and shows only in some areas rather mild intracellular edema and spongiosis. The underlying dermis, including the papillae, shows dilated capillaries and, around them, an infiltrate composed of neutrophils and a few eosinophils and mononuclear cells (Wolff).

In some instances, a few acantholytic cells are seen at the base of a pustule. They usually still show partial attachment to the epidermis but may lie free in the pustule among the neutrophils. Since the pustules in subcorneal pustular dermatosis do not form on the basis of acantholysis, and acantholytic cells appear only later, one may regard their presence as being due to secondary acantholysis caused probably by proteolytic enzymes present in the pustular content (Burns and Fine).

Histogenesis. *Electron microscopic examination* of the border of pustules has shown cytolytic changes in the upper epidermis, especially in the granular layer. Dissolution of the plasma membrane and of the cytoplasm of granular cells causes the formation of a subcorneal slit. The transepidermal migration of leukocytes and their subcorneal accumulation are regarded as events secondary to the cellular destruction in the stratum granulosum (Metz and Schröpl).

Differential Diagnosis. Histologic differentiation from impetigo usually is impossible, since, as a rule, bacteria cannot be demonstrated in the pustules of impetigo even with the use of a Gram stain. However, culturing of the contents of pustules may be helpful.

Histologic differentiation from pemphigus foliaceus or pemphigus erythematosus may also be impossible, since one observes in both diseases subcorneal blisters with acantholysis, which is usually but not always more pronounced in pemphigus foliaceus than in subcorneal pustular dermatosis. Thus, clinical information, immunofluorescence testing, and a therapeutic test with sulfones may be necessary for a decision to be reached.

Although subcorneal pustules occur in both pustular psoriasis and subcorneal pustular dermatosis, spongiform pustules occur only in pustular psoriasis. In subcorneal pustular dermatosis, the neutrophils pass the upper malpighian layer without being arrested there, as they are in pustular psoriasis (Sneddon and Wilkinson, 1979). The presence of spongiform pustules in a case clinically regarded as subcorneal pustular dermatosis is evidence in favor of a diagnosis of pustular psoriasis, but it does not indicate that subcorneal pustular dermatosis is a variant of pustular psoriasis, a view that has been expressed (Sanchez and Ackerman; Chimenti and Ackerman). It is possible, however, that some relationship exists between these two diseases, since, of 23 patients originally diagnosed as having subcorneal pustular dermatosis and followed, 7 showed spongiform pustules later on and were then regarded as having pustular psoriasis (Sanchez et al).

TRANSIENT ACANTHOLYTIC DERMATOSIS

In transient acantholytic dermatosis, a condition first described in 1970 (Grover), pruritic, discrete papules and occasionally also papulovesicles are present mainly on the chest, back, and thighs. Most patients are middle-aged or elderly men. Although, in the majority of patients, the disorder is transient, lasting from 2 weeks to 3 months, it can persist for several years (Chalet et al; Heaphy et al; Heenan and Quirk). For this reason, some authors have objected to the term *transient*. However, since most patients have a brief course, the allusion to transience remains valid (Chalet et al).

Histopathology.   Focal acantholysis is present. Since these foci are small, they are sometimes found only when step sections are obtained. The acantholysis may occur in five histologic patterns, two or more of which may be found in the same specimen (Chalet et al; Wolff et al; Heenan and Quirk). Most commonly seen are a pattern resembling pemphigus vulgaris, showing suprabasal acantholysis, and a pattern resembling Darier's disease, characterized by acantholytic dyskeratosis and the presence of corps ronds. In addition, there are a pattern resembling Hailey–Hailey disease, with suprabasal clefts and abundant acantholysis; a pattern resembling pemphigus foliaceus, with superficial acantholysis (Fig. 7-28); and a spongiotic pattern, in which acantholytic cells are present within spongiotic foci.

Histogenesis. *Immunofluorescence studies* in general have given negative results (Heaphy et al; Pehamberger et al). In one study, 5 of 11 patients showed abnormalities by immunofluorescence, but there was no consistent pattern (Bystryn).

Electron microscopic findings have shown intradesmosomal separation as described in pemphigus vulgaris (Kanzaki and Hashimoto), diminution in the number of desmosomes, and perinuclear aggregation of tonofilament bundles (Wolff et al). In the Darier type, cells showing the electron microscopic features of corps ronds may be seen (Grover and Duffy).

Differential Diagnosis.   In the four patterns that resemble other diseases, the decisive factors in the diagnosis are the limited extent of the histologic changes and the mixture of patterns. The clinical data also aid in the diagnosis. It is likely that cases reported as acute, eruptive Darier's disease (Fishman) and acute adult-onset Darier-like dermatosis (Gisslén and Mobacken) are instances of transient acantholytic dermatosis with a Darier-like pattern.

FRICTION BLISTERS

Friction blisters occur mainly on the soles, as a result of prolonged walking, and on the palms and the palmar

Fig. 7-28.   Transient acantholytic dermatosis
The pattern resembles pemphigus foliaceus, although acantholysis is more pronounced and extends deeper into the epidermis than in pemphigus foliaceus. Also, the lesion is quite small. (×200)

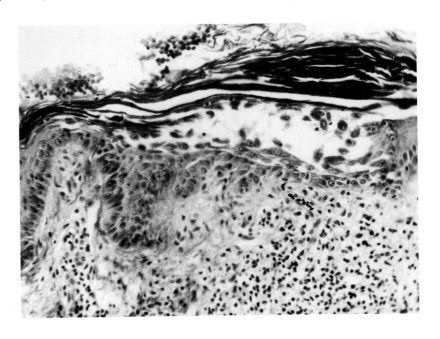

surfaces of the fingers, as a result of repetitive actions required in certain occupations or sports. They may occur also as self-inflicted artifacts (Brehmer-Anderson and Göransson).

Histopathology.   In both naturally occurring and experimentally produced friction blisters, intra-epidermal cleavage and blisters develop as a result of necrosis of keratinocytes in the stratum malpighii (Naylor). The cleavage lies always at the same level, the roof of the blister being composed of the stratum corneum, the stratum granulosum, and some amorphous cellular debris (Sulzberger et al). Most of the degenerated keratinocytes are located at the floor of the cleft. Their cytoplasm and nuclei stain only faintly. The deeper part of the epidermis consists of undamaged cells (Brehmer-Anderson and Göransson).

Histogenesis. Friction blisters are caused by shearing forces within the epidermis. They form only in sites in which the epidermis is both thick and firmly attached to the underlying tissue (Brehmer-Andersson and Göransson).

ELECTRIC BURNS

It is desirable that persons working in dermatopathology be familiar with the effects on the skin of an electric current such as is used during electrodesiccation or diathermy, because these modalities occasionally are used for removal of tumors. The effects on small specimens are so severe that usually no diagnosis other than electric burn can be made.

Histopathology.   The electrodesiccation or diathermy current causes a separation of the epidermis from the dermis. A diagnostic histologic feature is the fringe of elongated, degenerated cytoplasmic processes that protrudes from the lower end of the detached basal cells into the space separating the epidermis and the dermis (Fig. 7-29). The nuclei of the basal cells and often also of some of the higher-lying epidermal cells appear stretched in the same direction as the fringe of cytoplasmic processes. In addition, the upper portion of the dermis shows homogenization due to coagulation necrosis (Winer and Levin).

THERMAL BURNS

In the evaluation of thermal burns, the depth of penetration is of great importance with respect to whether healing can be expected, as in first- and second-degree burns, or whether grafting is indicated, as in third-degree burns.

Histopathology.   *First-degree burns* are those in which the deep parts of the epidermis, particularly the basal cell layer, remains viable and only the upper portion of the epidermis is affected by heat coagulation. In the affected areas, the nuclei appear either pyknotic and possess a perinuclear halo or, in a more advanced stage, stain faintly eosinophilic or not at all, appearing as "architectural ghosts" (Sevitt).

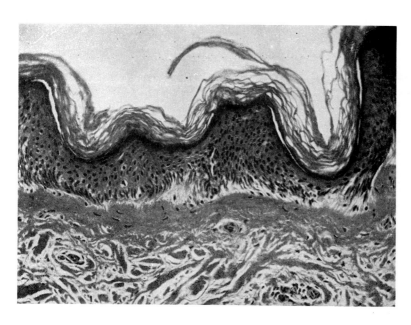

Fig. 7-29.   Blister caused by electrodesiccation
The subepidermal blister shows elongated, degenerated cytoplasmic processes protruding from the basal cells into the bulla cavity. Also, the nuclei of the basal cells appear markedly stretched. (×200)

Second-degree burns often show subepidermal blisters and are characterized by partial-thickness dermal necrosis, which leaves intact the lower portion of the cutaneous appendages from which re-epithelization can occur. One may distinguish between superficial and deep second-degree burns. Superficial second-degree burns are associated with necrosis of the surface epidermis and of only a small amount of superficial dermal collagen; in deep second-degree burns, much of the dermal collagen and the cutaneous appendages is injured (Foley). In partial-thickness dermal necrosis, the depth of epithelial damage in the cutaneous appendages is a good indicator of the depth of irreversible damage to the collagen, because, in the appendages, there generally is a fairly sharp border between heat-coagulated and relatively normal epithelium (Sevitt). At a later stage, an inflammatory reaction develops at the junction of the viable and nonviable tissue.

Third-degree burns show full-thickness dermal necrosis with destruction of all cutaneous appendages. The coagulation necrosis may even extend to the subcutaneous tissue and to the underlying muscle (Foley).

BIBLIOGRAPHY

Dermatitis (Eczema)

ACKERMAN AB, BREZA TS, CAPLAND L: Spongiotic simulants of mycosis fungoides. Arch Dermatol 109:218–220, 1974

BAER RL: Die Rolle der Langerhans-Zellen bei der Kontaktallergie. Hautarzt 27:554–558, 1976

BAER RL: Immunologic functions of Langerhans cells. J Dermatol (Tokyo) 5:257–263, 1978

BAER RL, ROSENTHAL SA, SIMS CF: The allergic eczema-like reaction and the primary irritant reaction. Arch Dermatol 76:549–560, 1957

BANDMANN HJ: Monocyten bei experimentellem Kontaktekzem. Hautarzt 18:122–133, 1967

BLOCK JB, EDGCOMB J, EISEN A, et al: Mycosis fungoides: Natural history and aspects of its relationship to other malignant lymphomas. Am J Med 34:228–235, 1963

BLUEFARB SM, ADAMS LA: Arteriovenous malformation with angiodermatitis. Arch Dermatol 96:176–181, 1967

BRAUN-FALCO O, BURG G: Celluläres Infiltrat und Capillaren bei Neurodermitis diffusa. Arch Dermatol Forsch 249:113–124, 1974

BRAUN-FALCO O, PETRY G: Feinstruktur der Epidermis bei chronischem nummulärem Ekzem. Arch Klin Exp Dermatol 222:219–241, 1965, and 224:63–80, 1966

BRAUN-FALCO O, WOLFF HH: Zur Ultrastruktur der menschlichen Epidermis bei der allergischen Epicutantestreaktion. Arch Dermatol Forsch 240:23–37, 1971

BYROM NA, STAUGHTON RCO, CAMPBELL MA et al: Thymosin-induced "null" cells in atopic eczema. Br J Dermatol 100:499–510

CALNAN CD: Eczema for me. Trans St John's Hosp Dermatol Soc 54:54–64, 1968

CARR RD, SCARPELLI DG, GREIDER M: Allergic contact dermatitis: Light and electron microscopy. Dermatologica 137:358–368, 1968

COHEN S: The role of cell-mediated immunity in the induction of inflammatory responses. Am J Pathol 88:501–528, 1977

CONSTANTINE VS: Current concepts in mycosis fungoides: Its nosology, diagnosis and treatment. Int J Dermatol 15:723–731, 1976

COOPER KD, WUEPPER KD, HANIFIN JM: T cell subset enumeration and functional analysis in atopic dermatitis. (Abstr) J Invest Dermatol 74:253, 1980

DILWORTH JA, MANDELL GL: Adults with chronic granulomatous disease of "childhood." Am J Med 63:233–243, 1977

DVORAK HF, MIHM MC, JR., DVORAK AM: Morphology of delayed-type hypersensitivity in man. J Invest Dermatol 67:391–401, 1976

EDELSON RL, LUTZNER MA, KIRKPATRICK CH et al: Morphologic and functional properties of the atypical T lymphocytes of the Sézary syndrome. Mayo Clin Proc 49:558–566, 1974

ELLIOTT ST, HANIFIN JM: Delayed cutaneous hypersensitivity and lymphocyte transformation. Arch Dermatol 115:36–39, 1979

EPSTEIN EH, JR., LEVIN DL, CROFT JD, JR., et al: Mycosis fungoides. Medicine (Baltimore) 15:61–72, 1972

EPSTEIN S: Chlorpromazine photosensitivity. Arch Dermatol 98:354–363, 1968

EPSTEIN WL: Immunologic (allergic) contact dermatitis. J Dermatol (Tokyo) 2:105–110, 1975

FRICHOT BC, III, ZELICKSON AS: Steroids, lysosomes and dermatitis. Acta Derm Venereal (Stockh) 52:311–319, 1972

FUKS ZY, BAGSHAW MA, FARBER EM: Prognostic signs and the management of mycosis fungoides. Cancer 32:1385–1395, 1973

HALL JB, SMITH JG, JR., BURNETT SC: The lysosome in contact dermatitis: A histochemical study. J Invest Dermatol 49:590–594, 1967

HILL HR, QUIE PG: Raised serum-IgE levels and defective neutrophil chemotaxis in three children with eczema and bacterial infections. Lancet 1:183–187, 1974

HOHENADL L, DE PAOLA D: Über Gewebsreaktionen nach parenteraler Zufuhr von Melanin unter besonderer Berücksichtigung der lipomelanotischen Reticulose. Frankfurt Z Pathol 69:374–383, 1958

HUNZIKER N, WINKELMANN RK: Cell populations in experimental contact dermatitis. Arch Dermatol 113:1543–1549, 1977

HURWITT E: Dermatopathic lymphadenitis. J Invest Dermatol 5:197–204, 1942

JACOBS JC, MILLER ME: Fatal familial Leiner's disease. Pediatrics 49:225–232, 1972

JONES HE, INOUYE JC, MCGERITY JL et al: Atopic disease and serum immunoglobulin-E. Br J Dermatol 92:17–25, 1975

JONES HE, LEWIS CW, MCMARLIN SL: Allergic contact sensitivity in atopic dermatitis. Arch Dermatol 107:217–222, 1973

KERL H, BURG G, BRAUN-FALCO O: Contact dermatitis in guinea pigs. Arch Dermatol Forsch 249:207–226, 1974

KOMURA J, OFUJI S: Ultrastructural studies of allergic contact dermatitis in man. Arch Dermatol Res 267:275–290, 1980

KRUEGER GG: Lymphokines in health and disease. Int J Dermatol 16:539–551, 1977

LAIPPLY TC: Lipomelanotic reticular hyperplasia of lymph nodes. Arch Intern Med 81:19–36, 1948

MACKIE RM, ALCORN MJ, STEVENSON RD et al: Wiscott-Aldrich syndrome with partial response to transfer factor. Br J Dermatol 98:567–571, 1978

MACKIE RM, COBB SJ, COCHRAN REI et al: Total and specific IgE levels in patients with atopic dermatitis. Clin Exp Dermatol 4:187–195, 1979

MEDENICA M, ROSTENBERG A: A comparative light and electron microscopic study of primary irritant contact dermatitis and allergic contact dermatitis. J Invest Dermatol 56:259–271, 1971

METZ J: Ultrastruktur der Spongiose beim allergischen Kontaktekzem. Dermatologica 141:315–320, 1970

METZ J, METZ G: Zur Ultrastruktur der Epidermis bei seborrhoischem Ekzem. Arch Dermatol Forsch 252:285–296, 1975

MIESCHER G: Abgrenzung des allergischen und toxischen Geschehens in morphologischer und funktioneller Sicht. Arch Klin Exp Dermatol 213:297–313, 1961

NICOLIS GD, HELWIG EB: Exfoliative dermatitis. Arch Dermatol 108:788–797, 1973

NEUMANN E, WINTER V: The character of cells with "altération cavitaire" (Leloir). Acta Derm Venereol (Stockh) 45:272–274, 1965

OGAWA M, BERGER PA, MC INTIRE OR et al: IgE in atopic dermatitis. Arch Dermatol 103:575–580, 1971

PINKUS H, MEHREGAN AH: The primary histologic lesion of seborrheic dermatitis and psoriasis. J Invest Dermatol 46:109–116, 1966

PROSE PH, SEDLIS E: Morphologic and histochemical studies of atopic eczema in infants and children. J Invest Dermatol 34:149–165, 1960

PROSE PH, SEDLIS E, BIGELOW M: The demonstration of lysosomes in the diseased skin of infants with infantile eczema. J Invest Dermatol 45:448–457, 1965

RAUSCH E, KAISERLING E, GOOS M: Langerhans cells and interdigitating reticulum cells in the thymus-dependent region in human dermatopathic lymphadenitis. Virchows Arch [Cell Pathol] 25:327–343, 1977

ROSEN FS: The primary immunodeficiencies: Dermatologic manifestations. J Invest Dermatol 67:402–411, 1976

SCHEFFER E, MEIJER CJLM, VAN VLOTEN WA: Dermatopathic lymphadenopathy and lymph node involvement in mycosis fungoides. Cancer 45:137–148, 1980

SILBERBERG I: Apposition of mononuclear cells to Langerhans cells in contact allergic reactions. Acta Derm Venereol (Stockh) 53:1–12, 1973

SILBERBERG I, BAER RL, ROSENTHAL SA: The role of Langerhans cells in contact allergy. Acta Derm Venereol (Stockh) 54:321–331, 1974

SILBERBERG-SINAKIN I: On Langerhans cells. Int J Dermatol 16:581–583, 1977

SILBERBERG-SINAKIN I, BAER RL, THORBECKE GJ: Langerhans cells: A review of their nature with emphasis on their immunologic functions. Prog Allergy 24:268–294, 1978

SILBERBERG-SINAKIN I, THORBECKE GJ, BAER RL et al: Antigen-bearing Langerhans cells in skin, dermal lymphatics and in the lymph nodes. Cell Immunol 25:137–151, 1976

STANLEY J, PEREZ D, GIGLI I et al: Hyperimmunoglobulin E syndrome. Arch Dermatol 114:765–767, 1978

STINGL G, GAZZE LA, CZERNECKI N, WOLFF K: Suppressor cell defect in atopic dermatitis patients. (Abstr) Arch Dermatol Res 267:199, 1980

STONE SP, MULLER SA, GLEICH GJ: IgE levels in atopic dermatitis. Arch Dermatol 108:806–811, 1973

STREILEIN JW, BERGSTRESSER PR: Langerhans cell function dictates induction of contact hypersensitivity or unresponsiveness to DNFB in Syrian hamsters. J Invest Dermatol 77:272–277, 1981

WESTON WL: Evaluation of cell mediated immunity. Int J Dermatol 14:699–707, 1975

WESTON WL: Disorders of phagocytic function. Arch Dermatol 112:1589–1596, 1976

WESTON WL, HUMBERT JR: Failure of fresh plasma in Leiner's disease. Arch Dermatol 113:233–234

WIEDMANN A: Die arterielle Genese des Ulcus cruris "varicosum." Hautarzt 5:85–91, 1954

WINKELMANN RK, PERRY HO, MULLER SA et al: The pre-Sézary erythroderma syndrome. Mayo Clin Proc 49:588–589,1974

Miliaria

DOBSON RL, LOBITZ WC, JR.: Some histochemical observations on the human eccrine sweat glands. II. The pathogenesis of miliaria Arch Dermatol 75:653–666, 1957

HÖLZLE E, KLIGMAN AM: The pathogenesis of miliaria rubra: Role of the resident microflora. Br J Dermatol 99:117–137, 1978

LOEWENTHAL LJA: The pathogenesis of miliaria. Arch Dermatol 84:2–17, 1961

LYONS RE, LEVINE R, AULD D: Miliaria rubra: A manifestation of staphylococcal disease. Arch Dermatol 86:282–286, 1962

O'BRIEN JP: The etiology of poral closure. J. Invest Dermatol 15:95–152, 1950

SHELLEY WB, HORVATH PN: Experimental miliaria in man. J Invest Dermatol 14:9–20, 1950

SINGH G: The role of bacteria in anhidrosis. Dermatologica 146:256–261, 1973

SULZBERGER MB, ZIMMERMAN HM: Studies on prickly heat. J Invest Dermatol 7:61–68, 1946

Erythema Toxicum Neonatorum

FREEMAN RG, SPILLER R, KNOX JM: Histopathology of erythema toxicum neonatorum. Arch Dermatol 82:586–589, 1960

POHLANDT F, HARNISCH R, MEIGEL WN et al: Zum Bild des Erythema toxicum neonatorum. Hautarzt 28:469–474, 1977

Transient Neonatal Pustular Melanosis

BARR RJ, GLOBERMAN LM, WERBER FA: Transient neonatal pustular melanosis. Int J Dermatol 18:636–638, 1979

RAMAMURTHY RS, REVERI M, ESTERLY NB et al: Transient neonatal pustular melanosis. J Pediatr 88:831–835, 1976

Acropustulosis of Infancy

JARRATT M, RAMSDELL W: Infantile acropustulosis. Arch Dermatol 115:834–836, 1979

KAHN G, RYWLIN AM: Acropustulosis of infancy. Arch Dermatol 115:831–833, 1979

Pemphigus

ASBOE-HANSEN G: Blister-spread induced by finger pressure, a diagnostic sign of pemphigus. J Invest Dermatol 34:5–9, 1960

BARRIÈRE H: Anticorps circulants et évolutivité du pemphigus. Ann Dermatol Venereol 107:849–850, 1980

BEUTNER EH, JORDON RE: Demonstration of skin antibodies in sera of pemphigus vulgaris patients by indirect immunofluorescent staining. Proc Soc Exp Biol Med 117:505–510, 1964

BEUTNER EH, PRIGENZI LS, HALE LS et al: Immunofluorescent studies of autoantibodies to intracellular areas of epithelia in Brazilian pemphigus foliaceus. Proc Soc Exp Biol Med 127:81–86, 1968

CIVATTE A: Diagnostic histopathologique de la dermatite polymorphe douloureuse ou maladie de Duhring-Brocq. Ann Dermatol Syph 3:1–30, 1943

CHORZELSKI T, JABLONSKA S, BLASZCZYK M: Immunopathological investigation in the Senear-Usher syndrome (coexistence of pemphigus and lupus erythematosus). Br J Dermatol 80:211–217, 1968

CRESWELL SN, BLACK MM, BHOGAL B et al: Correlation of circulating intercellular antibody titers in pemphigus with disease activity. Clin Exp Dermatol 6:477–483, 1981

EMMERSON RW, WILSON JONES E: Eosinophilic spongiosis in pemphigus. Arch Dermatol 97:252–257, 1968

FITZPATRICK RE, NEWCOMER VD: The correlation of disease activity and antibody titers in pemphigus. Arch Dermatol 116:285–290, 1980

FORMAN L: Pemphigus vegetans of Hallopeau. Arch Dermatol 114:627–628, 1978

FURTADO TA: Histopathology of pemphigus foliaceus. Arch Dermatol 80:66–71, 1959

GRAHAM JH, BINGUL O, BURGOON CB: Cytodiagnosis of inflammatory dermatoses. Arch Dermatol 87:118–127, 1963

HAENSCH R: Pemphigus herpetiformis. Hautarzt 30:418–422, 1979

HASHIMOTO K, LEVER WF: An electron microscopic study of pemphigus vulgaris of the mouth with special reference to the intercellular cement. J Invest Dermatol 48:540–552, 1967a

HASHIMOTO K, LEVER WF: The intercellular cement in pemphigus vulgaris: An electron microscopic study. Dermatologica 135:27–34, 1967b

HASHIMOTO K, LEVER WF: An ultrastructural study of cell junctions in pemphigus vulgaris. Arch Dermatol 101:287–298, 1970

HÖNIGSMANN H, HOLUBAR K, WOLFF K et al: Immunochemical localization of in vivo bound immunoglobulins in pemphigus vulgaris epidermis. Arch Dermatol Res 254:113–120, 1975

JABLONSKA S, CHORZELSKI TP, BEUTNER EH et al: Herpetiform pemphigus: A variable pattern of pemphigus. Int J Dermatol 14:353–359, 1975

JABLONSKA S, CHORZELSKI T, BLASZCZYK M et al: Pathogenesis of pemphigus erythematosus. Arch Dermatol Res 258:135–140, 1977

JUDD KP, LEVER WF: Correlation of antibodies in skin and serum with disease severity in pemphigus. Arch Dermatol 115:428–432, 1979

JUDD KP, MESCON H: Comparison of different epithelial substrates useful for indirect immunofluorescent testing of sera from patients with active pemphigus. J Invest Dermatol 72:314–316, 1979

KNIGHT AG, BLACK MM, DELANEY JJ: Eosinophilic spongiosis: Clinical, histologic and immunofluorescent correlation. Clin Exp Dermatol 1:141–153, 1976

LAGERHOLM B, FRITHZ A, BORGLUND E: Light and electron microscopic aspects of pemphigus herpetiformis (eosinophilic spongiosis) in comparison with other acantholytic disorders. Acta Derm Venereol (Stockh) 59:305–314, 1979

LEVER WF: Pemphigus and Pemphigoid. Springfield, IL, Charles C Thomas, 1965

LEVER WF: Pemphigus and pemphigoid: A review of the advances made since 1964. J Am Acad Dermatol 1:2–31, 1979

LEVER WF, HASHIMOTO K: The etiology and treatment of pemphigus and pemphigoid. J Invest Dermatol 53:373–389, 1969

MICHEL B, KO CS: Effect of pemphigus or bullous pemphigoid sera and leukocytes on normal skin in organ culture. (Abstr) J Invest Dermatol 62:541–542, 1974

NELSON CG: Pemphigus vegetans of Hallopeau. Arch Dermatol 114:627–628, 1978

NELSON CG, APISARNTHANARAX P, BEAN SF et al: Pemphigus vegetans of Hallopeau. Arch Dermatol 113:942–945, 1977

NEUMANN HAM, FABER WR: Pyodermite végétante of Hallopeau. Arch Dermatol 116:1169–1171, 1980

ORFANOS CE, GARTMANN H, MARKLE G: Zur Pathogenese des Pemphigus erythematosus. Arch Dermatol Res 240:317–333, 1971

OSTEEN FB, WHEELER CE, JR., BRIGGAMAN RA et al: Pemphigus foliaceus: Early clinical appearance as dermatitis herpetiformis

with eosinophilic spongiosis. Arch Dermatol 112:1148–1152, 1976

PEARSON RW, O'DONOGHUE M, KAPLAN SJ: Pemphigus vegetans: Its relationship to eosinophilic spongiosis and favorable response to dapsone. Arch Dermatol 116:65–68, 1980

PERRY HO: Pemphigus foliaceus. Arch Dermatol 83:52–72, 1961

PERRY HO, BRUNSTING LA: Pemphigus foliaceus. Arch Dermatol 91:10–23, 1965

RÖCKL H: Über die Pyodermite végétante von Hallopeau als benigne Form des Pemphigus vegetans von Neumann nebst einigen Bemerkungen zur Pyostomatitis vegetans von McCarthy. Arch Klin Exp Dermatol 218:574–582, 1964

RUZICKA T, GOETZ G: Beobachtungen bei der Pyodermite végétante Hallopeau. Z Hautkr 54:24–32, 1979

SCHILTZ JR, MICHEL B: Production of epidermal acantholysis in normal human skin in vitro by the IgG fraction from pemphigus serum. J Invest Dermatol 67:254–260, 1976

TAGAMI H, IMAMURA S, NOGUCHI S et al: Coexistence of peculiar pemphigus, myasthenia gravis and malignant thymoma. Dermatologica 152:181–190, 1976

TAPPEINER J, PFLEGER L: Pemphigus vulgaris–dermatitis herpetiformis. Arch Klin Exp Dermatol 214:415–431, 1962

THIVOLET J, BEYVIN A, ANDRÉ D: Anticorps "pemphiguslike" et "pemphigoidlike." Dermatologica 140:310–317, 1970

TUFFANELLI DL: Cutaneous immunopathology: Recent observations. J Invest Dermatol 65:143–153, 1975

TZANCK A: Le cytodiagnostic immédiat en dermatologie. Ann Dermatol Syph 8:205–218, 1948

WILGRAM GF, CAULFIELD JB, MADGIC EB: An electron microscopic study of acantholysis and dyskeratosis in pemphigus foliaceus. J Invest Dermatol 43:287–299, 1964

WINKELMANN RK, ROTH HL: Dermatitis herpetiformis with acantholysis or pemphigus with response to sulfonamides. Arch Dermatol 82:385–390, 1960

Bullous Pemphigoid

AHMED AR, CHU TM, PROVOST TT: Bullous pemphigoid: Clinical and serologic evaluation for associated malignant neoplasms. Arch Dermatol 113:969, 1977a

AHMED AR, MAIZE JC, PROVOST TT: Bullous pemphigoid: Clinical and immunologic follow-up after successful therapy. Arch Dermatol 113:1043–1046, 1977b

BEAN SF, MICHEL B, FUREY N et al: Vesicular pemphigoid. Arch Dermatol 112:1402–1406, 1976

BRAUN-FALCO O, RUPEC M: Elektronenmikroskopische Untersuchungen zur Dynamik der Acantholyse bei Pemphigus vulgaris. Arch Klin Exp Dermatol 230:1–12, 1967

CONNOR BL, MARKS R, WILSON JONES E: Dermatitis herpetiformis: Histologic discriminants. Trans St John's Hosp Dermatol Soc 58:191–198, 1972

DUBERTRET L, BERTRAUX B, FOSSE M et al: Cellular events leading to blister formation in bullous pemphigoid. Br J Dermatol 103:615–624, 1980

DVORAK AM, MIHM MC, JR., OSAGE JE et al: Bullous pemphigoid, an ultrastructural study of the inflammatory response. J Invest Dermatol 78:91–101, 1982

ENG AM, MONCADA B: Bullous pemphigoid and dermatitis herpetiformis. Histologic differentiation. Arch Dermatol 110:51–57, 1978

HODGE L, MARSDEN RA, BLACK MM et al: Bullous pemphigoid: The frequency of mucosal involvement and concurrent malignancy related to indirect immunofluorescence findings. Br J Dermatol 105:65–69, 1981

HOLUBAR K, WOLFF K, KONRAD K et al: Ultrastructural localization of immunoglobulins in bullous pemphigoid skin. J Invest Dermatol 64:220–227, 1975

JABLONSKA S, CHORZELSKI, T: Kann das histologische Bild die Grundlage zur Differenzierung des Morbus Duhring mit dem Pemphigoid und Erythema multiforme darstellen? Dermatol Wochenschr 146:590–603, 1963

JABLONSKA S, CHORZELSKI TP, BEUTNER EH et al: Dermatitis herpetiformis and bullous pemphigoid: Intermediate and mixed forms. Arch Dermatol 112:45–48, 1976

JAKUBOWICZ K, DABROWSKI J, MACIEJEWSKI W: Elektronenmikroskopische Untersuchungen bei bullösem Pemphigoid und Dermatitis herpetiformis Duhring. Arch Klin Exp Dermatol 238:272–284, 1970

JORDON RE, TRIFTSHAUSER CT, SCHROETER AL: Direct immunofluorescent studies of pemphigus and bullous pemphigoid. Arch Dermatol 103:486–491, 1971

KOBAYASI T: The dermo-epidermal junction in bullous pemphigoid. Dermatologica 134:157–165, 1967

KRESBACH H, HARTWAGNER E: Zur Differentialdiagnose zwischen Dermatitis herpetiformis Duhring und bullösem Pemphigoid. Z Hautkr 43:165–176, 1968

KUOKKANEN K, HELIN H: Pemphigoid vegetans. Arch Dermatol 117:56–57, 1981

LEVER, WF: Pemphigus. Medicine (Baltimore) 32:1–123, 1953

LEVER WF: Pemphigus and pemphigoid: A review of the advances made since 1964. J Am Acad Dermatol 1:2–31, 1979

LEVER WF, HASHIMOTO K: The etiology and treatment of pemphigus and pemphigoid. J Invest Dermatol 53:373–389, 1969

NAITO K, MORIOKA S, OGAWA H: The pathogenic mechanisms of bullous pemphigoid in blister formation. (Abstr) J Invest Dermatol 76:420, 1981

PERSON JR, ROGERS RS, III: Bullous and cicatricial pemphigoid: Clinical, histopathogenic, and immunopathologic correlations. Mayo Clin Proc 52:54–66, 1977

PERSON JR, ROGERS RS, III, PERRY HO: Localized pemphigoid. Br J Dermatol 95:531–534, 1976

ROOK AJ, WADDINGTON E: Pemphigus and pemphigoid. Br J Dermatol 65:425–431, 1953

SAMS WM, JORDON RD: Correlation of pemphigoid and pemphigus antibody with activity of disease. Br J Dermatol 84:7–13, 1971

SCHAUMBURG-LEVER G, ORFANOS CE, LEVER WF: Electron microscopic study of bullous pemphigoid. Arch Dermatol 106:662–667, 1972

SCHAUMBURG-LEVER G, RULE A, SCHMIDT-ULLRICH B et al: Ultrastructural localization of in vivo bound immunoglobulins in bullous pemphigoid. J Invest Dermatol 64:47–49, 1975

STONE SP, SCHROETER AL: Bullous pemphigoid and associated malignant neoplasms. Arch Dermatol 111:991–994, 1975

UEKI H, WOLFF HH, BRAUN-FALCO O: Cutaneous localization of human gammaglobulins in lupus erythematosus. Arch Dermatol Forsch 248:297–314, 1974

VAN DER MEER JB: Dermatitis herpetiformis: A specific (immunopathological?) entity. Thesis, University of Utrecht, The Netherlands, 1972

WEBER L, KRIEG T, MÜLLER PK et al: Immunofluorescent localization of type IV collagen and laminin in human skin and its application in junctional zone pathology. Br J Dermatol 106:267–273, 1982

WINKELMANN RK, SU WPD: Pemphigoid vegetans. Arch Dermatol 115:446–448, 1979

Cicatricial Pemphigoid

BEAN SF: Cicatricial pemphigoid: Immunofluorescent studies. Arch Dermatol 110:552–555, 1974

BEHLEN CH, MACKAY DM: Benign mucous membrane pemphigus with a generalized eruption. Arch Dermatol 92:566–567, 1965

BRAUN-FALCO O, WOLFF HH, PONCE E: Disseminiertes vernarbendes Pemphigoid. Hautarzt 32:233–239, 1981

BRAUNER GJ, JIMBOW K: Benign mucous membrane pemphigoid. Arch Dermatol 106:535–540, 1972

BRUNSTING LA, PERRY HO: Benign pemphigoid? A report of seven cases with chronic scarring, herpetiform plaques about the head and neck. Arch Dermatol 75:489–501, 1957

CAPUTO R, BELLONE AG, CROSTI C: Pathogenesis of the blister in cicatricial pemphigoid and in bullous pemphigoid. Arch Dermatol Forsch 247:181–192, 1973

DANTZIG P: Circulating antibodies in cicatricial pemphigoid. Arch Dermatol 108:264–266, 1973

GRIFFITH MR, FUKUYAMA K, TUFFANELLI D et al: Immunofluorescent studies in mucous membrane pemphigoid. Arch Dermatol 109:195–199, 1974

HANNO R, FOSTER DR, BEAN SF: Brunsting-Perry cicatricial pemphigoid associated with bullous pemphigoid. J Am Acad Dermatol 3:470–473, 1980

HARDY KM, PERRY HO, PINGREE GC et al: Benign mucous membrane pemphigoid. Arch Dermatol 104:467–475, 1971

JACOBY WD, JR., BARTHOLOME CW, RAMCHAND SC, et al: Cicatricial pemphigoid (Brunsting-Perry type). Case report and immunofluorescence findings. Arch Dermatol 114:779–781, 1978

KLEINE-NATROP HE, HAUSTEIN UF: "Benignes Schleimhautpemphigoid" mit rascher Erblindung und generalisierten vernarbenden Hautveränderungen. Hautarzt 19:6–12, 1968

LEVER WF: Pemphigus conjunctivae with scarring of the skin. Arch Dermatol Syph 46:875–880, 1942, and 49:113–117, 1944

LEVER WF: Pemphigus. Medicine (Baltimore) 32:1–123, 1953

MICHEL B, BEAN SF, CHORZELSKI T et al: Cicatricial pemphigoid of Brunsting-Perry: Immunofluorescent studies. Arch Dermatol 113:1403–1405, 1977

PROVOST TT, MAIZE JC, AHMED AR et al: Unusual subepidermal bullous diseases with immunologic features of bullous pemphigoid. Arch Dermatol 115:156–160, 1979

ROGERS RS, III, PERRY HO, BEAN SF et al: Immunopathology of cicatricial pemphigoid: Studies of complement deposition. J Invest Dermatol 68:39–43, 1977

SUSI FR, SHKLAR G: Histochemistry and fine structure of oral lesions of mucous membrane pemphigoid. Arch Dermatol 104:244–253, 1971

TAGAMI H, IMAMURA S: Benign mucous membrane pemphigoid. Arch Dermatol 109:711–713, 1974

Herpes Gestationis

CARRUTHERS JA, BLACK MM, RAMNARAIN N: Immunopathological studies in herpes gestationis. Br J Dermatol 96:35–43, 1977

CHORZELSKI TP, JABLONSKA S, BEUTNER EH et al: Herpes gestationis with identical lesions in the newborn. Arch Dermatol 112:1129–1131, 1976

HERTZ KC, KATZ SI, MAIZE J et al: Herpes gestationis: A clinicopathological study. Arch Dermatol 112:1543–1548, 1976

HÖNIGSMANN H, STINGL G, HOLUBAR K et al: Herpes gestationis: Fine structural pattern of immunoglobulin deposits in the skin in vivo. J Invest Dermatol 66:389–392, 1976

KATZ A, MINTA JO, TOOLE JWP et al: Immunopathologic study of herpes gestationis in mother and infant. Arch Dermatol 113:1069–1072, 1977

KOCSIS M, EEG TL, HUSBY G et al: Immunofluorescence studies in herpes gestationis. Acta Derm Venereol (Stockh) 55:25–29, 1975

LAWLEY TJ, STINGL G, KATZ SI: Fetal and maternal risk factors in herpes gestationis. Arch Dermatol 114:552–555, 1978

PIÉRARD J, THIERY M, KINT A: Histologie et ultrastructure de l'herpes gestationis. Arch Belg Derm Syph 25:321–335, 1969

PROVOST TT, TOMASI TB: Evidence for complement activation via the alternate pathway in skin diseases. J Clin Invest 52:1779–1787, 1973

REUNALA T, KARVONEN J, TIILIKAINEN A et al: Herpes gestationis. Br J Dermatol 96:563–568, 1977

SCHAUMBURG–LEVER G, SAFFOLD OE, ORFANOS CE et al: Herpes gestationis: Histology and ultrastructure. J Invest Dermatol 107:888–892, 1973

YAOITA H, GULLINO M, KATZ SI: Herpes gestationis: Ultrastructure and ultrastructural localization on in vivo-bound complement. J Invest Dermatol 66:383–388, 1976

Dermatitis Herpetiformis, Chronic Dermatosis of Childhood

CHORZELSKI TP, BEUTNER EH, JABLONSKA S et al: Immunofluorescence studies in the diagnosis of dermatitis herpetiformis and its differentiation from bullous pemphigoid. J Invest Dermatol 56:373–380, 1971

CHORZELSKI TP, JABLONSKA S: IgA linear dermatosis of childhood (chronic bullous disease of childhood). Br J Dermatol 101:535–542, 1979

CHORZELSKI T, JABLONSKA S: IgA-lineäre Dermatose. Hautarzt 32:546–547, 1981

CONNOR BL, MARKS R, WILSON JONES E: Dermatitis herpetiformis. Trans St. John's Hosp Dermatol Soc 58:191–198, 1972

DABROWSKI J, CHORZELSKI T, JABLONSKA S, et al: Immunoelectron microscopic studies in IgA linear dermatosis. Arch Dermatol Res 265:289–298, 1979

ENG AM, MONCADA B: Bullous pemphigoid and dermatitis herpetiformis. Arch Dermatol 110:51–57, 1974

ESTERLY NB, FUREY NL, KIRSCHNER BS et al: Chronic bullous dermatosis of childhood. Arch Dermatol 113:42–46, 1977

FABER WR, VAN JOOST T: Juvenile pemphigoid. Br J Dermatol 89:519–522, 1973

FRÖDIN T, GOTTHARD R, HED J et al: Gluten-free diet for dermatitis herpetiformis. Acta Derm Venereol (Stockh) 61:405–411, 1981.

HEADING RC, PATERSON WD, MCCLELLAND DBL et al: Clinical response of dermatitis herpetiformis skin lesions to a gluten-free diet. Br J Dermatol 94:509–514, 1976

HONEYMAN JF, HONEYMAN AR, DE LA PARRA MA et al: Polymorphic pemphigoid. Arch Dermatol 115:423–427, 1979

JABLONSKA S, CHORZELSKI T: Kann das histologische Bild die Grundlage zur Differenzierung des Morbus Duhring mit dem Pemphigoid und Erythema multiforme darstellen? Dermatol Wocherschr 146:590–603, 1963

JABLONSKA S, CHORZELSKI T: Dermatose à IgA linéaire. Ann Dermatol Venereol 106:651–655, 1979

JABLONSKA S, CHORZELSKI T: When and how to use sulfones in bullous diseases. Int J Dermatol 20:103–105, 1981

JABLONSKA S, CHORZELSKI TP, BEUTNER EH et al: Dermatitis herpetiformis and bullous pemphigoid: Intermediate and mixed forms. Arch Dermatol 112:45–48, 1976

JAKUBOWICZ K, DABROWSKI J, MACIEJEWSKI W: Elektronenmikroskopische Untersuchungen bei bullösem Pemphigoid und Dermatitis herpetiformis Duhring. Arch Klin Exp Dermatol 238:272–284, 1970

KATZ SI, STROBER W: The pathogenesis of dermatitis herpetiformis. (Review) J Invest Dermatol 70:63–75, 1978

KINT A, GEERTS ML, DE BRAUWERE D: Diagnostic criteria in dermatitis herpetiformis. Dermatologica 153:266–271, 1976

KRESBACH H, HARTWAGNER A: Zur Differentialdiagnose zwischen Dermatitis herpetiformis Duhring und bullösem Pemphigoid. Z Hautkr 43:165–176, 1968

LAWLEY TJ, STROBER W, YAOITA H et al: Small intestinal biopsies and HLA types in dermatitis herpetiformis patients with granular and linear IgA skin deposits. J Invest Dermatol 74:9–12, 1980

LEVER WF: Pemphigus and pemphigoid: A review of the advances made since 1964. J Am Acad Dermatol 1:2–31, 1979

MACVICAR DN, GRAHAM JH, BURGOON CF, JR.: Dermatitis herpetiformis, erythema multiforme and bullous pemphigoid: A comparative histopathological and histochemical study. J Invest Dermatol 41:289–300, 1963

MARKS JM: Dogma and dermatitis herpetiformis. Clin Exp Dermatol 2:189–207, 1977

MARSDEN RA, MCKEE PH, BHOGAL B et al: A study of benign chronic bullous dermatosis of childhood. Clin Exp Dermatol 5:159–172, 1980

MCGUIRE J, NORDLUND J: Bullous disease of childhood. Arch Dermatol 108:284–285, 1973

PEHAMBERGER H, KONRAD K, HOLUBAR K: Circulating IgA antibasement membrane antibodies in linear dermatitis herpetiformis (Duhring): Immunofluorescence and immunoelectronmicroscopic studies. J Invest Dermatol 69:490–493, 1977

PEHAMBERGER H, KONRAD K, HOLUBAR K: Juvenile dermatitis herpetiformis: An immunoelectron microscopic study. Br J Dermatol 101:271–277, 1979

PIÉRARD J: De l'aspect histologique des plaques érythémateuses de la dermatite herpétiforme de Duhring. Ann Dermatol Syph 90:121–133, 1963

PIÉRARD J, KINT A: Dermatite herpétiforme et pemphigoide bulleuse. Ann Dermatol Syph 95:391–404, 1968

REUNALA T: Gluten-free diet in dermatitis herpetiformis. Br J Dermatol 98:69–78, 1978

REUNALA T, BLOMQUIST K, TARPILA et al: Gluten-free diet in dermatitis herpetiformis. Br J Dermatol 97:473–480, 1977

SCHAUMBURG-LEVER G, ORFANOS CE, LEVER WF: Electron microscopic study of bullous pemphigoid. Arch Dermatol 106:662–667, 1972

SEAH PP, FRY L: Immunoglobulins in the skin in dermatitis herpetiformis and their relevance in diagnosis. Br J Dermatol 92:157–166, 1975

SEAH PP, FRY L, STEWART JS et al: Immunoglobulins in the skin in dermatitis herpetiformis and coeliac disease. Lancet 1:611–614, 1972

THUNE P, HUSBY G, FAUSA O et al: Immunological and gastrointestinal abnormalities in dermatitis herpetiformis. Int J Dermatol 18:136–141, 1979

TOLMAN MM, MOSCHELLA SL, SCHNEIDERMAN RN: Dermatitis herpetiformis: Specific entity or clinical complex? J Invest Dermatol 32:557–561, 1959

VAN DER MEER JB: Dermatitis herpetiformis: A specific (immunopathological?) entity. Thesis, University of Utrecht, The Netherlands, 1972

VAN DER MEER JB, REMME JJ, NELKINS MJJ et al: IgA antibasement membrane antibodies in a boy with pemphigoid. Arch Dermatol 113:1462, 1977.

YAOITA H, KATZ SI: Immunoelectronmicroscopic localization of IgA in skin of patients with dermatitis herpetiformis. J Invest Dermatol 67:502–506, 1976

YAOITA H, KATZ SI: Circulating IgA anti-basement membrane zone antibodies in dermatitis herpetiformis. J Invest Dermatol 69:558–560, 1977

Erythema Multiforme

ACKERMAN AB, PENNEYS NS, CLARK WH: Erythema multiforme exudativum: Distinctive pathological process. Br J Dermatol 84:554–566, 1971

BEDI TR, PINKUS H: Histopathological spectrum of erythema multiforme. Br J Dermatol 95:243–250, 1976

BRAUN-FALCO O: Histopathologie des Lyell-Syndromes. In Braun-Falco O, Bandmann HJ (eds): Das Lyell-Syndrom, pp 61–80. Bern, Hans Huber, 1970

BRAUN-FALCO O, WOLFF HH: Zur Ultrastruktur der Epidermis beim Lyell-Syndrom. Arch Klin Exp Dermatol 236:83–96, 1969

BUSHKELL LL, MACKEL SE, JORDON RE: Erythema multiforme: Direct immunofluorescence studies and detection of circulating immune complexes. J Invest Dermatol 74:372–374, 1980

HUFF JC, WESTON WL: Clinical and laboratory features of recurrent erythema multiforme. (Abstr) J Invest Dermatol 76:331, 1981

IMAMURA S, YANASE K, TANIGUCHI S et al: Erythema multiforme: Demonstration of immune complexes in the sera and skin lesions. Br J Dermatol 102:161–166, 1980

KAZMIEROWSKI JA, WUEPPER KD: Erythema multiforme: Immune complex vasculitis of the superficial cutaneous microvasculature. J Invest Dermatol 71:366–369, 1978

KOPF AW, GRUPPER C, BAER RL: Eruptive nevocytic nevi after severe bullous disease. Arch Dermatol 113:1080–1084, 1977

LYELL A: Toxic epidermal necrolysis: An eruption resembling scalding of the skin. Br J Dermatol 68:355–361, 1956

LYELL A: A review of toxic-epidermal necrolysis in Britain. Br J Dermatol 79:662–671, 1967

LYELL A: Toxic epidermal necrolysis (the scalded skin syndrome): A reappraisal. Br J Dermatol 100:69–86, 1979

MACVICAR DN, GRAHAM JH, BURGOON CF, JR.: Dermatitis herpetiformis, erythema multiforme, and bullous pemphigoid: A comparative histopathological and histochemical study. J Invest Dermatol 41:289–300, 1963

ORFANOS CE, SCHAUMBURG-LEVER G, LEVER WF: Dermal and epidermal types of erythema multiforme. Arch Dermatol 109:682–688, 1974

PRUTKIN L, FELLNER MJ: Erythema multiforme bullosum. Acta Derm Venereol (Stockh) 51:429–434, 1971

RUSSELL JONES R: Azathioprine therapy in the management of persistent erythema multiforme. Br J Dermatol 105:465–468, 1981

SHELLEY WB: Herpes simplex virus as a cause of erythema multiforme. JAMA 201:153–156, 1967

SONTHEIMER RD, GARIBALDI RA, KRUEGER GG: Stevens-Johnson syndrome associated with *Mycoplasma pneumoniae* infections. Arch Dermatol 114:241–244, 1978

TRITSCH H: Nekrolyse als histopathologisches Phänomen. Arch Klin Exp Dermatol 237:295–299, 1970

Graft-Versus-Host Disease

DE DOBBELEER GD, LEDOUX-CORBUSIER MH, ACHTERN GA: Graft versus host reaction: An ultrastructural study. Arch Dermatol 111:1597–1602, 1975

GLUCKSBERG H, STROB R, FEFER A et al: Clinical manifestations of graft-versus-host disease in human recipients of marrow from HL-A-matched sibling donors. Transplantation 18:295–304, 1975

GROGAN TH, ODOM RB, BURGESS JH: Graft-vs-host reaction. Arch Dermatol 113:806–812, 1977

HOOD AF, SOTER NA, RAPPEPORT J et al: Graft-vs-host reaction. Arch Dermatol 113:1087–1091, 1977

JANIN-MERCIER A, SAURAT JH, BOURGES M et al: The lichen planuslike and sclerotic phases of the graft versus host disease in man. Acta Derm Venereol (Stockh) 61:187–193, 1981

MASCARO JM, ROZMAN C, PALOU J et al: Acute and chronic graft-vs-host reaction in skin: Report of two cases. Br J Dermatol 102:461–466, 1980

MORHENN VB, MAIBACH HI: Graft vs. host reaction in a newborn. Acta Derm Venereol (Stockh) 54:133–136, 1974

PARKMAN R, RAPPEPORT J, ROSEN F: Human graft versus host disease. J Invest Dermatol 74:276–279, 1980

PECK GL, HERZIG GP, ELIAS PM: Toxic epidermal necrolysis in a patient with graft-vs-host reaction. Arch Dermatol 105:561–569, 1972

SAURAT JH, GLUCKMAN E, RUSSEL A et al: The lichen planus-like eruption after bone marrow transplantation. Br J Dermatol 93:675–681, 1975

SCHMITT D, THIVOLET J: Lymphocyte–epidermis interactions in malignant epidermotropic lymphomas. Acta Derm Venereol (Stockh) 60:1–11, 1980

SHULMAN HM, SALE GE, LERNER KG et al: Chronic cutaneous graft-versus-host disease in man. Am J Pathol 91:545–570, 1978

SPIELVOGEL RL, GOLTZ RW, KERSEY JH: Scleroderma-like changes in chronic graft vs host disease. Arch Dermatol 113:1424–1428, 1977

TSOI MS, STORB R, JONES E et al: Deposition of IgM and C at the dermoepidermal junction in acute and chronic cutaneous graft-vs-host disease in man. J Immunol 120:1485–1492, 1978

ULLMAN S: Immunoglobulins and complement in skin in graft-versus-host disease. Ann Intern Med 85:205, 1976

Subcorneal Pustular Dermatosis

BURNS RE, FINE G: Subcorneal pustular dermatosis. Arch Dermatol 80:72–80, 1959

CHIMENTI S, ACKERMAN AB: Is subcorneal pustular dermatosis of Sneddon and Wilkinson an entity *sui generis?* Am J Dermatopathol 3:363–376, 1981

METZ J, SCHRÖPL F: Elektronenmikroskopische Untersuchungen bei subcornealer pustulöser Dermatose. Arch Klin Exp Dermatol 236:190–206, 1970

SANCHEZ N, ACKERMAN, AB: Subcorneal pustular dermatosis: A variant of pustular psoriasis. Acta Derm Venereol (Stockh) 59, Suppl 85:147–151, 1979

SANCHEZ NP, PERRY HO, MULLER SA: On the relationship between subcorneal pustular dermatosis and pustular psoriasis. Am J Dermatopathol 3:385–386, 1981

SNEDDON IB, WILKINSON DS: Subcorneal pustular dermatosis. Br J Dermatol 68:385–394, 1956

SNEDDON IB, WILKINSON DS: Subcorneal pustular dermatosis. Br J Dermatol 100:61–68, 1979

WOLFF K: Ein Beitrag zur Nosologie der subcornealen pustulösen Dermatose (Sneddon-Wilkinson). Arch Klin Exp Dermatol 224:248–267, 1966

Transient Acantholytic Dermatosis

BYSTRYN JC: Immunofluorescence studies in transient acantholytic dermatosis (Grover's disease). Am J Dermatopathol 1:325–327, 1979

CHALET M, GROVER R, ACKERMAN AB: Transient acantholytic dermatosis. Arch Dermatol 113:431–435, 1977

FISHMAN HC: Acute eruptive Darier disease. Arch Dermatol 111:221–222, 1975

GISSLÉN H, MOBACKEN H: Acute adult-onset Darier-like dermatosis. Br J Dermatol 98:217–220, 1978

GROVER RW: Transient acantholytic dermatosis. Arch Dermatol 101:426–434, 1970

GROVER RW, DUFFY JL: Transient acantholytic dermatosis. J Cutan Pathol 2:111–127, 1975

HEAPHY MR, TUCKER SB, WINKELMANN RK: Benign papular acantholytic dermatosis. Arch Dermatol 112:814–821, 1976

HEENAN PJ, QUIRK CJ: Transient acantholytic dermatosis. Br J Dermatol 102:515–520, 1980

KANZAKI T, HASHIMOTO K: Transient acantholytic dermatosis with involvement of oral mucosa. J Cutan Pathol 5:23–30, 1978

PEHAMBERGER H, GSCHNAIT F, KONRAD K et al: Transient acantholytic dermatosis Grover. Z Hautkr 52:841–846, 1977

WOLFF HH, CHALET MD, ACKERMAN AB: Transitorische akantholytische Dermatose (Grover). Hautarzt 28:78–82, 1977

Friction Blisters

BREHMER-ANDERSON E, GÖRANSSON K: Friction blisters as a manifestation of pathomimia. Acta Derm Venereol (Stockh) 55:65–71, 1975

NAYLOR PFD: Experimental friction blisters. Br J Dermatol 67:327–342, 1955

SULZBERGER MB, CORTESE TA, JR., FISHMAN L et al: Studies on blisters produced by friction. J Invest Dermatol 47:456–465, 1966

Electric Burns

WINER LH, LEVIN GH: Changes in the skin as a result of electric current. Arch Dermatol 78:386–390, 1958

Thermal Burns

FOLEY FD: Pathology of cutaneous burns. Surg Clin North Am 50:1200–1210, 1970

SEVITT S: Histological changes in burned skin. In Burns: Pathology and Therapeutic Applications, pp 18–27. London, Butterworth & Co, 1957

Noninfectious Erythematous, Papular, and Squamous Diseases

8

URTICARIA

Urticaria is characterized by the presence of transient, recurrent wheals, that is, raised, erythematous areas of edema. It is usually accompanied by itching. Large wheals in which the edema extends to the subcutaneous tissue are referred to as angioedema.

In *hereditary angioedema,* a rare form of dominantly inherited angioedema, recurrent attacks of edema occur not only on the skin but also on the oral, laryngeal, and gastrointestinal mucosa. Itching is absent. Before treatment with danazol, a synthetic androgen, was available, death from sudden laryngeal edema could occur (Tappeiner et al).

Urticarial vasculitis is a syndrome consisting of recurrent episodes or urticaria often associated with arthralgia and abdominal pain and rarely with glomerulonephritis (Soter). The individual lesions of urticaria tend to persist for 1 to 3 days and may reveal faint purpura (Sams).

Histopathology. In the *common type of urticaria,* one observes dermal edema and a perivascular lymphocytic infiltrate that is usually sparse but may be dense and intermingled with eosinophils (Monroe et al). In angioedema, the edema and infiltrate extend into the subcutaneous tissue.

In *hereditary angioedema,* there is subcutaneous and submucosal edema without infiltrating inflammatory cells (Soter and Wasserman).

In *urticarial vasculitis,* the dermis shows a leukocytoclastic vasculitis characterized by fibrinoid deposits in the blood vessel walls, an infiltrate composed largely of neutrophils, many of which show fragmentation of their nuclei, and slight to moderate extravasation of erythrocytes (Soter et al). (For details about leukocytoclastic vasculitis, see p. 168.)

Histogenesis. Common urticaria often has no apparent cause. In some instances, however, it is caused by sensitivity to specific antigens such as certain foods and drugs and then is IgE-dependent, that is, it occurs as an anaphylactic reaction or type I reaction. In contrast, hereditary angioedema and urticarial vasculitis are complement-mediated (Soter and Wasserman).

On *electron microscopic examination,* common urticaria reveals mast cell and eosinophilic degranulation. Vascular deposits of immunoglobulins, complement, or fibrin are only rarely seen (Monroe et al).

Hereditary angioedema has a low serum level of the esterase inhibitor of the first component of complement (C1). Exhaustion of this inhibitor allows activation of C1. This leads to activation of C4 and C2, with the generation of a C2 fragment possessing kininlike activity and causing increased vasopermeability (Tappeiner et al).

In urticarial vasculitis, circulating immune complexes are found in about one half of the patients, and vascular deposits of immunoglobulins, complement, or fibrin in about one third of the patients (Monroe et al). In addition, some patients show hypocomplementemia (McDuffie et al; Soter et al).

PRURITIC URTICARIAL PAPULES AND PLAQUES OF PREGNANCY

A fairly common entity first described in 1979 (Lawley et al), pruritic urticarial papules and plaques of pregnancy (PUPPP) is an intensely pruritic eruption occurring in the third trimester of pregnancy. It shows a symmetric

136

distribution of papules, urticarial lesions, and some erythema-multiforme-like target lesions. The abdomen and the proximal parts of the extremities are most commonly involved. There may be no recurrences with subsequent pregnancies (Callen and Hanno).

Histopathology. The histologic findings are non-specific. One observes a moderately pronounced perivascular mononuclear infiltrate with a variable number of eosinophils.

Epidermal changes may be absent or present. If present, they consist of focal spongiosis and para-keratosis in association with mild acanthosis (Lawley et al; Callen and Hanno).

ERYTHEMA ANNULARE CENTRIFUGUM

In erythema annulare centrifugum, one observes one or, more commonly, several annular or serpiginous lesions with a red, raised, firm border that in the course of weeks extends peripherally. Some lesions may be as large as 10 cm in diameter. The process may go on for years, with new lesions appearing successively. The preferred site of the eruption is the trunk.

According to some authors, there exists, in addition to this deep form first described by Darier, a superficial form with less induration but with scaling along the ring-shaped or gyrate border (Ackerman; Bressler and Jones).

Histopathology. In the classic deep or indurated type, a cellular infiltrate showing a fairly sharply demarcated perivascular "coat-sleeve-like" arrangement is present in the middle and lower

portions of the dermis (Ellis and Friedman; Nordenskjöld and Wahlgren). The infiltrate consists of mononuclear cells, largely lymphocytes (Fig. 8-1).

In the superficial form, the histologic picture is rather nonspecific, showing a mild, superficial perivascular lymphohistiocytic infiltrate, slight spongiosis with microvesiculation, and focal para-keratosis (Ackerman; Bressler and Jones).

Differential Diagnosis. The rather striking "coat-sleeve-like" perivascular arrangement of the infiltrate seen in the deep form of erythema annulare centrifugum is encountered also in secondary syphilis. However, in secondary syphilis, numerous plasma cells usually are present, and the intima and endothelial cells are swollen (see p. 323).

ERYTHEMA GYRATUM REPENS

A very rare but clinically highly characteristic dermatosis first reported in 1952 (Gammel), erythema gyratum repens has been associated with a carcinoma in nearly all reported cases (Skolnick and Mainman) with only very few exceptions (Stankler). Clinically, there is a generalized, mildly itching eruption consisting of parallel red bands with an annular and serpiginous arrangement resembling the grain of wood. The bands often show peripheral scaling. The clinical picture changes daily, since the bands of erythema move about 1 cm per day.

Histopathology. The histologic picture is non-specific, showing mild patchy spongiosis and para-keratosis and a moderate, perivascular, lympho-cytic, histiocytic infiltrate (Gammel; Holt and Davies).

Fig. 8-1. Erythema annulare centrifugum
Throughout the dermis, thick perivascular sleeves of mononuclear cells, largely lymphocytes, are seen. (×100)

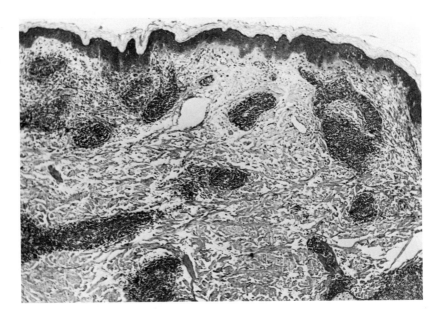

In one instance, eosinophils and melanophages were also seen in the dermal infiltrate (Leavell et al), and, in another, a dense and diffuse cellular infiltrate was seen in the papillary and subpapillary layers (Skolnick and Mainman).

Histogenesis. In one case, granular deposits of immunoglobulin G (IgG) and C3 were seen at the basement membrane zone, suggesting that erythema gyratum repens may have an immunologic pathogenesis (Holt and Davies).

ERYTHEMA DYSCHROMICUM PERSTANS

Erythema dyschromicum perstans, also called ashy dermatosis, is an extensive asymptomatic eruption. It begins with disseminated macules that, by peripheral extension and coalescence, form large patches with a polycyclic outline. Although the macules may at first be erythematous before assuming their characteristic bluish gray color, they often appear bluish gray from the very beginning. The disease progresses slowly, and the discoloration persists. The most common areas of involvement are the trunk, arms, and face. Most patients with this disorder are Latin American.

Histopathology. In the early active stage, many basal cells, but also some squamous cells in the lower epidermis, show vacuolization of their cytoplasm, leading to liquefaction degeneration. The upper dermis shows a mild to moderate perivascular infiltrate in the upper third of the dermis. This infiltrate consists of lymphocytes and histiocytes intermingled with melanophages (Knox et al). There may also be exocytosis of the infiltrate into the epidermis, and occasional colloid bodies resembling those seen in lichen planus may be present (Tschen et al). The only abnormality late lesions show is aggregates of melanophages (Knox et al).

Histogenesis. *Electron microscopic examination* reveals within the affected keratinocytes, as the ultrastructural counterpart of the liquefaction degeneration, many vacuoles delimited by a membrane. This is associated with widening of the intercellular spaces and retraction of desmosomes to either one cell or the other. Additional findings are discontinuities in the subepidermal basement membrane and the presence in the dermis of melanophages containing aggregates of melanosomes enclosed by a lysosomal membrane (Soter et al). It can be assumed that the liquefaction degeneration is the cause of the incontinence of pigment, as well as of the formation of the colloid bodies.

The presence of damage to the basal cell layer with formation of colloid bodies and pigmentary incontinence suggests a possible relationship of erythema dyschromicum perstans to lichen planus pigmentosus, also called lichen planus actinicus or subtropicus (Tschen et al) (see p. 154). However, lichen planus pigmentosus has a more pronounced lichenoid, that is, subepidermal, distribution of the infiltrate, and its lesions have a greater predilection to be located in exposed areas (Sanchez et al).

Differential Diagnosis. The histologic picture of erythema dyschromicum perstans is not diagnostic. Similar inflammation and pigmentary incontinence may be seen in drug eruptions, especially in fixed drug eruptions (Knox et al).

PRURIGO SIMPLEX

Erythematous urticarial papules that are intensely pruritic are seen in symmetric distribution, especially on the extensor surfaces of the extremities. In contrast with dermatitis herpetiformis, which prurigo simplex may resemble in clinical appearance, there is no grouping of lesions (Braun-Falco and von Eickstedt). In other cases, prurigo simplex greatly resembles arthropod bites (papular urticaria).

Histopathology. The histologic picture is nonspecific. Early papules show mild acanthosis, spongiosis with an occasional small spongiotic vesicle, and parakeratosis. The upper dermis contains a mild, chronic inflammatory infiltrate in a largely perivascular arrangement (Kocsard). An admixture of eosinophils is present in some cases (Braun-Falco and von Eickstedt; Rosen and Algra). Excoriated papules show partial absence of the epidermis; instead, they are covered with a crust containing degenerated nuclei of inflammatory cells (Braun-Falco and von Eickstedt). On serial sectioning, the histologic changes may be found to be centered around hair follicles, which then show spongiosis, mononuclear cell infiltration of the follicular infundibulum, and a perifollicular infiltrate (Uehara and Ofuji). In other instances, there is distinct sparing of the follicular structures (Rosen and Algra).

Differential Diagnosis. The diagnosis of dermatitis herpetiformis is easily excluded by the absence in prurigo simplex of microabscesses at the tips of papillae and of neutrophils, eosinophils, and nuclear dust in the dermal infiltrate. The histologic picture of prurigo simplex resembles that of a subacute dermatitis, except that the extent of its papular lesions is much more limited. Histologic differentiation from papular urticaria is not possible (Braun-Falco and von Eickstedt).

PRURIGO NODULARIS

In prurigo nodularis, there are discrete, raised, firm hyperkeratotic lesions, usually from 5 mm to 12 mm in size but occasionally larger. They occur chiefly on the extensor surfaces of the extremities and are intensely pruritic.

Histopathology. One observes pronounced hyperkeratosis and acanthosis. In addition, there may be papillomatosis and irregular downward proliferation of the epidermis (Fig. 8-2) approaching pseudocarcinomatous hyperplasia (Runne and Orfanos) (see p. 505). The dermis shows a nonspecific inflammatory infiltrate and a proliferation of nerves. Even with routine stains, one may occasionally observe hyperplasia of cutaneous nerves (Feuerman and Sandbank) or neuroid structures similar to the Verocay bodies in neurilemmoma (Runne and Orfanos). In other cases, silver stains or cholinesterase stains are necessary to demonstrate an increase in both size and number of the cutaneous nerves (Doyle et al).

Histogenesis. On *electron microscopic examination*, it is evident that the neural proliferation involves both axons and Schwann cells (Runne and Orfanos). Degenerative changes in these nerve structures, such as swelling of axons, are only rarely seen and, if present, are mild (Feuerman and Sandbank).

It is generally assumed that the neural proliferation in prurigo nodularis is a secondary phenomenon due to chronic traumatization by scratching. Still, it may well be that the extreme pruritus is related to the increased number of dermal nerves (Runne and Orfanos).

Differential Diagnosis. Multiple keratoacanthomas, which often show less of a central crater than solitary keratoacanthomas, may be difficult to distinguish from prurigo nodularis, since both show marked epithelial hyperplasia (Ereaux and Schopflocher).

PSORIASIS

Psoriasis may be divided into (1) psoriasis vulgaris, in which pustules are absent, (2) generalized pustular psoriasis, and (3) localized pustular psoriasis. Generalized pustular psoriasis includes the von Zumbusch type and, as variants, generalized acrodermatitis continua of Hallopeau (acral type of generalized pustular psoriasis) and impetigo herpetiformis (exanthematous type of generalized pustular psoriasis). There are three types of localized pustular psoriasis: (a) "psoriasis with pustules" (Schuppener), in which only one or a few of the areas of psoriasis show pustules and the tendency to change into a generalized pustular psoriasis is not great; (b) localized acrodermatitis continua of

Fig. 8-2. Prurigo nodularis
There are hyperkeratosis and considerable acanthosis with irregular downward proliferation of the epidermis approaching pseudocarcinomatous hyperplasia. (×100)

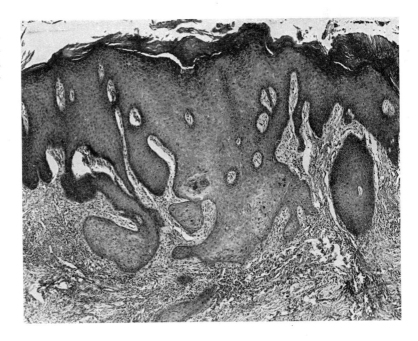

Hallopeau, which occasionally changes into generalized acrodermatitis continua; and (c) pustular psoriasis of the palms and soles, also called pustulosis palmaris et plantaris, which occasionally is seen in association with psoriasis vulgaris. The relationship of Reiter's disease to psoriasis will be discussed in the description of Reiter's disease.

Psoriasis Vulgaris

Psoriasis vulgaris is a chronic disorder characterized by brownish red papules and plaques. The lesions are sharply demarcated, dry, and usually covered with layers of fine, silvery scales. As the scales are removed by gentle scraping, fine bleeding points usually are seen, the so-called Auspitz sign. The scalp, sacral region, and extensor surfaces of the extremities are commonly involved, although, in some patients, the flexural and intertriginous areas are mainly affected. Involvement of the nails is common. In severe cases, the disease may affect the entire skin and present itself as generalized erythrodermic psoriasis. Pustules generally are absent in psoriasis vulgaris, although pustular psoriasis of the palms and soles occasionally occurs. Rarely, one or a few areas show pustules, and this is referred to as psoriasis with pustules. Also rarely, severe psoriasis vulgaris develops into generalized pustular psoriasis (see p. 145). Oral lesions do not occur in psoriasis vulgaris but may be seen in generalized pustular psoriasis.

Psoriatic arthritis chracteristically involves the terminal interphalangeal joints, but, not infrequently, the large joints are also affected, so that a clinical differentiation from rheumatoid arthritis often is impossible.

However, the rheumatoid factor, determined by latex fixation or the sheep red cell agglutination test, generally is absent.

Histopathology. The histologic picture of psoriasis vulgaris varies considerably with the stage of the lesion and usually is diagnostic only in early, scaling papules and near the margin of advancing plaques.

The earliest pinhead-sized macules or smooth-surfaced papules show a nonspecific histologic picture with a preponderance of dermal changes (Braun-Falco and Christophers; Ragaz and Ackerman). At first, there is capillary dilatation and edema in the papillary dermis, with a mononuclear infiltrate surrounding the capillaries. The mononuclear cells move into the lower portion of the epidermis, where slight spongiosis develops. Then focal changes occur in the upper portion of the epidermis, where granular cells become vacuolated and disappear, and parakeratosis forms above these focal changes. At this point, the phenomenon of the "squirting papillae" occurs (Pinkus and Mehregan): neutrophils are discharged intermittently from papillary capillaries and are attracted to the parakeratotic zones. The neutrophils clearly move rapidly, because they are usually seen only at the summits of some of the mounds of parakeratosis, which, since they form at various times, appear scattered through an otherwise orthokeratotic stratum corneum (Fig. 8-3). These parakeratotic mounds with their admixture of neutrophils represent the earliest manifestation of Munro mi-

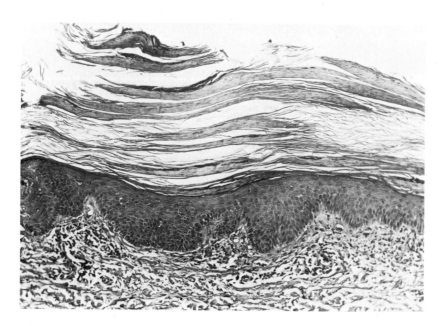

Fig. 8-3.   Psoriasis vulgaris
Earliest diagnostic lesion consisting of scattered parakeratotic mounds within an otherwise orthokeratotic stratum corneum. Some of the parakerototic mounds show degenerated neutrophils in their summits. ($\times 100$)

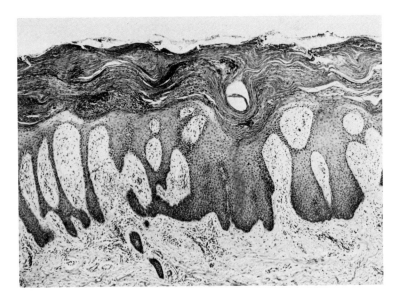

Fig. 8-4. Psoriasis vulgaris
Low magnification. The rete ridges show regular elongation with thickening in the lower portion. The papillae are elongated and edematous. In addition, there is marked parakeratosis. ($\times 50$)

croabscesses (Ragaz and Ackerman). At this stage, characterized clinically by an early, scaling papule, a histologic diagnosis of psoriasis can often be made. In some cases, when there is marked exudation of neutrophils, one finds neutrophils also in the uppermost portion of the spinous layer, where they may aggregate to form small spongiform pustules. Mononuclear cells remain confined to the lower epidermis, which, as more and more mitoses occur, becomes increasingly hyperplastic. The epidermal changes at first are focal but later on become confluent, leading clinically to the formation of plaques.

In the fully developed lesions of psoriasis, as best seen at the margin of enlarging plaques, the histologic picture is characterized by (1) regular elongation of the rete ridges with thickening in their lower portion, (2) elongation and edema of the papillae, (3) thinning of the suprapapillary portions of the stratum malpighii, with the occasional presence of a very small spongiform pustule, (4) the absence of granular cells, (5) parakeratosis, and (6) the presence of Munro microabscesses (Fig. 8-4). Of all the listed features, only the spongiform pustule and Munro microabscesses are truly diagnostic of psoriasis, and, in their absence, the diagnosis rarely can be made with certainty on a histologic basis. In detail, the changes in active psoriasis are as follows.

The rete ridges show considerable elongation and extend downward to a uniform level, resulting in regular acanthosis. They are often slender in their upper portion but show thickening ("clubbing") in their lower portion. Not infrequently,

neighboring rete ridges are seen to coalesce at their bases. There is as a rule neither intercellular nor intracellular edema in the rete ridges, in which even those cells that are located well above the basal layer show deep basophilia. Also, mitoses are not limited, as in normal skin, to the basal layer but are seen also in the two rows of cells above the basal layer (Van Scott and Ekel).

The papillae, in accordance with the elongation and basal thickening of the rete ridges, are elongated and club-shaped. They show edema, and the capillaries within them appear dilated and tortuous. A relatively mild inflammatory infiltrate is present in the upper dermis and the papillae. It consists only of mononuclear cells, except in early lesions, in which neutrophils are also present in the upper portion of the papillae (Pinkus and Mehregan).

The stratum malpighii overlying the papillae appears relatively thin in comparison with the markedly elongated rete ridges, and the cells in the upper stratum malpighii may appear enlarged and pale-staining as a result of intracellular edema. The epidermal cells located immediately beneath the parakeratotic stratum corneum may be intermingled with neutrophils (Fig. 8-5) (Gordon and Johnson). The histologic picture is then that of a small spongiform pustule of Kogoj. Although it is only a micropustule, it is nevertheless of the same type as the much larger macropustules seen in pustular psoriasis (see p. 145). Such a spongiform pustule, highly diagnostic for psoriasis and its variants, shows aggregates of neutrophils within the interstices of a spongelike network formed by degenerated and thinned epidermal cells (Rupec).

The horny layer in some instances consists entirely of parakeratotic cells, and, since, in the epidermis, a direct relationship exists between the absence of keratohyaline granules and the development of parakeratosis, there is concomitantly an absence of stratum granulosum. However, not infrequently, some orthokeratosis is present with underlying granular cells (see below).

Munro microabscesses (Fig. 8-5) are located within parakeratotic areas of the horny layer. They consist of accumulations of pyknotic nuclei of neutrophils that have migrated there from capillaries in the papillae through the suprapapillary epidermis. As a rule, Munro microabscesses are found easily in early lesions but are few in number or absent in old lesions (Burks and Montgomery).

An entirely typical histologic picture as described above is actually found in only a small percentage of biopsy specimens, even if only clinically typical lesions of psoriasis are examined. Thus, in a series of 107 lesions examined, only about one third exhibited extensive continuous parakeratosis. Nearly one third showed orthokeratosis to be more prevalent than parakeratosis, and some of these lesions had a completely orthokeratotic stratum corneum (Cox and Watson). Orthokeratosis often appears intermingled with parakeratosis. In such cases, one may see vertically adjoining areas of hyperkeratosis and parakeratosis, patchy parakeratosis, or, occasionally, alternating layers of orthokeratosis and parakeratosis. The latter pattern indicates a fluctuation in the intensity of the psoriasis.

The bleeding points that may be produced by gentle scraping of the skin correspond to the tips of papillae. They are attributable to the following histologic changes: parakeratosis, intracellular edema of the keratinocytes in the suprapapillary epidermis, and dilatation of the capillaries in the upper portion of the papillae.

The histologic picture of *erythrodermic psoriasis* in some instances shows enough of the characteristics of psoriasis to allow this diagnosis (Fig. 8-6). Frequently, however, the histologic appearance is indistinguishable from that of a chronic dermatitis (Abrahams et al).

Histogenesis. In active lesions of psoriasis, the rate of *epidermal cell replication* is markedly accelerated, as shown by the higher than normal number of mitotic figures and the greater number of premitotic cells labeled by tritiated thymidine (Weinstein and Van Scott). However, it is not fully established by which means this excessive replication comes about. Early calculations made it appear likely that, in psoriatic lesions, there was a great acceleration of the transit time of cells from the basal cell layer to the uppermost row of the squamous cell layer—from approximately 13 days in normal epidermis to only 2 days in the epidermis of active psoriatic lesions (Weinstein and Van Scott)—and that, in addition, the reproductive cell cycle was reduced from 457 hr for normal germinative cells to 37½ hr for psoriatic germi-

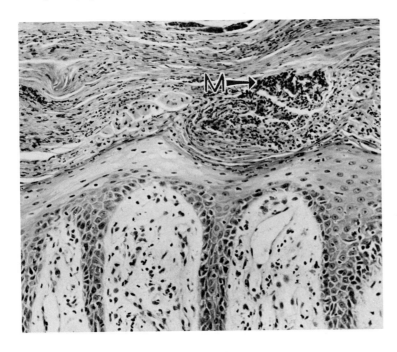

Fig. 8-5. Psoriasis vulgaris
High magnification. The suprapapillary portions of the stratum malpighii are thinned and composed of cells showing intracellular edema. The epidermal cells located immediately beneath the parakeratotic stratum corneum are intermingled with neutrophils, suggestive of a spongiform pustule of Kogoj. A Munro abscess (M.) is located within the parakeratotic horny layer. (×200)

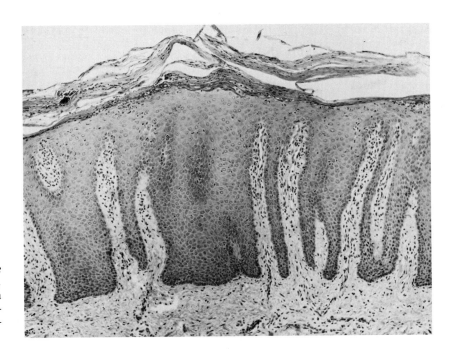

Fig. 8-6. Psoriasis vulgaris, erythrodermic type
A diagnosis of psoriasis is possible if there are, as in this instance, small aggregates of neutrophils in the uppermost rete malpighii resulting in small spongiform pustules of Kogoj. (×50)

native cells (Weinstein and Frost, 1971). More recent calculations, however, have shown that, in psoriatic lesions, the transit time of cells from the basal cell layer to the uppermost row of the squamous cell layer amounts to 5 days rather than to 2 days, as originally assumed (Goodwin et al) and that the reproductive cell cycles for normal germinative cells and for psoriatic germinative cells are 200 hours and about 100 hours, respectively (Gelfant). These figures thus indicate that there is not a 12-fold speeding up of the cell division cycle time of germinative cells in psoriatic epidermis, as originally assumed, but merely a twofold speeding up.

The most recently obtained figures make it appear unlikely that the moderately sped up transit time and cycle time could explain the greatly accelerated rate of epidermal replication in psoriasis. Evidence has been provided that there are noncycling cells in the germinative layer of the epidermis (Gelfant). The reproductive cell cycle is divided into four phases. Following mitosis, the M phase, the cell spends a fairly long period of time in an interphase, referred to as G1. It then enters the deoxyribonucleic acid (DNA) synthesis period, the S phase, during which it doubles its complement of DNA in preparation for mitosis. A short post-DNA synthesis period, referred to as G2, occurs before mitosis takes place (Weinstein and Frost, 1968). It is now fairly well established that there are three distinct populations of epidermal cells. First, there are cycling cells that actively move through the cell cycle, and then there are two categories of noncycling cells blocked in the G1 or the G2 period of the cell cycle that are capable of moving into the proliferative pool upon special stimulation. The increased epidermal cell proliferation in active lesions of psoriasis is believed to be brought about mainly by a

recruitment or a release of the two categories of noncycling cells (Gelfant). Although the theory of the existence of noncycling cells has found cautious acceptance, some authors believe that, in psoriasis, there is a release into mitosis largely of a noncycling G2 population (Rowe et al), whereas others believe that, if noncycling cells exist, they are primarily G1-blocked and released from the G1 population (Grove). The reason that there is no agreement lies in the present limitations inherent in cell kinetic analysis (Grove).

The mitotic activity within different lesions of psoriasis and even within the same lesion can vary considerably and seems to correlate with the degree of parakeratosis. Thus, psoriatic epidermis with 91% to 100% parakeratosis shows on the average 5 times as many mitotic figures as psoriatic epidermis with only 0% to 20% parakeratosis (Cox and Watson). Step sections of early "punctate" papules show a mitotically very active parakeratotic center surrounded by a zone with a thickened granular layer and a relatively low mitotic rate (Soltani and Van Scott).

Electron microscopic studies indicate that psoriatic keratinocytes in the stratum malpighii show significant abnormalities. The tonofilaments are decreased in number and in diameter and lack their normal aggregation. The size and number of keratohyaline granules is greatly reduced, and, occasionally, they are absent (Brody; Hashimoto and Lever). The horny cells also possess thin tonofilaments and often still contain organelles and a nucleus as parakeratotic cells. They often fail to form a marginal band and to lose their outer plasma membrane (Orfanos et al). The intercellular spaces between all epidermal cells are widened because of a deficiency in the glycoprotein-rich cell surface coat, so that intercellular adhesion is limited to the desmosomes (Mercer and Maibach; Orfanos et al). Electron microscopic studies thus have confirmed the view that the keratinocytes in psoriasis are defective and not just immature owing to accelerated epidermal proliferation. Although a correlation exists in psoriasis between an increased rate of mitosis and parakeratosis, rapid proliferation of the epidermis does not cause parakeratosis. Thus, prolonged application of vitamin A acid to normal guinea pig skin accelerates the rate of epidermal proliferation to a level equal to that found in psoriasis without, however, inducing parakeratosis (Christophers and Braun-Falco). Also, in epidermolytic hyperkeratosis, mitotic activity in the epidermis is equal to that of psoriasis, yet there is a well-developed granular layer (Frost and Van Scott).

The ultrastructure of the most characteristic histologic structure encountered in psoriasis, the spongiform pustule of Kogoj, is of interest. In the spongiform pustule, located in the uppermost portion of the stratum malpighii, neutrophils lie intercellularly, rather than intracellularly as was originally assumed on the basis of light microscopic studies. It is a multilocular pustule in which the spongelike network is composed of degenerated and flattened keratinocytes (Rupec). The transepidermal migration of neutrophils from "squirting papillae" to spongiform pustules and, further on, to Munro microabscesses can be explained by the chemotactic properties of soluble substances in psoriasis scales. When examined by a modified Boyden's chamber, all crude extracts of horny tissue studied, such as callus and scales of exfoliative dermatitis and of psoriasis vulgaris, show chemotactic activity for human peripheral blood leukocytes, but only the chemotactic activity of psoriasis scale extracts is highly potent (Tagami and Ofuji, 1976).

The ultrastructure of the capillary loops in the dermal papillae shows them to be different from normal capillary loops. Normal capillary loops have the appearance of arterial capillaries, that is, a homogeneous-appearing basement membrane and no bridged fenestrations between endothelial cells (see p. 35). In psoriasis, however, the capillary loops have the appearance of venous capillaries, that is, a wider lumen, bridged fenestrations between endothelial cells, and a multilayered basement membrane. This finding apparently is unique for psoriasis, indicating a greatly increased capillary permeability (Braverman and Yen).

Two theories that probably are interrelated have been advanced to explain the rapid rate of replication in the epidermis. These two theories suggest that "loss of contact inhibition of growth" among epidermal cells (Orfanos et al) and a disturbance in the function of the cyclic nucleotides (Vorhees et al) are responsible for the accelerated cellular proliferation. Electron microscopy has shown, as already mentioned (see p. 48), a nearly complete absence of the glycoprotein-rich cell surface coat in psoriatic stratum malpighii and, as a result of its absence, a decreased adhesiveness of the keratinocytes. Thus, it may be assumed that the psoriatic epidermis lacks the intercellular contact that is known to provide

inhibition of uncontrolled cellular proliferation in tissue culture (Orfanos et al). In addition, the greatly reduced cell surface coat shows reduced activities of cell membrane-bound enzymes, such as adenosine triphosphatase and phosphomonoesterase, and a lack of sensitivity of adenyl cyclase to specific stimulators, indicating that a latent defect of adenyl cyclase may exist in psoriasis (Mahrle and Orfanos). Since adenyl cyclase synthesizes adenosine 3',5'-monophosphate (cyclic AMP) from adenosine triphosphate it is likely that a deficiency of membrane-bound enzymes leads to a disturbance of the intracellular regulation of the two cyclic nucleotides cyclic AMP and guanosine 3',5'-monophosphate (cyclic GMP). Although, at first, a significant decrease in cyclic AMP was reported in involved psoriatic epidermis when compared with uninvolved psoriatic and control epidermis (Vorhees et al), the most recent results indicate that the content of cyclic AMP is decreased in both involved and uninvolved epidermis of patients with psoriasis when compared with control epidermis. In addition, cyclic GMP levels are more than twice as high in lesional epidermis as in uninvolved areas in the same patient. This suggests that cyclic nucleotides are involved in the pathophysiology of psoriasis (Marcelo et al).

Investigations into a possible *immunologic basis* for psoriasis have not been fruitful. Direct immunofluorescence testing usually is negative in psoriasis vulgaris, and, even if it is positive, there are various nonspecific patterns (Doyle et al). Of interest is the fact that stratum corneum antibodies are regularly found in the parakeratotic stratum corneum of all fully developed lesions of psoriasis. Generally, IgG deposits are found, but, often, so are other immunoglobulins and complement components as a result of in vivo binding of the stratum corneum antibodies (Jablonska et al, 1978, 1979). However, the immunofluorescence is not specific for psoriasis; identical or similar deposits are present in 30% of control specimens (Jablonska et al, 1978). Nor are the stratum corneum antibodies present in an immunologically bound form, since preincubation of tissue sections in acid citrate buffer does not affect the positive fluorescence for IgG in psoriasis lesions but prevents fluorescence for IgG in pemphigus lesions (Kimura and Nishikawa). Since stratum corneum antibodies are present in all human sera, as seen by indirect immunofluorescence, such depositions can occur when plasma proteins are deposited in a parakeratotic horny layer as a result of increased capillary permeability (Harrist and Mihm).

Differential Diagnosis.   Three histologic features are of great value in the diagnosis of psoriasis vulgaris: (1) mounds of parakeratosis with or without neutrophils at their summits within an orthokeratotic stratum corneum seen only in early papular lesions; (2) spongiform micropustules of Kogoj in the uppermost layers of the stratum malpighii; and (3) Munro microabscesses in the stratum corneum. Dilatation and tortuosity of capillaries in the papillae may also be of help in the diagnosis. All other features, such as acanthosis with elongation of the rete ridges and parakeratosis, can be found also in chronic dermatitis, which then may appear to be "psoriasiform." Although mild spongiosis may be seen in psoriasis in the lower epidermis, the presence of marked spongiosis and especially of coagulated serum as evidence of crusting in the stratum corneum are features speaking against psoriasis. Since spongiform pustules are rarely seen in psoriasis vulgaris and Munro microabscesses are seen only in early, active plaques, even a clinically typical lesion of psoriasis in many instances cannot be reliably differentiated from a chronic dermatitis.

Although Kogoj's spongiform pustule is highly diagnostic of the psoriasis group of diseases, including Reiter's disease, histologically typical spongiform pustules may occur in two other diseases: candidiasis, particularly if pustules are clinically present (Degos et al), and geographic tongue, or superficial migratory glossitis (Dawson, 1969). Aggregates of neutrophils with pyknotic nuclei within areas of parakeratosis may occur in conditions other than psoriasis, but they generally differ from Munro microabscesses by being larger and less well circumscribed and by often showing crusting.

Generalized Pustular Psoriasis (Including Acrodermatitis Continua and Impetigo Herpetiformis)

Basically, generalized pustular psoriasis of von Zumbusch, acrodermatitis continua of Hallopeau, and impetigo herpetiformis represent the same disease process (Soltermann; Lapière; Baker and Ryan; Wagner et al). There is considerable resemblance and overlapping in the clinical picture of these three diseases, and they have the same histologic appearance. They differ mainly in mode of onset and in distribution of the lesions. Clinically, all three diseases show groups of shallow pustules on an erythematous base, and all three quite frequently show oral pustules, particularly on the tongue (Wagner et al). Sudden exacerbations in association with chills and fever occur in all three diseases and, in the intervals between exacerbations, all three may show lesions having the clinical appearance of psoriasis.

Pustular psoriasis of von Zumbusch is generally diagnosed when the pustular eruption occurs in patients with pre-existing psoriasis either of the plaque type (Shelley and Kirschbaum) or of the erythrodermic type (Braverman et al).

Acrodermatitis continua of Hallopeau is the term used if the pustular eruption either is limited to the distal portions of the fingers and toes, as in the localized type

of acrodermatitis continua, or involves extensive areas of the skin in addition to the distal portions of the fingers and toes, as in the generalized type of acrodermatitis continua. The generalized type has been aptly referred to as the *acral type of generalized pustular psoriasis* (Baker and Ryan). On the fingers and toes, atrophy of the skin and permanent loss of the nails may occur.

Impetigo herpetiformis is diagnosed when the disease starts suddenly without any preceding lesions of psoriasis as an extensive eruption of pustules on an erythematous base. This type is also referred to as the *exanthematous type of generalized pustular psoriasis* (Baker and Ryan). It may occur repeatedly during successive pregnancies (Katzenellenbogen and Feuerman) but may also occur without any known cause. In some instances, the lesions are annular or gyrate and show a clinical resemblance to subcorneal pustular dermatosis (Resneck and Cram; Adler et al) (see p. 125).

Histopathology.   Whereas, in ordinary psoriasis, the spongiform pustule of Kogoj is a very small micropustule and is seen only in early, active lesions, it occurs as a macropustule in all three variants of generalized pustular psoriasis and represents their characteristic histologic lesion. The spongiform pustule forms through the migration of neutrophils from the papillary capillaries to the upper stratum malpighii, where they aggregate within the interstices of a spongelike network formed by degenerated and thinned epidermal cells (Fig. 8-7) (Rupec). As the size of the pustule increases, the epidermal cells in the center of the pustule undergo complete cytolysis, so that a large single cavity forms. At the periphery of the pustule, however, the network of thinned epidermal cells persists for a much longer time (Fig. 8-8). As the neutrophils of the spongiform pustule move up into the horny layer, they become pyknotic and assume the appearance of a large Munro abscess (Shelley and Kirschbaum; Muller and Kitzmiller).

Aside from the presence of large spongiform pustules, the epidermal changes in generalized pustular psoriasis are very much like those seen in psoriasis, consisting of parakeratosis and elongation of the rete ridges. The upper dermis contains an infiltrate of mononuclear cells, and neutrophils can often be seen migrating from the capillaries in the papillae into the epidermis (Kingery et al). The oral lesions show the same spongiform pustule formation as seen on the skin (Wagner et al).

In the healing stage, the lesions of all three types of generalized pustular psoriasis may present the same histologic appearance as ordinary psoriasis (Shelley and Kirschbaum).

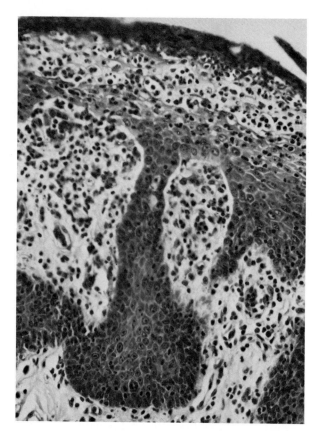

Fig. 8-7.   Generalized pustular psoriasis
Early state. There is acanthosis with elongation of the rete ridges. The upper stratum malpighii shows an early spongiform pustule formed through the migration of neutrophils from the papillary capillaries to the upper stratum malpighii, where they aggregate within the interstices of a spongelike network formed by degenerated and thinned epidermal cells. (×300)

Differential Diagnosis.   Because of the clinical and, particularly, the histologic, resemblance of the tongue lesions in pustular psoriasis to those seen in geographic tongue, it has been suggested that geographic tongue represents an abortive form of pustular psoriasis (Dawson, 1974) (see p. 476).

Localized Pustular Psoriasis (Including Pustulosis Palmaris et Plantaris)

In two of the three types of localized pustular psoriasis, "psoriasis with pustules" (Schuppener) (see p. 139) and localized acrodermatitis continua of Hallopeau (see p. 145), the histologic picture is the same as that described for generalized pustular psoriasis.

The third type of localized pustular psoriasis, pustulosis palmaris et plantaris, is a chronic, relapsing disorder occurring on either the palms or the soles or both. Crops of small, deep-seated pustules are seen within areas of erythema and scaling. In the earliest stage, the lesions may appear as vesicles or vesicopustules. During the subsiding stage, the pustules appear as brown macules. The sites of predilection are the midpalms and thenar eminences of the hands, and the heels and insteps of the feet (Ashhurst). In pustulosis palmaris et plantaris, in contrast to acrodermatitis continua of Hallopeau, the acral portions of the fingers and toes are spared.

Histopathology.   A fully developed pustule is large, intraepidermal in location, unilocular, and rounded on both sides (Fig. 8-9). It is elevated only slightly above the surface but extends into the underlying dermis. Many neutrophils are present within the cavity of the pustule. The epidermis surrounding the pustule shows slight acanthosis, and an inflammatory infiltrate can be seen beneath the pustule (Piérard and Kint, 1978). In many instances, one can observe typical, though small, spongiform pustules in the epidermal wall of the pustule, most commonly at the junction of the lateral walls and the overlying epidermis (Piérard and Kint, 1966, 1978; Lever; Uehara and Ofuji; Thorman and Heilesen). These spongiform pustules are identical with those seen in the walls of the pustules of generalized pustular psoriasis.

Very early lesions may show spongiosis and a mononuclear infiltrate in the lower epidermis overlying the tips of papillae (Uehara and Ofuji). This may be followed by the formation of an intraepidermal vesicle containing mostly mononuclear cells (Uehara and Ofuji; Piérard and Kint, 1978). Subsequently, as the vesicle expands, it becomes a pustule. There is a massive invasion of the cavity by neutrophils, which penetrate the intracellular spaces of the vesicle wall, where the histologic picture of spongiform pustules is then seen (Piérard and Kint, 1978).

Histogenesis. After the original description in 1930 of a localized pustular psoriasis as pustular psoriasis of the palms and soles (Barber), the view that the eruption represented psoriasis was abandoned and the term *pustular bacterid* introduced in 1935 (Andrews and Machacek). This designation became widely accepted, with the connotation that focal infections caused the eruption. Other authors have preferred the noncommittal term *pustulosis palmaris et plantaris*.

A relationship of pustulosis palmaris et plantaris with psoriasis is not generally accepted, although two facts favor a close relationship: (1) the relatively common occurrence of psoriasis in patients with pustulosis pal-

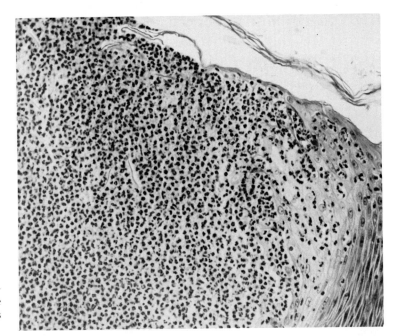

Fig. 8-8. Generalized pustular psoriasis
A fully developed pustule filled with neutrophils is shown. At the periphery of the pustule, shown to the right, the epidermis has a spongiform appearance. (×200)

Fig. 8-9. Localized pustular psoriasis: pustulosis palmaris et plantaris
A large intraepidermal unilocular pustule is present. On the floor and on the roof of the pustule, evidence of spongiform pustule formation can still be recognized. (×100)

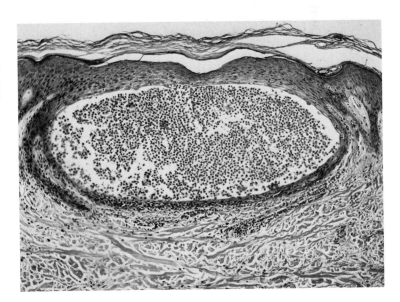

maris et plantaris, observed by various observers in 19%, 24%, and 48% of the patients, respectively (Everall; Enfors and Molin; Thomsen); and (2) the common presence of spongiform pustules in the walls of the pustules of pustulosis palmaris et plantaris. The argument that the primary occurrence of a mononuclear reaction in pustulosis palmaris et plantaris speaks against a relationship with psoriasis (Piérard and Kint, 1978) can be countered by the fact that a mononuclear infiltrate precedes the appearance of neutrophils in psoriasis as well (see p. 140). Also, a leukotactic factor identical to that noted in psoriasis (see p. 144) has been found in pustulosis palmaris et plantaris (Tagami and Ofuji, 1978).

REITER'S DISEASE

In typical cases, Reiter's disease consists of the triad of urethritis, arthritis, and conjunctivitis. Although, as a rule, the arthritis occurs in attacks and is followed by recovery, it progresses in some cases to cause permanent damage to the affected joints (Perry and Mayne; Khan and Hall). In about two thirds of the patients, cutaneous lesions are present. They have a predilection for the glans penis, the palms and soles, and the subungual areas. On the glans penis, not infrequently the only area of involvement, the usual appearance is that of a brownish red patch with central clearing, referred to as balanitis

147

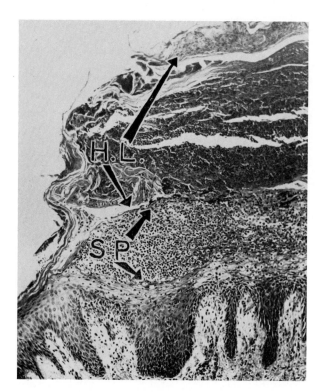

Fig. 8-10. Reiter's disease
Low magnification. There is a very thick parakeratotic horny layer (*H.L.*) permeated by numerous neutrophils. The upper stratum malpighii is the seat of a spongiform pustule (*SP*). The rete ridges are elongated, and the papillae show edema. (×100)

circinata. On the palms and the soles, early lesions consist of pustules. Gradually, the lesions on the palms and the soles become covered with thick horny crusts, and confluence of neighboring lesions leads to extensive horny excrescences. Occasionally, there are pustular or crusted hyperkeratotic lesions elsewhere on the skin that at first resemble pustular psoriasis but later may have the appearance of ordinary psoriasis (Perry and Mayne; Khan and Hall).

Histopathology. Early pustular lesions on the palms or soles show a spongiform macropustule in the upper epidermis (Fig. 8-10) (Weinberger et al; Perry and Mayne). In addition, one observes parakeratosis and elongation of the rete ridges.

As the lesions age, the parakeratotic horny layer overlying the spongiform pustule thickens considerably (Figs. 8-10, 8-11). This greatly thickened horny layer is the anatomic substrate for the horny excrescences seen clinically. The horny layer consists of parakeratotic cells intermingled with the pyknotic nuclei of neutrophils (Fig. 8-10).

In old lesions, spongiform pustules are no longer seen. The histologic picture usually is nonspecific, showing acanthosis and hyperkeratosis with only a few areas of parakeratosis, but, occasionally, the histologic picture resembles psoriasis (Perry and Mayne).

Histogenesis. The cause of Reiter's disease is not known. That the nature of the disease is infectious has not been proved. The former designation of the hyperkeratotic palmar and plantar lesions as *keratosis blennorrhagica*, referring to gonorrhea, was also erroneous. A close relationship to psoriasis has been assumed for the cutaneous lesions because of their clinical resemblance to psoriasis and the presence of spongiform pustules (Perry and Mayne). Similarly, the arthritis of Reiter's disease resembles psoriatic arthritis not only clinically but also because of the absence of the rheumatoid factor (Wright and Reed; Khan and Hall).

Differential Diagnosis. The early spongiform macropustule seen in Reiter's disease is indistinguishable from the spongiform macropustule seen in pustular psoriasis. Slightly older lesions often can be identified as representing Reiter's disease in contradistinction to psoriasis by the presence of a greatly thickened horny layer.

PARAPSORIASIS

Three types of parapsoriasis are recognized: the small plaque type of parapsoriasis en plaques, the large plaque type of parapsoriasis en plaques, and parapsoriasis variegata. All three are very chronic and usually asymptomatic.

The *small plaque type* of parapsoriasis en plaques is known also as xanthoerythrodermia perstans of Crocker (Goldberg) and as digitate dermatosis (Hu and Winkelmann). Pink to yellow, slightly scaling, oval or elongated, often fingerprintlike patches 1 cm to 5 cm in diameter are symmetrically distributed over the trunk and the proximal portions of the extremities. In some instances, cases diagnosed originally as representing the small plaque type later on show reticulate pigmentation and atrophy, requiring reclassification as the large plaque type (Fleischmajer et al; Samman).

The *large plaque type* of parapsoriasis en plaques is known also as atrophic parapsoriasis (Samman) and poikilodermatous parapsoriasis (Bardach and Raff). The patches are larger, more irregularly shaped, and less sharply defined than in the small plaque type. Although, in some instances, poikilodermatous changes do not develop (Bonvalet et al), usually telangiectasias, mottled hyperpigmentation, and atrophy either are present from the beginning (Samman) or develop after a certain length of time (Osmundsen; Heid et al). Ultimately, as the

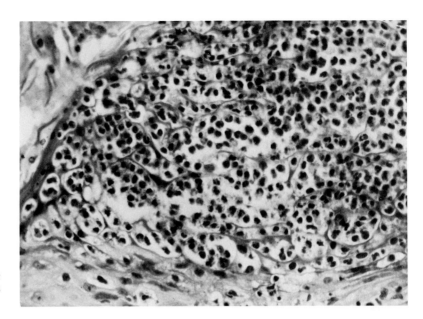

Fig. 8-11. Reiter's disease
High magnification of Figure 8-10. The spongiform nature of the pustule is very apparent. (×400)

result of extension and coalescence of the patches, the appearance may be that of poikiloderma atrophicans vasculare (Samman).

Parapsoriasis variegata, also known as parakeratosis variegata (Vella Briffa et al), as parapsoriasis lichenoides of Brocq (Musger), and as retiform parapsoriasis (Lambert and Everett), shows an extensive eruption of brownish red, slightly raised, flat, scaling papules in a netlike or zebralike pattern. Gradually, the papules undergo atrophy with formation of telangiectases and mottled pigmentation, so that the eruption assumes the appearance of poikiloderma atrophicans vasculare and thus greatly resembles the large plaque type of parapsoriasis en plaques.

Histopathology. The *small plaque type* of parapsoriasis in typical cases shows a nonspecific histologic picture consisting of a lymphocytic perivascular infiltrate and in some instances shows also focal epidermal involvement consisting of exocytosis, spongiosis, mild acanthosis, and parakeratosis (Hu and Winkelmann). However, in some instances, the infiltrate is more pronounced and resembles that seen in the large plaque type; such cases require inclusion in the large plaque category (Samman; Binazzi).

In the *large plaque type,* the histologic picture at the beginning is nonspecific. However, as the disease progresses toward atrophy, the infiltrate assumes a bandlike arrangement beneath a flattened epidermis that may be invaded by the infiltrate. There may be vacuolization of the basal cell layer, dilated capillaries, and pigmentary incontinence (Bardach and Raff). Thus, the histologic

picture resembles that seen generally in poikiloderma atrophicans vasculare (see p. 460). The important question is whether atypical cells are present in the dermal infiltrate or within the epidermis. Such atypical cells are characterized by large, irregularly shaped, hyperchromatic nuclei analogous to those of mycosis cells (see p. 739). In some cases, they are present, and in others not, the incidence increasing with time (Samman; Bonvalet et al).

In *parapsoriasis variegata,* the histologic picture closely resembles that of the large plaque type. In the early stage, the flat papules show a patchy rather than a bandlike infiltrate and the overlying epidermis may be markedly thinned. Small extravasations of red cells may be seen in the infiltrate (Musger). The presence of atypical nuclei has been observed in some cases (Vella Briffa et al) but not in all (Musger).

Relationship to Lymphoma. Since the division of parapsoriasis en plaques into a small plaque type and a large plaque type and the gradual acceptance of the term *digitate dermatosis* for the small plaque type, the relationship of parapsoriasis to mycosis fungoides has been greatly clarified. It is now generally accepted that the small plaque type, or digitate dermatosis, is a benign disorder and not related to mycosis fungoides (Samman; Hu and Winkelmann; Bonvalet et al; Heid et al). However, it must be conceded that, in some instances, a clinical or histologic distinction of the small plaque type from the large plaque type is difficult, so that only the subsequent course decides the issue (Samman).

In the other two types of parapsoriasis, the large

plaque type and parapsoriasis variegata, histologic and clinical transitions to mycosis fungoides occur. Clinical transition occurs, even with follow-up periods over many years, in only about 12% of the cases, that is, in 17 of 140 cases if four recent series are combined (Samman; Bonvalet et al; Binazzi; Heid et al). Very significant is the statement by Samman that, whereas clinical transition to mycosis fungoides occurred in only 8.5% of his patients with the large plaque type, "in over half the cases the histology pointed to a progression to malignancy; but that this has not occurred suggests that the body can maintain the status quo for a long time." It is a correct appraisal to state that mycosis fungoides does not develop from other diseases and that "names like parapsoriasis en plaques, poikiloderma vasculare atrophicans, and parapsoriasis variegata are simply descriptive terms for types of large patch lesions of mycosis fungoides" (Sanchez and Ackerman). Still, in the great majority of cases, mycosis fungoides presenting as parapsoriasis is biologically a benign disease perhaps analogous to the Woringer–Kolopp type of mycosis fungoides (see p. 747).

PITYRIASIS ROSEA

Pityriasis rosea is a self-limited disorder lasting from 4 to 7 weeks. The lesions, found chiefly on the trunk, consist of round to oval salmon-colored patches following the lines of cleavage and showing peripherally attached, thin, cigarette-paper-like scales.

Histopathology. The histologic picture is that of a subacute or chronic dermatitis (see p. 95). The infiltrate in the upper dermis consists predominantly of small mononuclear cells, with a few eosinophils and histiocytes. In some of the lesions, mononuclear cells are seen migrating from the upper dermis into the epidermis. Spongiosis and intracellular edema occur at sites at which the epidermis has been invaded by the cellular infiltrate (Fig. 8-12). Spongiotic vesicles are found in about half of the cases (Bunch and Tilley). Mild acanthosis and focal parakeratosis are also present.

PAPULAR ACRODERMATITIS OF CHILDHOOD (GIANOTTI–CROSTI SYNDROME)

Papular acrodermatitis of childhood, first described in 1955 (Gianotti), represents a primary infection with hepatitis B virus acquired through the skin or a mucous membrane. It is characterized by (1) a nonpruritic, erythematous, papular eruption on the face, extremities, and buttocks lasting about 3 weeks; (2) enlargement of subcutaneous lymph nodes; (3) acute hepatitis, usually anicteric, which lasts at least 2 months but only rarely progresses to chronic liver disease; and (4) hepatitis B surface antigenemia, subtype ayw, which may persist for a long time (Gianotti). Rarely, the disease is seen in adults (Claudy et al).

Histopathology. The histologic appearance of the papules is nonspecific. A moderately severe infiltrate of lymphocytes and histiocytes is present

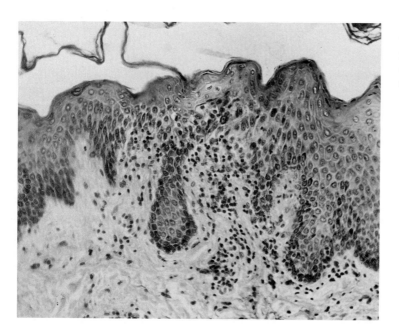

Fig. 8-12. Pityriasis rosea
The epidermis shows spongiosis and is invaded by an infiltrate of mononuclear cells. The upper dermis shows a chronic inflammatory infiltrate ($\times 200$)

in the upper dermis, mainly around capillaries, which exhibit endothelial swelling (Gianotti). In addition, focal spongiosis and parakeratosis with mild acanthosis may be present (Castellano et al).

Histogenesis. The surface antigen of the hepatitis B virus is detectable in the sera of all cases of papular acrodermatitis of childhood by radioimmunoassay and in nearly all cases by immunodiffusion. The surface antibody of the hepatitis B virus is not detected during the eruptive phase but is usually found 6 to 12 months later. All patients who become hepatitis B surface antigen-negative develop hepatitis B surface antibodies, suggesting that these antibodies play a role in the recovery from hepatitis. Since the disease is almost exclusively related to the subtype ayw of the hepatitis B virus, it is encountered mainly in Mediterranean countries, where this subtype is common (Gianotti).

MUCOCUTANEOUS LYMPH NODE SYNDROME (KAWASAKI'S DISEASE)

The mucocutaneous lymph node syndrome, first reported in 1967 (Kawasaki et al), is most common in Japan but also occurs elsewhere either sporadically or epidemically. Five of the following six criteria should be met to establish the diagnosis: (1) fever unresponsive to antibiotics; (2) conjunctivitis; (3) erythema and edema of the palms and soles, often followed by desquamation; (4) lesions of the lips and oral mucosa, such as erythema of lips and oropharynx, fissuring of lips, and "strawberry tongue"; (5) a polymorphous eruption; and (6) cervical lymphadenopathy. Scarlet fever must be excluded by a negative or unchanging antistreptolysin O titer (Schlossberg et al).

The rash appears on the third to the fifth day of illness, starting usually on the extremities and spreading over the trunk within two days. It then clears in less than a week (Kawasaki et al). Usually widespread, the rash has one of three patterns: diffuse scarlatiniform erythroderma, morbilliform, or multiform (Bitter et al).

Although most patients are infants or small children, young adults in rare instances can be affected (Schlossberg et al). The prognosis is good with the exception that 1% to 2% of the patients die of coronary arteritis and thrombosis (Kawasaki et al).

Histopathology. The histologic changes in the skin are nonspecific, consisting of a perivascular infiltrate or lymphocytes and histiocytes (Kawasaki et al).

Histogenesis. The cause of the mucocutaneous lymph node syndrome is unknown. There is no evidence of person-to-person transmission or of a common-source exposure among patients (Bell et al). Doubt has been expressed that Kawasaki's disease is a distinct syndrome, since the diagnostic criteria required for its diagnosis can be found in various other diseases, among them erythema multiforme, drug reactions, infectious mononucleosis, and infantile periarteritis nodosa (Weston and Huff).

LICHEN PLANUS

Lichen planus is a subacute or a chronic dermatosis characterized by small, polygonal, violaceous papules that may coalesce into plaques. As a rule, itching is pronounced, but it may be slight or absent. The disease usually is limited to a few areas, the sites of predilection being the flexor surfaces of the forearms, the legs, the glans penis, and the oral mucosa; however, in some cases, the eruption is very extensive.

The oral lesions of lichen planus are seen most commonly in the buccal region and usually consist of whitish papules often arranged in a reticular pattern. There may also be oral vesicles, erosions, and ulcers, occurring occasionally as the only manifestation of the disease (Shklar). The nails are involved in about 10% of the cases and then show roughening, longitudinal ridging, and, rarely, thinning and destruction (Samman).

A common variant is hypertrophic lichen planus, which is usually found on the shins and consists of thickened, often verrucous plaques. In contrast, vesicular lichen planus is rare. It shows vesicles situated on only some of the lesions (Sarkany et al; Saurat et al). It is different from so-called lichen planus pemphigoides in which there are bullae, rather than vesicles (see below).

Lichen planopilaris designates lichen planus with a follicular arrangement of some or all of the lesions. This type of lichen planus often affects the scalp. At first, there may be follicular papules or perifollicular erythema, but, with the loss of hair, irregularly shaped patches of atrophic alopecia develop on the scalp that are indistinguishable from those seen in pseudopelade of Brocq (Altman and Perry) (see p. 204). Other hairy areas, such as the axillae and the pubic region, may also be affected, but the alopecia in these areas is usually noncicatricial (Cram et al). Follicular papules may also be seen on the glabrous skin (Waldorf).

Ulcerative lichen planus, a rare but quite characteristic variant of lichen planus, shows bullae, erosions, and ulcerations on the feet and toes resulting in atrophic scarring and permanent loss of the toenails. It is usually associated with patches of atrophic alopecia of the scalp and with cutaneous and oral lesions of lichen planus (Cram et al; Male; Thormann; Weidner and Ummenhofer).

Lichen planus actinicus, or *pigmentosus,* has been described as occurring mainly in Middle Eastern countries, where between 20% and 30% of the cases of lichen planus are of this type (Katzenellenbogen; Dilaimy). The lesions develop on exposed parts, especially the face, and are annular, often showing a pigmented center and

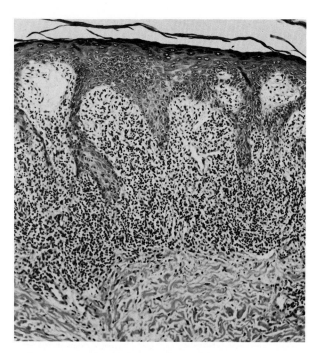

Fig. 8-13. Lichen planus, early lesion
There are hyperkeratosis, focal thickening of the granular layer, and acanthosis with irregular elongation of the rete ridges. The rete ridge in the center has a triangular sawtooth configuration. The basal layer has been invaded by the inflammatory infiltrate and appears "wiped out." The infiltrate is bandlike and sharply demarcated at its lower border. (× 100)

well-defined, slightly raised, pale margin. Pruritus is minimal or absent.

The *overlap syndrome lichen planus / lupus erythematosus* shows clinical features of both diseases. There are chronic, bluish red, somewhat atrophic patches most commonly on the acral portions of the extremities (Romero et al; Jamison et al).

In *twenty-nail dystrophy,* encountered usually in children, all nails are thin, ridged, roughened, and often also split. The nail changes thus resemble those seen in lichen planus (Scher et al; Wilkinson et al) (see above). However, other manifestations of lichen planus are absent.

Two diseases are associated with lichen planus more commonly than could be explained by chance: bullous pemphigoid and lichen nitidus. The association of lichen planus and bullous pemphigoid is known as *lichen planus pemphigoides.* The bullae are seen to arise from papules of lichen planus as well as from normal skin (Sobel et al; Saurat et al; Hintner et al). The simultaneous occurrence of lichen planus and lichen nitidus is frequent enough to have suggested to some authors that they are variants of the same disease (Waisman et al) (see p. 158).

Development of squamous cell carcinoma is a very exceptional occurrence in hypertrophic lichen planus of the leg (Kronenberg et al). It occurs occasionally on lesions of lichen planus situated on mucous surfaces or the vermilion border (Jänner et al; Male and Azambuja). The incidence of carcinoma of the oral mucosa in two large series was about 0.5% (Fulling; Holmstrup and Pindborg), with an additional 0.5% in one series having carcinoma in situ (Holmstrup annd Pindborg). The tendency toward development of carcinoma in ulcers of the feet in ulcerative lichen planus is fairly high, unless the ulcers are grafted (Male and Azambuja).

Histopathology. Typical papules of lichen planus show (1) hyperkeratosis, (2) focal hypergranulosis, (3) irregular acanthosis, (4) damage to the basal cell layer, and (5) a bandlike dermal infiltrate in close approximation to the epidermis (Fig. 8-13). This constellation of findings is sufficiently diagnostic that, in lichen planus, in contrast to psoriasis, for instance, a histologic diagnosis can be made in more than 90% of the cases (Ellis).

The horny layer is moderately thickened and contains very few if any parakeratotic cells, a fact that is important for the diagnosis.

The thickening of the stratum granulosum is irregular, showing so-called beading. The granular cells in the areas of thickening appear increased in size and contain coarser and more abundant keratohyaline granules than are observed normally. On step sectioning, the areas of hypergranulosis are found to be contiguous to intraepidermal adnexal structures, namely acrosyringia and acrotrichia (Ragaz and Ackerman).

The acanthosis in lichen planus affects the rete ridges as well as the stratum malpighii. The cells of the stratum malpighii often appear eosinophilic, possibly because of advanced keratinization. The rete ridges show irregular lengthening, and some of them are pointed at their lower end, giving them a saw-toothed appearance. The papillae between lengthened rete ridges are often dome-shaped (Gougerot and Civatte).

The cells of the basal layer are not clearly visible in early lesions, because the dense dermal infiltrate closely approximates ("hugs") the basal layer and extends between the basal cells. The border between the epidermis and the dermis thus appears hazy. Wherever recognizable, the basal cells in early lesions show liquefaction degeneration. In fully developed lesions, the lowest cell layer of the epidermis has the appearance of flattened squamous cells, giving the impression that the basal cell layer has been "wiped out."

The infiltrate in the upper dermis is bandlike

and, although ill defined at the dermal-epidermal junction, is quite sharply demarcated at its lower border. The infiltrate is composed almost entirely of lymphocytes intermingled with a few histiocytes. Mast cells are also present, whereas eosinophils and plasma cells are absent. Melanophages are seen in the upper dermis, often in considerable number, since, as a result of damage to the basal cells, the basal cells are incapable of storing melanin ("incontinence of pigment"; see Glossary).

In old lesions, the cellular infiltrate decreases in density, but the number of histiocytes increases. Also, in some areas in which a basal cell layer has reformed, the dermal infiltrate no longer lies in close approximation to the epidermis. In the late stage, some lesions may show considerable acanthosis, papillomatosis, and hyperkeratosis (*hypertrophic lichen planus*).

One frequently observes *colloid bodies* in the lower epidermis and especially in the upper dermis. They are referred to also as hyaline, cytoid, or Civatte bodies. In routinely stained sections, they have been found in 37% of the cases (Ellis). However, on direct immunofluorescence staining, they can be seen much more frequently, in 87% of the cases (Abell et al) (see below). Colloid bodies average 20 μm in diameter and have a homogeneous, eosinophilic appearance (Fig. 8-14). They are periodic acid-Schiff (PAS)-positive and diastase-resistant. They represent degenerated keratinocytes and, even though they are found most commonly in lichen planus, may occur in any disease in which damage to the basal cells occurs, such as lupus erythematosus (Ebner and Gebhart, 1977).

Occasionally, small areas of separation are seen between the epidermis and the dermis, and these are referred to as Max Joseph spaces (Ellis). In some instances, the separation increases to such an extent that subepidermal vesicles form (*vesicular lichen planus*; Fig. 8-15). These vesicles form as a result of damage to the basal cells (Sarkany et al). (See Classification of Blisters, p. 93.)

The *oral lesions* of lichen planus differ in their histologic appearance from those of the skin, as one would expect, since the oral mucosa normally shows parakeratosis without the presence of a granular layer (p. 11). Thus, the lesions of the mouth often show parakeratosis rather than hyperkeratosis, although alternate areas of both types of keratinization may be observed (Shklar). Also, rather than showing acanthosis, the epithelium often is thin. Ulcerations develop either through the rupture of vesicles or as a result of necrosis of the epithelium.

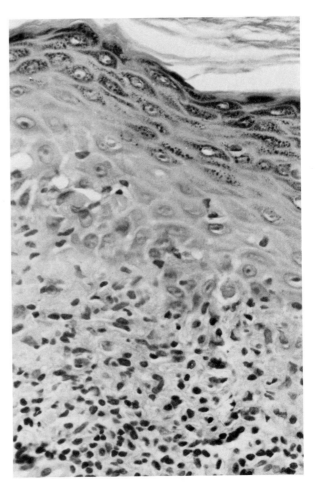

Fig. 8-14.   Lichen planus, colloid bodies
Two colloid bodies are present. The colloid body on the right side lies just below the epidermis. The hyaline body on the left side lies in the lowermost epidermis and contains a narrow crescent of degenerating nuclear material. (× 400)

Lichen Planopilaris. Early lesions of lichen planopilaris, whether obtained from the glabrous skin or from hairy areas, show, occasionally in association with a subepidermal infiltrate typical of lichen planus, a dense mononuclear infiltrate surrounding the hair follicle and the dermal hair papilla (Waldorf). Damage to the dermal hair papilla leads to obliteration of the hair. At first, the hair follicles are dilated and filled with a keratotic plug (Fig. 8-16) (Silver et al). Later on, however, the hair follicles and sebaceous glands are no longer present, the epidermis is flattened, and the dermis shows fibrosis and a mild perivascular infiltrate (Altman and Perry). At this stage, both the clinical

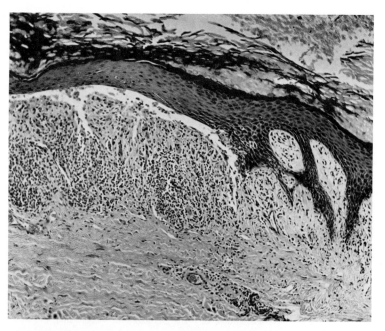

Fig. 8-15. Lichen planus, vesicular lesion
Separation of the epidermis from the dermis has taken place. (×100)

Fig. 8-16. Lichen planopilaris
There is a dilated hair follicle containing a keratotic plug. At the lower pole of the hair follicle is a dense chronic inflammatory infiltrate. In addition, there is a bandlike infiltrate beneath the epidermis. (×50)

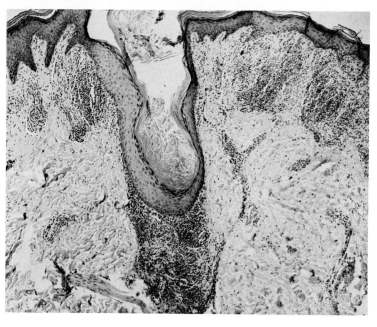

and the histologic findings are indistinguishable from those of pseudopelade of Brocq (see p. 204).

Ulcerative Lichen Planus. In ulcerative lichen planus, specimens taken from skin situated just outside an ulcer generally show active lichen planus (Cram et al; Male, 1970; Weidner and Ummenhofer).

Lichen Planus Actinicus. In some instances, the histologic picture of lichen planus actinus is compatible with lichen planus but with a tendency toward thinning of the epidermis in the center of the lesion (Dilaimy). In other cases, the resemblance to lichen planus is vague, and some similarity to lupus erythematosus exists (Katzenellenbogen); and, in still others, there is a "lichenoid tissue reaction" with only a slight resemblance to lichen planus (Verhagen and Koten). A relationship between lichen planus actinicus and erythema dyschromicum perstans has been postulated (Tschen et al) (see p. 138).

Overlap Syndrome Lichen Planus / Lupus Erythematosus. In some cases of the overlap syndrome, the histologic features and direct immunofluorescence findings are more consistent with lichen planus than with lupus erythematosus (Copeman et al). In others, the histologic findings are consistent with lichen planus, but the results of direct immunofluorescence testing favor lupus erythematosus (Davies et al). In still others, histologic features of lichen planus are found in some lesions and those of lupus erythematosus in others, so that it seems as if the two diseases coexist (Romero et al). It is thus evident that, in some instances, the overlap of the two diseases is such that a clear differentiation is impossible and only the subsequent evolution of the disease will make a diagnosis possible.

Twenty-Nail Dystrophy. Histologic data on twenty-nail dystrophy are available in only three cases. In one, the findings were interpreted as lichen planus (Scher et al). In the other two cases, however, the presence of spongiosis and parakeratosis was regarded as incompatible with a diagnosis of lichen planus (Wilkinson et al; Braun-Falco et al).

Lichen Planus Pemphigoides. In lichen planus pemphigoides, biopsies taken from bullae arising from skin not involved with lichen planus show subepidermal bullae with an infiltrate that is not bandlike and that contains eosinophils (Saurat et al). Direct immunofluorescence shows the presence of IgG and C3 in a linear arrangement at the dermal-epidermal border (Sobel et al; Saurat et al). On immunoelectron microscopy, C3 is seen to be localized within the lamina lucida, analogous to its location in bullous pemphigoid (Hintner et al). Circulating IgG antibodies have also been found (Sobel et al; Saurat et al). The findings thus are those of bullous pemphigoid (see p. 115).

Histogenesis. On *electron microscopy*, the primary damage in lichen planus seems to involve the basal keratinocytes, which, together with their desmosomes and hemidesmosomes, undergo degenerative changes (Medenica and Lorincz; Shklar et al). A secondary event is a dermal infiltrate that, on invading the epidermis, causes damage to the basement membrane such as fragmentation (EM 28). This may be followed by duplication and irregular folding of the basement membrane (Ebner and Gebhart, 1976). The dermal infiltrate contains mainly lymphocytes but also macrophages. Some of the lymphocytes have hyperconvoluted nuclei and appear indistinguishable from Sézary cells. Attachment sites between lymphocytes and macrophages are seen, suggesting operation of a cell-mediated immune mechanism (Medenica and Lorincz).

The possibility has been considered that the primary event in lichen planus is not damage to the basal keratinocytes but rather a delayed hypersensitivity reaction in which an as yet unidentified antigen, after having been processed in the Langerhans cells, attracts T lymphocytes, which, in turn destroy keratinocytes (Ragaz and Ackerman). This assumption is based on observations that the lymphocytes in the dermal infiltrate of lichen planus are principally T lymphocytes (Alano et al) and that the number of Langerhans cells in the epidermis is increased very early in the disease (Ragaz and Ackerman). The use of monoclonal antibodies for the identification of various types of T cells and of Langerhans cells has confirmed the T-cell nature of the infiltrate in lichen planus and has shown that most of the T cells in the infiltrate are of the helper/inducer subset. It also has demonstrated an increased number of Langerhans cells in the epidermis and their presence in the dermal infiltrate (Bhan et al).

The colloid or hyaline bodies are located largely in the papillary dermis but also in the lowermost epidermis (EM 28). They can be seen to develop from damaged keratinocytes through filamentous degeneration. This is followed by their discharge into the dermis, referred to as apoptosis (Hashimoto). The colloid bodies are filled with filaments 6 nm to 8 nm in diameter, the width of which is intermediate between that of tonofilaments, 4 nm to 6 nm in diameter, and that of keratin filaments, 8 nm to 10 nm in diameter, indicative of a premature transformation of tonofilaments into keratin filaments (Hashimoto). The use of antikeratin immune sera has resulted in intense staining of the colloid bodies (Gomes et al). Colloid bodies often still contain cell organelles, such as melanosomes and mitochondria, but only rarely contain nuclear material (Ebner and Gebhart, 1977). Fibrin deposits in the upper dermis are a common finding (EM 28). In the vesicular lesions of lichen planus, electron microscopic examination shows cytolysis of basal keratinocytes; the blister cavity is therefore situated either within the cytoplasm of basal cells (Ebner and Gebhart, 1976) or, after complete cytolysis of the basal cells, below the stratum spinosum (Ebner et al, 1973).

Labeling of lichen planus lesions with tritiated thymidine in vivo or in vitro has produced varied results. Whereas some authors have observed a reduced labeling index of epithelial cells within lesions showing a marked inflammatory response (Marks et al; Walker and Dolby), others have noted an increased labeling index not only in the epidermis but also in the eccrine ducts within the lesions (Ebner et al, 1977). Whether even an increased labeling index would result in increased epidermal proliferation is questionable, since not all labeled cells may complete mitosis and undergo cell division. It appears that even cells undergoing mitosis can degenerate into colloid bodies (El-Labban and Kramer). Reduced mitotic activity in lesions of lichen planus and the consequently prolonged retention of keratinocytes in the stratum malpighii within the epidermis would explain the increased size and eosinophilia of these cells.

DIRECT IMMUNOFLUORESCENCE TESTING. Colloid bodies are demonstrable in lichen planus by direct immunofluorescence staining in about 87% of the cases (Abell et al). They stain mainly with IgM but often also with IgG, IgA, C3, and fibrin. Although colloid bodies are found occasionally in many other conditions with damage to the basal cell layer, such as lupus erythematosus, they are highly suggestive of lichen planus if they are present in large numbers or arranged in clusters. Their staining is not an immunologic phenomenon; rather, they act as a filamentous sponge by which immunoglobulins, complement, and fibrin are absorbed (Black). Fibrin depositions can also be demonstrated very frequently by direct immunofluorescence. Usually, they are seen as granular or linear deposits at the dermal-epidermal junction, with irregular strands extending into the dermis (Abell et al). Only occasionally are there granular deposits of IgM (Baart de la Faille-Kuyper and Baart de la Faille) or linear deposits of C3 (Varelzidis et al) or of both IgG and C3 (Morel et al) in the basement membrane zone.

Differential Diagnosis. It should be borne in mind that parakeratosis is not a feature of lichen planus of the skin and that, if more than slight focal parakeratosis is present, a diagnosis of lichen planus should not be made on histologic grounds. Not infrequently, difficulties arise in the differentiation of lichen planus from chronic discoid lupus erythematosus, as the recognition of an "overlap syndrome" shows (see p. 155). Generally, however, lupus erythematosus shows hydropic degeneration of the basal cells during the entire course of the disease, rather than merely as a stage preceding the replacement of the basal cells by flattened squamous cells. Lupus erythematosus also usually shows (1) atrophy of the epidermis, rather than acanthosis with saw-tooth formations; (2) absence of eosinophilia of the cells in the stratum malpighii; (3) a patchy rather than a bandlike infiltrate; and (4) quite commonly, small areas of hemorrhage in the upper dermis. Direct immunofluorescence findings may also be helpful, since, in lupus erythematosus, linear deposits of immunoglobulins predominate in the lesions, whereas, in lichen planus, clusters of colloid bodies with positive immunofluorescence are found. It may be difficult to differentiate long-standing hypertrophic lichen planus from lichen simplex chronicus, because, in long-standing hypertrophic lichen planus, the basal layer may show hardly any residual damage, and the infiltrate may no longer be band-like (Haber and Sarkany). However, in the case of lichen planus, deeper sections still may show areas of damage to the basal layer.

On the lips and in the mouth, the differentiation of lichen planus from squamous cell carcinoma in situ ("dysplastic leukoplakia") may cause difficulties clinically as well as histologically. Both diseases may show hyperkeratosis and an inflammatory infiltrate close to the epidermis. Yet thorough study of the epidermis reveals some atypicality of the squamous cells in dysplastic leukoplakia. Furthermore, dysplastic leukoplakia is more apt than lichen planus to show irregular downward proliferation of the rete ridges and a conspicuous number of plasma cells.

Lichen planopilaris of the scalp must be differentiated in its early phase from chronic discoid lupus erythematosus, which also affects the hair follicles as well as the surface epidermis. Lupus erythematosus shows more prominent hydropic degeneration of the basal cells both in the epidermis and in the hair follicles without their replacement by squamous cells; in addition, it shows an interfollicular patchy infiltrate. In their late stages, both lichen planopilaris and lupus erythematosus are indistinguishable from pseudopelade of Brocq.

Benign lichenoid keratosis may show a histologic picture indistinguishable from that of lichen planus (see below).

BENIGN LICHENOID KERATOSIS

Originally described in 1966 as solitary lichen planus (Lumpkin and Helwig) and as solitary lichen planus like keratosis (Shapiro and Ackerman), benign lichenoid keratosis consists of a nonpruritic solitary papule or slightly indurated plaque. It usually measures 5 mm to 20 mm in diameter and its color varies from bright red to violaceous to brown. Its surface may be smooth or slightly verrucous (Goette). Benign lichenoid keratosis may occur in sun-exposed as well as in covered areas. It is a fairly common lesion, as shown by the fact that one report concerns 138 patients (Scott and Johnson).

Histopathology. Histologic examination shows a lichenoid tissue reaction that may be indistinguishable from lichen planus (Lumpkin and Helwig; Shapiro and Ackerman). As in lichen planus, there is dissolution of the basal cell layer and a bandlike mononuclear infiltrate "hugging" the epidermis. Colloid bodies are commonly seen (Goette). In contrast to lichen planus, however, parakeratosis is fairly common (Scott and Johnson). Although usually focal, at times parakeratosis is

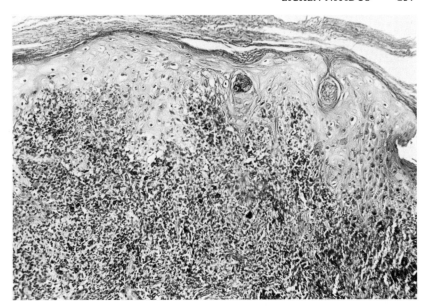

Fig. 8-17.   Benign lichenoid keratosis
A dense infiltrate lies in close approximation to an acanthotic epidermis. Except for the absence of hypergranulosis and the presence of parakeratosis, there is a considerable resemblance to lichen planus. (× 100)

prominent (Fig. 8-17) (Goette). Even though some keratinocytes may show pyknotic hyperchromatic nuclei, no definite nuclear atypicality is seen.

Histogenesis. Direct immunofluorescence examination has shown that the colloid bodies contain IgM and fibrinogen (Tegner). Benign lichenoid keratosis has been noted to involute spontaneously, indicating that it is not a tumor but instead probably represents a delayed hypersensitivity reaction (Berman et al).

KERATOSIS LICHENOIDES CHRONICA

A rare, chronic, progressive, asymptomatic dermatosis, keratosis lichenoides chronica was first described as lichen ruber moniliformis (Kaposi). It received its present name in 1972 (Margolis et al). It shows an extensive eruption of erythematous papulonodules covered with a thick, adherent scale and arranged often in a characteristic linear and occasionally in a netlike pattern. The designation *keratosis lichenoides striata* has therefore been suggested (Duperrat et al). Nodular infiltration of the epiglottis causing hoarseness may occur (Margolis et al; Duperrat et al).

Histopathology.   There is a "lichenoid tissue reaction" with areas of liquefaction degeneration or dissolution of the basal cell layer and a chronic inflammatory infiltrate that in some areas lies in close apposition to the epidermis (Margolis et al; Nabai and Mehregan). The epidermis shows areas of acanthosis as well as of atrophy covered by a hyperkeratotic horny layer showing focal parakeratosis (Petrozzi).

Differential Diagnosis.   Although the histologic picture may resemble that of lichen planus very closely, the presence of parakeratosis, of alternating areas of atrophy and acanthosis, and of a heavier infiltrate than usually seen in lichen planus may help in the differentiation. In addition, the clinical appearance is quite different from that of lichen planus.

LICHEN NITIDUS

Lichen nitidus is characterized by asymptomatic, flat-topped, flesh-colored papules 2 mm to 3 mm in size that may occur in groups but do not coalesce. Their sites of predilection are the penis, arms, and abdomen.

Histopathology.   Each papule of lichen nitidus consists of a circumscribed infiltrate closely attached to the lower surface of the epidermis. Most of the cells within the infiltrate are lymphocytes and histiocytes. Frequently, some of the latter have the appearance of epithelioid cells (Fig. 8-18). A few multinucleated giant cells may be present. The dermal infiltrate often extends to a slight degree into the overlying epidermis.

The epidermis above the infiltrate is flattened and shows either hydropic degeneration or absence of the basal cell layer. If the basal cell layer is absent, the overlying epidermis may become partially detached from the dermis (Ellis and Hill). The horny layer shows parakeratosis above the center of the infiltrate (Weiss and Cohen; Pinkus). Transepidermal perforation of the infiltrate through

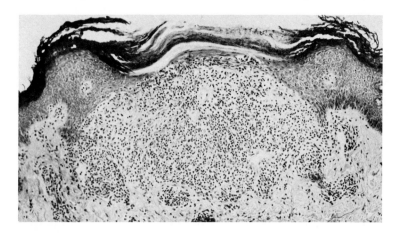

Fig. 8-18.   Lichen nitidus
A circumscribed nest of cells lies in close approximation to the epidermis. The infiltrate consists of lymphocytes, histiocytes, and epithelioid cells. The stratum malpighii above the infiltrate is flattened, and the horny layer is in part parakeratotic. (×100)

the thinned epidermis may occur (Bardach). At each lateral margin of the infiltrate, rete ridges tend to extend downward and seem to clutch the infiltrate in the manner of a claw clutching a ball.

RELATIONSHIP BETWEEN LICHEN PLANUS AND LICHEN NITIDUS. The view that lichen nitidus represents a variant of lichen planus has been supported by several authors because both diseases are occasionally present simultaneously (Ellis and Hill; Gougerot and Civatte). Furthermore, in cases of extensive lichen planus, some of the lesions, consisting of small miliary papules, may have a histologic appearance consistent with lichen nitidus (Ellis and Hill; Wilson and Bett). It seems likely that very early small papules of lichen planus can resemble lichen nitidus histologically by having a flattened epidermis, but they differ in their subsequent evolution (Gougerot and Civatte). The two are therefore different diseases. In particular, they differ in that, in lichen nitidus, the papule remains small and develops parakeratosis as well as epidermal flattening, whereas, in lichen planus, the papule develops acanthosis and hyperkeratosis (Weiss and Cohen). Also, whereas colloid bodies can be demonstrated by direct immunofluorescence in about 90% of the cases of lichen planus (see p. 156), no colloid bodies are seen in lichen nitidus (Waisman et al).

LICHEN STRIATUS

Lichen striatus is a fairly uncommon eruption that as a rule occurs in children but may be seen in adults (Reed et al). It manifests itself usually on one of the extremities as either a continuous or an interrupted band composed of erythematous papules, which may have a scaly surface. The eruption appears suddenly and usually involutes within a year. There is no itching.

Histopathology. A fairly heavy chronic inflammatory infiltrate is seen around the subpapillary vessels and usually also around some of the deeper vessels. The infiltrate extends into some of the papillae (Pinkus). The epidermal changes are secondary and consist of intercellular and intracellular edema often associated with some exocytosis and parakeratosis. In lichen striatus, in contrast to dermatitis, there is usually no acanthosis. Old lesions are apt to show a lichenoid pattern that in some areas may resemble the histologic picture of lichen planus (Reed et al; Stewart et al). The presence of a few large, eosinophilic, dyskeratotic keratinocytes in the granular or horny layer has been described in some cases (Staricco; Charles et al). They resemble the corps ronds of Darier's disease but usually are smaller in size.

Differential Diagnosis. The histologic picture of lichen striatus is nonspecific. Although, as a rule, lichen striatus shows no acanthosis, whereas inflammatory linear verrucous epidermal nevus (ILVEN) does show acanthosis, exceptions occur, and the two conditions thus cannot always be differentiated on histologic grounds (see below).

INFLAMMATORY LINEAR VERRUCOUS EPIDERMAL NEVUS

A persistent, linear, pruritic lesion, inflammatory linear verrucous epidermal nevus (ILVEN) is composed of erythematous, slightly verrucous, scaling papules arranged in one or several lines. Although the usual time of onset is early childhood, the disease may arise in adults (Hodge et al). The most common location is one of the lower extremities.

Histopathology. The histologic picture is essentially that of a nonspecific chronic dermatitis (Kaidbey and Kurban). One observes hyperkeratosis with foci of parakeratosis, moderate acanthosis, elongation of the rete ridges, and, occasionally, slight spongiosis (Altman and Mehregan). In some lesions, extensive parakeratosis is found (Altman and Mehregan; Hodge et al). In an occasional lesion, a somewhat characteristic histologic feature is seen consisting of a regular alternation of slightly raised, parakeratotic areas without a granular layer and slightly depressed, hyperkeratotic areas with a distinct granular layer (Dupré and Christol; Toribio and Quiñones). The dermis shows a chronic inflammatory infiltrate.

Histogenesis. The clinical appearance of lichen striatus and ILVEN may be indistinguishable. However, ILVEN, in contrast to lichen striatus, is pruritic and persistent. Histologically, lichen striatus tends toward a lichenoid pattern, and ILVEN toward a psoriasiform pattern. Nevertheless, the histologic picture in both is basically nonspecific. It has therefore been proposed that they are one and the same disease (Laugier and Olmos). Still, the clinical courses of the two are so different that it seems best to regard them as separate entities.

PITYRIASIS RUBRA PILARIS

Two forms of pityriasis rubra pilaris are recognized according to age of onset. When the disease begins in childhood, the presentation is usually typical; however, pityriasis rubra pilaris with onset in adult life may be difficult to differentiate from psoriasis on the basis of clinical appearance (Davidson et al). The primary lesions consist of follicular and nonfollicular papules. Follicular papules with a keratotic plug are seen best on the dorsal aspect of the proximal phalanges but are often recognizable also on the extensor surfaces of the wrists and forearms and occasionally elsewhere (Lamar and Gaethe). Through coalescence, the nonfollicular papules form scaling plaques. Ultimately, most of the body surface may be affected by a scaling erythroderma. Palmar and plantar erythema and hyperkeratosis are common.

Histopathology. In areas with follicular hyperkeratosis, a large follicular horn plug is seen surrounded by perifollicular parakeratosis (Brunsting and Sheard). Even in areas that do not show clinically visible follicular hyperkeratosis, one may find follicular horn plugs with perifollicular parakeratosis (Niemi et al). Elsewhere, there is diffuse hyperkeratosis with focal parakeratosis and mild irregular acanthosis. In the upper dermis, a mild chronic inflammatory infiltrate is observed around the blood vessels (Niemi et al).

Differential Diagnosis. In spite of an occasional close clinical resemblance to psoriasis, pityriasis rubra pilaris does not resemble psoriasis histologically.

BIBLIOGRAPHY

Urticaria
MCDUFFIE FC, SAMS MW JR, MALDONADO JE et al: Hypocomplementemia with cutaneous vasculitis and arthritis. Mayo Clin Proc 48:340–348, 1973
MONROE EW, SCHULZ CI, MAIZE JC et al: Vasculitis in chronic urticaria. J Invest Dermatol 76:103–107, 1981
SAMS WM JR: Necrotizing vasculitis. (Review) J Am Acad Dermatol 3:1–13, 1980
SOTER NA: Chronic urticaria as a manifestation of necrotizing venulitis. N Engl J Med 296:1440–1442, 1977
SOTER NA, AUSTEN KF, GIGLI I: Urticaria and arthralgias as manifestations of necrotizing angiitis (vasculitis). J Invest Dermatol 63:485–490, 1974
SOTER NA, WASSERMAN SI: Urticaria, angioedema. (Review) Int J Dermatol 18:517–532, 1979
TAPPEINER G, HINTNER H, GLATZL J et al: Hereditary angioedema: Treatment with danazol. Br J Dermatol 100:207–217, 1979

Pruritic Urticarial Papules and Plaques of Pregnancy
CALLEN JP, HANNO R: Pruritic urticarial papules and plaques of pregnancy (PUPPP). J Am Acad Dermatol 5:401–405, 1981
LAWLEY TJ, HERTZ HC, WADE TR et al: Pruritic urticarial papules and plaques of pregnancy. JAMA 241:1696–1699, 1979

Erythema Annulare Centrifugum
ACKERMAN AB: Histologic Diagnosis of Inflammatory Skin Diseases, pp 174–175, 231–233. Philadelphia, Lea & Febiger, 1978.
BRESSLER GS, JONES RE JR: Erythema annulare centrifugum. J Am Acad Dermatol 4:597–602, 1981
DARIER J: De l'érythème annulaire centrifuge. Ann Dermatol Syph 6:57–76, 1916
ELLIS F, FRIEDMAN AA: Erythema annulare centrifugum (Darier's). Arch Dermatol Syph 70:496–507, 1954
NORDENSKJÖLD A, WAHLGREN F: Erythema annulare centrifugum. Acta Derm Venereol (Stockh) 35:281–291, 1955

Erythema Gyratum Repens
GAMMEL JA: Erythema gyratum repens. Arch Dermatol 66:494–505, 1952
HOLT PJA, DAVIES MG: Erythema gyratum repens, an immunologically mediated dermatosis. Br J Dermatol 96:343–347, 1977
LEAVELL US, WINTERNITZ WW, BLACK JH: Erythema gyratum repens and undifferentiated carcinoma. Arch Dermatol 95:343–347, 1977
SKOLNICK M, MAINMAN ER: Erythema gyratum repens with metastatic adenocarcinoma. Arch Dermatol 111:227–229, 1975
STANKLER L: Erythema gyratum repens: Spontaneous resolution in a healthy man. Br J Dermatol 99:461, 1978

Erythema Dyschromicum Perstans
KNOX JM, DODGE BG, FREEMAN RG: Erythema dyschromicum perstans. Arch Dermatol 97:262–272, 1968
SANCHEZ NP, PATHAK MA, SATO SS et al: Circumscribed dermal melaninoses: Classification, light, histochemical, and electron microscopic studies on three patients with the erythema

dyschromicum perstans type. Int J Dermatol 21:25–31, 1982

SOTER NA, WAND C, FREEMAN RG: Ultrastructural pathology of erythema dyschromicum perstans. J Invest Dermatol 52:155–162, 1969

TSCHEN JA, TSCHEN EA, MCGAVRAN MH: Erythema dyschromicum perstans. J Am Acad Dermatol 2:295–302, 1980

Prurigo Simplex

BRAUN-FALCO O, VON EICKSTEDT UM: Beitrag zur Urticaria papulosa chronica. Hautarzt 8:534–540, 1957

KOCSARD E: The problem of prurigo. Australas J Dermatol 6:156–166, 1962

ROSEN T, ALGRA RJ: Papular eruption in black men. Arch Dermatol 116:416–418, 1980

UEHARA M, OFUJI S: Primary eruption of prurigo simplex subacuta. Dermatologica 153:49–56, 1976

Prurigo Nodularis

DOYLE JA, CONNOLLY SM, HUNZIKER N et al: Prurigo nodularis: A reappraisal of the clinical and histologic features. J Cutan Pathol 6:392–403, 1979

EREAUX LP, SCHOPFLOCHER P: Familial primary self-healing squamous epithelioma of skin. Arch Dermatol 91:589–594, 1965

FEUERMAN EJ, SANDBANK M: Prurigo nodularis. Histological and electron microscopical study. Arch Dermatol 111:1472–1477, 1975

RUNNE U, ORFANOS CE: Cutaneous neural proliferation in highly pruritic lesions of chronic prurigo. Arch Dermatol 113:787–791, 1977

Psoriasis

ABRAHAMS J, MCCARTHY JT, SANDERS SL: 101 cases of exfoliative dermatitis. Arch Dermatol 87:96–101, 1963

ADLER DJ, ROWER JM, HASHIMOTO K: Annular pustular psoriasis. Arch Dermatol 117:313, 1981

ANDREWS GC, MACHACEK GF: Pustular bacterids of the hands and feet. Arch Dermatol Syph 32:837–847, 1935

ASHHURST PJC: Relapsing pustular eruptions of the hands and feet. Br J Dermatol 776:169–180, 1964

BAKER H, RYAN TJ: Generalized pustular psoriasis. Br J Dermatol 80:771–793, 1968

BARBER HW: Acrodermatitis continua vel perstans (dermatitis repens) and psoriasis pustulosa. Br J Dermatol 42:500–518, 1930

BRAUN-FALCO O, CHRISTOPHERS E: Structural aspects of initial psoriatic lesions. Arch Dermatol Forsch 251:95–110, 1974

BRAVERMAN IM, COHEN I, O'KEEFE EO: Metabolic and ultrastructural studies in a patient with pustular psoriasis (Von Zumbusch). Arch Dermatol 105:189–196, 1972

BRAVERMAN IM, YEN A: Ultrastructure of the human dermal microcirculation. II. The capillary loops of the dermal papillae. J Invest Dermatol 68:44–52, 1977

BRODY I: The ultrastructure of the epidermis in psoriasis vulgaris as revealed by electron microscopy. J Ultrastruct Res 6:304–367, 1962

BURKS JW, MONTGOMERY H: Histopathologic study of psoriasis. Arch Dermatol Syph 48:479–493, 1943

CHRISTOPHERS E, BRAUN-FALCO O: Mechanism of parakeratosis. J Dermatol 82:268–275, 1970

COX AJ, WATSON W: Histologic variations in lesions of psoriasis. Arch Dermatol 106:503–506, 1972

DAWSON TAJ: Microscopic appearance of geographic tongue. Br J Dermatol 81:827–828, 1969

DAWSON TAJ: Tongue lesions in generalized pustular psoriasis. Br J Dermatol 91:419–424, 1974

DEGOS R, GARNIER G, CIVATTE J: Pustulose par *Candida albicans* avec lésions psoriasiformes rappelant le psoriasis pustuleux. Bull Soc Fr Dermatol Syph 69:231–233, 1962

DOYLE JA, MULLER SA, ROGERS RS III et al: Immunofluorescence in psoriasis. J Am Acad Dermatol 5:655–660, 1981

ENFORS W, MOLIN L: Pustulosis palmaris et plantaris. Acta Derm Venereol (Stockh) 51:289–294, 1971

EVERALL J: Intractable pustular eruption of the hands and feet. Br J Dermatol 69:269–272, 1957

FROST P, VAN SCOTT EJ: Ichthyosiform dermatoses. Arch Dermatol 94:113–126, 1966

GELFANT S: The cell cycle in psoriasis: A reappraisal. Br J Dermatol 95:577–590, 1976

GOODWIN P, HAMILTON S, FRY L: The cell cycle in psoriasis. Br J Dermatol 90:517–524, 1974

GORDON M, JOHNSON WC: Histopathology and histochemistry of psoriasis. Arch Dermatol 95:402–407, 1967

GROVE GL: Epidermal cell kinetics in psoriasis. Int J Dermatol 18:111–121, 1979

HARRIST TJ, MIHM MC JR: Cutaneous immunopathology. Hum Pathol 10:625–653, 1979

HASHIMOTO K, LEVER WF: Elektronenmikroskopische Untersuchungen der Hautveränderungen bei Psoriasis. Dermatol Wochenschr 152:713–722, 1966

JABLONSKA S, BEUTNER EH, BINDER WL et al: Immunopathology of psoriasis. Arch Dermatol Res 264:65–71, 1979

JABLONSKA S, CHORZELSKI TP, BEUTNER EH et al: Autoimmunity in psoriasis. Relation of disease activity and forms of psoriasis to immunofluorescence findings. Arch Dermatol Res 261:135–146, 1978

KATZENELLENBOGEN I, FEUERMAN EI: Psoriasis pustulosa and impetigo herpetiformis: Single or dual entity? Acta Derm Venereol (Stockh) 46:86–94, 1966

KIMURA S, NISHIKAWA T: An immunohistochemical analysis of the deposited immunoglobulins or fibrinogen in parakeratotic psoriatic horny layer and pemphigus skin lesions. Arch Dermatol Res 261:55–62, 1978

KINGERY FAJ, CHINN HD, SAUNDERS TS: Generalized pustular psoriasis. Arch Dermatol 84:912–919, 1961

LAPIÈRE S: Les dermatoses à pustules spongiformes multiloculaires. Ann Dermatol Syph 88:481–506, 1961

LEVER WF: In discussion to Pay D: Pustular psoriasis. Arch Dermatol 99:641–642, 1969

MAHRLE G, ORFANOS CE: Ultrastructural localization and differentiation in normal and psoriatic epidermis. Br J Dermatol 93:495–507, 1975

MARCELO CL, DUELL EA, STAWISKI MA et al: Cyclic nucleotide levels in psoriatic and normal keratomed epidermis. J Invest Dermatol 72:20–24, 1979

MERCER EH, MAIBACH HI: Intercellular adhesion and surface coats of epidermal cells in psoriasis. J Invest Dermatol 51:215–221, 1968

MULLER SA, KITZMILLER KW: Generalized pustular psoriasis. Acta Derm Venereol (Stockh) 42:504–512, 1962

ORFANOS CE, SCHAUMBURG-LEVER G, MAHRLE G et al: Alterations of cell surfaces as a pathogenetic factor in psoriasis. Arch Dermatol 107:38–46, 1973

PIÉRARD J, KINT A: Les "bactérides pustuleuses" d'Andrews. Arch Belg Derm Syph 22:83–101, 1966

PIÉRARD J, KINT A: La pustulose palmo-plantaire chronique et recidivante. Ann Dermatol Venereol 105:681–688, 1978

PINKUS H, MEHREGAN AH: The primary histologic lesion of seborrheic dermatitis and psoriasis. J Invest Dermatol 46:109–116, 1966.

RAGAZ A, ACKERMAN AB: Evolution, maturation, and regression of lesions of psoriasis. Am J Dermatopathol 1:199–214, 1979

RESNECK JS, CRAM DL: Erythema annulare-like pustular psoriasis. Arch Dermatol 108:687–688, 1973

ROWE L, DIXON W, FORSYTHE A: Mitoses in normal and psoriatic epidermis. Br J Dermatol 98:293–299, 1978

RUPEC M: Zur Ultrastruktur der spongiformen Pustel. Arch Klin Exp Dermatol 239:30–49, 1970

SCHUPPENER HJ: Ausdrucksformen pustulöser Psoriasis. Dermatol Wochenschr 138:841–854, 1958

SHELLEY WB, KIRSCHBAUM JO: Generalized pustular psoriasis. Arch Dermatol 84:73–78, 1961

SOLTANI K, VAN SCOTT EJ: Patterns and sequence of tissue changes in incipient and evolving lesions of psoriasis. Arch Dermatol 106:484–490, 1972

SOLTERMANN W: Familiäre Psoriasis pustulosa unter dem Bilde der Impetigo herpetiformis. Dermatologica 116:313–330, 1958

TAGAMI H, OFUJI S: Leukotactic properties of soluble substances in psoriatic scales. Br J Dermatol 95:1–8, 1976

TAGAMI H, OFUJI S: A leukotactic factor in the stratum corneum of pustulosis palmaris et plantaris. Acta Derm Venereol (Stockh) 58:401–405, 1978

THOMSEN K: Pustulosis palmaris et plantaris treated with methotrexate Acta Derm Venereol (Stockh) 51:397–400, 1971

THORMAN J, HEILESEN B: Recalcitrant pustular eruptions of the extremities. J Cutan Pathol 2:19–24, 1975

UEHARA M, OFUJI S: The morphogenesis of pustulosis palmaris et plantaris. Arch Dermatol 109:518–520, 1974

VAN SCOTT EJ, EKEL TW: Kinetics of hyperplasia in psoriasis. Arch Dermatol 88:373–381, 1963

VORHEES JJ, DUELL EA, BASS LJ et al: Decreased cyclic AMP in the epidermis of lesions of psoriasis. Arch Dermatol 105:695–701, 1972

WAGNER G, LUCKASEN JR, GOLTZ RW: Mucous membrane involvement in generalized pustular psoriasis. Arch Dermatol 112:1010–1014, 1976

WEINSTEIN GD, FROST P: Abnormal cell proliferation in psoriasis. J Invest Dermatol 50:254–259, 1968

WEINSTEIN GD, FROST P: Methotrexate for psoriasis. Arch Dermatol 103:33–38, 1971

WEINSTEIN GD, VAN SCOTT EJ: Autoradiographic analysis of turnover times of normal and psoriatic epidermis. J Invest Dermatol 45:257–262, 1965

Reiter's Disease

KHAN MY, HALL WH: Progression of Reiter's syndrome to psoriatic arthritis. Arch Intern Med 116:911–917, 1965

PERRY HO, MAYNE JG: Psoriasis and Reiter's syndrome. Arch Dermatol 92:129–136, 1965

WEINBERGER HW, ROPES MW, KULKA JP et al: Reiter's syndrome, clinical and pathologic observations. (Review) Medicine (Baltimore) 41:35–91, 1962

WRIGHT V, REED WB: The link between Reiter's syndrome and psoriatic arthritis. Ann Rheum Dis 23:12–20, 1964

Parapsoriasis

BARDACH H, RAFF M: Poikilodermatische Parapsoriasis. Hautarzt 28:542–546, 1977

BINAZZI M: Some research on parapsoriasis and lymphoma. Arch Dermatol Res 258:17–23, 1977

BONVALET D, COLAU-GOHM K, BELAICH S et al: Les différentes formes du parapsoriasis en plaques. Ann Dermatol Venereol 104:18–25, 1977

FLEISCHMAJER R, PASCHER F, SIMS CF: Parapsoriasis en plaques and mycosis fungoides. Dermatologica 131:149–160, 1965

GOLDBERG LC: Xantho-erythrodermia (Crocker). Arch Dermatol 88:901–907, 1963

HEID E, DESVAUX J, BRÄNDLE J et al: Der Verlauf der Parapsoriasis en plaques (Brocq'sche Krankheit). Z Hautkr 52:658–662, 1977

HU CH, WINKELMANN RK: Digitate dermatosis. A new look at symmetrical small plaque parapsoriasis. Arch Dermatol 107:65–69, 1973

LAMBERT WE, EVERETT MA: The nosology of parapsoriasis. (Review) J Am Acad Dermatol 5:373–395, 1981

MUSGER A: Zur Frage der nosologischen Stellung der Parapsoriasis lichenoides Brocq. Hautarzt 17:280–284, 1966

OSMUNDSEN PE: Parapsoriasis en plaques. Acta Derm Venereol (Stockh) 48:345–354, 1968

SAMMAN PD: The natural history of parapsoriasis en plaques (chronic superficial dermatitis) and prereticulotic poikiloderma. Br J Dermatol 87:405–411, 1972

SANCHEZ JL, ACKERMAN AB: The patch stage of mycosis fungoides. Am J Dermatopathol 1:5–26, 1979

VELLA BRIFFA D, WARIN AP, CALNAN CD: Parakeratosis variegata: A report of two cases and their treatment with PUVA. Clin Exp Dermatol 4:537–541, 1979

Pityriasis Rosea

BUNCH LW, TILLEY JC: Pityriasis rosea. Arch Dermatol 84:79–86, 1961

Papular Acrodermatitis of Childhood (Gianotti–Crosti Syndrome)

CASTELLANO A, SCHWEITZER R, TONG MJ et al: Papular acrodermatitis of childhood and hepatitis B infection. Arch Dermatol 114:1530–1532, 1978

CLAUDY AL, ORTONNE JP, TREPO C et al: Acrodermatite papuleuse de l'adulte. Ann Dermatol Venereol 104:190–194, 1977

GIANOTTI F: Papular acrodermatitis of childhood and other papulovesicular acro-located syndromes. (Review) Br J Dermatol 100:49–59, 1979

Mucocutaneous Lymph Node Syndrome (Kawasaki's Disease)

BELL DM, BRINK EW, NITZKIN JL et al: Kawasaki syndrome. N Engl J Med 304:1568–1575, 1981

BITTER JJ, FRIEDMAN SA, PALTZIK RL et al: Kawasaki's disease appearing as erythema multiforme. Arch Dermatol 115:71–72, 1979

KAWASAKI T, KOSAKI F, OWAKA S et al: A new infantile febrile mucocutaneous lymph node syndrome (MLNS) prevailing in Japan. Pediatrics 54:271–276, 1974

SCHLOSSBERG D, KANDRA J, KREISER J: Possible Kawasaki disease in a 20-year-old woman. Arch Dermatol 115:1435–1436, 1979

WESTON WL, HUFF JC: The mucocutaneous lymph node syndrome: A critical re-examination. Clin Exp Dermatol 6:167–178, 1981

Lichen Planus

ABELL E, PRESBURY DG, MARKS R et al: The diagnostic significance of immunoglobulin and fibrin deposition in lichen planus. Br J Dermatol 93:17–24, 1975

ALANO A, ORTONNE JP, SCHMIDT D et al: Lichen planus: Study with antihuman T lymphocytes antigen serum on frozen tissue sections. Br J Dermatol 98:601–604, 1978

ALTMAN J, PERRY HO: The variations and course of lichen planus. (Review) Arch Dermatol 84:179–191, 1961

BAART DE LA FAILLE-KUYPER EH, BAART DE LA FAILLE H: An immunofluorescence study of lichen planus. Br J Dermatol 90:365–371, 1974

BHAN AK, HARRIST TJ, MURPHY GF et al: T cell subsets and Langerhans cells in lichen planus: In situ characterization using monoclonal antibodies. Br J Dermatol 105:617–622, 1981

BLACK MM: What is going on in lichen planus? Clin Exp Dermatol 2:303–310, 1977

BRAUN-FALCO O, DORN M, NEUBERT U et al: Trachyonychie: 20 Nägel-Dystrophie. Hautarzt 32:17–22, 1981

COPEMAN PWM, SCHROETTER AL, KIERLAND RR: An unusual variant of lupus erythematosus or lichen planus. Br J Dermatol 83:269–272, 1970

CRAM DL, KIERLAND RR, WINKELMANN RK: Ulcerative lichen planus of the feet. Arch Dermatol 93:692–701, 1966

DAVIES MG, GORKIEWICZ A, KNIGHT A et al: Is there a relationship between lupus erythematosus and lichen planus? Br J Dermatol 96:145–154, 1977

DILAIMY M: Lichen planus subtropicus. Arch Dermatol 112:1251–1253, 1976

EBNER H, ERLACH E, GEBHART W: Untersuchungen über die Blasenbildung beim Lichen ruber planus. Arch Dermatol Forsch 247:193–205, 1973

EBNER H, GEBHART W: Epidermal changes in lichen planus. J Cutan Pathol 3:167–174, 1976

EBNER H, GEBHART W: Light and electron microscopic studies on colloid and other cytoid bodies. Clin Exp Dermatol 2:311–322, 1977

EBNER H, GEBHART W, LASSMANN H et al: The epidermal cell proliferation in lichen planus. Acta Derm Venereol (Stockh) 57:133–136, 1977

EL-LABBAN NG, KRAMER IRH: Civatte bodies and the actively dividing epithelial cells in oral lichen planus. Br J Dermatol 90:13–23, 1974

ELLIS FA: Histopathology of lichen planus based on analysis of one hundred biopsies. J Invest Dermatol 48:143–148, 1967

FULLING HJ: Cancer development in oral lichen planus. Arch Dermatol 108:667–669, 1973

GOMES MA, STAQUET MJ, THIVOLET J: Staining of colloid bodies by keratin antisera in lichen planus. Am J Dermatopathol 3:341–347, 1981

GOUGEROT H, CIVATTE A: Critères cliniques et histologiques des lichens plans cutanés et muqueux: Délimitation. Ann Dermatol Syph 80:5–29, 1953

HABER H, SARKANY I: Hypertrophic lichen planus and lichen simplex. Trans St John's Hosp Dermatol Soc 41:61–65, 1958

HASHIMOTO K: Apoptosis in lichen planus and several other dermatoses. Acta Derm Venereol (Stockh) 56:187–210, 1976

HINTNER H, TAPPEINER G, HÖNIGSMANN H et al: Lichen planus and bullous pemphigoid. Acta Derm Venereol (Stockh) 59, Suppl 85:71–76, 1979

HOLMSTRUP P, PINDBORG JJ: Erythroplakic lesions in relation to oral lichen planus. Acta Derm Venereol (Stockh) 59, Suppl 85:77–84, 1979

JAMISON TH, COOPER NM, EPSTEIN WV: Lichen planus and discoid lupus erythematosus. Overlap syndrome. Arch Dermatol 114:1039–1042, 1978

JÄNNER M, MUISSUS E, ROHDE B: Lichen planus als fakultative Präkanzerose. Dermatol Wochenschr 153:513–518, 1967

KATZENELLENBOGEN I: Lichen planus actinicus (Lichen planus in subtropical countries). Dermatologica 124:10–20, 1962

KRONENBERG K, FRETZIN D, POTTER B: Malignant degeneration of lichen planus. Arch Dermatol 104:304–307, 1971

MALE O: Über die ulzerös-atrophisierende Form des Lichen ruber planus. Z Hautkr 45:17–28, 1970

MALE O, AZAMBUJA R: Diagnostische und therapeutische Probleme beim Lichen ruber ulcerosus. Z Hautkr 50:403–412, 1975

MARKS R, BLACK M, WILSON JONES E: Epidermal cell kinetics in lichen planus. Br J Dermatol 88:37–45, 1973

MEDENICA M, LORINCZ A: Lichen planus: An ultrastructural study. Acta Derm Venereol (Stockh) 57:55–62, 1977

MOREL P, PERRON J, CRICKX B et al: Lichen plan avec dépôts linéaires d'IgG et de C3 à la jonction dermo-épidermique. Dermatologica 163:117–124, 1981

RAGAZ A, ACKERMAN AB: Evolution, maturation, and regression of lesions of lichen planus. Am J Dermatopathol 3:5–25, 1981

ROMERO RW, NESBITT LT JR, REED RJ: Unusual variant of lupus erythematosus or lichen planus. Arch Dermatol 113:741–748, 1977

SAMMAN PD: The nails in lichen planus. Br J Dermatol 73:288–292, 1961

SARKANY I, CARON GA, JONES HH: Lichen planus pemphigoides. Trans St John's Hosp Dermatol Soc 50:50–55, 1964

SAURAT JH, GUINEPAIN MT, DIDIERJEAN L et al: Coexistence d'un lichen plan et d'un pemphigoide bulleuse. Ann Dermatol Venereol 104:368–374, 1977

SCHER RK, FISCHBEIN R, ACKERMAN AB: Twenty-nail dystrophy. A variant of lichen planus. Arch Dermatol 114:612–613, 1978

SHKLAR G: Erosive and bullous oral lesions of lichen planus. Arch Dermatol 97:411–416, 1968

SHKLAR G, FLYNN E, SZABO G: Basement membrane alterations in oral lichen planus. J Invest Dermatol 70:45–50, 1978

SILVER H, CHARGIN L, SACHS PM: Follicular lichen planus (Lichen planopilaris). Arch Dermatol 67:346–354, 1953

SOBEL S, MILLER R, SHATIN H: Lichen planus pemphigoides. Arch Dermatol 112:1280–1283, 1976

THORMANN J: Ulcerative lichen planus of the feet. Arch Dermatol 110:753–755, 1974

TSCHEN JA, TSCHEN EA, MCGAVRAN MH: Erythema dyschromicum perstans. J Am Acad Dermatol 2:295–302, 1980

VARELZIDIS A, TOSCA A, PERISSIOS A et al: Immunohistochemistry in lichen planus. Dermatologica 159:137–144, 1979

VERHAGEN ARHB, KOTEN JW: Lichenoid melanodermatitis. A clinicopathological study of 51 Kenyan patients with so-called tropical lichen planus. Br J Dermatol 101:651–658, 1979

WAISMAN M, DUNDON BC, MICHEL B: Immunofluorescent studies in lichen nitidus. Arch Dermatol 107:200–203, 1973

WALDORF DS: Lichen planopilaris. Arch Dermatol 93:684–691, 1966

WALKER DM, DOLBY AE: Labelling index in the mucosal lesions of lichen planus. Br J Dermatol 91:549–556, 1974

WEIDNER F, UMMENHOFER B: Lichen ruber ulcerosus (dystrophicans). Z Hautkr 54:1008–1017, 1979

WILKINSON JD, DAWBER RPR, BOWERS RP et al: Twenty-nail dystrophy of childhood. Br J Dermatol 100:217–221, 1979

Benign Lichenoid Keratosis

BERMAN A, HERSZENSON S, WINKELMANN RK: The involuting lichenoid plaque. Arch Dermatol 118:93–96, 1982

GOETTE DK: Benign lichenoid keratosis. Arch Dermatol 116:780–782, 1980

LUMPKIN LR, HELWIG EB: Solitary lichen planus. Arch Dermatol 93:54–55, 1966

SCOTT MA, JOHNSON WC: Lichenoid benign keratosis. J Cutan Pathol 3:217–221, 1976

SHAPIRO L, ACKERMAN AB: Solitary lichen planus-like keratosis. Dermatologica 132:386–392, 1966

TEGNER E: Solitary lichen planus simulating malignant lesions. Acta Derm Venereol (Stockh) 59:263–266, 1979

Keratosis Lichenoides Chronica

DUPERRAT B, CARTON FX, DENOEUX JP et al: Kératose lichénoide striée. Ann Dermatol Venereol 104:564–566, 1977

KAPOSI M: Lichen ruber moniliformis. Vrtljschr Dermatol 13:571–582, 1886

MARGOLIS MG, COOPER GA, JOHNSON SAM: Keratosis lichenoides chronica. Arch Dermatol 105:739–743, 1972

NABAI H, MEHREGAN AH: Keratosis lichenoides chronica. J Am Acad Dermatol 2:217–220, 1980

PETROZZI JW: Keratosis lichenoides chronica. Arch Dermatol 112:709–711, 1976

Lichen Nitidus

BARDACH H: Perforating lichen nitidus. J Cutan Pathol 8:111–116, 1981

ELLIS FA, HILL WF: Is lichen nitidus a variety of lichen planus? Arch Dermatol Syph 38:568–573, 1938

GOUGEROT H, CIVATTE A: Critères cliniques et histologiques des lichens plans cutanés et muqueux: délimitation. Ann Dermatol Syph 80:5–29, 1953

PINKUS H: Lichenoid tissue reactions. Arch Dermatol 197:840–846, 1973

WAISMAN M, DUNDON BC, MICHEL B: Immunofluorescent studies in lichen nitidus. Arch Dermatol 107:200–203, 1973

WEISS RM, COHEN AD: Lichen nitidus of the palms and soles. Arch Dermatol 104:538–540, 1971

WILSON HTH, BETT DCH: Miliary lesions in lichen planus. Arch Dermatol 83:920–923, 1961

Lichen Striatus

CHARLES CR, JOHNSON BL, ROBINSON TA: Lichen striatus. J Cutan Pathol 1:265–274, 1974

PINKUS H: Lichen striatus and lichen planus. J Invest Dermatol 11:9–17, 1948

REED RJ, MEEK T, ICHINOSE H: Lichen striatus: A model for the histologic spectrum of lichenoid reactions. J Cutan Pathol 2:1–18, 1975

STARICCO RG: Lichen striatus. Arch Dermatol 79:311–324, 1959

STEWART WM, LAURET P, PIETRINI P et al: Lichen striatus. Critères histologiques. Ann Dermatol Venereol 104:132–135, 1977

Inflammatory Linear Verrucous Epidermal Nevus

ALTMAN J, MEHREGAN AH: Inflammatory linear verrucose epidermal nevus. Arch Dermatol 104:385–389, 1971

DUPRÉ A, CHRISTOL B: Inflammatory linear verrucose epidermal nevus. Arch Dermatol 113:767–769, 1977

HODGE SJ, BARR JM, OWEN LG: Inflammatory linear verrucose epidermal nevus. Arch Dermatol 114:436–438, 1978

KAIDBEY KH, KURBAN AK: Dermatitic epidermal nevus. Arch Dermatol 104:166–171, 1971

LAUGIER P, OLMOS L: Naevus linéaire inflammatoire (NEVIL) et lichen striatus. Deux aspects d'une même affection. Bull Soc Fr Dermatol Syph 83:48–53, 1976

TORIBIO J, QUIÑONES PA: Inflammatory linear verrucose epidermal nevus. Dermatologica 150:65–69, 1975

Pityriasis Rubra Pilaris

BRUNSTING LA, SHEARD C: Dark adaptation in pityriasis rubra pilaris. Arch Dermatol Syph 43:42–61, 1941

DAVIDSON CL JR, WINKELMANN RK, KIERLAND RK: Pityriasis rubra pilaris. Arch Dermatol 100:175–178, 1969

LAMAR LM, GAETHE G: Pityriasis rubra pilaris. Arch Dermatol 89:515–522, 1964

NIEMI KM, KOUSA M, STORGARDS K et al: Pityriasis rubra pilaris. Dermatologica 152:109–118, 1976

9 Vascular Diseases

NONINFLAMMATORY PURPURAS

Purpura represents a hemorrhage into the skin. Lesions less than 3 mm in diameter are called *petechiae*. Larger lesions are called *ecchymoses*. Purpura occurs as the result of either noninflammatory or inflammatory changes within or around blood vessel walls.

Noninflammatory purpura occurs (1) on the basis of deficient collagen formation around capillaries in *senile purpura* and in *scurvy*; (2) on the basis of sensitivity phenomena without vascular occlusion in *idiopathic thrombocytopenic purpura* and possibly in *autoerythrocyte sensitization;* and (3) on the basis of sensitivity phenomena with vascular occlusion in *coumarin necrosis,* in *thrombotic thrombocytopenic purpura,* and in *purpura fulminans.*

Senile Purpura

In senile purpura, well-defined ecchymoses are present on the dorsa of the forearms and hands of the elderly. Prolonged ingestion of corticosteroids is a predisposing factor.

Histopathology. The capillaries within the areas of extravasations appear fairly normal. However, the dermis in which the capillaries are located is altered. It shows solar elastosis in its upper portion (see p. 271) and atrophy in its lower portion, where the collagen is present largely as individual fibers rather than as bundles of fibers (Tattersall and Seville).

Scurvy

In scurvy, caused by a deficiency of ascorbic acid, the purpura usually consists of perifollicular petechiae, especially on the lower extremities. In addition, broken off "corkscrew hairs" are seen in association with follicular hyperkeratosis. In long-standing scurvy, extensive ecchymoses may be present over the shins (Walker).

Histopathology. Extravasations of red cells are found predominantly in the vicinity of hair follicles without evidence of capillary changes or signs of inflammation. Extensive extravasations usually show deposits of hemosiderin both within and outside of macrophages (Walker). In many instances, intrafollicular keratotic plugs are seen.

Histogenesis. In scurvy, there is both a decreased and an abnormal formation of collagen. On *electron microscopic examination,* the dermal fibroblasts appear shrunken and show a decreased amount of rough-surfaced endoplasmic reticulum (Hashimoto et al). In the vicinity of the fibroblasts, one observes increased amounts of extracellular filamentous or amorphous material that has failed to polymerize into collagen fibrils with normal periodicity (Ross and Benditt). The extravasation of red cells is caused by (1) vacuolar degeneration of endothelial cells, (2) junctional separation of adjoining endothelial cells, and (3) detachment of the basement membrane

164

from the endothelium in capillaries and small venules (Hashimoto et al).

Idiopathic Thrombocytopenic Purpura

In idiopathic thrombocytopenic purpura, petechiae and often ecchymoses as well are present as a result of a greatly reduced platelet count. In addition, there may be hemorrhages from the nose, mouth, or uterus.

Histopathology. Extravasations of red cells without evidence of inflammation are seen in the dermis.

Histogenesis. Most patients with idiopathic thrombocytopenic purpura have a circulating antiplatelet factor, usually an immunoglobulin G (IgG) antibody, directed toward a platelet-associated antigen. It coats the platelets, causing accelerated platelet destruction by macrophages, especially in the spleen (McMillan). Also, as *electron microscopic examination* has shown, the experimental reduction of platelets in the blood streams results in widened intercellular spaces in the endothelial lining of capillaries and defects in the capillary basement membrane. These two factors account for the extravasation of blood in thrombocytopenic purpura (Gore et al).

Autoerythrocyte Sensitization Syndrome

First described in 1955 (Gardner and Diamond), the autoerythrocyte sensitization syndrome occurs as recurrent attacks in persons with hysterical personality patterns, almost invariably women, although it has also been observed in a man (Shustik). The lesions begin as red, raised, tender nodules and progress to large, painful ecchymoses.

Histopathology. Numerous extravasated red cells are present in the dermis and the subcutaneous fat. There is no evidence of vasculitis, but, in a few instances, a mild perivascular infiltrate of mononuclear cells has been found (Ratnoff and Agle). At a later stage, one finds in the dermis, in addition to decomposing red cells, hemosiderin, macrophages, and fibroblasts (Waldorf and Lipkin).

Histogenesis. It is undecided whether the syndrome has an organic basis or is factitial in origin. Several suspected organic causes have been described. It has been observed that typical bruises can be induced in patients with the syndrome by the intradermal injection of their sonicated erythrocytes (Pearson and Mazza) and that the presence of phosphatidyl-L-serine in their erythrocyte stroma is responsible (Groch et al). Other investigators have found morphologic abnormalities of erythrocytes on electron microscopic examination (Oei et al). A possible immunologic etiology has been suspected because, on direct immunofluorescence examination, granular deposits of IgM, the third component of complement (C3), factor B, and properdin have been observed at the dermal-epidermal border of the lesions (Pinnas et al).

In favor of a factitial origin are the findings that intradermal injections of autologous red cells do not necessarily reproduce the lesions (Shustick); patients in whom the lesions were regarded as reproduced were not always closely observed for possible manipulation of the lesions (Stocker et al); and, in several patients, multiple injections of their own blood led to lesions only in areas they were told were sites of injection of their own blood but not to lesions in areas they were told were sites of injection of donor blood (Stocker et al; Vakilzadeh and Bröcker).

Coumarin Necrosis

In rare instances, patients receiving loading doses of coumarin congeners, such as dicumarol or warfarin (Coumadin), show between the third and tenth days of therapy one or several areas of ecchymosis that progress rapidly to central blistering and necrosis (Jones and Cunningham). The extent of necrosis varies greatly. If it is extensive, death may ensue as the result of septicemia or renal failure (Lacy and Goodwin).

Histopathology. The primary event is extensive occlusion of dermal and subcutaneous capillaries, venules, and small arterioles with fibrin and platelet thrombi without signs of inflammation (Jones and Cunningham; Schleicher and Fricker). This results in hemorrhagic infarcts, necrosis of the dermis, and subepidermal bullae due to dermal necrosis (Fig. 9-1).

Histogenesis. The necrosis is regarded by many authors as a toxic effect of coumarin on the vascular endothelium (Nalbandian et al). The possibility of a fall in the level of factor VII following a loading dose of coumarin has been considered, since low levels of factor VII can cause intravascular thrombosis (Jones and Cunningham). Although continued coumarin therapy does not aggravate the lesions, resumption of therapy with loading doses can lead to new lesions (Schleicher and Fricker).

Differential Diagnosis. Histologically, the lesions of coumarin necrosis are identical with those found in purpura fulminans (Friedenberg et al). However, purpura fulminans has different clinical characteristics, may have extracutaneous lesions,

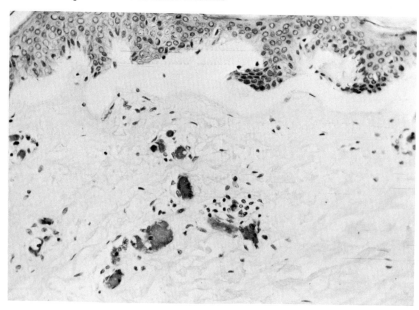

Fig. 9-1. Coumarin necrosis
An early lesion shows occlusion of several dermal vessels by fibrin and platelet thrombi without signs of inflammation. In addition, there is a large subepidermal bulla. (×100)

is associated with disseminated intravascular coagulation, and, in contrast to coumarin necrosis, responds to heparin therapy (see below).

Purpura Fulminans

Purpura fulminans is characterized by the sudden occurrence of large areas of ecchymosis associated with hypotension, fever, and disseminated intravascular coagulation. The areas of ecchymosis are located mainly on the extremities. Large hemorrhagic bullae may overlie the ecchymoses, and some of the ecchymotic areas may undergo necrosis. Purpura fulminans occurs most commonly in children recovering from an infection, such as scarlet fever or varicella, but it may occur without a preceding illness (Cram and Soley) and in adults (Spicer and Rau). The lesions progress rapidly with severe systemic toxicity. The disease used to have a very high mortality; however, treatment for shock and then with heparin has reduced the mortality rate to about 18% (Spicer and Rau).

Histopathology. In the dermis and the subcutaneous tissue, blood vessels in the vicinity of areas of necrosis are occluded by platelet–fibrin thrombi. No inflammation surrounds the blood vessels. There are large areas of hemorrhage in which one finds focal necrosis of the walls of small blood vessels (Spicer and Rau). The epidermis and portions of the dermis often show necrosis. At sites of bullae, the epidermis is detached from the necrotic dermis.

In addition to the skin and the subcutaneous tissue, some internal organs occasionally show thrombosis of small vessels and hemorrhagic necrosis, particularly the intestines, bladder, brain, and serosal surfaces (Chambers et al; Spicer and Rau).

Histogenesis. Purpura fulminans represents a consumption coagulopathy. As a result of disseminated intravascular coagulation, there is depletion of platelets, fibrinogen, prothrombin, and various coagulation factors. The administration of heparin inhibits the coagulation cascade and thus inhibits the development of intravascular thrombosis (Spicer and Rau). As far as the cause of purpura fulminans is concerned, it is assumed that, in cases following an infectious disease, a circulating bacterial endotoxin, by virtue of its antigenicity, causes damage to the vascular endothelium (Case Records, Massachusetts General Hospital).

Differential Diagnosis. The histologic findings in coumarin necrosis are identical with those seen in purpura fulminans (see p. 165).

Thrombotic Thrombocytopenic Purpura

A rare syndrome, thrombotic thrombocytopenic purpura usually has an acute and fulminant course, although some patients have recurrent episodes of several months' duration (Ridolfi and Bell). The disorder is characterized by widespread thrombotic occlusions in the microcirculation in which platelets are consumed. It appears possible that deficiency of a plasma factor is the cause. Although the mortality rate used to be 80% (Myers et al), plasma therapy by exchange, pheresis, or infusion has been found to control the disease (Ridolfi and Bell; Myers et al; Byrnes and Khurana).

Thrombotic thrombocytopenic purpura has five major manifestations: (1) thrombocytopenic purpura, (2) microangiopathic hemolytic anemia often associated with jaundice, (3) fluctuating neurologic signs, (4) severe renal involvement, and (5) fever. Extensive thrombosis of small blood vessels causes small hemorrhages in many organs of the body, including occasionally the skin (Luttgens). In particular, melena, hematuria, and hemoptysis may occur.

Cutaneous manifestations aside from jaundice consist of petechiae and ecchymoses due to the thrombocytopenia. In addition, there may be areas of hemorrhagic necrosis that may be covered by large bullae (Luttgens).

Histopathology. The cutaneous lesions and sometimes even areas of the skin free of lesions show occlusion of capillaries by an amorphous, eosinophilic, periodic acid-Schiff (PAS)-positive material containing platelets and fibrin (Beigelman). This may be accompanied by endothelial proliferation (Bone et al). There is a striking absence of inflammatory changes in and around the vessels. In addition, as a result of the thrombocytopenic purpura, the skin shows more or less extensive extravasations of red cells.

In the absence of diagnostic findings in the skin, it may be possible to establish the diagnosis of thrombotic thrombocytopenic purpura by demonstrating the presence of thrombi in the small blood vessels through random biopsy of a lymph node (Ruffolo et al), through aspiration of bone marrow (Ruffolo et al), or through biopsy of the gingiva, a highly vascular tissue (Goldenfarb and Finch).

Autopsy reveals the widespread presence of thrombi in the small blood vessels of many organs, especially the kidneys, adrenals, spleen, pancreas, myocardium, and brain (Ruffolo et al).

Histogenesis. *Electron microscopic examination* of the thrombi reveals that they are composed of platelet aggregates and small amounts of intermixed fibrin (Myers et al). In addition, they may contain red cells and leukocytes (Bone et al).

There is platelet consumption in the occluding platelet thrombi. Coagulation studies usually fail to show evidence of disseminated intravascular coagulation (Myers et al). The primary lesion is believed to be a vascular endothelial injury followed by the adherence of platelets and fibrin at the site of the vascular injury (Bone et al).

INFLAMMATORY PURPURA (VASCULITIS)

The following types of purpura are caused by inflammatory changes in the walls of blood vessels, that is, by a vasculitis: (1) leukocytoclastic vasculitis, or anaphylactoid purpura, and (2) mixed cryoglobulinemia, both of which show a neutrophilic type of vasculitis; (3) pityriasis lichenoides et varioliformis of Mucha–Habermann and (4) purpura pigmentosa chronica, both representing a lymphocytic type of vasculitis. Two other types of purpura will be discussed elsewhere: bacterial purpura, which is usually caused by meningococci (see p. 294), gonococci (see p. 296), *Mycobacterium leprae* (see p. 308), or rickettsia (see p. 310), and purpura due to drug allergy (see p. 259).

Leukocytoclastic Vasculitis (Anaphylactoid Purpura)

Leukocytoclastic vasculitis, also called allergic or necrotizing vasculitis (Sams et al, 1975), has as its most common primary lesion purpuric papules known as palpable purpura. It is characterized histologically by damage to the small cutaneous vessels and an infiltrate of neutrophils showing fragmentation of nuclei (karyorrhexis or leukocytoclasis). It can be divided into an acute type, the Henoch–Schönlein type, which frequently is associated with systemic manifestations, and a chronic type, the Gougerot–Ruiter type, in which systemic manifestations usually are absent (Winkelmann and Ditto). Intermediate cases between these two types also occur.

In the acute Henoch-Schönlein type, petechiae and often ecchymoses are present in association with papular and urticarial lesions. One also frequently observes erythema. In some cases, vesicles and bullae are seen, causing a marked resemblance to erythema multiforme (Gammon and Wheeler). Some of the lesions may ulcerate, in which case fever and malaise are present. Systemic manifestations are frequent and may consist of arthralgia (Schönlein's purpura), crises of abdominal pain with melena (Henoch's purpura), hematuria due to either focal or diffuse glomerulonephritis, and, in rare instances, dyspnea due to pulmonary infiltrates (McCoombs). In severe cases referred to as hypersensitivity angiitis (Zeek) and characterized by marked pulmonary and renal involvement, death occurs within a few days or weeks, usually with renal failure as the cause. As a rule, Henoch-Schönlein purpura lasts about 4 weeks, but recurrences develop in about 40% of the cases (Allen et al). Even though the renal lesions often are reversible, death from either acute or chronic renal failure occurs in some patients (Ansell).

In the chronic Gougerot-Ruiter type of leukocytoclastic vasculitis, the eruption is often polymorphous. Petechiae are present in most but not all patients and are limited largely to the lower legs, occurring only occasionally on the thighs and arms. Other cutaneous manifestations are macules, papules, nodules, blisters, and ulcers. The eruption often shows remissions and exacerbations (Ruiter).

Three clinical variants of leukocytoclastic vasculitis are *urticarial vasculitis, hypergammaglobulinemic purpura of Waldenström,* and *systemic rheumatoid vasculitis.* Urticarial vasculitis shows urticarial wheals that persist longer than in the usual form of urticaria, while purpura is faint or absent (see p. 136). Hypergammaglobulinemic purpura is mild and chronic and is characterized by petechiae, usually on the lower legs, in association with a polyclonal hypergammaglobulinemia (Olmstead et al). Systemic rheumatoid vasculitis may develop in patients with long-standing rheumatoid arthritis. It is chronic and may be fatal. Purpuric lesions are present in some patients; however, digital infarcts and cutaneous ulcers are the usual cutaneous manifestations (Scott et al).

Histopathology.   The histologic changes in leukocytoclastic vasculitis of the skin are the same in the acute and the chronic types, except that extravasation of red cells is less pronounced in the chronic type and may even be absent. The two outstanding features in leukocytoclastic vasculitis are vascular changes and a cellular infiltrate containing many neutrophils.

Vascular changes are found only in small blood vessels and are limited to the dermis, except in relatively rare cases of the chronic type that have nodular lesions (see below). The dermal vessels show swelling of their endothelial cells and deposits of strongly eosinophilic strands of fibrin within and around their walls. The deposits of fibrin and the marked edema combine to give the walls of blood vessels and the perivascular collagen a smudgy appearance referred to as fibrinoid degeneration. Actual necrosis of the perivascular collagen, however, is seen only rarely in conjunction with ulcerative lesions (Winkelmann and Ditto). If the vascular changes are severe, swelling of the endothelial cells may result in occlusion of the lumen.

The cellular infiltrate is present predominantly around the dermal blood vessels but often also within the vascular walls, so that the outline of the blood vessels may appear indistinct (Fig. 9-2). The infiltrate consists mainly of neutrophils and of varying numbers of eosinophils and mononuclear cells. A characteristic feature is the presence of many scattered nuclear fragments, referred to as nuclear dust, resulting from the disintegration of neutrophils (karyorrhexis or leukocytoclasis). In addition to its perivascular location, the infiltrate is found scattered through the upper dermis in association with fibrin deposits between and within collagen bundles. As a rule, extensive extravasations of erythrocytes are present; however, they may be slight or absent in chronic cases of allergic vasculitis. Vesicles, if present, usually form subepidermally (Ruiter and Hadders). Often, the detached epidermis is necrotic. The ulcers seen in occasional cases are the result of vascular necrosis and subsequent cutaneous infarction (Winkelman and Ditto).

In old lesions, the number of neutrophils may

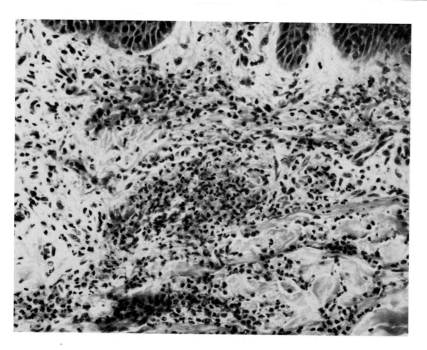

Fig. 9-2.   Leukocytoclastic vasculitis (anaphylactoid purpura) The capillaries show swelling of the endothelial cells and deposition of fibrinoid material around them. A rather severe inflammatory infiltrate is present, especially around the capillaries. It is composed largely of neutrophils, many of which show fragmentation of nuclei (karyorrhexis). No extravasation of erythrocytes is present, probably as a result of occlusion of the capillaries. (×200)

be decreased and the number of mononuclear cells increased so that, in some instances, mononuclear cells predominate (Gower et al).

The nodular lesions occasionally seen in chronic leukocytoclastic vasculitis and referred to as nodular dermal allergid of Gougerot (Gougerot and Duperrat; Laymon) show extension of involvement to the small vessels present at the dermal-subcutaneous border. Like the dermal vessels, these vessels show an infiltrate composed largely of neutrophils and deposits of fibrin within and around their walls. In contrast to periarteritis nodosa, medium-sized arteries are not involved.

Visceral Lesions. In the rapidly fatal cases of hypersensitivity angiitis, a widespread vasculitis of small blood vessels is found in many organs (Zeek). Otherwise, the only organ that is frequently affected is the kidney, with involvement in about 40% of the cases of the acute Henoch-Schönlein type of leukocytoclastic vasculitis. There may be either a focal or a diffuse glomerulitis characterized by occlusion of lobules of glomeruli by fibrinoid material (Ansell). Occasionally, the small intestine shows focal areas of vasculitis during crises of abdominal pain (Ansell).

Leukocytoclastic vasculitis occurs as part of allergic granulomatosis and of Wegener's granulomatosis (Winkelmann and Ditto). In addition, it is seen in the cutaneous lesions of systemic polyarteritis nodosa (see p. 178).

Histogenesis. *Electron microscopic studies* have shown that leukocytoclastic vasculitis affects blood vessels of the size and appearance of postcapillary venules having a minimal smooth muscle coat and numerous pericytes (Sams et al, 1976). The endothelial cells are sometimes so severely swollen that the lumen is obstructed (Ruiter and Molenaar). The endothelial cells show a large number of pinocytotic vesicles, which are indicative of an increased metabolic and phagocytotic activity (Sams et al, 1976). The basement membrane is thickened and has a spongelike appearance, because it consists of several layers, with deposition of fibrin between the layers (Ruiter and Molenaar). Large amounts of fibrin are present also around the vascular walls in close association with collagen fibrils (Ruiter and Molenaar). Neutrophils are seen around the vessels together with nuclear fragments and cytoplasmic debris (Perrot et al). It is thus evident that, basically, the vasculitis is not "necrotizing," but rather that this light microscopic image is evoked by the presence of abundant amounts of fibrin within the walls and around the venules. In addition to fibrin, immune complexes are demonstrable by electron microscopy in lesions less than 24 hr old as electron-dense amorphous deposits in the walls of postcapillary venules (Braverman and Yen). In involved skin, immune complexes are also present within cytoplasmic vacuoles of neutrophils, indicating their phagocytosis and removal by neutrophils.

Direct immunofluorescence examination of early lesions less than 24 hr old shows in the majority of cases in the walls of blood vessels complement components, particularly C3, frequently in association with IgM or IgA. In the clinically normal skin of the patients, C3 is somewhat less frequently and IgM and IgA only rarely demonstrable (Sams et al, 1975). It is not surprising that only C3 can be demonstrated in some patients, since C3 is the amplification step in the complement cascade, and several hundred or thousand more C3 molecules may be bound in the vessel walls than C1q, which is bound molecule for molecule to immunoglobulin (Sams et al, 1975). The detection of C1q and C4 in some patients in the absence of factor B or properdin indicates that the classic rather than the alternative complement pathway is activated. The frequent absence of complement and immunoglobulins in lesions older than 24 hr is the result of their lysosomal destruction (see below).

The intradermal injection of histamine into the uninvolved skin of patients with leukocytoclastic vasculitis in most cases increases vascular permeability, thereby inducing a lesion of vasculitis preceded by increased deposits of C3 and immunoglobulins. The increase in deposits of C3 and immunoglobulins is apparent after 1 hr to 4 hr and precedes the appearance of neutrophilic infiltration and of clinical lesions (Gower et al). This finding supports the contention that deposition of immune complexes within vessel walls is responsible for the appearance of leukocytoclastic vasculitis. The complement activation is chemotactic for neutrophils. Disintegration of neutrophils leads to the release of lysosomal enzymes, including elastase and collagenase, which cause vascular damage and tissue destruction as well as removal of the immune complexes (Wolff et al). Circulating immune complexes can be found in most patients with leukocytoclastic vasculitis, the exception being patients with only cutaneous vasculitis of just a few weeks' duration (Herrmann et al).

Leukocytoclastic vasculitis thus represents an immune complex disorder, a type III immune reaction analogous to the *Arthus phenomenon*. The Arthus phenomenon occurs in sensitized animals at the site of an intradermal injection of the specific antigen to which they have been sensitized. Histologically, like leukocytoclastic vasculitis, the Arthus phenomenon shows leukocytoclasis; immunologically, it shows as the primary event the vascular deposition of antigen–antibody complexes followed by complement-dependent leukocytic infiltration (Cochrane). In the Arthus reaction in the guinea pig, immune complexes form within 20 min of intradermal challenge and are removed within 8 hr to 18 hr (Cream et al).

Although the *etiology* is not apparent in most instances of leukocytoclastic vasculitis, the disorder is known to occur in association with streptococcal tonsillitis or hepatitis B disease. It also occurs as a drug allergy and in association with systemic lupus erythematosus and mixed cryoglobulinemia (Gower et al). For a discussion of the relationship between mixed cryoglobulinemia and leukocytoclastic vasculitis, see below.

Cryoglobulinemia

Two types of cryglobulinemia are recognized: the relatively uncommon monoclonal variety, and the mixed or multicomponent variety.

Cryoglobulins are immunoglobulins that precipitate at cold temperatures and redissolve on rewarming. When a cryoglobulin determination is to be made, it is important that the blood be kept at 37°C until after the red blood cells have been spun down to prevent a rapidly precipitable cryoglobulin from being lost with the red blood cells (Sams).

Monoclonal Cryoglobulinemia

Monoclonal cryoglobulinemia, either IgG or IgM cryoglobulin or cryo-Bence Jones protein, may occur in multiple myeloma, Waldenström's macroglobulinemia, lymphoma, and lymphocytic leukemia. Very rarely, cryoglobulins of the IgG type are found in relatively high concentrations in essential monoclonal cryoglobulinemia.

Essential monoclonal cryoglobulinemia shows purpuric lesions and ulcerations that in some cases are limited to the legs (Ellis; Baughman and Sommer) but may be widespread (Koda et al). There may also be ulcerations of fingers and toes and occasionally gangrene (McKenzie et al). Although only cutaneous vessels are affected in some cases, the vessels of the renal glomeruli, of the brain, and of the lungs can also be involved, resulting in death (Ellis; McKenzie et al).

Histopathology. In the involved areas, the dermal vessels contain in their lumina an amorphous eosinophilic substance consisting largely of precipitated cryoglobulin (Fig. 9-3). This intracapillary precipitate is visible in hematoxylin-eosin-stained sections (Ellis); however, it is best demonstrated by the PAS stain (Baughman and Sommer). Some capillaries are densely filled with erythrocytes, and extensive extravasations of red cells are present. Vascular changes similar to those in the dermis may be present in the subcutaneous tissue (McKenzie et al). Although an inflammatory infiltrate is absent in some lesions (Baughman and Sommer), a mild to moderately severe perivascular lymphocytic infiltrate is present in others (Koda et al). There is, however, no evidence of vasculitis.

Histogenesis. Although in some patients the disease is aggravated by exposure to cold weather (Koda et al), in others it is not affected by cold temperature (Ellis; Baughman and Sommer). Rather, the intravascular precipitates form on the basis of hyperviscosity of the serum caused by the cryoglobulin. Hyperviscosity is also responsible for the renal precipitates (Moroz and Rose).

Mixed Cryoglobulinemia

In mixed cryoglobulinemia, the cryoprecipitate consists of two and occasionally three cryoglobulins, with one cryoglobulin acting as an antibody against the other. Such cryoglobulins are therefore circulating immune complexes (Cream). The most common combination is IgG–IgM, but other combinations also exist. Mixed cryoglobulinemia may occur in association with autoimmune diseases, such as systemic lupus erythematosus,

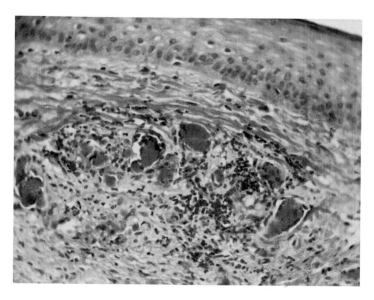

Fig. 9-3.   Essential monoclonal cryoglobulinemia
Dilated capillaries contain in their lumina an amorphous eosinophilic substance consisting largely of precipitated cryoglobulin. (× 200)

rheumatoid arthritis, Sjögren's syndrome, hepatitis B infection, and leukocytoclastic vasculitis. In addition, there is a distinct clinical syndrome, essential mixed cryoglobulinemia, in which there is no identifying underlying disease (Fauci).

Essential mixed cryoglobulinemia is characterized by chronic dependent palpable purpura, arthralgia, and, sometimes, a diffuse proliferative glomerulonephritis.

Histopathology. The cutaneous lesions of mixed cryoglobulinemia are indistinguishable histologically from those seen in leukocytoclastic vasculitis (Nir et al) (see p. 168).

Histogenesis. The cutaneous vasculitis and the glomerulonephritis are caused by the deposition in the cutaneous vessel walls and in the glomeruli of immune complexes principally made up of IgM rheumatoid factor cryoglobulin and IgG cryoglobulin, demonstrable by direct immunofluorescence (Fauci).

Pustulosis Acuta Generalisata

First described in 1974 (Tan), pustulosis acuta generalisata shows, subsequent to a streptococcal tonsillitis, a sudden widespread eruption of sterile pustules up to 8 mm in size. The greatest number of pustules is found on the distal parts of the extremities. Spontaneous clearing occurs after 1 to 4 weeks.

Histopathology. A unilocular large intraepidermal pustule is filled with neutrophils (Braun-Falco et al). In the dermis beneath the pustule, a leukocytoclastic vasculitis with fibrin deposits in the vessel walls is seen (Ishikawa et al). Extravasation of red cells has been described in only one case (Tan).

Histogenesis. Direct immunofluorescence testing has revealed in all cases deposits of C3 in the vessel walls and in some cases deposits of IgM as well (Ishakawa et al).

Pityriasis Lichenoides

Pityriasis lichenoides occurs in two forms, which differ in severity. Transitions between the two forms occur (Nasemann et al; Marks et al). Both are chronic and asymptomatic, with crops of self-healing lesions that on histologic examination show a lymphocytic vasculitis or perivasculitis.

The milder form, called *pityriasis lichenoides chronica,* is characterized by recurrent crops of brownish red papules, mainly on the trunk, that are covered with a scale and show a slow evolution.

The more severe form, called *pityriasis lichenoides et varioliformis acuta* (PLEVA) and referred to also as Mucha–Habermann disease, consists of a fairly extensive eruption, mainly on the trunk, characterized by papules that develop into papulonecrotic, occasionally hemorrhagic lesions. Within a few weeks, individual lesions heal with little or no scarring. Although the individual lesions follow an acute course, the disorder is chronic, extending over several months or even years because of the continuous development of new lesions. In occasional patients, some lesions increase in size to necrotic ulcers 1 cm to 2 cm in diameter that heal with atrophic scarring. Very rarely, patients with PLEVA have a sudden, severe flare-up of their disease characterized by innumerable coalescent ulcerations associated with high fever. After a few months, the flare-up subsides (Degos et al; Burke et al; Auster et al).

Lymphomatoid papulosis combines the clinical features of PLEVA with a histologic infiltrate suggestive of lymphoma. Many but not all observers regard it as a variant of PLEVA (see Histogenesis). A few scattered ulceronecrotic lesions are seen quite commonly in lymphomatoid papulosis, in addition to papulonecrotic lesions (Black and Wilson Jones). The course is protracted. The malignant histologic appearance thus contrasts with the benign clinical course, which is characterized by spontaneous healing of individual lesions. Still, in two cases, death from lymphoma, with cutaneous lesions of lymphoma, occurred after 7 and 18 years, respectively (Kawada et al; Black and Wilson Jones), and, in one case, visceral lymphoma developed after 40 years (Dupont).

Histopathology. In the mild form, pityriasis lichenoides chronica, one observes a perivascular infiltrate composed largely of mononuclear cells. The infiltrate does not invade the walls of the vessels, and extravasations of red cells thus do not occur (Szymanski). The infiltrate extends into the papillae and the epidermis, where one observes spongiosis and a thickened, parakeratotic horny layer. Occasionally, there are degenerative changes in the epidermis with swelling and degeneration of some of the malpighian cells, so that the histologic picture approaches that of PLEVA (Piérard and Van Steenbergen).

In PLEVA, the more severe form, one observes vascular changes consisting of a pronounced mononuclear infiltrate around capillaries, with the capillaries showing endothelial swelling and permeation of their walls by the infiltrate. This usually results in only mild, focal extravasations of erythrocytes representing a lymphocytic vasculitis (Piérard and Van Steenbergen; Szymanski). There often is marked exocytosis of lymphoid cells. As a fairly characteristic feature of the disease, a few erythrocytes often are seen "trapped" within the epidermis (Fig. 9-4). Pronounced intercellular and intracellular edema may occur in the epidermis, leading to degeneration and necrosis of the epidermis (Nasemann et al). Finally, as a result of disintegration of the epidermis, erosion or even ulceration may occur.

In general, PLEVA differs from leukocytoclastic vasculitis by the absence of neutrophils, of nuclear dust, and of fibrinoid deposits around the capillaries. In some cases, however, especially those with ulcers, these features are present to some extent (Burke et al; Muller and Schulze).

In *lymphomatoid papulosis*, one observes scattered through the cellular infiltrate of PLEVA varying numbers of large, atypical cells with hyperchromatic, irregularly shaped nuclei resembling those seen in mycosis fungoides (Fig. 9-5) (Black and Wilson Jones). They may be so large and atypical that they resemble the cells of metastatic carcinoma or malignant melanoma (Macauley). In other instances, multinucleated cells resembling Reed–Sternberg giant cells are present (Valentino and

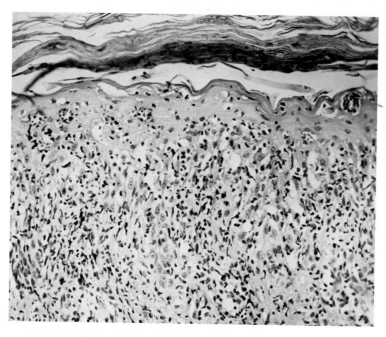

Fig. 9-4. Pityriasis lichenoides et varioliformis acuta
A pronounced mononuclear infiltrate is present in the dermis and is seen invading the epidermis. The epidermis, which appears pale-staining because of its degeneration, contains small accumulations of erythrocytes. (×200)

Fig. 9-5. Lymphomatoid papulosis
The dermal infiltrate contains numerous cells with large, hyperchromatic, irregularly shaped nuclei that have an atypical appearance. (*Left*) Low magnification. (×100) (*Right*) Higher magnification. (×400)

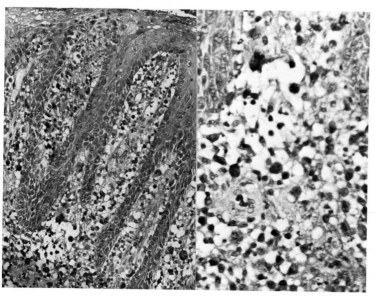

Helwig; Schimpf and Pons). In such cases, the presence of vasculitis, the diapedesis of red cells into the dermis and the epidermis, and clinical data aid in arriving at the right diagnosis (Valentino and Helwig).

Histogenesis. *Direct immunofluorescence studies* of the chronic and the acute varioliform types of pityriasis lichenoides have shown deposits of IgM and C3 in the vessel walls and along the dermal-epidermal junction in many but by far not in all cases. Authors who have examined only purpuric lesions (Clayton and Haffenden) or varioliform lesions (Hayashi) have detected such deposits much more frequently than authors who have also included cases of the chronic type (Thivolet et al; Faber and van Joost). Vascular deposits of IgM and C3 have been noted also in lymphomatoid papulosis (Harrist et al). The fluorescence in pityriasis lichenoides appears to be most intense in blood vessels that are affected by inflammatory infiltrates and show fibrinoid changes of their walls (Hayashi). Thus, evidence that pityriasis lichenoides represents an immune complex vasculitis is seen only in severely affected blood vessels.

Four views exist on the nosologic position of lymphomatoid papulosis: (1) it represents a variant of PLEVA; (2) it represents an independent entity; (3) it belongs to the group of T-cell lymphomas; and (4) it represents a T-cell pseudolymphoma. In favor of a close relationship to PLEVA are the facts that (a) lymphomatoid papulosis is indistinguishable from PLEVA in its clinical appearance and course (Muller and Schulze); (b) aside from atypical cells, the histologic picture is the same in both diseases (Valentino and Helwig; Black); and (c) approximately 7% of biopsies from patients with pityriasis lichenoides have a small number of large, abnormal-appearing mononuclear cells, so that it seems that the difference between the two diseases is only a matter of degree (Marks et al). Some authors, however, regard lymphomatoid papulosis as an independent entity either on the basis of the presence of atypical cells and the development of lymphoma in a few instances (Macaulay; Feuerman and Sandbank; Balaich et al) or because of the absence of vasculitis in some cases (Jimbow et al; Piérard et al). The possibility that lymphomatoid papulosis, like mycosis fungoides and Sézary's syndrome, represents a T-cell lymphoma has been proposed, because, in cell suspensions, 90% or more of the cells form rosettes with sheep red blood cells (Edelson). Some authors believe, however, that, even though the infiltrate of lymphomatoid papulosis, like that of mycosis fungoides, is seen on examination with monoclonal antibodies to consist largely of helper T lymphocytes, lymphomatoid papulosis, because of its benign course, represents a cutaneous T-cell pseudolymphoma (Burg et al). In favor of this view is also the observation that the apparently atypical cells seen on electron microscopic examination are similar to those seen during in vitro blastogenesis induced by various mitogens and thus are the result of a reactive lymphocytic hyperplasia (Jimbow

et al; Brehmer-Andersson). In the few instances in which lymphomatoid papulosis seems to coexist with mycosis fungoides (Fine et al; Brehmer-Andersson; Thomsen and Schmidt), it is likely that the lymphomatoid papulosis represents a variant of mycosis fungoides (Brehmer-Andersson; Black).

Differential Diagnosis. The resemblance of the atypical cells of lymphomatoid papulosis to Reed–Sternberg cells has led to a mistaken diagnosis of cutaneous Hodgkin's disease (Szur et al), especially in cases in which Hodgkin's disease of lymph nodes has also been present (Rubin; Gordon et al). However, primary cutaneous Hodgkin's disease does not occur, and, when Hodgkin's disease involves the skin secondarily, the infiltrate is usually more extensive and involves mainly the deep portions of the dermis and the subcutaneous fat.

Purpura Pigmentosa Chronica (Majocchi–Schamberg Disease)

Four diseases constitute purpura pigmentosa chronica: purpura annularis telangiectodes of Majocchi, progressive pigmentary dermatosis of Schamberg, pigmented purpuric lichenoid dermatitis of Gougerot and Blum, and eczematidlike purpura of Doucas and Kapetanakis. They are closely related to one another, so that they often cannot be differentiated on clinical or histologic grounds. Therefore, their separation into different entities is not warranted (Randall et al). The term *purpura pigmentosa chronica* appears suitable for this disease.

Clinically, the primary lesion consists of purpuric puncta appearing in groups and extending slowly, so that patches of various sizes form. Gradually, telangiectatic puncta may appear as a result of capillary dilatation, and pigmentation as a result of hemosiderin deposits. In some cases, telangiectasia predominates (Majocchi's disease), and in others, pigmentation (Schamberg's disease). Not infrequently, clinical signs of inflammation are present, such as erythema, papules, and scaling (Gougerot–Blum disease) or papules, scaling, and lichenification (eczematidlike purpura). The disorder is often limited to the lower extremities, but it may be extensive. Mild pruritis may be present. There are no systemic symptoms.

A localized variant of purpura pigmentosa chronica is *lichen aureus*, in which one or a few patches are present, usually on the legs. The patches are composed of closely set, flat papules of a rust, copper, or orange color (Waisman and Waisman). In some cases, petechiae are present within the patches (Maciejewski et al).

Histopathology. The basic process is a lymphocytic type of vasculitis limited to the upper dermis. In early lesions, the capillaries of the upper dermis, including those located in the papillae, show swelling of their endothelial cells. Small amounts of extravasated red cells usually are found in the vicinity of the capillaries (Fig. 9-6). A cellular infiltrate, consisting largely of lymphocytes and histiocytes, is present in the upper dermis, especially in the vicinity of the capillaries (Randall et al). In some instances, the infiltrate invades the epidermis and provokes mild spongiosis of the stratum malpighii and patchy parakeratosis. This is seen particularly in some cases of pigmented purpuric lichenoid dermatitis of Gougerot and Blum (Randall et al) and eczematidlike purpura of Doucas and Kapetanakis (Mosto and Casala).

In old lesions, the capillaries often show dilatation of their lumen and proliferation of their endothelium. Extravasated red cells may no longer be present, but one frequently finds hemosiderin, though in varying amounts. The inflammatory infiltrate is less pronounced than in the early stage.

Histogenesis. On *electron microscopic examination*, purpura pigmentosa chronica shows swelling and vacuoli-

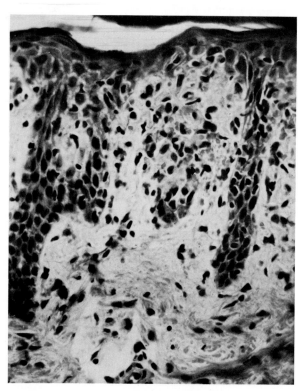

Fig. 9-6.   Purpura pigmentosa chronica (Majocchi–Schamberg disease)
The capillaries of a papilla show swelling of their endothelial cells and are surrounded by extravasated erythrocytes and a lymphoid infiltrate. (× 400)

zation of endothelial cells and multiplication of the vascular basement membrane. The infiltrate contains some Langerhans cells in addition to lymphocytes and macrophages (Haustein and Klug). The lymphocytes are frequently seen in apposition to macrophages and Langerhans cells, suggesting a transfer of antigen to T lymphocytes as seen in delayed hypersensitivity reactions (Klug and Haustein).

Direct immunofluorescence testing has in some cases failed to show any vascular deposits of immunoglobulins or complement (Verburgh-van der Zwan and Manuel; Maciejewski et al); however, in other cases, deposits of C3 and occasionally also of immunoglobulins have been found (Iwatsuki et al).

Differential Diagnosis. Purpura pigmentosa chronica may resemble stasis dermatitis because inflammation, dilatation of capillaries, extravasation of erythrocytes, and deposits of hemosiderin occur in both. However, in stasis dermatitis, the process extends much deeper into the dermis, and more pronounced epidermal changes and fibrosis of the dermis are present (see p. 99). Leukocytoclastic vasculitis differs from purpura pigmentosa chronica by the predominance of neutrophils and the presence of nuclear dust in the infiltrate and by the deposits of fibrinoid material within and around the walls of dermal vessels.

GRANULOMA FACIALE

Granuloma faciale, first described in 1945 (Wigley) and also called granuloma faciale eosinophilicum, consists occasionally of one but usually of several asymptomatic, soft, brownish red, slowly enlarging patches. Their surface appears normal except for dilatation of the follicular openings. The lesions are nearly always limited to the face. In rare instances, a few lesions are present also on the trunk (Lever et al; Rusin et al).

Histopathology. A dense polymorphous infiltrate is found (Fig. 9-7) that, although it is located mainly in the upper half of the dermis, extends in some areas into the lower dermis and occasionally even into the subcutaneous tissue. Quite characteristically, the infiltrate does not invade the epidermis or the pilosebaceous appendages but is separated from them by a narrow "grenz" zone of normal collagen (Lever; Pfleger and Tappeiner). The pilosebaceous appendages are well preserved.

The polymorphous infiltrate consists in large part of neutrophils and eosinophils, but mononuclear cells, that is, lymphocytes and histiocytes, as well as plasma cells and mast cells are also present. Frequently, the nuclei of some of the

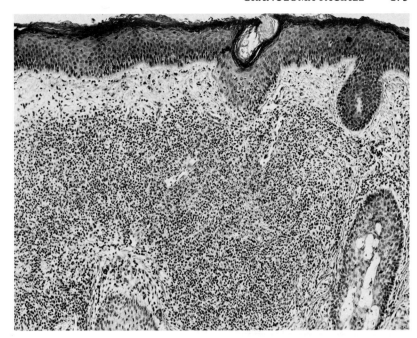

Fig. 9-7. Granuloma faciale
A dense infiltrate containing many eosinophils is present in the dermis. The infiltrate does not invade the epidermis or the sebaceous gland shown on the right but is separated from them by a zone of normal collagen. (×100)

neutrophils are fragmented, especially in the vicinity of the capillaries, thus forming nuclear dust (Pinkus; Johnson et al). There is evidence of vasculitis, since many capillaries are dilated and show strongly eosinophilic fibrinoid material within and around their walls (Fig. 9-8). A few extravasated red cells are often seen. In many cases, deposits of hemosiderin are present in the upper dermis as a result of extravasation of red cells (Johnson et al). The presence of foam cells has been noted in a few instances (Lever; McCarthy).

Areas of fibrosis are present in some lesions, but their presence does not necessarily relate to the age of the lesion and does not indicate a tendency of the lesion to regress, which it seldom does.

Histogenesis. *Direct immunofluorescence testing* shows extensive granular or bandlike deposits of IgG, complement, and, less consistently, IgM and IgA along the basement membrane zone, as well as in and around the walls of vessels (Schroeter et al; Nieboer and Kalsbeek). In addition, heavy fibrillar deposits of fibrin are present in and around the walls of vessels and throughout the cellular infiltrate. Granuloma faciale thus can be regarded as a chronic form of leukocytoclastic vasculitis (Nieboer and Kalsbeek). Immunofluorescence of the eosinophilic infiltrate is also seen, but this is a nonspecific phenomenon, since the granules of eosinophils are fluorophilic (Katz et al).

Electron microscopic studies show degenerative changes in most of the eosinophils, such as granules without crystalline cores. Also, many granules are seen outside

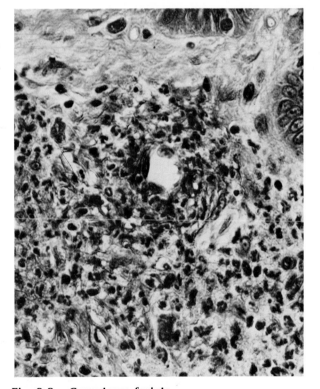

Fig. 9-8. Granuloma faciale
Two types of cells, eosinophils and histiocytes, predominate in the inflammatory infiltrate. Some nuclei in the infiltrate are fragmented. The capillary shown is dilated and shows strongly eosinophilic fibrinoid material within and around its wall. (×400)

of eosinophils. Histiocytes, some of them with foamy cytoplasm, contain many lysosomes that digest cellular material (Schnitzler et al).

Differential Diagnosis.   The arrangement and the composition of the infiltrate in granuloma faciale result in a diagnostic histologic picture. Granuloma faciale shares with erythema elevatum diutinum the presence of vasculitis and of a dense inflammatory infiltrate containing numerous neutrophils. However, erythema elevatum diutinum differs from granuloma faciale by the nearly complete absence of eosinophils and by the lack of a grenz zone of normal collagen beneath the epidermis.

ERYTHEMA ELEVATUM DIUTINUM

Erythema elevatum diutinum, a rare disorder, shows persistent brownish red to purple papules, nodules, and plaques located in symmetric distribution on the extensor surfaces of the extremities, on the elbows and knees, and on the dorsa of the hands and feet. The lesions at first are soft, but later they become hard as the result of fibrosis. During the early phase of the disease or during exacerbations, some patients show areas of erythema with vesicles and bullae (Herzberg; Wolff). Even later on, bullae may be seen on some of the plaques (Vollum).

Extracellular cholesterosis, originally described as a lipoidosis (Urbach et al), is now regarded as erythema elevatum diutinum with secondary lipid deposits (Herzberg; Laymon).

Histopathology.   In its early stage, erythema elevatum diutinum shows a dense, predominantly perivascular infiltrate composed largely of neutrophils intermingled with varying numbers of lymphocytes and histiocytes and few eosinophils. Some of the neutrophils show fragmentation of their nuclei, so-called nuclear dust (Cream et al; Katz et al; Wolff et al, 1978a). There is widespread vasculitis characterized by swelling of the endothelial cells and deposits of strongly eosinophilic fibrinoid material within and around the vessel walls (Mraz and Newcomer). Occasionally, one also sees a few extravasated erythrocytes (Herzberg). The bullae that are present in some patients arise subepidermally (Vollum).

In the late fibrotic stage, the cellular infiltrate is less pronounced, but, even then, neutrophils often predominate (Mraz and Newcomer). The capillaries may still show deposits of fibrinoid material or merely fibrous thickening.

The lipid material that may be present in lesions of the late fibrotic stage has been deposited as a secondary event in damaged tissue. It is doubly refractile and therefore probably consists largely of cholesterol esters (Herzberg). It may be located entirely extracellularly (Urbach et al; Mraz and Newcomer) or both extracellularly and intracellularly (Herzberg; Wolff et al, 1978a).

Histogenesis.   *Electron microscopic examination* has resulted in findings similar to those in leukocytoclastic vasculitis (see p. 169). One observes endothelial swelling and the presence of decomposing neutrophils and of deposits of fibrin within and around the walls of venules. Aggregates of lipid have been seen both extracellularly and within histiocytes. In the latter case, the lipid substances are located both within and outside of lysosomal membranes (Wolff et al, 1978a).

Direct immunofluorescence studies have revealed perivascular deposits of IgG, IgA, IgM, complement, fibrin, transferrin, and alpha-2-macroglobulin (Cream et al). Since some of these substances, such as transferrin and alpha-2-macroglobin, are not involved in immune reactions, it was originally assumed that the deposits were not specific but had leaked out because of damage to the vessels (Cream et al).

Experimental production of lesions in patients with erythema elevatum diutinum, however, has shown that the vasculitis represents an immune reaction. Intradermal injections into normal skin of either streptokinase–streptodornase (Katz et al) or streptococcal antigen (Wolff et al, 1978b) have shown a leukocytoclastic vasculitis on biopsy 4 hr to 6 hr later (Katz et al). Electron microscopic examination has suggested the following sequence of events after the injection of streptococcal antigen. First, immune complexes are deposited in the vessel walls (Wolff et al, 1978b), and then neutrophils infiltrate the vessel walls, phagocytize immune complexes, and disintegrate. This sequence of events is the same as shown in the experimental production of lesions in leukocytoclastic vasculitis through the intradermal injection of histamine (see p. 169).

Additional findings that speak for an immune complex etiology for erythema elevatum diutinum are the finding of C1q binding activity in the serum (Katz et al) and the occasional association with an IgA monoclonal gammopathy (Wolff; Katz et al), an IgG monoclonal gammopathy (Kövary et al), or a mixed IgG–IgM cryoglobulinemia (Morrison et al). It appears likely that elicitation of an immune reaction by bacterial antigens is the initial event in erythema elevatum diutinum (Wolff et al, 1978b).

ACUTE FEBRILE NEUTROPHILIC DERMATOSIS (SWEET'S SYNDROME)

First described in 1964 (Sweet), acute febrile neutrophilic dermatosis shows tender, raised, dark red plaques that usually are from 0.5 cm to 2 cm in diameter but may be larger. They are found mainly on the face and extremities and only rarely on the trunk. The eruption, which has a sudden onset and is associated with fever and leuko-cytosis, may last from 1 to 8 months, and there may be recurrences. Most patients are women. In about one third of the patients, vesicles or pustules are seen on some of the plaques (Goldman and Moschella).

The occurrence of acute febrile neutrophilic dermatosis in patients with acute myelogenous leukemia has been repeatedly observed (Klock and Oken; Raimer and Duncan).

Histopathology. There is a dense perivascular infiltrate composed largely of neutrophils (Fig. 9-9). Some of the neutrophils show leukocytoclasia (Crow et al). In addition, there are some mononuclear cells, such as lymphocytes and histiocytes, and, rarely, a few eosinophils (Crow et al). Although the capillaries may show endothelial swelling, there is no evidence of a true vasculitis, such as deposits of fibrinoid material around the capillaries or extravasation of red cells (Goldman and Moschella). The upper dermis shows edema, which in some instances results in subepidermal blisters (Evans and Evans). In occasional instances, multiple intraepidermal vesicles are seen (Greer et al; Klock and Oken).

Histogenesis. *Direct immunofluorescence studies* have revealed the presence of intracellular IgM and IgE in the neutrophils present in the dermal infiltrate. This finding suggests that neutrophils are recruited to the skin by the local deposition of immunoglobulins (Nunzi et al).

Differential Diagnosis. Erythema elevatum diutinum and acute febrile neutrophilic dermatosis have in common a prevalence of neutrophils with nuclear dust and the presence of subepidermal blisters, but acute febrile neutrophilic dermatosis lacks perivascular fibrin deposits.

POLYARTERITIS NODOSA, BENIGN CUTANEOUS PERIARTERITIS NODOSA

Polyarteritis nodosa represents a severe necrotizing inflammation of small and medium-sized arteries. The most commonly affected arteries are those of the gastrointestinal tract, mesentery, and kidney. The central nervous system is rarely affected, and the lungs almost never (Zeek). The skin is involved in about half of the cases of systemic polyarteritis nodosa (Cohen et al). The cutaneous involvement in systemic polyarteritis must be distinguished from that seen in benign cutaneous periarteritis nodosa.

Polyarteritis nodosa follows an intermittent course and used to be uniformly fatal within a few months to a few years; however, with present-day therapy, which

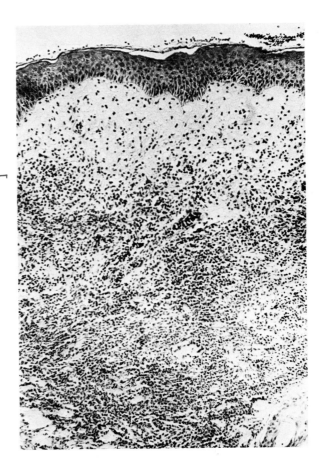

Fig. 9-9. Acute febrile neutrophilic dermatosis (Sweet's syndrome)
Beneath a zone of edema in the upper dermis, a dense infiltrate composed largely of neutrophils is seen. (× 100)

consists mainly of corticosteroids, half of the patients survive (Cohen et al). The clinical symptoms depend on the sites of involvement. The most common clinical manifestations are fever, weakness, abdominal pain, hypertension, and cardiac insufficiency. There may be sensory–motor polyneuropathy and painful polymyositis. Renal insufficiency is the most common cause of death, followed by gastrointestinal bleeding and bowel infarction resulting in perforation (Cohen et al).

The cutaneous lesions of systemic polyarteritis nodosa are usually limited to the lower extremities and consist of purpura and erythema. The areas of purpura may show bullae and, as a result of acute infarction, ulcers (Diaz-Perez and Winkelmann). The lesions thus show a clinical resemblance to those seen in severe leukocytoclastic vasculitis. In addition, there may be extensive livedo reticularis (Ketron and Bernstein). Cutaneous–subcutaneous nodules are very rarely encountered; none was seen in a series of 31 patients who had systemic polyarteritis nodosa with skin involvement (Cohen et al).

Benign cutaneous periarteritis nodosa is a distinct clinical entity in which cutaneous lesions predominate and there is no visceral involvement. In some instances, fever, peripheral neuropathy (Borrie), myalgia (Kint and Van Herpe), or arthralgia (Diaz-Perez and Winkelmann) is present. Painful cutaneous or subcutaneous nodules appear in crops, mainly on the lower extremities. In addition, focal livedo reticularis and cutaneous ulcerations are often present. After many years' duration, the disease gradually subsides. Since nodules are regularly present in the benign cutaneous form and only very rarely encountered in the systemic form, they are suggestive of a good prognosis (Borrie).

Histopathology.   The characteristic lesion of systemic polyarteritis nodosa is a panarteritis of medium-sized and small arteries. The term *nodosa* is based on the fact that the arteritis is focal and thus can cause nodose swellings (Zeek).

Even though in systemic polyarteritis nodosa the arteries in many viscera show the characteristic changes, involvement in the skin, the subcutaneous tissue, and the skeletal muscle is limited to the small vessels (Patalano and Sommers; Cohen et al). Thus, a diagnosis of systemic polyarteritis nodosa by biopsy of the skin or muscle is not possible. Even on autopsy, most of the arteries in the subcutaneous fat appear normal, and only an occasional artery shows the characteristic changes of polyarteritis nodosa (Ketron and Bernstein).

The cutaneous lesions of systemic polyarteritis nodosa show a widespread leukocytoclastic vas-culitis. It may differ from the leukocytoclastic vasculitis seen in anaphylactoid purpura by showing actual necrosis of the vessel walls (Borrie) or occlusion of vessels by thrombi with only little perivascular infiltration (Ketron and Bernstein). In the absence of diagnostic findings in the skin, subcutaneous fat, and muscle, a diagnosis of systemic polyarteritis nodosa can often be established by a renal biopsy, which may show, in addition to glomerular lesions, arteritis or arteriolitis with necrosis of the vessel walls (Patalano and Sommers).

Benign Cutaneous Periarteritis Nodosa.   The cutaneous and subcutaneous nodules in benign cutaneous periarteritis nodosa show the same histologic picture as that seen in the visceral lesions of systemic polyarteritis nodosa, that is, a panarteritis. Several stages of development may be found in different lesions of the same patient. Early lesions show degeneration of the arterial wall with deposition of fibrinoid material (Fig. 9-10) (Borrie). There is partial to complete destruction of the external and internal elastic laminae. An infiltrate present within and around the arterial wall is composed largely of neutrophils showing evidence of leukocytoclasia, although it often also contains some eosinophils (Diaz-Perez and Winkelmann). At a later stage, intimal proliferation and thrombosis lead to complete occlusion of the lumen (Fig. 9-11). This then leads to ischemia and ulceration. The infiltrate by that time also contains

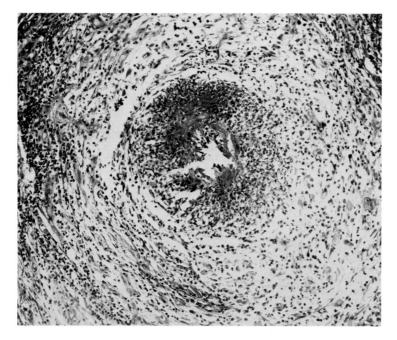

Fig. 9-10.   Benign cutaneous periarteritis nodosa
Early stage. An artery located in the lower dermis shows degeneration of the vessel wall with deposition of fibrinoid material. An infiltrate is present within and around the arterial wall. ($\times 200$)

lymphocytes and macrophages and extends far into the tissue surrounding the artery. In the healing stage, there is fibroblastic proliferation extending into the perivascular area (Fauci). The small vessels of the middle and upper dermis show only a nonspecific lymphocytic perivascular infiltrate.

Histogenesis. *Direct immunofluorescence testing* of lesions of benign cutaneous periarteritis nodosa has shown in most instances deposits of either IgM or C3 in vessel walls and only rarely deposits of both immunoreactants. In some instances, the deposits are seen only in the superficial, uninvolved, small vessels rather than in the deep, involved artery (Diaz-Perez et al).

VASCULITIS WITH GRANULOMATOSIS

There are three systemic diseases in which a necrotizing vasculitis is seen in association with necrotizing granulomas. In allergic granulomatosis (Churg–Strauss syndrome), about two thirds of the patients have cutaneous lesions, in Wegener's granulomatosis, about one half, and in lymphomatoid granulomatosis, about one third.

Allergic Granulomatosis

Allergic granulomatosis, or the Churg–Strauss syndrome, was recognized as an entity separate from polyarteritis nodosa in 1951 (Churg and Strauss). It differs from polyarteritis nodosa by (1) respiratory symptoms, usually asthma, preceding the onset of allergic granulomatosis, often by many years; (2) pronounced eosinophilia both in the circulating blood and in the lesions; (3) the presence of pulmonary infiltrations, in contrast to their absence in polyarteritis nodosa; (4) the involvement of small arteries and veins, rather than of small and medium-sized arteries; and (5) the presence of palisading granulomas with central necrosis extravascularly in the connective tissue.

As in polyarteritis nodosa, present-day treatment of allergic granulomatosis, mainly with corticosteroids, has reduced the mortality from close to 100% to about 50% (Chumbley et al). The most common causes of death are related to the cardiovascular system; in contrast to polyarteritis nodosa, renal failure is rare (Chumbley et al).

Cutaneous lesions are present in about two thirds of the patients (Strauss et al; Chumbley et al). They are of two types: (1) hemorrhagic lesions varying from petechiae to extensive ecchymoses, sometimes accompanied by necrotic ulcers and often associated with areas of erythema (similar to Henoch-Schönlein purpura), and (2) cutaneous–subcutaneous nodules. The most common sites of skin lesions are the extremities, but, not infre-

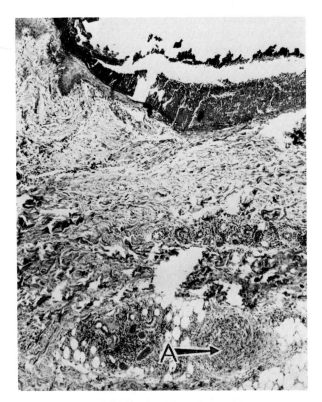

Fig. 9-11. Benign cutaneous periarteritis nodosa Late stage. An artery (*A*) located at the cutaneous–subcutaneous border is occluded as the result of intimal proliferation and thrombosis. Above the artery is an ulcer, probably caused by the occlusion of the artery. (×50)

quently, the trunk also shows involvement. In some instances, the petechiae and ecchymoses are generalized (Strauss et al).

Histopathology. The areas of cutaneous hemorrhage show a leukocytoclastic vasculitis similar to that seen also in anaphylactoid purpura and in systemic polyarteritis nodosa; however, in addition to neutrophils, lymphocytes, and histiocytes, eosinophils are present in much greater number than generally seen in leukocytoclastic vasculitis. Extensive deposits of fibrin are seen around vessels and on collagen fibers, giving them a "smudgy" appearance. In some instances, the dermis shows a granulomatous reaction around degenerated collagen fibers consisting predominantly of radially arranged histiocytes and, frequently, multinucleated giant cells. The central portion of the granulomas contains not only degenerated collagen fibers but also disintegrated cells, particularly eosinophils. The latter are in some instances so numerous that their nuclear debris imparts a bluish tinge to the center of the granuloma (Strauss et al). These granulomas are a characteristic histologic feature and are referred to as extravascular Churg–Strauss granulomas (Crotty et al).

Inflammatory and degenerative changes are found also in the subcutaneous tissue. There, the granulomas may attain considerable size through expansion and conglomeration, thus giving rise to the clinically apparent cutaneous–subcutaneous nodules. The palisading granulomas are embedded in a diffuse inflammatory exudate rich in eosinophils (Strauss et al). The presence of granulomas in the dermis and in subcutaneous nodules is of significant diagnostic value (Churg and Strauss). In a few instances, the histologic features of polyarteritis have been observed in the medium-sized muscular arteries of the deep dermis and subcutaneous tissue (Crotty et al).

Differential Diagnosis.   Since the histologic features of polyarteritis (periarteritis) do not occur in the skin in association with systemic polyarteritis nodosa but only in benign cutaneous periarteritis nodosa (see p. 176), the occurrence of polyarteritis in the skin or subcutaneous tissue in connection with a severe systemic illness points toward a diagnosis of allergic granulomatosis.

Wegener's Granulomatosis

Wegener's granulomatosis is characterized by the following triad: (1) necrotizing granulomatous lesions, mainly in the upper and lower respiratory tract, such as the nose, nasal sinuses, nasopharynx, glottis, trachea, bronchi, and lungs, but often also in other viscera; (2) extensive necrotizing vasculitis involving small arteries and veins, present almost always in the lungs and, more or less widely disseminated, at other sites; and (3) focal necrotizing glomerulitis, often associated with interstitial necrotizing vasculitis and granulomas in the extraglomerular tissue (Godman and Churg; Fauci and Wolff).

The disease begins in two thirds of the patients with upper respiratory tract symptoms, whereas, in one third, the lungs are the first organ involved (Eisner and Harper). Once rapidly fatal because of renal involvement, Wegener's granulomatosis can often be put into sustained clinical remission with cyclophosphamide (Cupps and Fauci). Two variants exist in the usual clinical course of Wegener's granulomatosis: a limited form and a protracted superficial form. In the limited form of Wegener's granulomatosis, renal lesions do not develop and patients thus stay alive in spite of the presence of massive pulmonary and extrapulmonary lesions, including cutaneous lesions (Carrington and Liebow; Cassan et al). In the protracted superficial form, localized ulcerated lesions of the upper respiratory tract or of the skin of the face remain localized for months or years without treatment (Fienberg).

Cutaneous lesions are present in the early stage of the disease in about one fourth of the patients, and at the height of the disease in about one half of the patients (Reed et al). Oral lesions occur in a large number of patients. The cutaneous lesions may consist of papulonecrotic lesions (Reed et al), nodules with central ulceration (Knoth et al), ulcers (Godman and Churg), and, especially in the later stage of the disease, petechial or ecchymotic lesions (Hu et al). Subcutaneous nodules are only rarely encountered (Fauci and Wolff). Oral lesions, analogous to lesions of the respiratory tract, consist of ulcers, especially on the palate, buccal mucosa, and gums (Reed et al).

Histopathology.   The two types of lesions, necrotizing granulomas and necrotizing vasculitis, are seen also in involved skin. The granulomas are characterized by variously sized, often confluent areas of necrosis surrounded by a polymorphous infiltrate containing neutrophils, lymphoid cells, and plasma cells but only rarely a few eosinophils. Epithelioid cells are few or absent. Multinucleated giant cells, however, are common (Godman and Churg). The necrotizing vasculitis, involving small arteries and veins, is characterized by fibrinous deposits and a polymorphous inflammatory infiltrate with nuclear dust and a prevalence of neutrophils (Hu et al). Whereas both types of lesions are seen in some areas, only one type of lesion is present in others (Fauci and Wolff).

Although histologic examination in some instances shows only nonspecific inflammation, some correlation exists between the types of clinical and histologic lesions. Papulonecrotic lesions usually show a necrotizing vasculitis with thrombosis of the lumen. The thrombosis explains the frequent presence of central ulceration (Reed et al). Occasionally, however, necrotizing granulomas are also present (Kraus et al). Purpuric lesions generally show a necrotizing vasculitis with thrombosis and subsequent extravasation of erythrocytes (Hu et al). Cutaneous ulcers and cutaneous and subcutaneous nodules show necrotizing granulomas either with or without necrotizing vasculitis (Knoth et al; Kraus et al; Fauci and Wolff). In rare instances only do the necrotizing granulomas resemble those seen in allergic granulomatosis, consisting of a small central area of collagen degeneration surrounded by radially arranged histiocytes. They differ, however, in that, in Wegener's granulomatosis, the disintegrating cells in the center of the granuloma are not eosinophils, as in allergic granulomatosis, but neutrophils (Hu et al).

Differential Diagnosis. Allergic granulomatosis and Wegener's granulomatosis have in common the presence of extensive necrotizing vasculitis and necrotizing granulomas. They also have similar cutaneous lesions. However, allergic granulomatosis is almost always preceded by asthma, lacks lesions in the upper respiratory tract, and rarely shows severe renal involvement. Histologically, both the vasculitis and the granulomas in allergic granulomatosis show a predominance of eosinophils, and the granulomas show palisading of histiocytes around the central area of necrosis, whereas in Wegener's granulomatosis, giant cells predominate in the necrotizing granulomas.

Lymphomatoid Granulomatosis

Like Wegener's granulomatosis, lymphomatoid granulomatosis, first described in 1972 (Liebow et al), is a serious systemic disease affecting primarily the lungs with vasculitis and a granulomatous necrotizing infiltrate. However, lymphomatoid granulomatosis differs from Wegener's granulomatosis clinically by the absence of glomerulitis and lesions in the upper respiratory tract and histologically by the presence of a dense polymorphous infiltrate, which, especially in advanced lesions, contains some lymphoid cells with pleomorphic, hyperchromatic nuclei suggestive of atypia (James et al). Involvement of the central nervous system occurs in about 20% of the patients. Without adequate treatment, the disease is fatal in about two thirds of the patients, the median time of survival being only 14 months. Most of the deaths reported in the past were due to extensive destruction of pulmonary parenchyma, while malignant lymphoma supervened in about 15% of the patients (Katzenstein et al). By means of adequate treatment with cyclophosphamide and prednisone, more than half of the patients can be cured. Those not cured nearly all die of lymphoma; it seems, however, that the development of lymphoma may be prevented by early recognition and prompt treatment (Fauci et al).

Cutaneous lesions are found in more than one third of the patients. They usually appear simultaneously with the pulmonary lesions, although they may precede or follow involvement of the lung by several months (Katzenstein et al). They consist of erythematous papules, plaques, and subcutaneous or dermal nodules with a tendency to ulcerate (Minars et al; MacDonald and Sarkany; Rosen and Chernoski). If present, cutaneous lesions are often extensive. They resemble the cutaneous lesions seen in Wegener's granulomatosis; however, purpuric lesions do not occur.

Histopathology. The skin lesions show a polymorphous cellular infiltrate that is most pronounced in the deep layers of the dermis around the cutaneous appendages. It is composed of lymphocytes, plasma cells, and histiocytes. Only in some cases are there large, hyperchromatic nuclei and frequent mitoses (Liebow et al; Rosen and Chernoski; James et al). Vasculitis is present but may not be clearly in evidence in areas of heavy infiltration; it is seen best in areas in which the infiltrate is scanty. In instances of involvement of the subcutaneous fat, foci of fat necrosis with a foreign body giant cell reaction are present, suggestive of vaso-occlusive disease with infarction of the fat (Liebow et al). In some instances, particularly in areas of ulceration, obvious evidence of vasculitis may be seen in the dermis, especially in the deep vessels. There, one may see swollen endothelial cells, fibrinoid deposits in the vascular wall, and, occasionally, organized thrombi (Minars et al; MacDonald and Sarkany). Small aggregates of epithelioid cells or of multinucleated giant cells in the dermis are seen only in exceptional cases (MacDonald and Sarkany).

Differential Diagnosis. In lesions showing a heavy polymorphous infiltrate intermingled with large hyperchromatic nuclei, the resemblance of lymphomatoid granulomatosis to mycosis fungoides is great (Liebow et al). Search for evidence of vasculitis is then essential.

MIDLINE GRANULOMA OF THE FACE

First described in 1933 (Stewart), midline granuloma of the face begins insidiously with edema of the nose and congestion of the nasal passages. This is followed by perforation of the nasal septum, ulcerations of the hard palate, and extensive mutilating destruction in the center of the face. Unless a cure is achieved by radiation therapy in the early stage (Fauci et al; Simonis-Blumenfrucht et al; Lober et al), the disease is fatal, usually within 12 to 18 months of onset.

On autopsy, lesions are found to be limited to the facial structures in about half of the cases; in the other half, more or less widespread dissemination of lesions is present (Fechner and Lamppin). The most common sites of dissemination are cervical and mediastinal lymph nodes, the lungs, and the gastrointestinal tract (Spear and Walker; Resnick and Skerrett; Kassel et al).

Histopathology. In the early stage of the disease, and in superficial biopsies, histologic examination often shows a nonspecific chronic inflammatory infiltrate (Stewart; Kassel et al). The infiltrate involves and obliterates small blood vessels and clusters around blood vessels at the periphery of the infiltrate (Crissman). Occasionally in the early stage, but more often in advanced lesions, one observes cells with large hyperchromatic nuclei scattered through the nonspecific infiltrate (Resnick and Skerrett; Simonis-Blumenfrucht et al; Lober et al). Even though the number of such atypical-appearing nuclei often increases with the duration of the disease, they always remain scattered (Crissman). Similar scattered atypical nuclei are generally found on autopsy in visceral lesions as well (Spear and Walker; Kassel et al).

Histogenesis. The fact that atypical nuclei are present in the infiltrate that are suggestive of lymphoma but differ from the cohesive pattern of growth usually observed in that disorder has suggested to some authors that midline granuloma of the face represents a special type of lymphoma. It has been regarded as a *polymorphic reticulosis* (Eichel and Mabery) and referred to also as midline malignant reticulosis (Kassel et al). It has been pointed out that the cells with atypical nuclei resemble the mycosis cells of mycosis fungoides, which are also often difficult to detect in early lesions (Kassel et al).

Since lymphomatoid granulomatosis was described in 1972 (Liebow et al), the considerable histologic resemblance, if not identity, of midline granuloma of the face and lymphomatoid granulomatosis has become apparent (DeRemee et al, 1978). Both have scattered "malignant-appearing" mononuclear cells with a background of polymorphous inflammatory cells (Crissman). Involvement of the lung, if it occurs in midline granuloma of the face, is histologically as well as clinically indistinguishable from that seen in lymphomatoid granulomatosis (DeRemee et al, 1978; Crissman). Even though both diseases may represent a form of hypersensitivity vasculitis expressed by transformed lymphocytes (Crissman), it is best to regard them as separate diseases because of their different initial clinical presentations and, based on this, their entirely different treatments.

Differential Diagnosis. Although Wegener's granulomatosis may start in the upper respiratory tract, it differs from midline granuloma of the face by the presence of necrotizing granulomas surrounded by multinucleated giant cells and by the absence of atypical mononuclear cells (DeRemee et al, 1976).

TEMPORAL GIANT CELL ARTERITIS

Temporal arteritis affects large or medium-sized elastic arteries in the temporal region (Goodman). It may be unilateral or bilateral and may be associated with involvement of other cranial arteries, including cerebral and retinal arteries. It occurs in elderly persons and is characterized clinically by unilateral or bilateral tender-

ness or pain of the forehead. There may be erythema and edema of the skin overlying the involved arteries, and, occasionally, there are ulcerations of the scalp that may be linear or extensive (Hitch). The involved temporal artery and its branches may be palpable. Because of the rather frequent involvement of the retinal arteries, sudden visual impairment in one or both eyes is common. Unless death occurs on the basis of involvement of cerebral arteries, the arteritis usually resolves.

Histopathology. Since the arteritis is often focal, palpation is advisable for identification of an area of tenderness or nodularity for biopsy (Goodman). Unless one is sure that the main branch of the arteria temporalis is occluded, the biopsy should not be carried out on it, because it may result in a large ischemic ulceration. It is preferable to select a side branch of the artery for biopsy (Foged). Involved arteries show a panarteritis that is unevenly distributed (Hitch). The primary event is degeneration of the internal elastic lamina followed by digestion of the degenerated portions of the internal elastic lamina by macrophages that evolve into multinucleated giant cells (Luger and Wuketich). However, giant cells may be absent (Hitch). There is an infiltrate of mononuclear cells and plasma cells between the intima and media and thickening of the intima by fibrinoid degeneration and fibrosis, so that the lumen of the artery is reduced and may even be obliterated in some areas (Kinmont and McCallum).

Differential Diagnosis. In temporal giant cell arteritis, in contrast to periarteritis nodosa, there is no frank necrosis of the arterial wall. The presence of giant cells is of diagnostic importance. For the demonstration of damage to the internal elastic lamina, an elastic tissue stain is necessary.

MALIGNANT ATROPHIC PAPULOSIS (DEGOS' DISEASE)

A rare but characteristic disease first recognized as a distinct entity in 1942 (Degos et al), malignant atrophic papulosis begins with crops of asymptomatic, slightly raised, yellowish red papules that gradually develop an atrophic porcelain-white center. Most of the papules are situated on the trunk and the proximal portions of the extremities. In rare instances, lesions occur also on the bulbar conjuctiva and the oral mucosa. In the majority of cases, systemic manifestations develop from a few weeks to several years after the onset of the cutaneous lesions. The systemic disease usually consists of recurrent attacks of abdominal pain and ends in death from intestinal perforations. Less commonly, death occurs as a result of cerebral infarctions (Winkelmann et al). According to a recent review, 64% of 76 cases had internal lesions (Metz et al). However, in view of the long interval in some cases between cutaneous and systemic manifestations, it appears likely that most, if not all, cases reported as having only cutaneous lesions develop systemic lesions sooner or later (Degos). The longest reported period of follow-up without the appearance of visceral lesions is 14 years (Black and Wilson Jones).

Histopathology.   The essential finding in the skin is a cone-shaped ischemic infarct, the broad base of which is located at the epidermis. The infarct is the result of endovasculitis in an arteriole located at the apex of the infarct. Usually, serial sections are required to find the affected arteriole, which occasionally may be missed despite use of this method (Muller and Landry). Since the affected arteriole is often located in the subcutaneous fat, the biopsy specimen should include adequate

amounts of subcutaneous tissue (Muller and Landry).

In the early stage of the endovasculitis, one observes fibrinoid degeneration of the intima and swelling of the endothelial cells. At a later stage, fibrosis of the intima and proliferation of endothelial cells are seen (Metz et al; Howsden et al). Occlusion occurs in some instances through subendothelial fibrosis but more often as a result of thrombosis (Muller and Landry). The wall of the vessel often is infiltrated by lymphocytes and histiocytes (Olmos and Laugier).

The ischemic infarct in an early lesion shows swelling of the dermal collagen and an accumulation of mucin (Feuerman et al; Black and Wilson Jones). In a late lesion, one finds marked atrophy of the stratum malpighii associated with slight hyperkeratosis (Fig. 9-12). Within the infarct, the collagen, as a result of necrobiosis, has a homogeneous, smudged appearance and is nearly com-

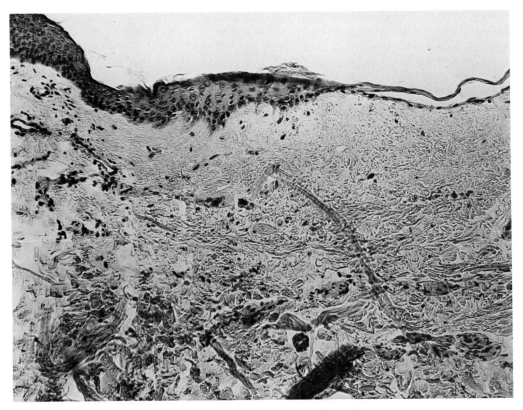

Fig. 9-12.   Malignant atrophic papulosis (Degos' disease)
The margin of a lesion is shown. Within the lesion, which consists of an ischemic infarct, the stratum malpighii is markedly atrophic. As a result of necrobiosis, the collagen has a homogeneous, smudged appearance and is nearly completely devoid of nuclei. ($\times$ 140) (Courtesy of Ruben Nomland, M.D., and Jack M. Layton, M.D.)

pletely devoid of nuclei (Howsden et al). Blood vessels and appendages are necrotic or absent. In such late lesions, mucin is no longer seen within the necrobiotic area but rather only at its margins, where there is a moderately dense perivascular infiltrate of mononuclear cells (Black and Wilson Jones).

The mucin present first within the necrobiotic area and later at its periphery contains acid mucopolysaccharides. Consequently, it stains with alcian blue but not with PAS and shows metachromasia with toluidine blue at pH 3.0 (Feuerman et al).

On autopsy, vascular lesions are seen most commonly in the small intestine (Degos; Strole et al). In some instances, vascular changes are found also in other organs, such as the brain, the kidneys, and the myocardium (Strole et al; Olmos and Laugier; Metz et al). In rare instances, the brain is the only site of internal involvement (Winkelmann et al).

On gross examination, the lesions of the small intestine, analogous to those seen in skin, are found to consist of scattered white patches representing subserosal ischemic infarcts. Areas of ulceration and perforation are also found. On histologic examination, the arterioles or small arteries at the sites of the subserosal infarcts are occluded either by subendothelial fibrosis or by thrombosis (Feuerman et al; Strole et al).

Histogenesis. In several instances, *direct immunofluorescence examination* has shown deposits of IgM or IgG in association with C3 in the affected vessel deep in the dermis, suggesting an immunologic basis for the endovasculitis (Frank et al; Metz et al).

On *electron microscopic examination,* "paramyxovirus-like" structures have been found in endothelial cells and fibroblasts (Olmos and Laugier; Stahl et al). As in lupus erythematosus, they probably represent degenerative changes (see p. 455) (Stahl et al).

Differential Diagnosis.

Lesions that both clinically and histologically resemble those of malignant atrophic papulosis may occur in systemic lupus erythematosus (Dubin and Stawiski; Black and Hudson). Therefore, a diagnosis of malignant atrophic papulosis should be made only after systemic lupus erythematosus has been excluded (Black and Hudson).

ATROPHIE BLANCHE

In atrophie blanche, a condition first described in 1929 (Milian), one observes on the lower portions of the legs,

particularly on the ankles and the dorsa of the feet, irregularly outlined, whitish atrophic areas showing hyperpigmentation and telangiectatic vessels at their periphery. In addition, there are in many cases small, painful ulcers with a tendency to recur. These ulcers may precede as well as follow the development of the whitish atrophic areas (Nelson; Gray et al). Petechiae are also seen in some instances (Schroeter et al; Stiefler and Bergfeld).

Histopathology.   The histologic findings differ somewhat with the type of lesion examined, that is, whether it is an early, active lesion in the vicinity of an ulcer or an inactive, atrophic lesion (Gray et al). However, in all stages, vascular changes are the decisive factor. In an early, active lesion, eosinophilic fibrinoid material is present in the walls of dermal vessels and lumina, producing partial to complete occlusion (Gray et al; Metz and Sturm). This fibrinoid material is PAS-positive and diastase-resistant. In addition, there is usually infarction with hemorrhage and an inflammatory infiltrate in the dermis and often necrosis of the epidermis as well.

In the atrophic lesions of atrophie blanche, the epithelium is thinned, and the dermis is sclerotic, with little, if any, cellular infiltrate. The walls of the dermal vessels show thickening and hyalinization of the intima (Nelson; Bard and Winkelmann). Like the fibrin in early lesions, the hyaline material is PAS-positive and diastase-resistant. In addition, there is endothelial proliferation. Even in atrophic lesions, vascular lumina may be occluded with fibrinoid material (Bard and Winkelmann). Subsequently, there may be recanalization (Miura and Torinuki). In some cases, the vessels in the superficial dermis are predominantly affected (Gray et al); in others, the vessels in the middle and lower parts of the dermis are mostly affected (Bard and Winkelmann).

Histogenesis.   In all cases of atrophie blanche tested, *direct immunofluorescence studies* have revealed the presence of immunoglobulins, especially IgM, of complement components, and of fibrin in the vascular walls of the lesions (Schroeter et al; Posternak et al). This suggests an immune pathogenesis.

It is likely that the fibrin found in the dermal vessels of early lesions and the hyalin present in atrophic lesions are basically the same substance, since both are PAS-positive and diastase-resistant and direct immunofluorescence testing has shown that the hyaline deposits stain positively for fibrin. Inflammatory changes, if present at all, are a secondary event (Nelson; Metz and Sturm). Thus, a vasculitis in the true sense does not exist, as the designation *segmental hyalinizing vasculitis* (Bard and Winkelmann) might suggest.

Differential Diagnosis. A histologic differentiation of atrophie blanche from stasis dermatitis usually is possible, since stasis dermatitis shows only slight thickening of the capillary walls.

CUTANEOUS CHOLESTEROL EMBOLISM

In patients with severe arteriosclerosis of the abdominal aorta, cholesterol crystals may become detached from atheromatous plaques. This may occur spontaneously from time to time, after a surgical procedure such as grafting of an aneurysm, or after translumbar aortography. The cholesterol crystals result in microemboli with ensuing skin lesions on the lower extremities. There may be extensive livedo reticularis, purple discoloration, and even distal gangrene of the toes, as well as small, painful ulcerations on the legs (Deschamps et al). Occasionally, there are also a few nodules (Stewart et al) or indurated plaques (Fisher and Kistner). A typical feature is the presence of adequate distal pulsation, indicating that the ischemia is arteriolar rather than arterial (Stewart et al).

Histopathology. A deep biopsy through a mottled area of livedo reticularis or, if present, of a nodule or indurated plaque reveals biconvex, needle-shaped cholesterol clefts within the lumina of arterioles. The clefts are surrounded by multinucleated foreign body giant cells and fibrous tissue occluding the arterioles (Deschamps et al; Stewart et al).

SCLEROSING LYMPHANGITIS OF THE PENIS

Sclerosing lymphangitis of the penis is characterized by the sudden appearance of a nearly asymptomatic, firm, cordlike, subcutaneous lesion partially encircling the penis in the coronal sulcus. Spontaneous resolution takes place in 2 to 6 weeks (Nickel and Plumb).

Histopathology. An early lesion shows a dilated lymphatic collecting vessel containing a fibrin thrombus, which, as evidence of beginning recanalization, contains sprouts of endothelial cells (Marsch and Stüttgen). At a later stage, in the process of organization, the thrombus is replaced by connective tissue containing histiocytes, fibroblasts, and lymphocytes together with blood capillaries (Kandil and Al-Kashlan). With reopening of the lumen, the lymphatic vessel shows thickening and fibrosis of its wall (Nickel and Plumb).

BIBLIOGRAPHY

Noninflammatory Purpuras

BEIGELMAN PM: Variants of the platelet thrombosis syndrome and their relationship to disseminated lupus. Arch Pathol 51:213–223, 1951

BONE RC, HENRY JE, PETTERSON J et al: Respiratory dysfunction in thrombotic thrombocytopenic purpura. Am J Med 65:262–270, 1978

BYRNES JJ, KHURANA M: Treatment of thrombotic thrombocytopenic purpura with plasma. N Engl J Med 297:1386–1389, 1977

Case Records of the Massachusetts General Hospital, Case 29-1969: Purpura fulminans. N Engl J Med 281:153–162, 1969

CHAMBERS WN, HOLYOKE JB, WILSON RF: Purpura fulminans. N Engl J Med 247:933–935, 1952

CRAM DL, SOLEY RL: Purpura fulminans. Br J Dermatol 80:323–327, 1968

FRIEDENBERG WR, WEST M, MIECH DJ et al: Atypical purpura fulminans with benign monoclonal gammopathy. Arch Dermatol 114:578–580, 1978

GARDNER FH, DIAMOND LK: Autoerythrocyte sensitization: Form of purpura producing painful bruising following autosensitization to red blood cells in certain women. Blood 10:675–690, 1955

GOLDENFARB PB, FINCH SC: Thrombotic thrombocytopenic purpura. JAMA 226:644–647, 1973

GORE J, TAKADA M, AUSTIN J: Ultrastructural basis of experimental thrombocytopenic purpura. Arch Pathol 90:197–205, 1970

GROCH GS, FINCH SC, ROGOWAY W et al: Studies in the pathogenesis of autoerythrocyte sensitization syndrome. Blood 28:19–34, 1966

HASHIMOTO K, KITABCHI AE, DUCKWORTH WC et al: Ultrastructure of scorbutic human skin. Acta Derm Venereol (Stockh) 50:9–21, 1970

JONES RR, CUNNINGHAM J: Warfarin skin necrosis, the role of factor VII. Br J Dermatol 101:561–565, 1979

LACY JP, GOODWIN RR: Warfarin-induced necrosis of the skin. Ann Intern Med 82:381–382, 1975

LUTTGENS WF: Thrombotic thrombocytopenic purpura with extensive hemorrhagic gangrene of the skin and subcutaneous tissue. Ann Intern Med 46:1207–1212, 1957

MCMILLAN R: Chronic idiopathic thrombocytopenic purpura. N Engl J Med 304:1135–1147, 1981

MYERS TJ, WAKEM CJ, BALL ED et al: Thrombotic thrombocytopenic purpura: Combined treatment with plasmapheresis and antiplatelet agents. Ann Intern Med 92:149–155, 1980

NALBANDIAN RM, MADER JJ, BARRETT JL et al: Petechiae, ecchymoses, and necrosis of skin induced by coumarin congeners. JAMA 192:603–608, 1965

OEI SH, DE VRIES E, CATS A et al: Abnormal circulating red blood cells in the painful bruising syndrome. Arch Dermatol Res 263:227–233, 1978

PEARSON B, MAZZA JJ: Gardner-Diamond syndrome with multiple glomus tumors. Arch Dermatol 111:893–895, 1975

PINNAS JL, TAN EM, TEPLITZ RL et al: Autosensitization to DNA: Evidence for an immunologic basis. J Invest Dermatol 72:157–160, 1979

RATNOFF OD, AGLE D: Psychogenic purpura: A re-evaluation of the syndrome of autoerythrocyte sensitization. Medicine (Baltimore) 47:475–500, 1968

RIDOLFI RL, BELL WR: Thrombotic thrombocytopenic purpura. (Review) Medicine (Baltimore) 60:413–428, 1981

ROSS R, BENDITT EP: Wound healing and collagen formation. IV. Distortion of ribosomal patterns of fibroblasts in scurvy. J Cell Biol 22:365–389, 1964

RUFFOLO EH, PEASE GL, COOPER T: Thrombotic thrombocytopenic purpura. Arch Intern Med 110:78–82, 1962

SCHLEICHER SM, FRICKER MP: Coumarin necrosis. Arch Dermatol 116:444–445, 1980

SHUSTIK C: Gardner-Diamond's syndrome in a man. Arch Intern Med 137:1621–1622, 1977

SPICER TE, RAU JM: Purpura fulminans. Am J Med 61:566–571, 1976

STOCKER WW, MCINTYRE OR, CLENDENNING WE: Psychogenic purpura. Arch Dermatol 113:606–609, 1977

TATTERSALL RN, SEVILLE R: Senile purpura. Q J Med 19:151–159, 1950

VAKILZADEH F, BRÖCKER EB: Syndrom der blauen Flecken. Hautarzt 32:309–312, 1981

WALDORF DS, LIPKIN G: Sensitization to erythrocytes. JAMA 203:597–599, 1968

WALKER A: Chronic scurvy. Br J Dermatol 80:625–630, 1968

Inflammatory Purpuras (Vasculitis)

ALLEN DM, DIAMOND LK, HOWELL DA: Anaphylactoid purpura in children (Schönlein-Henoch syndrome). Am J Dis Child 99:833–854, 1960

ANSELL BM: Henoch-Schönlein purpura with particular reference to the prognosis of the renal lesion. Br J Dermatol 82:211–215, 1970

AUSTER BL, SANTA CRUZ DJ, EISEN AZ: Febrile ulceronecrotic Mucha-Habermann disease with interstitial pneumonitis. J Cutan Pathol 6:66–76, 1979

BAUGHMAN RD, SOMMER RG: Cryoglobulinemia presenting as "factitial ulceration." Arch Dermatol 94:725–731, 1966

BELAICH S, DEGOS R, CIVATTE J et al: La papulose lymphomatoide. Ann Dermatol Syph 99:483–492, 1972

BLACK MM: "Classical" lymphomatoid papulosis. A variant of pityriasis lichenoides. Am J Dermatopathol 3:175–176, 1981

BLACK MM, WILSON JONES E: "Lymphomatoid" pityriasis lichenoides: A variant with histologic features simulating a lymphoma. Br J Dermatol 86:329–347, 1972

BRAUN-FALCO O, LUDERSCHMIDT C, MACIEJEWSKI W et al: Pustulosis acuta generalisata. Hautarzt 29:371–377, 1978

BRAVERMAN IM, YEN A: Demonstration of immune complexes in spontaneous and histamine-induced lesions and in normal skin of patients with leukocytoclastic angiitis. J Invest Dermatol 64:105–112, 1975

BREHMER-ANDERSSON E: Lymphomatoid papulosis. Am J Dermatopathol 3:169–174, 1981

BURG G, HOFFMANN-FEZER G, NIKOLOWSKI J et al: Lymphomatoid papulosis: A cutaneous T-cell pseudolymphoma. Acta Derm Venereol (Stockh) 61:491–496, 1981

BURKE DP, ADAMS RM, ARUNDELL FD: Febrile ulceronecrotic Mucha-Habermann's disease. Arch Dermatol 100:200–206, 1969

CLAYTON R, HAFFENDEN G: An immunofluorescence study of pityriasis lichenoides. Br J Dermatol 99:491–493, 1978

COCHRANE GG: Mediators of the Arthus and related reactions. Prog Allergy 11:1–35, 1967

CREAM JJ: Cryoglobulins in vasculitis. Clin Exp Immunol 10:117–126, 1972

CREAM JJ, BRYCESON ADM, RYDER G: Disappearance of immunoglobulin and complement from the Arthus reaction and its relevance to studies of vasculitis in man. Br J Dermatol 84:106–109, 1971

DEGOS R, DUPERRAT B, DANIEL F: Le parapsoriasis ulcéronécrotique hyperthermique. Ann Dermatol Syph 93:481–496, 1966

DUPONT A: Transformation maligne très tardive d'une réticulose papuleuse à évolution prolongée (lymphomatoid papulosis). Ann Dermatol Syph 100:141–146, 1965

EDELSON RL: Cutaneous T-cell lymphoma: Clues of a skin-thymus interaction. J Invest Dermatol 67:419–424, 1976

ELLIS FA: The cutaneous manifestations of cryoglobulinemia. Arch Dermatol 89:690–697, 1964

FABER WR, VAN JOOST T: Pityriasis lichenoides, an immune complex disease? Acta Derm Venereol (Stockh) 60:259–261, 1980

FAUCI AS: The spectrum of vasculitis. Ann Intern Med 89:660–676, 1978

FEUERMAN EJ, SANDBANK M: Lymphomatoid papulosis. Arch Dermatol 105:233–235, 1972

FINE RM, MELTZER HD, RUDNER EJ: Lymphomatoid papulosis eventuating in mycosis fungoides. South Med J 67:1492–1497, 1974

GAMMON WR, WHEELER CE, JR: Urticarial vasculitis. (Review) Arch Dermatol 115:76–80, 1979.

GORDON RA, LOCKINGBILL DP, ABT AB: Skin infiltration in Hodgkin's disease. Arch Dermatol 116:1038–1040, 1980

GOUGEROT H, DUPERRAT B: The nodular dermal allergides of Gougerot. Br J Dermatol 66:283–286, 1954

GOWER RG, SAMS WM JR, THORNE EG et al: Leukocytoclastic vasculitis: Sequential appearance of immunoreactants and cellular changes in serial biopsies. J Invest Dermatol 69:477–484, 1977

HARRIST TJ, BHAN AK, MURPHY GF et al: Lymphomatoid papulosis and lymphomatoid granulomatosis. (Abstr) J Invest Dermatol 76:326, 1981

HAUSTEIN UF, KLUG H: Elektronenmikropische Untersuchungen zur Purpura pigmentosa progressiva. Dermatol Monatsschr 162:806–816, 1976

HAYASHI T: Pityriasis lichenoides et varioliformis acuta: Immunohistopathologic study. J Dermatol 4:173–178, 1977

HERRMANN WA, KAUFFMANN RH, VAN ES LA et al: Allergic vasculitis. Arch Dermatol Res 269:179–187, 1980

ISHIKAWA H, NAMEKI H, HATTORI A: Akutes generalisiertes pustulöses Bakterid. Hautarzt 30:144–148, 1979

IWATSUKI K, AOSKIMA T, TAGAMI H et al: Immunofluorescence study in purpura pigmentosa chronica. Acta Derm Venereol (Stockh) 60:341–348, 1980

JIMBOW K, KATO M, SUGIYAMA S: Immunohistochemical and electron microscopic characterization of lymphomatoid papulosis. J Dermatol 5:113–125, 1978

KAWADA A, ANEKOJI K, MIYAMOTO M et al: Unusual manifestation of malignant reticulosis of the skin: Cutaneous lesion simulating parapsoriasis guttata. Dermatologica 138:369–378, 1969

KLUG H, HAUSTEIN UF: Ultrastructure of macrophage-lymphocyte interaction in purpura pigmentosa progressiva. Dermatologica 153:209–217, 1976

KODA H, KANAIDE A, MASAKAZU A et al: Essential IgG cryoglobulinemia with purpura and cold urticaria. Arch Dermatol 114:784–786, 1978

LAYMON CW The nodular dermal allergid. Arch Dermatol 82:163–170, 1960

MACAULAY WL: Lymphomatoid papulosis. Int J Dermatol 17:204–212, 1979

MACIEJEWSKI W, BANDMANN HJ, KLAWITER M: Lichen purpuricus (lichen aureus). Hautarzt 30:440–442, 1979

MARKS R, BLACK M, WILSON JONES E: Pityriasis lichenoides. Br J Dermatol 86:215–222, 1972

MCCOOMBS RP: Systemic "allergic" vasculitis. JAMA 194:1059–1063, 1965

MCKENZIE AW, EARLE JHO, LOCKEY E et al: Essential cryoglobulinemia. Br J Dermatol 73:22–29, 1961

MOROZ LA, ROSE B: The cryopathies. In Samter M (ed): Immunological Diseases, 3rd ed, Vol 1, pp 570–591. Boston, Little, Brown, 1978

MOSTO SJ, CASALA AM: Disseminated pruriginous angiodermatitis (itching purpura). Arch Dermatol 91:351–356, 1965

MULLER SA, SCHULZE TW JR: Mucha-Habermann disease mistaken for reticulum cell sarcoma. Arch Dermatol 103:423–427, 1971

NASEMANN T, MARKOWSKI R, JAKUBOWICZ K: Zur histologischen Differentialdiagnose der Pityriasis lichenoides et varioliformis acute Mucha-Habermann. Hautarzt 17:395–399, 1966

NIR MA, PIAK AI, SCHREIBMAN S et al: Mixed IgG-IgM cryoglobulinemia with follicular pustular purpura. Arch Dermatol 109:539–542, 1974

OLMSTEAD AD, ZONE JJ, LASALLE B et al: Immune complexes in the pathogenesis of hypergammaglobulinemic purpura. J Am Acad Dermatol 3:174–179, 1980

PERROT H, LEUNG TK, LEUNG J et al: Étude ultrastructurale des lesions vasculaires dermiques du trisyndrome de Gougerot (vasculite leucocytoclasique). Arch Dermatol Forsch 241:44–55, 1971

PIERARD GE, ACKERMAN AB, LAPIERE CM: Follicular lymphomatoid papulosis. Am J Dermatopathol 2:173–180, 1980

PIÉRARD J, VAN STEENBERGEN EP: A propos du parapsoriasis varioliforme et de son histologie. Ann Dermatol Syph 84:630–646, 1957

RANDALL SJ, KIERLAND RR, MONTGOMERY H: Pigmented purpuric eruptions. Arch Dermatol Syph 64:177–191, 1951

RUBIN J: Cutaneous Hodgkin's disease. Cancer 42:1219–1221, 1978

RUITER M: Arteriolitis (vasculitis) "allergica" cutis (superficialis). A new dermatological concept. Dermatologica 129:217–231, 1964

RUITER M, HADDERS HN: Predominantly cutaneous form of necrotizing angiitis. J Pathol Bacteriol 77:71–77, 1959

RUITER M, MOLENAAR I: Ultrastructural changes in arteriolitis (vasculitis) allergica cutis superficialis. Br J Dermatol 83:14–26, 1970

SAMS WM JR: Necrotizing vasculitis. (Review) J Am Acad Dermatol 3:1–13, 1980.

SAMS WM JR, CLAMAN HN, KOHLER PF et al: Human necrotizing vasculitis: Immunoglobulins and complement in vessel walls of cutaneous lesions and normal skin. J Invest Dermatol 64:441–445, 1975

SAMS WM JR, THORNE EG, SMALL P et al: Leukocytoclastic vasculitis. (Review) Arch Dermatol 112:219–226, 1976

SCHIMPF A, PONS F: Zum Krankheitsbild des Pseudolymphoma cutis ("lymphomatoid papulosis" Macaulay). Z Hautkr 48:913–917, 1973

SCOTT DGI, BACON PA, TRIBE CR: Systemic rheumatoid vasculitis. Medicine 60:288–297, 1981

SZUR L, HARRISON CV, LEVENER GM et al: Primary cutaneous Hodgkin's disease. Lancet 7:1016–1020, 1970

SZYMANSKI FJ: Pityriasis lichenoides et varioliformis acuta. Arch Dermatol 79:7–16, 1959

TAN SH: Acute generalized pustular bacterid. Br J Dermatol 91:209–215, 1974

THIVOLET J, FAURE M, CHOUVET B: Immunofluorescence study of pityriasis lichenoides. Br J Dermatol 101:237, 1979

THOMSEN K, SCHMIDT M: Letter: Lymphomatoid papulosis. Arch Dermatol 113:232–233, 1977

VALENTINO LA, HELWIG EB: Lymphomatoid papulosis. Arch Pathol 96:409–416, 1973

VERBURGH-VAN DER ZWAN N, MANUEL HR: Lichen purpuricus. Dermatologica 152:347–351, 1976

WAISMAN M, WAISMAN M: Lichen aureus. Arch Dermatol 112:696–697, 1976

WINKELMANN RK, DITTO WB: Cutaneous and visceral syndromes of necrotizing or "allergic" angiitis. Medicine (Baltimore) 43:59–89, 1964

WOLFF HH, MACIEJEWSKI W, SCHERER R et al: Immunoelectron-microscopic examination of early lesions in histamine induced immune complex vasculitis in man. Br J Dermatol 99:13–24, 1978

ZEEK PM: Periarteritis nodosa and other forms of necrotizing angiitis. N Engl J Med 248:764–772, 1953

Granuloma Faciale

JOHNSON WC, HIGDON RS, HELWIG EB: Granuloma faciale. Arch Dermatol 79:42–52, 1959

KATZ SI, GALLIN JI, HERTZ KC et al: Erythema elevatum diutinum. Medicine (Baltimore) 56:443–455, 1977

LEVER WF: Eosinophilic granuloma of the skin: Its relation to erythema elevatum diutinum and eosinophilic granuloma of the bone. Arch Dermatol 55:194–211, 1947

LEVER WF, LANE CG, DOWNING JG et al: Eosinophilic granuloma of the skin. Arch Dermatol 58:430–438, 1948

MCCARTHY PL: Granuloma faciale. Arch Dermatol 77:458–459, 1958

NIEBOER C, KALSBEEK GL: Immunofluorescence studies in granuloma eosinophilicum faciale. J Cutan Pathol 5:68–75, 1978

PFLEGER L, TAPPEINER S: Über das eosinophile Granulom des Gesichtes. Arch Dermatol Syph (Berlin) 193:1–13, 1951

PINKUS H: Granuloma faciale. Dermatologica 105:85–99, 1952

RUSIN LJ, DUBIN HV, TAYLOR WB: Disseminated granuloma faciale. Arch Dermatol 112:1575–1577, 1976

SCHNITZLER L, VERRET JL, SCHUBERT B: Granuloma faciale. Ultrastructural study of three cases. J Cutan Pathol 4:123–173, 1977

SCHROETER AL, COPEMAN PWM, JORDON RE et al: Immunofluorescence of cutaneous vasculitis associated with systemic disease. Arch Dermatol 104:254–259, 1945

WIGLEY JEM: ? Sarcoid of Boeck. ? Eosinophilic granuloma. Br J Dermatol 57:68–69, 1945

Erythema Elevatum Diutinum

CREAM JJ, LEVINE GM, CALNAN DD: Erythema elevatum diutinum. Br J Dermatol 84:393–399, 1971

HERZBERG JJ: Die extracelluläre Cholesterinose (Kerl-Urbach), eine Variante des Erythema elevatum diutinum. Arch Klin Exp Dermatol 205:477–496, 1958

KATZ SI, GALLIN JI, HERTZ KC et al: Erythema elevatum diutinum. Medicine (Baltimore) 56:443–455, 1977

KÖVARY PM, DHONAN H, HAPPLE R: Paraproteinemia in erythema elevatum diutinum. Arch Dermatol Res 260:153–158, 1977

LAYMON CW: Erythema elevatum diutinum. Arch Dermatol 85:22–28, 1962

MORRISON JGL, HULL PR, FOURIE E: Erythema elevatum diutinum, cryoglobulinaemia, and fixed urticaria on cooling. Br J Dermatol 97:99–104, 1977

MRAZ JP, NEWCOMER VD: Erythema elevatum diutinum. Arch Dermatol 96:235–246, 1967

URBACH E, EPSTEIN E, LORENZ K: Extrazelluläre Cholesterinose. Arch Dermatol Syph (Berlin) 166:243–272, 1932

VOLLUM DI: Erythema elevatum diutinum—vesicular lesions and sulphone response. Br J Dermatol 80:178–183, 1968

WOLFF HH, MACIEJEWSKI W, SCHERER R: Erythema elevatum diutinum. I. Electron microscopy of a case with extracellular cholesterosis. Arch Dermatol Res 261:7–16, 1978a

WOLFF HH, SCHERER R, MACIEJEWSKI W et al: Erythema elevatum diutinum. II. Immunoelectronmicroscopical study of leukocytoclastic vasculitis within the intracutaneous test reaction induced by streptococcal antigen. Arch Dermatol Res 261:17–26, 1978b

WOLFF K: Erythema elevatum diutinum. Z Hautkr 46:257, 1971

Acute Febrile Neutrophilic Dermatosis (Sweet's Syndrome)

CROW KD, KERDEL-VEGAS F, ROOK A: Acute febrile neutrophilic dermatosis. Sweet's syndrome. Dermatologica 139:123–134, 1969

EVANS S, EVANS CC: Acute febrile neutrophilic dermatosis. Two cases. Dermatologica 143:153–159, 1971

GOLDMAN GC, MOSCHELLA SL: Acute febrile neutrophilic dermatosis (Sweet's syndrome). Arch Dermatol 103:654–660, 1971

GREER KE, PRUITT JL, BISHOP GF: Acute febrile neutrophilic

dermatosis (Sweet's syndrome). Arch Dermatol 111:1461–1463, 1975

KLOCK JC, OKEN RL: Febrile neutrophilic dermatosis in acute myelogenous leukemia. Cancer 37:922–927, 1976

NUNZI E, COVATO F, DALLEGRI F et al: Immunopathological studies on a case of Sweet's syndrome. Dermatologica 163:393–400, 1981

RAIMER SS, DUNCAN C: Febrile neutrophilic dermatosis in acute myelogenous leukemia. Arch Dermatol 114:413–414, 1978

SWEET RD: An acute febrile dermatosis. Br J Dermatol 76:349–356, 1964

Polyarteritis Nodosa, Benign Cutaneous Periarteritis Nodosa

BORRIE P: Cutaneous polyarteritis nodosa. Br J Dermatol 87:87–95, 1972

COHEN RD, CONN DL, ILSTRUP DM: Clinical features, prognosis, and response to treatment in polyarteritis. Mayo Clin Proc 55:146–155, 1980

DIAZ-PEREZ JL, SCHROETER AL, WINKELMANN RK: Cutaneous periarteritis nodosa. Arch Dermatol 116:56–58, 1980

DIAZ-PEREZ JL, WINKELMANN RK: Cutaneous periarteritis nodosa. Arch Dermatol 110:407–414, 1974

FAUCI AS: The spectrum of vasculitis. Ann Intern Med 89:660–676, 1978

KETRON LW, BERNSTEIN JC: Cutaneous manifestations of periarteritis nodosa. Arch Dermatol Syph 40:929–944, 1939

KINT A, VAN HERPE L: Cutaneous periarteritis nodosa. Dermatologica 158:185–189, 1979

PATALANO VJ, SOMMERS SC: Biopsy diagnosis of periarteritis nodosa. Arch Pathol 72:1–7, 1961

ZEEK PM: Periarteritis nodosa: A critical review. Am J Clin Pathol 22:777–790, 1952

Vasculitis with Granulomatosis: Allergic Granulomatosis, Wegener's Granulomatosis, Lymphomatoid Granulomatosis

CARRINGTON CB, LIEBOW AA: Limited forms of angiitis and granulomatosis of Wegener's type. Am J Med 41:497–527, 1966

CASSAN SM, COLES DT, HARRISON EG JR: The concept of limited forms of Wegener's granulomatosis. Am J Med 49:366–379, 1970

CHUMBLEY LC, HARRISON EG JR, DEREMEE RA: Allergic granulomatosis and angiitis (Churg-Strauss syndrome). Report and analysis of 30 cases. Mayo Clin Proc 52:477–484, 1977

CHURG J, STRAUSS L: Allergic granulomatosis, allergic angiitis, and periarteritis nodosa. Am J Pathol 27:277–301, 1951

CROTTY CP, DEREMEE RA, WINKELMANN RK: Cutaneous clinico-pathologic correlation of allergic granulomatosis. J Am Acad Dermatol 5:571–581, 1981

CUPPS TR, FAUCI AS: Wegener's granulomatosis. Int J Dermatol 19:76–80, 1980

EISNER B, HARPER FB: Disseminated Wegener's granulomatosis with breast involvement. Arch Pathol 87:545–547, 1969

FAUCI AS, HAYNES BF, COSTA J et al: Lymphomatoid granulomatosis. Prospective clinical and therapeutic experience over 10 years. N Engl J Med 306:68–74, 1982

FAUCI AS, WOLFF SM: Wegener's granulomatosis: Studies in 18 patients and a review of the literature. Medicine (Baltimore) 52:535–561, 1973

FIENBERG R: The protracted superficial phenomenon in pathergic (Wegener's) granulomatosis. Hum Pathol 12:458–467, 1981

GODMAN GC, CHURG J: Wegener's granulomatosis. Arch Pathol 58:533–553, 1954

HU CH, O'LAUGHLIN S, WINKELMANN RK: Cutaneous manifestations of Wegener's granulomatosis. Arch Dermatol 113:175–182, 1977

JAMES WD, ODOM RB, KATZENSTEIN ALA: Cutaneous manifestations of lymphomatoid granulomatosis. Arch Dermatol 117:196–202, 1981

KATZENSTEIN ALA, CARRINGTON CB, LIEBOW AA: Lymphomatoid granulomatosis. A clinico-pathologic study of 152 cases. Cancer 43:360–373, 1979.

KNOTH W, BENEKE G, KUNTZ E: Zur Kenntnis der Wegenerschen Granulomatose. Hautarzt 16:289–294, 1965

KRAUS Z, VORTEL V, FINGERLAND A et al: Unusual cutaneous manifestations in Wegener's granulomatosis. Acta Derm Venereol (Stockh) 45:288–294, 1965

LIEBOW AA, CARRINGTON CRB, FRIEDMAN PJ: Lymphomatoid granulomatosis. Hum Pathol 3:457–558, 1972

MACDONALD DM, SARKANY I: Lymphomatoid granulomatosis. Clin Exp Dermatol 1:163–173, 1976

MINARS N, KAY S, ESCOBAR MR: Lymphomatoid granulomatosis of the skin. Arch Dermatol 111:493–496, 1975

REED WB, JENSEN AK, KONWALER BE et al: The cutaneous manifestations in Wegener's granulomatosis. Acta Derm Venereol (Stockh) 43:250–264, 1963

ROSEN T, CHERNOSKI ME: Lymphomatoid granulomatosis. Int J Dermatol 18:497–498, 1979

STRAUSS L, CHURG J, ZAK FG: Cutaneous lesions of allergic granulomatosis. A histopathologic study. J Invest Dermatol 17:349–359, 1951

Midline Granuloma of the Face

CRISSMAN JD: Midline malignant reticulosis and lymphomatoid granulomatosis. Arch Pathol 103:561–564, 1979

DEREMEE RA, MCDONALD TJ, HARRISON EG JR et al: Wegener's granulomatosis. Mayo Clin Proc 51:777–781, 1976

DEREMEE RA, WEILAND LH, MCDONALD TJ: Polymorphic reticulosis, lymphomatoid granulomatosis. Two diseases or one? Mayo Clin Proc 53:634–640, 1978

EICHEL BS, MABERY TE: The enigma of the lethal midline granuloma. Laryngoscope 78:1367–1386, 1968

FAUCI AS, JOHNSON RE, WOLFF SM: Radiation therapy of midline granuloma. Ann Intern Med 84:140–147, 1974

FECHNER RE, LAMPPIN DW: Midline malignant reticulosis. A clinicopathologic entity. Arch Otolaryngol 95:467–476, 1972

KASSEL SH, ECHEVARRIA RE, GUZZO FP: Midline malignant reticulosis (so-called lethal midline granuloma). Cancer 23:920–935, 1969

LIEBOW AA, CARRINGTON CRB, FRIEDMAN PJ: Lymphomatoid granulomatosis. Hum Pathol 3:457–558, 1972

LOBER CW, KAPLAN RJ, WEST WH: Midline granuloma. Arch Dermatol 118:52–54, 1982

RESNICK N, SKERRETT PV: Lethal midline granuloma of the face. Arch Intern Med 103:116–123, 1959

SIMONIS-BLUMENFRUCHT A, MESTDAGH C, LUSTMAN F et al: Le granulome malin centro-facial. Dermatologica 158:153–162, 1979

SPEAR GS, WALKER WG: Lethal midline granuloma (granuloma gangrenescens) at autopsy. Bull Johns Hopkins Hosp 99:313–332, 1956

STEWART JP: Progressive lethal granulomatous ulceration of the nose. J Laryngol Otol 48:657–674, 1933

Temporal Giant Cell Arteritis

FOGED EK: Chronische Ulzeration nach Biopsie der Arteria temporalis. Hautarzt 32:647–648, 1981

GOODMAN BW JR: Temporal arteritis. (Review) Am J Med 67:839–852, 1979

HITCH JM: Dermatologic manifestations of giant-cell (temporal, cranial) arteritis. Arch Dermatol 101:409–415, 1970

KINMONT PDC, MCCALLUM DI: Skin manifestations of giant-cell arteritis. Br J Dermatol 76:299–308, 1964

LUGER A, WUKETICH S: Kopfschwartennekrose bei temporaler Riesenzellarteriitis. Dermatol Wochenschr 153:89–98, 1967

Malignant Atrophie Papulosis (Degos' Disease)

BLACK MM, HUDSON PM: Atrophie blanche lesions closely resembling malignant atrophic papulosis (Degos' disease) in systemic lupus erythematosus. Br J Dermatol 95:649–652, 1976

BLACK MM, WILSON JONES E: Malignant atrophic papulosis (Degos syndrome). Br J Dermatol 85:290–292, 1971

DEGOS R: Malignant atrophic papulosis. (Review) Br J Dermatol 100:21–35, 1979

DEGOS R, DELORT J, TRICOT R: Dermatite papulo-squameuse atrophiante. Bull Soc Fr Dermatol Syph 49:148–150, 281, 1942

DUBIN HV, STAWISKI MA: Systemic lupus erythematosus resembling malignant atrophic papulosis. Arch Intern Med 134:321–323, 1974

FEUERMAN EJ, DOLLBERG L, SALVADOR O: Malignant atrophic papulosis with mucin in the dermis. Arch Pathol 90:310–315, 1970

FRANK H, METZ J, MÜLLER E: Papulosis atrophicans maligna (Degos). Hautarzt 25:432–437, 1974

HOWSDEN SM, HODGE SJ, HERNDON JH et al: Malignant atrophic papulosis of Degos. Arch Dermatol 112:1582–1588, 1976

METZ J, AMSCHLER A, HENKE M: Morbus Degos (papulosis atrophicans maligna). Hautarzt 31:108–110, 1980

MULLER SA, LANDRY M: Malignant atrophic papulosis (Degos disease). Arch Dermatol 112:357–363, 1976

OLMOS L, LAUGIER P: Ultrastructure de la maladie de Degos. (Review) Ann Dermatol Venereol 104:280–293, 1977

STAHL D, THOMSEN K, HOU-JENSEN K: Malignant atrophic papulosis. Arch Dermatol 114:1687–1689, 1978

STROLE WE JR, CLARK WH JR, ISSELBACHER KJ: Progressive arterial occlusive disease (Köhlmeyer-Degos). N Engl J Med 276:195–201, 1967

WINKELMANN RK, HOWARD FM JR, PERRY HO et al: Malignant papulosis of skin and cerebrum. Arch Dermatol 87:54–62, 1963

Atrophie Blanche

BARD IW, WINKELMANN RK: Livedo vasculitis. Arch Dermatol 96:489–499, 1967

GRAY HR, GRAHAM JH, JOHNSON W et al: Atrophie blanche: Periodic painful ulcers of the lower extremities. Arch Dermatol 93:187–193, 1966

METZ J, STURM G: Atrophie blanche (sog. Capillaritis alba). Hautarzt 25:103–109, 1974

MILIAN G: Les atrophies cutanées syphilitiques. Bull Soc Fr Dermatol Syph 36:865–871, 1929

MIURA T, TORINUKI W: Clinical course of atrophie blanche. J Dermatol 4:259–262, 1977

NELSON LM: Atrophie blanche en plaque. Arch Dermatol 72:242–251, 1955.

POSTERNAK F, ORUSCO M, OLMOS L et al: Livedoid vasculitis (vascularite hyalinisante segmentaire). Ann Dermatol Venereol 104:50–52, 1977

SCHROETER AL, DIAZ-PEREZ JL, WINKELMANN RK et al: Livedo vasculitis (the vasculitis of atrophie blanche). Arch Dermatol 111:188–193, 1976

STIEFLER RE, BERGFELD WF: Atrophie blanche. (Review) Int J Dermatol 21:1–7, 1982

Cutaneous Cholesterol Embolism

DESCHAMPS P, LEROY D, MANDARD JC et al: Livedo reticularis and nodules due to cholesterol embolism in the lower extremities. Br J Dermatol 97:93–97, 1077

FISHER DA, KISTNER RL: Atherothrombotic emboli in the lower extremities. Arch Dermatol 104:533–537, 1971

STEWART WM, LAURET P, TESTART J et al: Les manifestations cutanées des embolies de cristaux de cholestérol. Ann Dermatol Venereol 104:5–11, 1977

Sclerosing Lymphangitis of the Penis

KANDIL E, AL-KASHLAN IM: Non-venereal sclerosing lymphangitis of the penis. Acta Derm Venereol (Stockh) 50:309–312, 1970.

MARSCH WC, STÜTTGEN G: Sclerosing lymphangitis of the penis: A lymphangiofibrosis thrombotica occlusiva. Br J Dermatol 104:687–695, 1981

NICKEL WR, PLUMB RT: Non-venereal sclerosing lymphangitis of the penis. Arch Dermatol 86:761–763, 1962

Systemic Diseases with Cutaneous Manifestations

10

ANGIOIMMUNOBLASTIC LYMPHADENOPATHY

A disorder first described in 1975 (Lukes and Tindle; Frizzera et al), angioimmunoblastic lymphadenopathy has a fairly rapid onset, with fever and malaise, and shows a generalized lymphadenopathy. It is frequently associated with hepatosplenomegaly, polyclonal hypergammaglobulinemia, and Coombs'-positive hemolytic anemia. Approximately 40% of the patients have skin lesions. The course is variable: in some patients, the disorder is chronic and is followed by remission; in others, the disease follows an acute course, with death often caused by severe infection; and in still others, the disease eventuates in a rapidly progressing lymphoma (Nathwani et al).

The skin eruption consists in most instances of a pruritic generalized maculopapular eruption and occasionally of a petechial eruption. Quite frequently, the skin eruption precedes other clinical symptoms (Bernstein et al).

Histopathology. The histologic picture in the lymph nodes is diagnostic, whereas, in the skin lesions, it is at best only suggestive (Seehafer et al).

In the *lymph nodes*, one observes (1) a polymorphous cellular infiltrate that effaces the nodal architecture and is composed of small and large lymphocytes, immunoblasts, and plasma cells, with varying numbers of intermingled histiocytes and eosinophils; (2) arborizing vascular proliferations

showing endothelial cell hyperplasia; and (3) interstitial depositions of an amorphous, eosinophilic material representing cellular detritus (Matloff and Neiman).

In the *skin*, the maculopapular eruption in some cases shows only a nonspecific perivascular infiltrate (Bernstein et al). In others, one observes, as in the lymph nodes, a fairly dense infiltrate together with vascular proliferation (Matloff and Neiman; Lessana-Leibowitch et al). In still others, the dermal vessels show evidence of vasculitis together with a lymphohistiocytic infiltrate (Seehafer et al). In patients with petechial lesions, the vasculitis is more pronounced and is associated with extravasation of erythrocytes (Seehafer et al). In cases with development of an immunoblastic lymphoma, the skin is only occasionally involved and then is infiltrated with large lymphoid cells (Nathwani et al) (see p. 737).

Histogenesis. The basic process appears to be a nonneoplastic hyperimmune proliferation of the B-cell system resulting from a decrease in suppressor T-cell influence on B cells (Bernstein et al). The defect in T-cell function explains the increased susceptibility to overwhelming infections. Whether or not immunoblastic lymphoma will develop cannot be predicted from the initial histologic features in the lymph nodes. Multiple clusters or islands of compactly arranged, large lymphoid cells constitute the initial histologic evidence of immunoblastic lymphoma (Nathwani et al).

SINUS HISTIOCYTOSIS WITH MASSIVE LYMPHADENOPATHY

First described in 1969 (Rosai and Dorfman), sinus histiocytosis with massive lymphadenopathy is benign and generally self-limited. It is characterized by pronounced cervical lymphadenopathy. Other lymph node groups and, rarely, extranodal sites may also be involved. In about 10% of the cases, one or several skin lesions consisting of papules or nodules are present (Thawerani et al). In one patient, massive skin infiltrations were reported (Lampert and Lennert).

Histopathology. The histologic picture in the lymph nodes is diagnostic; the cutaneous lesions may or may not be diagnostic.

In the *lymph nodes*, the sinuses are greatly dilated and are crowded with inflammatory cells, particularly histiocytes. Some of the histiocytes have an abundant, foamy cytoplasm containing phagocytized lymphocytes or other blood cells (Rosai and Dorfman; Lampert and Lennert).

The *skin* contains a polymorphous infiltrate in which histiocytes with abundant cytoplasm are the most important element. Some have a foamy cytoplasm, which is suggestive of lipid accumulation, and an occasional foam cell may exhibit the features of a Touton giant cell. In about half of the cases with skin lesions, phagocytized lymphocytes can be identified within the cytoplasm of the histiocytes (Thawerani et al).

NECROLYTIC MIGRATORY ERYTHEMA (GLUCAGONOMA SYNDROME)

This characteristic eruption was first described in 1942 in a patient with an islet cell type of pancreatic carcinoma (Becker et al). It was given the name *necrolytic migratory erythema* in 1973 (Wilkinson). It is seen most commonly, but not exclusively, in association with a glucagon-secreting alpha-cell tumor of the pancreas and is caused by an amino acid deficiency (see Histogenesis).

The eruption may precede all other symptoms of pancreatic carcinoma by several years (Domen et al). Removal of the carcinoma before metastases have occurred results in a complete cure with clearing of the dermatosis (Sweet; Binnick et al).

The manifestations of the glucagonoma syndrome consist, aside from the cutaneous and mucosal lesions, of weight loss, anemia, mild adult-onset diabetes or, in its absence, glucose intolerance, and extreme elevation of the serum glucagon level (Leichter).

The cutaneous lesions are situated mainly on the face, perineum, genitals, shins, ankles, and feet and consist of erythema, erosions, and flaccid vesicular–pustular lesions that rupture easily. There is peripheral spreading with central clearing resulting in circinate lesions. Rapid healing together with the continuous development of new lesions result in daily fluctuations of the eruption (Wilkinson). Cheilitis and glossitis also exist.

Histopathology. It is important that biopsies be taken from the edge of very early lesions, because only there are the characteristic epidermal changes

Fig. 10-1. Necrolytic migratory erythema (glucagonoma syndrome)
The lower portion of the stratum malpighii appears essentially normal, whereas the upper portion shows necrolysis or "sudden death." The necrolytic portion appears eosinophilic with pyknotic nuclei. (×100)

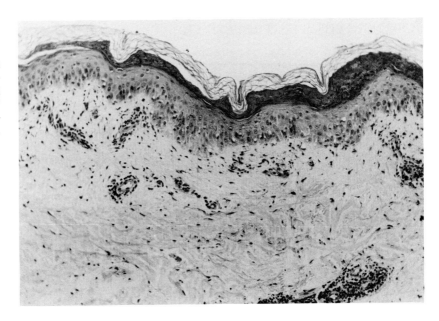

evident. Whereas the lower half or two thirds of the stratum malpighii appear normal, the upper layers show abrupt necrolysis or "sudden death" (Fig. 10-1) (Wilkinson). This results in the formation of a cleft or vesicle. The detached necrolytic portion appears pale and eosinophilic, and the nuclei show pyknosis (Kahan et al). Subsequently, neutrophils invade the detached portion of the epidermis, which assumes the appearance of a crust. In other areas, no true blister forms, but the necrolytic cells of the upper stratum malpighii show a very pronounced intracellular edema and absence of a granular layer (Sweet; Pedersen et al).

Histogenesis. The existence of a glucagonoma is not an absolute prerequisite for the development of necrolytic migratory erythema, since this disorder has been observed in a patient with hyperglucagonemia due to hepatic cirrhosis (Doyle et al). Moreover, not even hyperglucagonemia is required, since necrolytic migratory erythema has been described in patients with malabsorption (Goodenberger et al). It appears very likely that the eruption is the result of a deficiency in amino acids, which are required in large amounts for the synthesis of glucagon. Thus, all patients with glucagonoma in whom determinations of serum amino acid levels were carried out had low levels (Mallinson et al; Pedersen et al; Norton et al), and, in a patient who had an unresectable glucagonoma together with necrolytic migratory erythema and markedly decreased serum amino acid levels, the infusion of amino acids caused rapid clearing of the cutaneous lesions (Norton et al). The situation thus is similar to that in Hartnup's disease, in which an aminoaciduria and the resultant deficiency of tryptophan causes the cutaneous manifestations (see p. 433).

ACRODERMATITIS ENTEROPATHICA

Acrodermatitis enteropathica, first described in 1942 (Danbolt and Closs), is transmitted as an autosomal recessive trait. It is caused by defective intestinal absorption of zinc (Moynahan). It starts as a rule in infancy and is characterized (1) by a cutaneous eruption most pronounced in the periorificial areas and the distal portions of the extremities, (2) by diarrhea, and (3) by diffuse partial alopecia. The cutaneous lesions of acrodermatitis enteropathica consist of areas of erythema associated with vesicles and pustules and with scaling and crusting. Paronychia and stomatitis are common. An acquired form of acrodermatitis enteropathica may occur in patients receiving total intravenous hyperalimentation if the zinc content of the hyperalimentation solution is low (Bernstein and Leyden).

Histopathology. The histologic picture is nonspecific. Generally, the lesions have the appearance of a chronic dermatitis (Tompkins and Livingood). The epidermis may be infiltrated with neutrophils, which subsequently accumulate as crusts in the horny layer (van Vloten and Bos). Vesicles, if present, are intraepidermal in location (Graves et al). Contrary to the findings in two published reports, acantholysis does not occur in acrodermatitis enteropathica. In one instance, the patient probably had benign familial pemphigus (Piper), and in the other pemphigus foliaceus (Juljulian and Kurban).

Histogenesis. Defective intestinal absorption of zinc has been demonstrated in children with acrodermatitis enteropathica by means of the oral administration of ^{65}Zn and a whole-body counting assay (Weissman et al). This defect results in plasma zinc levels well below the normal range of 68 μg/dl to 112 μg/dl (Weston et al). Oral administration of zinc sulfate results in rapid and complete resolution of the disease (Campo and McDonald).

INTESTINAL BYPASS SYNDROME

An intermittent eruption may appear after jejunal–ileal bypass surgery for morbid obesity. The lesions are present mainly on the extremities and consist of a large number of macules and papules that may develop into vesiculopustules and undergo central necrosis. Polyarthritis, malaise, and fever are often associated with the eruption (Morrison and Fourie; Ely).

Histopathology. In early lesions, the dermis contains a massive infiltrate of neutrophils showing leukocytoclasia. In some instances, there is evidence of a necrotizing vasculitis with fibrin deposits within and around the vessel walls (Morrison and Fourie; Goldman et al); in other cases, vascular damage is slight or absent (Ely). In early lesions, there may be papillary edema with a subepidermal vesicle, which, however, soon becomes a pustule through extension of the dermal neutrophilic infiltrate into the vesicle (Ely). As the lesion heals, the dermal mass of neutrophilic debris is extruded through the epidermis.

Histogenesis. This syndrome appears to be an immune complex disease, since in most patients serum immune complexes are found with the Raji cell technic (Utsinger). Most patients also have serum cryoproteins. Direct *immunofluorescence testing* has shown deposits of immunoglobulins and complement along the dermal-epidermal junction. The possible role of *Escherichia coli* in causing the disease is suggested by the presence of both *E. coli* antigens and anti-*E. coli* antibody in the serum cryoproteins and of *E. coli* antigen in the deposits at the dermal-epidermal junction (Utsinger).

HYPEREOSINOPHILIC SYNDROME

The hypereosinophilic syndrome is characterized by a persistent idiopathic eosinophilia associated with a diffuse infiltration of various organs by eosinophils (Chusid et al). There may be hepatosplenomegaly, as well as cardiovascular, pulmonary, neurologic, or dermatologic abnormalities (Kazmierowski et al). The major cause of disability and death is cardiac dysfunction due to hypereosinophilic cardiomyopathy with cardiomegaly (Parillo et al).

Cutaneous manifestations are encountered in about half of the patients and consist of pruritic, erythematous papules and/or urticaria and angioedema. A skin eruption may be the only manifestation of the hypereosinophilic syndrome (Nir and Westfried). In other patients, however, an abnormal echocardiogram is found in addition to the skin lesions (Kazmierowski et al).

Histopathology. The cutaneous lesions show a predominantly perivascular infiltrate of mature eosinophils and mononuclear cells (Kazmierowski et al; Nir and Westfried).

Differential Diagnosis. Bone marrow examination is necessary to rule out eosinophilic leukemia (see p. 749).

APHTHOSIS (BEHÇET'S SYNDROME)

Aphthosis commonly occurs in the mouth as recurrent ulcers. Usually they are small, but occasionally they consist of fairly large, irregularly shaped ulcers measuring more than 1 cm in diameter.

Behçet's syndrome represents the maximal variant within the spectrum of aphthosis (Levinsky and Lehner; Luderschmidt et al). First described in 1937 (Behçet), it consists of an association of oral aphthae with recurrent ulcers on the external genitals and with uveitis, thus forming the so-called triple syndrome. However, the uveitis is frequently absent. Instead, there may be additional manifestations.

Rather frequent cutaneous manifestations seen in Behçet's syndrome are widely scattered papules that often become pustules (Civatte and Belaich) and painful nodose lesions on the legs resembling erythema nodosum (Tokoro et al). There may be arthralgia or nonmigratory arthritis, especially of the large joints, and recurrent superficial or deep migratory thrombophlebitis, especially of the lower limbs (Chajek and Fainaru). Systemic manifestations include pneumonitis and gastrointestinal ulcerations. There may be recurrent attacks of central nervous system lesions, such as meningoencephalitis, cranial nerve palsies, and cerebellar and spinal cord lesions, occasionally causing death (O'Duffy and Goldstein).

Histopathology. The diagnosis of aphthosis and of Behçet's disease is made on the basis of clinical rather than histologic findings. However, according to most observers, the common denominator in all systems is a vasculitis (James). In oral and cutaneous lesions, the vasculitis may be leukocytoclastic (Maciejewski and Bandmann; Luderschmidt et al) or lymphocytic (Lehner, 1969a; Nethercott and Lester). Some authors have noted the presence of vasculitis in late lesions but not in early lesions (Civatte and Belaich) and, according to some observers, vasculitis is absent (Haim). It can thus be concluded that vasculitis is a finding in many but not all lesions.

Histogenesis. Cellular as well as humoral immunologic factors seem to play a role in aphthosis and Behçet's syndrome. For a cellular immunogenesis speak phenomena of lymphocyte transformation and lymphocyte cytotoxity. Thus, it has been found that incubation with homogenates of normal oral mucosa causes a much higher rate of transformation in the peripheral lymphocytes of patients with aphthosis than in normal lymphocytes (Lehner, 1967); it has also been found that lymphocytes of patients with aphthosis exert a cytotoxic effect in vitro in that they reduce the survival time of normal oral epithelial cells to a much greater degree than that of lymphocytes of patients with other types of oral lesions (Rogers et al).

Speaking in favor of a humoral mechanism in the pathogenesis are (1) the presence of circulating antibodies directed against oral and other mucosal epithelial cells (Lehner, 1969b); (2) the finding of elevated levels of immune complexes, the highest levels being in patients with systemic manifestations (Levinsky and Lehner; Gupta et al); and (3) the frequent demonstration through direct immunofluorescence testing of the deposition of immunoglobulins and complement components within and around blood vessel walls and/or in the subepithelial zone (Ullman and Gorlin; Maciejewski and Bandmann; Luderschmidt et al; Van Hale et al).

CROHN'S DISEASE (REGIONAL ENTERITIS)

Crohn's disease, first described in 1932, is characterized by segmental inflammation of the intestinal tract. Its etiology is unknown. Nearly half of the patients with Crohn's disease have perianal lesions (McCallum and Kinmont), which, in rare instances, represent the first manifestation of the disease (Haustein). They may consist of ulcers, fissures, sinus tracts arising from perianal abscesses, or granulomatous vegetations (Korting). They may extend to the perineum, buttocks, crural folds, or abdominal wall. Also, lesions may appear in laparotomy scars, ileostomies, or colostomies. In rare instances, lesions of "metastatic" Crohn's disease arise in distant areas such as the retroauricular region (McCallum and Gray) or the legs (Witkowski et al). About 6% of patients with Crohn's disease have oral ulcerations at some time in their illness (Croft and Wilkinson). Tender, recurrent nodules with the clinical appearance of erythema nodosum also occur occasionally.

Histopathology. Perianal, cutaneous, and oral lesions have the same histologic appearance as the intestinal lesions. They consist of noncaseating granulomas composed of epithelioid and giant cells and are surrounded by variable numbers of mononuclear cells (Korting; Haustein; Witkowski et al).

Histologic examination of the erythema-nodosumlike lesion may show one of three patterns: classic erythema nodosum with septal panniculitis (McCallum and Kinmont); noncaseating granulomas, as seen in metastatic Crohn's disease (Witkowski et al); or fibrinoid necrosis of deep dermal vessels with narrowing and even occlusion of their lumens and surrounding inflammatory reaction, which may be in part granulomatous (Verbov and Stansfeld; Burgdorf and Orkin).

Differential Diagnosis.   The absence of caseation in the granulomas of Crohn's disease aids in their differentiation from tuberculosis.

PYODERMA GANGRENOSUM

In pyoderma gangrenosum, first described in 1930 (Brunsting et al), one or several ulcers are present. The lesions begin as a pustule or fluctuant nodule with subsequent breakdown. As the ulcer enlarges peripherally, the skin at the margin of the ulcer is purplish red and undermined. A variety of systemic diseases may be found in association with pyoderma gangrenosum. Still, about half of the patients with pyoderma gangrenosum have no associated disease (Hickman and Lazarus). Among the systemic diseases are chronic rheumatoidlike polyarthritis (Lazarus et al), ulcerative colitis (Perry and Brunsting), and myelogenous leukemia (Perry and Winkelmann). In patients with myelogenous leukemia, the ulcers usually are superficial and show purplish bullae at their periphery (Pye and Choudhury), but the same appearance may be found in cases of pyoderma gangrenosum that are not associated with leukemia (Crow and Bowers).

Histopathology.   The histologic appearance of pyoderma gangrenosum is not diagnostic. At the onset, when a pustule or fluctuant nodule is present, there is a fairly well circumscribed abscess composed largely of neutrophils (Holt et al). In cases showing bullae at the periphery, one observes, in addition to a dense infiltrate of neutrophils in the upper dermis, a multilocular intraepidermal bulla (Pye and Choudhury).

A fully developed ulcer shows no epidermis, necrosis and an acute inflammatory infiltrate in the upper dermis, and a chronic inflammatory infiltrate in the lower dermis. Occasionally, a few foreign body giant cells are present (Stathers et al). The cellular infiltrate may extend deep into the

subcutaneous tissue. The epidermis at the edge of an ulcer may show hyperplasia.

Considerable variation exists among reports on vascular involvement. Involvement of blood vessels has not been found by some authors (Kresbach; van der Sluis) or has been described as consisting only of minimal endothelial proliferation (Perry and Brunsting; Haim and Friedman-Birnbaum). However, other authors have observed varying degrees of vascular damage, particularly vessel wall necrosis (Sönnichsen et al), and still others have observed fibrinoid necrosis of vessels with leukocytoclasis (Stolman et al). Of interest is the observation that a lymphocytic vasculitis is regularly found when the biopsy specimen is taken from the erythematous border of the ulcer. In addition to a perivascular lymphocytic infiltrate, fibrinoid necrosis of vessels is seen in this location, often in association with vessel infarction and thrombosis (Schroeter and Su).

Histogenesis.   Even though the cause of pyoderma gangrenosum is unknown, immunologic abnormalities have been found in a significant number of patients. Immunoelectrophoresis has revealed in some cases the presence of a monoclonal gammopathy. In most instances, an abnormal immunoglobulin A (IgA) component has been found (van der Sluis); however, some authors have reported an IgG gammopathy (Imhof et al) or an IgM gammopathy (Cream). Other patients have shown defects in their delayed hypersensitivity reactions (Lazarus et al) or diminished monocyte or neutrophil chemotaxis (Norris et al). Nevertheless, direct immunofluorescence studies have failed to demonstrate deposits of immunoglobulins or complement in the skin, and no evidence of circulating immune complexes has been found (Holt et al). The good response of patients with pyoderma gangrenosum to the systemic administration of corticosteroids suggests that the disease has an immunogenic etiology (Holt et al). However, it is not clear why clofazimine is often effective in treating the disorder (Michaelsson et al).

HISTIOCYTIC CYTOPHAGIC PANNICULITIS

An apparently always fatal systemic disease first described in 1980 (Winkelmann and Bowie), histiocytic cytophagic panniculitis starts with widely distributed painful subcutaneous nodules associated with malaise and fever. Hepatosplenomegaly, pancytopenia, and progressive liver dysfunction develop. Death occurs in association with hemorrhage from the gastrointestinal, urinary, and respiratory tracts and into the skin. In addition, there are jaundice and liver failure.

Histopathology.   The subcutaneous nodules show the fatty tissue infiltrated by histiocytes and inflammatory cells, followed by fat necrosis and hemorrhage. The histiocytes appear benign but show marked phagocytic activity. Some histiocytes are so stuffed with erythrocytes, leukocytes, and cell particles that they have the appearance of a bean bag (Winkelmann and Bowie).

Autopsy reveals the presence of cytophagic histiocytes also in the liver, spleen, lymph nodes, bone marrow, myocardium, lungs, and gastrointestinal tract. The liver shows fatty degeneration and hepatocellular necrosis (Crotty and Winkelmann; Csató et al).

Differential Diagnosis. Histiocytic cytophagic panniculitis shares with malignant histiocytosis the presence of fever, hepatosplenomegaly, pancytopenia, jaundice, and purpura (see p. 748). However, in malignant histiocytosis, one observes papular and nodular lesions of the skin rather than panniculitis. Histologically, the presence of malignant, atypical histiocytes separates malignant histiocytosis from histiocytic cytophagic panniculitis.

BIBLIOGRAPHY

Angioimmunoblastic Lymphadenopathy
BERNSTEIN JE, SOLTANI K, LORINCZ AL: Cutaneous manifestations of angioimmunoblastic lymphadenopathy. Cancer 41:578–606, 1978
FRIZZERA G, MORAN EM, RAPPAPORT H: Angio-immunoblastic lymphadenopathy. Am J Med 59:803–817, 1975
LESSANA-LEIBOWITCH M, MIGNOT L, BLOCH C et al: Manifestations cutanées des lymphadénopathies angio-immunoblastiques. Ann Dermatol Venereol 104:603–610, 1977
LUKES RJ, TINDLE BH: Immunoblastic lymphadenopathy. N Engl J Med 292:1–8, 1975
MATLOFF RB, NEIMAN RS: Angioimmunoblastic lymphadenopathy. Arch Dermatol 114:92–94, 1978
NATHWANI BN, RAPPAPORT H, MORAN EM et al: Malignant lymphoma arising in angioimmunoblastic lymphadenopathy. Cancer 41:578–606, 1978
SEEHAFER JR, GOLDBERG NC, DICKEN CH et al: Cutaneous manifestations of angioimmunoblastic lymphadenopathy. Arch Dermatol 116:41–45, 1980

Sinus Histiocytosis with Massive Lymphadenopathy
LAMPERT F, LENNERT K: Sinus histiocytosis with massive lymphadenopathy. Cancer 37:783–789, 1976
ROSAI J, DORFMAN RF: Sinus histiocytosis with massive lymphadenopathy. Arch Pathol 87:63–70, 1969
THAWERANI H, SANCHEZ RL, ROSAI J et al: The cutaneous manifestations of sinus histiocytosis with massive lymphadenopathy. Arch Dermatol 114:191–197, 1978

Necrolytic Migratory Erythema (Glucagonoma Syndrome)
BECKER SW, KAHN D, ROTHMAN S: Cutaneous manifestations of internal malignant tumors. Arch Dermatol Syph 45:1069–1080, 1942
BINNICK AN, SPENCER SK, DENNISON WL JR et al: Glucagonoma syndrome. Arch Dermatol 113:749–754, 1977

DOMEN RE, SHAFFER MB JR, FINKE J et al: The glucagonoma syndrome. Arch Intern Med 140:262–263, 1980
DOYLE JA, SCHROETER AL, ROGERS RS III: Hyperglucagonemia and necrolytic migratory erythema in cirrhosis, possible pseudoglucagonoma syndrome. Br J Dermatol 101:581–587, 1979
GOODENBERGER DM, LAWLEY TJ, STROBER W et al: Necrolytic migratory erythema without glucagonoma. Arch Dermatol 115:1429–1432, 1979
KAHAN RS, PEREZ-FIGAREDO RA, NEIMANIS A: Necrolytic migratory erythema. Arch Dermatol 113:792–797, 1977
LEICHTER SB: Clinical and metabolic aspects of glucagonoma. Medicine (Baltimore) 59:100–113, 1980
MALLINSON CN, BLOOM SR, WARIN AP et al: A glucagonoma syndrome. Lancet 2:1–5, 1974
NORTON JA, KAHN CR, SCHIEBINGER R et al: Amino acid deficiency and the skin rash associated with glucagonoma. Ann Intern Med 91:213–215, 1979
PEDERSEN NB, JONSSON L, HOLST JJ: Necrolytic migratory erythema and glucagon cell tumour of the pancreas: The glucagonoma syndrome. Acta Derm Venereol (Stockh) 56:391–395, 1976
SWEET RD: A dermatosis specifically associated with a tumor of pancreatic alpha cells. Br J Dermatol 90:301–308, 1974
WILKINSON DS: Necrolytic migratory erythema with carcinoma of the pancreas. Trans St John's Hosp Dermatol Soc 59:244–250, 1973

Acrodermatitis Enteropathica
BERNSTEIN B, LEYDEN JL: Zinc deficiency and acrodermatitis after intravenous hyperalimentation. Arch Dermatol 114:1070–1072, 1978
CAMPO AG JR, MCDONALD CJ: Treatment of acrodermatitis enteropathica with zinc sulfate. Arch Dermatol 112:687–689, 1976
DANBOLT N, CLOSS K: Akrodermatitis enteropathica. Acta Derm Venereol (Stockh) 23:127–169, 1942
GRAVES K, KESTENBAUM T, KALIVAS J: Hereditary acrodermatitis enteropathica in an adult. Arch Dermatol 116:562–564, 1980
JULJULIAN HH, KURBAN AK: Acantholysis: A feature of acrodermatitis enteropathica. Arch Dermatol 103:105–106, 1971
MOYNAHAN EJ: Acrodermatitis enteropathica: A lethal inherited human zinc-deficiency disorder. Lancet 2:399–400, 1974
PIPER EL: Acrodermatitis enteropathica in an adult. Arch Dermatol 76:221–224, 1957
TOMPKINS RR, LIVINGOOD CS: Acrodermatitis enteropathica persisting into adult life. Arch Dermatol 99:190–195, 1969
VAN VLOTEN WA, BOS LP: Skin lesions in acquired zinc deficiency due to parenteral nutrition. Dermatologica 156:175–183, 1978
WEISSMAN K, HOE S, KNUDSEN L et al: Zinc absorption in patients suffering from acrodermatitis enteropathica and in normal adults assessed by whole-body counting technique. Br J Dermatol 101:573–579, 1979
WESTON WL, HUFF C, HUMBERT JR et al: Zinc correction of defective chemotaxis in acrodermatitis enteropathica. Arch Dermatol 113:422–425, 1977

Intestinal Bypass Syndrome
ELY PH: The bowel bypass syndrome: A response to bacterial peptidoglycans. J Am Acad Dermatol 2:473–487, 1980
GOLDMAN JA, CASEY HL, DAVIDSON ED et al: Vasculitis associated with intestinal bypass surgery. Arch Dermatol 115:725–727, 1979
MORRISON JGL, FOURIE ED: A distinctive skin eruption following small-bowel by-pass surgery. Br J Dermatol 102:467–471, 1980

UTSINGER PD: Systemic immune complex disease following intestinal bypass surgery: Bypass disease. J Am Acad Dermatol 2:488–495, 1980

Hypereosinophilic Syndrome

CHUSID MJ, DALE DC, WEST BC et al: The hypereosinophilic syndrome. Medicine (Baltimore) 54:1–27, 1975

KAZMIEROWSKI JA, CHUSID MJ, PARILLO JE et al: Dermatologic manifestations of the hypereosinophilic syndrome. Arch Dermatol 114:531–535, 1978

NIR MA, WESTFRIED M: Hypereosinophilic dermatitis. Dermatologica 162:444–450, 1981

PARILLO JE, BORER JS, HENRY WL et al: The cardiovascular manifestations of the hypereosinophilic syndrome. Am J Med 67:572–582, 1979

Aphthosis (Behçet's Syndrome)

BEHÇET H: Über rezidivierende, aphthöse, durch ein Virus verursachte Geschwüre am Mund, am Auge und an den Genitalien. Dermatol Wochenschr 105:1152–1157, 1937

CHAJEK T, FAINARU M: Behçet's disease. Report of 41 cases and a review of the literature. Medicine (Baltimore) 54:179–196, 1975

CIVATTE J, BELAICH S: Histopathologie des aphtes cutanés au cours du syndrome de Behçet. Ann Dermatol Syph 103:135–140, 1976

GUPTA RC, O'DUFFY JD, MCDUFFIE FC et al: Circulating immune complexes in active Behçet's disease. Clin Exp Immunol 34:213–218, 1978

HAIM S: The pathogenesis of lesions in Behçet's disease. Dermatologica 158:31–37, 1979

JAMES DG: Behçet's syndrome. N Engl J Med 301:431–432, 1979

LEHNER T: Stimulation of lymphocyte transformation by tissue homogenates in recurrent oral ulceration. Immunology 13:159–166, 1967

LEHNER T: Pathology of recurrent oral ulceration and oral ulceration in Behçet's syndrome. J Pathol 97:481–494, 1969a

LEHNER T: Characterization of mucosal antibodies in recurrent aphthous ulceration and Behçet's syndrome. Arch Oral Biol 14:443–453, 1969b

LEVINSKY RJ, LEHNER T: Circulating soluble immune complexes in recurrent oral ulceration and Behçet's syndrome. Clin Exp Immunol 32:193–198, 1978

LUDERSCHMIDT C, WOLFF HH, SCHERER R: Aphthen: Histologische, immunofluoreszenz- und immunelektronenmikroskopische Studie zur Pathogenese. Hautarzt 32:364–369, 1981

MACIEJEWSKI W, BANDMANN HJ: Immune complex vasculitis in a patient with Behçet's syndrome. Arch Dermatol Res 264:253–256, 1979

NETHERCOTT J, LESTER RS: Azathioprine therapy in incomplete Behçet syndrome. Arch Dermatol 110:432–434, 1974

O'DUFFY JD, GOLDSTEIN NP: Neurologic involvement in seven patients with Behçet's disease. Am J Med 61:170–177, 1976

ROGERS RS III, SAMS WM JR, SHORTER RG: Lymphocytotoxicity in recurrent aphthous stomatitis. Arch Dermatol 109:361–363, 1974

TOKORO Y, SETO T, ABE Y et al: Skin lesions in Behçet's disease. Int J Dermatol 16:227–244, 1977

ULLMAN S, GORLIN RJ: Recurrent aphthous stomatitis. Arch Dermatol 114:955–956, 1978

VAN HALE HM, ROGERS RS III, DOYLE JA et al: Immunofluorescence microscopic studies of recurrent aphthous stomatitis. Arch Dermatol 117:779–781, 1981

Crohn's Disease (Regional Enteritis)

BURGDORF W, ORKIN M: Granulomatous perivasculitis in Crohn's disease. Arch Dermatol 117:674–675, 1981

CROFT CB, WILKINSON AR: Ulceration of the mouth, pharynx and larynx. Br J Surg 59:249–252, 1972

CROHN BB, GINZBURG L, OPPENHEIMER GD: Regional ileitis; Pathologic and clinical entity. JAMA 99:1323–1329, 1932

HAUSTEIN UF: Perianale granulomatöse Vegetationen als diagnostischer Wegweiser zur Enterocolitis regionalis Crohn. Dermatol Monatsschr 162:826–832, 1976

KORTING GW: Zur perianalen Erscheinungsweise der Crohnschen Krankheit. Hautarzt 19:553–556, 1968

MCCALLUM DI, GRAY WM: Metastatic Crohn's disease. Br J Dermatol 95:551–554, 1976

MCCALLUM DI, KINMONT PDC: Dermatologic manifestations of Crohn's disease. Br J Dermatol 80:1–8, 1968

VERBOV J, STANSFELD AG: Cutaneous polyarteritis nodosa and Crohn's disease. Trans St John's Hosp Dermatol Soc 58:261–268, 1972

WITKOWSKI JA, PARISH LC, LEWIS JE: Crohn's disease, noncaseating granulomas on the legs. Acta Derm Venereol (Stockh) 57:181–183, 1977

Pyoderma Gangrenosum

BRUNSTING LA, GOECKERMAN WE, O'LEARY PA: Pyoderma (ecthyma) gangrenosum. Arch Dermatol 22:655–680, 1930

CREAM JJ: Pyoderma gangrenosum with monoclonal IgM red cell agglomerating factor. Br J Dermatol 84:223–226, 1971

CROW KD, BOWERS RE: Bullous hemorrhagic ulceration, a variant of pyoderma gangrenosum. Trans St John's Hosp Dermatol Soc 60:142–151, 1974

HAIM S, FRIEDMAN-BIRNBAUM R: Pyoderma gangrenosum in immunosuppressed patients. Dermatologica 153:44–48, 1976

HICKMAN JG, LAZARUS GS: Pyoderma gangrenosum: A reappraisal of associated systemic disease. Br J Dermatol 102:235–237, 1980

HOLT PJA, DAVIES MG, SAUNDERS KC et al: Pyoderma gangrenosum. Medicine (Baltimore) 59:114–133, 1980

IMHOF JW, SCHUTTER GJNV, HART HC et al: Monoclonal gammopathy (IgG) and chronic ulcerative dermatitis (phagedenic pyoderma). Acta Med Scand 186:289–292, 1969

KRESBACH H: Ein Beitrag zum Problem der sogenannten Pyodermia ulcerosa. Arch Klin Exp Dermatol 208:128–159, 1959

LAZARUS GS, GOLDSMITH LA, ROCKLIN RE et al: Pyoderma gangrenosum, altered delayed hypersensitivity, and polyarthritis. Arch Dermatol 105:46–51, 1972

MICHAELSSON G, MOLIN L, ÖHMAN S et al: Clofazimine, a new agent for the treatment of pyoderma gangrenosum. Arch Dermatol 112:344–349, 1976

NORRIS DA, WESTON WL, THORNE EG et al: Pyoderma gangrenosum. Arch Dermatol 114:906–911, 1978

PERRY HO, BRUNSTING LA: Pyoderma gangrenosum. Arch Dermatol 75:380–386, 1957

PERRY HO, WINKELMANN RK: Bullous pyoderma gangrenosum and leukemia. Arch Dermatol 106:901–905, 1972

PYE RJ, CHOUDHURY C: Bullous pyoderma as a presentation of acute leukemia. Clin Exp Dermatol 2:33–38, 1977

SCHROETER AL, SU WPD: The vasculitis of pyoderma gangrenosum. (Abstr) Arch Dermatol 116:1388, 1980

SÖNNICHSEN N, SCHULZE P, AUDRING H: Diagnostik und Therapie der Dermatitis ulcerosa. Dermatol Monatsschr 166:667–678, 1980

STATHERS GM, ABBOTT LG, MCGUINNESS AE: Pyoderma gangrenosum in association with regional enteritis. Arch Dermatol 95:375–380, 1967

STOLMAN LP, ROSENTHAL D, YAWORSKY R et al: Pyoderma gangrenosum and rheumatoid arthritis. Arch Dermatol 111:1020–1023, 1975

VAN DER SLUIS I: Two cases of pyoderma (ecthyma) gangraenosum associated with the presence of an abnormal serum protein (IgA-paraprotein). Dermatologica 132:409–424, 1966

Histiocytic Cytophagic Panniculitis

CROTTY CP, WINKELMANN RK: Cytophagic histiocytic panniculitis with fever, cytopenia, liver failure, and terminal hemorrhagic diathesis. J Am Acad Dermatol 4:181–194, 1981

CSATÓ M, SZEKEVES L, FRECSKA I et al: Zytophagische Pannikulitis. Hautarzt 32:370–371, 1981

WINKELMANN RK, BOWIE EJW: Hemorrhagic diathesis associated with benign histiocytic, cytophagic panniculitis and systemic histiocytosis. Arch Intern Med 140:1460–1463, 1980

Inflammatory Diseases of the Epidermal Appendages and of Cartilage

11

ACNE VULGARIS

Acne vulgaris occurs predominantly during adolescence and in early adulthood. It affects mainly the face, the upper back, and the upper chest. Clinically, two types of lesions occur: comedones and inflammatory lesions. A comedo can be located either in an open follicle as a "blackhead" or in a closed follicle as a "whitehead." Inflammatory lesions only rarely develop at sites of open comedones; they tend to arise in either a closed comedo or a microcomedo that is visible only in histologic sections. An inflammatory lesion begins either as a follicular papule that may evolve into a pustule or as a nodule that may evolve into a cyst.

Histopathology. A comedo contains keratinized cells, sebum, and some microorganisms, but, in routinely prepared sections, one sees only keratinized cells, since the xyline used in processing has removed the lipid material. The black color at the tip of open comedones is due to melanin (see below).

The follicular papules of acne are characterized by a predominantly lymphocytic infiltrate arranged around a follicle containing either a closed comedo or a microcomedo. On careful searching, one may find small areas of disintegration of the follicular wall (Strauss and Kligman).

Pustules as well as nodules form after the follicular wall has ruptured and the contents of the comedo have been extruded into the dermis. If the resulting aggregation of neutrophils is small and superficial, a pustule results, but, if the aggregation is large and deep, a nodule forms. In addition to

neutrophils, there are also mononuclear cells and foreign body giant cells. Frequently, keratin particles are seen near giant cells. In the process of healing, sheaths of cells grow out from the epidermis or the appendageal structures in an attempt to encapsulate the inflammatory reaction (Strauss and Kligman).

Histogenesis. The primary lesion of acne is the comedo. A comedo begins to form as a result of an increased rate of proliferation of the epithelium in the lower portion of the infundibulum, called the infrainfundibulum. This hyperproliferation of horny cells can be measured by ^{3}H-thymidine and ^{3}H-histidine incorporation technics in microcomedones, which are clinically invisible but can easily be identified histologically in biopsy specimens from apparently normal skin of acne patients (Plewig). Not only is there an increased production of horn cells, but, as the result of a change in the intercellular substance, the horn cells adhere to one another and fill the infundibulum as a lamellar horn mass intermingled with sebum and bacterial colonies. The widening of the infundibulum with horn masses leads to a closed comedo, or whitehead, for which there are two possibilities of further development. Either the hyperkeratosis extends to the upper portion of the infundibulum and distends its opening, so that an open comedo or blackhead forms, or the wall of the infundibulum undergoes further distention and thinning until it ruptures (Plewig and Kligman).

Although the precise cause of acne is not known, three factors contribute to its development: androgens, sebum, and *Propionibacterium acnes* (formerly called *Corynebacterium acnes*).

In regard to *androgens*, even though sebaceous secretion is androgen-stimulated, there is no evidence of overproduction of androgens in most patients with acne vulgaris (Förström). In some women with acne vulgaris, however, elevated plasma testosterone levels are found (Förström et al), often in association with ovarian dysfunction (Steinberger). The occurrence of acne vulgaris in the polycystic ovary syndrome or Stein-Leventhal syndrome is well established (Strauss and Pochi, 1969). It is also significant that skin with acne converts testosterone to dihydrotestosterone at a higher rate than normal skin (Sansone and Reisner; Hay and Hodgkins). This indicates that, even though acne vulgaris usually is not a systemic hormonal disorder, it may be caused by a hormonal disturbance in its target organ, the sebaceous gland.

In regard to *sebum*, even though sebum excretion is not consistently increased in patients with acne vulgaris, it is possible that the hyperkeratinization of the infrainfundibulum, the first step in the formation of a comedo, is brought on by the irritant effect of sebum (Cunliffe and Tan). It also appears significant that the oral administration of 13-cis retinoic acid, which often improves acne vulgaris, greatly decreases sebum production (Strauss).

In regard to *P. acnes*, even though the population of *P. acnes* is not consistently greater on affected skin than on normal skin (Leyden et al; Cove et al), this organism has widely been regarded as important in the pathogenesis of acne vulgaris. At one time, the view was widely held that, through its lipolytic enzymes, *P. acnes* hydrolyzed the triglycerides of sebum into free fatty acids and glycerol and that the free fatty acids induced marked inflammation and in this way caused erosion and disruption of the follicular wall, thereby allowing the follicular content to enter the dermis (Strauss and Pochi, 1965). However, there is no direct evidence that free fatty acids in physiologic concentrations are inflammatory (Puhvel and Sakamoto). Furthermore, the abnormal keratinization in the infrainfundibulum that results in the formation of comedones is unrelated to the presence of *P. acnes* (Lavker et al). It is possible, however, that immunologic reactions to *P. acnes* contribute to the inflammatory response in acne lesions. It has been shown that patients with acne vulgaris not only have elevated serum antibody levels and increased immediate hypersensitivity reactions to *P. acnes*, but also exhibit cell-mediated immunity to *P. acnes*. The existence of cell-mediated immunity is demonstrable through an increased transformation of lymphocytes in vitro on exposure to *P. acnes* antigen (Puhvel et al). Furthermore, a good correlation exists between the delayed skin test reactivity to *P. acnes* and the severity of inflammation in lesions of acne vulgaris (Kersey et al).

The beneficial effect of the systemic or topical administration of antibiotics is widely attributed to their suppressive effect on *P. acnes* (Akers et al); however, there are studies throwing doubt on this supposition. Thus, the oral administration of tetracycline, although clinically effective, does not necessarily reduce the population of *P. acnes* (Cove et al); similarly, the topical application of erythromycin, though it substantially improves the disease, does not depress *P. acnes* counts in open comedones (Resh and Stoughton).

The difference in melanin content between open and closed comedones is due to the fact that, in closed comedones, the melanocytes normally present in the upper portion of the infundibulum produce very little melanin, whereas, in open comedones, numerous large, enzymatically active melanocytes are present (Kaidbey and Kligman).

ACNE ROSACEA

Acne rosacea affects mainly the center of the face but occasionally also the sides of the face. Three types of acne rosacea occur, sometimes together: the erythematous telangiectatic type, the glandular hyperplastic type, and the papular type. The erythematous telangiectatic type often shows, besides erythema and telangiectasia, follicular pustules. The glandular hyperplastic type causes an enlargement of the nose called rhinophyma. The papular type shows numerous moderately firm, slightly raised papules 1 mm to 3 mm in diameter that are usually associated with erythema. Formerly, some cases of papular acne rosacea were mistakenly diagnosed as rosacealike tuberculid because of the presence on histologic examination of granulomatous "tuberculoid" formations (see Histogenesis below).

Histopathology. In the erythematous telangiectatic type of acne rosacea, a nonspecific inflammatory infiltrate is present in the dermis, often arranged around dilated capillaries. The follicular pustules show aggregations of neutrophils, usually high in the follicle but occasionally leading to total destruction of the follicle (Marks and Harcourt-Webster).

In the glandular hyperplastic type of acne rosacea, the sebaceous glands are increased in size and number. The sebaceous ducts are dilated and filled with keratinous material. In addition, the capillaries are dilated, and a chronic inflammatory infiltrate is present in the upper dermis (Marks and Harcourt-Webster).

In the papular type of acne rosacea, the papules usually show merely a nonspecific chronic inflammatory infiltrate. However, in about 10% of the cases, one finds, in addition, foci of a granulomatous infiltrate (Laymon and Schoch; Marks and Harcourt-Webster). In most of these cases, one finds islands composed of epithelioid cells and a few giant cells that are surrounded by a "round-cell" infiltrate, resulting in a "tuberculoid" picture. Caseation is generally absent (Mullanax and Kierland; Erlach et al). In some cases, one may find islands

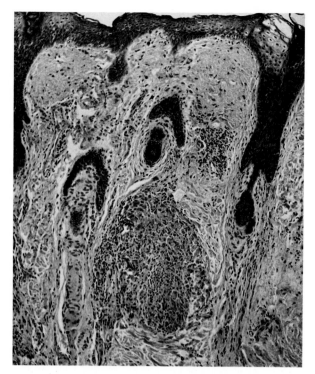

Fig. 11-1. Acne rosacea, papular type
An epithelioid cell tubercle showing no necrosis and only a very slight inflammatory infiltrate at its periphery is present, resembling sarcoidosis. Formerly, a lesion of this type was diagnosed as *rosacealike tuberculid*. (× 100)

of epithelioid cells with only a slight admixture of lymphoid cells, as seen in sarcoidosis; occasionally, such "naked" tubercles predominate in the infiltrate (Fig. 11-1) (Laymon; Veien et al).

Histogenesis. The presence of granulomatous, "tuberculoid" formations in the lesions of papular acne rosacea at one time was interpreted as evidence of the existence of a tuberculid. Such cases were diagnosed either as *rosacealike tuberculid*, a term introduced in 1917 (Lewandowsky), or as *micropapular tuberculid,* a term chosen in 1940 (Laymon and Michelson) for the purpose of differentiating this disorder from the lupoid or macropapular tuberculid or lupus miliaris disseminatus faciei (see below). The realization that well-developed tuberculoid structures can occur in acne rosacea was first given expression in 1948 (Laymon and Schoch) and 1949 (Snapp) and this view is now generally accepted.

The presence of granulomatous formations in acne rosacea is usually explained as a foreign body reaction against keratinized cells of disintegrating hair structures. The possibility that the granulomas represent a delayed hypersensitivity reaction to the mite *Demodex folliculorum* was considered in one report in which 10 of 20 biopsy specimens of granulomatous acne rosacea showed intact

or fragmented *Demodex* (Grosshans et al). However, other authors (Ecker and Winkelmann; Erlach et al) have doubted the role of *Demodex*, since they have encountered it only very rarely. Because of the presence of phagocytized elastic fibers in some giant cells, the question has been raised as to whether granulomatous acne rosacea might not be a foreign body reaction against elastotic material (Erlach et al).

Differential Diagnosis.   Inasmuch as the histologic picture of granulomatous acne rosacea can mimic the histologic picture of lupus vulgaris or of sarcoidosis, it is advisable never to make a diagnosis of tuberculosis or sarcoidosis on biopsy specimens obtained from the face without adequate supporting evidence.

Lupus Miliaris Disseminatus Faciei

In lupus miliaris disseminatus faciei, a condition also referred to as acne agminata (Scott and Calnan), discrete, reddish papules are seen on the face, singly or in groups. Papules are often also present on the eyelids and the upper lip, areas in which lesions of acne rosacea are rarely seen (Ueki and Masuda). Also, the erythema and telangiectasias that are so characteristic of acne rosacea are absent. Still, in some cases, features of acne rosacea may be present. In one follow-up study, the eruption of lupus miliaris disseminatus faciei was followed by acne rosacea either of the papular or of the erythematous type in 7 of 13 patients (Strauss).

Histopathology.   The histologic picture is regarded as highly characteristic, since it shows fairly large "tubercles" composed of epithelioid cells and some giant cells showing in their center a large area of "caseation" necrosis that has an amorphous appearance. At the periphery of the "tubercles," varying amounts of a chronic inflammatory infiltrate are seen (Fig. 11-2) (Scott and Calnan; Simon; Pinkus and Mehregan).

Histogenesis. Even though nothing could look more tuberculous than the histology of "acne agminata," there is "not a single piece of evidence, apart from the histology, to support a tuberculous etiology" (Scott and Calnan). The etiology is obscure, but some affinity to acne rosacea is likely.

DISSEMINATE INFUNDIBULOFOLLICULITIS

Disseminate infundibulofolliculitis, an eruption first described in 1968 (Hitch and Lund), consists of firm, closely set, skin-colored, follicular papules having the appearance of exaggerated cutis anserina. The trunk and proximal portions of the extremities are the areas of predilection. The eruption may be recurrent or persistent (Owen and Wood). It occurs almost exclusively in blacks.

Histopathology. The histologic findings, although not specific, are characteristic. There is spongiosis of the uppermost portion of the hair follicle, the so-called infundibulum. The adjoining dermis shows a fairly mild chronic inflammatory infiltrate. Exocytosis of inflammatory cells from the dermis into the spongiotic areas is usually seen (Hitch and Lund, 1968, 1972). Some follicles show infundibular keratin plugging and there may be suprafollicular parakeratosis (Owen and Wood).

EOSINOPHILIC PUSTULAR FOLLICULITIS

A rare condition first described in 1970 in Japan (Ofuji et al), eosinophilic pustular folliculitis has since been described in several European countries. The dermatosis is characterized by erythematous patches with largely follicular papules and pustules. The patches have a tendency toward central healing and peripheral extension. There are exacerbations and remissions, but the patient's general health is not affected. The most commonly involved areas are the face, trunk, and arms. Occasionally, lesions are present in nonfollicular areas such as the palms and soles (Ishibashi et al). Involvement of hair follicles in the scalp may produce some scarring there (Orfanos and Sterry). Moderate leukocytosis and eosinophilia are often present.

Histopathology. In follicular lesions, the hair follicles, and often also the sebaceous glands, are infiltrated mainly by eosinophils and by some mononuclear cells and neutrophils. This results in spongiosis, and even in some destruction, especially in the upper portion of the hair follicle, the infundibulum (Ofuji et al; Orfanos and Sterry). In addition, the epidermis outside the hair follicles shows infiltration by eosinophils leading to spongiosis and intraepidermal abscesses filled with eosinophils (Holst). Also, the dermis shows a perivascular infiltrate containing mainly eosinophils (Guillaume et al).

Differential Diagnosis. The eosinophilic follicular pustules of erythema toxicum neonatorum histologically resemble those of eosinophilic pustular folliculitis, but the clinical appearance is quite different (Ofuji et al).

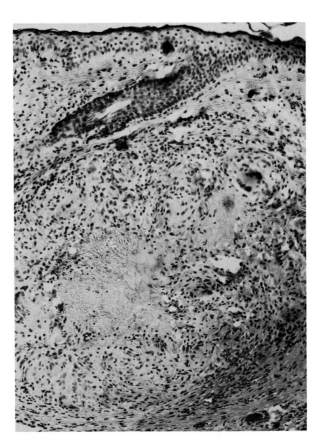

Fig. 11-2. Lupus miliaris disseminatus faciei
A large ''tubercle'' composed of epithelioid cells and some giant cells shows in its center a large area of ''caseation'' necrosis. At the periphery, an inflammatory infiltrate is present. (× 100)

EOSINOPHILIC CELLULITIS (WELLS' SYNDROME)

Eosinophilic cellulitis, a rare dermatosis first described in 1971 (Wells), is characterized by recurrent episodes of sudden outbreaks of erythematous cutaneous swellings that often are painful or pruritic. Some blistering may be present. The swellings spread rapidly over 2 or 3 days and are followed by indolent indurations requiring from 4 to 8 weeks to resolve. Peripheral blood eosinophilia is regularly present.

Histopathology. In the early acute stage, one observes a dense cellular infiltrate composed predominantly of eosinophils, many of which show degranulation (Wells and Smith). The infiltrate extends into the subcutaneous tissue and may even extend into the underlying muscle (Spigel and Winkelmann). Blisters, if present, are subepidermal and contain many eosinophils (Wells). Lesions from 1 to 3 weeks old show, in addition to eosinophils, elongated areas of fibrinoid necrosis of the dermal collagen surrounded by eosinophils and histiocytes (Nielson et al). These elongated areas of collagen necrosis, with their bright red, granular deposits of fibrin, are referred to as flame figures (Wells and Smith). On resolution, few eosinophils are found, but large, pale histiocytes are grouped around the flame-shaped areas together with some giant cells, thus forming small phagocytic granulomas (Wells; Marks).

TRICHORRHEXIS INVAGINATA (NETHERTON'S SYNDROME)

Trichorrhexis invaginata is a nearly always autosomal recessively inherited condition that occurs almost exclusively in females. The scalp hair of affected persons is short, sparse, and brittle. Trichorrhexis invaginata usually is found in association with ichthyosis linearis circumflexa, which is characterized by migratory polycyclic lesions of erythema (Hurwitz et al) (see p. 60). In a few instances, however, as in the original case described in 1958 (Netherton), trichorrhexis invaginata has been found in association with lamellar ichthyosis (see p. 61).

Histopathology. On histologic examination of a scalp biopsy or on microscopic examination of a plucked hair, trichorrhexis invaginata, or bamboo hair, shows invagination of the distal portion of the hair shaft (as "ball") into its proximal portion (as "cup") (Altman and Stroud).

Histogenesis. Invagination of the hair results from a transient defect in the keratinization of both hair shaft and inner root sheath in the keratogenous zone of the hair, so that the inner root sheath no longer can act as a splint, and the distal portion of the hair is wedged into its proximal portion (Julius and Keeran).

TRICHOSTASIS SPINULOSA

Trichostasis spinulosa is a common follicular condition in elderly persons that occurs on the skin of the face. It may be clinically inapparent to the naked eye (Goldschmidt et al). In some instances, however, it manifests itself as slightly raised follicular spines resembling comedones (Braun-Falco and Vakilzadeh). The same condition occurs occasionally on the trunk and limbs and may also affect young persons (Sarkany and Gaylarde).

Histopathology. Each affected hair follicle contains in its infundibular portion numerous hairs,

usually between 6 and 20, enveloped in a keratinous sheath (Sarkany and Gaylarde).

Histogenesis. The retained hairs are telogen or club hairs of the vellus type that have all been produced successively by the same hair matrix and have not been shed. It appears likely that the retention is a result of hyperkeratotic changes in the follicular infundibulum leading to partial obstruction, which prevents the expulsion of small club hairs to the skin surface (Goldschmidt et al).

ALOPECIA AREATA

Alopecia areata is characterized by the complete or nearly complete absence of hair in one or several circumscribed areas. There is no visible evidence of inflammation, and the follicular openings are preserved. The scalp is the most common site of lesions. In most cases, there is complete regrowth of hair. In occasional instances, the entire scalp is involved (alopecia totalis) as well as other hair-bearing portions of the skin (alopecia universalis). In such cases, the loss of hair often is permanent.

Histopathology. The characteristic finding in alopecia areata is the presence of miniature hair structures. They are either dystrophic early anagen hair structures or dystrophic telogen hair structures. Early anagen hair structures usually predominate in lesions of alopecia areata of recent onset, and dystrophic telogen hair structures in longstanding alopecia areata (Swanson et al). Yet early anagen hairs may constitute as many as 75% of the hair structures in some cases of alopecia areata of many years' duration (Van Scott).

Early anagen hair structures appear diminutive. The bulb of such early anagen hairs is located, on the average, only 2 mm below the skin surface, rather than 3.5 mm, as is the bulb of mature anagen hair (Van Scott). Keratinization of the small hairs in the miniature hair follicles is incomplete, the hair shaft being composed largely of nucleated cells. However, a small internal root sheath is generally present.

Dystrophic telogen hair structures either contain no hair or show only a small dystrophic hair. Such telogen hair follicles have moved into the upper portion of the dermis. They possess a thin cord of epithelium at their base and are surrounded by a thick, folded fibrous root sheath (Fig. 11-3). (For a discussion of the normal hair cycle, see also p. 28.)

The sebaceous glands vary in size: they may be normal in size or may be atrophic, independent of the duration of the hair loss (Goos). The dermis surrounding the miniature hair structures in alopecia areata is infiltrated with a variable number of lymphocytes. The amount of the inflammatory infiltrate in cases of long duration is apt to be less than in cases of recent onset (Van Scott). The inflammatory cells often invade the matrix of the bulb and the outer root sheath of early anagen hairs. The infiltrate is also present, but somewhat less severe, in the thick, folded fibrous root sheath surrounding telogen hair structures. It is seen extending to the surface epidermis only in early, rapidly advancing cases, in which it then may cause spongiosis of the lower portion of the surface epidermis (Goos). The inflammatory infiltrate around early anagen hair bulbs appears loosely arranged, surrounding them like a "swarm of bees" (Kalkoff and Macher).

Histogenesis. Transverse sections through lesions of alopecia areata at the level of the sebaceous glands show a normal number of pilar units, albeit of a decreased diameter (Swanson et al). The number of circulating T lymphocytes is significantly reduced in nearly all patients with alopecia areata (Brown et al), supporting the assumption that an autoimmune process is responsible for the disorder. Repeated applications of dinitrochlorobenzine (DNCB) on the scalp of patients with alopecia areata previously sensitized to this hapten not only stimulates regrowth of hair but also increases the T-cell population in the blood. This indicates that the mechanism for hair regrowth in alopecia areata treated by DNCB is not irritation but rather an immune T-cell-dependent response (Van Neste et al).

Differential Diagnosis.   For differentiation from trichotillomania, see below.

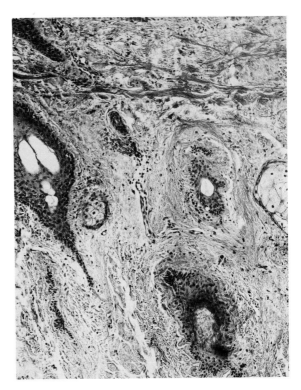

Fig. 11-3.   Alopecia areata, scalp
Three miniature telogen hair structures without hairs are shown. The two structures in the center are each surrounded by a thick fibrous root sheath. The hair structure on the left shows an epithelial cord extending downward into a thickened fibrous root sheath. (×50)

TRICHOTILLOMANIA

Although the temporary hair loss resulting from compulsive hair-pulling does not result in well-demarcated patches of alopecia as usually seen in alopecia areata, differentiation between the two conditions on clinical grounds can be almost impossible, since alopecia areata occasionally also show the "moth-eaten" type of thinning of the hair that is characteristic of trichotillomania.

Histopathology.   The most characteristic feature of trichotillomania is the presence of normally growing hairs among empty hair follicles in a noninflammatory dermis (Muller and Winkelmann). Many of the empty hair follicles show evidence of changing into the catagen state, with transformation of the lower follicular epithelium into a cord of undifferentiated basaloid cells (Mehregan). Evidence of traumatic damage is often seen on the retained portion of partially extracted hairs, such as clefts separating the cells of the hair matrix (Lachapelle and Pierard) and trichomalacia. In the latter condition, the hair shaft within the lower follicular duct appears small, wavy, amorphous, and sometimes corkscrewlike (Mehregan; Lachapelle and Pierard). If the trauma of extraction is severe, one may observe separation of the follicular epithelium from the surrounding sheath of connective tissue and areas of intraepithelial and parafollicular hemorrhage (Mehregan).

Differential Diagnosis.   A histologic differentiation of alopecia areata from trichotillomania is usually possible; alopecia areata, in contrast to trichotillomania, shows many miniature hair structures and a loosely arranged perifollicular inflammatory infiltrate.

PSEUDOPELADE OF BROCQ
(ALOPECIA CICATRISATA)

In pseudopelade of Brocq, also referred to as alopecia cicatrisata, one finds scattered through the scalp irregularly defined and confluent patches of alopecia. In the early stage these patches of alopecia may show mild perifollicular erythema and scaling, but, in the late stage, they show smooth atrophy without any signs of inflammation. Characteristically, a few solitary hairs often persist for a long time within the patches of atrophy.

Although pseudopelade of Brocq generally occurs without any accompanying manifestations, it has been seen in several instances in association with ulcerative lichen planus of the feet (Cram et al; Male) (see p. 151). Also, it is a regular manifestation of the rare Graham Little syndrome. The latter shows, in association with pseudopelade of Brocq, follicular, horny papules that may be grouped or widely disseminated (Kubba and Rook). In addition, there may be nonscarring partial alopecia of the pubic region, axillae, and eyebrows (Spier and Keilig; Pagès et al; Waldorf) and, very rarely, typical, nonfollicular lesions of lichen planus of the skin (Silver et al) or even of the scalp (Gay Prieto). The alopecia may precede by months or years the appearance of the follicular papules on the trunk and limbs (Kubba and Rook).

Histopathology. In the early stage of pseudopelade of Brocq, one finds a moderately severe, predominantly perifollicular infiltrate composed of mononuclear cells. The infiltrate is present around the upper and middle thirds of the hair follicles but spares the lower third (Miescher and Lenggenhager). It invades the walls of the follicles and the sebaceous glands. A mild inflammatory infiltrate is occasionally seen also around the subpapillary vessels (Laymon) and slight follicular hyperkeratosis may be present (Miescher and Lenggenhager). The infiltrate destroys the hair follicles and the sebaceous glands.

In the late stage, there is extensive fibrosis of the dermis with only traces of an inflammatory infiltrate. The follicles and the sebaceous glands are absent, but fibrous cords are often present at the sites of the destroyed hair follicles. They contain a heavy elastic fiber component and therefore are best demonstrated by an elastic tissue stain (Pinkus). The epidermis usually appears normal, with well-developed rete ridges.

Histogenesis. Different opinions exist about the nature of pseudopalade of Brocq, particularly about its relationship to lichen planopilaris. Some authors (Laymon; Miescher and Lenggenhager; Keining and Rathjens; Ronchese; Pinkus) maintain that pseudopelade of Brocq differs clinically and histologically from lichen planopilaris and represents a separate disease entity.

Several other authors have denied the existence of pseudopelade of Brocq as an autonomous disease on the basis of the fact that it represents the atrophic, final "pseudopeladic" stage of several scarring diseases, not only lichen planopilaris and the Graham Little syndrome, but also chronic discoid lupus erythematosus, morphea, and folliculitis decalvans (Degos et al; Juon; Gay Prieto). However, it can be maintained that, in their active phase, chronic discoid lupus erythematosus, morphea, and folliculitis decalvans are quite distinct from pseudopelade of Brocq. This then leaves, aside from an occasional association of pseudopelade of Brocq with ulcerative lichen planus of the feet, lichen planopilaris and the Graham Little syndrome as the two diseases in which the scalp lesions are indistinguishable clinically as well as histologically from pseudopelade of Brocq throughout their course.

Several persuasive arguments speak in favor of the view that pseudopelade of Brocq is a monosymptomatic form of lichen planopilaris and the Graham Little syndrome and that the Graham Little syndrome is an expression of lichen planopilaris (Spier and Keilig; Waldorf; Silver et al; Altman and Perry; Cram et al). There are the findings that (1) pseudopelade of Brocq is regularly present in the Graham Little syndrome; (2) the lesions both in the scalp and on the skin are primarily follicular, leading to destruction of the hair follicle; and (3) all three diseases only rarely show histologically typical lichen planus with involvement of the surface epidermis, although this has been observed occasionally in the cutaneous lesions of the trunk or extremities (Spier and Keilig; Silver et al; Altman and Perry) and the scalp (Gay Prieto; Altman and Perry). Rather, the histologic picture of both the scalp lesions and lesions outside the scalp shows a perifollicular mononuclear infiltrate leading to destruction of the hair (Spier and Keilig; Waldorf). An explanation for the relative rarity of the finding of histologically typical lichen planus in the lesions of lichen planopilaris, the Graham Little syndrome, and pseudopelade of Brocq, whether they are located in the scalp or elsewhere on the skin, is the fairly rapid course of the process of destruction of individual hair follicles, so that often only residual nonspecific inflammation or the end result, that is, fibrosis and absence of pilosebaceous structures, is seen.

Differential Diagnosis. In typical cases of discoid lupus erythematosus, in contrast to pseudopelade of Brocq, the inflammatory infiltrate not only is located around hair follicles and sebaceous glands but also is distributed in a patchy fashion throughout the dermis. In addition, the basal layer of the epidermis, and often also the basal layer of the outer root sheath, shows liquefaction degeneration. There is also more pronounced hyperkeratosis not limited to the follicles.

Circumscribed scleroderma is characterized by thickening and homogenization of the collagen bundles extending into the subcutaneous tissue.

Folliculitis decalvans, which represents a folliculitis of the scalp, in its early stage shows intrafollicular pustules. Often, the perifollicular infiltrate contains a good number of plasma cells, which are absent in alopecia cicatrisata (Miescher and Lenggenhager).

ALOPECIA MUCINOSA

Alopecia mucinosa, also referred to as follicular mucinosis, was first described in 1957 (Pinkus). The disorder shows two types of lesions: grouped follicular papules and red, raised, boggy, occasionally nodular plaques. The two types may occur together. The lesions are devoid of hair, but, except, in the scalp or eyebrows, this is not a conspicuous feature. A primary or idiopathic benign form and a secondary symptomatic form, secondary usually to lymphoma, are recognized.

The primary form, which is more common than the secondary form, is either localized to the head and neck or disseminated, with lesions occurring also on the trunk and limbs. Usually, the lesions resolve spontaneously within 2 months to 2 years, but occasionally, especially in middle-aged or elderly persons, they persist for many years (Emmerson). When the process is widespread and presenting plaques, distinction between the primary and secondary types can be difficult, since the resemblance to mycosis fungoides, clinically and histologically, may be considerable (Kim and Winkelmann). An apparent transition of primary alopecia mucinosa into mycosis fungoides has been described only rarely (Kim and Winkelmann; Plotnick and Abbrecht).

The secondary form, secondary to lymphoma, usually mycosis fungoides, is seen predominantly in elderly persons. It consists of plaques that as a rule are widely disseminated but in rare instances are localized (Binnick et al). From the beginning, the clinical and histologic appearance is that of mycosis fungoides or lymphoma (Emmerson).

In a few instances, follicular mucinosis has been observed in other diseases, such as chronic discoid lupus erythematosus (Cabré and Korting) and angiolymphoid hyperplasia (Wolff et al).

Histopathology. The histologic picture is characterized by mucinous changes in the outer root sheath and sebaceous glands. One observes accumulation of mucin between the cells, which often appear spindle-shaped or stellate and lose their coherence, so that the epithelium appears to have undergone reticular degeneration (Fig. 11-4). This may be followed by the formation of cystic spaces partially filled with mucin (Fig. 11-5) (Johnson et al). Occasionally, however, no mucin is found, probably, because it was removed during fixation on account of its solubility in water (Braun-Falco).

The mucin consists of acid mucopolysaccharides

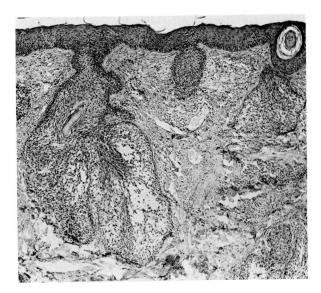

Fig. 11-4. Alopecia mucinosa
The pilosebaceous follicle on the left shows "reticular" degeneration of its cells associated with the presence of mucin. (×40) (Armed Forces Institute of Pathology, No. 57-13780)

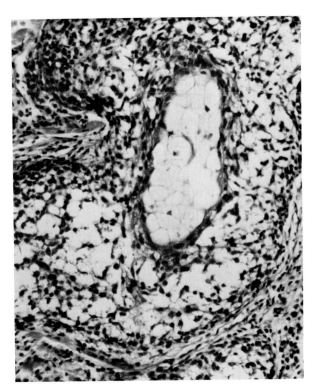

Fig. 11-5. Alopecia mucinosa
The outer root sheath contains cystic spaces as a result of mucinous degeneration of its cells. The sebaceous lobule in the center as yet shows no degeneration. (×100)

that stain metachromatically with the Giemsa stain or toluidine blue and stain with alcian blue. The mucin is largely removed by hyaluronidase. The periodic acid-Schiff (PAS) reaction demonstrates a moderate amount of positive material throughout the involved pilosebaceous apparatus. Most of this material, however, is digested by diastase, an indication that it is glycogen (Johnson et al).

The inflammatory infiltrate in the primary form of alopecia mucinosa is variable in its intensity, but it may be pronounced, especially in boggy, nodular plaques. The infiltrate consists of lymphocytes and histiocytes with a moderate number of eosinophils (Emmerson). In cases with a very dense infiltrate, differentiation from mycosis fungoides may be difficult. Repeat excisions for biopsy are then advisable, since instances of transition into mycosis fungoides have been observed (Kim and Winkelmann; Plotnick and Abbrecht).

Histogenesis. *Electron microscopic examination* of affected outer root sheath cells shows that the mucin is produced by a secretory function of these cells. Their cytoplasm shows a prominent, dilated rough-surfaced endoplasmic reticulum containing fine, granular, filamentous material that is secreted into the intercellular spaces (Ishibashi).

FOX–FORDYCE DISEASE

Fox–Fordyce disease occurs almost exclusively in women. It is characterized by the presence of discrete, firm, follicular, pruritic papules in areas in which apocrine glands are found, namely, in the axillae, the areolae, and the pubic region.

Histopathology.   Fox–Fordyce disease represents an "apocrine miliaria" (Shelley and Levy). The primary event is the formation of a keratotic plug in the uppermost portion of the hair follicle, the infundibulum. This keratotic plug obstructs the ostium of the apocrine duct as it emerges from the follicular wall. A spongiotic vesicle is located within the follicular wall where the apocrine duct has ruptured. The formation of this "apocrine sweat retention vesicle" is followed by acanthosis of the infundibulum and by an inflammatory infiltrate occupying the dermis outside the infundibulum and extending to the vesicle within the follicular wall. Since the vesicle within the follicular wall is small, it can usually be found only when step sections are studied (Mevorah et al; Macmillan and Vickers).

Histogenesis. In Fox–Fordyce disease, complete apocrine anhidrosis exists. Whereas the intradermal injection of a 1:1000 solution of epinephrine into an area of the axilla normally causes apocrine sweat to appear at the follicular orifices, this is not observed in patients with Fox–Fordyce disease (Shelley and Levy).

CHONDRODERMATITIS NODULARIS HELICIS

In chondrodermatitis nodularis helicis, one or, rarely, several nodules are found usually on the apex of the helix of the ear. Occasionally, a nodule may be located instead on the antihelix. The nodules are very tender. They usually measure less than 1 cm in diameter and show in their center either crusting or ulceration. There is no tendency toward spontaneous involution.

Histopathology.   The epidermis overlying the nodule shows irregular acanthosis with hyper- and parakeratosis. In the center, an ulcer is usually seen that may be narrow like a channel or large. It is filled with necrotic dermal debris and covered by a crust (Fig. 11-6) (Goette). The dermis in the center of the lesion shows degenerated homogeneous collagen devoid of nuclei. On both sides of the degenerated collagen, there is richly vascularized granulation tissue composed of lymphocytes, plasma cells, histiocytes, and fibroblasts (Newcomer et al; Shuman and Helwig). Within the vascularized granulation tissue, structures resembling those seen in glomus tumors may be seen occasionally. One may regard these structures as reactive, hyperplastic changes in arteriovenous anastomoses that are normally present in the ear (Haber).

The perichondrium is thickened, and the impression is produced that perichondrial cells migrate upward into the area of dermal necrosis (Leonforte). Frequently, but not always, changes in the cartilage occur. When present, they may vary from merely a diminution in the number of nuclei to focal degeneration. If the degenerative changes are severe, focal calcification and ossification may occur (Garcia e Silva et al).

Histogenesis. It was originally assumed that the primary event in chondrodermatitis nodularis helicis was degeneration of the cartilage. However, several authors (Newcomer et al; Shuman and Helwig; Goette) have pointed out that degenerative changes in the aural cartilage similar to those that may be seen in chondrodermatitis nodularis helicis are commonly found in elderly persons and, furthermore, that changes in the aural cartilage may be absent in chondrodermatitis nodularis helicis. It is now assumed that the initial damage in chondrodermatitis nodularis helicis occurs in the dermis, and that the basically poor blood supply of the ear in conjunction with solar elastosis and repeated minor traumas is probably responsible for the dermal degeneration. The central epidermal channel or ulcer forms for the purpose of transepidermal elimination of the degenerated dermal collagen (Leonforte; Goette; Santa Cruz). Persistence of the lesion can be ascribed to the fact that degenerated perichondrial cells, and in some instances degenerated cartilaginous cells as well, replenish the area of dermal necrosis (Leonforte). It appears possible that the glomoid proliferation of capillaries is responsible for the great tenderness of the lesion (Santa Cruz).

RELAPSING POLYCHONDRITIS

Relapsing polychondritis is an episodic, yet generally progressive inflammation of cartilaginous structures throughout the body. The most common clinical features are bilateral auricular chondritis, polyarthritis, nasal chondritis, ocular inflammation, and respiratory tract chondritis. The mortality is about 25%, usually either from respiratory tract involvement or from cardiac valvular involvement (McAdam et al).

The involvement of the ears and nose consists of intermittent attacks of painful erythema and edema. Ultimately, the ears become soft and flabby because of degeneration of the cartilage, and the nose assumes a saddle-nose deformity (Thurston and Curtis).

Cutaneous lesions occur occasionally. They consist of purpuric or erythema-nodosum-like lesions (McAdam et al; Weinberger and Myers).

Histopathology. Histologically, one observes chondrolysis associated with perichondritis. The overlying dermis of the ear usually appears normal. In early lesions, only the marginal chondrocytes appear degenerated, showing vacuolization, nuclear pyknosis, and loss of their basophilia caused by the release of chondroitin sulfate from their matrix and resulting in faint eosinophilic staining (Valenzuela et al). An elastic tissue stain shows clumping and destruction of the cartilaginous elastic fibers (Feinerman et al). A dense inflammatory infiltrate is present in the perichondrium encroaching upon the cartilage. It contains neutrophils, lymphocytes, and plasma cells as well as macrophages. With succeeding attacks, increasingly more chondrocytes are destroyed and phagocytized and replaced by fibrous tissue (Barranco et al).

Histologic examination of cutaneous lesions has shown a vasculitis with occlusion of vessel lumina and an infiltrate of lymphocytes and eosinophils (Weinberger and Myers). This may be associated with a systemic vasculitis or with an arteritis of the aorta or large arteries (McAdam et al).

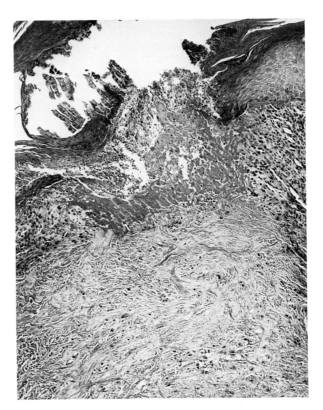

Fig. 11-6. Chondrodermatitis nodularis helicis
The epidermis shows an ulcer that is covered by a crust. Through the ulcer, necrotic dermal debris is being eliminated. On the right, richly vascularized granulation tissue is visible. (×50)

Histogenesis. Circulating antibodies to type II collagen have been detected in patients with relapsing perichondritis. Type II collagen is found exclusively in cartilage and constitutes over 50% of the proteins of cartilage. The antibodies are generally found only in patients with active disease (Foidart and Katz). In addition, circulating immune complexes can often be demonstrated (Foidart et al). Furthermore, direct immunofluorescence testing has shown granular deposits of immunoglobulins and complement along the chondrofibrous junction (Valenzuela et al). These findings suggest that circulating antibodies to type II collagen play an important role in the pathogenesis of relapsing polychondritis (Foidart and Katz).

BIBLIOGRAPHY

Acne Vulgaris
AKERS WA, ALLEN AM, BURNETT JW et al: Systemic antibiotics for treatment of acne vulgaris. Arch Dermatol 111:1630–1636, 1975
COVE JH, CUNLIFFE WJ, HOLLAND KT: Acne vulgaris. Is the bacterial population size significant? Br J Dermatol 102:277–288, 1980

CUNLIFFE WJ, TAN SG: Acne and the sebaceous glands. (Review) Int J Dermatol 15:337–343, 1976

FÖRSTRÖM L: The influence of sex hormones on acne. Acta Derm Venereol (Stockh) Suppl 89:27–31, 1980

FÖRSTRÖM L, MUSTAKALLIO KK, DESSYPRIS A et al: Plasma testosterone levels and acne. Acta Derm Venereol (Stockh) 54:369–371, 1974

HAY JB, HODGKINS MB: Metabolism of androgens by human skin in acne. Br J Dermatol 91:123–133, 1974

KAIDBEY KH, KLIGMAN AM: Pigmentation in comedones. Arch Derm 109:60–62, 1974

KERSEY P, SUSSMAN M, DAHL M: Delayed skin test reactivity to *Proprionibacterium acnes* correlates with severity of inflammation in acne vulgaris. Br J Dermatol 103:651–655, 1980

LAVKER RM, LEYDEN JJ, MCGINLEY KT: The relationship between bacteria and the abnormal follicular keratinization in acne vulgaris. J Invest Dermatol 77:325–330, 1981

LEYDEN JJ, MCGINLEY KJ, MILLS OH et al: Proprionibacterium levels in patients with and without acne vulgaris. J Invest Dermatol 65:382–384, 1975

PLEWIG G: Morphologic dynamics of acne vulgaris. Acta Derm Venereol (Stockh) Suppl 89:9–16, 1980

PLEWIG G, KLIGMAN AM: Acne: Morphogenesis and Treatment. Berlin, Springer-Verlag, 1975

PUHVEL SM, AMIRIAN D, WEINTRAUB J et al: Lymphocyte transformation in subjects with nodulo-cystic acne. Br J Dermatol 97:205–211, 1977

PUHVEL SM, SAKAMATO M: A reevaluation of fatty acids as inflammatory agents in acne. J Invest Dermatol 68:93–97, 1977

RESH W, STOUGHTON RB: Topically applied antibiotics in acne vulgaris. Arch Dermatol 112:182–184, 1976

SANSONE G, REISNER RM: Differential rates of conversion of testosterone to dihydrotestosterone in acne and in normal human skin—A possible pathogenic factor in acne. J Invest Dermatol 56:366–372, 1971

STEINBERGER E, RODRIGUEZ-RIGAU LJ, SMITH KD et al: The menstrual cycle and plasma testosterone levels in women with acne. J Am Acad Dermatol 4:54–58, 1981

STRAUSS JS: In discussion of Zachariae H: Topical vitamin-A-acid in acne. Acta Derm Venereol (Stockh) Suppl 89:68, 1980

STRAUSS JS, KLIGMAN AM: The pathologic dynamics of acne vulgaris. Arch Dermatol 82:779–790, 1960

STRAUSS JS, POCHI PE: Intracutaneous injection of sebum and comedones. Arch Dermatol 92:443–456, 1965

STRAUSS JS, POCHI PE: Recent advances in androgen metabolism and their relation to the skin. Arch Dermatol 100:621–636, 1969

Acne Rosacea

ECKER RI, WINKELMANN RK: Demodex granuloma. Arch Dermatol 115:343–344, 1979

ERLACH E, GEBHART W, NIEBAUER G: Zur Pathogenese der granulomatösen Rosacea. Z Hautkr 51:459–464, 1976

GROSSHANS EM, KREMER M, MALEVILLE J: Demodex folliculorum und die Histogenese der granulomatösen Rosacea. Hautarzt 25:166–177, 1974

LAYMON CW: Lupoid rosacea. Arch Dermatol 63:409–418, 1951

LAYMON CW, MICHELSON HE: The micropapular tuberculid. Arch Dermatol Syph 42:625–640, 1940

LAYMON CW, SCHOCH EP JR: Micropapular tuberculid and rosacea. Arch Dermatol Syph 58:286–300, 1948

LEWANDOWSKY F: Über rosacea-ähnliche Tuberkulide des Gesichtes. Korresp-Bl Schweiz Ärz 47:1280–1282, 1917

MARKS R, HARCOURT-WEBSTER JN: Histopathology of rosacea. Arch Dermatol 100:683–691, 1969

MULLANAX MG, KIERLAND RR: Granulomatous rosacea. Arch Dermatol 101:206–211, 1970

PINKUS H, MEHREGAN AH: A Guide to Dermatohistopathology, 2nd ed, p 298–299. New York, Appleton-Century-Crofts, 1976

SCOTT KW, CALNAN CD: Acne agminata. Trans St John's Hosp Dermatol Soc 53:60–69, 1967

SIMON N: Ist der Lupus miliaris disseminatus tuberkulöser Ätiologie? Hautarzt 26:625–630, 1975

SNAPP RH: Lewandowsky's rosacea-like eruption. J Invest Dermatol 13:175–190, 1949

STRAUSS H: Katamnestische Untersuchungen von Fäilen mit Tuberkulid. Arch Dermatol Syph (Berlin) 198:417–434, 1954

UEKI H, MASUDA T: Lupus miliaris disseminatus faciei. Hautarzt 30:553–555, 1979

VEIEN NK, STAHL D, BRODTHAGEN H: Granulomatous rosacea treated with tetracycline. Dermatologica 163:267–269, 1981

Disseminate Infundibulofolliculitis

HITCH JM, LUND HZ: Disseminate and recurrent infundibulofolliculitis. Arch Dermatol 97:432–435, 1968

HITCH JM, LUND HZ: Disseminate and recurrent infundibulofolliculitis. Arch Dermatol 105:580–583, 1972

OWEN WR, WOOD C: Disseminate and recurrent infundibulofolliculitis. Arch Dermatol 115:174–175, 1979

Eosinophilic Pustular Folliculitis

GUILLAUME JC, DUBERTRET L, COSNES A et al: Folliculite à éosinophiles (maladie d'Ofuji). Ann Dermatol Venereol 106:347–350, 1979

HOLST R: Eosinophilic pustular folliculitis. Br J Dermatol 95:661–664, 1976

ISHIBASHI A, NISHIYAMA Y, MIYATA C et al: Eosinophilic pustular folliculitis (Ofuji). Dermatologica 149:240–247, 1974

OFUJI S, OGINO A, HORIO T et al: Eosinophilic pustular folliculitis. Acta Derm Venereol (Stockh) 50:195–203, 1970

ORFANOS CE, STERRY W: Sterile eosinophile Pustulose. Dermatologica 157:193–205, 1978

Eosinophilic Cellulitis (Wells' Syndrome)

MARKS R: Eosinophilic cellulitis. Aust J Dermatol 21:10–12, 1980

NIELSEN T, SCHMIDT H, SØGAARD H: Eosinophilic cellulitis (Wells' syndrome) in a child. Arch Dermatol 117:427–429, 1981

SPIGEL GT, WINKELMANN RK: Wells' syndrome. Arch Dermatol 115:611–613, 1979

WELLS GC: Recurrent granulomatous dermatitis with eosinophilia. Trans St John's Hosp Dermatol Soc 57:46–56, 1971

WELLS GC, SMITH NP: Eosinophilic cellulitis. Br J Dermatol 100:101–109, 1979

Trichorrhexis Invaginata (Netherton's Syndrome)

ALTMAN J, STROUD J: Netherton's syndrome and ichthyosis linearis circumflexa. Psoriasiform ichthyosis. Arch Dermatol 100:550–558, 1969

HURWITZ S, KIRSCH N, MCGUIRE I: Reevaluation of ichthyosis and hair shaft abnormalities. Arch Dermatol 103:266–271, 1971

JULIUS CE, KEERAN M: Netherton's syndrome in a male. Arch Dermatol 104:422–424, 1971

NETHERTON EW: A unique case of trichorrhexis nodosa: "Bamboo hairs." Arch Dermatol 78:483–487, 1958

Trichostasis Spinulosa

BRAUN-FALCO O, VAKILZADEH F: Trichostasis spinulosa. Hautarzt 18:501–504, 1967

GOLDSCHMIDT H, HOJYO-TOMOKA MT, KLIGMAN AM: Trichostasis spinulosa. Hautarzt 26:299–303, 1975

SARKANY J, GAYLARDE PM: Trichostasis spinulosa and its management. Br J Dermatol 84:311–315, 1971

Alopecia Areata

BROWN AC, OLKOWSKI ZL, MCLAREN JR: Thymus lymphocytes of the peripheral blood in patients with alopecia areata. Arch Dermatol 113:688, 1977

GOOS M: Zur Histopathologie der Alopecia areata. Arch Dermatol Forsch 240:160–172, 1971

KALKOFF KW, MACHER E: Über das Nachwachsen der Haare bei der Alopecia areata und maligna nach intracutaner Hydrocortisoninjektion. Hautarzt 9:441–451, 1958

SWANSON NA, MITCHELL AJ, LEAHY MS et al: Topical treatment of alopecia areata. Arch Dermatol 117:384–387, 1981

VAN NESTE D, DEBRUYÈRE M, BREUILLARD F: Immunotherapy of alopecia areata. Arch Dermatol Res 266:323–325, 1979

VAN SCOTT EJ: Morphologic changes in pilosebaceous units and anagen hairs in alopecia areata. J Invest Dermatol 31:35–43, 1958

Trichotillomania

LACHAPELLE JM, PIERARD GE: Traumatic alopecia in trichotillomania. J Cutan Pathol 4:51–67, 1977

MEHREGAN AH: Trichotillomania. Arch Dermatol 102:129–133, 1970

MULLER SA, WINKELMANN RK: Trichotillomania. Arch Dermatol 105:535–540, 1972

Pseudopelade of Brocq (Alopecia Cicatrisata)

ALTMAN J, PERRY HO: The variations and course of lichen planus. Arch Dermatol 84:179–191, 1961

CRAM DL, KIERLAND RR, WINKELMANN RK: Ulcerative lichen planus of the feet. Arch Dermatol 93:692–701, 1966

DEGOS R, RABUT R, DUPERRAT B et al: L'état pseudo-peladique. Réflexions à propos de cent cas d'alopécies cicatricielles en aires, d'apparence primitive du type pseudopelade. Ann Dermatol Syph 81:5–26, 1954

GAY PRIETO J: Pseudopelade of Brocq: Its relationship to some forms of cicatricial alopecias and to lichen planus. J Invest Dermatol 24:323–335, 1955

JUON M: Le problème des états pseudopeladiques ou pseudo-peladoides dans le cadre des alopécies cicatricielles. Dermatologica 133:66–75, 1966

KEINING E, RATHJENS B: Versuch einer Abgrenzung des Graham Little-Syndroms. Dermatol Wochenschr 132:1016–1023, 1955

KUBBA R, ROOK A: The Graham-Little syndrome: Follicular keratosis with cicatricial alopecia. Br J Dermatol 93, Suppl 11:53–55, 1975

LAYMON CW: The cicatricial alopecias. J Invest Dermatol 8:99–122, 1947

MALE O: Über die ulzerös-atrophisierende Form des Lichen ruber planus. Z Hautkr 45:17–28, 1970

MIESCHER G, LENGGENHAGER R: Über Pseudopelade Brocq. Dermatologica 94:122–130, 1947

PAGÈS E, LAPEYRE J, MISSON R: Syndrome de Lassueur-Graham-Little. Ann Dermatol Syph 88:272–278, 1961

PINKUS H: Differential patterns of elastic fibers in scarring and non-scarring alopecias. J Cutan Pathol 5:93–104, 1978

RONCHESE F: Pseudopelade. Arch Dermatol 82:336–343, 1960

SILVER H, CHARGIN L, SACHS PM: Follicular lichen planus (lichen planopilaris). Arch Dermatol 67:346–354, 1953

SPIER HW, KEILIG W: Lichen ruber follicularis decalvans (Graham Little-Syndrom) und seine Beziehungen zur Pseudopelade Brocq. Hautarzt 4:457–467, 1953

WALDORF DS: Lichen planopilaris. Arch Dermatol 93:684–691, 1966

Alopecia Mucinosa

BINNICK AN, WAX FD, CLENDENNING WE: Alopecia mucinosa of the face associated with mycosis fungoides. Arch Dermatol 114:791–792, 1978

BRAUN-FALCO O: In the discussion of Zambal Z: Ablagerungen in der Haut bei Alopecia mucinosa. Arch Klin Exp Dermatol 237:155, 1970

CABRÉ J, KORTING GW: Zum symptomatischen Charakter der "Mucinosis follicularis": Ihr Vorkommen beim Lupus erythematodes chronicus. Dermatol Wochenschr 149:513–518, 1964

EMMERSON RW: Follicular mucinosis. Br J Dermatol 81:395–413, 1969

ISHIBASHI A: Histogenesis of mucin in follicular mucinosis. An electron microscopic study. Acta Derm Venereol (Stockh) 56:163–171, 1976

JOHNSON WC, HIGDON RS, HELWIG EB: Alopecia mucinosa. Arch Dermatol 79:395–406, 1959

KIM R, WINKELMANN RK: Follicular mucinosis (alopecia mucinosa). Arch Dermatol 85:490–498, 1962

PINKUS H: Alopecia mucinosa. Arch Dermatol 76:419–426, 1957

PLOTNICK H, ABBRECHT M: Alopecia mucinosa and lymphoma. Arch Dermatol 92:137–141, 1965

WOLFF HH, KINNEY J, ACKERMAN AB: Angiolymphoid hyperplasia with follicular mucinosis. Arch Dermatol 114:229–232, 1978

Fox–Fordyce Disease

MACMILLAN DC, VICKERS HR: Fox–Fordyce disease. Br J Dermatol 84:181, 1971

MEVORAH B, DUBOFF GS, WASS RW: Fox–Fordyce disease in prepubescent girls. Dermatologica 136:43–56, 1968

SHELLEY WB, LEVY EJ: Apocrine sweat retention in man. II. Fox–Fordyce disease (apocrine miliaria). Arch Dermatol 73:38–49, 1956

Chondrodermatitis Nodularis Helicis

GARCIA E SILVA L, MARTINS O, DA SILVA PICOTO A: Bone formation in chondrodermatitis nodularis helicis. J Dermatol Surg Oncol 6:582–585, 1980

GOETTE DK: Chondrodermatitis nodularis chronica helicis: A perforating necrobiotic granuloma. J Am Acad Dermatol 2:148–154, 1980

HABER H: Chondrodermatitis nodularis chronica helicis. Hautarzt 11:122–127, 1960

LEONFORTE JE: Le nodule douloureux de l'oreille: Hyperplasie épidermique avec élimination transépithéliale. Ann Dermatol Venereol 106:577–581, 1979

NEWCOMER VD, STEFFEN CG, STERNBERG TH et al: Chondrodermatitis nodularis chronica helicis. Arch Dermatol 68:241–255, 1953

SANTA CRUZ DJ: Chondrodermatitis nodularis helicis: A transepidermal perforating disorder. J Cutan Pathol 7:70–76, 1980

SHUMAN R, HELWIG EB: Chondrodermatitis helicis. Am J Clin Pathol 24:126–144, 1954

Relapsing Polychondritis

BARRANCO VP, MINOR DB, SOLOMON H: Treatment of polychondritis with dapsone. Arch Dermatol 112:1286–1288, 1976

FEINERMAN LK, JOHNSON WC, WEINER J et al: Relapsing polychondritis. Dermatologica 140:369–377, 1970

FOIDART JM, ABE S, MARTIN GR et al: Antibodies to type II collagen in relapsing polychondritis. N Engl J Med 299:1203–1207, 1978

FOIDART JM, KATZ SI: Relapsing polychondritis. Am J Dermatopathol 1:257–260, 1979

MCADAM LP, O'HANLAN MA, BLUESTONE R et al: Relapsing polychondritis: Prospective study of 23 patients and a review of the literature. Medicine 55:193–215, 1976

THURSTON CS, CURTIS AC: Relapsing polychondritis. Arch Dermatol 93:664–669, 1966

VALENZUELA R, COOPERRIDER PA, GOGATE P et al: Relapsing polychondritis. Hum Pathol 11:19–22, 1980

WEINBERGER A, MYERS AR: Relapsing polychrondritis associated with cutaneous vasculitis. Arch Dermatol 115:980–981, 1979

Inflammatory Diseases Due to Physical Agents and Foreign Substances

12

POLYMORPHOUS LIGHT ERUPTION

Polymorphous light eruption represents an abnormal reaction to sunlight. The onset is any time after puberty. Only exposed areas are affected. Its occurrence in the temperate zone is confined to the period from late spring to early autumn (Calnan and Meara). The eruption appears from 4 hr to 24 hr after exposure to the sun. When protected from direct sunlight, it subsides within a few days. Four types of eruptions may be seen in exposed areas: a papular type, a papulovesicular type, a plaque type, and a diffuse erythematous type. Not infrequently, several of these four types of eruption are present together.

In the papular type, scattered edematous papules are present. In the papulovesicular type, the papules are associated with vesicles and crusting. Lesions of the plaque type are red, slightly edematous, and indurated. They show a close clinical resemblance to the early lesions of chronic discoid lupus erythematosus as well as to those of Jessner's lymphocytic infiltration of the skin. The lesions of the diffuse erythematous type have the clinical appearance of lupus erythematosus, except for their strict limitation to sun-exposed areas.

In polymorphous light eruption, the sunburn spectrum, or UVB, comprising rays in the range from 290 nm to 320 nm, makes up the clinical action spectrum (Fisher et al). In most instances, polymorphous light eruption responds well to treatment with antimalarial drugs of the 4-aminoquinoline group, such as chloroquine.

Histopathology. In the papular, the papulovesicular, and the diffuse erythematous types of eruption, the histologic picture is nonspecific (Meara et al).

In the plaque type, the histologic picture shows a patchy infiltrate of lymphoid cells resembling that seen in early lesions of lupus erythematosus, except that the infiltrate is apt to be arranged around blood vessels rather than around the pilosebaceous structures, and liquefaction degeneration of the cells of the basal layer is absent (Fig. 12-1) (Wright and Winer). Yet differentiation is not always possible, since, in early lesions of discoid lupus erythematosus, hydropic degeneration of the basal layer may be absent (see p. 447). In addition, the plaque type of polymorphous light eruption must be differentiated from Jessner's lymphocytic infiltration, lymphoma, and pseudolymphoma of Spiegler–Fendt. (For a discussion of this differentiation, see p. 449.)

Histogenesis. Phototesting with wavelengths shorter than 320 nm is valuable in establishing the existence of light sensitivity, but it does not rule out lupus erythematosus, since approximately one third of patients with lupus erythematosus give positive phototests with short ultraviolet rays (Fisher et al). However, immunofluorescence testing usually permits a distinction, since on direct testing, deposits of immunoglobulins and complement are found in lesions of lupus erythematosus but not in those of polymorphous light eruption (Chorzelski et al; Fisher et al). On the other hand, testing for the presence of antinuclear antibodies is of limited value; if undilated serum is used, the test is nearly always negative in polymorphous light eruption, but it is negative also in nearly one half of the patients with discoid lupus erythematosus (Peterson and Fusaro).

Differential Diagnosis. Before accepting polymorphous light eruption as the diagnosis, it is necessary to exclude not only lupus erythematosus

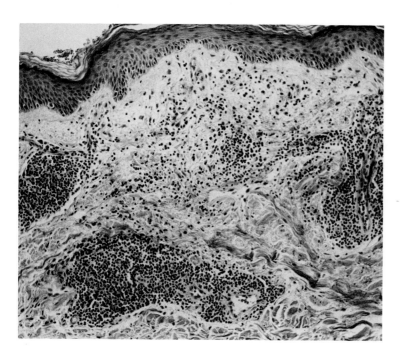

Fig. 12-1. Polymorphous light eruption, plaque type
A patchy infiltrate of lymphoid cells is present in the dermis, as in discoid lupus erythematosus. However, there is no hydropic degeneration of the basal cells. ($\times 100$)

and the other above-mentioned diseases but also porphyria of the papular and papulovesicular types. (For a discussion of the latter differentiation, see p. 418.)

Actinic Prurigo

Actinic prurigo, also referred to as Hutchinson's summer prurigo, differs sufficiently from polymorphous light eruption to be regarded as a separate entity. It is common among American Indians (Everett et al; Scheen et al) but occurs also in Europe, especially in England (Meara et al; Calnan and Meara).

Actinic prurigo, in contrast to polymorphous light eruption, almost always has its onset before puberty. It shows primarily prurigolike papules, but there may also be eczematous patches. Although worst in the summer, lesions are often present throughout the year, and they often involve covered as well as exposed parts of the skin. It thus represents a chronic disease. Skin testing for photosensitivity has yielded inconsistent results (Scheen et al). There is no response to treatment with antimalarials (Everett et al).

Histopathology.   The findings are nonspecific and are those of a subacute or chronic dermatitis. One observes irregular acanthosis, a lymphocytic infiltrate in the dermis, and often also epidermal spongiosis and overlying crusting (Everett et al; Scheen et al).

HYDROA VACCINIFORME

In hydroa vacciniforme, vesicles and papulovesicles develop on an erythematous base in sun-exposed areas of the body. As the vesicles undergo necrosis, they first become umbilicated and then crusted (Jaschke et al). The disorder usually starts in early childhood and tends to improve in adolescence. Generally, there are no active lesions during the winter months (McGrae and Perry). There is a good response to treatment with drugs of the 4-aminoquinoline group.

Histopathology.   The earliest lesion is an intraepidermal vesicle that is multilocular owing to reticular degeneration. The underlying dermis may show hemorrhage and thrombosis of the vessels in addition to inflammation (Bickers et al). Subsequently, one finds at the site of the blister necrosis of the epidermis and of the subjacent dermis (Fig. 12-2). The area of necrosis in the dermis appears homogeneous and eosinophilic. A cellular infiltrate surrounds the area of necrosis (McGrae and Perry).

Histogenesis. It is generally agreed that hydroa vacciniforme represents a disease entity apart from polymorphous light eruption because of its different clinical and histologic appearance, which is characterized by umbilicated vesicles, necrosis, and scarring (McGrae and Perry; Jaschke et al; Bickers et al). The action spectrum is not known, since it has not been possible to reproduce the lesions of hydroa vacciniforme with artificial light sources (McGrae and Perry; Jaschke et al; Bickers et al).

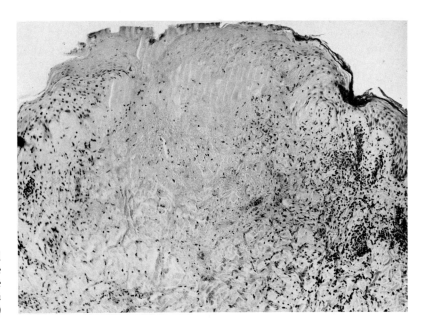

Fig. 12-2. Hydroa vacciniforme
There is necrosis of the epidermis and of the subjacent dermis at the site previously occupied by a blister. The area of necrosis is walled off by a chronic inflammatory infiltrate. ($\times 100$)

Differential Diagnosis. Even though erythropoietic protoporphyria shows more edema than hydroa vacciniforme, and only rarely vesicles, this diagnosis should always be excluded by appropriate porphyrin studies (p. 416).

CHRONIC PHOTOSENSITIVITY DERMATITIS, ACTINIC RETICULOID

The terms *chronic photosensitivity dermatitis* and *actinic reticuloid* refer to a spectrum of chronic photosensitivity reactions varying from a localized lichenified dermatitis of exposed sites to the fully developed picture of actinic reticuloid. Intermediate stages between these two extremes occur both clinically and histologically (Frain-Bell et al, 1974). Both conditions occur almost entirely in elderly men.

Patients with actinic reticuloid at first show erythema and lichenified plaques only in exposed areas, but the eruption gradually spreads to cover most of the skin surface as a generalized erythroderma. The exposed skin may show considerable thickening resulting in deep furrows (Ive et al). Itching is severe. The eruption clears slowly when the patient is confined to a darkened room illuminated by incandescent bulbs rather than by fluorescent lighting (Ive et al; Johnson et al).

Histopathology. In chronic photosensitivity dermatitis, the histologic changes are mild and nonspecific, consisting of spongiosis, patchy parakeratosis, and a superficial, perivascular infiltrate of mononuclear cells, often with an admixture of eosinophils (Frain-Bell et al, 1974).

In actinic reticuloid, the infiltrate is dense and bandlike in the upper part of the dermis and may extend into the lower dermis. The cells of the infiltrate are largely lymphoid cells and histiocytes, with an admixture of eosinophils and plasma cells. However, the similarity to mycosis fungoides is often great, not only as a result of the density of the infiltrate, but also because of the presence of hyperchromatic nuclei resembling mycosis cells and their invasion into the epidermis, where they may form aggregates resembling Pautrier microabscesses (Ive et al; Degos et al; Johnson et al; Guardiola and Sánchez; Brody and Bergfeld). Also, in several patients, circulating Sézary cells were found exceeding 10% of the total white blood cell count (Johnson et al; Neild et al).

In spite of its clinical and histologic resemblance to mycosis fungoides, actinic reticuloid is benign and reversible. There are three reports of lymphoma developing in patients with actinic reticuloid: in one patient in the skin of the groin (Jensen and Sneddon), and in two patients in the lymph nodes (Thomsen; Perrot et al). It is significant, however, that the disease did not eventuate in mycosis fungoides in any of the reported patients.

Histogenesis. In the original report published in 1969 (Ive et al), it was stressed that the action spectrum in actinic reticuloid lay in the longwave ultraviolet radiation range (UVA), between 320 nm and 400 nm, and frequently extended into the visible range. Since then, however, it has become evident that short ultraviolet wavelengths (UVB), which are between 290 nm and

320 nm, also frequently produce abnormal morphologic responses (Frain-Bell et al; Johnson et al).

Many patients with photosensitivity dermatitis or actinic reticuloid have been found to have a contact allergic sensitivity to oleoresin extracts from *Compositae* plants (Frain-Bell and Johnson), and some patients are sensitive to chrysanthemum oleoresin extract (Frain-Bell et al, 1979).

ERYTHEMA AB IGNE

Prolonged exposure to moderate heat emanating from fireplaces, radiators, or heating pads causes a persistent reticular erythema with or without pigmentation. The shins and buttocks are the most common sites.

Histopathology. The epidermis appears flattened. On staining with hematoxylin-eosin, the collagen bundles are seen to be reduced in thickness, and the fibers appear fragmented and disrupted. There is no basophilia as seen in solar elastosis (Shahrad and Marks). On staining for elastic tissue, a great increase in the amount of elastic fibers is seen in the upper dermis and the midportion of the dermis (Finlayson et al; Johnson and Butterworth). There is, however, no homogenization with loss of fibrous structure as seen in solar elastosis (Shahrad and Marks). In most cases, melanin granules are found in the upper dermis, and in some cases hemosiderin as well.

The development of "thermal keratoses" and of in situ carcinoma of the Bowen type has been reported to occur on the shins (Shahrad and Marks; Arrington and Lockman).

Differential Diagnosis. The absence of basophilic staining of the collagen and of homogenization of the elastic fibers differentiates erythema ab igne from solar (actinic) degeneration (see p. 271).

RADIATION DERMATITIS

An early (acute) stage and a late (chronic) stage of radiation dermatitis are recognized. Early radiation dermatitis develops after large doses of x-radiation or radium. Erythema develops within about a week. This may heal with desquamation and pigmentation. If the dose was high enough, painful blisters may develop at the site of erythema. In that case, healing usually takes place with atrophy, telangiectasia, and irregular hyperpigmentation. Subsequent to very large doses, ulceration occurs, generally within 2 months. Such an ulcer may heal ultimately with severe atrophic scarring, or it may not heal.

Late (chronic) radiation dermatitis occurs from a few months to many years after the administration of fractional doses of x-rays or radium. The skin shows atrophy, telangiectasia, and irregular hyper- and hypopigmentation. Ulceration, as well as foci of hyperkeratosis, may be seen within the areas of atrophy. Squamous cell carcinomas or basal cell epitheliomas may develop. The former tend to arise in areas of severe radiation damage, and the latter in areas in which the radiation damage is rather mild (Lazar and Cullen).

Histopathology. In *early radiation dermatitis*, there is intracellular edema of the epidermis with pyknosis of the nuclei. The cells of the hair follicles, sebaceous glands, and sweat glands also show degenerative changes. An inflammatory infiltrate is seen throughout the dermis and may permeate the epidermis. Some of the blood vessels are dilated, whereas others, especially large ones in the deep portions of the dermis, show edema of their walls, endothelial proliferation, and even thrombosis (Epstein). The collagen bundles show edema. In cases with blisters, the degenerated epidermis is detached from the dermis, and, if ulceration is present, not only the epidermis but also the upper dermis have undergone necrosis. The area of necrosis is then surrounded by neutrophils.

In *late radiation dermatitis*, the epidermis is irregular, showing atrophy in some areas and variable hyperplasia in others. Hyperkeratosis is common. The cells of the stratum malpighii show degenerative changes, such as edema and homogenization. In addition, they may show a disorderly arrangement and individual cell keratinization. Some of the nuclei may be atypical. The epidermis may also show irregular downward growth and may even grow around telangiectatic vessels, which thus may become nearly enclosed in the epidermis (Fig. 12-3).

In the dermis, the collagen bundles are swollen and often show hyalinization. They may stain irregularly and appear faintly eosinophilic in some areas and deeply eosinophilic in others. In response to the degeneration of collagen, new collagen may form throughout the dermis. Striking and rather typical changes may be observed on the blood vessels. Those located in the deep portions of the dermis often show fibrous thickening of their walls, so that the lumen may be nearly or entirely occluded (Fig. 12-4). Some of the vessels show thrombosis and recanalization. In contrast, the vessels of the upper dermis may show telangiectasia. Also, there may be lymphedema in the subepidermal region. Hair structures and sebaceous glands are absent, but the sweat glands usually are preserved at least in part, except in areas of severe injury.

In severe cases of late radiation dermatitis, ulceration occurs. The deep-lying, large blood vessels in the regions of such ulcers often show complete occlusion.

Squamous cell carcinomas arising in late radiation dermatitis often show a high degree of malignancy with a tendency to metastasize. Frequently, they are of the spindle cell type (Sims and Kirsch) (see p. 501). Basal cell epitheliomas tend to be less invasive and destructive (Anderson and Anderson; Totten et al). The occurrence of a fibrosarcoma is rare. A few quite convincing cases of fibrosarcoma have been reported (Blom-Ides; Maggiora et al); however, in most instances, the diagnosis of spindle cell squamous cell carcinoma cannot be ruled out conclusively, because differentiation between this type of carcinoma and fibrosarcoma may be nearly impossible (see p. 612).

Differential Diagnosis.   The epidermal changes of late radiation dermatitis may be similar to those of either an atrophic or a hyperplastic solar keratosis. However, the dermal changes differ. In solar keratosis, there is basophilic degeneration of the collagen limited to the upper dermis, whereas, in late radiation dermatitis, degenerative changes of the collagen extend deep into the dermis.

Subcutaneous Fibrosis After Megavoltage Radiotherapy

Supervoltage radiation permits the concentration of the dose to be centered well below the skin surface at the site of deep tumors. It may lead, however, to the development of subcutaneous fibrosis several months after radiotherapy. In order for recurrent tumor to be ruled out, a deep biopsy, including muscle, is needed.

Histopathology.   Histologic examination shows a band of fibrosis overlying degenerated skeletal

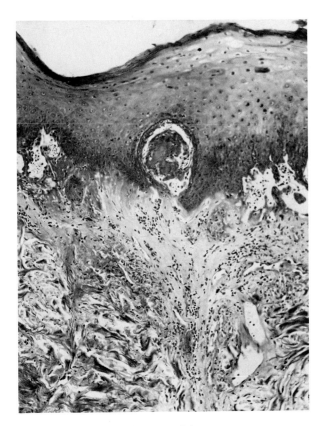

Fig. 12-3.   Late radiodermatitis
The epidermis shows irregular acanthosis and downward growth around a telangiectatic blood vessel. The collagen shows degeneration. ($\times 100$)

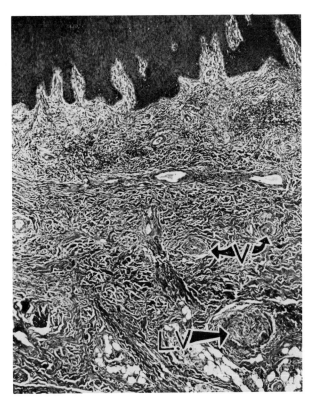

Fig. 12-4.   Late radiodermatitis
The walls of the vessels ($V.$) show fibrotic thickening. A large vessel ($L.V.$) at the junction of dermis and subcutis shows thrombosis. The collagenous bundles of the dermis appear sclerotic. ($\times 50$)

muscle. The blood vessels show thickening of the walls and endothelial proliferation (James and Odom).

CALCANEAL PETECHIAE (BLACK HEEL)

An asymptomatic, pigmented, macular lesion is found on one or both heels immediately above the hyperkeratotic border of the foot. The margin of the lesion is ill defined and speckled. The lesion is traumatic in origin and is caused by any sport, such as basketball, tennis, or football, that leads to slamming of the foot against the shoe. The importance of the lesion lies in its resemblance to a malignant melanoma.

Histopathology. Extravasated erythrocytes may be found in the dermal papillae (Crissey and Peachey). Often, however, the histologic changes are limited to the stratum corneum, where one observes rounded collections of amorphous, yellow brown material representing lysed red blood cells (Vakilzadeh and Happle). The amorphous material does not stain blue with Perls' stain, as hemosiderin would do. However, positive peroxidase and benzidine reactions prove that the material is derived from hemoglobin (Kirton and Price).

Histogenesis. Small foci of hemorrhages move from the tips of the dermal papillae into the epidermis and are found in the thick keratin layer of the heel (Mehregan). The Perls' stain for iron is negative because of the absence of phagocytosis of the lysed red blood cells in the stratum corneum (Rufli).

SCABIES

Scabies, caused by the itch mite *Acarus scabiei*, presents burrows as its characteristic lesion. The burrows, which are produced by female mites, occur mainly on the palms, the palmar and lateral aspects of the fingers, the web spaces between the fingers, the flexor surfaces of the wrists, the nipples of women, and the genitals of men. They appear as fine, tortuous, blackish threads a few millimeters long. Often, a vesicle is visible near the blind end of the burrow. The mite is situated in this vesicle and often is visible as a tiny gray speck. In addition, a papular pruritic eruption is present, usually without recognizable burrows. It is most pronounced on the abdomen, the lower portions of the buttocks, and the anterior axillary folds. In some patients, itching nodules persist for several months after successful treatment. They are found most commonly on the scrotum and represent lesions that at one time harbored mites but no longer contain them.

In a rare variant, so-called Norwegian scabies, innumerable mites are present. Patients with this variant show widespread erythema, hyperkeratosis, and crusting but no obvious burrows.

Histopathology. A definitive diagnosis of scabies can be made only by demonstration of the mite. For this purpose, a very superficial epidermal shave biopsy of an early papule or, preferably, of an entire burrow may be carried out with a scalpel blade (Martin and Wheeler). Local anesthesia is not required. The biopsy specimen is placed on a glass slide, and a drop of immersion oil and then a coverslip are placed on top of it.

Histologic examination of a specimen containing a burrow reveals that the burrow in almost its entire length is located within the horny layer. Only the extreme, blind end of the burrow, where the female mite is situated, extends into the stratum malpighii (Hejazi and Mehregan). The mite has a rounded body and measures about 400 μm in length (Fig. 12-5) (Orkin and Maibach). Spongiosis is present in the stratum malpighii near the mite to such an extent that formation of a vesicle is often the result. Even if no mite is found in the sections, the presence of eggs within the horny layer is indicative of scabies (Fernandez et al). The dermal infiltrate in sections containing mites shows

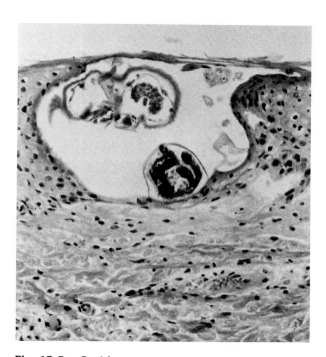

Fig. 12-5. Scabies
A female mite is located within a subcorneal burrow. (× 400)

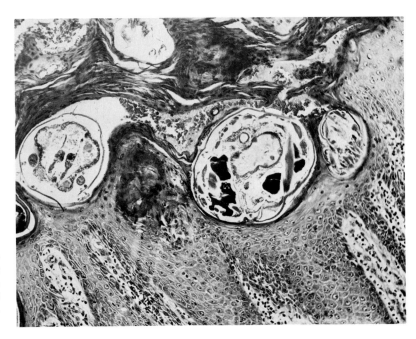

Fig. 12-6. Scabies (Norwegian scabies)
Multiple subcorneal burrows containing female mites are present. There are also hyperkeratosis, acanthosis, and a marked dermal cellular infiltrate. (×200) (Courtesy of Robert N. Buchanan, Jr., M.D.)

varying numbers of eosinophils (Falk and Eide). Papular lesions not containing mites show a nonspecific picture in which eosinophils generally are absent (Falk and Eide).

The persistent nodules of scabies show a dense, chronic inflammatory infiltrate in which eosinophils may be present (Fernandez et al) or absent (Falk and Eide). The blood vessels may have thickened walls, and there may even be vasculitis with fibrinoid deposits and inflammatory cells within the vessel walls (Fernandez et al). Atypical mononuclear cells may be found, and, in some instances, the nodules show, as in persistent arthropod bites or stings (see p. 220), a histologic picture resembling lymphoma (Thomsen et al). Mites are hardly ever found.

In Norwegian scabies, the thickened horny layer is riddled with innumerable mites, so that nearly every section shows several parasites (Fig. 12-6) (Fernandez et al).

Histogenesis. Both cell-mediated and humoral hypersensitivity are activated in scabies. For cell-mediated hypersensitivity speaks the acute eczematoid reaction in the epidermis and for humoral hypersensitivity, the presence of immunoglobulin M (IgM) and the third component of complement (C3) in vessel walls and occasionally also along the dermal-epidermal junction (Hoefling and Schroeter). Intradermal testing with an extract prepared from adult female scabies mites shows a positive reaction indicative of the humoral or immediate type of hypersensitivity only in patients who have had scabies within the preceding year (Falk and Bolle). Norwegian scabies is seen generally in persons who have a congenital or iatrogenic impairment of their immune responses but also in the mentally deficient and the physically debilitated (Dick et al).

SUBCUTANEOUS DIROFILARIASIS

Subcutaneous infection of humans by *Dirofilaria* is rare. The infection, transmitted by mosquitoes, may occur throughout the southern, eastern, and midwestern states of the United States (Billups et al). One or, occasionally, several well-defined, firm, slightly red, tender nodules 1 cm to 2 cm in diameter are present (Payan).

Histopathology. The subcutaneous nodule shows in its center a tightly convoluted worm seen in multiple transverse and diagonal sections. Transverse sections measure 125 μm to 250 μm in diameter (Fisher et al; Billups et al). The worm, often partially degenerated, possesses a thick, laminated cuticle (Payan). It is embedded in eosinophilic, fibrinoid material and surrounded by an inflammatory reaction that includes mononuclear cells, many eosinophils, and, often, foreign body giant cells (Fisher et al; Payan).

Histogenesis. The usual hosts of *Dirofilaria* are dogs, in whom the worm causes so-called heartworm disease. From these animals, mosquitoes may transmit microfilariae to humans, who act as terminal hosts (Billups et al).

ONCHOCERCIASIS

Onchocerciasis is common in certain regions of Central America, Venezuela, and tropical Africa. It is transmitted by black flies; through their proboscis, the infective larvae of *Onchocerca* enter the human skin. They mature to the adult stage in the subcutaneous tissue. The adult filariae or worms become clinically apparent as asymptomatic subcutaneous nodules called onchocercomas, of which there are usually only a few, ranging in size from 0.5 cm to 2 cm. The adult worms do not cause any harm; however, their progeny, consisting of millions of microfilariae, live in the dermis and the aqueous humor of the eyes, where they provoke inflammatory changes after several years. Clinically, onchocercal dermatitis is characterized by itching, edema, lichenification, and pigment shifting. Later on, the skin becomes atrophic. In the eyes, iritis may result in blindness. On slit lamp examination, the microfilariae in the anterior chamber of the eyes may be seen to be moving actively (Connor et al).

Histopathology.   The onchocercomas show at their periphery a chronic inflammatory infiltrate and fibrosis. Their center consists of dense fibrous tissue containing transverse and diagonal sections of adult worms measuring from 100 μm to 500 μm in their transverse diameter (Fig. 12-7). Some of them are alive at the time of biopsy. Dead worms are surrounded by an inflammatory reaction containing foreign body giant cells. Microfilariae, hatched by female worms, are seen occasionally within lymphatic vessels of the onchocercomas, through which they are disseminated in the skin.

They measure from 5 μm to 9 μm in diameter and from 150 μm to 360 μm in length (Piers and Fasal).

In onchocercal dermatitis, numerous microfilariae are seen within the dermis. They are found in greatest number close to the epidermis. In early infections, reactive changes in the dermis are minimal, but, in the course of years, chronic inflammatory cells and eosinophils accumulate around the vessels, and, ultimately, fibrosis of the dermis and flattening of the epidermis result (Connor et al).

Histogenesis. The slow development of the cutaneous and also of the ocular changes suggests that microfilariae, as they gradually disintegrate, act as a source of foreign protein and that the dermatitis and iritis are the result of a delayed hypersensitivity (Connor et al).

SCHISTOSOMIASIS

Schistosomiasis is acquired through exposure to a schistosome pathogenic to humans that has been discharged by a freshwater snail and is in the cercarial stage. The cercariae burrow through the skin and migrate to venous plexuses, where they mature. The initial penetration causes a pruritic papular eruption referred to as swimmer's itch. Several weeks after penetration, the schistosomes have matured into worms 15 mm to 25 mm in length. The female then releases thousands of eggs. Their release may be accompanied by urticaria and a serum-sickness-like syndrome (Wood et al; Walther).

Three species of *Schistosoma* are pathogenic to humans. *Schistosoma mansoni* is common in the Caribbean islands

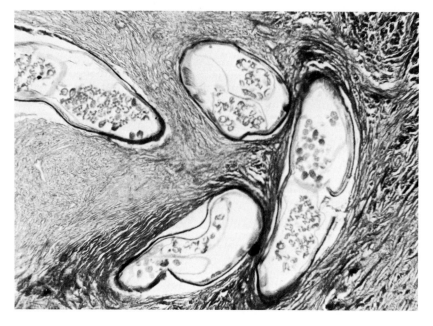

Fig. 12-7.   Onchocerciasis
Transverse and diagonal sections of the adult filaria *Onchocerca* are located in the subcutis within a dense fibrous tissue. (× 50)

and in Africa, and *S. japonicum* in Eastern Asia. Their usual habitats are the portal circulation and mesenteric venules, with discharge of the eggs with the stool. *S. haematobium* is found in Africa and the Near East. Its habitats are the pelvic and vesical venules, with passage of the eggs with the urine. *S. mansoni* and *S. japonicum*, through granulomas in the liver, may cause portal hypertension and esophageal varices, and *S. haematobium*, through granulomas in the bladder, may lead to hematuria and hydronephrosis (Mahmoud). In Africa, mixed infections with both *S. mansoni* and *S. haematobium* are not uncommon (Wood et al).

Specific cutaneous involvement may occur as papular, ulcerative, granulomatous, and fistulous lesions in the genital and perirectal skin secondary to the deposition of ova in dermal vessels contiguous to pelvic vessels (Torres; Walther). In rare instances, there is "ectopic" involvement of the skin elsewhere when ova have become dislodged from their natural habitat in the venous circulation. One observes in such cases either slightly erythematous grouped papules (Wood et al) or, rarely, a solitary plaque (Jacyk et al).

Histopathology.   In genital and perirectal lesions, numerous ova are found within a granulomatous infiltrate or within microabscesses (Torres). The ova measure up to 1 mm in their greatest dimension and possess a chitinous outer shell staining positively with the periodic acid-Schiff (PAS) stain. The presence and position of a spine on the shell of the ova permits their classification within the tissue. *S. haematobium* ova have a spine in the apical position, whereas the spine of *S. mansoni* ova is on the lateral aspect (Fig. 12-8), and *S. japonicum* ova have no spine. Ova may be seen crossing the epithelium toward the surface. In rare instances, one may also see adult worms within distended blood vessels in the dermis (Torres).

In ectopic papules or plaques, many palisading, necrotizing granulomas extend throughout the dermis and may cause perforation of the epidermis. Within the necrotic area, one or several ova may be seen (Fig. 12-8). The infiltrate at the periphery of the necrotic area shows epithelioid cells, histiocytes, lymphocytes, and numerous plasma cells (Wood et al); in some instances, it also shows eosinophils and giant cells (Jacyk et al).

SUBCUTANEOUS CYSTICERCOSIS

The pork tapeworm *Taenia solium* develops in the human intestinal tract following the ingestion of inadequately cooked pork containing *T. solium* larvae. The tapeworm discharges its eggs in the feces. When these eggs are ingested by humans, they hatch, and larvae are borne by blood or lymph to various tissues, where they develop

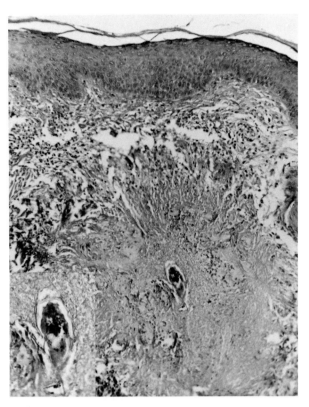

Fig. 12-8.   Schistosomiasis
An ovum of *S. mansoni* showing a spine on its lateral aspect is located within an area of necrosis. (×100) *Inset* shows the ovum at a higher magnification. (×200)

into cysticerci. These organisms are encountered most often in the subcutaneous tissue, eye, brain, skeletal muscle, and heart (Raimer and Wolf).

Clinically, one or several, or, rarely, numerous firm, asymptomatic nodules are present in the subcutaneous tissue. They usually measure 1 cm to 2 cm in diameter (Tschen et al). They persist for many years. In some patients with subcutaneous cysticercosis, there is either a preceding or a simultaneous intestinal infection with *T. solium* (taeniosis) (Schlossberg and Mader.).

Histopathology.   A thick, fibrous capsule surrounds a cystic cavity containing clear fluid and a white, irregularly shaped membranous structure representing a cysticercus larva and referred to as *Cysticercus cellulosae* (King et al).

ARTHROPOD BITES AND STINGS

Mosquito bites evoke an early toxic response that is urticarial and a later allergic response that is characterized by papules (Bandmann and Bosse).

Stings of bees, wasps, or hornets may produce one of three types of reaction: an acute necrotic response, a subacute inflammatory response, or a chronic lymphoid response (Horen). The latter is referred to as a persistent arthropod sting. The bites of ticks may similarly result in persistent papular or nodular lesions that cause a diagnostic problem clinically as well as histologically.

Hypersensitivity to insect bites, especially from fleas, mosquitoes, or bedbugs, may result in papular urticaria (see below).

Histopathology. Mosquito bites show mainly neutrophils during the early toxic response and a mononuclear infiltrate of lymphoid cells and plasma cells during the later allergic response. Eosinophils are few or absent (Bandmann and Bosse).

The acute necrotic response and the subacute inflammatory response to the stings of bees, wasps, or hornets have a nonspecific histologic appearance. In contrast, the chronic lymphoid response to these stings and also to the bites of ticks often has a pseudolymphomatous appearance.

In the chronic lymphoid response, the dermis presents a dense inflammatory infiltrate that may even extend into the subcutaneous fat. It consists of lymphoid cells and histiocytes with an admixture of eosinophils and plasma cells. Some of the cells may show hyperchromatic nuclei. Multinucleated cells may also occur (Allen). Frequently, one finds large lymphoid follicles with germinal centers (Winer and Strakosch; Allen; Tobias). In the case of tick bites, parts of the tick are occasionally found in the dermis.

Differential Diagnosis. In the chronic lymphoid response, the dense infiltrate and the presence of hyperchromatic nuclei may suggest mycosis fungoides, or the multinucleated cells, if present, may suggest Hodgkin's disease because of their resemblance to Reed–Sternberg cells. However, the presence of lymphoid follicles like those seen in lymphocytoma (Spiegler–Fendt pseudolymphoma) points toward a benign, reactive process such as arthropod bites or stings.

Papular Urticaria

Papular urticaria, also known as lichen urticatus, is the result of hypersensitivity to bites from certain insects, especially mosquitoes, fleas, and bedbugs. One observes edematous papules and papulovesicles, which, because of severe itching, usually are excoriated. The eruption is more commonly found in children than adults, and, if caused by mosquitoes, is limited to the summer months. The lesions of papular urticaria are clinically and often also histologically indistinguishable from those of prurigo simplex (see p. 138).

Histopathology. The stratum malpighii shows intercellular and intracellular edema and occasionally a spongiotic vesicle. A chronic inflammatory infiltrate is present around the vessels of the dermis, often extending into the lower dermis and containing a significant admixture of eosinophils (Shaffer et al).

Differential Diagnosis. Eosinophils, if present in significant numbers, speak in favor of a diagnosis of papular urticaria rather than prurigo simplex.

ERYTHEMA CHRONICUM MIGRANS, LYME DISEASE

Erythema chronicum migrans used to occur predominantly in Europe (Hellerström; Degos et al; Flanagan) and only rarely in the United States (Scrimenti). Recently, however, the occurrence of small endemic clusters of erythema chronicum migrans were described in the United States as Lyme disease or Lyme arthritis, first around Lyme, Connecticut, but then also elsewhere (Steere and Malawista; Reik et al).

Erythema chronicum migrans forms around a tick bite as a gradually expanding, edematous, red ring, clearing spontaneously after several weeks. The tick responsible for this dermatosis is *Ixodes ricinus* in Europe and *I. dammini* in the United States (Hardin et al). Lyme disease begins in 95% of the cases with erythema chronicum migrans, which is followed after several weeks or months by attacks of arthritis in 59% and by neurologic or cardiac involvement in 18% (Hardin et al).

Histopathology. Both the tick bite and the surrounding ring of erythema chronicum migrans show edema of the papillary dermis and a heavy mononuclear infiltrate around blood vessels and cutaneous appendages. The tick bite shows, in addition, spongiosis of the epidermis (Steere et al).

Histogenesis. A rickettsial genesis is assumed for the European type of erythema chronicum migrans, since the presence of antirickettsial antibodies has been demonstrated (Degos et al). In addition, rickettsialike bodies have been seen on *electron microscopy* in macrophages both free in the cytoplasm and within phagolysosomes. They measure about 7 nm by 10 nm in diameter, show a thick capsule, and contain ribosomelike particles (Sandbank and Feuerman). The presence of circulating immune complexes has been demonstrated in patients with Lyme disease (Hardin et al).

ACANTHOMA FISSURATUM

Acanthoma fissuratum may occur at any location along the retroauricular fold or on the sides or in the center of the nasal bridge. It is caused by pressure of the spectacle frame or its ear pieces. Characteristically, there is a small nodule showing a central furrow or fissure. The lesion may be asymptomatic or tender. Healing occurs often but not invariably after correction of the ill-fitting spectacles (Tennstedt and Lachapelle). Clinically, the lesion is often mistaken for a basal cell epithelioma.

Histopathology. The epidermis of the nodule shows considerable acanthosis, which may be so marked as to amount to pseudocarcinomatous hyperplasia (Epstein). Sections across the fissure show either a depressed area of markedly thinned epidermis (MacDonald and Martin) or a true epidermal separation filled with keratin and degenerated inflammatory cells (Tennstedt and Lachapelle). The dermal collagen underlying the fissure appears hyalinized (McDonald and Martin).

Histogenesis. The epidermal separation filled with debris and the underlying degenerated collagen show considerable resemblance to chondrodermatitis nodularis helicis (Tennstedt and Lachapelle) (see p. 206). It is possible that, in acanthoma fissuratum as in chondrodermatitis helicis, there is an attempt at eliminating collagen that has become degenerated.

FOREIGN BODY REACTIONS

Some foreign substances, when injected or implanted accidentally into the skin, produce a focal, nonallergic foreign body reaction. Other foreign substances produce in persons specifically sensitized to them a focal allergic response. In addition, certain substances formed within the body may produce a nonallergic foreign body reaction when deposited in the dermis or the subcutaneous tissue. Such endogenous foreign body reactions are produced, for instance, by urates in gout and by keratinous material in pilomatricoma, as well as in ruptured epidermal and trichilemmal cysts.

Histopathology. A *nonallergic* foreign body reaction typically shows macrophages and giant cells around the foreign material. In addition, lymphoid cells and plasma cells are present in most types of foreign body reactions. The presence of giant cells gives foreign body reactions the appearance of a granuloma. In some instances, epithelioid cells that have developed from macrophages are also present (see p. 52). Frequently, some of the foreign material is seen near macrophages and giant cells, a finding that of course is of great diagnostic value. Substances producing nonallergic foreign body reactions are, for instance, silk and nylon sutures (Fig. 12-9), wood, paraffin and other oily substances, silicone gel, talc, surgical glove starch powder, cactus spines, and human hair. Some of these substances—nylon sutures, wood, talc, surgical glove starch powder, and sea-urchin spines—are doubly refractile on polarizing examination (see p. 45). Double refraction often is very helpful in localizing foreign substances.

An *allergic* granulomatous reaction to a foreign body typically shows a tuberculoid pattern consisting of epithelioid cells with or without giant cells and with or without caseation necrosis. Phagocytosis of the foreign substance is slight or

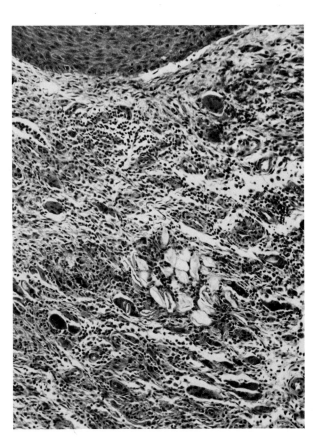

Fig. 12-9.   Foreign body granuloma caused by a nylon suture
The nylon suture is located in the center of the field. Around it is a severe inflammatory infiltrate containing numerous foreign body giant cells. (× 100)

absent. Substances that in sensitized persons produce an allergic granulomatous reaction are, for instance, zirconium, beryllium, and certain dyes used in tattoos. Some substances that at first act as foreign material may later on, after sensitization has occurred, act as allergens, as in the case of sea-urchin spines and silica.

A histologic decision as to whether a granuloma is of the foreign body type or of the allergic type is usually but by no means always possible. A granuloma of the allergic type, being a manifestation of delayed hypersensitivity, resembles tuberculosis or sarcoidosis and shows many epithelioid cells and relatively few giant cells. In contrast, a nonallergic foreign body granuloma shows macrophages and few or no epithelioid cells but many giant cells (Epstein et al, 1962, 1963).

Nonallergic Foreign Body Reactions

Paraffinoma

Foreign body reactions following injections of oily substances—for instance, mineral oil (paraffin), cottonseed oil, sesame oil, or camphor oil—occur as irregular, plaquelike indurations of the skin and subcutaneous tissue. Ulceration may develop. The interval between the time of injection and the development of induration or ulceration may be many years (Rupec et al).

The misleading term *sclerosing lipogranuloma* was given to paraffinoma of the male genitalia because of the disproved assumption that it was a local reactive process following injury to adipose tissue (Smetana and Bernhard).

Histopathology. Paraffinomas have a "Swiss cheese" appearance because of the presence of numerous ovoid or round cavities showing great variation in size (Fig. 12-10). These cavities represent spaces occupied by the oily substance (Oertel and Johnson). The spaces between the cavities are taken up in part by fibrotic connective tissue and in part by a cellular infiltrate of macrophages, and lymphoid cells. Some of the macrophages have the appearance of foam cells. Variable numbers of multinucleated foreign body giant cells are present.

In frozen sections of paraffinoma, the foreign material stains orange with Sudan IV or oil red O, though less so than neutral fat. If the foreign substance consists of paraffin or other mineral oils rather than vegetable oils, the osmic acid stain is negative (Best et al; Newcomer et al), as are the bromine-silver stain (Urbach et al) and the phospholipid reaction of Baker (Rupec et al). The reason for the negative staining is that osmic acid, bromine-silver, and the Baker reaction stain only substances containing unsaturated carbon links, which are present in animal and vegetable lipids but not in mineral oil.

Differential Diagnosis. Spontaneous lipogranulomas, such as lipogranulomatosis of Rothmann–Makai, in contrast to paraffinoma, show positive staining of their lipid substances with osmic acid, bromine-silver, and the phospholipid reaction.

Silicone Granuloma

Implantable bags filled with silicone gel are used for augmentation mammoplasty. The gel contains vegetable oil and fatty acids in addition to silicone. Even minor trauma may cause rupture of a bag and leakage of the silicone gel into the surrounding tissue, resulting in

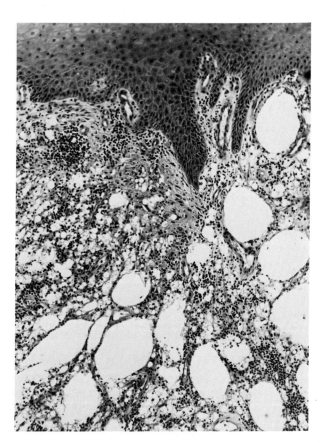

Fig. 12-10.   Lipid granuloma caused by the injection of mineral oil (paraffinoma)
The many large and small ovoid or round cavities that give the section a "Swiss cheese" appearance represent spaces that were filled with mineral oil (paraffin). (×200)

subcutaneous fibrotic nodules that may gradually migrate to adjoining tissues.

Histopathology. As in paraffinoma, numerous ovoid or round cavities of varying sizes are seen, resulting in a "Swiss cheese" appearance. Between the cavities lies a cellular infiltrate consisting of macrophages, lymphocytes, and multinucleated giant cells (Mason and Apisarnthanarax). In addition, varying degrees of fibrosis are present.

Talc Granuloma

Talc granulomas may arise when powdered talc (magnesium silicate) is introduced into open wounds.

Histopathology. Histologic examination reveals many large giant cells intermingled with macrophages and some epithelioid cells. With polarized light, numerous white birefringent particles are seen in many cells (Macher; Tye et al).

Histogenesis. The presence of talc can be confirmed by x-ray diffraction studies (Tye et al).

Starch Granuloma

Starch granulomas result from the accidental contamination of wounds with surgical glove powder. Such powder consists of cornstarch that has been treated with epichlorhydrin so that the powder can be autoclaved. As a result of this treatment, the powder acts as a foreign body.

Histopathology. A foreign body reaction with multinucleated giant cells is present. Scattered through the infiltrate, one observes starch granules as ill-defined ovoid basophilic structures measuring 10 μm to 20 μm in diameter. Most of the granules are seen within the foreign body giant cells. They react with PAS and methenamine silver and, on examination in polarized light, are birefringent, showing a Maltese cross configuration (Leonard).

Cactus Granuloma

Cactus granulomas show within days or weeks after the injury papules from which cactus spines may still protrude. They are extruded spontaneously within a few months.

Histopathology. The papules show, in addition to macrophages and epithelioid cells, many giant cells. Sharply marginated spicules are seen both within giant cells and lying free in the dermis. The spicules are PAS-positive (Winer and Zeilenga). The lesions represent nonallergic foreign body granulomas.

Interdigital Pilonidal Sinus

In barbers, the implantation of human hair in the interdigital web spaces may cause small, asymptomatic or slightly tender openings (Joseph and Gifford). Similar lesions have been observed in dog groomers (Price and Popkin).

Histopathology. Histologic examination reveals a sinus tract lined by epidermis and containing one or several hairs, thus resembling a hair follicle. Either the sinus tract encases the hair completely, or, if the hair extends deeper than the sinus tract, one finds at the lower end of the hair a foreign body giant cell reaction intermingled with inflammatory cells (Joseph and Gifford; Goebel and Rupec).

Allergic Foreign Body Reactions

Sea-Urchin Granuloma

Injuries from the spines of sea urchins occur most commonly on the hands and feet. Even if the friable spines have been only incompletely removed, the wounds tend to heal after spontaneous extrusion of most of the foreign material (Rocha and Fraga; Haneke and Kölsch). However, in some persons, violaceous nodules appear at the sites of injury after a latent period of 2 to 12 months (Kinmont).

Histopathology. The nodules are composed largely of epithelioid cell and giant cells (Rocha and Fraga). Doubly refractile material may be present in the granulomas (Haneke and Kölsch). If remnants of a spine are still present, they are surrounded by a wall of leukocytes and many large foreign body giant cells (Haneke and Kölsch).

Histogenesis. The appearance of sarcoidlike granulomas after a latent interval of months in only a small proportion of the injured patients suggests a delayed hypersensitivity reaction (Kinmont). The spines of sea urchins, in addition to the calcified material, contain remnants of epithelial cells (Kinmont). The double refraction that may be found in the granulomas may be due to the presence of a small amount of silica in the calcified spines (Haneke and Kölsch).

Silica Granuloma

Silica (silicon dioxide) contained in soil and glass frequently contaminates accidental wounds, in which it sets up a foreign body reaction of limited duration followed by fibrosis (Epstein et al, 1955). In the vast majority of cases, silica causes no further trouble. In exceptional cases, a delayed-hypersensitivity granulomatous reaction occurs at the site of the old scar many years later (Eskeland et al). The latency period may be as long as 29 years (Sommerville and Milne) or 40 years (Degos and Civatte). When this reaction occurs, indurated nodules develop in the skin and in the subcutaneous tissue.

Histopathology. In silica granuloma, numerous epithelioid cell tubercles are present that contain multinucleated giant cells but only a minimal admixture of lymphoid cells, resulting in a pattern greatly resembling that of sarcoidosis (Sommerville and Milne; Arzt; Epstein; Degos and Civatte). However, the diagnosis of sarcoidosis is easily excluded by the presence, especially within giant cells, of crystalline particles varying in size from barely visible to 100 µm in length; they represent silica crystals. When examined with polarized light, these particles are doubly refractile (Sommerville and Milne; Epstein). Furthermore, spectrographic analysis reveals the presence of silicon (Arzt).

Histogenesis. According to some authors (Shelley and Hurley, 1960; Epstein et al, 1963), the long interval between injury and the appearance of the silica granuloma is caused by the very slow conversion of the large particles of silica introduced into the tissue to colloidal silica. These authors found by means of intradermal injections of silica particles of various sizes that only silica in colloidal form with a particle size between 1 nm and 100 nm produces a reaction. Since the injection of colloidal silica regularly produced a granulomatous reaction, it was concluded that the development of silica granuloma represents a foreign body reaction rather than an allergic phenomenon. This reasoning, however, has been called erroneous (Eskeland et al), inasmuch as injections of colloidal silica elicit a foreign body reaction in all persons, whereas silica granuloma occurs in only a few.

Zirconium Granuloma

Deodorant sticks containing zirconium lactate and creams containing zirconium oxide may cause a persistent eruption composed of soft, reddish brown papules in the areas to which they have been applied.

Histopathology. Histologic examination shows large aggregates of epithelioid cells forming tubercles without caseation. A few giant cells and a moderate lymphoid cell infiltrate are present (LoPresti and Hambrick). Thus, the histologic picture is indistinguishable from that of sarcoidosis. Because of the small size of the zirconium particles, they cannot be detected on examination with polarized light (Williams and Skipworth). Their presence, however, can be demonstrated by spectrographic analysis (Baler).

Histogenesis. It is evident that zirconium granulomas develop on the basis of an allergic sensitization to zirconium, since (1) they occur only in persons sensitized to zirconium (Shelley and Hurley, 1958), (2) they consist of epithelioid cell granulomas, and (3) autoradiographic analysis of experimentally induced lesions in sensitized individuals reveals no zirconium within epithelioid cells, a fact that favors the theory that granulomas are formed on the basis of a delayed hypersensitivity reaction (Epstein et al, 1962).

Systemic Berylliosis

Up to 1949, beryllium-containing compounds were widely used in the manufacture of fluorescent light tubes. Two diseases resulted from this: (1) systemic berylliosis developed in some workers in plants manufacturing the tubes through inhalation of these compounds; and (2) purely local beryllium granulomas occurred in persons who cut themselves on broken fluorescent tubes. For a discussion of local beryllium granuloma, see below.

Systemic berylliosis primarily shows pulmonary involvement, which results in death in about one third of the patients (Stoeckle et al). Beryllium may reach the skin through the blood circulation and cause cutaneous granulomas. However, this is a rare event, having been observed in one series in only 4 instances among 535 patients with systemic berylliosis (Stoeckle et al). The granulomas consist of only a few papular lesions over which the skin remains intact.

Histopathology. The cutaneous granulomas of systemic berylliosis are indistinguishable from sarcoidosis, showing very slight or no caseation (Stoeckle et al).

Histogenesis. Systemic berylliosis develops on the basis of a delayed hypersensitivity reaction. This has been shown by means of in vitro testing: when exposed to beryllium oxide in vitro, the lymphocytes of patients with systemic berylliosis undergo blastogenic transformation (Hanifin et al) and produce macrophage migration inhibitory factor (MIF) (Henderson et al).

Local Beryllium Granuloma

Local beryllium granulomas were observed some years ago from cuts with fluorescent light tubes, which at that time were coated with a mixture containing zinc–beryllium silicate (Neave et al).

The cutaneous granulomas following laceration show as their first sign incomplete healing of the laceration, followed by swelling, induration and tenderness, and, finally, central ulceration (Dutra).

Histopathology. The cutaneous granulomas following laceration, in contrast to the cutaneous granulomas of systemic berylliosis, show pronounced necrosis, which may affect the entire center of the lesion (Fig. 12-11) (Neave et al). Often, a collar of lymphoid cells surrounds some of the epithelioid cell islands, giving them the appearance of true tubercles. The epidermis shows acanthosis and possibly ulceration. No particles of beryllium are seen in histologic sections, but its presence in the lesions can be demonstrated by spectrographic analysis (Dutra).

Tattoo Granuloma

Allergic reactions to tattoos have been observed most commonly with cinnabar, a red dye containing mercuric sulfide, but occasionally also with chrome green, a tervalent chrome compound, and with cobalt blue. The reactions can be one of two types, either an allergic dermatitis or an allergic granulomatous reaction.

Histopathology. Ordinarily, tattoos show diffusely scattered granules of dye that seem to be located not only within macrophages but also extracellularly in the dermis without any inflammatory reaction (Rostenberg et al).

In cases of *allergic dermatitis,* such as may occur against mercuric sulfide (Madden) or against chrome green (Rostenberg et al), a pronounced inflammatory infiltrate is present in the dermis that is composed largely of lymphoid cells but that also contains histiocytes, eosinophils, and a few plasma cells. The tattoo granules are found predominantly in macrophages. The epidermis shows acanthosis and spongiosis. In some instances, the allergic reaction is lichenoid in character, showing great resemblance either to lichen planus (Winkelmann and Harris) or to hypertrophic lichen planus (Clarke and Black). In others, the infiltrate is massive and patchy and thus may be difficult to differentiate from lymphoma or pseudolymphoma, except for the presence of coarse tattoo pigment granules (Blumental et al).

In cases of an *allergic granulomatous reaction,* as has been observed with mercuric sulfide (Sulzberger and Tolmach), chrome green (Loewenthal), and cobalt blue (Björnberg), the reaction may be either of the tuberculoid type (Björnberg) or of the sarcoidal type (Loewenthal). In the tuberculoid type of granuloma, one finds, in addition to epithelioid cells and giant cells, lymphoid cells and occasionally central necrosis in the granulomas. In

Fig. 12-11. Beryllium granuloma caused by laceration with a fluorescent light bulb
There is a large area of caseation necrosis surrounded by a tuberculoid granulomatous infiltrate. ($\times 100$)

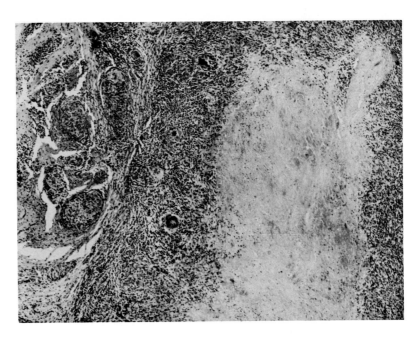

the sarcoidal type, the infiltrate consists almost entirely of epithelioid cell granulomas, as in sarcoidosis (Madden; Sulzberger and Tolmach). The occurrence of a sarcoidal type of reaction in tattoos of patients with systemic sarcoidosis has been repeatedly reported (Weidman et al; Dickinson). Tattoo granules are found scattered throughout the infiltrate in both the tuberculoid type and the sarcoidal type of reaction.

Histogenesis. *Electron microscopic examination* of tattoo marks without an allergic reaction shows that most tattoo granules are located within macrophages, where they often lie within membrane-bound lysosomes. In addition, some tattoo granules are found free in the dermis (Abel et al).

BIBLIOGRAPHY

Polymorphous Light Eruption

CALNAN CD, MEARA RH: Actinic prurigo (Hutchinson's summer prurigo). Clin Exp Dermatol 2:365–372, 1977

CHORZELSKI T, JABLONSKA S, BLASZCZYK M: Immunopathologic investigations in lupus erythematosus. J Invest Dermatol 52:333–338, 1969

EVERETT MA, LAMB JH, MINOR D: Light-sensitive eruptions in American Indians. Arch Dermatol 83:243–248, 1961

FISHER DA, EPSTEIN, JH, KAY DN et al: Polymorphous light eruption and lupus erythematosus. Arch Dermatol 101:458–461, 1970

MEARA RH, MAGNUS IA, GRICE K et al: Hutchinson's summer prurigo. Trans St John's Hosp Dermatol Soc 57:87–97, 1971

PETERSON WC JR, FUSARO RM: Antinuclear factor in light sensitivity and lupus erythematosus. Arch Dermatol 87:563–565, 1963

SCHEEN SR III, CONNOLLY SM, DICKEN CH: Actinic prurigo. J Am Acad Dermatol 5:183–190, 1981

WRIGHT ET, WINER LH: Histopathology of ellergic solar dermatitis. J Invest Dermatol 34:103–106, 1960

Hydroa Vacciniforme

BICKERS DR, DEMAR LK, DELEO V et al: Hydroa vacciniforme. Arch Dermatol 114:1193–1196, 1978

JASCHKE E, REINKEN L, FRISCH A: Hydroa vacciniforme Bazin. Hautarzt 26:11–27, 1975

MCGRAE JD, PERRY HO: Hydroa vacciniforme. Arch Dermatol 87:618–625, 1963

Chronic Photosensitivity Dermatitis, Actinic Reticuloid

BRODY R, BERGFELD WF: Actinic reticuloid. Int J Dermatol 20:374–379, 1981

DEGOS R, CIVATTE J, AKHOUND-ZADEH et al: Actino-réticulose. Photo-allergie avec infiltrat hématodermique. Ann Dermatol Syph 97:121–134, 1970

FRAIN-BELL W, HETHERINGTON A, JOHNSON BE: Contact allergic sensitivity to chrysanthemum and the photosensitivity dermatitis and actinic reticuloid syndrome. Br J Dermatol 101:491–501, 1979

FRAIN-BELL W, JOHNSON BE: Contact allergic sensitivity to plants and the photosensitivity dermatitis and actinic reticuloid syndrome. Br J Dermatol 101:503–512, 1979

FRAIN-BELL W, LAKSHMIPATHI T, ROGERS J et al: The syndrome of chronic photosensitivity dermatitis and actinic reticuloid. Br J Dermatol 91:617–634, 1974

GUARDIOLA A, SÁNCHEZ JL: Actinic reticuloid. Int J Dermatol 19:154–158, 1980

IVE FA, MAGNUS IA, WARIN RP et al: "Actinic reticuloid," a chronic dermatosis associated with severe photosensitivity and the histologic resemblance to lymphoma. Br J Dermatol 81:469–485, 1969

JENSEN NE, SNEDDON IB: Actinic reticuloid with lymphoma. Br J Dermatol 82:287–291, 1970

JOHNSON SC, CRIPPS DJ, NORBACK DH: Actinic reticuloid. A clinical, pathologic, and action spectrum study. Arch Dermatol 115:1078–1083, 1979

NEILD VS, HAWK JLM, EADY RAJ et al: Actinic reticuloid with Sézary cells. Clin Exp Dermatol 7:143–148, 1982

PERROT H, FRIONNET M, FRANCES C et al: Sarcome ganglionnaire généralisé au cours de l'évolution d'une actino-réticulose. Ann Dermatol Venereol 105:33–40, 1978

THOMSEN K: The development of Hodgkin's disease in a patient with actinic reticuloid. Clin Exp Dermatol 2:109–113, 1977

Erythema ab Igne

ARRINGTON JH III, LOCKMAN DS: Thermal keratoses and squamous cell carcinoma in situ associated with erythema ab igne. Arch Dermatol 115:1226–1228, 1979

FINLAYSON GR, SAMS WM JR, SMITH JG JR: Erythema ab igne: A histopathological study. J Invest Dermatol 46:104–108, 1966

JOHNSON WC, BUTTERWORTH T: Erythema ab igne. Arch Dermatol 104:128–131, 1971

SHAHRAD P, MARKS R: The wages of warmth: Changes in erythema ab igne. Br J Dermatol 97:179–186, 1977

Radiation Dermatitis

ANDERSON NP, ANDERSON HE: Development of basal cell epithelioma as a consequence of radiodermatitis. Arch Dermatol Syph 63:586–596, 1951

BLOM-IDES C: Sarcoma in Röntgenoderma. Acta Derm Venereol (Stockh) 30:47–49, 1950

EPSTEIN E: Radiodermatitis. Springfield, IL, Charles C Thomas, 1962

JAMES WD, ODOM RB: Late subcutaneous fibrosis following megavoltage radiotherapy. J Am Acad Dermatol 3:616–618, 1980

LAZAR P, CULLEN SI: Basal cell epithelioma and chronic radiodermatitis. Arch Dermatol 88:172–175, 1963

MAGGIORA A, BUJARD E, JADASSOHN W: Beitrag zur Frage des Röntgensarkoms. Dermatol Wochenschr 147:209–215, 1963

SIMS CF, KIRSCH N: Spindle-cell epidermoid epithelioma simulating sarcoma in chronic radiodermatitis. Arch Dermatol Syph 57:63–68, 1948

TOTTEN RS, ANTYPES PG, DUPERTUIS SM et al: Pre-existing roentgen-ray dermatitis in patients with skin cancer. Cancer 10:1024–1030, 1957

Calcaneal Petechiae (Black Heel)

CRISSEY JT, PEACHEY JC: Calcaneal petechiae. Arch Dermatol 83:501, 1961

KIRTON V, PRICE MW: "Black heel." Trans St John's Hosp Dermatol Soc 51:80–84, 1965

MEHREGAN AH: Perforating dermatoses: A clinicopathologic review. Int J Dermatol 16:19–27, 1977

RUFLI T: Hyperkeratosis haemorrhagica. Hautarzt 31:606–609, 1980

VAKILZADEH F, HAPPLE R: Die Tennisferse (Black Heel). Z Hautkr 49:285–288, 1974

Scabies

DICK GF, BURGDORF WHC, GENTRY WC JR: Norwegian scabies in Bloom's syndrome. Arch Dermatol 115:212–213, 1979

FALK ES, BOLLE R: In vivo demonstration of specific immunological hypersensitivity to scabies mite. Br J Dermatol 103:367–373, 1980

FALK ES, EIDE TJ: Histologic and clinical findings in human scabies. Int J Dermatol 20:600–605, 1981

FERNANDEZ N, TORRES A, ACKERMAN AB: Pathological findings in human scabies. Arch Dermatol 113:320–324, 1977

HEJAZI N, MEHREGAN AH: Scabies. Histological study of inflammatory lesions. Arch Dermatol 111:37–39, 1975

HOEFLING KK, SCHROETER AL: Dermatoimmunopathology of scabies. J Am Acad Dermatol 3:237–240, 1980

MARTIN WC, WHEELER CE JR: Diagnosis of human scabies by epidermal shave biopsy. J Acad Dermatol 1:335–337, 1979

ORKIN M, MAIBACH HI: This scabies pandemic. N Engl J Med 298:496–498, 1978

THOMSON J, COCHRANE T, COCHRAN R et al: Histology simulating reticulosis in persistent nodular scabies. Br J Dermatol 90:421–429, 1974

Subcutaneous Dirofilariasis

BILLUPS J, SCHENKEN JR, BEAVER PC: Subcutaneous dirofilariasis in Nebraska. Arch Pathol 104:11–13, 1980

FISHER BK, HOMAYOUNI M, ORIHEL TC: Subcutaneous infections with *Dirofilaria*. Arch Dermatol 89:837–840, 1964

PAYAN HM: Human infection with *Dirofilaria*. Arch Dermatol 114:593–594, 1978

Onchocerciasis

CONNOR DH, WILLIAMS PH, HELWIG EB et al: Dermal changes in onchocerciasis. Arch Pathol 87:193–200, 1969

PIERS F, FASAL P: Onchocerciasis. In Simons RDGP (ed): Handbook of Tropical Dermatology, Vol 2, pp 950–962. Amsterdam, Elsevier Press, 1953

Schistosomiasis

JACYK WK, LAWANDE RW, TULPULE SS: Unusual presentation of extragenital cutaneous schistosomiasis mansoni. Br J Dermatol 103:205–208, 1980

MAHMOUD AA: Schistosomiasis. N Engl J Med 297:1329–1331, 1977

TORRES VM: Dermatologic manifestations of schistosomiasis mansoni. Arch Dermatol 112:1539–1542, 1976

WALTHER RR: Chronic papular dermatitis of the scrotum due to *Schistosoma mansoni*. Arch Dermatol 115:869–870, 1979

WOOD MG, SROLOVITZ H, SCHETMAN D: Schistosomiasis. Arch Dermatol 112:690–695, 1976

Subcutaneous Cysticercosis

KING DT, GILBERT DJ, GUREVITCH AW et al: Subcutaneous cysticercosis. Arch Dermatol 115:236, 1979

RAIMER S, WOLF JE JR: Subcutaneous cysticercosis. Arch Dermatol 114:107–108, 1978

SCHLOSSBERG D, MADER JT: *Cysticercus cellulosae* cutis. Arch Dermatol 114:459–460, 1978

TSCHEN EH, TSCHEN EA, SMITH EB: Cutaneous cysticercosis treated with metrifonate. Arch Dermatol 117:507–509, 1981

Arthropod Bites and Stings

ALLEN AC: Persistent "insect bites" (dermal eosinophilic granulomas) simulating lymphoblastomas, histiocytoses, and squamous cell carcinomas. Am J Pathol 24:367–375, 1948

BANDMAN HJ, BOSSE K: Histologie des Mückenstiches (*Aedes aegypti*). Arch Klin Exp Dermatol 231:59–67, 1967

HOREN WP: Insect and scorpion sting. JAMA 221:894–898, 1972

SHAFFER B, JACOBSEN C, BEERMAN H: Histopathologic correlation of lesions of papular urticaria and positive skin test reactions to insect antigens. Arch Dermatol 70:437–442, 1954

TOBIAS N: Tickbite granuloma. J Invest Dermatol 12:255–259, 1949

WINER LH, STRAKOSCH EA: Tickbites—*Dermacentor variabilis* (Say). J Invest Dermatol 4:249–258, 1941

Erythema Chronicum Migrans, Lyme Disease

DEGOS R, TOURAINE R, AROUETTE J: L'erythema chronicum migrans. Ann Dermatol Syph 89:247–260, 1962

FLANAGAN BP: Erythema chronicum migrans Afzelius in Americans. Arch Dermatol 86:410–411, 1962

HARDIN JA, STEERE AC, MALAWISTA SE: Immune complexes and the evolution of Lyme arthritis. N Engl J Med 301:1358–1363, 1979

HELLERSTRÖM S: Erythema chronicum migrans Afzelius with meningitis. Acta Derm Venereol (Stockh) 31:227–234, 1951

REIK L, STEERE AC, BARTENHAGEN NH et al: Neurologic abnormalities of Lyme disease. Medicine (Baltimore) 58:281–294, 1979

SANDBANK M, FEUERMAN EJ: Ultrastructural observation of rickettsia-like bodies in erythema chronicum migrans. J Cutan Pathol 6:253–264, 1979

SCRIMENTI RJ: Erythema chronicum migrans. Arch Dermatol 102:104–105, 1970

STEERE AC, MALAWISTA SE: Cases of Lyme disease in the United States: Locations correlated with distribution of *Ixodes dammini*. Ann Intern Med 91:730–733, 1979

STEERE AC, MALAWISTA SE, HARDIN JA et al: Erythema chronicum migrans and Lyme arthritis. Ann Intern Med 86:685–698, 1977

Acanthoma Fissuratum

EPSTEIN E: Granuloma fissuratum of the ears. Arch Dermatol 91:621–622, 1965

MACDONALD DM, MARTIN SJ: Acanthoma fissuratum: Spectacle frame acanthoma. Acta Derm Venereol (Stockh) 55:485–488, 1975

TENNSTEDT D, LACHAPELLE JM: Acanthome fissuré. Ann Dermatol Venereol 106:219–225, 1979

Foreign Body Reactions

ABEL EA, SILBERBERG I, QUEEN D: Studies of chronic inflammation in a red tattoo by electron microscopy and histochemistry. Acta Derm Venereol (Stockh) 52:453–461, 1972

ARZT L: Foreign body granulomas and Boeck's sarcoid. J Invest Dermatol 24:155–166, 1955

BALER GR: Granulomas from topical zirconium in poison ivy dermatitis. Arch Dermatol 91:145–148, 1965

BEST EW, MASON HL, DEWEERD JW et al: Sclerosing lipogranuloma of the male genitalia produced by mineral oil. Proc Mayo Clin 28:623–631, 1953

BJÖRNBERG A: Allergic reaction to cobalt in light blue tattoo markings. Acta Derm Venereol (Stockh) 41:259–263, 1961

BLUMENTAL G, OKUN MR, PONITCH JA: Pseudolymphomatous reaction to tattoos. J Am Acad Dermatol 6:485–488, 1982

CLARKE J, BLACK MM: Lichenoid tattoo reactions. Br J Dermatol 100:451–454, 1979

DEGOS R, CIVATTE J: Das Silikosegranulom der Haut. Hautarzt 10:106–110, 1959

DICKINSON JA: Sarcoidal reactions in tattoos. Arch Dermatol 100:315–319, 1969

DUTRA FR: Beryllium granulomas of the skin. Arch Dermatol Syph 60:1140–1147, 1949

EPSTEIN E: Silica granuloma of the skin. Arch Dermatol 71:24–35, 1955

EPSTEIN E, GERSTL B, BERK M et al: Silica pregranuloma. Arch Dermatol 71:645–647, 1955

EPSTEIN WL, SKAHEN JR, KRASNOBROD H: Granulomatous hypersensitivity to zirconium: Localization of allergen in tissue and its role in formation of epithelioid cells. J Invest Dermatol 38:223–232, 1962

EPSTEIN WL, SKAHEN JR, KRASNOBROD H: The organized epithelioid cell granuloma: Differentiation of allergic (zirconium) from colloidal (silica) types. Am J Pathol 43:391–405, 1963

ESKELAND G, LANGMARK F, HUSBY G: Silicon granuloma of the skin and subcutaneous tissue. Acta Pathol Microbiol Scand (A) Suppl 248:69–73, 1974

GOEBEL M, RUPEC M: Interdigitaler pilonidaler Sinus. Dermatol Wochenschr 153:341–345, 1967

HANEKE E, KÖLSCH I: Seeigelgranulome. Hautarzt 31:159–160, 1980

HANIFIN JM, EPSTEIN WL, CLINE MJ: In vitro studies of granulomatous hypersensitivity to beryllium. J Invest Dermatol 55:284–288, 1970

HENDERSON WR, FUKUYAMA K, EPSTEIN WL et al: In vitro demonstration of delayed hypersensitivity in patients with berylliosis. J Invest Dermatol 58:5–8, 1972

JOSEPH HL, GIFFORD H: Barber's interdigital pilonidal sinus. Arch Dermatol 70:616–624, 1954

KINMONT PDC: Sea-urchin sarcoidal granuloma. Br J Dermatol 77:335–343, 1965

LEONARD DD: Starch granulomas. Arch Dermatol 107:101–103, 1973

LOEWENTHAL LJA: Reactions in green tattoos. Arch Dermatol 82:237–243, 1960

LOPRESTI PJ, HAMBRICK GW: Zirconium granuloma following treatment of Rhus dermatitis. Arch Dermatol 92:188–191, 1965

MACHER E: Die Bedeutung des Talkumgranuloms in der Dermatologie. Hautarzt 4:529–533, 1954

MADDEN JF: Reactions in tattoos. Arch Dermatol Syph 40:256–262, 1939

MASON J, APISARNTHANARAX P: Migratory silicone granuloma. Arch Dermatol 117:366–367, 1981

NEAVE HJ, FRANK SB, TOLMACH J: Cutaneous granulomas following laceration by fluorescent light bulbs. Arch Dermatol Syph 61:401–406, 1950

NEWCOMER VD, GRAHAM JH, SCHAFFERT RR et al: Sclerosing lipogranuloma resulting from exogenous lipids. Arch Dermatol 73:361–372, 1956

OERTEL VC, JOHNSON FB: Sclerosing lipogranuloma of male genitalia. Arch Pathol 101:321–326, 1977

PRICE SM, POPKIN GL: Barber's interdigital hair sinus. A case report in a dog groomer. Arch Dermatol 112:523, 1976

ROCHA G, FRAGA S: Sea urchin granuloma of the skin. Arch Dermatol 85:406–408, 1962

ROSTENBERG A JR, BROWN RA, CARO MR: Discussion of tattoo reactions with report of a case showing a reaction to a green color. Arch Dermatol Syph 62:540–547, 1950

RUPEC M, TREECK W, BRAUN-FALCO O: Zum Paraffingranulom. Dermatol Wochenschr 151:129–140, 1965

SHELLEY WB, HURLEY HJ: The allergic origin of zirconium deodorant granulomas. Br J Dermatol 70:75–101, 1958

SHELLEY WB, HURLEY HJ: The pathogenesis of silica granulomas in man: A non-allergic colloidal phenomenon. J Invest Dermatol 34:107–123, 1960

SMETANA HF, BERNHARD W: Sclerosing lipogranuloma. Arch Pathol 50:296–325, 1950

SOMMERVILLE J, MILNE JA: Pseudotuberculoma silicoticum. Br J Dermatol 62:105–108, 1950

STOECKLE JD, HARDY HL, WEBER AL: Chronic beryllium disease. Am J Med 46:545–557, 1967

SULZBERGER MB, TOLMACH JA: Allergische Aufflammungs-Reaktionen in roten Tätowierungen. Hautarzt 10:110–114, 1959

TYE MJ, HASHIMOTO K, FOX F: Talc granulomas of the skin. JAMA 198:1370–1372, 1966

URBACH F, WINE SS, JOHNSON WC et al: Generalized pararfinoma (sclerosing lipogranuloma). Arch Dermatol 103:277–285, 1971

WEIDMAN AI, ANDRADE R, FRANKS AG: Sarcoidosis. Arch Dermatol 94:320–325, 1966

WILLIAMS RM, SKIPWORTH GB: Zirconium granulomas of the glabrous skin following treatment of Rhus dermatitis. Arch Dermatol 80:273–276, 1959

WINER LH, ZEILENGA RH: Cactus granuloma of the skin. Arch Dermatol 72:566–569, 1955

WINKELMANN RK, HARRIS RB: Lichenoid delayed hypersensitivity reactions in tattoos. J Cutan Pathol 6:59–65, 1979

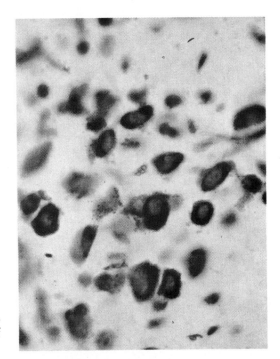

Urticaria pigmentosa. Methylene blue stain. Numerous basophilic granules are present in the cytoplasm of the mast cells. (See p. 81.) (×800)

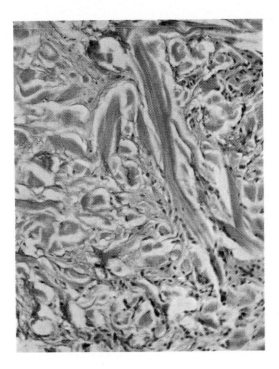

Granuloma annulare. Foci of incomplete degeneration of collagen show partially degenerated and partially normal collagen bundles. Fine threads and granules of mucinous material are located at the sites of collagen degeneration. (See p. 235.) (×150)

Noninfectious Granulomas

13

SARCOIDOSIS

Sarcoidosis is a systemic granulomatous disease of undetermined etiology. A distinction is made between the rare subacute, transient type of sarcoidosis and the usual chronic, persistent type.

In subacute, transient sarcoidosis, one encounters erythema nodosum in association with hilar adenopathy, fever, and often also migrating polyarthritis and acute iritis. The disease subsides in almost all patients within a few months without sequelae. Cutaneous manifestations other than erythema nodosum do not occur (Putkonen; James et al). Occasionally, there is enlargement of some of the subcutaneous lymph nodes, such as the submental or cervical lymph nodes (Wood et al).

In chronic, persistent sarcoidosis, cutaneous lesions are encountered in about one third of the patients who are seen in medical departments (Maycock et al). In contrast to this, cutaneous lesions are the only manifestation of sarcoidosis in about one fourth of the patients with sarcoidosis seen in dermatological departments, since in three combined series 25 of 104 patients had lesions limited to the skin (Umbert and Winkelmann; Veien; Hanno et al). The most common type of cutaneous lesion consists of brownish red or purplish papules and plaques. Through central clearing, annual or circinate lesions may result. When the papules or plaques are situated on the nose, cheeks, and ears, the term *lupus pernio* is applied. A rather rare form of sarcoidosis is the lichenoid form, in which small, papular lesions may be widespread (Thal), limited to a few areas (Brunner and Robin), or arranged within well-demarcated patches (Thal; Nozaki).

Very rare manifestations of sarcoidosis are erythrodermic, ichthyosiform, and ulcerating lesions. In erythrodermic sarcoidosis, the erythroderma may be generalized (Morrison) or may consist of extensive, sharply demarcated, brownish red, slightly scaling patches with little or no palpable infiltration (Lever and Freiman). In ichthyosiform sarcoidosis, areas of ichthyosis are found on the lower extremities (Kelly) but at times also elsewhere on the skin (Kauh et al). In ulcerating sarcoidosis, ulcers are seen most commonly on the legs (Hopf and Krebs) and may be associated with extensive cutaneous atrophy (Chevrant-Breton et al).

Subcutaneous nodules of sarcoidosis are quite rare. They may occur either in association with cutaneous lesions (Lever and Freiman) or alone (Clayton and Wood; Gross et al).

The occasional coexistence of granuloma annulare with systemic sarcoidosis is of interest and suggests an immunologic relationship (Umbert and Winkelmann).

Histopathology. The lesions of erythema nodosum occurring in subacute, transient sarcoidosis have the same histologic appearance as "idiopathic" erythema nodosum (Wood et al).

Like lesions in other organs, the cutaneous lesions of chronic, persistent sarcoidosis are characterized by the presence of circumscribed granulomas of epithelioid cells, so-called epithelioid cell tubercles showing little or no necrosis.

The papules, plaques, and lupus-pernio-type lesions show variously sized aggregates of epithelioid cells scattered irregularly through the dermis with occasional extension into the subcutaneous tissue (Barrie and Bogoch). In the erythrodermic form, the infiltrate shows rather small granulomas

229

of epithelioid cells in the upper dermis intermingled with numerous monocytes and lymphocytes (Lever and Freiman; Wigley and Musso), and, rarely, also giant cells (Morrison). Typical epithelioid cell tubercles are found in the ichthyosiform lesions (Kauh et al), in ulcerated areas (Hopf and Krebs), and in areas of atrophy (Chevrant-Breton et al). In subcutaneous nodules, epithelioid cell tubercles lie in the subcutaneous fat (Gross et al).

In typical lesions of sarcoidosis of the skin, the well-demarcated islands of epithelioid cells contain only few, if any, giant cells (Fig. 13-1). A slight to moderate admixture of lymphoid cells is usually present, particularly at the margins of the epithelioid cell granulomas (Fig. 13-2). Occasionally, a slight degree of coagulation necrosis showing eosinophilic staining is found in the center of some of the granulomas (Barrie and Bogoch). If a reticulum stain is employed, one sees a network of reticulum fibers surrounding and permeating the epithelioid cell granulomas (Fig. 13-3). In old lesions, one can observe within the epithelioid cell

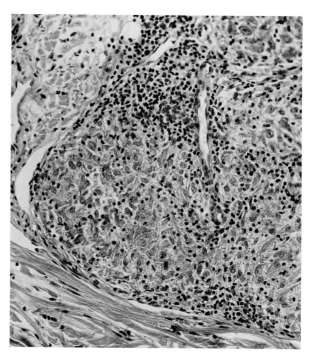

Fig. 13-2. Sarcoidosis
High magnification of Figure 13-1. The island of epithelioid cells is sharply demarcated. A "sprinkling" of lymphoid cells is present at the margin of the island. Histochemical stains have shown the presence of lysosomal enzymes in most of the lymphoid cells, which thus appear as monocytes and not lymphocytes. ($\times 200$)

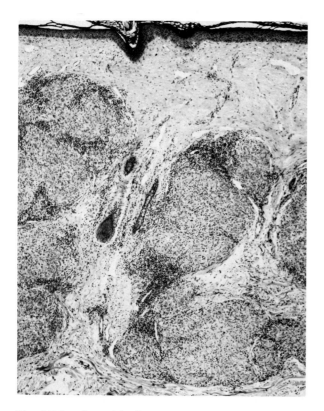

Fig. 13-1. Sarcoidosis
Low magnification. There are large islands of epithelioid cells with only a slight admixture of lymphoid cells. ($\times 50$)

granulomas not only reticulum fibers, but also some collagen fibers that are resistant to silver impregnation (Barrie and Bogoch). A moderate number of giant cells is often found in old lesions. These giant cells are apt to be quite large and irregular in shape; occasionally, they contain Schaumann bodies or asteroid bodies. Schaumann bodies are round or oval, laminated, and calcified, especially at their periphery. They stain dark blue because of the presence of calcium. Asteroid bodies (Fig. 13-4) stain best with phosphotungstic acid-hematoxylin, which stains the center brownish red and the spikes blue (Lever and Freiman). Neither of the two bodies is specific for sarcoidosis; they have been observed also in other granulomas, such as tuberculosis, leprosy, and berylliosis. If the granulomas of sarcoidosis involute, fibrosis extends from the periphery toward the center, with gradual disappearance of the epithelioid cells (Barrie and Bogoch).

Systemic Lesions. A diagnosis of chronic, persistent sarcoidosis should not be made on the

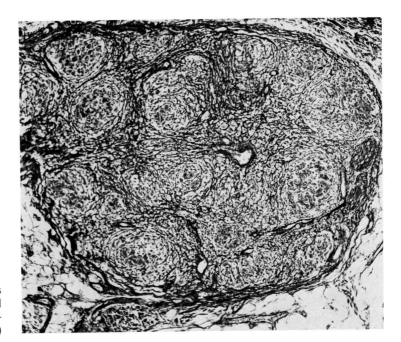

Fig. 13-3. Sarcoidosis
Foot's reticulum stain. Reticulum fibers surround and permeate the epithelioid cell granuloma. At the margin of the granuloma, collagen fibers are also seen. (×100)

Fig. 13-4. Sarcoidosis
A large giant cell contains an asteroid body. (×400)

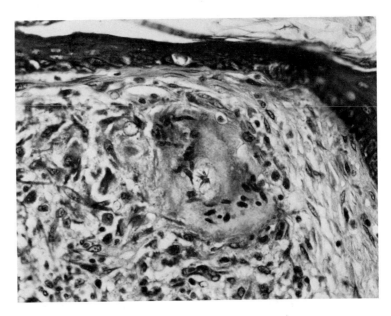

basis of clinical and radiologic manifestations alone, because sarcoidosis may resemble, among other diseases, tuberculosis and deep fungal infections. Since material for a Kveim test (see below) often is not available, a biopsy is essential for the diagnosis. In contrast, the symptom complex of the acute, transient type of sarcoidosis is unique, so that a biopsy may not be required.

The chronic, persistent type of sarcoidosis often is widespread even in the absence of symptoms. If skin lesions are present, they are the obvious site for biopsy. If there are no cutaneous lesions and no palpable lymph nodes or other lesions present near the surface, transbronchial lung biopsy under fluoroscopic guidance with local anesthesia is the procedure of choice for obtaining histologic confirmation, even in patients without positive x-ray findings (Koerner et al). However, random biopsy of a minor salivary gland from the lower lip (Nessan and Jacoway) or of the gastrocnemius muscle (Israel and Sones) may be carried out first.

The lungs are the most common organ to produce clinical manifestations in the chronic, persistent type of sarcoidosis, doing so in about 50% of the cases (James et al). The lesions may be either nodular or disseminated with extensive parenchymal fibrosis of the lungs. In the latter type of involvement, cavities form not infrequently, and aspergillosis with pulmonary hemorrhage may ensue (Israel and Ostrow).

In about 25% of the patients, ocular manifestations, consisting most commonly of a chronic iridocyclitis, occur. Splenomegaly exists in about 17%. In about 12%, osseous granulomas are present, most commonly in the phalanges of the fingers and toes but in some instances in the skull (Bodie et al), appearing in roentgenograms as circumscribed lytic lesions. About 8% of the patients have involvement of large salivary glands, usually of the parotid gland (James et al). In about 5%, one encounters paresis of a cranial nerve, most commonly of the facial nerve (James et al). Asymptomatic enlargement of the hilar lymph nodes is present in 70%, of peripheral lymph nodes in 30%, and of the liver in 20% of the patients (Maycock et al; James et al).

Sarcoidosis, although usually a benign disease, may lead to death. The mortality rate of sarcoidosis lies between 5% and 6% (Maycock et al; James et al). The most common cause of death from sarcoidosis is insufficiency of the right side of the heart resulting from massive involvement of the lungs with parenchymal fibrosis. Rather rare is death from pulmonary hemorrhage (see above) or from tuberculosis superimposed on sarcoidosis of the lungs. Another possible fatal complication is renal insufficiency resulting from hypercalcemia and hypercalciuria (Longcope and Freiman) or from sarcoidal glomerulonephritis (McCoy and Fisher). In very rare instances only, death results from massive involvement of the myocardium (Roberts et al) or of the liver (Mistilis et al). Hypopituitarism from involvement of either the pituitary gland or the hypothalamus is also a rare fatal complication (Selenkow et al).

Histogenesis. In sarcoidosis, a particular state of host reactivity exists that is characterized by an impairment in some delayed hypersensitivity reactions. Thus, there may be (1) depression of the phytohemagglutinin-stimulated transformation of lymphocytes into blast cells in vitro, measured by the percentage of lymphocytes that, as an indication of deoxyribonucleic acid (DNA) synthesis, are labeled with tritiated thymidine (Langner et al); (2) a weakened response to skin tests with tuberculin and other antigens such as are used in testing for mumps, pertussis, trichophytosis, and candidiasis (Sones and Israel); (3) failure to reject homografts (Elton and Andrew); and (4) failure of potent allergens, such as dinitrochlorobenzene and paradinitrodiphenylaniline, to induce contact sensitivity (Epstein and Maycock). In contrast to the frequent depression in delayed or cellular hypersensitivity, the immediate or humoral hypersensitivity is unimpaired.

The cause of the impaired cellular immunity, or *anergy*, in sarcoidosis is not known. The number of circulating T cells is reduced in only a few patients with sarcoidosis. It appears likely that the anergy in sarcoidosis is not due to a deficiency, but rather to an active suppression. It is likely that suppressor T cells are responsible for this active suppression (Kantor et al).

The Kveim test, which consists of the intradermal injection of a heat-sterilized suspension of sarcoidal tissue, preferably spleen or lymph nodes, is useful; however, unfortunately, material for this test often is unavailable. The test is positive in about 80% of the patients with sarcoidosis, with false-positive reactions in less than 2% (Siltzbach et al). For evaluation of this test, histologic examination of the test site 6 to 8 weeks after the injection is required. In the case of a positive reaction, this shows well-defined epithelioid cell granulomas, as in sarcoidosis (Rupec et al). If the histologic examination is carried out prior to the 6 weeks necessary for the development of the epithelioid cell granuloma, the prevalence of pregranulomatous monocytes and the presence of necrosis may interfere with evaluation of the test (Steigleder et al; Rupec et al). It is not known whether the Kveim test represents an isomorphic effect or a specific hypersensitivity to a cellular protein present in human sarcoidal tissue (Danbolt).

Histochemical examination of sarcoidal granulomas has shown that most of the lymphoid cells present at the periphery of the granulomas, like the epithelioid cells, show positive staining with alpha-naphthyl acetate esterase and acid phosphatase, indicating that they are monocytes from which the epithelioid cells develop (Mustakallio and Niemi; Hundeiker). This finding has been confirmed with the use of an immunologic marker that is specific for monocytes, such as erythrocytes coated with immunoglobulin G antibody (IgG EA) (Bjerke et al).

Electron microscopic examination has similarly indicated that many of the round cells at the periphery of granulomas, formerly regarded as lymphocytes, possess lysosomes in which acid phosphatase and other lysosomal enzymes are present (see p. 53). Thus, they are blood monocytes from which the epithelioid cells develop. The epithelioid cells fail to show any evidence of bacterial fragments, unlike the macrophages seen in granulomas caused by mycobacteria, although they contain both electron-light and electron-dense lysosomes (EM 29), some autophagic vacuoles, and complex, laminated residual bodies (Azar and Lunardelli). The giant cells form through the coalescence of epithelioid cells with partial fusion of their plasma membranes (see p. 52 for details). The Schaumann bodies probably form from laminated residual bodies of lysosomes. The asteroid bodies consist of collagen showing the typical 64-nm to 70-nm periodicity. It seems likely that the collagen is trapped between epithelioid cells during the stage of giant cell formation (Azar and Lunardelli).

Differential Diagnosis. The histologic differentiation of lesions of sarcoidosis from lupus vulgaris may be very difficult, and it is occasionally impossible. There is no absolute histologic criterion by which the two diseases can be differentiated with certainty. However, as a rule, the infiltrate in sarcoidosis lies scattered throughout the dermis, whereas the infiltrate in lupus vulgaris is located close to the epidermis. Furthermore, sarcoidosis usually shows only few lymphoid cells at the periphery of the granulomas, giving them the appearance of "naked" epithelioid cell tubercles, whereas lupus vulgaris often shows a marked inflammatory reaction around and between the granulomas. Also, the granulomas of sarcoidosis usually show much less central necrosis than the granulomas of lupus vulgaris (Civatte). The epidermis in sarcoidosis is either normal or atrophic, whereas in lupus vulgaris, in addition to atrophy, there may be areas of ulceration, acanthosis, and pseudocarcinomatous hyperplasia. Aside from the Kveim test, tuberculin tests as well as immunologic testing may be helpful. Tissue culture and guinea pig inoculations should be done in a search for tubercle bacilli, even though bacilli often cannot be found in lupus vulgaris (see p. 300).

The granulomas occurring in systemic berylliosis and in response to the local application of zirconium (occasionally incorporated into deodorant sticks and into creams) are indistinguishable from the granulomas seen in sarcoidosis. Clinical data are necessary for their differentiation (Epstein and Allen).

Tuberculoid leprosy may also be difficult to distinguish from sarcoidosis; only 7% of the cases of tuberculoid leprosy show acid-fast bacilli, and then only a few, so that they may easily be overlooked (Azulay). The most likely place to find bacilli is within degenerated dermal nerves, since, as a rule, the epithelioid cell granulomas of tuberculoid leprosy form around dermal nerves that are undergoing necrosis. Thus, the epithelioid cell granulomas of tuberculoid leprosy show central necrosis more often than those of sarcoidosis. Also, the granulomas of tuberculoid leprosy, in contrast

with those of sarcoidosis, follow nerves and therefore often appear elongated (Wiersema and Binford).

CHEILITIS GRANULOMATOSA (MIESCHER–MELKERSSON–ROSENTHAL SYNDROME)

Cheilitis granulomatosa is characterized by a chronic, often somewhat fluctuating swelling, usually of one lip but occasionally of both lips. Associated with this may be recurrent facial pareses and a lingua plicata (Hornstein). One occasionally observes, either in addition to or sometimes in place of swelling of the lips, swelling of the forehead, the chin, the cheeks, the eyelids, or the tongue (Wagner and Oberste-Lehn). In rare instances, enlargement of cervical or submental lymph nodes is present (Hornstein; Klaus and Brunsting). Chronic swelling of the vulva or of the foreskin has been described as a genital counterpart of cheilitis granulomatosa (Westermark and Henriksson).

Histopathology. In the skin, one observes diffuse or focal accumulations of either a tuberculoid or a lymphoid-plasma-cellular infiltrate. Usually, both types of infiltrate are seen, and there are occasionally also small "naked" epithelioid cell granulomas, as in sarcoidosis (Miescher; Hornstein; Laymon; Krutchkoff and James; Westermark and Henriksson). The infiltrate may extend to the underlying muscle (White et al). Lymph nodes, if involved, show the same histologic features as the skin, including the occasional presence of epithelioid cell granulomas (Hering and Scheid).

Histogenesis. The cause of the disorder is unknown. A relationship to sarcoidosis, originally assumed by some authors (Hering and Scheid), does not exist. The granulomas may represent a foreign body reaction arising in response to degenerative changes in the tissue, especially the subcutaneous fat (Laymon).

CHEILITIS GLANDULARIS

Cheilitis glandularis is characterized by persistent swelling of the lower lip and occasionally also of the upper lip. When the lip is squeezed, droplets of a mucoid fluid emerge from the mucosa of the lip and from the vermilion border. Not infrequently, rupture of one of the dilated mucous ducts leads to the formation of mucous cysts (Weir and Johnson) (see p. 617). In about 20% of the cases, squamous cell carcinoma of the lower vermilion border develops (Michalowski).

Histopathology. Numerous large salivary glands and dilated ducts are present in the vermilion border and in the neighboring mucosa of one or both lips, that is, in areas in which salivary glands are normally absent or present in only small numbers (Ruelens-van Haeverbeek). An infiltrate of lymphoid cells, histiocytes, and plasma cells surrounds the acini of the salivary glands. Their ducts are dilated and contain eosinophilic material (Schweich), which represents sialomucin (see p. 618).

GRANULOMA ANNULARE

The lesions of granuloma annulare consist of small, firm, asymptomatic nodules that are flesh-colored or pale red and are often grouped in a ringlike or circinate fashion. There usually are several lesions, but there may be just one, or there may be many. The lesions are found most commonly on the hands and feet. Though chronic, they subside after a number of years. Unusual variants of granuloma annulare include (1) a generalized form, consisting of hundreds of papules that are either discrete or confluent but only rarely show an annular arrangement (Dicken et al; Haim et al); (2) perforating granuloma annulare, with umbilicated lesions occurring usually in a localized distribution (Owens and Freeman; Gattlen and Delacrétaz), and rarely in a generalized distribution (Duncan et al); (3) erythematous granuloma annulare, showing slightly edematous and infiltrated, erythematous patches on which subsequently scattered papules may arise (Selmanowitz et al; Ogino and Tamaki); and (4) subcutaneous granuloma annulare, in which subcutaneous nodules occur, especially in children, either alone (Beatty) or in association with intradermal lesions (Draheim et al; Rubin and Lynch; Kerl). The subcutaneous nodules have the same clinical appearance as rheumatoid nodules (see p. 240).

A certain correlation between generalized papular granuloma annulare and diabetes mellitus has been observed by several authors (Romaine et al; Haim et al).

Histopathology. The histologic picture of granuloma annulare is characterized by focal degeneration of collagen and by reactive inflammation and fibrosis. The epidermis appears normal, except in the rare instances of perforating granuloma annulare (see below). The degeneration of collagen consists either of large foci of complete collagen degeneration or of small foci of incomplete collagen degeneration. Most commonly, one observes only scattered small foci of incomplete collagen degeneration. Less commonly, there are one or several large foci of complete collagen degeneration usually intermingled with small foci of incomplete collagen degeneration. Very rarely, the infiltrate consists of epithelioid cell nodules in association with small foci of incomplete collagen degeneration (Umbert and Winkelmann).

Foci of complete degeneration consist of large, well-demarcated areas of collagen degeneration surrounded by histiocytes in a palisading or radial arrangement and an infiltrate containing lymphoid cells and fibroblasts (Fig. 13-5). Within the area of complete collagen degeneration, the collagen appears pale and homogeneous and contains only a few pyknotic nuclei. Mucin can be seen within the area of complete collagen degeneration between the collagen bundles; it usually can be recognized even with hematoxylin-eosin staining as bluish, stringy material but stains better still with Giemsa,

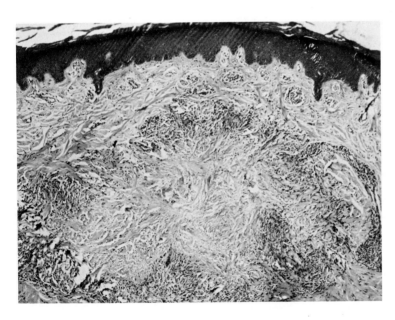

Fig. 13-5. Granuloma annulare
There is a large, sharply demarcated focus of complete collagen degeneration containing only very few nuclei. It is surrounded by an infiltrate composed largely of histiocytes in a palisading arrangement. (×50)

alcian blue, or colloidal iron. The mucin stains metachromatically with the Giemsa stain or toluidine blue (Gray et al).

Foci of incomplete degeneration consist of usually small, ill-defined areas in which some of the collagen bundles appear normal while others are found in various stages of degeneration ranging from a slight decrease in the degree of eosinophilic staining to disappearance and replacement by basophilic mucinous material. In addition, an infiltrate of lymphoid cells, histiocytes, and fibroblasts is seen, often in a single-row alignment, in the spaces between the partially degenerated and partially normal collagen bundles. Also, new collagen is being laid down. In areas thus affected, the collagen bundles present an irregular, disorderly arrangement (Fig. 13-6). The mucinous material consists of fine, basophilic threads and granules (see Plate 1, facing p. 228).

The epithelioid cell nodules seen on rare occasions in granuloma annulare usually contain some giant cells and a rim of lymphoid cells (Gray et al; Umbert and Winkelmann). They resemble the epithelioid cell nodules of sarcoidosis but show in their vicinity foci of incomplete collagen degeneration, thus allowing differentiation from sarcoidosis.

Vascular changes in granuloma annulare are variable but generally are not regarded as conspicuous (Wood and Beerman). In some instances, however, one can find, aside from endothelial swelling and thickening of vessel walls, fibrinoid deposits in vessel walls and occlusion of vascular lumina (Dahl et al). Occasionally, a few isolated, "naked" giant cells with irregularly arranged nuclei are present (Gray et al). Not infrequently, on staining for lipids, small deposits of lipid material are encountered extracellularly in areas of collagen degeneration (Gray et al; Wood and Beerman).

Among the variants of granuloma annulare mentioned, the usual histologic picture is found in the generalized form (Dicken et al) and the erythematous form (Ogino and Tamaki). In perforating granuloma annulare, foci of complete collagen degeneration surrounded by palisading histiocytes are located directly beneath the epidermis. Part of the degenerated collagen is released through a "transepidermal elimination canal" (Owens and Freeman; Duncan et al; Gattlen and Delacrétaz). In some instances, the elimination is transfollicular (Bardach). In other instances of perforating granuloma annulare, however, there is merely a central ulcer rather than true transepidermal elimination (Delaney et al).

The subcutaneous nodules of granuloma annulare show multiple large foci or complete collagen degeneration with peripheral palisading of histiocytes. The foci of degeneration in this disorder differ from those seen in dermal lesions of granuloma annulare. Whereas the dermal foci show homogeneous, pale staining of the collagen with deposits of basophilic mucin, the subcutaneous

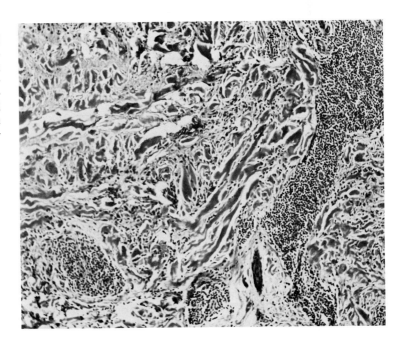

Fig. 13-6. Granuloma annulare
In the left upper quadrant is an ill-defined area of incomplete degeneration of collagen. Some of the collagen bundles are in various stages of degeneration; others appear normal. Note the disorderly arrangement of the collagen bundles. Peripheral to the area of collagen degeneration is a marked perivascular inflammatory infiltrate. (×100)

foci show strongly eosinophilic staining as a result of fibrinoid degeneration (Beatty; Kerl). Peripheral to the foci of fibrinoid degeneration and the palisading rim of histiocytes is a chronic inflammatory infiltrate (Draheim et al; Rubin and Lynch). The histologic appearance is identical with that of rheumatoid nodules (see p. 240).

Histogenesis. *Electron microscopic examination* reveals degeneration of both collagen and elastic fibers in the necrobiotic areas of granuloma annulare (Haustein; Wolff and Maciejewski; Umbert and Winkelmann). The collagen fibrils show swelling, loss of electron density, cross striation, and, in some areas, degradation to granular and amorphous material. Deposits of mucin and fibrin are apparent. The histiocytes in the vicinity of areas of degeneration show few primary and secondary lysosomes, an indication of low phagocytic activity (Umbert and Winkelmann). In contrast, fibroblasts at the periphery of areas of degeneration appear active and have a well-developed rough endoplasmic reticulum (Wolff and Maciejewski). No significant vascular changes have been noted (Haustein; Wolff and Maciejewski). Inasmuch as some foci of necrobiosis are seen without a cellular infiltrate, it is possible that focal collagen alteration represents the primary event (Wolff and Maciejewski).

Direct immunofluorescence studies have shown as the only consistent finding the presence of fibrin in necrobiotic areas (Kleinhans and Knoth; Nieboer and Kalsbeek; Thyresson et al). Blood vessel deposits of IgM and the third component of complement (C3) have been observed by some investigators (Dahl et al), but others have found them only rarely (Thyresson et al) or not at all (Nieboer and Kalsbeek). Thus, the existence of an immune complex vasculitis in granuloma annulare (Dahl et al) appears unlikely.

Differential Diagnosis. The changes in the type of granuloma annulare that has small areas of incomplete collagen degeneration may be so inconspicuous as to be easily overlooked. However, the presence of single rows of fibroblasts between collagen bundles and some disorder in the arrangement of the collagen bundles should raise suspicion and set off a search for foci of collagen degeneration.

The type of granuloma annulare that shows multiple, fairly conspicuous areas of incomplete collagen degeneration may greatly resemble necrobiosis lipoidica, in which a similar pattern of collagen degeneration may be present (see below). In fact, all the histologic and histochemical features seen in necrobiosis lipoidica may sometimes occur in granuloma annulare (Ellis and Kirby-Smith; Wood and Beerman; Gray et al). However, necrobiosis lipoidica differs from granuloma annulare as a rule by (1) the presence of a larger number of giant cells, (2) more pronounced vascular changes, (3) more extensive degeneration of collagen, often associated with hyalinization (4) more extensive deposits of lipids, and (5) smaller amounts or an absence of mucin (Laymon and Fisher).

Differentiation of subcutaneous granuloma annulare from rheumatoid nodules is not possible on clinical or histologic grounds. Thus, in the absence of any rheumatoid disease, it is best to regard such nodules as subcutaneous granuloma annulare (Kerl) (see p. 240).

In spite of the histologic differences usually present in these three diseases, it stands out that granuloma annulare, necrobiosis lipoidica, and rheumatoid nodules have a common histologic pattern based on a focal degeneration of collagen. This suggests a similar pathogenesis (Wood and Beerman).

NECROBIOSIS LIPOIDICA

In necrobiosis lipoidica, one observes clinically one or several sharply but irregularly demarcated patches, usually on the shins. They appear yellowish in the center and violaceous at the periphery. Whereas the periphery of the lesions may show slight induration, the center of the lesions gradually becomes atrophic and shows telangiectases, and it may break down to form an ulcer. In addition to the shins, lesions may be present elsewhere on the legs, particularly the calves. In about 15% of the cases, lesions are present also in areas other than the legs, especially on the hands, fingers, forearms, face, and scalp. However, necrobiosis lipoidica with lesions exclusively outside the legs occurs in less than 2% of the patients (Muller and Winkelmann, 1966a).

Lesions located in areas other than the legs may appear raised and firm and may have a papular, nodular, or plaquelike appearance without atrophy, so that they clinically resemble granuloma annulare (Muller and Winkelmann, 1966a; Balabanow et al). Involvement of the scalp with large, atrophic patches occurs occasionally; it has been observed not only in association with lesions on the shins and elsewhere (Williams; Mehregan and Pinkus; Mackey) but also, rarely, as the only lesion present (Forman; Gaethe; Metz and Metz).

In rare instances, transfollicular elimination of necrobiotic material takes place in necrobiosis lipoidica. Clinically, one observes in such cases hyperkeratotic plugs 2 mm to 3 mm in diameter distributed over the lesion (Parra; Garcia e Silva et al).

About three quarters of the patients with necrobiosis are female, and approximately two thirds have diabetes mellitus (Muller and Winkelmann, 1966a) (see also Histogenesis).

Histopathology.   On histologic examination, the epidermis may be normal, but it is often atrophic and may be absent owing to ulceration of the lesion. Two types of reaction may be observed in the dermis, a necrobiotic and a granulomatous type. Cases with the latter type of reaction at one time were referred to as granulomatosis disciformis (Miescher and Leder). However, combinations of the two types of reaction and transitions between them occur so frequently that they are now regarded as variants of the same process. Furthermore, at one time, the necrobiotic type of reaction was regarded as typical for the diabetic type of necrobiosis lipoidica, and the granulomatous type of reaction as typical for the nondiabetic type. Although this is true to some extent, there are so many exceptions that the histologic appearance cannot be correlated with the presence or absence of diabetes in any specific case (Gray et al; Muller and Winkelmann, 1966b). A large proportion of lesions of necrobiosis lipoidica located in areas other than the legs show a predominantly granulomatous reaction.

In the *necrobiotic* type of reaction, poorly defined areas of necrobiosis of collagen, often quite large, are seen throughout the dermis but especially in the lower portions (Fig. 13-7). The collagen bundles in these areas appear split up, amorphous, and anuclear. The areas of necrobiosis, because of the presence of fibrin, are periodic acid-Schiff (PAS)-positive and diastase-resistant (Gray et al). Quite frequently, deposits of mucin are present within the areas of necrobiosis. They are usually inconspicuous and are seen more distinctly on staining with the Giemsa stain or alcian blue (Gray et al; Muller and Winkelmann, 1966b). Frequently, young collagen fibers are seen near the areas of collagen degeneration. Because of the continuous process of degeneration and regeneration, the collagen fibers and bundles extend in various directions, resulting in considerable disorder of the collagen. In many areas, the collagen bundles appear thickened, hyalinized, and deeply eosinophilic and lie in close approximation to one another.

At the margin of the areas of necrobiosis, as well as scattered through the dermis and often extending into the subcutaneous fat, one finds a cellular infiltrate composed of lymphoid cells, histiocytes, fibroblasts, and occasional groups of epithelioid cells. In some areas, the infiltrate is arranged in a palisading fashion around the areas of necrobiosis. Scattered foreign body giant cells frequently are present and are of considerable diagnostic value (Fig. 13-8) (Gray et al). Whereas some of the giant cells lie by themselves as "naked" giant cells, others lie intermingled with histiocytes and epithelioid cells, giving the infiltrate a granulomatous appearance (Laymon and Fisher). Cases with conspicuous granuloma formation are intermediate between the necrobiotic and the granulomatous types of necrobiosis lipoidica (see below).

The blood vessels, particularly in the middle

Fig. 13-7.   Necrobiosis lipoidica, necrobiotic type of reaction
Much of the collagen appears degenerated. An inflammatory infiltrate is scattered through the areas of degeneration. A vessel in the center shows intimal thickening. (×100)

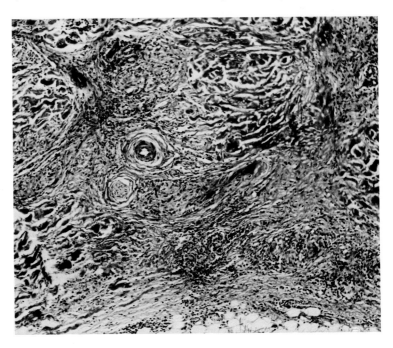

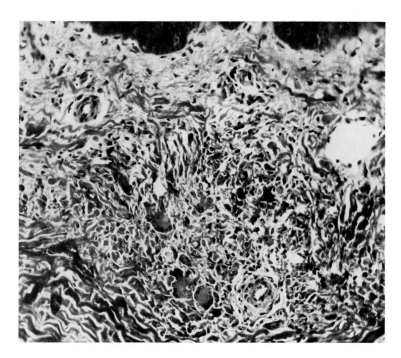

Fig. 13-8.   Necrobiosis lipoidica, necrobiotic type of reaction
Several foreign body giant cells are located within an area of collagen degeneration. Two fibrotic vessels are present. (×200)

and lower dermis, often exhibit thickening of their walls with proliferation of their endothelial cells. The process may lead to partial and, occasionally, even to complete occlusion of the lumen. The thickened walls appear heavily infiltrated with PAS-positive, diastase-resistant material (Wood and Beerman). Vascular changes of this type are seen particularly near areas in which the collagen bundles appear thickened and hyalinized. Whereas the vascular changes often are conspicuous in lesions of the lower legs, they usually are mild or absent elsewhere (Metz and Metz).

Staining for lipids with scarlet red frequently, but not always, reveals numerous granules of lipid extracellularly in areas of necrobiosis of collagen. In rare instances, a few foam cells are also noted (Nicholas; Metz and Metz). On staining with scarlet red, the extracellular lipid deposits stain a rusty brown, in contrast with the neutral fat in the subcutaneous layer and the fat in the sebaceous glands, which stain orange red. The lipid deposits probably consist of neutral fat, phospholipids, and small amounts of free cholesterol (Hildebrand et al). Cholesterol esters cannot be present in significant amounts, since the granules only rarely show double refraction (Laymon and Fisher; Mehregan and Pinkus).

In the *granulomatous* type of reaction, the dermis contains scattered granulomatous foci composed of histiocytes, epithelioid cells, and giant cells

(Fig. 13-9). Asteroid bodies within the giant cells are present in some instances (Smith and Wansker). Aside from the granulomatous foci, one observes a mild to moderately severe inflammatory infiltrate and, often, extensive hyalinization of the collagen. However, areas of necrobiosis and deposits of lipids are not conspicuous and occasionally are even absent (Miescher and Leder; Muller and Winkelmann, 1966a). Also, vascular changes usually are mild. In some lesions of necrobiosis lipoidica, especially those located on the scalp, the predominance of epithelioid cells and giant cells causes considerable resemblance to sarcoidosis (Fig. 13-10) (Williams; Mehregan and Pinkus).

In cases of necrobiosis lipoidica with transfollicular elimination of necrobiotic material, one observes necrotic material either at the base or within the infundibulum of dilated hair follicles (Parra; Garcia e Silva et al).

Histogenesis. Some authors have expressed their belief that the necrobiosis of collagen is due to vascular changes and that, in cases in which clinical or latent diabetes exists, the diabetes is the cause of the vascular changes (Hildebrand et al; Knoth and Füller; Bauer et al). However, even though vascular changes are a prominent feature in many lesions of necrobiosis lipoidica, they are absent in about one third of the lesions (Muller and Winkelmann, 1966b). Also, the affected vessels are often situated in the lower layers of the dermis and are of a much larger caliber than the type of vessel affected by

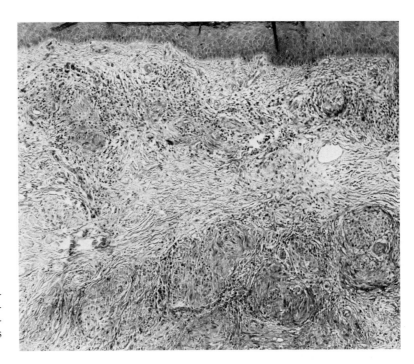

Fig. 13-9.   Necrobiosis lipoidica, granulomatous type
The dermis contains scattered granulomas composed of histiocytes, epithelioid cells, and giant cells. There is fibrosis but only slight focal necrobiosis of the collagen. (×100)

diabetic microangiopathy (Bauer et al). Thus, it appears quite possible that vascular changes, if present, are a part of the process of necrobiosis, hyalinization, and fibrosis of collagen. This would also explain why, when they occur, vascular changes are much more pronounced on the legs, where the vascular walls normally contain a greater amount of collagen than in other areas. Many authors therefore regard focal degeneration of collagen as the primary event in necrobiosis lipoidica, a feature that represents the primary event also in granuloma annulare and rheumatoid nodules (Wood and Beerman).

About two thirds of the patients with necrobiosis lipoidica have clinical evidence of diabetes mellitus. Occasionally, diabetes develops many years after the appearance of the cutaneous lesions (Muller and Winkelmann, 1966a). Furthermore, half of 38 patients with "nondiabetic" necrobiosis lipoidica tested showed an abnormal cortisone glucose tolerance test (Komisaruk; Narva et al; Muller and Winkelmann, 1966c; Mobacken et al). However, this still leaves a significant number of patients with necrobiosis lipoidica without evidence of diabetes. Only long-range follow-up studies will prove or disprove the postulate that diabetes mellitus will occur in all nondiabetic patients with necrobiosis lipoidica who attain sufficient age (Muller and Winkelmann, 1966a).

Direct immunofluorescence studies have shown that necrobiotic areas invariably contain fibrinogen. Deposits of IgM and C3 have been found in the vessel walls of about 50% of the patients tested (Ullman and Dahl). Analogous findings have been described in granuloma annulare (Dahl et al; see p. 236) and have been interpreted as being suggestive of an immune complex vasculitis.

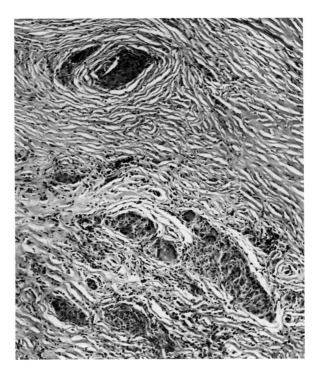

Fig. 13-10.   Necrobiosis lipoidica, granulomatous type
Islands containing epithelioid cells and giant cells are closely surrounded by hyalinized bundles of collagen. (×200)

The deposition of lipids extracellularly in necrobiotic areas and, rarely, within foam cells is generally regarded as a secondary event, because the lesions occasionally contain no lipids (Leifer). It probably represents a "lipid phanerosis" secondary to collagen degeneration (Gertler).

Differential Diagnosis. As already pointed out, differentiation of necrobiosis lipoidica from granuloma annulare may be difficult (see p. 236). However, this difficulty is rarely encountered in lesions of necrobiosis lipoidica located on the shins because, in that location, hyalinization of collagen and thickening of vessel walls usually are pronounced, and, as a rule, more giant cells, more lipid, and less mucin are present than in granuloma annulare. However, lesions of necrobiosis lipoidica in locations other than the shins may be histologically indistinguishable from granuloma annulare (Wood and Beerman; Gray et al; Muller and Winkelmann, 1966a).

Occasionally, the granulomatous type of necrobiosis lipoidica shows well-defined granulomas containing epithelioid cells and giant cells, so that the histologic picture resembles that of sarcoidosis (Mehregan and Pinkus; Muller and Winkelmann, 1966b). However, hyalinization of the collagen and often also the presence of foci of necrobiosis and of extracellular lipids aid in the differential diagnosis (Mehregan and Pinkus).

For a discussion of differentiation of necrobiosis lipoidica from annular elastolytic granuloma, see p. 241.

RHEUMATOID NODULES

Subcutaneous rheumatoid nodules occur most commonly in rheumatoid arthritis and rheumatic fever (Watt and Baumann). In rare instances, their occurrence in systemic lupus erythematosus has also been described (Hahn et al; Dubois et al). The nodules develop near bony structures, often in the vicinity of a joint, and they may or may not be attached to the overlying skin. Their size usually varies from a few millimeters to 2 cm, but they may be larger (Bennett et al).

Subcutaneous nodules that are indistinguishable both clinically and histologically from rheumatoid nodules but that are not accompanied by a rheumatoid disease occur occasionally in children (Beatty; Kerl) and rarely in adults (Lowney and Simons; Kerl). Whereas rheumatoid arthritis occasionally develops subsequently in adults, it does not seem to do so in children (Lowney and Simons). However, intradermal lesions of granuloma annulare have appeared subsequently in some children as well as in some adults (Kerl). It is therefore best to regard such nodules as subcutaneous granuloma annulare in all children and in most adults (see p. 235).

Histopathology. A rheumatoid nodule shows several sharply but irregularly demarcated foci of fibrinoid collagen degeneration surrounded by histiocytes in a palisade arrangement. In the intermediary stroma of the nodule, one observes a chronic inflammatory infiltrate with proliferation of blood vessels and fibrosis (Fig. 13-11) (Watt and Baumann). Staining for lipids frequently reveals droplets of lipid in the necrotic centers. Occasionally, intercellular as well as intracellular deposits of lipid are seen in the surrounding zone of palisading histiocytes (Kerl). Although, in general, inflammatory changes prevail in the nodules of rheumatic fever and degenerative and proliferative changes predominate in the nodules of rheumatoid arthritis, this difference is nevertheless based on the age of the lesion. Thus, young nodules of rheumatoid arthritis have an appearance similar to those of rheumatic fever (Bennett et al).

ANNULAR ELASTOLYTIC GRANULOMA

In annular elastolytic granuloma, one or several annular lesions with an elevated, red border and hypopigmented center are present mainly on the face. The lesions may extend to the scalp, and, in some instances, similar lesions are present also on the neck and extremities. The annular lesions undergo slow peripheral extension, and, if several lesions are present, they may coalesce, resulting in a serpiginous border. After persisting for several years, the lesions usually resolve without residual scarring.

This disorder was first described in 1967 as atypical, annular necrobiosis lipoidica (Dowling and Wilson Jones). Even then it was recognized that the elastic tissue is lost in areas of the infiltrate and phagocytized by giant cells. Because of the absence of necrobiosis, the dermatosis was regarded in 1973 as Miescher's granuloma of the face (Mehregan and Altman). Then, in 1975, it was called actinic granuloma (O'Brien). However, subsequent studies have revealed only moderate, if any, solar elastosis in the skin surrounding the lesions. Therefore, the designation of *annular elastolytic giant cell granuloma* was proposed in 1979 (Hanke et al).

Histopathology. Histologic examination reveals as the outstanding feature numerous large giant cells often containing prominent asteroid bodies. In addition, there is an infiltrate of histiocytes, lymphocytes, and scattered groups of epithelioid cells (Wilson Jones). Necrobiosis or vascular changes are absent, and there are no deposits of mucin or lipids (Hanke et al).

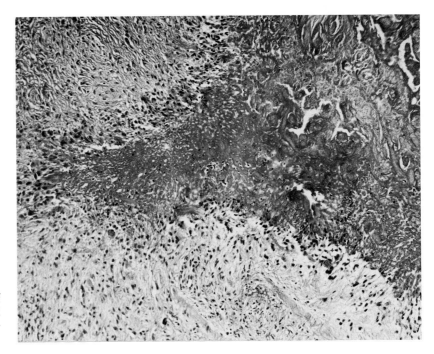

Fig. 13-11. Subcutaneous nodule of rheumatoid arthritis
There is a large, central zone of fibrinoid degeneration surrounded by histiocytes in a palisade arrangement. (×100)

The elastic tissue changes are appreciated best when the biopsy incision is made radially across the elevated border of the lesion (O'Brien). Elastic tissue stains then reveal an abrupt loss of elastic material in the granulomatous infiltrate. Fragments of elastic fibers can frequently be identified within the multinucleated giant cells (Dowling and Wilson Jones; O'Brien), and the asteroid bodies stain like elastic fibers with acid orcein (Mehregan and Altman). The hypopigmented center of the lesion shows a lack of elastic tissue with little or no inflammation.

Differential Diagnosis. Annular elastolytic granuloma differs from granuloma annulare by the absence of collagen degeneration and mucin. In addition, giant cells are rarely prominent in granuloma annulare and, in particular, do not contain asteroid bodies. Differentiation of annular elastolytic granuloma from the granulomatous type of necrobiosis lipoidica is more difficult, since multinucleated giant cells, even with asteroid bodies, and absence of lipid deposition can occur in the latter as well as in the former. However, a radial biopsy will demonstrate not only the destruction of elastic tissue in the granulomatous zone but also its absence in the hypopigmented center in annular elastolytic granuloma.

GRANULOMA GLUTEALE INFANTUM

Granuloma gluteale infantum, first described in 1971 (Tappeiner and Pfleger), shows asymptomatic, round to oval, smooth, raised nodules, reddish blue in color, from a few millimeters to a few centimeters in diameter, and irregularly distributed over the region of the skin that is covered by diapers (Tappeiner and Pfleger; Uyeda et al; Simmons). Although usually seen in infants, it has also been described in aged women wearing diapers because of incontinence (Maekawa et al).

Histopathology. A dense polymorphous inflammatory infiltrate is seen throughout the dermis. It contains various types of mononuclear cells as well as neutrophils and eosinophils (Simmons). In addition, there may be microabscesses composed of neutrophils and eosinophils, as well as extravasations of erythrocytes together with a proliferation of capillaries (Tappeiner and Pfleger). In a few instances, staining with the PAS reaction has revealed spores and pseudohyphae consistent with the presence of *Candida albicans* in the stratum corneum (Delacrétaz et al).

Histogenesis. In nearly all patients described in the literature, the development of granuloma gluteale infantum has been preceded by a diaper dermatitis, which only in some instances has been associated with a *Candida albicans* infection (Uyeda). Almost all patients have received topical applications of fluorinated corticosteroid preparations for a prolonged period of time, and this is regarded by several authors as a possible cause (Altmeyer; Simmons). However, in some instances, only dusting powder had been used (Maekawa et al); in such cases, the prolonged wearing of plastic diapers would seem to be responsible. In any case, it appears very likely that exogenous factors are the cause of the eruption (Tappeiner and Pfleger).

BIBLIOGRAPHY

Sarcoidosis

AZAR HA, LUNARDELLI C: Collagen nature of asteroid bodies of giant cells in sarcoidosis. Am J Pathol 57:81–92, 1969

AZULAY RD: Histopathology of skin lesions in leprosy. Int J Lepr 39:244–250, 1971

BARRIE HJ, BOGOCH A: The natural history of the sarcoid granuloma. Am J Pathol 29:451–469, 1953

BJERKE JR, KROGH HR, MATRE R: In situ identification of mononuclear cells in cutaneous infiltrates in discoid lupus erythematosus, sarcoidosis and secondary syphilis. Acta Derm Venereol (Stockh) 61:371–380, 1981

BODIE BF, KHEIR SM, OMURA EF: Calvarial sarcoid mimicking metastatic disease. J Am Acad Dermatol 3:401–405, 1980

BRUNNER MJ, ROBIN M: Lichen-scrofulosorum-like lesions associated with sarcoidosis. Arch Dermatol Syph 60:1212–1214, 1949

CHEVRANT-BRETON J, REVILLON L, PONY JC et al: Sarcoidose à manifestations cutanées extensives ulcéreuses et atrophiantes. Ann Dermatol Venereol 104:805–810, 1977

CIVATTE J: Sarcoidose et infiltrats tuberculoides. Ann Dermatol Syph 90:5–28, 1963

CLAYTON R, WOOD PL: Subcutaneous nodular sarcoid. Dermatologica 149:51–54, 1974

DANBOLT N: Kveim's reaction and its significance in sarcoidosis research. Acta Derm Venereol (Stockh) 42:354–362, 1962

ELTON RF, ANDREW JH: Homograft survival in sarcoidosis. Arch Dermatol 94:403–405, 1966

EPSTEIN WL, ALLEN JR: Granulomatous hypersensitivity after use of zirconium-containing poison oak lotion. JAMA 190:940–942, 1964

EPSTEIN WL, MAYCOCK RL: Induction of allergic contact dermatitis in patients with sarcoidosis. Proc Soc Exp Biol Med 96:786–788, 1957

GROSS MD, ANDRIACCI F, GORDON R et al: Nodular subcutaneous sarcoidosis. Arch Dermatol 113:1442–1443, 1977

HANNO R, NEEDELMAN A, EIFERMAN RA et al: Cutaneous sarcoidal granulomas and the development of systemic sarcoidosis. Arch Dermatol 117:203–207, 1981

HOPF B, KREBS A: "Ulcera cruris" als seltene Form einer Sarkoidose. Dermatologica 149:55–62, 1974

HUNDEIKER M: Zur Abstammung der Zellen des Sarkoidosegranuloms. Hautarzt 20:164–167, 1969

ISRAEL HL, OSTROW A: Sarcoidosis and aspergilloma. Am J Med 47:243–250, 1969

ISRAEL HL, SONES M: Selection of biopsy procedures for sarcoidosis diagnosis. Arch Intern Med 113:255–260, 1964

JAMES DG, SILTZBACH LE, SHARMA OP et al: A tale of two cities. A comparison of sarcoidosis in London and New York. Arch Intern Med 123:187–191, 1969

KANTOR FS, DWYER JM, MANGI RJ: Sarcoid. J Invest Dermatol 67:470–476, 1976

KAUH YC, GOODY HE, LUSCOMBE HA: Ichthyosiform sarcoidosis. Arch Dermatol 114:100–101, 1978

KELLY AP: Ichthyosiform sarcoid. Arch Dermatol 114:1551–1552, 1978

KOERNER SK, SAKOWITZ AJ, APPELMAN RI et al: Transbronchial lung biopsy for the diagnosis of sarcoidosis. N Engl J Med 293:268–270, 1975

LANGNER A, MOSKALEWSKA K, PRONIEWSKA M: Studies on the mechanism of lymphocyte transformation inhibition in sarcoidosis. Br J Dermatol 81:829–834, 1969

LEVER WF, FREIMAN DG: Sarcoidosis: A report of a case with erythrodermic lesions, subcutaneous nodes and asteroid inclusion bodies in giant cells. Arch Dermatol Syph 57:639–654, 1948

LONGCOPE WT, FREIMAN DG: A study of sarcoidosis. Medicine (Baltimore) 31:1–132, 1952

MAYCOCK RL, BERTRAND P, MORISON CE et al: Manifestations of sarcoidosis. Am J Med 35:67–74, 1963

MCCOY RC, FISHER CC: Glomerulonephritis associated with sarcoidosis. Am J Pathol 68:339–358, 1972

MISTILIS SP, GREEN JR, SCHIFF L: Hepatic sarcoidosis with portal hypertension. Am J Med 36:470–477, 1964

MORRISON JGL: Sarcoidosis in a child, presenting as an erythroderma with keratotic spines and palmar pits. Br J Dermatol 95:93–97, 1976

MUSTAKALLIO KK, NIEMI M: Histochemie der Lysosomenzyme des Sarkoidosegranuloms. Dermatol Wochenschr 152:1454–1455, 1966

NESSAN VJ, JACOWAY JR: Biopsy of minor salivary glands in the diagnosis of sarcoidosis. N Engl J Med 301:922–924, 1979

NOZAKI T: Sarcoidosis with lichenoid type eruption. Jpn J Dermatol 82:47–54, 1972

PUTKONEN T: Symptomenkomplex der beginnenden Sarkoidose. Dermatol Wochenschr 152:1455–1456, 1966

ROBERTS WC, MCALLISTER HA JR, FERRANS VJ: Sarcoidosis of the heart. Am J Med 63:86–108, 1977

RUPEC M, KORB G, BEHREND H: Feingewebliche Untersuchungen zur Entwicklung des positiven Kveim-Tests. Arch Klin Exp Dermatol 237:811–818, 1970

SELENKOW HA, TYLER HR, MATSON DD et al: Hypopituitarism due to hypothalamic sarcoidosis. Am J Med Sci 238:456–460, 1959

SILTZBACH LE, JAMES DG, NEVILLE E et al: Course and prognosis of sarcoidosis around the world. Am J Med 57:847–852, 1974

SONES M, ISRAEL HL: Altered immunologic reactions in sarcoidosis. Ann Intern Med 40:260–268, 1954

STEIGLEDER GK, SILVA A JR, NELSON CT: Histopathology of the Kveim test. Arch Dermatol 84:828–834, 1961

THAL M: Klinik der lichenoiden Form des Boeck'schen Sarcoids. Dermatologica 111:87–92, 1955

UMBERT P, WINKELMANN RK: Granuloma annulare and sarcoidosis. Br J Dermatol 97:481–486, 1977

VEIEN NK: Cutaneous sarcoidosis treated with levamisole. Dermatologica 154:185–189, 1977

WIERSEMA JP, BINFORD CH: The identification of leprosy among epithelioid cell granulomas of the skin. Int J Lepr 40:10–32, 1972

WIGLEY JEM, MUSSO LA: A case of sarcoidosis with erythrodermic lesions. Br J Dermatol 63:398–407, 1951

WOOD BT, BEHLEN CHII, WEARY PE: The association of sarcoidosis, erythema nodosum and arthritis. Arch Dermatol 94:406–408, 1966

Cheilitis Granulomatosa (Miescher–Melkersson–Rosenthal Syndrome)

HERING H, SCHEID P: Kritische Bemerkungen zum Melkersson–Rosenthal–Syndrom als Teilbild des Morbus Besnier–Boeck–Schaumann. Arch Dermatol Syph (Berlin) 197:344–382, 1954

HORNSTEIN O: Über die Pathogenese des sogenannten Melkersson–Rosenthal Syndroms (einschliesslich der "Cheilitis granulomatosa" Miescher). Arch Klin Exp Dermatol 212:570–605, 1961

KLAUS SN, BRUNSTING LA: Melkersson's syndrome (persistent swelling of the face, recurrent facial paralysis and lingua plicata): Report of a case, Proc Mayo Clin 34:365–370, 1959

KRUTCHKOFF D, JAMES R: Cheilitis granulomatosa. Arch Dermatol 114:1203–1206, 1978

LAYMON CW: Cheilitis granulomatosa and Melkersson–Rosenthal syndrome. Arch Dermatol 83:112–118, 1963

MIESCHER G: Über essentielle granulomatöse Makrocheilie (Cheilitis granulomatosa). Dermatologica 91:57–85, 1945

WAGNER G, OBERSTE-LEHN H: Zur Kenntnis der Symptomatologie der Granulomatosis idiopathica. Z Hautkr 32:166–176, 1963

WESTERMARK P, HENRIKSSON TG: Granulomatous inflammation of the vulva and penis, a genital counterpart to cheilitis granulomatosa. Dermatologica 158:269–274, 1979

WHITE IR, SOUTERYRAND P, MACDONALD DM: Granulomatous cheilitis (Miescher). Clin Exp Dermatol 6:391–397, 1981

Cheilitis Glandularis

MICHALOWSKI R: Cheilitis glandularis, heterotopic salivary glands and squamous cell carcinoma of the lips. Br J Dermatol 74:455–449, 1962

RUELENS-VAN HAEVERBEEK A: A propos de la cheilite glandulaire de Puente. Arch Belg Dermatol Syph 25:147–150, 1969

SCHWEICH L: Cheilitis glandularis simplex (Puente and Acevedo). Arch Dermatol 89:301–302, 1964

WEIR TW, JOHNSON WC: Cheilitis glandularis. Arch Dermatol 103:433–437, 1971

Granuloma Annulare

BARDACH HG: Granuloma annulare with transfollicular perforation. J Cutan Pathol 4:99–104, 1977

BEATTY EC JR: Rheumatic-like nodule occurring in nonrheumatic children. Arch Pathol 68:154–159, 1959

DAHL MV, ULLMAN S, GOLTZ RW: Vasculitis in granuloma annulare. Arch Dermatol 113:463–467, 1977

DELANEY TJ, GOLD SC, LEPPARD B: Disseminated perforating granuloma annulare. Br J Dermatol 89:523–526, 1973

DICKEN CH, CARRINGTON SG, WINKELMANN RK: Generalized granuloma annulare. Arch Dermatol 99:556–563, 1969

DRAHEIM JH, JOHNSON LC, HELWIG EB: A clinico-pathological analysis of "rheumatoid" nodules occurring in 54 children. Am J Pathol 35:678, 1959

DUNCAN WC, SMITH JD, KNOX JM: Generalized perforating granuloma annulare. Arch Dermatol 108:570–572, 1973

ELLIS FA, KIRBY-SMITH H: Necrobiosis lipoidica and granuloma annulare. Arch Dermatol Syph 45:40–60, 1942

GATTLEN JM, DELACRÉTAZ J: Le granulome annulaire perforant. Dermatologica 151:368–375, 1975

GRAY HR, GRAHAM JH, JOHNSON WC: Necrobiosis lipoidica: A histopathological and histochemical study. J Invest Dermatol 44:369–380, 1965

HAIM S, FRIEDMAN-BIRNBAUM R, SHAFRIR A: Generalized granuloma annulare: Relationship to diabetes mellitus as revealed in 8 cases. Br J Dermatol 83:302–305, 1970

HAUSTEIN UF: Zur Ultrastruktur des Granuloma annulare. Dermatol Monatsschr 162:289–299, 1976

KERL H: Knotige rheumatische Hautmanifestationen und ihre Differentialdiagnose. Z Hautkr 47:193–208, 1972

KLEINHANS D, KNOTH W: Immunhistochemischer Fibrin-Nachweis beim Granuloma anulare. Arch Dermatol Res 258:231–234, 1977

LAYMON CW, FISHER I: Necrobiosis lipoidica (diabeticorum?). A

histologic study and comparison with granuloma annulare. Arch Dermatol Syph 59:150–167, 1949

NIEBOER C, KALSBEEK GL: Direct immunofluorescence studies in granuloma annulare, necrobiosis lipoidica and granulomatosis disciformis Mieschner. Dermatologica 158:427–432, 1979

OGINO A, TAMAKI E: Atypical granuloma annulare. Dermatologica 156:97–100, 1978

OWENS DW, FREEMAN RG: Perforating granuloma annulare. Arch Dermatol 103:64–67, 1971

ROMAINE R, RUDNER EJ, ALTMAN J: Papular granuloma annulare and diabetes mellitus. Arch Dermatol 98:152–154, 1968

RUBIN M, LYNCH FW: Subcutaneous granuloma annulare. Arch Dermatol Syph 93:416–420, 1966

SELMANOWITZ VJ, VANDOW JE, DIRECTOR W: Atypical granuloma annulare. Arch Dermatol 93:454–456, 1966

THYRESSON HN, DOYLE JA, WINKELMANN RK: Granuloma annulare. Histopathologic and direct immunofluorescence study. Acta Derm Venereol (Stockh) 60:261–263, 1980

UMBERT P, WINKELMANN RK: Histologic, ultrastructural, and histochemical studies of granuloma annulare. Arch Dermatol 113:1681–1686, 1977

WOLFF HH, MACIEJEWSKI W: The ultrastructure of granuloma annulare. Arch Dermatol Res 259:225–234, 1977

WOOD MG, BEERMAN H: Necrobiosis lipoidica, granuloma annulare, and rheumatoid nodule. J Invest Dermatol 34:139–147, 1960

Necrobiosis Lipoidica

BALABANOW K, DURMISCHEV A, KARAJACHEV G: Ein Fall von Nekrobiosis lipoidica diabeticorum mit ungewöhnlicher Lokalisation. Z Hautkr 47:217–224, 1972

BAUER MF, HIRSCH P, BULLOCK WK et al: Necrobiosis lipoidica diabeticorum. A cutaneous manifestation of diabetic microangiopathy. Arch Dermatol 90:558–566, 1964

DAHL MV, ULLMAN S, GOLTZ RW: Vasculitis in granuloma annulare. Arch Dermatol 113:463–467, 1977

FORMAN L: Necrobiosis lipoidica diabeticorum of the scalp. Proc R Soc Med 47:658–659, 1954

GAETHE G: Necrobiosis lipoidica diabeticorum of the scalp. Arch Dermatol 89:865–866, 1964

GARCIA E SILVA L, CAPITÃO-MOR M, DE CARVALHO I: Nécrobiose lipoidique perforante. Ann Dermatol Venereol 108:891–896, 1981

GERTLER W: Die nosologische Stellung der Granulomatosis (tuberculoides) pseudosklerodermiformis symmetrica chronica (Gottron). Dermatol Wochenschr 141:241–258, 1960

GRAY HR, GRAHAM JH, JOHNSON WC: Necrobiosis lipoidica: A histopathological and histochemical study. J Invest Dermatol 44:369–380, 1965

HILDEBRAND AG, MONTGOMERY H, RYNEARSON EH: Necrobiosis lipoidica diabeticorum. Arch Intern Med 66:851–878, 1940

KNOTH W, FÜLLER R: Zur Patho- und Histogenese der Nekrobiosis lipoidica "diabeticorum." Arch Dermatol Syph (Berlin) 199:109–133, 1955

KOMISARUK E: Cortisone glucose tolerance test in necrobiosis lipodica. Arch Dermatol 90:208–210, 1964

LAYMON CW, FISHER I: Necrobiosis lipoidica (diabeticorum?). Arch Dermatol Syph 59:150–167, 1949

LEIFER W: Necrobiosis lipoidica diabeticorum in a nondiabetic person. Arch Dermatol Syph 44:717–719, 1941

MACKEY JP: Necrobiosis lipoidica diabeticorum involving scalp and face. Br J Dermatol 93:729–730, 1975

MEHREGAN AH, PINKUS H: Necrobiosis lipoidica with sarcoid reaction. Arch Dermatol 83:143–145, 1961

METZ G, METZ J: Extracrurale Manifestion der Necrobiosis lipoidica. Isolierter Befall des Kopfes. Hautarzt 28:359–363, 1977

MIESCHER G, LEDER M: Granulomatosis disciformis chronica et progressiva. Dermatologica 97:25–34, 1948

MOBACKEN H, GISSLEN H, JOHANNISSON G: Granuloma annulare. Acta Derm Venereol (Stockh) 50:440–444, 1970

MULLER SA, WINKELMANN RK: Necrobiosis lipoidica diabeticorum. Arch Dermatol 93:272–281, 1966a

MULLER SA, WINKELMANN RK: Necrobiosis lipoidica diabeticorum. Arch Dermatol 94:1–10, 1966b

MULLER SA, WINKELMANN RK: Necrobiosis lipoidica diabeticorum. Results of glucose tolerance tests in nondiabetic patients. JAMA 195:433–436, 1966c

NARVA WM, BENOIT FL, RINGROSE EJ: Necrobiosis lipoidica diabeticorum with apparently normal carbohydrate tolerance. Arch Intern Med 115:718–722, 1965

NICHOLAS L: Necrobiosis lipoidica diabeticorum with xanthoma cells. Arch Dermatol Syph 48:606–611, 1943

PARRA CA: Transepithelial elimination in necrobiosis lipoidica. Br J Dermatol 96:83–86, 1977

SMITH JG JR, WANSKER BA: Asteroid bodies in necrobiosis lipoidica. Arch Dermatol 74:276–279, 1956

ULLMAN S, DAHL MV: Necrobiosis lipoidica. Arch Dermatol 113:1671–1673, 1977

WILLIAMS RM: Necrobiosis lipoidica diabeticorum with alopecia showing sarcoid-like reaction. Arch Dermatol 79:366–368, 1959

WOOD MG, BEERMAN H: Necrobiosis lipoidica, granuloma annulare, and rheumatoid nodule. J Invest Dermatol 34:139–147, 1960

Rheumatoid Nodules

BEATTY EC: Rheumatic-like nodules occurring in nonrheumatic children. Arch Pathol 68:154–159, 1959

BENNETT GA, ZELLER JW, BAUER W: Subcutaneous nodules of rheumatoid arthritis and rheumatic fever. Arch Pathol 30:70–89, 1940

DUBOIS EL, FRIOU GJ, CHANDOR S: Rheumatoid nodules and rheumatoid granulomas in systemic lupus erythematosus. JAMA 220:515–518, 1972

HAHN BH, YARDLEY JH, STEVENS MD: Rheumatoid "nodules" in systemic lupus erythematosus. Ann Intern Med 72:49–58, 1970

KERL H: Knotige rheumatische Hautmanifestationen und ihre Differentialdiagnose. Z Hautkr 47:193–208, 1972

LOWNEY ED, SIMONS HM: "Rheumatoid" nodules of the skin. Arch Dermatol 88:853–858, 1963

WATT TL, BAUMANN RR: Pseudoxanthomatous rheumatoid nodules. Arch Dermatol 95:156–160, 1967

Annular Elastolytic Granuloma

DOWLING GB, WILSON JONES E: Atypical (annular) necrobiosis lipoidica of the face and scalp. Dermatologica 135:11–26, 1967

HANKE CW, BAILIN PL, ROENIGK HH JR: Annular elastolytic giant cell granuloma. J Am Acad Dermatol 1:413–421, 1979

MEHREGAN AH, ALTMAN J: Miescher's granuloma of the face. Arch Dermatol 107:62–64, 1973

O'BRIEN JP: Actinic granuloma. Arch Dermatol 111:460–466, 1975

WILSON JONES E: Necrobiosis lipoidica presenting on the face and scalp. Trans St John's Hosp Dermatol Soc 57:203–220, 1971

Granuloma Gluteale Infantum

ALTMEYER P: Die Bedeutung fluorierter Glucocorticoide in der Aetiopathogenese des Granuloma glutaeale infantum (Tappeiner und Pfleger). Z Hautkr 48:621–626, 1973

DELACRÉTAZ J, GRIGORIU D, DE CROUSAZ H et al: Candidose nodulaire de la région inguino-génitale et des fesses (granuloma glutaeale infantum). Dermatologica 144:144–155, 1972

MAEKAWA Y, SAKAZAKI Y, HAYASHIBARA T: Diaper area granuloma of the aged. Arch Dermatol 114:382–383, 1978

SIMMONS IJ: Granuloma gluteale infantum. Aust J Dermatol 18:20–24, 1977

TAPPEINER J, PFLEGER L: Granuloma glutaeale infantum. Hautarzt 22:383–388, 1971

UYEDA K, NAKAYASU K, TAKAISHI Y: Kaposi sarcoma-like granuloma on diaper dermatitis. Arch Dermatol 107:605–607, 1973

Inflammatory Diseases of the Subcutaneous Fat

14

CLASSIFICATION OF PANNICULITIS

No generally agreed upon classification of panniculitis exists, because certain forms of panniculitis are regarded by some as an entity and by others as merely a variant. Nevertheless, there exist several well-established forms of panniculitis with established etiologies. Among those that will be discussed in this chapter are subcutaneous nodular fat necrosis in pancreatitis, factitial panniculitis, cold panniculitis, sclerema neonatorum, and subcutaneous fat necrosis of the newborn. Other forms, among them histiocytic cytophagic panniculitis (see p. 194), subcutaneous sarcoidosis (see p. 229), subcutaneous granuloma annulare (see p. 235), and lupus erythematosus panniculitis (see p. 455), are discussed in other chapters.

The problem of classification concerns the remainder of nodose lesions, which occur predominantly on the lower legs. With the exception of acute erythema nodosum, these nodose lesions are chronic and show variations of their histologic picture on the basis of duration, so that different histologic interpretations can be made during different stages (Pierini at al). In most instances of panniculitis, an early stage of nonspecific inflammation with varying degrees of vascular changes is followed by a stage that is characterized by phagocytosis of fat and a more or less pronounced granulomatous reaction, and by a final stage of fibrosis. Since different areas of the same lesion may show different stages, a punch biopsy often is insufficient for adequate evaluation. Instead, a scalpel excision of an entire node or at least a large part of it is generally required. Often, therefore, when merely a small specimen is submitted, only a diagnosis of panniculitis without further classification can be rendered (Winkelmann and Förström). But even with adequate histologic material, it may be difficult to assign every case to a recognized entity, and only adequate follow-up will make a diagnosis possible.

A simplified classification of panniculitis recognizes an acute and a chronic form of erythema nodosum and includes under the latter subacute nodular migratory panniculitis (Vilanova and Piñol Aguadé). Erythema induratum is also clearly an entity, since, in its late stage, it shows areas of necrosis, in contrast to erythema nodosum. Nodular vasculitis (Montgomery et al) can be classified as a variant of erythema induratum. Additional entities with characteristic histologic features are superficial migratory thrombophlebitis and Weber–Christian disease. It appears doubtful, however, that lipogranulomatosis subcutanea of Rothmann and Makai qualifies as an entity; most cases described as such can be assigned to erythema nodosum, to erythema induratum, or to Weber–Christian disease.

Because of this difficulty in assigning every case of panniculitis to one of the recognized entities, some cases will have to be called nonspecific panniculitis or nondefinite panniculitis (Niemi et al).

ERYTHEMA NODOSUM

An acute form and a chronic form of erythema nodosum exist that differ in their clinical manifestations but not in their histologic characteristics.

In the *acute form* of erythema nodosum, the lesions consist of tender, red or livid red nodes raised slightly above the level of the skin. They vary from 1 cm to 5 cm in diameter and usually are confined to the anterior surface of the lower legs, although they may occur elsewhere, especially on the calves, thighs, and forearms. Without breaking down, they generally involute within a few weeks, although, as a result of the intermittent appearance of new lesions, the disease may extend over several months.

In the *chronic form* of erythema nodosum, also referred to as erythema nodosum migrans (Bäfverstedt), one or several red, subcutaneous nodules are found on the lower legs. Tenderness is slight or absent. Through peripheral extension, the nodules change into plaques. Old plaques often show central clearing. The duration of the disease may be from a few months to a few years.

Histopathology.   The histologic changes are present mainly in the subcutaneous tissue. The dermis merely shows a moderate amount of a perivascular, chronic inflammatory infiltrate.

The typical histologic picture in early lesions of *acute erythema nodosum* consists of septal inflammation together with inflammation of the septal blood vessels. Only rarely is the septal inflammation predominantly neutrophilic (Förström and Winkelmann, 1977). Usually, it is lymphohistio-cytic with only a slight admixture of neutrophils. Edema and fibrinoid degeneration are seen in the septal collagen (Winkelmann and Förström). The type and degree of vessel involvement are variable, but vessel changes are usually found, provided the specimen is sufficiently large and contains adequate amounts of septal tissue. Such a specimen can usually be obtained only by scalpel excision and not with a biopsy punch. Whereas, in some cases, only small vessels show invasion by an inflammatory infiltrate with or without extravasation of erythrocytes (Zabel), involvement of medium-sized veins is often also observed, particularly on step sectioning (Fig. 14-1). Such veins only rarely show thrombophlebitis with hemorrhage (Winkelmann and Förström); more commonly, there is endothelial proliferation and separation of the muscular laminae of the venous wall by edema and a mixed inflammatory infiltrate (Löfgren and Wahlgren). Involvement of fat lobules is often limited to their periphery, where the infiltrate is seen extending from the septal tissue between individual fat cells in a lacelike fashion (Fig. 14-1). Necrosis of the fatty tissue does not occur.

In the late stage of acute erythema nodosum, neutrophils usually are absent. Lymphocytes and histiocytes predominate, and giant cells are present, often in significant numbers. In some instances, one finds small nodules in which histiocytes are lying in either a radial or a palisadelike arrangement around a small central fissure

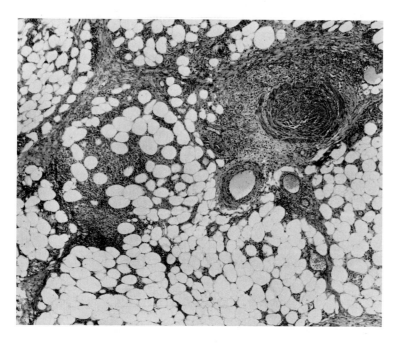

Fig. 14-1.   Erythema nodosum
A chronic inflammatory infiltrate extends from an interlobular septum into a fat lobule in a lacelike fashion. A medium-sized vein shows invasion of its wall by an inflammatory infiltrate and intimal proliferation. (×50)

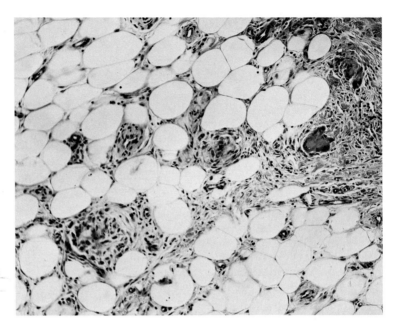

Fig. 14-2. Erythema nodosum
An old lesion shows two small nodules composed of histiocytes and, to the right, several giant cells of the foreign body type. (×200)

(Fig. 14-2) (Miescher). The giant cells usually show an irregular arrangement of their nuclei. They may lie alone or in association with a few histiocytes. True granulomas with epithelioid cells, however, are encountered very rarely.

In *chronic erythema nodosum,* the findings generally are the same as in the late stage of acute erythema nodosum. However, granuloma formation often is more pronounced and vascular changes less so. Thus, in some instances, one finds numerous granulomatous nodules composed of epithelioid cells and giant cells and devoid of caseation (Förström and Winkelmann, 1975). Although significant degrees of vasculitis have been observed by some authors (Vilanova and Piñol Aguadé; Fine and Meltzer), others have found them to be slight or absent (Hannuksela; Förström and Winkelmann, 1975).

Histogenesis. Although the cause of erythema nodosum often cannot be established, streptococcal tonsillitis is the most common among the known causes. In such cases, either beta-hemolytic streptococci can be cultured from the throat, or the patient has an elevated antistreptolysin-O titer (Favour and Sosman). In addition, primary infections with coccidioidomycosis or histoplasmosis can elicit an attack of erythema nodosum (Medeiros et al). The disorder may also be part of the symptom complex of subacute, transient sarcoidosis, which consists, in addition to lesions of the acute form of erythema nodosum, of hilar adenopathy, fever, arthralgia, and, often, acute iritis (see p. 229). Furthermore, erythema nodosum may occur in association with regional enteritis

(see p. 194) and Behçet's disease (see p. 193). Allergy to some drugs, such as sulfathiazole (Miescher), gold sodium thiomalate (Stone et al), and the contraceptive drugs (Salvatore and Lynch), may occasionally cause erythema nodosum as well.

A rather common cause of erythema nodosum in Northern Europe is infection with *Yersinia enterocolitica.* Gastrointestinal symptoms precede the onset of the cutaneous lesions by about 2 weeks, and a high serum antibody titer for *Yersinia enterocolitica* agglutinins is found (Debois et al).

Direct immunofluorescence studies have only very rarely shown deposits of immunoglobulins in the vessel walls of erythema nodosum (Niemi et al). Thus, it is unlikely that an immune complex vasculitis exists in this disorder, in spite of the conspicuous involvement of blood vessels found both by light and by electron microscopy. On *electron microscopic examination,* there is evidence of vasculitis consisting of damage to endothelial cells and infiltration of vessel walls by inflammatory cells, especially lymphocytes (Haustein and Klug).

Differential Diagnosis.   For a discussion of differentiation from erythema induratum, see p. 250. In cases of erythema nodosum showing severe vascular involvement, the possibility of benign cutaneous periarteritis nodosa must be excluded. In the latter disease, medium-sized arteries rather than veins or small-caliber blood vessels are affected, and there is necrosis of the walls of involved arteries (see p. 178). Superficial migratory thrombophlebitis, unlike erythema nodosum, shows a large vein in the center of the lesion.

SUPERFICIAL MIGRATORY THROMBOPHLEBITIS

Multiple, tender, erythematous nodules are found in superficial migratory thrombophlebitis, usually on the lower legs but occasionally also on the arms (Ruiter). After several days, a cordlike induration a few centimeters long can often be felt (Schuppli). As the old lesions gradually resolve, new nodules usually erupt. Recurrent migratory thrombophlebitis may occur as a manifestation of Behçet's disease (see p. 193).

Histopathology. A large vein at the border between the dermis and the subcutaneous tissue that is well endowed with thick muscular and elastic layers shows an inflammatory infiltrate permeating all layers of its wall. A thrombus usually occludes the entire lumen (Fig. 14-3) (Röckl). The inflammatory infiltrate extends only a short distance into the tissue surrounding the vein (Montgomery et al). In early lesions, the infiltrate shows a fairly large number of neutrophils, whereas, later, it is composed mainly of lymphocytes, histiocytes, and a few giant cells (Ruiter). When recanalization of the lumen takes place, intravasal and intramural granulomas with giant cells are often seen (Röckl). These giant-cell-containing granulomas aid in the phagocytosis of the thrombus (Schuppli).

ERYTHEMA INDURATUM

The lesions in erythema induratum consist of chronic, painless but somewhat tender, deep-seated subcutaneous infiltrations on the lower legs, especially the calves. Gradually, the infiltrations extend to the surface,

forming bluish red plaques that often ulcerate before healing with atrophic scars. Recurrences are common and often are precipitated by the onset of cold weather. Women are more commonly affected than men.

Histopathology. In early lesions, the histologic changes are limited to the subcutaneous tissue (Fig. 14-4), but, in lesions that are farther advanced, the infiltrate extends into the dermis. The histologic picture is characterized by a granulomatous, tuberculoid infiltrate, vascular changes, and areas of caseation necrosis.

The infiltrate may be largely nonspecific; however, if the lesion is at least a few weeks old and an adequate specimen has been taken for biopsy, the infiltrate usually shows a granulomatous, tuberculoid structure, at least in some areas. Sometimes, it is necessary to carry out step sections throughout the block of tissue to find areas with a granulomatous, tuberculoid structure. In such areas, one finds epithelioid and giant cells, occasionally in a tubercle arrangement (Fig. 14-5). In areas of nonspecific infiltration, lymphoid and plasma cells predominate. Both the tuberculoid and nonspecific infiltrates extend between the fat cells, largely replacing them.

Vascular changes are extensive and usually severe. Arteries and veins of small and medium size show invasion of their walls by a dense inflammatory infiltrate, leading to endothelial swelling and edema of the vessel walls (Montgomery et al; Eberhartinger; Schneider and Undeutsch). Thrombosis and occlusion of the lumen result

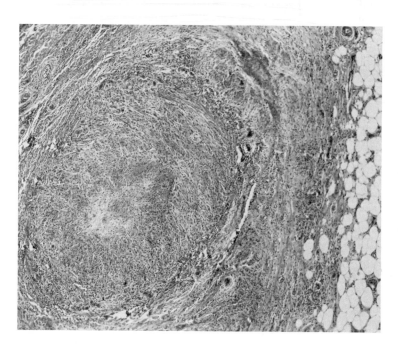

Fig. 14-3. Superficial migratory thrombophlebitis
A large vein shows an inflammatory infiltrate permeating all layers of its wall. The infiltrate contains several giant cells. The lumen of the vein is occluded by a thrombus. ($\times 50$)

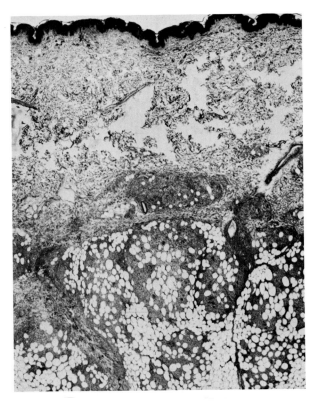

Fig. 14-4.   Erythema induratum
Low magnification. The infiltrate is limited to the sub-cutaneous fat, where it is located between the fat cells, in part replacing them. (×25)

Fig. 14-5.   Erythema induratum
High magnification. The infiltrate in the area shown is tuberculoid in appearance, being composed largely of epithelioid cells and giant cells. Many of the small vessels show proliferation of their walls. (×200)

(Fig. 14-6). The occlusion may lead to caseation necrosis.

Caseation necrosis is a fairly late development and therefore is lacking in about half of the cases in which a biopsy is carried out (Andersen; Förström and Hannuksela). In lesions in which ulceration has taken place, caseation necrosis usually is extensive. In areas of caseation necrosis, the fat cells may still be partially preserved, whereas the invading infiltrate between the fat cells has been transformed into an amorphous, finely granular, eosinophilic material in which some pyknotic nuclei are present.

Cases showing evidence of vasculitis but only minor tuberculoid changes and little or no caseation necrosis have been called nodular vasculitis and have been regarded as a "nontuberculous" type of erythema induratum (Montgomery et al). However, abandonment of the tuberculous etiology for erythema induratum (see below) has made this subdivision unnecessary. In reality, nodular vasculitis represents merely an early or a mild manifestation of erythema induratum (Eberhartinger).

Histogenesis. Because of the presence of a tuberculoid infiltrate and, often, of caseation necrosis, erythema induratum has been regarded by many authors as a form of tuberculosis, or at least as a tuberculid (Andersen; Förström and Hannuksela). Against the assumption that erythema induratum is a manifestation of tuberculosis

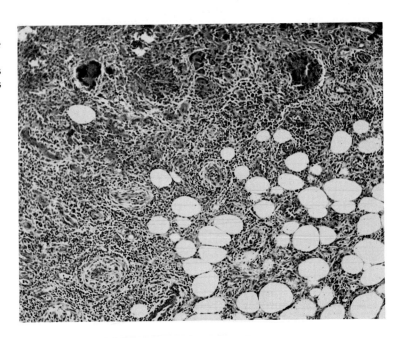

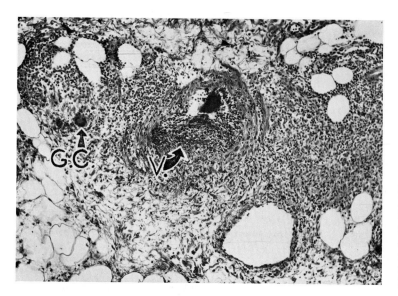

Fig. 14-6. Erythema induratum
High magnification. A large vessel (*V.*) in the subcutaneous fat is invaded by inflammatory cells and thrombosed. At the right of the vessel, the inflammatory infiltrate is nonspecific; at the left are epithelioid cells and a Langhans type of giant cell (*G.C.*). (×200)

are the findings that neither inoculation of tissue from lesions into guinea pigs (Telford) nor culturing of such tissue (Eberhartinger; Andersen) has resulted in the isolation of tubercle bacilli and that erythema induratum responds to treatment with corticosteroids (Eberhartinger; Van der Lugt). Against the assumption that erythema induratum is a tuberculid are the findings that active tuberculosis occurs with no greater frequency in patients with erythema induratum than in the general population (Eberhartinger) and that, although many patients with erythema induratum in a survey done in Vienna showed sensitivity to testing with old tuberculin, about 60% of the patients failed to react to a high dilution of 1:10,000 (Eberhartinger).

Several authors have expressed their belief that the primary event in erythema induratum is a vasculitis of subcutaneous arteries and veins (Eberhartinger; Schneider and Undeutsch). Any fat necrosis that occurs following vascular damage can develop a tuberculoid appearance (Telford).

Differential Diagnosis. Histologic differentiation of erythema induratum from erythema nodosum rarely causes difficulties, even though vascular changes and giant cells may occur in both. In erythema nodosum, the infiltrate is much less massive than in erythema induratum, caseation is regularly absent, and tuberculoid structures are rarely encountered, even though giant cells and histiocytes occur. Also, the vascular changes are less pronounced than in erythema induratum.

Lesions of erythema induratum showing a pronounced tuberculoid infiltrate, extensive caseation, and ulceration may resemble scrofuloderma. However, scrofuloderma shows no significant vascular changes, and tubercle bacilli can usually be found

on staining with the Ziehl–Neelsen stain and on culturing.

For a discussion of differentiation of erythema induratum from gummatous syphilis, see p. 324.

RELAPSING FEBRILE NODULAR NONSUPPURATIVE PANNICULITIS (WEBER–CHRISTIAN DISEASE)

Weber–Christian disease is characterized by the appearance of crops of tender nodules and plaques in the subcutaneous fat, usually in association with mild fever. The lower extremities are predominantly involved, but lesions can also occur on the trunk, the upper extremities, and, rarely, on the face (Pambor et al). As the lesions involute, they may leave a depression in the skin. The overlying skin as a rule shows no involvement other than mild erythema. In occasional instances, the nodules liquefy, the overlying skin breaks down, and an oily liquid is discharged (liquefying panniculitis).

The disease occurs most frequently in middle-aged women, although it has been seen in both sexes and at all ages, including the neonatal period (Hendricks et al). In general, the prognosis is good, with the attacks gradually becoming less severe and ultimately ceasing (Albrectsen). However, if systemic panniculitis is present, the disease may be fatal (Achten et al; Ciclitira et al).

Histopathology. The subcutaneous lesions of Weber–Christian disease pass through three stages. The first two stages occur while there is induration clinically. During the third stage, depression of the skin may develop. The first stage is found only rarely on histologic examination, because it is usually of short duration, although it occasionally persists for several days (Hendricks et al). It is even possible that it does not always occur. Most sections show a combination of the changes of the second and the third stages. In some cases, however, a biopsy has shown only a nonspecific picture of inflammatory cells without a significant number of foam cells, on the presence of which the diagnosis depends (Pinals).

In the first (acute inflammatory) stage, one observes degeneration of fat cells accompanied by an inflammatory infiltrate composed of neutrophils, lymphocytes, and histiocytes. Neutrophils may predominate (Fig. 14-7, *top*) (Ungar; Lever). Abscess formation does not occur.

In the second (macrophagic) stage, the infiltrate consists predominantly of histiocytes. A few lymphocytes and plasma cells are also present. Many

Fig. 14-7.   Relapsing febrile nodular suppurative panniculitis

(*Top*) First stage. An acute inflammatory infiltrate composed predominantly of neutrophils is seen between the fat cells. (×100) (*Bottom*) Second and third stages. The left side and the center of the field show the second stage, which consists of foam cells (macrophages) invading and digesting the fat cells. The right side shows the third stage, which consists of replacement of the foam cells by fibrotic connective tissue. (×100)

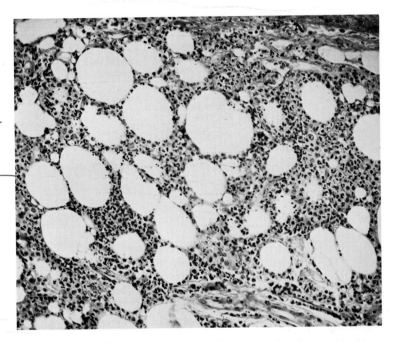

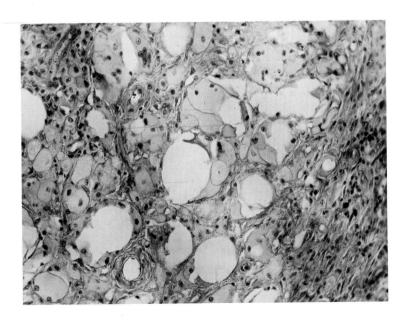

histiocytes in the vicinity of fat cells have the appearance of foam cells (macrophages) as a result of digesting fat from degenerated fat cells. Many foam cells are quite large, and some of them are multinucleated. In some areas, numerous macrophages with foamy cytoplasm replace the fat cells completely (Fig. 14-7, *bottom*). A few foreign body type giant cells without foamy cytoplasm may also be present (Kooij).

In the third (fibrotic) stage, fibroblasts intermingled with lymphocytes and some plasma cells gradually replace the foam cells. Collagen is laid down with resulting fibrosis.

The epidermis and dermis show no involvement except in the rare cases of liquefying panniculitis (see below). In some cases, the large subcutaneous vessels show mild changes, such as endothelial proliferation, as well as edema and thickening of their walls (Cummins and Lever; Steinberg).

In cases of liquefying panniculitis (Shaffer; Binkley; Hoyos et al), the second (macrophagic) stage is followed by liquefaction of the foam cell infiltrate instead of by fibrosis. One finds an amorphous matrix in which foam cells, as well as lymphocytes and neutrophils, are situated (Achten et al).

Systemic Lesions. Among the 27 autopsies on record, death in 9 patients was due to an intercurrent disease (Achten et al). In the remaining 18 cases, four types of lesions were described: (1) involvement of perivisceral adipose tissue, including mesenteric and omental fat (Spain and Foley; Mostofi and Engleman); (2) involvement of intravisceral adipose tissue, which causes focal necroses in liver or spleen (Miller and Kritzler; Mostofi and Engleman) and may be followed by an invasion of macrophages, resulting in enlargement of these organs (Steinberg; Arnold and Bainborough) and, in some instances, in hepatic failure either with jaundice (Ciclitira et al) or without jaundice (Miller and Kritzler); (3) involvement of bone marrow, resulting in interference with its hematopoietic activity (Steinberg); and (4) accumulation of large amounts of oily fluid in either the peritoneal or pleural cavity (Steinberg; Achten et al).

Among the nonfatal extracutaneous manifestations, painful osteolytic lesions have been repeatedly described. On histologic examination, the bone lesions have shown fat necrosis, chronic inflammation, fat-laden macrophages, and multinucleated giant cells (Pinals).

Histogenesis. The cause of Weber–Christian disease is unknown. An immune mechanism may be responsible for the damage to the adipose tissue (Allen-Mersh). However, there is no reason to doubt the existence of the disease as an entity, as has been done (MacDonald and Feiwel; Förström and Winkelmann). It is of course necessary to rule out the presence of lupus panniculitis (see p. 455), factitial panniculitis (see p. 253), and pancreatic panniculitis (see p. 253), but, in most instances, this can be done without great difficulty.

Differential Diagnosis. The histologic appearance of Weber–Christian disease is diagnostic during the second stage; in no other condition is there such preponderance of foam cells in the subcutaneous fat. In rare instances, the infiltrate in erythema nodosum may show a marked preponderance of neutrophils, and then it resembles that seen during the first stage of Weber–Christian disease (Förström and Winkelmann); however, the first stage of Weber–Christian disease is of short duration, so that histologic examination of an old lesion would no longer show it.

The subcutaneous nodular fat necrosis occurring in pancreatic disease may resemble Weber–Christian disease clinically, but it differs histologically by showing more pronounced necrosis of the fat cells and the presence of "ghostlike" cells having thick, shadowy walls and no nuclei (see below).

Before its recognition as an entity, histiocytic phagocytic panniculitis was diagnosed on several occasions as Weber–Christian disease (Winkelmann and Bowie). Even though panniculitis is the initial clinical feature in both diseases, histologic examination in histiocytic phagocytic panniculitis shows pronounced phagocytosis of erythrocytes, leukocytes, and cell particles by histiocytes, resulting in "bean-bag" cells, rather than phagocytosis of fat, resulting in foam cells (see p. 194).

PANNICULITIS ROTHMANN–MAKAI

The term *panniculitis Rothmann–Makai* was proposed in 1945 as the designation for a "heterogeneous group of cases of idiopathic panniculitis that do not fit into any of the distinctly defined syndromes, such as Weber–Christian syndrome, erythema nodosum, or erythema induratum" (Baumgartner and Riva). These authors cited as examples cases reported by Rothmann and by Makai, as well as a case of their own. Thus, this diagnostic term is based entirely on negative criteria (Schuppli). It therefore seems better to refer to such unclassifiable cases as nonspecific panniculitis or nondefinite panniculitis (Niemi et al) (see p. 245).

In spite of the vagueness of the concept, cases referred to as panniculitis of Rothmann–Makai or lipogranulomatosis subcutanea, the term used by Makai, have appeared sporadically in the literature up to the present time. Some of these cases are difficult to assign to any established entity and, on histologic examination, show necrosis of fatty tissue and noncaseating granulomas (Undeutsch and Berger; Burford and Clarke; Chan). Other cases, however, can be regarded as only minor variants of one of the established entities: Weber–Christian panniculitis (Pambor et al), erythema nodosum (Laymon and Peterson), or erythema induratum (Röckl and Thiess).

SUBCUTANEOUS NODULAR FAT NECROSIS IN PANCREATIC DISEASE

Subcutaneous nodules may occur on the basis of fat necrosis in patients with either pancreatitis or pancreatic cancer. The pretibial region is the most common site of the nodules, but they may occur also on the thighs, the buttocks, and elsewhere. The nodules usually are tender and red and may be fluctuant (Cannon et al), but they only rarely discharge an oily substance through fistular ducts (de Graciansky). Although abdominal pain is almost always present in cases of pancreatitis (Bennett and Petrozzi), it is quite commonly absent in cases of pancreatic carcinoma when the nodules first appear. However, in both pancreatitis and pancreatic carcinoma, arthralgic pain, especially in the ankles, is a common early symptom and thus of great diagnostic importance (Osborne; Szymanski and Bluefarb; Hughes et al).

Histopathology.   The histologic appearance of the subcutaneous nodules in pancreatic disease is characteristic in most instances (Szymanski and Bluefarb; Hughes et al). Multiple foci of fat necrosis are present. They consist of "ghostlike" fat cells having thick, shadowy walls and no nuclei (Szymanski and Bluefarb). Basophilic deposits of calcium may be seen as granules in the cytoplasm of necrotic fat cells, as lamellar formations around individual fat cells, and as patchy deposits at the periphery of foci of fat necrosis (Cannon et al). A polymorphous infiltrate consisting of neutrophils, lymphoid cells, histiocytes, foam cells, and foreign body giant cells surrounds the foci of fat necrosis (Mullin et al).

Systemic Lesions.   Fat necrosis may be widespread. The symptoms of arthralgia are due to periarticular fat necrosis (Mullin et al). On autopsy, necrosis of the fat is found in the pancreas and the peripancreatic tissue and often also in the fatty tissue of many other areas, such as the peritoneum, omentum, mesentery, and the pericardial and perirenal fat (Auger), as well as in the mediastinum and bone marrow (Cannon et al).

In cases with carcinoma of the pancreas, the tumor is usually of the acinar cell type (Auger; Osborne; de Graciansky) and only rarely of the islet cell type (Millns et al).

Histogenesis.   Trypsin, amylase, and lipase are released from the pancreas. The values for serum amylase and serum lipase usually are elevated; however, this elevation is temporary and thus may not be found in all cases. Peak amylase levels generally occur 2 to 3 days after the appearance of new nodules (Hughes et al). Lipase may be found also in tissue affected by subcutaneous fat necrosis (Millns et al).

It is believed that trypsin causes changes in the permeability of the subcutaneous blood and lymph vessels and that the fat necrosis is then produced by lipase (Hughes et al). Resistance of the fat cell membrane to this lipolytic enzyme results in the formation of "ghost cells" with shadowy cell walls (Bennett and Petrozzi). The fatty acids formed by lipolysis readily combine with calcium to form calcium soaps (Levine and Lazarus).

Differential Diagnosis.   For a discussion of differentiation of fat necrosis from Weber–Christian disease, see p. 252.

FACTITIAL PANNICULITIS

Factitial panniculitis results from the surreptitious injection of various substances into the subcutaneous tissue. It often causes a bizarre clinical and histologic picture that defies diagnosis until self-inoculation is suspected and proved. The substances used usually are organic materials, drugs, or oily materials (Förström and Winkelmann). Among the organic materials are milk (Ackerman et al) and feces (Sullivan and Trosow); among the drugs are meperidine hydrochloride, or Demerol (Förström and Winkelmann), and pentazocine, or Talwin (Parks et al); and among the oily materials are mineral oil, or paraffin, (Oertel and Johnson) and silicone (Winer et al). Clinically, one observes in some cases nodules that may undergo liquefaction and then discharge pus or a thick fluid (Ackerman et al) and in other cases indurated areas, ulcers, or scars (Parks et al).

Histopathology.   The injection of organic materials and drugs results in a variable, nonspecific histologic picture. There may be acute inflammation with aggregation of neutrophils and focal necrosis of fat (Ackerman et al), or there may be areas of hemorrhage, chronic inflammation with large giant cells, and fibrosis (Parks et al). Absence of vessel involvement is characteristic for factitial panniculitis. In some cases, birefringent particles can be identified in polarized light (Förström and Winkelmann).

The injection of oily materials or silicone causes the highly characteristic histologic picture known as paraffinoma, in which there are oil cysts of varying size surrounded by fibrosis and inflammation, giving the tissue a Swiss-cheese-like appearance (Oertel and Johnson; Winer et al) (see also p. 221).

COLD PANNICULITIS

Cold panniculitis occurs predominantly in infants as red, indurated plaques or nodules on the face following exposure to severe cold (Haxthausen; Rotman). In some instances, similar nodules have been seen on one or both cheeks of infants who had eaten a popsicle that had rested intermittently against the subsequently involved sites (Duncan et al; Epstein and Oren). The plaques or nodules appear from 1 to 3 days after exposure and subside spontaneously within 2 weeks.

In rare instances, similar lesions have occurred in older children and in adults on the face and also on the legs (Haxthausen; Solomon and Beerman). In addition, several cases of equestrian cold panniculitis have been described in women who have ridden horses for several hours daily throughout the winter. The location of the lesions is the upper outer thighs (Beacham et al).

Histopathology. At the onset of the reaction to cold, an infiltrate of lymphoid and histiocytic cells is observed around the blood vessels at the dermal–subdermal junction. At the height of the reaction, on the third day, some of the fat cells in the subcutaneous tissue have ruptured and coalesced into cystic structures (Duncan et al; Beacham et al). A rather marked inflammatory infiltrate is present around the cystic structures and between the fat cells. Besides lymphoid and histiocytic cells, a few neutrophils and eosinophils may be present (Solomon and Beerman). In addition, stringy mucinous material has been noted (Beacham et al).

Histogenesis. Applying an ice cube to the skin for 50 sec produces nodules of cold panniculitis in all newborn infants and in 40% of infants 6 months old but only occasionally in 9-month-old infants (Epstein and Oren). It is known that the fatty acids of the subcutaneous fat are more highly saturated in the newborn than in the adult and that the fat therefore solidifies more readily at lower temperatures in infants than in adults (see also under Sclerema Neonatorum).

SCLEREMA NEONATORUM

Sclerema neonatorum, a very rare disorder, is characterized by a diffuse, rapidly spreading hardening of the entire subcutaneous fat of infants during the first few days of life. The entire skin has a waxlike appearance and feels cold, tight, and indurated. Death usually occurs within a few days. On autopsy, the subcutaneous tissue appears greatly thickened, hardened, and lardlike. Most infants with sclerema neonatorum are cyanotic at birth, have difficulty maintaining their body temperature, and have a major debilitating illness (Kellum et al).

Histopathology. The subcutaneous tissue owes its thickening in sclerema neonatorum to an increase in the size of the fat cells and to the presence of wide, intersecting fibrous bands (Kellum et al). Many of the fat cells are filled with rosettes of fine, needlelike clefts. In frozen sections, these clefts are found to be occupied by crystals. The crystals fail to stain with fat stains but are doubly refractile in the polarizing microscope (Zeek and Madden). In most instances, there is no evidence of fat necrosis or inflammation (Kellum et al). In only some cases, one can see fat necrosis and an inflammatory reaction with giant cells (Zeek and Madden; Flory), but these changes are much less extensive and less pronounced than in subcutaneous fat necrosis of the newborn.

Systemic Lesions. In most cases of sclerema reported, the changes in the fatty tissue were found to be limited to the subcutaneous fat when an autopsy was performed (Kellum et al). In two cases of sclerema, however, autopsy revealed lesions in the visceral fat that were histologically identical with those observed in the subcutaneous fat. In one of these cases (Zeek and Madden), the lesions were widely distributed, whereas, in the other case (Flory), they were limited to the perirenal and retroperitoneal fat.

Histogenesis. The subcutaneous fat of the normal newborn, in comparison to adult subcutaneous fat, has greater amounts of saturated fatty acids, lower amounts of unsaturated fatty acids, a higher melting point, and a higher solidification point. The alterations in the subcutaneous fatty acids of infants with sclerema neonatorum represent an exaggeration of the normal newborn pattern. Thus, the increased ratio of saturated to unsaturated fatty acids in the subcutaneous triglycerides could be responsible for the physical changes of the subcutaneous fat in sclerema neonatorum (Kellum et al). The increased ratio of saturated to unsaturated fatty acids is probably due to defective enzyme mechanisms to unsaturate fatty acid chains (Kellum et al). As x-ray diffraction has shown, the doubly refractile crystals in the fat cells consist of triglycerides (Horsfield and Yardley).

SUBCUTANEOUS FAT NECROSIS OF THE NEWBORN

Subcutaneous fat necrosis of the newborn does not represent a localized form of sclerema neonatorum, as was assumed by some authors in the past, but differs from it clinically, as well as histologically, and in its prognosis.

In subcutaneous fat necrosis of the newborn, nodules and plaques usually appear within a few days of birth. Some of the nodules discharge a caseous material (Oswalt et al). Although the patient's general health is usually not affected and the nodules disappear spontaneously after a few weeks or months, some infants are severely ill (Wesener) and may even die (Oswalt et al). In 15 reported instances, the subcutaneous fat necrosis was associated with hypercalcemia, and 3 patients died (Thomsen).

Histopathology. Histologic examination shows areas of fat necrosis in the subcutaneous tissue infiltrated by inflammatory cells and foreign body giant cells. Many of the remaining fat cells, as well as the giant cells, contain needle-shaped clefts that often lie in a radial arrangement (Fig. 14-8) (Tsuji). In frozen sections, the clefts are seen to contain doubly refractile crystals. Calcium deposits are scattered through the necrotic fat (Noojin et al). In some instances, extensive areas of calcification are present that may require several years to involute (Wesener).

Histogenesis. *Electron microscopic examination* shows that the phagocytosis of fat crystals starts with the invasion of fat cells by cytoplasmic projections of macrophages. Subsequently, fat crystals are seen within the cytoplasm of macrophages and of foreign body giant cells, which result from the fusion of macrophages (Tsuji).

The cause of subcutaneous fat necrosis of the newborn

is not known. It is not likely that trauma plays a role in the development of the lesions, since the disease has been found even at birth in a child delivered by cesarean section (Tsuji).

Differential Diagnosis. Even though needle-shaped clefts are found in the fat cells of both diseases, sclerema neonatorum differs from subcutaneous fat necrosis of the newborn by (1) the presence of either little or no fat necrosis, inflammation, or giant cell infiltration, (2) the absence of calcium deposits, and (3) the presence of wide fibrous bands in the subcutaneous tissue (Kellum et al).

CONGENITAL LYMPHEDEMA

Congenital lymphedema is found most commonly on one or both lower extremities. It may be associated with edema in other areas, such as one or both arms (Dubin et al), the face, or the scrotum and penis (Rufli). The lymphedema is hereditary in only a small fraction of cases and is then referred to as Milroy's disease (Rosenberg).

In rare instances, lymphangiosarcoma develops secondary to congenital lymphedema (Dubin et al) (see p. 643).

Histopathology. In congenital lymphedema, the collagen bundles of the dermis appear homogenized and widened (Tappeiner). The subcutaneous tissue is permeated by thick strands of collagen,

Fig. 14-8. Subcutaneous fat necrosis of the newborn
Several fat cells contain needle-shaped clefts in a radial arrangement. These clefts are indicative of fat crystals. The fat crystals themselves are not visible, because lipids have been extracted by the processing of the tissue. An inflammatory infiltrate containing many foreign body giant cells is present between the fat cells. (×400)

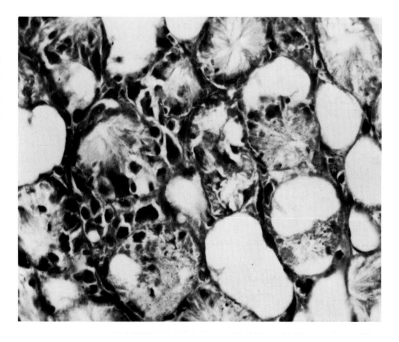

and, as evidence of edema, there are empty spaces devoid of endothelial lining (Rosenberg).

Histogenesis. As a rule, the lymphatic vessels are so severely hypoplastic or aplastic that no vessel can be found on the dorsum of the foot, and lymphangiography cannot be carried out (Rufli; Dubin et al).

PROGRESSIVE LIPODYSTROPHY

Progressive lipodystrophy shows progressive disappearance of the subcutaneous fat in certain areas of the body. Most cases are of the cephalothoracic type, involving the face, the neck, the upper extremities, and the upper trunk. In other cases, atrophy of the fat extends from the crest of the ilium downward. In lipoatrophic diabetes, there is generalized rather than localized loss of fat.

Histopathology. The involved regions show a complete lack of subcutaneous fat. The dermis lies directly on the fascia or muscle (Taylor and Honeycutt).

BIBLIOGRAPHY

Classification of Panniculitis
MONTGOMERY H, O'LEARY PA, BARKER NW: Nodular vascular diseases of the legs. JAMA 128:335–341, 1945
NIEMI KM, FÖRSTRÖM L, HANNUKSELA M et al: Nodules on the legs. Acta Derm Venereol (Stockh) 57:145–154, 1977
PIERINI LE, ABULAFIA J, WAINFELD S: Idiopathic lipogranulomatous hypodermitis. Arch Dermatol 98:290–298, 1968
VILANOVA X, PIÑOL AGUADÉ J: Subacute nodular migratory panniculitis. Br J Dermatol 71:45–50, 1959
WINKELMANN RK, FÖRSTRÖM L: Observations in the histopathology of erythema nodosum. J Invest Dermatol 65:441–446, 1975

Erythema Nodosum
BÄFVERSTEDT B: Erythema nodosum migrans. Acta Derm Venereol (Stockh) 48:381–384, 1968
DEBOIS J, VANDEPITTE J, DEGREEF H: *Yersinia enterocolitica* as a cause of erythema nodosum. Dermatologica 156:65–78, 1978
FAVOUR CB, SOSMAN MC: Erythema nodosum. Arch Intern Med 80:435–453, 1947
FINE RM, MELTZER HD: Chronic erythema multiforme. Arch Dermatol 100:33–38, 1969
FÖRSTRÖM L, WINKELMANN RK: Granulomatous panniculitis in erythema nodosum. Arch Dermatol 111:335–340, 1975
FÖRSTRÖM L, WINKELMANN RK: Acute panniculitis. Arch Dermatol 113:909–917, 1977
HANNUKSELA M: Erythema nodosum migrans. Acta Derm Venereol (Stockh) 53:313–317, 1973
HAUSTEIN UF, KLUG H: Ultrastrukturelle Untersuchungen der Blutgefässe beim Erythema nodosum. Dermatol Monatsschr 163:13–22, 1977
LÖFGREN S, WAHLGREN F: On the histopathology of erythema nodosum. Acta Derm Venereol (Stockh) 29:1–13, 1949

MEDEIROS AA, MARTY SD, TOSH FE et al: Erythema nodosum and erythema multiforme as clinical manifestations of histoplasmosis in a community outbreak. N Engl J Med 274:415–420, 1966
MIESCHER G: Zur Histologie des Erythema nodosum. Acta Derm Venereol (Stockh) 27:447–468, 1947
NIEMI KM, FÖRSTRÖM L, HANNUKSELA M et al: Nodules on the legs. Acta Derm Venereol (Stockh) 57:145–154, 1977
SALVATORE MA, LYNCH PJ: Erythema nodosum, estrogens, and pregnancy. Arch Dermatol 116:557–558, 1980
STONE RL, CLAFLIN A, PENNEYS NS: Erythema nodosum following gold sodium thiomalate therapy. Arch Dermatol 107:602–604, 1973
VILANOVA X, PIÑOL AGUADÉ J: Subacute nodular migratory panniculitis. Br J Dermatol 71:45–50, 1959
WINKELMANN RK, FÖRSTRÖM L: New observations in the histopathology of erythema nodosum. J Invest Dermatol 65:441–446, 1975
ZABEL M: Zur Histopathologie des Erythema nodosum. Z Hautkr 52:1253–1258, 1977

Superficial Migratory Thrombophlebitis
MONTGOMERY H, O'LEARY PA, BARKER NW: Nodular vascular diseases of the legs. JAMA 128:335–341, 1945
RÖCKL H: Die Bedeutung der Histopathologie für die Diagnostik knotiger Unterschenkel-Dermatosen. Hautarzt 19:540–547, 1968
RUITER M: Über die sogenannte Thrombophlebitis migrans. Arch Dermatol Syph (Berlin) 197:22–36, 1953
SCHUPPLI R: Zur Ätiologie der Phlebitis saltans. Hautarzt 10:466–467, 1959

Erythema Induratum
ANDERSEN S LA C: Erythema induratum (Bazin) treated with isoniazid. Acta Derm Venereol (Stockh) 50:65–68, 1970
EBERHARTINGER C: Das Problem des Erythema induratum Bazin. Arch Klin Exp Dermatol 217:196–254, 1963
FÖRSTRÖM L, HANNUKSELA M: Antituberculous treatment of erythema induratum Bazin. Acta Derm Venereol (Stockh) 50:143–147, 1970
MONTGOMERY H, O'LEARY PA, BARKER NW: Nodular vascular diseases of the legs. JAMA 128:335–341, 1945
SCHNEIDER W, UNDEUTSCH W: Vasculitiden des subcutanen Fettgewebes. Arch Klin Exp Dermatol 221:600–610, 1965
TELFORD ED: Lesions of the skin and subcutaneous tissue in diseases of the peripheral circulation. Arch Dermatol Syph 36:952–963, 1937
VAN DER LUGT L: Some remarks about tuberculosis of the skin and tuberculids. Dermatologica 131:266–275, 1965

Relapsing Febrile Nodular Nonsuppurative Panniculitis (Weber–Christian Disease)
ACHTEN G, MORIAME-ROUSSEL N, WANET J et al: Panniculite liquéfiante idiopathique à évolution fatale. Ann Dermatol Venereol 104:693–696, 1977
ALBRECTSEN B: The Weber-Christian syndrome, with particular reference to etiology. Acta Derm Venereol (Stockh) 40:474–484, 1960
ALLEN-MERSH TG: Weber-Christian panniculitis and auto-immune disease: A case report. J Clin Pathol 29:144–149, 1976
ARNOLD HA, BAINBOROUGH AR: Weber-Christian disease with viscereal involvement. Can Med Assoc J 89:1138–1142, 1963
BINKLEY JS: Relapsing febrile nodular nonsuppurative panniculitis. JAMA 113:113–116, 1939

CICLITIRA PJ, WIGHT DGD, DICK AP: Systemic Weber-Christian disease. Br J Dermatol 103:685–692, 1980

CUMMINS LJ, LEVER WF: Relapsing febrile nodular nonsuppurative panniculitis (Weber-Christian disease). Arch Dermatol Syph 38:415–426, 1938

FÖRSTRÖM L, WINKELMANN RK: Acute panniculitis. Arch Dermatol 113:909–917, 1977

HENDRICKS WM, AHMAD M, GRATZ E: Weber-Christian syndrome in infancy. Br J Dermatol 98:175–186, 1978

HOYOS N, SHAFFER B, BEERMAN H: Liquefying nodular panniculitis. Arch Dermatol 94:436–439, 1966

KOOIJ R: Weber-Christian disease, a form of spontaneous panniculitis. Dermatologica 101:332–344, 1950

LEVER WF: Nodular nonsuppurative panniculitis (Weber-Christian disease). Arch Dermatol 59:31–35, 1949

MACDONALD A, FEIWEL M: A review of the concept of Weber-Christian panniculitis with a report of five cases. Br J Dermatol 80:355–361, 1968

MILLER JL, KRITZLER RA: Nodular nonsuppurative panniculitis. Arch Dermatol Syph 47:82–96, 1943

MOSTOFI FK, ENGLEMAN E: Fatal relapsing febrile nonsuppurative panniculitis. Arch Pathol 43:417–426, 1947

PAMBOR M, KEMNITZ P, THEURING F: Panniculitis nodularis febrilis "nonsuppurativa" (Morbus Pfeifer-Weber-Christian) mit foudroyant-letalem Verlauf nach langjährigem afebrilem Bestehen. Dermatol Monatsschr 155:330–339, 1969

PINALS RS: Nodular panniculitis associated with an inflammatory bone lesion. Arch Dermatol 101:359–363, 1970

SHAFFER B: Liquefying nodular panniculitis. Arch Dermatol Syph 38:535–544, 1938

SPAIN DM, FOLEY JM: Nonsuppurative panniculitis (Weber-Christian's disease). Am J Pathol 20:783–787, 1944

STEINBERG B: Systemic nodular panniculitis. Am J Pathol 29:1059–1073, 1953

UNGAR H: Relapsing febrile nodular inflammation of adipose tissue (Weber-Christian syndrome): Report of a case with autopsy. J Pathol Bacteriol 58:175–185, 1946

WINKELMANN RK, BOWIE EJW: Hemorrhagic diathesis associated with benign histiocytic, cytophagic panniculitis and systemic histiocytosis. Arch Intern Med 140:1460–1463, 1980

Panniculitis Rothmann–Makai

BAUMGARTNER W, RIVA G: Panniculitis, die herdförmige Fettgewebsentzündung. Helv Med Acta 12 (Suppl 14):3–69, 1945

BURFORD JC, CLARKE DM: Lipogranulomatosis subcutanea of Rothmann-Makai. Aust J Dermatol 13:117, 1972

CHAN HL: Panniculitis (Rothmann-Makai), with good response to tetracycline. Br J Dermatol 92:351–354, 1975

LAYMON CW, PETERSON WC JR: Lipogranulomatosis subcutanea (Rothmann-Makai). Arch Dermatol 90:288–292, 1964

MAKAI E: Über Lipogranulomatosis subcutanea. Klin Wochenschr 7:2343–2346, 1928

NIEMI KM, FÖRSTRÖM L, HANNUKSELA M et al: Nodules on the legs. Acta Derm Venereol (Stockh) 57:145–154, 1977

PAMBOR M, KEMNITZ P, THEURING F: Panniculitis nodularis febrilis "nonsuppurativa" (Morbus Pfeifer-Weber-Christian) mit foudroyant-letalem Verlauf nach langjährigem afebrilem Bestehen. Dermatol Monatsschr 155:330–339, 1969

RÖCKL H, THIESS W: Herdförmige chronisch rezidivierende Krankheitszustände des subcutanen Fettgewebes. Zur Histopathogenese der Lipogranulomatosis. Hautarzt 8:58–65, 1957

ROTHMANN M: Über Entzündung und Atrophie des subcutanen Fettgewebes. Virchows Arch Pathol Anat 136:159–169, 1894

SCHUPPLI R: Die Panniculitis Typus Rothmann-Makai. In Marchionini A (ed): Handbuch der Haut- und Geschlechtskrankheiten, Vol II/2, p. 127. Berlin, Springer-Verlag, 1965

UNDEUTSCH W, BERGER HE: Lipogranulomatosis Rothmann-Makai, eigenständiges Krankheitsbild oder polyätiologisches Syndrom? Hautarzt 21:221–225, 1970

Subcutaneous Nodular Fat Necrosis in Pancreatic Disease

AUGER C: Acinous cell carcinoma of the pancreas with extensive fat necrosis. Arch Pathol 43:400–405, 1947

BENNETT RG, PETROZZI JW: Nodular subcutaneous fat necrosis. A manifestation of silent pancreatitis. Arch Dermatol 111:896–898, 1975

CANNON JR, PITHA JV, EVERETT MA: Subcutaneous fat necrosis in pancreatitis. J Cutan Pathol 6:501–506, 1979

DE GRACIANSKY P: Weber-Christian syndrome of pancreatic origin. Br J Dermatol 79:278–283, 1967

HUGHES PSH, APISARNTHANARAX P, MULLINS JF: Subcutaneous fat necrosis associated with pancreatic disease. Arch Dermatol 111:506–509, 1975

LEVINE N, LAZARUS GS: Subcutaneous fat necrosis after paracentesis. Report of a case in a patient with acute pancreatitis. Arch Dermatol 112:993–994, 1976

MILLNS JL, EVANS HL, WINKELMANN RK: Association of islet cell carcinoma of the pancreas with subcutaneous fat necrosis. Am J Dermatopathol 1:273–280, 1979

MULLIN GT, CAPERTON EM JR, CRESPIN SR et al: Arthritis and skin lesions resembling erythema nodosum in pancreatic disease. Ann Intern Med 68:75–87, 1968

OSBORNE RR: Functioning acinous cell carcinoma of the pancreas accompanied with widespread focal fat necrosis. Arch Intern Med 85:933–943, 1950

SZYMANSKI FJ, BLUEFARB SM: Nodular fat necrosis and pancreatic disease. Arch Dermatol 83:224–229, 1961

Factitial Panniculitis

ACKERMAN AB, MOSHER DT, SCHWAMM HA: Factitial Weber-Christian syndrome. JAMA 198:731–736, 1966

FÖRSTRÖM L, WINKELMANN RK: Factitial panniculitis. Arch Dermatol 110:747–750, 1974

OERTEL YC, JOHNSON FB: Sclerosing lipogranuloma of the male genitalia. Arch Pathol 101:321–326, 1977

PARKS, DL, PERRY HO, MULLER SA: Cutaneous complications of pentazocine injections. Arch Dermatol 104:231–235, 1971

SULLIVAN M, TROSOW A: Multiple subcutaneous abscesses produced by the hypodermic injection of feces. South Med J 42:402–404, 1949

WINER LH, STEINBERG TH, LEHMAN R et al: Tissue reactions to injected silicone liquids. Arch Dermatol 90:588–593, 1964

Cold Panniculitis

BEACHAM BE, COOPER PH, BUCHANAN S et al: Equestrian cold panniculitis in women. Arch Dermatol 116:1025–1027, 1980

DUNCAN WC, FREEMAN RG, HEATON CL: Cold panniculitis. Arch Dermatol 94:722–724, 1966

EPSTEIN EH JR, OREN ME: Popsicle panniculitis. N Engl J Med 282:966–967, 1970

HAXTHAUSEN H: Adiponecrosis e frigore. Br J Dermatol 53:83–89, 1941

ROTMAN H: Cold panniculitis in children. Arch Dermatol 94:720–721, 1966

SOLOMON LM, BEERMAN H: Cold panniculitis. Arch Dermatol 88:897–900, 1963

Sclerema Neonatorum

FLORY CM: Fat necrosis of the newborn. Arch Pathol 45:278–288, 1948

HORSFIELD GI, YARDLEY HJ: Sclerema neonatorum. J Invest Dermatol 44:326–332, 1965

KELLUM RE, RAY TL, BROWN GR: Sclerema neonatorum. Arch Dermatol 97:372–380, 1968

ZEEK P, MADDEN EM: Sclerema adiposum neonatorum of both internal and external adipose tissue. Arch Pathol 41:166–174, 1946

Subcutaneous Fat Necrosis of the Newborn

KELLUM RE, RAY TL, BROWN GR: Sclerema neonatorum. Arch Dermatol 97:372–380, 1968

NOOJIN RO, PACE BF, DAVIS HG: Subcutaneous fat necrosis of the newborn: Certain etiologic considerations. J Invest Dermatol 12:331–334, 1949

OSWALT GC JR, MONTES LF, CASSADY G: Subcutaneous fat necrosis of the newborn. J Cutan Pathol 5:193–199, 1978

THOMSEN RJ: Subcutaneous fat necrosis of the newborn and idiopathic hypercalcemia. Arch Dermatol 116:1155–1158, 1980

TSUJI T: Subcutaneous fat necrosis of the newborn. Light and electron microscopic studies. Br J Dermatol 95:407–416, 1976

WESENER G: Zur Klinik und Therapie der Adiponecrosis subcutanea neonatorum. Arch Klin Exp Dermatol 206:531–536, 1957

Congenital Lymphedema

DUBIN HV, CREEHAN EP, HEADINGTON JT: Lymphangiosarcoma and congenital lymphedema of the extremity. Arch Dermatol 110:608–614, 1974

ROSENBERG WA: Hereditary edema of the legs (Milroy's disease). Arch Dermatol Syph 42:1113–1121, 1940

RUFLI T: Primäres, kongenitales Lymphödem (Syndrom von Nonne-Milroy-Meige). Dermatologica 150:210–211, 1975

TAPPEINER J: Störungen der Lymphzirkulation als diagnostisches Problem des Dermatologen. Hautarzt 20:412–418, 1969

Progressive Lipodystrophy

TAYLOR WB, HONEYCUTT WM: Progressive lipodystrophy and lipoatrophic diabetes. Arch Dermatol 84:31–36, 1961

Eruptions Due to Drugs

15

Allergic reactions to drugs may cause various eruptions identical in their clinical appearance to cutaneous diseases occurring also as idiopathic entities. For instance, drugs may cause urticaria, erythema multiforme, erythema nodosum, dermatitis, including generalized exfoliative dermatitis, folliculitis, and purpura due to either allergic vasculitis or thrombocytopenia. The histologic picture is the same in these diseases, whether they are due to a drug or occur in their idiopathic form.

Several histologic changes more or less typical for drug eruptions will be discussed in this chapter.

DRUG-INDUCED VASCULITIS

A drug-induced vasculitis can be caused by numerous drugs, among the most common of which are ampicillin, chlorothiazide, phenylbutazone, and sulfonamides. Although drug-induced vasculitis can be of the leukocytoclastic type (Winkelmann and Ditto; van Joost et al), it is in most instances lymphocytic (Mullick et al).

Two distinct groups of patients with drug-induced lymphocytic vasculitis can be recognized. In one group, the lymphocytic vasculitis is limited to the skin and is present predominantly over the extremities. In such cases, the eruption is apt to be maculopapular rather than purpuric, and it clears promptly when the drug is withdrawn. In the other group, the lymphocytic vasculitis involves all areas of the skin, and purpuric lesions are common. In addition, multiple organ systems are often involved, especially the heart, liver, and kidneys, and death may thus occur (Mullick et al).

Histopathology. In drug-induced leukocytoclastic vasculitis, leukocytes predominate, and the vessel walls show fibrinoid deposits (Winkelmann and Ditto) (see p. 168). In drug-induced lymphocytic vasculitis, an infiltrate of mononuclear cells and of eosinophils is found in the walls and around the involved small vessels of the skin without evidence of fibrinoid deposits (Mullick et al) (see p. 173).

FIXED DRUG ERUPTION

Fixed drug eruptions are circumscribed lesions that recur persistently at the same site with each administration of the allergenic drug. The most common type of fixed drug eruption consists of one or several slightly elevated, erythematous patches that may become bullous and, on healing, leave pigmented areas. Fixed drug eruptions occur most commonly after the ingestion of either phenolphthalein, one of the barbiturates, or phenylbutazone.

Histopathology. The histologic changes observed in fixed drug eruption suggest that it is a variant of erythema multiforme (see p. 122). Just as in erythema multiforme, the reaction may be predominantly dermal or epidermal or may take place in both the dermis and the epidermis. The latter type of reaction is the most common.

The frequent presence of hydropic degeneration of the basal cell layer leads to "pigmentary incontinence," which is characterized by the presence of large amounts of melanin within macrophages in the upper dermis (Tarnowski). In addition, scattered dyskeratotic keratinocytes with eosinophilic cytoplasm and pyknotic nuclei are frequently seen in the epidermis (Furuya et al). Bullae form by detachment of the epidermis from the dermis (Stritzler and Kopf). Not infrequently, the epidermis shows extensive colliquation necrosis, even in areas in which it has not yet become detached (Tritsch et al).

Histogenesis. On *electron microscopic examination,* the dyskeratotic keratinocytes are filled with thick, homogenized tonofilaments and show only sparse remnants of organelles and nuclei. They resemble the dyskeratotic cells seen in the epidermal type of erythema multiforme (see p. 123) and in the acute type of graft-versus-host disease (see p. 124) (de Dobbeleer and Achten).

The serum of patients with fixed drug eruption has mitogenic properties when it is obtained during the active phase of the disease and added to an autologous lymphocyte culture (Gimenez-Camarasa et al).

BULLAE AND SWEAT GLAND NECROSIS IN DRUG-INDUCED COMA

Patients who are in a coma due to an accident, illness, or a suicidal dose of a narcotic drug may within a few hours show areas of erythema at sites of pressure. Subsequently, usually within 24 hr, vesicles and bullae develop in the areas of erythema. The incidence of bullae depends on the severity of the coma and thus is highest in patients who subsequently die. In addition to coma from narcotic drugs, coma caused by carbon monoxide poisoning can also produce the lesions (Leavell et al). The bullae are located at sites subjected to pressure, such as the hands, wrists, scapulae, sacrum, knees, legs, ankles, and heels.

Histopathology. The epidermis shows varying degrees of necrosis. In areas of complete necrosis of the epidermis, the bullae arise subepidermally, but, in areas of only diminished viability showing eosinophilia of the cytoplasm and decreased staining of the nuclei, small intraepidermal vesicles may be seen (Mandy and Ackerman). Where the epidermis is necrotic in its upper layers but not in its lower layers, even large bullae can form intraepidermally (Achten et al). Blisters may also form in a suprabasal location and may contain some acantholytic cells (Herschthal and Robinson).

The secretory cells of the sweat glands show necrosis characterized by eosinophilic homogenization of their cytoplasm and by pyknosis or absence of their nuclei (Achten et al). The sweat ducts usually appear less severely damaged but may also show pale staining or necrosis similar to that of the secretory cells (Brehmer-Andersson and Pedersen). It is of interest that the sweat gland necrosis is limited to areas in which there are skin lesions. In patients who survive, the necrotic sweat gland epithelium is replaced by normal-appearing epithelial cells within about 2 weeks (Mandy and Ackerman). In many instances, the pilosebaceous units are also affected with sebaceous gland necrosis and occasional necrosis of the outer and inner root sheaths (Arndt et al).

The dermis beneath the bullae, and occasionally also the dermis around the sweat glands, contains a sparse polymorphous infiltrate composed of neutrophils, eosinophils, lymphoid cells, and histiocytes. In addition, some extravasated erythrocytes are often present (Mandy and Ackerman).

Histogenesis. The necrosis of the epidermis and sweat glands is a result of both generalized and local hypoxia (Mandy and Ackerman; Achten et al). The bullae, in turn, are the result of epidermal damage. Coma, whether the result of an accident, an illness, or a drug, causes generalized hypoxia by depressing blood circulation and respiration. In the case of poisoning with carbon monoxide, its binding to hemoglobin acts as an additional factor (Leavell et al). Pressure causes local hypoxia by decreasing local blood flow (Mandy and Ackerman).

DRUG-INDUCED PHOTOSENSITIVITY

A distinction is made between photoallergic and phototoxic drug eruptions. Photoallergic drug eruptions, in contrast to phototoxic drug eruptions, represent a cell-mediated, delayed immunologic response.

Photoallergic Drug Eruption

In photoallergy, light is required for the allergic reaction to occur. The role of light consists in altering either the hapten itself or the avidity with which the hapten combines with the carrier protein to form a complete photoantigen (Harber and Baer). Among the photoallergenic drugs are the sulfonamides; the thiazides, such as chlorothiazide (Diuril, a diuretic and antihypertensive agent) and tolbutamide (Orinase, an oral antidiabetic agent), both of which are aromatic sulfonamides; griseofulvin; and the phenothiazines, such as chlorpromazine, a psychosedative. A photoallergic drug eruption causes a photocontact dermatitis in all light-exposed areas. Like any allergic contact dermatitis, it causes itching (Hägermark et al).

Histopathology. The histologic appearance of a photocontact dermatitis is that of an allergic contact dermatitis and, as such, shows epidermal spongiosis and microvesiculation, a perivascular lymphoid cell infiltrate, and exocytosis (Willis and Kligman) (see p. 96).

Phototoxic Drug Eruption

If given in sufficiently large doses, certain internally administered drugs, in association with exposure to sunlight, may produce a phototoxic dermatitis, which represents an intensified sunburn and as such does not cause any itching (Hägermark et al). Among the drugs known to elicit a phototoxic response are all drugs capable of producing a photoallergic reaction, provided that they are given in sufficiently high concentrations (Harber and Baer). Other commonly prescribed phototoxic drugs are certain tetracyclines, such as demeclocycline hydrochloride (Declomycin) and doxycycline (Vibramycin) (Frost et al), and the psoralens.

Histopathology. A phototoxic drug eruption does not have a diagnostic histologic appearance. There merely is a nonspecific dermal inflammatory infiltrate.

Chlorpromazine Pigmentation

When chlorpromazine is given in high doses for several years as a tranquilizer to psychiatric patients, it may produce in exposed areas of the skin a slate-gray discoloration resembling the discoloration seen in argyria. Exposed parts of the bulbar conjunctivae may show brownish pigmentation (Hays et al).

Histopathology. The amount of melanin in the basal layer of the epidermis may be normal (Hays et al; Zelickson) or increased (Hashimoto et al). Considerable accumulations of pigment are found throughout the dermis within macrophages, especially in the vicinity of the capillaries. The pigment has the staining properties of melanin in that it stains black with the Fontana–Masson silver stain and is decolorized by hydrogen peroxide (Hays et al).

In patients who have been on prolonged medication with chlorpromazine and who have died of unrelated causes, autopsy may reveal in many internal organs melaninlike material that stains black with the Fontana–Masson silver stain and can be decolorized by hydrogen peroxide. This material is found throughout the entire mononuclear–phagocyte system and, to a lesser degree, in the parenchymal cells of the liver, kidneys, and endocrine glands, in myocardial fibers, and in cerebral neurons (Greiner and Nicolson).

Histogenesis. *Electron microscopic examination* has confirmed the presence of many melanosome complexes within the lysosomes of dermal macrophages. In addition, round or bizarrely shaped bodies may be seen measuring 0.2 μm to 3 μm in diameter and possessing such great electron density that no internal structure is recognizable (Zelickson; Hashimoto et al). These bodies are located in macrophages, endothelial cells, pericytes, Schwann cells, and fibroblasts, usually within lysosomes. At times, both electron-dense bodies and melanosome complexes are found within the same lysosome.

The electron-dense bodies have been interpreted either as a drug metabolite of chlorpromazine (Zelickson) or as a lipoprotein complex that is conjugated with chlorpromazine or its metabolites (Hashimoto et al). It has become apparent, however, that the dense bodies histochemically react like melanin (Greiner and Nicolson). Furthermore, chlorpromazine binds to melanin with a high degree of selectivity, with chlorpromazine acting as the electron donor and melanin as the acceptor (Blois). Thus, it seems likely that the electron-dense bodies represent complexes of melanin with chlorpromazine. It is apparent that, in contrast to melanin, the chlorpromazine–melanin complexes are not metabolized by the human body. Since these complexes are found also within neutrophils and monocytes of the circulating blood, it can be assumed that the phototoxic action of sunlight acting on the large amounts of chlorpromazine present in the skin leads to an increased production of melanin and to the formation of the chlorpromazine–melanin complexes. These complexes are subsequently carried from the dermis by way of the circulating blood to the various internal organs (Satanove).

Minocycline Pigmentation

The prolonged administration of minocycline, a semisynthetic derivative of tetracycline, customary especially for acne, may result in two distinct varieties of cutaneous pigmentation. One type is a diffuse pigmentation in sun-exposed areas (Simons and Morales). The second type is localized and arises either in areas of cutaneous inflammation, such as acne lesions and acne scars (Basler and Kohnen), or as patchy pigmentation on the legs and feet (McGrae and Zelickson; Sato et al; Leroy et al).

Histopathology. In the type of pigmentation arising in sun-exposed areas, melanin is present in increasing amounts in the basal portion of the epidermis and is seen also within macrophages in the upper dermis (Simons and Morales).

In the second type of pigmentation, occurring in acne lesions or in a patchy distribution on the legs and feet, the pigment is seen at all levels of the dermis, largely in a perivascular location. It stains with the Perls' stain, which is specific for iron, and with the Fontana–Masson stain. However, in contrast with melanin, there is no diminution in the intensity of pigmentation after attempts at bleaching with hydrogen peroxide (McGrae and Zelickson). No birefrigence is seen on examination with a polarizing microscope, but dark-field examination causes bright refractiveness of the pigment. This finding contrasts with the fact that neither hemosiderin nor melanin shows dark-field refractiveness (McGraw and Zelickson).

Histogenesis. Whereas the first type of pigmentation represents a phototoxic phenomenon, it appears likely that the second type of pigmentation is caused by a minocycline–hemosiderin complex (Fenske and Millns). On *electron microscopy*, the electron-dense iron-containing particles of the second type of pigmentation are found largely within macrophages, either within phagosomes or free in the cytoplasm (McGraw and Zelickson; Sato et al; Leroy et al). Electron x-ray microanalysis has confirmed the presence of iron within the electron-dense particles (Sato et al).

PENICILLAMINE-INDUCED DERMATOSES

The prolonged administration of penicillamine can cause alterations in collagen and elastic tissue that may result in areas of atrophy of the skin, including anetoderma, and in lesions of elastosis serpiginosa perforans. Damage to the intercellular substance of the epidermis may induce pemphigus.

Penicillamine-Induced Atrophy of the Skin

Patients on prolonged penicillamine therapy may show atrophic crinkling, or wrinkling, of the skin of the face and neck (Greer et al), light blue, atrophic macules resembling anetoderma (Davis), easy vulnerability of the skin resulting in small hemorrhages into the skin followed by milia (Katz; Bardach and Gebhart), or small, white papules at sites of venipuncture in the antecubital fossae (Greer et al).

Histopathology. The atrophic wrinkling and the atrophic macules resembling anetoderma show diminution or absence of elastic tissue (Davis). The areas of easy vulnerability of the skin and the papules at sites of venipuncture show either diminution (Bardach and Gebhart) or degeneration and homogenization of collagen (Katz; Greer et al).

Histogenesis. The formation of elastic tissue and collagen involves the participation of aldehydes to produce stable cross links. By reacting with aldehydes to form thiazolidine compounds, penicillamine impairs the formation of such stable cross links (Charles).

Penicillamine-Induced Elastosis Perforans Serpiginosa

Elastosis perforans serpiginosa may occur in patients receiving prolonged treatment with penicillamine (Guilaine et al; Pass et al; Kirsch and Hukill; Bardach et al). Although the clinical picture does not differ from that of idiopathic elastosis perforans serpiginosa (see p. 276), the histologic and electron microscopic features of the altered elastic fibers do.

Histopathology. In comparison to the idiopathic type of elastosis perforans serpiginosa, the penicillamine-induced type, on staining for elastic tissue, shows less hyperplasia of elastic fibers in the papillary dermis, except in areas of active transepidermal elimination (Bardach et al). However, in the middle and deep layers of the dermis, a greater number of hyperplastic elastic fibers is present than in idiopathic elastosis perforans serpiginosa. These fibers have an appearance that is specific for penicillamine-induced elastosis perforans serpiginosa: they show lateral budding, with the buds arranged perpendicular to the principal fibers (Guilaine et al). The coarse elastic fibers thus show a serrated, saw-tooth-like border (Kirsch and Hukill) and have been aptly compared to the twigs of a bramble bush (Hashimoto et al). Similar changes in individual elastic fibers are observed also in nonlesional skin (Bardach et al).

Histogenesis. On *electron microscopic examination*, the affected elastic fibers show an inner core that closely resembles a normal elastic fiber with dark microfibrils embedded in electron-lucent elastin. Peripheral to this, a wide, homogeneous, electron-lucent coat is seen that has the appearance of elastin and shows numerous saclike protuberances bulging outward between the adjacent collagen fibers (Kirsch and Hukill; Bardach et al).

Penicillamine-Induced Pemphigus

The occurrence of pemphigus in patients receiving penicillamine is not uncommon. The great majority of cases of penicillamine-induced pemphigus are pemphigus foliaceus, with only two cases of pemphigus vulgaris on record (Degos et al; From and Frederiksen). Most cases of pemphigus start between 6 and 12 months after institution of penicillamine therapy. In most instances, the pemphigus subsides shortly after penicillamine has been discontinued. In other instances, however, it is still present 1 to 2 years after discontinuance of penicillamine, despite treatment (Marsden et al), and, in one reported instance, it was fatal (Sparrow).

Histopathology. Histologic examination reveals a picture of either pemphigus foliaceus or pemphigus vulgaris identical with that seen in spontaneously arising cases (see pp. 110 and 105).

Histogenesis. *Direct immunofluorescence testing* has been positive for intercellular antibodies in all cases tested (From and Frederiksen; Kristensen and Wadskov). It is not known how penicillamine induces pemphigus, but it is assumed that penicillamine, possibly by the action of its sulfhydryl groups, alters the intercellular substance into an antigenic structure with subsequent antibody formation (Marsden et al; Kristensen and Wadskov).

DRUG-INDUCED LUPUS ERYTHEMATOSUS

Several drugs may induce a syndrome identical to systemic lupus erythematosus. The drugs that do this most commonly are procainamide, which is used against cardiac arrhythmia, hydralazine, an antihypertensive drug, and diphenylhydantoin (Dilantin), an anticonvulsive drug. It is likely that the development of a systemic-lupus-erythematosus-like syndrome in a patient under medication with these drugs represents the uncovering of a latent systemic lupus erythematosus rather than an allergic reaction (Alarcon-Segovia et al).

Drug-induced systemic lupus erythematosus is clinically, pathologically, and serologically indistinguishable from spontaneously arising systemic lupus erythematosus. However, cutaneous and renal manifestations are rarer in drug-induced than in spontaneous systemic lupus erythematosus, and pleuropulmonary manifestations are somewhat more common (Dubois). Usually, but not always, when the medication is discontinued, the clinical and laboratory manifestations subside (Dubois). Nevertheless, death can occur, especially as a result of renal involvement (Whittle and Ainsworth).

Histopathology. The histologic picture of the cutaneous lesions is the same as in systemic lupus erythematosus (see p. 450).

Histogenesis. Antinuclear antibodies are nearly always present as well as anti-single-stranded deoxyribonucleic acid (DNA) antibodies. However, anti-double-stranded DNA antibodies are usually absent. Hypocomplementemia is rare. Also, the occurrence of a "lupus band" on direct immunofluorescence testing of normal-appearing skin is uncommon (Grossman et al).

HALOGEN ERUPTIONS

Ingestion of bromides may cause, besides a pustular eruption, the formation of vegetating, papillomatous plaques called *bromoderma*. The plaques, which usually occur on the lower extremities, often show pustules at their periphery (Teller). Although bromoderma often appears only after prolonged intake of bromides, it has been reported to arise within 8 days (Schirren and Wehrmann).

Iododerma, usually seen on the face, begins as a rule with multiple pustules that rapidly coalesce into vegetating plaques (Perroud and Delacrétaz). Like bromoderma, the plaques of ioderma often show pustules at their periphery, but they usually show less papillomatous proliferation and a softer consistency than bromoderma, and they often ulcerate (Teller). Iododerma is frequently associated with fever. Although the eruption usually arises after prolonged ingestion of iodides, it may start within a few days, especially in patients with chronic nephritis (Kimmig; Freund). Iododerma may also start within a few days after a second urography (Heydenreich and Larsen) or a second lymphography (Perroud and Delacrétaz) for which iodine-containing compounds have been used.

Fluoroderma has been described as occurring after the frequent application of a fluoride gel to the teeth for the purpose of preventing caries during tumor radiation therapy to the face (Blasik and Spencer). The lesions consist of scattered papules and nodules on the neck and in the preauricular regions.

Histopathology. The histologic picture in the halogen eruptions is suggestive rather than diagnostic. The difference between bromoderma and iododerma lies largely in the epidermal changes, which usually are much more pronounced in bromoderma, although there is some overlapping. The dermal changes are essentially the same and vary with the age of the lesion.

In early lesions, the dermis in both bromoderma and iododerma shows a dense infiltrate of neutrophils, which, in areas of dermal necrosis, show nuclear dust (Rosenberg et al). There may be intradermal abscesses (Goos). Eosinophils are present in most cases and may be numerous (Leibl). Extensive extravasations of erythrocytes may also be seen (Teller). At a later stage, the proportion of lymphoid cells and histiocytes increases, and the histiocytes may show abundant cytoplasm (Perround and Delacrétaz) or large nuclei (Jones et al). The blood vessels are increased in number and dilated, and they may show proliferation of their endothelium.

The epidermal changes in bromoderma are often pronounced. In addition to papillomatosis, one may observe considerable downward proliferation, occasionally to such a degree as to produce the picture of pseudocarcinomatous hyperplasia. Frequently, intraepidermal abscesses are present in the surface epidermis as well as in the downward proliferations of the epidermis (Fig. 15-1) (Goos). The intraepidermal abscesses are filled with neutrophils, eosinophils, and some desquamated keratinocytes, most of which appear necrotic, although some resemble acantholytic cells (Schirren and Wehrmann). Some epithelial islands in the upper dermis, instead of enclosing an abscess, are filled with keratin (Leibl).

In iododerma, the epidermis may be partially absent as a result of ulceration. At the margin of the ulcers, one may find intraepidermal abscesses (Teller). In old lesions, pseudocarcinomatous hyperplasia may be encountered (Perroud and Delacrétaz).

Fluoroderma has been described only as a mild eruption, but it shares with iododerma and bromoderma the presence of eosinophils, neutrophils, and erythrocytes in the dermis and of microabscesses in the epidermis (Blasik and Spencer).

Histogenesis. Even though there is often a very long interval between the first ingestion of iodides or bromides and the appearance of the eruption, there can be no doubt that halogen eruptions are an allergic phenomenon; once a person has become sensitized, the eruption recurs within a few days upon the readministration of iodides (Jones et al) or bromides (Leibl).

It appears likely that halogen eruptions arise on the basis of delayed hypersensitivity. In one reported case of iododerma, the patient's lymphocytes underwent blastogenic transformation on exposure to ^{131}I-labeled serum albumin (Rosenberg et al).

Differential Diagnosis. Intraepidermal abscesses occur in blastomycosis and pemphigus vegetans as well as in the halogen eruptions. However, blastomycosis is easily differentiated by its numerous giant cells and the presence of yeast cells within them. In contrast, differentiation from pemphigus vegetans may cause difficulties, especially since eosinophils often are prominent in halogen eruptions as well. Generally, pemphigus vegetans shows a less extensive dermal infiltrate that only rarely contains neutrophils. Also, in pemphigus vegetans, acantholysis usually is pronounced, whereas, in halogen eruptions, it is rarely seen and, if present, is slight, since it is only a secondary acantholysis.

ARGYRIA

Argyria is caused by prolonged ingestion of silver salts or their prolonged application to the mucous membranes of the upper respiratory tract. It is characterized by a slate-gray discoloration of the skin, especially in the exposed areas, and, often, of the oral mucosa and conjunctivae. On laparotomy, many internal organs may

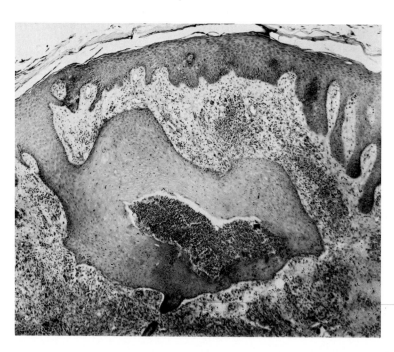

Fig. 15-1. Bromoderma
There is downward proliferation of the epidermis, which encloses a large abscess. The dermis contains a dense inflammatory infiltrate. (×50)

show a bluish discoloration, including the pancreas, stomach, liver, spleen, intestines, and peritoneum (Marshall and Schneider).

Histopathology.   Silver is found in the dermis extracellularly as fine, small, round, brownish black granules that appear fairly uniform in size. In contrast, silver is not seen in the epidermis or its appendages. The silver granules measure less than 1 μm in diameter and lie singly as well as in groups. Although visible in routine stains, they stand out much more clearly when sections are examined with a dark-field microscope. The silver granules then appear as brilliantly refractile, white particles against a dark background. Also, many more granules can be seen by this method than with direct illumination.

The silver granules are present in greatest number in the basement membrane zone, or membrana propria, surrounding the sweat glands (Fig. 15-2). They are also seen in high concentrations in the connective tissue sheaths around the hair follicles and sebaceous glands, in the walls of capillaries, in the arrectores pilorum, and in the nerves (Hill and Montgomery). Silver granules are also found in the dermal papillae and scattered diffusely through the dermis. Elastic tissue stains reveal a predilection of the granules for elastic fibers, which explains the presence of fingerlike chains of granules projecting into the dermal papillae (Hill and Mont-

gomery). The silver granules also show an affinity for areas of solar elastosis (Schröpl et al).

In addition to silver, there is an increase in the amounts of melanin, particularly in the exposed skin. Increased amounts of melanin are present in some cases only in the epidermis (Mehta et al); in other cases, melanin is found also within melanophages scattered throughout the upper dermis (Hill and Montgomery).

Comparing the amounts of silver granules in discolored, exposed skin with that found in non-discolored, or only slightly discolored, unexposed skin, several investigators have found equal quantities of silver in the same patient (Habermann; Gaul and Staud; Hill and Montgomery).

Deposits of silver are found also in internal organs. Thus, a gastric biopsy has shown silver granules in the connective tissue, and a liver biopsy has revealed silver deposited in portal areas and around central veins (Marshall and Schneider). Analogous to the marked involvement of the basement membrane zone around the sweat glands, the basement membrane zone around the seminiferous tubules of the testes is particularly rich in silver granules (Prose).

Histogenesis. On *electron microscopy,* the silver granules lie in most instances almost entirely extracellularly within the dermis (Mehta et al; Hönigsmann et al). The silver granules consist of aggregates of microgranules, which

Fig. 15-2. Argyria
Silver granules are present in the membrana propria of the sweat glands. In some places, the granules are so dense that they form a solid black band. (×400)

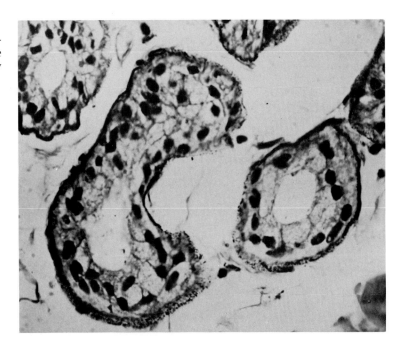

measure from 30 nm to 40 nm in diameter (Hönigsmann et al; Nasemann et al; Reymond et al) and can appear rounded or ovoid but mostly are irregularly shaped (Hönigsmann et al). The silver granules, in contrast to their rather uniform size on light microscopy, vary considerably in size when seen on electron microscopy. Although most of them measure between 200 nm and 400 nm in diameter (Mehta et al; Nasemann et al), some reach a size of 1000 nm (Prose; Reymond et al).

The silver granules are located predominantly in the basement membrane (basal lamina) that surrounds sweat glands, endothelial cells, nerve fibers, and smooth muscle cells (Hönigsmann et al). Their affinity for the subepidermal basement membrane and the basement membrane surrounding hair follicles and sebaceous glands is less pronounced (Mehta et al). The apparent diffuse distribution of silver granules throughout the dermis, as seen by light microscopy, is related to the elastic fibers; no granules are seen in the vicinity of collagen fibrils. In the elastic fibers, the granules are located only in the vicinity of microfibrils rather than free in the amorphous substance, the elastin (Hönigsmann et al). Rarely, a few granules are seen in the intercellular spaces of the epidermis and of hair follicles (Nasemann et al).

Although silver granules may be seen occasionally free in the cytoplasm of macrophages (Johansson et al), most authors have only rarely observed silver granules within lysosomes of macrophages (Hönigsmann et al) or fibroblasts (Mehta et al). However, in cases of recent onset, the main location of the silver granules is intracellular, within lysosomes of macrophages and fibroblasts (Reymond et al). It can thus be concluded that silver is at first phagocytized by macrophages and fibroblasts, but, since these cells are unable to perform complete degradation of the silver, it is discharged into the tissue (Reymond et al). Apparently, the silver is somewhat altered, probably through the loss of its protein carrier, so that, after its discharge, it no longer stimulates phagocytosis (Hönigsmann et al).

The increase in the amount of melanin in the basal cell layer and occasionally also in the upper dermis can be explained by the fact that the presence of silver in the skin stimulates melanocytic activity. Silver is assumed to act either by increasing oxidative processes (Robert and Zürcher) or by reacting with epidermal sulfhydryl groups, thus reducing the inhibition that these groups normally exert on the enzyme system governing melanin synthesis (Buckley). It is well known that melanocytic activity is stimulated not only by deposits of silver in the skin but also by deposits of other heavy metals, such as iron in hemochromatosis (see p. 432) and mercury in mercury pigmentation (see below).

The question arises whether the slate-gray pigmentation of argyria is caused solely by the deposits of silver, by the increase in the amount of melanin, or by both the silver and the melanin. The fact that pigmentation is more pronounced in sun-exposed areas of the skin probably cannot be explained solely by increased deposition of silver granules in areas of solar elastosis, as

has been suggested (Schröpl et al). Also, the amount of silver present has been found to be the same in exposed and unexposed skin (see p. 265). The amount of melanin can be assumed to be greater in sun-exposed areas of the skin than in unexposed areas. Still, the increase in melanin is moderate and is often limited to the epidermis, so that it would not cause the slate-gray hue that results from the Tyndall effect of deeply deposited pigment. It thus appears most likely that both the deposits of silver and the increase in melanin contribute to the pigmentation (Czitober et al). Also, the fact that in argyria many internal organs may have a bluish color (Marshall et al) indicates that silver can cause discoloration.

Differential Diagnosis. Histologic differentiation of argyria from other kinds of pigmentation rarely causes any difficulty because of the uniform size and characteristic distribution of the silver granules. The easiest procedure proving that the granules contain silver is placement of sections into a solution consisting of 1% potassium ferricyanide in 20% sodium thiosulfate; this will result in decolorization of silver (Pearse). Positive identification of the silver deposits in histologic sections can be accomplished by means of neutron-activation analysis (Czitober et al; Schröpl et al).

MERCURY PIGMENTATION

Regular application of a mercury-containing cream to the face and neck over many years may produce a slate-gray pigmentation of the skin in the areas to which the cream has been applied. Generally, the pigmentation is most pronounced on the eyelids, in the nasolabial folds, and in the folds of the neck (Lamar and Bliss).

Histopathology. Irregular, brownish black granules are found in the upper dermis, partially free in the dermis and partially within macrophages (Lüders et al). In rare instances, granules are seen also in the basal cell layer of the epidermis (Nasemann et al). Dark-field examination of sections reveals the granules to be brilliantly refractile (Burge and Winkelmann). On staining with silver nitrate, the amount of melanin in the basal layer of the epidermis may be found to be within normal limits (Lüders et al) or increased (Burge and Winkelmann).

Histogenesis. As seen by *electron microscopy*, the mercury particles measure approximately 14 nm in diameter and are aggregated into irregular granules up to 340 nm in size. Many granules are associated with elastic fibers, whereas others are situated free among the collagen fibers and in macrophages either within lysosomes or free in the cytoplasm (Burge and Winkelmann). If present in the epidermis, the mercury granules lie in the intercellular spaces of the basal cell layer (Nasemann et al).

Since, clinically, the pigmentation is most pronounced in skin folds that are protected from the sun, and, histologically, there may be no increase in the amount of melanin, it can be concluded that most of the pigmentation is caused by the presence of mercury rather than melanin.

Differential Diagnosis. Mercury pigmentation differs from a tattoo by the more superficial location of the granules and by refractility of the granules on dark-field examination. Positive identification of the granules as mercury can be made by submission of unstained sections to neutron-activation analysis (Burge and Winkelmann).

ARSENICAL KERATOSIS AND CARCINOMA

Inorganic arsenic was a frequently used oral medication for a number of dermatoses until evidence accumulated in the 1930s that, besides its long-known tendency to form arsenical keratoses on the palms and soles, inorganic arsenic quite frequently causes carcinoma of the skin (Montgomery). In the 1950s, it became apparent that inorganic arsenic could cause visceral carcinoma. The most common form in which inorganic arsenic has been administered was Fowler's solution containing 1% potassium arsenite.

A rare cause for an "epidemic" occurrence of arsenical keratoses and carcinomas is the presence of arsenic in well water, as reported in a study of 428 patients from Taiwan (Yeh).

Arsenical keratoses of the palms and soles, consisting of verrucous papules without surrounding inflammation, are a common manifestation of prolonged arsenic ingestion. Thus, in a follow-up study of 262 patients who had been taking Fowler's solution for 6 to 26 years prior to this study, arsenical keratoses of the palms and soles were observed in 40%, and arsenic-induced carcinomas of the skin in 8% (Fierz). In the study from Taiwan, 80% of the 428 patients with arsenical carcinomas of the skin had arsenical keratoses of the palms and soles (Yeh). The minimal latent period between the beginning of arsenic intake and the onset of arsenical keratoses of the palms and soles has been found to be 2½ years, and the average latent period 6 years (Fierz).

Cutaneous carcinomas following arsenic ingestion are usually multiple, and about three quarters of them are located on the trunk (Yeh). They consist of erythematous, scaling, occasionally crusted patches that slowly increase in size. Carcinomas can also arise in arsenical keratoses of the palms and soles (Fierz; Yeh). The average latency between the beginning of arsenic intake and the onset of carcinoma has been found to be 18 years, with a spread from 3 to 40 years (Neubauer).

Visceral carcinoma can be caused by arsenic intake, but the actual incidence is difficult to determine because of the long latent period, which may vary from 13 to 50 years, with an average of 24 years (Sommers and McManus). The most common locations appear to be the bronchi and the genitourinary system (Sommers and McManus; Fierz).

Since Bowen's disease is the most common cutaneous carcinoma produced by arsenic, the possibility of a relationship between Bowen's disease and visceral carcinoma is of interest. This association, first pointed out in 1959 (Graham and Helwig), appears to be greatest in those cases of Bowen's disease in which the lesions are located in unexposed areas and thus are not caused by sun exposure. In one report, an association with internal carcinoma was found in about one third of the cases (Peterka et al). It has been suggested that arsenic is the common denominator in such cases, causing both Bowen's disease and internal carcinoma. However, subsequent studies have shown no significant relationship between Bowen's disease in covered areas and internal malignancy (Andersen et al); or, if such a relationship has been found to exist, no arsenic ingestion has been found in most of the patients (Callen and Headington).

Histopathology. In *arsenical keratoses* of the palms and soles, one may find in some instances only hyperkeratosis and acanthosis, without evidence of nuclear atypicality (Yeh). However, on cutting deeper into the tissue block, atypicality may become apparent. Whereas some arsenical keratoses show only mild nuclear atypicality, the findings in others are those of a squamous cell carcinoma in situ and are analogous to Bowen's disease or a solar keratosis. One observes disorder in the arrangement of the squamous cells and nuclear atypicalities, such as hyperchromasia, clumping, or dyskeratosis (Hundeiker and Petres). Atrophy of the epidermis and basophilic degeneration of the upper dermis, as seen in some solar keratoses, are absent in arsenical keratoses. Evidence of development into an invasive squamous cell carcinoma may be seen in some arsenical keratoses (Fierz; Hundeiker and Petres; Yeh).

The type of *cutaneous carcinoma* that follows arsenic ingestion can be either squamous cell carcinoma or basal cell epithelioma, usually as multiple lesions. Squamous cell carcinomas usually occur as in situ lesions analogous to Bowen's disease, and basal cell epitheliomas occur as superficial basal cell epitheliomas, although invasive squamous cell carcinomas and basal cell epitheliomas occur occasionally. Invasive tumors may arise de novo or may develop within pre-existing lesions of Bowen's disease or superficial basal cell epithelioma.

A matter of controversy has been the question as to whether arsenical carcinomas occur more commonly as lesions of Bowen's disease or as superficial basal cell epitheliomas. For many years, it was accepted that lesions of Bowen's disease were the usual reaction (Montgomery and Waisman). However, two recent publications stated that superficial basal cell epitheliomas are far more prevalent than lesions of Bowen's disease (Fierz; Ehlers), although, in two other publications, Bowen's disease was found to be much more common (Hundeiker and Petres; Yeh). The most likely explanation for this discrepancy appears to be that, in many instances, lesions of Bowen's disease have been misinterpreted as superficial basal cell epithelioma (Hundeiker and Petres). The distinction can indeed be difficult; one author who found mainly superficial basal cell epitheliomas conceded that 25% of them showed "squamous metaplasia" (Ehlers), and another author has proposed the concept of "combined forms" consisting of a "mixture of superficial basal cell epithelioma and intraepidermal carcinoma" (Yeh). It appears likely that lesions designated as superficial basal cell epithelioma with squamous metaplasia or as combined forms represent lesions of Bowen's disease. (For histologic descriptions of Bowen's disease and superficial basal cell epithelioma, see pp. 496 and 569, respectively.)

Histogenesis. In vitro experiments concerning the effects of inorganic arsenic on human epidermal cells have shown that arsenic depresses premitotic DNA replication. Furthermore, incubation with inorganic arsenic and subsequent exposure of the cell cultures to ultraviolet light causes interruption of the enzymatic "dark repair mechanism" in the epidermal cells. Among other enzymes, arsenic seems to block predominantly DNA polymerase by attaching itself to sulfhydryl groups. The damaging effect of arsenic on DNA may explain its carcinogenic effect (Jung and Trachsel).

PHENYTOIN-INDUCED PSEUDOLYMPHOMA SYNDROME

Phenytoin (Dilantin) may cause a pseudolymphoma syndrome characterized by generalized lymphadenopathy, hepatosplenomegaly, fever, arthralgia, and eosinophilia. The cutaneous lesions usually consist of a generalized erythematous, macular or papular, pruritic eruption (Schreiber and McGregor; Charlesworth). In one reported instance, however, two cutaneous nodules were present (Adams).

Histopathology. The generalized cutaneous eruption usually shows a nonspecific histologic picture, although, in one instance, it was suggestive of mycosis fungoides because of the presence of Pautrier microabscesses (Schreiber and McGregor).

In the patient with cutaneous nodules, the infiltrate suggested a cutaneous lymphoma of the non-Hodgkin's type, because large masses of lymphocytes were present in the dermis as well as in the subcutaneous tissue (Adams).

The enlarged subcutaneous lymph nodes in some cases may show merely reactive hyperplasia (Charlesworth) but in other cases may be suggestive of lymphoma as a result of the complete loss of normal architecture (Schreiber and McGregor).

BIBLIOGRAPHY

Drug-Induced Vasculitis
MULLICK FG, MCALLISTER HA JR, WAGNER BM et al: Drug related vasculitis. Hum Pathol 10:313–325, 1979
VAN JOOST T, ASGHAR SS, CORMANE RH: Skin reactions caused by phenylbutazone. Arch Dermatol 110:929–933, 1974
WINKELMANN RK, DITTO WB: Cutaneous and visceral syndromes of necrotizing or "allergic" angiitis: A study of 38 cases. J Invest Dermatol 43:59–89, 1964

Fixed Drug Eruption
DE DOBBELEER G, ACHTEN G: Fixed drug eruption, ultrastructural study of dyskeratotic cells. Br J Dermatol 96:239–244, 1977
FURUYA T, SEKIDO N, ISHIHARA F: Beitrag zum fixen Arzneimittelexanthem. Arch Klin Exp Dermatol 225:375–383, 1966
GIMENEZ-CAMARASA JM, GARCIA-CALDERON P, DE MORAGAS JM: Lymphocyte transformation test in fixed drug eruption. N Engl J Med 292:819–821, 1975
STRITZLER C, KOPF AW: Fixed drug eruption caused by 8-chlorotheophylline in Dramamine with clinical and histologic studies. J Invest Dermatol 34:319–330, 1960
TARNOWSKI WM: Fixed drug eruption due to tetracyclines. Acta Derm Venereol (Stockh) 50:117–118, 1970
TRITSCH H, ORFANOS C, LUCKERATH, J: Nekrolytische Arznei-Exantheme. Hautarzt 19:24–29, 1968

Bullae and Sweat Gland Necrosis in Drug-Induced Coma
ACHTEN G, LEDOUX-CORBUSIER M, THYS JP: Intoxication à l'oxyde de carbone et lésions cutanées. Ann Dermatol Syph 98:421–428, 1971
ARNDT KA, MIHM MC JR, PARRISH JA: Bullae: A cutaneous sign of a variety of neurologic diseases. J Invest Dermatol 60:312–320, 1973
BREHMER-ANDERSSON E, PEDERSEN NB: Sweat gland necrosis and bullous skin changes in acute drug intoxication. Acta Derm Venereol (Stockh) 49:157–162, 1969
HERSCHTHAL D, ROBINSON MJ: Blisters of the skin in coma induced by amitriptyline and chloracepate dipotassium. Arch Dermatol 115:499, 1979
LEAVELL UW, FARLEY CH, MCINTIRE JS: Cutaneous changes in a patient with carbon monoxide poisoning. Arch Dermatol 99:429–433, 1969
MANDY S, ACKERMAN AB: Characteristic traumatic skin lesions in drug-induced coma. JAMA 213:253–256, 1970

Drug-Induced Photosensitivity
BASLER RSW, KOHNEN PW: Localized hemosiderosis as a sequala of acne. Arch Dermatol 114:1695–1697, 1978

BLOIS MS JR: On chlorpromazine binding in vivo. J Invest Dermatol 45:475–481, 1965

FENSKE NA, MILLNS JL: Cutaneous pigmentation due to minocycline hydrochloride. J Am Acad Dermatol 3:308–310, 1980

FROST P, WEINSTEIN GP, GOMEZ EC: Phototoxic potential of minocycline and doxycycline. Arch Dermatol 105:681–683, 1972

GREINER AC, NICOLSON GA: Pigmentary deposit in viscera associated with prolonged chlorpromazine therapy. Can Med Assoc J 91:627–635, 1964

HÄGERMARK Ö, WENNERSTEN G, ALMEYDA J: Cutaneous side effects of phenothiazines. Br J Dermatol 84:605–607, 1971

HARBER LC, BAER RL: Pathogenic mechanisms of drug-induced photosensitivity. J Invest Dermatol 58:327–342, 1972

HASHIMOTO K, WIENER W, ALBERT J et al: An electron microscopic study of chlorpromazine pigmentation. J Invest Dermatol 47:296–306, 1966

HAYS, GB, LYLE CB JR, WHEELER CE JR: Slate-grey color in patients receiving chlorpromazine. Arch Dermatol 90:471–476, 1964

LEROY JP, DORVAL JC, DEWITTE JD et al: Deux cas de pigmentation cutanée au cours de traitements par la minocycline. Ann Dermatol Venereol 108:871–875, 1981

MCGRAE JD JR, ZELICKSON AS: Skin pigmentation secondary to minocycline therapy. Arch Dermatol 116:1262–1265, 1980

SATANOVE A: Pigmentation due to phenothiazines in high and prolonged doses. JAMA 191:263–268, 1965

SATO S, MURPHY GF, BERNARD JD et al: Ultrastructural and x-ray microanalytical observations on minocycline-related hyperpigmentation of the skin. J Invest Dermatol 77:264–271, 1981

SIMONS JJ, MORALES A: Minocycline and generalized cutaneous pigmentation. J Am Acad Dermatol 3:244–247, 1980

WILLIS I, KLIGMAN AM: The mechanism of photoallergic contact dermatitis. J Invest Dermatol 51:378–384, 1968

ZELICKSON AS: Skin pigmentation and chlorpromazine. JAMA 194:670–672, 1965

Penicillamine-Induced Dermatoses

BARDACH H, GEBHART W: Penicillamininduzierte dermolytische Dermatose bei einer Patientin mit Morbus Wilson. Dermatologica 162:473–483, 1981

BARDACH A, GEBHART W, NIEBAUER G: "Lumpy-bumpy" elastic fibers in the skin and lungs of a patient with penicillamine-induced elastosis perforans serpiginosa. J Cutan Pathol 6:243–252, 1979

CHARLES R: In discussion of Davis W: Wilson's disease and penicillamine-induced anetoderma. Arch Dermatol 113:976, 1977

DAVIS W: Wilson's disease and penicillamine-induced anetoderma. Arch Dermatol 113:976, 1977

DEGOS R, TOURAINE R, BELAICH S et al: Pemphigus chez un malade traité par pénicillamine pour maladie de Wilson. Bull Soc Fr Dermatol Syph 76:751–753, 1969

FROM E, FREDERIKSEN P: Pemphigus vulgaris following D-penicillamine. Dermatologica 152:358–362, 1976

GREER KE, ASKEW FC, RICHARDSON DR: Skin lesions induced by penicillamine. Arch Dermatol 112:1267–1269, 1976

GUILAINE J, BENHAMON JP, MOLAS G: Élastome perforant verruciforme chez un malade traité par pénicillamine pour maladie de Wilson. Bull Soc Fr Dermatol Syph 79:450–453, 1972

HASHIMOTO K, MCEVOY B, BELCHER R: Ultrastructure of penicillamine-induced skin lesions. J Am Acad Dermatol 4:300–315, 1981

KATZ R: Penicillamine-induced skin lesions. Arch Dermatol 95:196–198, 1967

KIRSCH N, HUKILL PB: Elastosis perforans serpiginosa induced by penicillamine. Arch Dermatol 113:630–635, 1977

KRISTENSEN JK, WADSKOV S: Penicillamine-induced pemphigus foliaceus. Acta Derm Venereol (Stockh) 57:69–71, 1977

MARSDEN RA, RYAN TJ, VANHEGAN RI et al: Pemphigus foliaceus induced by penicillamine. Br Med J 2:1423–1424, 1976

PASS F, GOLDFISCHER S, STERNLIEB I et al: Elastosis perforans serpiginosa during penicillamine therapy for Wilson disease. Arch Dermatol 108:713–715, 1973

SPARROW GP: Penicillamine pemphigus and the nephrotic syndrome occurring simultaneously. Br J Dermatol 98:103–105, 1978

Drug-Induced Lupus Erythematosus

ALARCON-SEGOVIA D, WAKIN KG, WORTHINGTON JW et al: Clinical and experimental studies on the hydralazine syndrome and its relationship to systemic lupus erythematosus. Medicine (Baltimore) 46:1–33, 1967

DUBOIS EL: Procainamide induction of a systemic lupus erythematosus-like syndrome. Medicine (Baltimore) 48:217–228, 1969

GROSSMAN J, CALLERAME ML, CONDEMI JJ: Skin immunofluorescence studies on lupus erythematosus and other antinuclear antibody-positive diseases. Ann Intern Med 80:496–500, 1974

WHITTLE TS JR, AINSWORTH SK: Procainamide-induced systemic lupus erythematosus. Arch Pathol 100:469–474, 1976

Halogen Eruptions

BLASIK LG, SPENCER SK: Fluoroderma. Arch Dermatol 115:1334–1335, 1979

FREUND F: Zur Klinik der vegetierenden Jodausschläge unter besonderer Berücksichtigung des Schleimhautbefalles. Arch Dermatol Syph (Berlin) 198:352–362, 1954

GOOS M: Bromoderma tuberosum mit Erhöhung der sauren Serumphosphatase. Hautarzt 22:30–32, 1971

HEYDENREICH G, LARSEN PO: Iododerma after high dose urography in an oliguric patient. Br J Dermatol 97:567–569, 1977

JONES LE, PARISER H, MURRAY PF: Recurrent iododerma. Arch Dermatol 78:353–358, 1958

KIMMIG J: Ursache und Behandlung des Jododerma tuberosum. Hautarzt 2:78–79, 1951

LEIBL K: Bromoderma tuberosum. Dermatol Wochenschr 137:681–686, 1958

PERROUD H, DELACRÉTAZ J: Iodides végétantes. Ann Dermatol Venereol 104:154–156, 1977

ROSENBERG FR, EINBINDER J, WALZER RA et al: Vegetating iododerma. Arch Dermatol 105:900–905, 1972

SCHIRREN C, WEHRMANN R: Experimentelle Untersuchunger zur Ausscheidung von Brom bei Bromoderma tuberosum. Arch Klin Exp Dermatol 217:50–59, 1963

TELLER H: Bromoderma und Jododerma tuberosum. Dermatol Wochenschr 143:273–282, 1961

Argyria

BUCKLEY WR: Localized argyria. Arch Dermatol 88:531–539, 1963

CZITOBER H, FRISCHAUF H, LEODOLTER I: Quantitative Untersuchungen bei universeller Argyrose mittels Neutronenaktivierungsanalyse. Virchows Arch Abt A 350:44–51, 1970

GAUL LE, STAUD AH: Clinical spectroscopy: Seventy cases of generalized argyrosis following organic and colloidal silver medication, including a biospectrometric analysis of ten cases. JAMA 104:1387–1490, 1935

HABERMANN R: Über Argyria cutis nach Silbersalvarsan und den Wert der Leuchtbildmethode E. Hoffmanns für ihren Nachweis. Dermatol Ztschr 40:65–80, 1923

HILL WR, MONTGOMERY H: Argyria. Arch Dermatol Syph 44:588–599, 1941

HÖNIGSMANN H, KONRAD K, WOLFF K: Argyrose (Histologie und Ultrastruktur). Hautarzt 24:24, 1973

JOHANSSON EA, KANERVA L, NIEMI KM et al: Generalized argyria. Clin Exp Dermatol 7:169–176, 1982

MARSHALL JP, SCHNEIDER RP: Systemic argyria secondary to topical silver nitrate. Arch Dermatol 113:1077–1079, 1977

MEHTA AC, DAWSON-BUTTERWORTH K, WOODHOUSE MA: Argyria. Electron microscopic study of a case. Br J Dermatol 78:175–179, 1966

NASEMANN T, ROGGE T, SCHAEG G: Licht- und elektronenmikroskopische Untersuchungen bei der Hydrargyrose und der Argyrose der Haut. Hautarzt 25:534–540, 1974

PEARSE AGE: Histochemistry, Theoretical and Applied, 3rd ed, p. 1151. Edinburgh, Churchill Livingston, 1972

PROSE PH: An electron microscopic study of human generalized argyria. Am J Pathol 42:293–299, 1963

REYMOND JL, STOEBNER P, AMBLARD P: Argyrie cutanée. Ann Dermatol Venereol 107:251–255, 1980

ROBERT P, ZÜRCHER H: Pigmentstudien. I. Über den Einfluss von Schwermetallverbindungen, Hämin, Vitaminen, mikrobiellen Toxinen, Hormonen und weiteren Stoffen auf die Dopamelaninbildung in vivo. Dermatologica 100:217–241, 1950

SCHRÖPL F, OEHLSCHLAEGEL G, DRABNER, J: Schwermetallnachweis in der Haut bei Argyrose mittels Neutronenaktivierungsanalyse. Arch Klin Exp Dermatol 231:398–407, 1968

Mercury Pigmentation

BURGE KM, WINKELMANN RK: Mercury pigmentation. An electron microscopic study. Arch Dermatol 102:51–61, 1970

LAMAR LM, BLISS BO: Localized pigmentation of the skin due to topical mercury. Arch Dermatol 93:450–453, 1966

LÜDERS G, FISCHER H, HENSEL U: Hydrargyrosis cutis mit allgemeinen Vergiftungserscheinungen nach langdauernder Anwendung quecksilberhaltiger Kosmetica. Hautarzt 19:61–65, 1968

NASEMANN T, ROGGE T, SCHAEG G: Licht- und elektronenmikroskopische Untersuchungen bei der Hydrargyrose und der Argyrose der Haut. Hautarzt 25:534–540, 1974

Arsenical Keratosis and Carcinoma

ANDERSEN SL, NIELSEN H, REYMANN F: Relationship between Bowen's disease and internal malignant tumors. Arch Dermatol 108:367–370, 1973

CALLEN JP, HEADINGTON J: Bowen's and non-Bowen's squamous intraepidermal neoplasia of the skin. Arch Dermatol 116:422–426, 1980

EHLERS G: Klinische und histologische Untersuchungen zur Frage arzneimittelbedingter Arsen-Tumoren. Z Hautkr 43:763–774, 1968

FIERZ U: Katamnestische Untersuchungen über die Nebenwirkungen der Therapie mit anorganischem Arsen bei Hautkrankheiten. Dermatologica 131:41–58, 1965

GRAHAM JH, HELWIG EB: Bowen's disease and its relationship to systemic cancer. Arch Dermatol 80:133–159, 1959

HUNDEIKER M, PETRES J: Morphogenese und Formenreichtum der arseninduzierten Präkanzerosen. Arch Klin Exp Dermatol 231:355–365, 1968

JUNG EG, TRACHSEL B: Molekularbiologische Untersuchungen zur Arsencarcinogenese. Arch Klin Exp Dermatol 237:819–826, 1970

MONTGOMERY H: Arsenic as an etiologic agent in certain types of epithelioma. Arch Dermatol 32:218–233, 1935

MONTGOMERY H, WAISMAN M: Epithelioma attributable to arsenic. J Invest Dermatol 4:365–383, 1941

NEUBAUER O: Arsenical cancer. Br J Cancer 1:192–249, 1947

PETERKA ES, LYNCH FW, GOLTZ RW: An association between Bowen's disease and internal cancer. Arch Dermatol 84:623–629, 1961

SOMMERS SC, MCMANUS RG: Multiple arsenical cancers of skin and internal organs. Cancer 6:347–359, 1953

YEH S: Skin cancer in chronic arsenicism. Hum Pathol 4:469–485, 1973

Phenytoin-Induced Pseudolymphoma Syndrome

ADAMS JD: Localized cutaneous pseudolymphoma associated with phenytoin therapy: A case report. Aust J Dermatol 22:28–29, 1981

CHARLESWORTH EN: Phenytoin-induced pseudolymphoma syndrome. Arch Dermatol 113:477–480, 1977

SCHREIBER MM, MCGREGOR JG: Pseudolymphoma syndrome. A sensitivity to anticonvulsant drugs. Arch Dermatol 97:297–300, 1968

Degenerative Diseases

16

SOLAR (ACTINIC) ELASTOSIS

Senile changes in areas of the skin not regularly exposed to sunlight manifest themselves clinically only in thinning of the skin and a decrease in the amount of subcutaneous fat. In contrast, there often are pronounced changes in the exposed skin of elderly persons, especially persons with a fair complexion. These changes, however, are the result of chronic sun exposure rather than of age. In exposed areas, especially on the face, the skin shows wrinkling and furrowing as well as thinning. In addition, there may be an irregular distribution of pigment. In the nuchal region, the skin, after many years of exposure to the sun, may appear thickened and furrowed. This is referred to as cutis rhomboidalis nuchae.

Histopathology. In skin not regularly exposed to sunlight, the only histologic change of old age consists of a diminution in the number and diameter of the elastic fibers, particularly in the superficial dermis (Mitchell).

In skin exposed to the sun, especially in persons with a fair complexion, hyperplasia of the elastic tissue is usually evident on histologic examination by the age of 30, even though the skin may clinically appear normal. No white person past 40 years of age has normal elastic tissue in the skin of the face (Kligman). The elastic fibers may appear not only increased in number and thicker but also curled and tangled.

In patients with clinically evident solar elastosis of the exposed skin, staining with hematoxylin–eosin reveals in the upper dermis basophilic de-generation of the collagen separated from a somewhat atrophic epidermis by a narrow band of normal collagen. In the areas of basophilic degeneration, the bundles of eosinophilic collagen have been replaced by amorphous basophilic granular material (Plate 2, facing p. 324).

With elastic tissue stains, the areas of basophilic degeneration stain like elastic tissue and therefore are referred to as elastotic material (Fig. 16-1). The elastotic material usually consists of aggregates of thick, interwoven bands in the upper dermis, but, in areas of severe solar degeneration, the elastotic material may have an amorphous rather than a fibrous appearance and may extend into the lower portions of the dermis rather than being confined to upper dermis (Mitchell).

On staining with silver nitrate, the distribution of melanin in the basal cell layer may appear irregular in that areas of hyperpigmentation alternate with areas of hypopigmentation (Mitchell).

Histogenesis. *Electron microscopic examination* of areas of solar (actinic) elastosis shows elastotic material as the main component. Even though this elastotic material resembles elastic tissue in its chemical composition (see p. 272), it differs significantly in appearance from aged elastic fibers as seen in unexposed, aged skin. Instead of showing amorphous electron-lucent elastin and aggregates of electron-dense microfibrils (see p. 32 and EM 13), the thick fibers of elastotic material show two structural components: a fine granular matrix of medium electron density and, within this matrix, homogeneous, electron-dense, irregularly shaped inclusions (Nürnber-

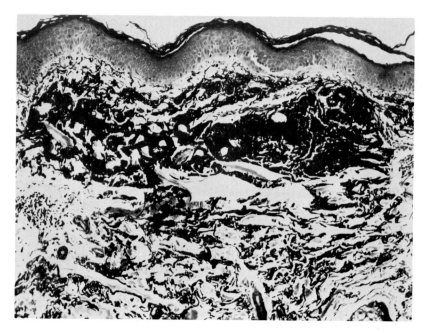

Fig. 16-1. Solar (actinic) degeneration
Elastic tissue stain. In the upper dermis, separated from the epidermis by a narrow band of normal collagen, there are aggregates of thick, interwoven bands of elastotic material staining like elastic tissue. (×100)

ger et al) (EM 30). The inclusions seem to develop by means of a condensation process in the granular matrix. The respective proportion for each of the two components can vary between 30% and 70% of the volume (Marsch et al). Microfibrils as seen in normal or aged elastic fibers are absent. The number and size of elastotic fibers is greatly increased over the number and size of elastic fibers found in normal or aged skin. Extensive amorphous material can be seen around the elastotic fibers and also among the collagen fibrils (EM 30). Collagen fibrils are diminished in number, with those present often showing a diminished electron density, a diminished contrast in cross striation, and a splitting up into filaments at their ends (Braun-Falco). The fibroblasts show the characteristics of actively synthesizing cells in that they possess an extensive rough endoplasmic reticulum containing amorphous to fine granular material that is excreted into the extracellular space (Ebner). Often, strands of fine granular material are discernible between the surface of active fibroblasts and masses of elastotic material (Nürnberger et al).

It can thus be concluded that the elastotic material is newly formed as the result of an altered function of fibroblasts, which are no longer capable of producing normal elastic fibers or collagen. The elastotic material is not regarded as a degeneration product of pre-existing elastic fibers. Neither is it formed by the incorporation of degraded collagen into elastotic material, a process that was once thought to explain the great increase in the bulk of elastotic fibers as well as the disappearance of collagen (Mitchell).

The elastotic material that histochemically stains like elastic tissue resembles elastic tissue with respect to its chemical composition and its physical and enzymatic reactions. Thus, (1) the amino acid composition of the elastotic tissue resembles that of elastin and differs significantly from that of collagen. In particular, the elastotic material, like elastic tissue, has a much lower content of hydroxyproline than collagen (Smith et al). (2) The elastotic material in unfixed sections shows the same brilliant autofluorescence as do elastic fibers on examination with the fluorescence microscope (Niebauer and Stockinger). (3) Both the elastotic material and elastic tissue are susceptible to elastase digestion (Findley).

The elastotic material contains a large amount of acid mucopolysaccharides, as indicated by staining with alcian blue. A significant portion of these acid mucopolysaccharides may be sulfated since prior incubation with hyaluronidase removes only 50% to 75% of the alcian-blue-positive staining. The basophilia of the elastotic material, however, is not affected by incubation with hyaluronidase (Sams and Smith).

The irregular distribution of melanin in the epidermis seen in some patients with solar degeneration, when studied by electron microscopy, is found to be caused largely by an impairment of pigment transfer from melanocytes to keratinocytes. Whereas some keratinocytes contain many melanosomes, others contain few or no melanosomes. The latter are surrounded by dendrites laden with melanosomes (Olsen et al).

Differential Diagnosis.   For a discussion of differentiation of solar elastosis from pseudoxanthoma elasticum, see p. 75.

Nodular Elastosis with Cysts and Comedones (Favre–Racouchot Syndrome)

Some patients with pronounced solar elastosis of the facial skin show, especially lateral to the eyes, multiple comedones as well as yellowish nodules that measure up to 4 mm in diameter and contain a central comedo.

A variant of nodular elastosis with cysts and comedones is the *actinic comedonal plaque.* It is found as a solitary plaque on sun-damaged skin of either the arms or the face. The plaque shows small nodules and dilated follicles (Eastern and Martin).

Histopathology. In addition to pronounced solar elastosis, one observes dilated pilosebaceous openings and large, round cysts that are lined by a flattened epidermis and represent greatly extended hair follicles (Favre and Racouchot; Helm). Both the dilated pilosebaceous openings and the cysts are filled with layered horny material and a lipoid substance similar to sebum. The sebaceous glands are atrophic. Abundant melanin is embedded in the superficial lamellae of the comedones, explaining the black color of the "blackheads." Since the comedones are open rather than closed, they do not tend to become inflamed (Fanta and Niebauer) (see Acne Vulgaris, p. 198).

The histologic findings in actinic comedonal plaque are quite similar to those of nodular elastosis, showing dilated pilosebaceous openings and large, round cysts (Eastern and Martin).

KYRLE'S DISEASE

Kyrle's disease and three unrelated diseases together form a group of perforating dermatoses with transepidermal elimination (Table 16-1). The other three diseases are perforating folliculitis, elastosis perforans serpiginosa, and reactive perforating collagenosis. The latter two diseases have so typical a histologic picture that they are easily diagnosed. In contrast, Kyrle's disease and perforating folliculitis may be difficult to differentiate clinically as well as histologically, except in sections showing the site of perforation.

Kyrle's disease is a rare disorder. Thus, in 1968, in a publication reporting five new cases of it, only 12 of the 45 cases recorded in the literature up to that time were accepted as valid examples of the disease (Carter and Constantine). It is of interest that, in turn, these five cases have been regarded by other authors as instances not of Kyrle's disease but of perforating folliculitis, a disease that was rather common in the late 1960s (Pinkus and Mehregan).

Kyrle's disease, described in 1916 as hyperkeratosis follicularis et parafollicularis in cutem penetrans (Kyrle), is characterized by a more or less extensive eruption of hyperkeratotic papules 2 mm to 8 mm in size containing a central, cone-shaped plug that can be removed with the aid of a curette. The papules may be follicular or extrafollicular in location and may coalesce into verrucous plaques. The extensor surfaces of the extremities are the most common sites of involvement. Quite frequently, diabetes is associated with Kyrle's disease (Carter and Constantine), and a rather high incidence of the disease has been reported among patients with

TABLE 16-1.   Group of Four Diseases Forming Perforations of Epidermis with Subsequent Transepidermal Elimination

	Primary Defect	Type of Epidermal Disruption	Eliminated Material
Kyrle's Disease	Focus of dyskeratotic, rapidly proliferating cells in epidermis	Rapid proliferation causes parakeratotic column in epidermal invagination and ultimate exhaustion of supply of cells in dyskeratotic focus, resulting in disruption	Elimination of granulomatous focus as basophilic debris into epidermal invagination
Perforating Folliculitis	Hyperkeratotic plug in hair follicle containing a curled-up hair	Hair causes perforation	Elimination of basophilic debris and eosinophilic elastic fibers into the hair follicle
Elastosis Perforans Serpiginosa	Formation of numerous coarse elastic fibers in dermal papillae	Formation of narrow winding channels through acanthotic epidermis	Elimination of basophilic debris and eosinophilic elastic fibers into narrow channels
Reactive Perforating Collagenosis	Trauma causes subepidermal focus of necrobiotic basophilic collagen	Overlying epidermis develops areas of disruption	Elimination of necrobiotic basophilic collagen bundles into cup-shaped epidermal depression

chronic renal failure who are receiving hemodialysis (Hood et al).

Histopathology. A heavy keratotic, partly parakeratotic plug occupies an invagination of the epidermis. It is possible that some of the plugs occupy hair follicles, but the invaginations often merely resemble hair follicles. Basophilic debris that does not stain like elastic tissue is present within most plugs (Fig. 16-2) (Thyresson; Constantine and Carter). The parakeratotic material within each plug extends downward to the epidermis of the invagination, reaching the epidermis usually at the deepest point of the invagination as a

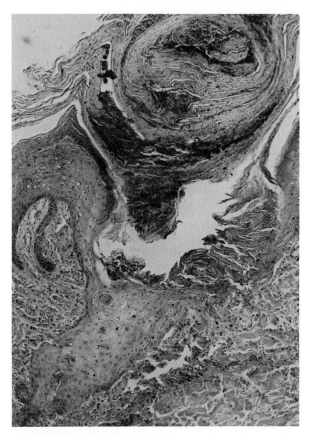

Fig. 16-2. Kyrle's disease
A heavy keratotic, partly parakeratotic plug containing basophilic debris lies in an invagination of the epidermis. On the left side of the invagination, where there are no granular cells, a parakeratotic column arises from epidermal cells that appear vacuolated and dyskeratotic. On the right side of the invagination, there is a disruption of the epidermal cells. Thus, the plug is in direct contact with the dermis, which, in this area, shows degeneration with inflammatory and foreign body giant cells. (×100) (Courtesy of Joseph M. Hitch, M.D.)

parakeratotic column (Tappeiner et al) but occasionally also at other sites (Constantine and Carter). The epidermal invagination shows a well-developed granular layer, except at the point(s) at which the parakeratotic cells of the plug are in contact with the epidermis of the invagination. At sites at which there is no granular layer, one observes within the epidermal invagination of early lesions a focus of vacuolated dyskeratotic cells extending to the basal cell layer; at a later stage, one finds a focus where epidermal cells are absent and the keratotic plug has penetrated into the dermis through the area of disruption of epidermal cells. Wherever the keratotic plug has penetrated into the dermis, one observes fragments of parakeratotic keratin in the dermis together with a rather pronounced granulomatous reaction composed of inflammatory and foreign body giant cells (Thyresson; de Graciansky et al; Abele and Dobson). The epidermal cells bordering the site of perforation proliferate and surround the granulomatous focus in the dermis. Subsequently, the granulomatous material is moved upward by the continuing epidermal cell proliferation around it and ultimately forms the basophilic debris within the keratotic plug (Constantine and Carter; Aram et al). Although the granulomatous focus in the dermis may show a mild degree of collagen degeneration, there is no degeneration of the elastic tissue (Abele and Dobson). Neither is there an increase in the amount of elastic tissue in the dermis, although it may occasionally appear increased beneath the keratotic invaginations as a result of compression (Haensch et al).

It should be pointed out that perforation of the keratotic plug is a stage that is not always reached. Thus, absence of perforation does not rule out Kyrle's disease. In cases without perforation, no basophilic debris is found in the keratotic plug; nevertheless, parakeratotic cells are present in the plug, and, at least at one site of the epidermal invagination, there are dyskeratotic cells, although it may require serial sections to find this site (Constantine and Carter).

Histogenesis. The primary event is a disturbance of epidermal keratinization characterized by the formation of dyskeratotic foci and acceleration of the process of keratinization. This leads to the formation of keratotic plugs with areas of parakeratosis (Constantine and Carter; Tappeiner et al; Bardach). Because the rapid rate of differentiation and keratinization exceeds the rate of cell proliferation, the parakeratotic column gradually extends deeper into the abnormal epidermis, resulting ultimately in perforation of the parakeratotic column into the dermis. Perforation thus is not the cause of Kyrle's disease, as originally thought (Kyrle), but rather represents the consequence or final event of the abnormally sped up keratinization. A certain similarity exists between the parakeratotic column in Kyrle's disease and that seen in porokeratosis Mibelli (Tappeiner et al). In both conditions, a parakeratotic column forms as the result of rapid and faulty keratinization of dyskeratotic cells, but, whereas in Kyrle's disease the dyskeratotic cells are used up and disruption of the epithelium occurs, the clone of dyskeratotic cells can maintain itself in porokeratosis Mibelli by extending peripherally.

Differential Diagnosis. For differentiation of Kyrle's disease from perforating folliculitis, see below and Table 16-1; for differentiation from elastosis perforans serpiginosa, see p. 277 and Table 16-1.

PERFORATING FOLLICULITIS

Perforating folliculitis, first described in 1968 (Mehregan and Coskey), was a fairly common disorder in the late 1960s and early 1970s, but since then has almost entirely disappeared (see Histogenesis) (Mehregan).

One observes erythematous papules 2 mm to 8 mm in diameter with a central keratinous plug that can be removed. Even though perforating folliculitis shows some clinical resemblance to Kyrle's disease, it differs from it in that the papules always are follicular, show no tendency to coalesce, and are limited to the extensor surfaces of the extremities and the buttocks.

Histopathology. Within a dilated hair follicle, one finds orthokeratotic and parakeratotic material that is intermingled with basophilic debris composed of degenerated collagen and inflammatory cells and with brightly eosinophilic, degenerated elastic fibers. In addition, a curled-up hair is often (but not always) seen. One or several small areas of perforation of the follicular epithelium are present within the infundibular region some distance above the level of the sebaceous glands (Fig. 16-3). At the sites of perforation, the dermis shows a focal inflammatory infiltrate containing degenerated collagen and, as a characteristic feature, degenerated elastic fibers that have lost their orceinophilic staining property and stain brightly eosinophilic (Mehregan and Coskey; Streitmann). This focus of inflammation and degeneration in the dermis is then surrounded by proliferating follicular epithelium and is thus moved upward into the follicular cavity and ultimately eliminated through the follicular opening to the surface. Staining for elastic tissue shows no increase in the number of elastic fibers in the dermis.

Histogenesis. It is likely that the perforations in perforating folliculitis are caused by a hair, since a portion of a curled-up hair is often seen close to or within the area of perforation or even in the dermis, surrounded by a foreign body granuloma (Mehregan and Coskey).

The frequent occurrence of this dermatosis in the late 1960s and early 1970s, followed by its virtual disappearance, as well as the distribution of the lesions, suggest that the eruption is related to some chemical in clothing. The reaction appears to be due to a primary irritant acting on the hair follicle. This causes follicular hyperkeratosis and retention of the hair shaft in the follicle and results in a breakdown of the follicular wall as a consequence of mechanical irritation by the curled-up hair (Mehregan).

Differential Diagnosis. In Kyrle's disease, the keratinous plug may be extrafollicular in location, the perforation usually is present deep in the invagination at the bottom of the keratinous plug, and, above all, no eosinophilic degeneration of

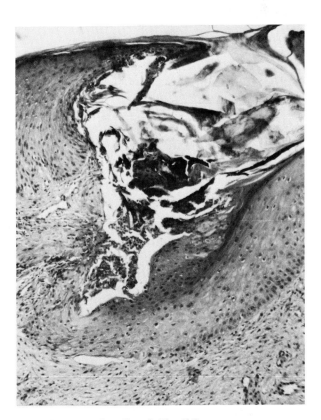

Fig. 16-3. Perforating folliculitis
A greatly dilated hair follicle contains keratotic material intermingled with basophilic debris. On the left side, a perforation of the follicular epithelium is seen within the infundibular region. Degenerated dermal material is eliminated through this perforation. ($\times 50$)

elastic fibers is found. For a discussion of the differential diagnosis of perforating folliculitis from elastosis perforans serpiginosa, see below.

ELASTOSIS PERFORANS SERPIGINOSA

In elastosis perforans serpiginosa, a fairly rare disorder first described in 1953 (Lutz) and 1955 (Miescher), hyperkeratotic scaling papules 2 mm to 5 mm in diameter are found grouped or arranged in an annular or circinate fashion. The lesions usually are confined to one area, most commonly the nape of the neck, the face, or the upper extremities; in rare instances, the lesions are widely disseminated (Rasmussen; Pedro and Garcia). Not infrequently, elastosis perforans serpiginosa is associated with Down's syndrome or with a disorder of the connective tissue, such as Ehlers–Danlos syndrome type IV, osteogenesis imperfecta, pseudoxanthoma elasticum, or Marfan's syndrome (Mehregan).

The development of lesions with the clinical appearance of elastosis perforans serpiginosa has been reported in patients receiving treatment with penicillamine. The histologic picture is distinct and differs from that of idiopathic elastosis perforans serpiginosa (see p. 262).

Histopathology.   The essential features of elastosis perforans serpiginosa are hyperplasia and transepidermal elimination of elastic tissue. Usually, the diagnosis can be suspected already from hematoxylin-eosin-stained sections, requiring staining for elastic tissue only for confirmation.

The characteristic histologic change is the presence of narrow transepidermal channels, which may be straight, wavy, or corkscrew-shaped. In their lowest portion, the channels are often surrounded by proliferating epidermis that engulfs the entrance to the channels like a pair of pincers (Fig. 16-4) (Schneider and Bock). In their lower portion, the channels are filled with bluish-staining necrobiotic masses consisting of a mixture of degenerated epithelial cells, numerous pyknotic nuclei of inflammatory cells, and brightly eosinophilic fibers representing degenerated elastic fibers (Mehregan). In their upper portion, the channels often contain keratotic material as well. The upper dermis contains a chronic inflammatory infiltrate and often, especially near the entrance to the channels, multinucleated giant cells.

On staining for elastic tissue, the great increase in the amount and size of the elastic fibers in the uppermost dermis and particularly in the dermal papillae becomes apparent and makes differentiation from any other dermatosis easy, since it is pathognomonic for elastosis perforans serpiginosa (Fig. 16-5). In their lowest portion, the transepidermal channels may still show some elastic fibers staining with elastic tissue stains, but, as they are extruded, the elastic fibers lose their ability to react with elastic tissue stains. Instead, in addition to staining eosinophilic with hematoxylin-eosin, they stain with the Giemsa stain (Whyte and Winkelmann).

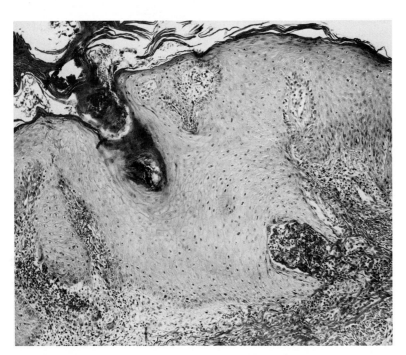

Fig. 16-4.   Elastosis perforans serpiginosa
Hematoxylin-eosin stain. The upper and lower portions of a narrow channel winding through the epidermis are shown. The upper portion of the channel contains basophilic necrotic material with a small keratotic plug on top. The lower portion of the channel contains, in addition to basophilic necrotic material, degenerated elastic fibers. (×100)

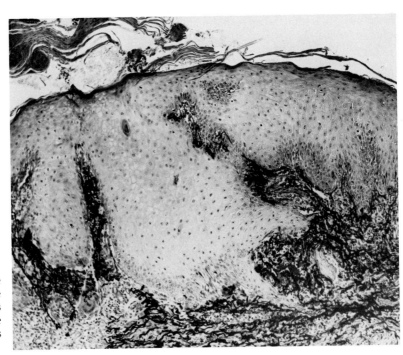

Fig. 16-5. Elastosis perforans serpiginosa
Elastic tissue stain. The great increase in both the amount and the size of the elastic fibers in the uppermost dermis and particularly in the dermal papillae is pathognomonic for elastosis perforans serpiginosa. (×100)

Histogenesis. That the orceinophilic material present in the uppermost dermis and the dermal papillae is elastic tissue has been established through digestion of this material by elastase (Whyte and Winkelmann) and by electron microscopic studies (Cohen and Hashimoto). On *electron microscopy,* the elastic fibers in the uppermost dermis appear much longer and thicker and show branching. In addition, there are many young, very small elastic fibers that are surrounded by numerous microfibrils. The fibroblasts possess an abundant rough endoplasmic reticulum with dilated cisternae, indicating increased synthetic activity (Meves and Vogel). Besides degenerated elastic fibers being eliminated through transepidermal channels, individual normal-appearing elastic fibers are eliminated passively through the epidermis as a result of the upward movement of the keratinocytes (Tsambaos and Berger).

Since the elastic fibers show no obvious abnormality within the dermis except hyperplasia, it is conceivable that the thickened elastic fibers act as a mechanical irritant and provoke an epidermal response in the form of hyperplasia. The epidermis then envelops the irritating material and eliminates it through transepidermal channels. The degeneration of the elastic fibers within the channels probably is secondary to the effect of proteolytic enzymes set free by degenerating inflammatory cells (Mehregan).

Although the invaginated epidermis surrounding the keratinous plugs within the upper portion of the channels may suggest pilosebaceous follicles, and although the winding channels through which the altered elastic tissue is extruded may suggest intraepidermal sweat ducts, it seems that, as a rule, the extrusion occurs without any relationship to these structures (Whyte and Winkelmann).

Differential Diagnosis. Both Kyrle's disease and perforating folliculitis share with elastosis perforans serpiginosa the presence of a central keratotic plug and of a perforation through which degenerated material is eliminated. In addition, perforating folliculitis, like elastosis perforans serpiginosa, shows the elimination of degenerated eosinophilic elastic fibers. However, neither of the two diseases shows the great increase in elastic tissue that is seen in elastosis perforans serpiginosa in the uppermost dermis and particularly in the dermal papillae on staining with elastic tissue stains.

REACTIVE PERFORATING COLLAGENOSIS

A rare dermatosis, reactive perforating collagenosis may show autosomal recessive inheritance and thus has been reported to occur in siblings (Weiner; Kanan). The lesions usually begin to appear in infancy or childhood but may first arise in adulthood (Mohri et al), in which case they may be associated with severe diabetes mellitus and chronic renal insufficiency (Poliak et al). The lesions consist of small papules that gradually grow in size and become unbilicated with an adherent, firm plug, reaching a diameter of 5 mm to 10 mm. They involute within 6 to 10 weeks. However, new lesions continue to appear, frequently as a result of minor trauma. The lesions are often haphazardly distributed and usually are discrete, but they may be linear at sites of trauma.

A variant of reactive perforating collagenosis exists that is referred to as collagenoma perforans verruciforme (Woringer and Laugier). The clinical and histologic features of the individual lesions are similar to those of reactive perforating collagenosis. However, there is only a single episode, without any familial background, and the trauma is much more pronounced, such as lacerations caused by broken glass (Woringer and Laugier) or abrasions resulting from a fall (Delacrétaz and Gattlen).

Histopathology. Early, nonumbilicated, small papules show an area of necrobiotic, deeply basophilic collagen in the papillary dermis. As the basophilic collagen bundles are gradually eliminated through one or several areas of epidermal disruption, the epidermis forms a cup-shaped depression (Mehregan).

Older, umbilicated lesions, in which the basophilic collagen has already been largely eliminated through perforations in the epidermis, show within the cup-shaped central area of depression an accumulation of parakeratotic keratin, basophilic collagen, and numerous pyknotic nuclei of inflammatory cells corresponding to the adherent plug seen clinically. The epidermis at the base of the plug appears atrophic and shows interruptions through which basophilic bundles of collagen extending in a vertical direction are still extruded from the underlying dermis (Fig. 16-6) (Mehregan et al; Bovenmyer). Once the supply of degenerated collagen is exhausted, the epidermis begins to

regenerate, closing the areas of interruptions (Mehregan).

The basophilic bundles of collagen that are extruded stain red with the van Gieson method. Elastic tissue stains show no increase in the number of elastic fibers in the dermis and no elastic fibers in the keratotic plug or in the areas of disruption in the epidermis. At the periphery of the cup-shaped depression, the epidermis may show hyperplasia (Woringer and Laugier; Fretzin et al).

Histogenesis. The basic process in reactive perforating collagenosis consists of the transepidermal elimination of histochemically altered collagen. Nevertheless, as seen by *electron microscopy*, the collagen fibrils appear intact, with regular periodicity (Fretzin et al).

PERFORATING CALCIFIC ELASTOSIS

In perforating calcific elastosis, also referred to as periumbilical perforating pseudoxanthoma elasticum, a gradually enlarging, well-demarcated, hyperpigmented patch may be seen in the periumbilical region of middle-aged, multiparous women. The patch is in some instances atrophic with discrete keratotic papules (Hicks et al); in other instances, it has a verrucous border (Lund and Gilbert), and, in still others, it has a fissured, verrucous surface throughout (Schwartz and Richfield). The size of the patch varies from 2 cm to 14 cm.

Histopathology. Numerous altered elastic fibers are seen in the reticular dermis. They are short, thick, and curled and contain calcium, as shown

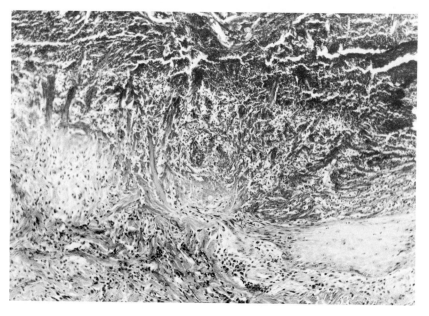

Fig. 16-6. Reactive perforating collagenosis
Basophilic bundles of collagen extending in a vertical direction are being extruded from the dermis through a perforation in the epidermis. (×100)

by a positive von Kossa stain. They are thus indistinguishable from the elastic fibers seen in pseudoxanthoma elasticum (see p. 75). As in pseudoxanthoma elasticum, the elastic fibers are visible even in sections stained with hematoxylin-eosin owing to their basophilia (Hicks et al). In contrast to pseudoxanthoma elasticum, however, the altered elastic fibers in perforating calcific elastosis are extruded to the surface either through the epidermis in a wide channel (Lund and Gilbert) or through a tunnel in the hyperplastic epidermis that ends in a keratin-filled crater (Hicks et al).

HYPERKERATOSIS LENTICULARIS PERSTANS (FLEGEL'S DISEASE)

A rare dermatosis first described in 1958 (Flegel), hyperkeratosis lenticularis perstans consists of asymptomatic, flat, hyperkeratotic papules from 1 mm to 5 mm in size located predominantly on the dorsa of the feet and on the lower legs. Removal of the adherent, horny scale causes slight bleeding. In addition to the central horny scale, larger papules often have a peripherally attached collarette of fine scaling. In two reported instances, extensive papular lesions were present on the oral mucosa (van de Staak et al). The disorder starts in late life and persists indefinitely. An autosomal dominant transmission has been noted in several instances (Bean, 1972; Beveridge and Langlands; Frenk and Tapernoux).

Histopathology. In some instances, the histologic picture is nonspecific, showing hyperkeratosis with occasional areas of parakeratosis, irregular acanthosis intermingled with areas of flattening of the stratum malpighii, and vascular dilation with a moderate amount of perivascular round cell infiltration (Bean, 1969). It seems, however, that if the specimen is obtained from a well-developed, markedly hyperkeratotic lesion, a fairly characteristic, although not diagnostic, histologic picture may be seen. Such a lesion shows a greatly thickened horny layer overlying a flattened stratum malpighii with thinning or even absence of the granular layer. Acanthosis is seen at the periphery. In some instances, owing to the central depression, the epidermis at the periphery forms a papillomatous elevation resembling a church spire (Flegel; Raffle and Rogers; Krinitz and Schäfer). The dermal infiltrate is composed largely of lymphoid cells and is located as a narrow band fairly close to the epidermis with a rather sharp demarcation at its lower border.

Histogenesis. On *electron microscopic examination*, the absence of membrane-coating granules was noted in some cases and regarded as the primary lesion of hyperkeratosis lenticularis perstans (Frenk and Tapernoux; van de Staak et al). However, in subsequent studies, the absence of membrane-coating granules (Ikai et al) or their reduction in number (Lindemayr and Jurecka) was found to be limited to the atrophic portion of the epidermis and was therefore regarded as secondary to a decrease in the thickness of the granular layer. In one case, membrane-coating granules were present but lacked a lamellate internal structure (Squier et al).

ACRODERMATITIS CHRONICA ATROPHICANS

Acrodermatitis chronica atrophicans occurs on the extremities, usually over their extensor surfaces. There is an initial inflammatory stage that is followed after weeks or months by an atrophic stage. The affected areas of the skin in the initial stage appear reddish and slightly edematous, but they gradually become atrophic and then present a bluish red or brownish, atrophic, wrinkled appearance. Because of the decrease in the thickness of the dermis and subcutaneous fat at the sites of atrophy, the subcutaneous veins are clearly visible. In some cases, areas of fibrous thickening develop within the atrophic skin. They may manifest themselves as indurated bands, especially in the ulnar or tibial region, as plaques, especially on the dorsa of the feet, or as nodules near joints.

Histopathology. In the initial inflammatory stage, the histologic picture usually is nonspecific, consisting of a largely perivascular chronic inflammatory infiltrate; however, in some instances, the initial stage already shows a bandlike infiltrate in the upper reticular dermis (Nasemann). In the early atrophic stage, the histologic findings are diagnostic. One observes atrophy of the epidermis with absence of the rete ridges. Directly beneath the epidermis is a narrow zone of connective tissue separating a bandlike chronic inflammatory infiltrate from the epidermis (Montgomery and Sullivan; Burgdorf et al). In addition, one finds scattered areas of inflammatory infiltration throughout the dermis, especially around the blood vessels, and in the subcutaneous fat. The infiltrate is composed predominantly of lymphoid cells, but it also contains histiocytes (Montgomery and Sullivan). In some instances, it is rich in plasma cells (Burgdorf et al). The entire dermis shows interstitial edema separating the bundles of collagen into fibers. In addition, there is a marked decrease in the amount of collagen. Ultimately, the dermis measures only one half or a quarter of its normal thickness (Fig. 16-7). There is a gradual loss of elastic tissue until, finally, it is completely absent (Korting et al).

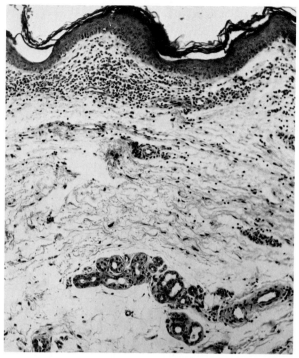

Fig. 16-7.   Acrodermatitis chronica atrophicans
There is atrophy of the stratum malpighii. A bandlike infiltrate is separated from the epidermis by a narrow zone of normal collagen. The dermis shows interstitial edema and atrophy of the collagen bundles. Because of this atrophy, the thickness of the dermis is markedly decreased, and the sweat glands lie unusually close to the epidermis. (× 100)

The hairs and sebaceous glands undergo atrophy early in the disease and are absent in the atrophic stage. However, as a rule, the sweat glands are preserved until very late in the process of atrophy. Because of the thinness of the dermis, the sweat glands lie unusually close to the epidermis (Montgomery and Sullivan). The subcutaneous tissue also undergoes atrophy, with a decrease in the number and size of the fat cells.

After the disorder has lasted for several years, an atrophic stage is reached in which the findings are no longer diagnostic; one sees merely an atrophic epidermis and atrophy of the dermis and subcutaneous fat without an inflammatory infiltrate.

The indurated bands and plaques show thickening of the collagen bundles, so that they may be indistinguishable from scleroderma (Montgomery and Sullivan). The fibrous nodules show coarse, hyalinized collagen bundles, sometimes in an onionlike arrangement (Hardmeier).

Histogenesis. Acrodermatitis chronica atrophicans appears to be caused by a group B arbovirus, with the *Ixodes ricinus* wood tick serving as the major vector. The incidence of acrodermatitis chronica atrophicans corresponds to the occurrence of *I. ricinus*. Thus, it is most common in central Europe and is very rare in native Americans with no history of travel abroad (Burgdorf et al). Penicillin and other antibiotics are a very effective treatment during the inflammatory stage.

PRETIBIAL PIGMENTED PATCHES IN DIABETES

Circumscribed, round to oval, pigmented, often slightly depressed macules from 2 mm to 10 mm in diameter are found on the shins in about 17% of adults with diabetes but also in about 3% of adults without diabetes (Bauer et al). The role of trauma in the development of these lesions is difficult to evaluate. Most patients give no specific history of trauma. However, the pretibial area is particularly exposed to frequent trauma (Kerl).

In rare instances, patients with diabetes show similar pigmented patches widely distributed over their skin, either in addition to patches in the pretibial region (Schneider et al) or without them (Bauer and Levan).

Histopathology. The findings are not diagnostic. The upper dermis shows a mild perivascular infiltrate of lymphoid and histiocytic cells, an increase in the number of capillaries, fibroblastic proliferation, and small amounts of hemosiderin (Fisher and Danowski; Kerl). The capillaries often show thickening of their walls, with greater than usual deposits of a periodic acid-Schiff (PAS)-positive, diastase-resistant material in a fibrillary pattern representing neutral mucopolysaccharides in the basement membrane.

Histogenesis. On *electron microscopy*, the fibrillar PAS-positive, diastase-resistant material corresponds to an increase in the thickness and number of layers of the pericapillary basement membrane (Auböck). Although this is a characteristic finding in diabetic microangiopathy, it is not specific for it and, in the skin, can be a nonspecific reaction of the vascular wall to perivascular inflammation.

Differential Diagnosis. Since proliferation of capillaries with thickening of their walls, deposits of hemosiderin, and fibrosis may occur in any mild dermal inflammation, the diagnosis of pretibial pigmented patches and their association with diabetes must be based on clinical rather than on histologic considerations. The pretibial pigmented patches differ from necrobiosis lipoidica by showing neither necrobiosis nor giant cells.

BULLOSIS DIABETICORUM

In rare instances, patients with diabetes show spontaneously arising bullae. They are located usually on the
hands and feet but occasionally also on the arms (Cantwell and Martz) or legs (Bernstein et al). The bullae can
attain a fairly large size and are slow to heal. Ulceration
may occur at the site of bullae (Lejman et al). The
coexistence of bullosis diabeticorum and pretibial pigmented patches has been observed (Kurwa et al; Kerl
and Kresbach).

Histopathology. In some instances, the bullae
are unilocular and show a subepidermal location
(Kurwa et al; Bernstein et al; James et al). In other
instances, the blisters are intraepidermal in location
and are either unilocular (Allen and Hadden) or
multilocular (Kerl and Kresbach). In most instances, the epidermis of the bullae, whether subepidermal or intraepidermal, shows pronounced
necrolytic changes (Kerl and Kresbach; Lejman et
al). One often finds thickening of the walls of
superficial blood vessels with an increase in the
amount of PAS-positive material (Kerl and Kresbach; Lejman et al; James et al). Dermal inflammation generally is mild.

Histogenesis. On *electron microscopic examination,* subepidermal bullae arise in the lamina lucida (Bernstein et
al). Direct immunofluorescence in some instances has
shown deposits of immunoglobulin M (IgM), complement, and fibrinogen in the superficial dermal vessels
(James et al). Because of the frequent presence of epidermal necrosis, it is likely that the bullae arise as a
result of trophic damage to the epidermis (Kerl and
Kresbach).

LICHEN SCLEROSUS ET ATROPHICUS

Lichen sclerosus et atrophicus is much more common
in women than in men. In both men and women, the
genitals are the most frequent, and often the only, site
of involvement. Involvement of the genitals in women
is known as *kraurosis vulvae* (see p. 283) and in men as
balanitis xerotica obliterans (see p. 283). Cutaneous lesions
outside the genital region may be seen either in association with genital lesions or alone.

The extragenital, cutaneous lesions of lichen sclerosus
et atrophicus consist of flat-topped white macules that
tend to coalesce to form white patches. Often, small,
comedolike follicular plugs are seen on their surface. As
the term *sclerosus* indicates, the lesions may feel somewhat indurated. Although usually limited in extent and
confined to the trunk, lichen sclerosus et atrophicus
occasionally occurs as an extensive eruption (Gottschalk
and Cooper). A patch of lichen sclerosus et atrophicus,
whether solitary or part of an extensive eruption, may
become bullous and show hemorrhagic areas (Di Silverio
and Serri).

Of interest is the occasional coexistence of lichen
sclerosus et atrophicus and morphea. In extensive cases
of morphea, lichen sclerosus et atrophicus may become
superimposed on some of the lesions. It is then best
recognized by the presence of follicular plugging (Wallace). The two diseases may coexist from the very
beginning even in fairly localized eruptions (Uitto et al).
However, the mere presence of induration in a lesion
of lichen sclerosus et atrophicus does not necessarily
indicate an association with morphea (Steigleder and
Raab).

Histopathology. In cutaneous lesions of lichen
sclerosus et atrophicus, one observes (1) hyperkeratosis with follicular plugging, (2) atrophy of
the stratum malpighii with hydropic degeneration
of basal cells, (3) pronounced edema and homogenization of the collagen in the upper dermis, and
(4) an inflammatory infiltrate in the middermis
(Fig. 16-8).

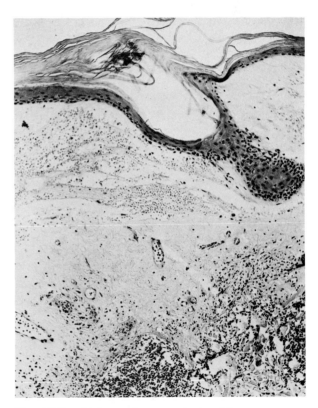

**Fig. 16-8. Lichen sclerosus et atrophicus,
cutaneous lesion**
There are hyperkeratosis with follicular plugging, atrophy of the stratum malpighii, marked lymphedema of
the upper dermis, and an inflammatory infiltrate in the
middermis. The edema in the subepidermal dermis is
so marked that a bulla has resulted. (×100)

The hyperkeratosis is so marked that the horny layer is often thicker than the atrophic stratum malpighii, which may be reduced to a few layers of flattened cells. The cells of the basal layer show hydropic degeneration. The rete ridges often are completely absent, although they may persist in a few areas and even show some irregular downward proliferation. In such proliferations, hydropic degeneration of the basal cells usually is pronounced.

Beneath the epidermis is a broad zone of pronounced lymphedema. Within this zone, the collagenous fibers are swollen and homogeneous and contain only a few nuclei. They stain poorly with eosin and other connective tissue stains. The blood and lymph vessels are dilated, and there may be areas of hemorrhage. Elastic fibers are sparse and, in old lesions, are absent within the area of lymphedema (Steigleder and Raab). In areas of severe lymphedema, clinically visible bullae may form; they are found in subepidermal location (Gottschalk and Cooper). In addition, shrinkage within the area of lymphedema may occur during the process of dehydration of the specimen, resulting in the formation of pseudobullae, which often are located intradermally (Piper).

Except in lesions of long duration, an inflammatory infiltrate is present in the dermis. The younger the lesion, the more superficial is the location of the infiltrate. In very early lesions and at the periphery of somewhat older lesions, the infiltrate may be found in the uppermost dermis, in direct apposition to the basal layer (Miller). Soon, however, a narrow zone of edema and homogenization of the collagen displaces the inflammatory infiltrate farther down, so that, in well-developed lesions, the infiltrate is found in the middermis. The infiltrate can be patchy, but it is often bandlike (Laymon). It consists largely of lymphoid cells intermingled with some histiocytes. In old lesions in which the infiltrate is slight or absent, the collagen bundles in the lower dermis may appear swollen, homogeneous, and hyperchromatic, as in scleroderma (Fig. 16-9).

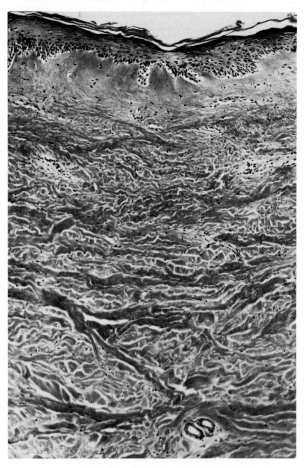

Fig. 16-9.   Lichen sclerosus et atrophicus, cutaneous lesion
In this old lesion, only a very slight inflammatory infiltrate is seen. However, hydropic degeneration of the basal cells and lymphedema of the upper dermis are present. The collagen bundles in the lower dermis appear swollen, homogeneous, and hyperchromatic, as in scleroderma. (×50)

Histogenesis. *Electron microscopic studies* suggest that the primary change consists of a degeneration of collagen fibrils, which often lack cross striation and, in cross sections, sometimes have the appearance of empty tubes (Mann and Cowan). In many fibroblasts, the cisternae of the endoplasmic reticulum are dilated and empty, which is indicative of reduced collagen synthesis (Klug and Sönnichsen). In some areas, however, new immature collagen fibrils are seen, recognizable by their variable but reduced diameter of 40 nm to 80 nm (Kint and Geerts). Considerable edema often separates the basal cells from one another (Klug and Sönnichsen). Thus, the hydropic degeneration of the basal cells observed by light microscopy in reality is intercellular edema. In addition, however, the basal cells themselves show degenerative changes (Mann and Cowan). There is a nearly complete absence of melanosomes within the keratinocytes. This is the result either of degeneration and disappearance of the melanocytes (Mann and Cowan) or of inhibition of the transfer of melanosomes from the melanocytes to the keratinocytes (Klug and Sönnichsen).

Differential Diagnosis.   Very early lesions may resemble lichen planus because of the apposition of the inflammatory infiltrate to the basal layer.

However, the basal cells are not replaced by flattened squamous cells, as in lichen planus, but appear hydropic, and a subepidermal zone of edema has usually already begun to form in some areas in lichen sclerosus et atrophicus.

Old lesions of lichen sclerosus et atrophicus with thickening and hyperchromasia of the collagen bundles in the lower dermis and only a slight inflammatory infiltrate may resemble morphea. Nevertheless, the epidermis in morphea, although it may be thin, shows neither hydropic degeneration of the basal cells nor follicular plugging, and the upper dermis shows no zone of edema (Steigleder and Raab). Still, in lesions in which lichen sclerosus et atrophicus develops either secondarily to morphea or simultaneously with it, there may be, in addition to the epidermal and subepidermal changes of lichen sclerosus et atrophicus, changes indicative of morphea in the lower dermis and in the subcutaneous fat, such as binding down of sweat glands by collagen and extension of newly formed and faintly staining collagen into the subcutaneous fat (see p. 462) (Bergfeld and Lesowitz; Uitto et al).

Kraurosis Vulvae

Lichen sclerosus et atrophicus of the vulva, often referred to as kraurosis vulvae, is characterized by sharply demarcated, whitish lesions that involve most of the vulva, including the labia majora and minora, and often extend to the perineum, the perianal region, and the inguinal folds. Atrophy of the labia and narrowing of the vaginal orifice ensue. In contrast with lichen sclerosus et atrophicus of the skin, which rarely itches, there is often severe pruritus in the vulvar region. Only about one fifth of the patients with lesions in the vulvar region have cutaneous lesions of lichen sclerosus et atrophicus (Wallace). Lichen sclerosus et atrophicus of the vulva may occur in prepubertal children. Whereas the lesions usually progress in adults, there often is improvement with time in children (Clark and Muller; Wallace).

Although lichen sclerosus et atrophicus of the skin never undergoes malignant degeneration, lichen sclerosus et atrophicus of the vulva can progress to squamous cell carcinoma. In a review of 465 cases from the literature, the incidence was found to be 3%, and in 107 personally observed cases, the incidence was 6% (Hart et al). Another large series of 290 cases showed development of carcinoma in 4% of the cases (Wallace). It has been suggested that the development of squamous cell carcinoma in lichen sclerosus et atrophicus of the vulva may actually be lower than the cited incidence of 3% to 6%, since in 5 of 6 patients having both carcinoma and lichen sclerosus et atrophicus of the vulva in one series (Hart et al), and in 8 of 9 patients in another series

(Suurmond), it was carcinoma of the vulva associated with mild, unnoticed lichen sclerosus et atrophicus that made the patient seek medical advice (Hart et al). Nevertheless, when patients presenting with squamous cell carcinoma of the vulva were examined, 61% of 85 patients in one series (Wallace) and 45% of 20 patients in another (Suurmond) showed evidence of lichen sclerosus et atrophicus of the vulva. This finding makes long-range follow-up of all patients with lichen sclerosus et atrophicus of the vulva highly advisable.

Histopathology. Kraurosis vulvae shows the same histologic picture as lichen sclerosus et atrophicus of the skin, with the exception that lesions on the mucous membranes show no keratotic plugs (Fig. 16-10) (Barker and Gross). Irregular downward proliferations of the epithelium in which the basal cells show considerable hydropic degeneration are seen more often and more extensively than on the skin (Fig. 16-11).

Areas of squamous hyperplasia adjacent to the atrophic epidermis can be found in about one third of the patients with lichen sclerosus et atrophicus of the vulva (Fig. 16-12) (Hart et al). Such areas may show varying degrees of "dysplasia" in the form of disorderly arrangement of the cells and enlarged, hyperchromatic nuclei. Transition of such areas into carcinoma is said to be rare, since carcinoma, if it occurs, arises adjacent to but separate from areas of lichen sclerosus et atrophicus (Hart et al). It is difficult to decide whether this allows the conclusion that "the lichen sclerosus et atrophicus was not likely to have been directly responsible for the development of the carcinoma" (Hart et al). It seems possible that, in the process of development of a carcinoma, the characteristic features of lichen sclerosus et atrophicus, such as atrophy of the epidermis and homogenization of the upper dermis, subside.

Balanitis Xerotica Obliterans

Balanitis xerotica obliterans, the term applied to lichen sclerosus et atrophicus of the glans penis and prepuce, shows white, atrophic, slightly edematous areas that, in uncircumcised patients, usually result in phimosis. Extragenital lesions may occur in association with lichen sclerosus et atrophicus of the penis (Wallace), but this is rare (Post and Jänner). Prepubertal occurrence was observed in 4% in a series of 117 cases (Post and Jänner).

Squamous cell carcinoma may supervene (Bart and Kopf). This occurred in 2 of 44 patients in one series (Wallace) but in none of 77 patients in another series who had a prolonged follow-up period (Post and Jänner).

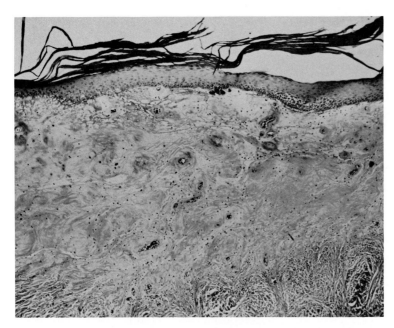

Fig. 16-10.   Lichen sclerosus et atrophicus of the vulva (kraurosis vulvae)
There are hyperkeratosis, atrophy of the stratum malpighii, and marked lymphedema of the upper dermis with homogenization of the collagen. ($\times 100$)

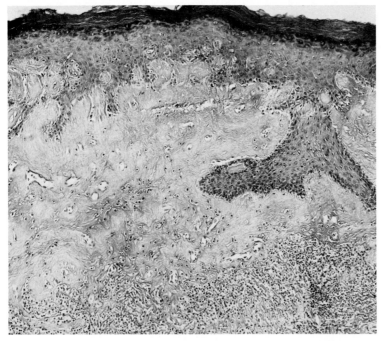

Fig. 16-11.   Lichen sclerosus et atrophicus of the vulva (kraurosis vulvae)
The upper dermis shows edema and homogenization of the collagen with a band-like inflammatory infiltrate beneath the zone of edema. In addition, there is irregular downward proliferation of the rete ridges with hydropic degeneration of the basal cells. The latter feature is typical of lichen sclerosus et atrophicus and speaks against carcinoma in situ. ($\times 100$)

Histopathology.   The histologic picture is that of lichen sclerosus et atrophicus. Because of the absence of follicles in the area of involvement, no keratotic plugging occurs (Laymon; Post and Jänner; Bart and Kopf).

STRIAE DISTENSAE

Striae distensae occur most commonly on the abdomen, the buttocks, and the thighs as well as in the inguinal region. They consist of bands of thin, wrinkled skin that at first are reddish, then purple, and finally white.

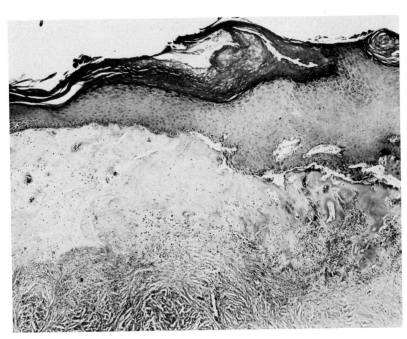

Fig. 16-12.   Lichen sclerosus et atrophicus of the vulva (kraurosis vulvae)
On the right side, squamous hyperplasia has developed with features of early carcinoma in situ. (×100)

Histopathology. The epidermis is thin and flattened. There is a decrease in the thickness of the dermis. The collagen fibers lie separated from one another rather than united into collagen bundles (Epstein et al). Elastic fibers are absent in the center of the lesion, whereas they appear curled and clumped at the periphery (Chernosky and Knox). In old striae, as a result of regeneration, one observes in the upper dermis many rather straight collagen bundles arranged parallel to the skin surface and intermingled with numerous fairly straight and thin elastic fibers. Beneath this area, absence of elastic fibers persists (Pinkus et al).

Histogenesis. Striae distensae occur in conditions associated with an increased production of glucocorticoids by the adrenal glands. Among these are pregnancy, obesity, adolescence, and, especially, Cushing's disease (Hauser; Epstein et al). In obesity, the increased adrenocortical activity is a consequence of the obesity, and the production of glucocorticoids returns to normal when the body weight is reduced (Simkin and Arce). Similarly, the occurrence of striae in nonobese adolescents, as noted in 35% of the girls and 15% of the boys examined, is associated with an increase in 17-ketosteroid excretion (Sisson). Striae may also form owing to prolonged intake of corticosteroids. Occasionally, striae develop following the prolonged local application of corticosteroid creams to the skin under occlusive dressings (Chernosky and Knox) and, if the creams are of high potency, even without occlusion (Epstein et al). The action of the glucocorticoids consists of an antianabolic effect suppressing both fibroblastic and epidermal activity, as tissue culture studies have shown (Klehr). Thus, even though stretching of the skin initiates striae, stretching is of significance only insofar as the localization and direction of the striae are concerned (Hauser; Shuster).

WRINKLING DUE TO MIDDERMAL ELASTOLYSIS

Wrinkling due to middermal elastosis is a rare disorder first described in 1977 (Shelley and Wood). It occurs in middle-aged women and consists of widespread, large areas of fine wrinkling. The wrinkling may be associated with small, soft, papular lesions consisting of tiny perifollicular protrusions, leaving the hair follicle itself as an indented center (Brenner et al). Some of the lesions may be preceded by urticaria (Shelley and Wood) or erythematous patches (Delacrétaz et al).

Histopathology. There is a selective absence of elastic tissue strictly limited to the middermis of involved areas (Shelley and Wood). The perifollicular protrusions around indented hair follicles are due to preservation of a thin layer of elastic tissue in the immediate vicinity of hair follicles. This causes the hair follicles to appear retracted while the perifollicular skin protrudes (Brenner et al).

MACULAR ATROPHY (ANETODERMA)

Macular atrophy, or anetoderma, is characterized by atrophic patches located mainly on the upper trunk. The skin of the patches is thin and bluish white and bulges slightly. The lesions may give the palpating finger the same sensation as a hernial orifice. Two types of macular atrophy are generally distinguished: the Jadassohn type, in which the atrophic lesions initially appear red and, on histologic examination, show an inflammatory infiltrate, and the Schweninger–Buzzi type, which clinically and histologically is noninflammatory from the beginning. However, not every case can be clearly assigned to one or the other of these two types; some clinically noninflammatory cases show an inflammatory infiltrate in early lesions when examined histologically (Deluzenne).

It appears dubious that a secondary form of macular atrophy exists occurring in the course of various diseases, such as syphilis, lupus erythematosus, and leprosy (Deluzenne). In some cases, coexistence is coincidental (Edelson and Grupper); in others, the "macular atrophy" represents the atrophic stage of the preceding disease (Ryll-Nardzewski et al). One instance of macular atrophy has been observed after prolonged treatment with penicillamine (see p. 262) (Davis).

Histopathology. Early, erythematous lesions of the Jadassohn type (Miller et al; Kossard et al) and some lesions of cases reported as the Schweninger–Buzzi type (Feldman) show a moderately pronounced perivascular infiltrate of mononuclear cells. In a few instances, however, the early inflammatory lesions show a perivascular infiltrate in which neutrophils and eosinophils predominate and nuclear dust is present, resulting in a histologic picture of leukocytoclastic vasculitis (Neumann and Vacátko; Cramer).

The elastic tissue may still appear normal in the early stage of an erythematous lesion (Miller et al). Usually, however, it is already decreased or even absent within the lesion. In cases with a decrease in the amount of elastic tissue, mononuclear cells may be seen adhering to elastic fibers (Kossard et al).

Long-standing, noninflammatory lesions usually show as the only abnormality an absence of elastic tissue, so that the sections appear normal when stained with hematoxylin-eosin (Miller et al; Kossard et al). In some cases, however, the collagen bundles appear swollen and homogenized (Duperrat; Korting et al).

Histogenesis. *Electron microscopic examination* of lesions containing only fragments of elastic fibers shows processes of macrophages surrounding these fragments.

Isolated elastic fibers that are unassociated with macrophages have a highly irregular margin (Kossard et al).

On *direct immunofluorescence examination*, the most striking finding is the presence of deposits of the third component of complement (C3) on autofluorescent elastic fibers. In addition, both C3 and IgM are seen in a granular pattern in the basement membrane zone (Kossard et al). These findings suggest that an immune mechanism plays a role in the destruction of the elastic fibers.

ACRO-OSTEOLYSIS

The term *acro-osteolysis* refers to lytic changes on the distal phalanges. Three types are recognized: (1) familial; (2) idiopathic, nonfamilial; and (3) occupational, associated with exposure to vinyl chloride gas.

The *familial type* affects mainly the phalanges of the feet and is associated with recurrent ulcers on the soles (Meyerson and Meier).

The *idiopathic type* affects largely the distal phalanges of the fingers, causing shortening of the fingers. It may be associated with Raynaud's phenomenon. Only one case has been described with cutaneous lesions consisting of numerous yellowish papules 2 mm to 4 mm in size and showing a linear distribution and coalescence into plaques, mainly on the arms (Meyerson and Meier).

Occupational acro-osteolysis, like the idiopathic type, causes shortening of the fingers due to osteolysis. This is often associated with Raynaud's phenomenon and progressive thickening of the skin of the hands and forearms simulating scleroderma. There may be erythema of the hands, and the thickening may consist of papules and plaques (Markowitz et al). The skin of the face may show diffuse induration (Veltmann et al). In addition, there may be thrombocytopenia, portal fibrosis, and impaired hepatic and pulmonary function (Fine).

Histopathology. The histologic changes in the papules and plaques of idiopathic and occupational acro-osteolysis consist of thickening of the dermis, with swelling and homogenization of the collagen bundles indistinguishable from scleroderma. Staining for elastic tissue shows disorganization of the elastic fibers, which appear thin and fragmented (Meyerson and Meier; Markowitz et al; Veltmann et al).

Histogenesis. Vinyl chloride disease is an immune-complex disorder associated with hyperimmunoglobulinemia, cryoglobulinemia, and evidence of in vivo activation of complement (Fine). The immunologic nature of the disease explains why less than 3% of the workers exposed to vinyl chloride gas develop the disease (Markowitz et al).

ULERYTHEMA OF EYEBROWS AND CHEEKS

Ulerythema of the eyebrows, referred to as ulerythema ophryogenes, starts in childhood with redness and thinning of the hair in the lateral portions of the eyebrows and ends with atrophy of the skin and hair loss in these areas (Davenport). Its inheritance is autosomal dominant, and it is commonly associated with Noonan's syndrome, which consists of congenital stenosis of the pulmonary artery valves in association with short stature and hypertelorism (Pierini and Pierini).

Ulerythema of the cheeks, referred to as folliculitis ulerythematosa reticulata, also is dominantly inherited and starts in childhood. Located on the cheeks are at first horny follicular plugs with an erythematous halo; upon disappearance of the plugs, there is perifollicular atrophy (Pierini and Pierini). As the result of numerous follicular pits, this atrophy on the cheeks has a honeycomb appearance (MacKee and Cipollaro).

Histopathology. The histologic findings are not diagnostic. In the early stage in both conditions, one observes hyperkeratosis of the pilosebaceous infundibulum surrounded by mild, nonspecific inflammation. Later on, there is atrophy of the sebaceous glands and hair follicles together with dermal fibrosis (Davenport; Pierini and Pierini).

In some cases of ulerythema of the cheeks, dense subepidermal aggregates of normal-appearing elastic fibers have been observed (Rozum et al; Pullmann and Gartmann). In contrast to solar elastosis, there is no basophilic staining of the areas.

BIBLIOGRAPHY

Solar (Actinic) Elastosis

BRAUN-FALCO O: Die Morphogenese der senil-aktinischen Elastose. Arch Klin Exp Dermatol 235:138–160, 1969

EASTERN JS, MARTIN S: Actinic comedonal plaque. J Am Acad Dermatol 3:633–636, 1980

EBNER H: Über die Entstehung des elastotischen Materials. Z Hautkr 44:889–894, 1969

FANTA D, NIEBAUER G: Aktinische (senile) Komedonen. Z Hautkr 51:791–797, 1976

FAVRE M, RACOUCHOT J: L'élastéidose cutanée nodulaire à kystes et à comédons. Ann Dermatol Syph 78:681–702, 1951

FINDLEY GH: On elastase and the elastic dystrophies of the skin. Br J Dermatol 66:16–24, 1954

HELM F: Nodular cutaneous elastosis with cysts and comedones (Favre-Racouchot syndrome). Arch Dermatol 84:666–668, 1961

KLIGMAN AM: Early destructive effect of sunlight on human skin. JAMA 210:2377–2380, 1969

MARSCH WC, SCHOBER E, NÜRNBERGER F: Zur Ultrastruktur und Morphogenese der elastischen Faser und der aktinischen Elastose. Z Hautkr 54:43–46, 1979

MITCHELL RE: Chronic solar dermatosis: A light and electron microscopic study of the dermis. J Invest Dermatol 48:203–220, 1967

NIEBAUER G, STOCKINGER L: Über die senile Elastose. Arch Klin Exp Dermatol 221:122–143, 1965

NÜRNBERGER F, SCHOBER E, MARSCH WC et al: Actinic elastosis in black skin. Arch Dermatol Res 262:7–14, 1978

OLSEN RL, NORDQUIST J, EVERETT MA: The role of epidermal lysosomes in melanin physiology. Br J Dermatol 83:189–199, 1970

SAMS WM JR, SMITH JG JR: The histochemistry of chronically sun-damaged skin. J Invest Dermatol 37:447–453, 1961

SMITH JG JR, DAVIDSON E, SAMS WM JR et al: Alterations in human dermal connective tissue with age and chronic sun damage. J Invest Dermatol 39:347–350, 1962

Kyrle's Disease

ABELE DC, DOBSON RL: Hyperkeratosis penetrans (Kyrle's disease). Arch Dermatol 83:277–283, 1961

ARAM H, SZYMANSKI FJ, BAILEY WE: Kyrle's disease. Arch Dermatol 100:453–456, 1969

BARDACH H: Dermatosen mit transepithelialer Perforation. Arch Dermatol Res 257:213–226, 1976

CARTER VH, CONSTANTINE VS: Kyrle's disease. I. Clinical findings in five cases and review of literature. Arch Dermatol 97:624–632, 1968

CONSTANTINE VS, CARTER VH: Kyrle's disease. II. Histopathologic findings in five cases and review of the literature. Arch Dermatol 97:633–639, 1968

DE GRACIANSKY P, BOULLE S, BOULLE M: et al: La maladie de Kyrle. Ann Dermatol Syph 82:8–33, 1955

HAENSCH R, HETTWER H, MEISEL U: Morbus Kyrle (Hyperkeratosis follicularis et parafollicularis penetrans). Z Hautkr 54:99–106, 1978

HOOD AF, HARDEGEN GL, ZARATE AR et al: Kyrle's disease in patients with chronic renal failure. Arch Dermatol 118:85–88, 1982

KYRLE J: Hyperkeratosis follicularis et parafollicularis in cutem penetrans. Arch Dermatol Syph (Berlin) 123:466–493, 1916

PINKUS H, MEHREGAN AH: A Guide to Dermatohistopathology, 3rd ed, p 209. New York, Appleton-Century-Crofts, 1981

TAPPEINER J, WOLFF K, SCHREINER E: Morbus Kyrle. Hautarzt 20:296–310, 1969

THYRESSON N: Hyperkeratosis follicularis et parafollicularis in cutem penetrans. Acta Derm Venereol (Stockh) 31:287–289, 1951

Perforating Folliculitis

MEHREGAN AH: Perforating dermatoses: A clinicopathologic review. Int J Dermatol 16:19–27, 1977

MEHREGAN AH, COSKEY RJ: Perforating folliculitis. Arch Dermatol 97:394–399, 1968

STREITMANN B: Ein Beitrag zu den das Follikelepithel durchbrechenden Prozessen. Z Hautkr 45:195–200, 1970

Elastosis Perforans Serpiginosa

COHEN AS, HASHIMOTO K: Electron microscopic observations on the lesions of elastosis perforans serpiginosa. J Invest Dermatol 35:15–19, 1960

LUTZ W: Keratosis follicularis serpiginosa. Dermatologica 106:318–320, 1953

MEHREGAN AH: Elastosis perforans serpiginosa. A review of the literature and report of 11 cases. Arch Dermatol 97:381–393, 1968

MEVES C, VOGEL C: Elektronenmikroskopische Untersuchungen an einem Fall von Elastosis perforans serpiginosa. Dermatologica 145:210–221, 1972

MIESCHER G: Elastoma intrapapillare perforans verruciforme. Dermatologica 110:254–266, 1955

PEDRO SD, GARCIA RL: Disseminate elastosis perforans serpiginosa. Arch Dermatol 109:84–85, 1974

RASMUSSEN JE: Disseminated elastosis perforans serpiginosa in four mongoloids. Br J Dermatol 86:9–13, 1972

SCHNEIDER W, BOCK HD: Elastosis perforans serpiginosum. Hautarzt 27:117–121, 1976

TSAMBAOS D, BERGER H: Elastosis perforans serpiginosa. Licht- und elektronenmikroskopische Befunde. Z Hautkr 55:563–577, 1979

WHYTE HJ, WINKELMANN RK: Elastosis perforans (Perforating elastosis). J Invest Dermatol 35:113–122, 1960

Reactive Perforating Collagenosis

BOVENMYER DA: Reactive perforating collagenosis. Arch Dermatol 102:313–317, 1970

DELACRÉTAZ J, GATTLEN JM: Transepidermal elimination of traumatically altered collagen. Dermatologica 152:65–71, 1976

FRETZIN DF, BEAL DW, JAO W: Light and ultrastructural study of reactive perforating collagenosis. Arch Dermatol 116:1054–1058, 1980

KANAN MW: Familial reactive perforating collagenosis and intolerance to cold. Br J Dermatol 91:405–414, 1974

MEHREGAN AH: Perforating dermatoses: A clinicopathologic review. Int J Dermatol 16:19–27, 1977

MEHREGAN AH, SCHWARTZ OD, LIVINGOOD CS: Reactive perforating collagenosis. Arch Dermatol 96:277–282, 1967

MOHRI S, SANO T, FUKUDA S: An adult case of reactive perforating collagenosis. J Dermatol (Tokyo) 7:363–369, 1980

POLIAK SC, LEBWOHL MG, PARRIS A et al: Reactive perforating collagenosis associated with diabetes mellitus. N Engl J Med 306:81–84, 1982

WEINER AL: Reactive perforating collagenosis. Arch Dermatol 102:540–544, 1970

WORINGER F, LAUGIER P: Collagenoma perforans verruciforme. Dermatol Wochenschr 147:64–68, 1963

Perforating Calcific Elastosis

HICKS J, CARPENTER CL JR, REED PJ: Periumbilical perforating pseudoxanthoma elasticum. Arch Dermatol 115:300–303, 1979

LUND HZ, GILBERT CF: Perforating pseudoxanthoma elasticum. Arch Pathol 100:544–546, 1976

SCHWARTZ RA, RICHFIELD DF: Pseudoxanthoma elasticum with transepidermal elimination. Arch Dermatol 114:279–280, 1978

Hyperkeratosis Lenticularis Perstans (Flegel's Disease)

BEAN SF: Hyperkeratosis lenticularis perstans. Arch Dermatol 99:705–709, 1969

BEAN SF: The genetics of hyperkeratosis lenticularis perstans. Arch Dermatol 106:72, 1972

BEVERIDGE GW, LANGLANDS AO: Familial hyperkeratosis lenticularis perstans associated with tumours of the skin. Br J Dermatol 88:453–458, 1973

FLEGEL H: Hyperkeratosis lenticularis perstans. Hautarzt 9:362–364, 1958

FRENK E, TAPERNOUX B: Hyperkeratosis lenticularis perstans (Flegel). Dermatologica 153:253–262, 1976

IKAI K, MURAI T, FUKUDA S et al: An ultrastructural study of the epidermis in hyperkeratosis lenticularis perstans. Acta Derm Venereol (Stockh) 58:363–365, 1978

KRINITZ K, SCHÄFER I: Hyperkeratosis lenticularis perstans. Dermatol Monatsschr 157:438–446, 1971

LINDEMAYR H, JURECKA W: Retinoid acid in the treatment of hyperkeratosis lenticularis perstans Flegel. Acta Derm Venereol (Stockh) 62:89–91, 1982

RAFFLE EJ, ROGERS J: Hyperkeratosis lenticularis perstans. Arch Dermatol 100:423–428, 1969

SQUIER CA, EADY RAJ, HOPPS RM: The permeability of epidermis lacking normal membrane-coating granules: An ultrastructural tracer study of Kyrle-Flegel disease. J Invest Dermatol 70:361–364, 1978

VAN DE STAAK WJBM, BERGERS AMG, BOUGAARTS P: Hyperkeratosis lenticularis perstans (Flegel). Dermatologica 161:340–346, 1980

Acrodermatitis Chronica Atrophicans

BURGDORF WHC, WORRET WI, SCHULTKA O: Acrodermatitis chronica atrophicans. Int J Dermatol 18:595–601, 1979

HARDMEIER T: Zur Histopathologie der fibroiden Knoten bei Akrodermatitis chronica atrophicans. Arch Klin Exp Dermatol 232:373–383, 1968

KORTING GW, HOEDE N, HOLZMANN H: Zur Frage des Elastikaverhaltens bei einigen sklerosierenden und atrophisierenden Hautkrankheiten. Hautarzt 20:351–361, 1969

MONTGOMERY H, SULLIVAN RR: Acrodermatitis atrophicans chronica. (Review) Arch Dermatol Syph 51:32–47, 1945

NASEMANN T: In Südafrika erworbene Acrodermatitis chronica atrophicans Herxheimer. Z Hautkr 55:310–312, 1980.

Pretibial Pigmented Patches in Diabetes

AUBÖCK L: Elektronenmikroskopische Untersuchungen der prätibialen Pigmentflecke. Z Hautkr 46:624–634, 1971

BAUER M, LEVAN NE: Diabetic dermangiopathy. A spectrum including pigmented pretibial patches and necrobiosis lipoidica diabeticorum. Br J Dermatol 83:528–535, 1970

BAUER MF, LEVAN NE, FRANKEL A. et al: Pigmented pretibial patches. Arch Dermatol 93:282–286, 1966

FISHER ER, DANOWSKI TS: Histologic, histochemical, and electron microscopic features of the skin spots of diabetes mellitus. Am J Clin Pathol 50:547–554, 1968

KERL H: Zur Frage der prätibialen Pigmentflecke bei Diabetes mellitus (Diabetische Dermopathie). Z Hautkr 46:619–624, 1971

SCHNEIDER HG, SCHNEIDER H, THORMANN T: Generalisierte diabetische Dermangiopathie. Z Hautkr 55:441–447, 1980

Bullosis Diabeticorum

ALLEN GE, HADDEN DR: Bullous lesions of the skin in diabetes (bullosis diabeticorum). Br J Dermatol 82:216–220, 1970

BERNSTEIN JE, MEDENICA M, SOLTANI K et al: Bullous eruption of diabetes mellitus. Arch Dermatol 115:324–325, 1979

CANTWELL AR JR, MARTZ W: Idiopathic bullae in diabetics. Bullosis diabeticorum. Arch Dermatol 96:42–44, 1967

JAMES WD, ODOM RB, GOETTE DK: Bullous eruption of diabetes mellitus. Arch Dermatol 116:1191–1192, 1980

KERL H, KRESBACH : Zu einigen Aspekten der "Bullosis diabeticorum." Hautarzt 25:60–65, 1974

KURWA A, ROBERTS P, WHITEHEAD R: Concurrence of bullous and atrophic skin lesions in diabetes mellitus. Arch Dermatol 103:670–675, 1971

LEJMAN K, CHORZELSKI TP, STARZYCKI Z: Bullöse Hautveränderungen mit nachfolgender Umwandlung in nekrotische Geschwüre bei Diabetes mellitus. Dermatol Monatsschr 163:790–793, 1977

Lichen Sclerosus et Atrophicus

BARKER LP, GROSS PL: Lichen sclerosus et atrophicus of the female genitalia. Arch Dermatol 85:362–373, 1962

BART RS, KOPF AW: Squamous cell carcinoma arising in balanitis xerotica obliterans. J Dermatol Surg Oncol 4:556–558, 1978

BERGFELD WF, LESOWITZ SA: Lichen sclerosus et atrophicus. Arch Dermatol 101:247–248, 1970

CLARK JA, MULLER SA: Lichen sclerosus et atrophicus in children. Arch Dermatol 95:476–482, 1967

DI SILVERIO A, SERRI F: Generalized bullous and hemorrhagic lichen sclerosus et atrophicus. Br J Dermatol 93:215–217, 1975

GOTTSCHALK HR, COOPER ZK: Lichen sclerosus et atrophicus with bullous lesions and extensive involvement. Arch Dermatol 55:433–440, 1947

HART WR, NORRIS HJ, HELWIG EB: Relation of lichen sclerosus et atrophicus of the vulva to development of carcinoma. Obstet Gyn 45:369–377, 1975

KINT A, GEERTS ML: Lichen sclerosus et atrophicus. An electron microscopic study. J Cutan Pathol 2:30–34, 1975

KLUG H, SÖNNICHSEN N: Elektronenoptische Untersuchungen bei Lichen sklerosus et atrophicus. Dermatol Monatsschr 158:641–654, 1972

LAYMON CM: Lichen sclerosus et atrophicus and related disorders. Arch Dermatol Syph 64:620–627, 1961

MANN PR, COWAN MA: Ultrastructural changes in four cases of lichen sclerosus et atrophicus. Br J Dermatol 89:223–231, 1973

MILLER RF: Lichen sclerosus et atrophicus with oral involvement. Arch Dermatol 76:43–55, 1957

PIPER HG: Lichen sklerosus et atrophicus partim bullosus. Dermatol Wochenschr 143:137–144, 1961

POST B, JÄNNER M: Lichen sclerosus et atrophicus penis. Z Hautkr 50:675–681, 1975

STEIGLEDER GK, RAAB WP: Lichen sclerosus et atrophicus. Arch Dermatol 84:219–226, 1961

SUURMOND D: Lichen sclerosus et atrophicus of the vulva. Arch Dermatol 90:143–152, 1964

UITTO J, SANTA CRUZ DJ, BAUER EA, et al: Morphea and lichen sclerosus et atrophicus. J Am Acad Dermatol 3:271–279, 1980

WALLACE HJ: Lichen sclerosus et atrophicus. (Review) Trans St John's Hosp Dermatol Soc 57:9–30, 1971

Striae Distensae

CHERNOSKY ME, KNOX JM: Atrophic striae after occlusive corticosteroid therapy. Arch Dermatol 90:15–19, 1964

EPSTEIN NW, EPSTEIN WL, EPSTEIN JH: Atrophic striae in patients with inguinal intertrigo. Arch Dermatol 87:450–457, 1963

HAUSER W: Zur Frage der Entstehung der Striae cutis atrophicae. Dermatol Wochenschr 138:1291–1295, 1958

KLEHR N: Striae cutis atrophicae. Morphokinetic examinations in vitro. Acta Derm Venereol (Stockh) 59, Suppl 85:105–108, 1979

PINKUS H, KEECH MK, MEHREGAN AH: Histopathology of striae distensae with special reference to striae and wound healing in the Marfan syndrome. J Invest Dermatol 46:283–292, 1966

SHUSTER S: The cause of striae distensae. Acta Derm Venereol (Stockh) 59, Suppl 85:161–169, 1979

SIMKIN B, ARCE R: Steroid excretion in obese patients with colored abdominal striae. N Engl J Med 266:1031–1035, 1962

SISSON WR: Colored striae in adolescent children. J Pediatr 45:520–530, 1954

Wrinkling Due to Middermal Elastolysis

BRENNER W, GSCHNAIT F, KONRAD K et al: Non-inflammatory dermal elastolysis. Br J Dermatol 99:335–338, 1979

DELACRÉTAZ J, PERROUD H, VULLIEMIN JF: Cutis laxa acquise. Dermatologica 155:233–234, 1977

SHELLEY WB, WOOD MG: Wrinkles due to idiopathic loss of middermal elastic tissue. Br J Dermatol 97:441–445, 1977

Macular Atrophy (Anetoderma)

CRAMER HJ: Zur Histopathogenese der Dermatitis atrophicans maculosa. Dermatol Wochenschr 147:230–237, 1963

DAVIS W: Wilson's disease and penicillamine-induced anetoderma. Arch Dermatol 113:976, 1977

DELUZENNE R: Les anétodermies maculeuses. Ann Dermatol Syph 83:618–630, 1956

DUPERRAT B: Anétodermie type Schweninger-Buzzi. Bull Soc Fr Derm Syph 61:11, 1954

EDELSON Y, GRUPPER C: Anétodermie maculeuse et lupus érythémateux. Bull Soc Fr Derm Syph 77:753–756, 1970

FELDMAN S: Macular atrophy (Schweninger and Buzzi type). Arch Dermatol Syph 38:117–118, 1938

KORTING GW, CABRÉ J, HOLZMANN H: Zur Kenntnis der Kollagenveränderungen bei der Anetodermie vom Typus Schweninger-Buzzi. Arch Klin Exp Dermatol 218:274–297, 1964

KOSSARD S, KRONMAN KR, DICKEN CH et al: Inflammatory macular atrophy: Immunofluorescent and ultrastructural findings. J Am Acad Dermatol 1:325–334, 1979

MILLER WM, RUGGLES CW, RIST TE: Anetoderma. Int J Dermatol 18:43–45, 1979

NEUMANN E, VACÁTKO S: Kutane Form der Arteritis als Vorläufer einer Atrophia maculosa. Dermatol Wochenschr 140:1008–1012, 1959

RYLL-NARDZEWSKI C, KUDEJKO T, KUDEJKO J: Remarques sur le lupus érythémateux profond de Kaposi-Irgang et sur l'anétodermie érythématoide. Ann Dermatol Syph 87:627–636, 1960

Acro-osteolysis

FINE RM: Acro-osteolysis: Vinyl chloride induced "scleroderma." Int J Dermatol 15:676–677, 1976

MARKOWITZ SS, MCDONALD CJ, FETHIERE W et al: Occupational acroosteolysis. Arch Dermatol 106:219–223, 1972

MEYERSON LB, MEIER GC: Cutaneous lesions in acroosteolysis. Arch Dermatol 106:224–227, 1972

VELTMANN G, LANGE CE, STEIN G: Die Vinylkrankheit. Hautarzt 29:177–182, 1978

Ulerythema of Eyebrows and Cheeks

DAVENPORT DD: Ulerythema ophryogenes. Arch Dermatol 89:74–80, 1964

MACKEE GM, CIPOLLARO AC: Folliculitis ulerythematosa reticulata. Arch Dermatol 57:281–292, 1948

PIERINI DO, PIERINI AM: Keratosis pilaris atrophicans faciei (ulerythema ophryogenes): A cutaneous marker in the Noonan syndrome. Br J Dermatol 100:409–416, 1979

PULLMANN H, GARTMANN H: Folliculitis ulerythematosa reticulata. Z Hautkr 56:1473–1477, 1981

ROZUM LT, MEHREGAN AH, JOHNSON SAM: Folliculitis ulerythematosa reticulata. Arch Dermatol 106:388–389, 1972

17 Bacterial Diseases

IMPETIGO

Two types of impetigo occur: impetigo contagiosa, or nonbullous impetigo, usually caused by group A streptococci, and bullous impetigo, including the staphylococcal scalded-skin syndrome, usually caused by phage group II staphylococci.

Impetigo Contagiosa

Impetigo contagiosa is primarily an endemic disease of pre-school-age children that may occur in epidemics. Very early lesions consist of vesicopustules that rupture quickly and are followed by heavy, yellowish crusts. Most of the lesions are located in exposed areas. An occasional sequela is acute glomerulonephritis. As a rule, however, the nephritis following impetigo contagiosa has a favorable long-term prognosis (Kaplan et al).

Histopathology.   The vesicopustule arises in the upper layers of the epidermis above, within, or below the granular layer (see Classification of Bullae, p. 93). It contains numerous neutrophils (Fig. 17-1). Not infrequently, a few acantholytic cells can be observed at the floor of the vesicopustule (Steigleder). Occasionally gram-positive cocci can also be found within the vesicopustule.

The stratum malpighii underlying the bulla shows spongiosis, and neutrophils can be seen migrating through it. The upper dermis contains a moderately severe inflammatory infiltrate of neutrophils and lymphoid cells.

At a later stage, when the bulla has ruptured, the horny layer is absent, and a crust composed of serous exudate and the nuclear debris of neutrophils may be seen covering the stratum malpighii.

Histogenesis. In the United States, group A streptococci are the most frequently recovered organisms in cases of impetigo contagiosa, either alone or in association with *Staphylococcus aureus. S. aureus* is the only organism isolated in less than 10% of the cases. It is believed that, in such instances, "bactericidin" produced by the secondary "colonizing" staphylococci has killed the streptococci (Peter and Smith). In other countries, however, such as Great Britain, *S. aureus* is the organism most commonly recovered, and it is therefore regarded as the main pathogen (Noble et al).

Differential Diagnosis.   A histologic differentiation of impetigo contagiosa from subcorneal pustular dermatosis is impossible (Ellis). The presence of a few acantholytic cells may lead to confusion with pemphigus foliaceus; but, aside from the fact that the number of acantholytic cells in impetigo is small, this disease differs from pemphigus foliaceus by the presence of numerous neutrophils in the bulla cavity.

Bullous Impetigo, Staphylococcal Scalded-Skin Syndrome

Phage group II staphylococci may produce bullous impetigo and the staphylococcal scalded-skin syndrome.

290

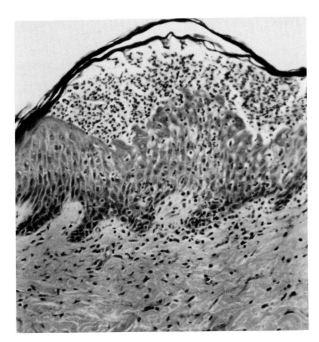

Fig. 17-1. Impetigo contagiosa
A subcorneal pustule containing numerous neutrophils is present. The underlying stratum malpighii shows spongiosis, and neutrophils are seen migrating through it. (×200)

Bullous impetigo occurs mainly in the newborn and in infants and young children. Occasionally, it is seen in adults, particularly in those with a deficiency in cell-mediated immunity (Levine and Norden; Reid et al). It is characterized by vesicles that rapidly progress to flaccid bullae with little or no surrounding erythema. The contents of the bullae are clear, at least at first; later on, they may be turbid. Bullous impetigo may spread and become generalized, so that clinical distinction from staphylococcal scalded-skin syndrome may be impossible (Elias et al). An important difference, however, is that cultures from intact bullae of bullous impetigo, unlike those of the staphylococcal scalded-skin syndrome, grow phage group II staphylococci.

Staphylococcal scalded-skin syndrome, first described more than 100 years ago (Ritter von Rittershain) and also known as Ritter's disease, occurs largely in the newborn and infants and rarely in children. It hardly ever occurs in adults, except in the presence of a severe underlying disease (Ridgway and Lowe; Pachinger). The disease begins abruptly with diffuse erythema and fever. Large, flaccid bullae filled with clear fluid form and rupture almost immediately. Large sheets of superficial epidermis separate and exfoliate. The disease runs an acute course and is fatal in less than 4% of all cases in children (Elias et al). Most fatalities occur in neonates with generalized lesions. In contrast, in the rare cases of staphylococcal scalded-skin syndrome occurring in adults, the prognosis is much worse, with a mortality rate exceeding 50%. Death is usually related to the coexistent disease or to immunosuppressive therapy given for it (Ridgway and Lowe). Both bullous impetigo and staphylococcal scalded-skin syndrome are transmissible and can cause epidemics in nurseries, where they may occur together (Melish and Glasgow). An important difference between the two diseases is that no phage group II staphylococci can be grown from the bullae of the staphylococcal scalded-skin syndrome, in contrast to the bullae of bullous impetigo. Absence of phage group II staphylococci from the bullae of staphylococcal scalded-skin syndrome is due to the fact that these staphylococci are present at a distant focus. Usually, the distant focus is extracutaneous and consists of a purulent conjunctivitis, rhinitis, or pharyngitis (Elias et al). Rarely, the distant focus consists of a cutaneous infection (Pachinger) or a septicemia (Ridgway and Lowe). The bullae are caused by a staphylococcal toxin referred to as exfoliatin (see Histogenesis).

Histopathology. In both bullous impetigo and staphylococcal scalded-skin syndrome, the cleavage plane of the bulla, like that in impetigo contagiosa, lies in the uppermost epidermis either below or, less commonly, within the granular layer. A few acantholytic cells are often seen adjoining the cleavage plane (Elias et al). In contrast to impetigo contagiosa, however, there are few or no inflammatory cells within the bulla cavity. In bullous impetigo, the upper dermis may show a polymorphous infiltrate, whereas, in the staphylococcal scalded-skin syndrome, also the dermis is usually free of inflammation (Elias and Levy).

Histogenesis. When cultures of phage group II staphylococci obtained either from the bullae of bullous impetigo or from the distant sites of infection in staphylococcal scalded-skin syndrome, or the exotoxin exfoliatin isolated from such cultures, are injected subcutaneously into newborn mice, they produce generalized exfoliation with intraepidermal cleavage, largely at the level of the stratum granulosum (Melish and Glasgow; Melish et al). The reason that only neonate mice develop generalized exfoliation is that adult mice excrete test doses of exfoliatin rapidly, within a few hours, whereas newborn mice excrete exfoliatin slowly. This probably is due to the fact that the newborn kidney is not fully developed (Fritsch et al). The ability of human adult kidneys to excrete exfoliatin produced by phage group II staphylococci explains the rarity of staphylococcal scalded-skin syndrome in adults.

Electron microscopy shows that the cleavage plane of lesions in humans as well as in mice is at the interface between the spinous and granular layers, with some upward extension into the lower granular layer. Splitting occurs without damage to adjacent acantholytic keratinocytes (Elias et al). Exfoliatin appears to act primarily on the intercellular substance, since, in studies carried out on newborn mice, the intercellular spaces widened and microvilli formed before the desmosomes separated within their interdesmosomal contact zone (Wuepper et al; Dimond et al).

Differential Diagnosis. Both staphylococcal scalded-skin syndrome and severe erythema multiforme of the toxic epidermal necrolysis or Lyell type show clinically extensive detachment of the epidermis and thus may clinically resemble one another. This resulted in confusion in the past, so that, at one time, both diseases were referred to as Lyell's disease or toxic epidermal necrolysis. However, the two diseases can be easily differentiated histologically; in severe erythema multiforme, the entire, or nearly the entire, epidermis detaches itself, with considerable necrosis of the epidermal cells (see p. 123), whereas, in staphylococcal scalded-skin syndrome, only the uppermost portion of the epidermis becomes detached, with relatively slight damage to the underlying epidermal cells (Dimond and Wuepper).

In fulminating cases in which rapid differentiation between the two diseases is required, one may obtain a freshly made peel of skin by eliciting the Nikolsky phenomenon. The peel is placed in normal saline solution and frozen in it to form a block. Sections cut with a cryostat and stained with hematoxylin-eosin then show the histologic differences just described (Amon and Dimond). In addition, a Tzanck smear may be obtained from the denuded base, fixed with 95% methyl alcohol for 1 min, and then stained with the Giemsa or Wright stain for 5 min. In the staphylococcal scalded-skin syndrome, the smear shows elongated epithelial cells with relatively small nuclei, as seen in the upper epidermis, and no inflammatory cells. In contrast, in severe erythema multiforme of the toxic epidermal necrolysis type, the smear shows either cuboidal cells with relatively large nuclei, as seen in the lower epidermis, or inflammatory cells, or both (Amon and Dimond; Dimond and Wuepper).

Ecthyma

Ecthyma is essentially ulcerated impetigo contagiosa. It occurs chiefly below the knees but occasionally also on the arms. It is clearly streptococcal in origin, since skin cultures are nearly always positive for group A streptococci. In addition, coagulase-positive staphylococci as secondary invaders can frequently be cultured from lesions (Kelly et al).

Histopathology. A nonspecific ulcer is seen with numerous neutrophils both in the dermis and in the serous exudate at the floor of the ulcer.

ERYSIPELAS

Erysipelas is an acute superficial cellulitis of the skin caused by group A streptococci. It is characterized by the presence of a well-demarcated, slightly indurated, dusky red area with an advancing, palpable border. In some persons, erysipelas has a tendency to recur periodically in the same areas.

Histopathology. The dermis shows marked edema and dilatation of the lymphatics and capillaries. There is a diffuse infiltrate, composed chiefly of neutrophils, that extends throughout the dermis and occasionally into the subcutaneous fat. It shows a loose arrangement around dilated blood and lymph vessels. If sections are stained with the Giemsa or Gram stain, streptococci are found in the tissue and within lymphatics.

In cases of recurring erysipelas, the lymph vessels of the dermis and subcutaneous tissue show fibrotic thickening of their walls with partial or complete occlusion of the lumen (Tappeiner and Pfleger).

ACUTE SUPERFICIAL FOLLICULITIS (IMPETIGO BOCKHART)

Impetigo Bockhart, caused by staphylococci, is characterized by an eruption of small pustules, many of which are pierced by a hair.

Histopathology. Impetigo Bockhart presents a subcorneal pustule situated in the opening of a hair follicle. The upper portion of the hair follicle is surrounded by a considerable inflammatory infiltrate composed predominantly of neutrophils.

ACUTE DEEP FOLLICULITIS (FURUNCLE)

A furuncle is caused by staphylococci and consists of a tender, red, perifollicular swelling terminating in the discharge of pus and of a necrotic plug.

Histopathology. A furuncle shows an area of perifollicular necrosis containing fibrinoid material and many neutrophils. At the deep end of the necrotic plug, in the subcutaneous tissue, is a large abscess. A Gram stain shows small clusters of staphylococci in the center of the abscess (Pinkus).

CHRONIC SUPERFICIAL FOLLICULITIS

Acne varioliformis, or acne necrotica, is characterized by recurrent, small, indolent, follicular papules and pustules on the forehead and in the scalp. The lesions undergo central necrosis and usually heal with small, pitted scars (Stritzler et al).

Acne necrotica miliaris of the scalp is a diminutive variety of acne varioliformis. Because of the superficial location of the necrosis, no hair loss ensues (Montgomery).

Histopathology. The histologic changes in both acne varioliformis and acne necrotica miliaris consist of an intrafollicular subcorneal pustule and an acute perifollicular infiltrate. A superficial perifollicular abscess may form, leaving a small area of necrosis. In the case of acne varioliformis, but not in the case of acne necrotica miliaris, the area of necrosis often is sufficiently large to result in healing with fibrosis and scar formation (Montgomery).

CHRONIC DEEP FOLLICULITIS

Folliculitis barbae is a deep-seated infection of the bearded region in men. There are follicular papules and pustules followed by erythema, crusting, and boggy infiltration of the skin. Abscesses may or may not be present. Scarring and permanent hair loss usually ensue.

Folliculitis decalvans occurs predominantly in men. Scattered through the scalp are bald, atrophic areas showing follicular postules at their periphery. In some instances, other hairy areas such as the bearded and pubic regions and the axillae (Bogg), as well as the eyebrows and eyelashes (Suter), are also involved. Through peripheral spreading, the atrophic areas gradually increase in size (Laymon and Murphy).

Folliculitis keloidalis nuchae represents a chronic folliculitis on the nape of the neck of men that causes hypertrophic scarring. In early cases, one observes follicular papules, pustules, and, occasionally, abscesses. The lesions are replaced gradually by indurated fibrous nodules.

Histopathology. In early lesions of all three forms of chronic deep folliculitis, one observes a perifollicular infiltrate composed largely of neutrophils but also containing lymphoid cells, histiocytes, and plasma cells. The infiltrate develops into a perifollicular abscess leading to destruction of the hair and hair follicle. Older lesions show chronic granulation tissue containing numerous plasma cells, as well as lymphoid cells and fibroblasts (Meinhof and Braun-Falco). Often, foreign body giant cells are present around remnants of hair follicles, and particles of keratin may be located near the giant cells (Moyer and Williams). As healing takes place, fibrosis is seen. If there is hypertrophic scar formation, as in folliculitis keloidalis nuchae, numerous thick bundles of sclerotic collagen are present.

PSEUDOFOLLICULITIS OF THE BEARD

Pseudofolliculitis of the beard represents a foreign body inflammatory reaction surrounding an ingrown beard hair. It occurs in men with curly hair, especially blacks, who shave closely. Clinically, one observes follicular papules and pustules resembling a bacterial folliculitis.

Histopathology. As a result of its curvature, the advancing sharp free end of the hair, as it approaches the skin, causes an invagination of the epidermis accompanied by inflammation and, often, an intraepidermal microabscess. As the hair enters the dermis, a more severe inflammatory reaction develops with downgrowth of the epidermis in an attempt to ensheath the hair. This is accompanied by abscess formation within the pseudofollicle and a foreign body giant cell reaction at the tip of the invading hair (Strauss and Kligman).

FOLLICULAR OCCLUSION TRIAD (HIDRADENITIS SUPPURATIVA, ACNE CONGLOBATA, PERIFOLLICULITIS CAPITIS ABSCEDENS ET SUFFODIENS)

The three diseases included into the follicular occlusion triad have a similar pathogenesis and similar histopathologic findings (Pillsbury et al). Quite frequently, two of the three diseases, and occasionally all three diseases, are encountered in the same patient (McMullan and Zeligman; Moyer and Williams; Hyland and Kheir). All three diseases represent a chronic, recurrent, deep-seated folliculitis resulting in abscesses and followed by the formation of sinus tracts and scarring.

In *hidradenitis suppurativa*, the axillary and anogenital regions are affected. An acute and a chronic form can be distinguished (Dvorak et al). In the acute form, red, tender nodules form that become fluctuant and heal after discharging pus. In the chronic form, deep-seated abscesses lead to the discharge of pus through sinus tracts. Severe scarring results (Brunsting).

Acne conglobata, an entity different from acne vulgaris, occurs mainly on the back, buttocks, and chest and only rarely on the face or the extremities. In addition to comedones, fluctuant nodules discharging pus or a mucoid material occur, as well as deep-seated abscesses that discharge through interconnecting sinus tracts (Strauss).

In *perifolliculitis capitis abscedens et suffodiens,* nodules and abscesses as described for acne conglobata occur in the scalp (Moschella et al).

Histopathology. Early lesions in all three diseases of the follicular occlusion triad show a perifolliculitis with an extensive infiltrate composed of neutrophils, lymphoid cells, and histiocytes. Abscess formation results and leads to the destruction first of the pilosebaceous structures and later also of the other cutaneous appendages. In response to this destruction, granulation tissue containing lymphoid and plasma cells, as well as foreign body giant cells, infiltrates the area near the remnants of hair follicles. As the abscesses extend deeper into the subcutaneous tissue, draining sinus tracts develop that are lined with epidermis. In areas of healing, extensive fibrosis may be seen (Hyland and Kheir).

Histogenesis. The common initiating event in the three diseases of the follicular occlusion triad appears to be follicular hyperkeratosis leading to retention of follicular products (Curry et al). Thus, the designation *hidradenitis suppurativa* is a misnomer, since involvement of apocrine as well as of eccrine glands represents a secondary phenomenon and is the result of extension of the inflammatory process into deep structures.

It appears doubtful that the diseases comprising the follicular occlusion triad are caused primarily by bacterial infection, since cultures from unopened abscesses often are negative (Moyer and Williams).

The beneficial effect of the internal administration of corticosteroids suggests that the three diseases represent antigen–antibody reactions resulting in tissue breakdown. Defects in cell-mediated immunity exist in some patients with hidradenitis suppurativa (Djawari and Hornstein) but not in others (Dvorak et al).

BLASTOMYCOSISLIKE PYODERMA (PYODERMA VEGETANS)

Two entirely different diseases have been described under the term *pyoderma vegetans* or *pyodermite végétante of Hallopeau*. One disease, now referred to as pemphigus vegetans of Hallopeau, shows the typical intercellular immunofluorescence of the pemphigus group on direct immunofluorescence testing (see p. 110). The other disease represents a vegetating tissue reaction, possibly secondary to bacterial infection (Su et al). In order to emphasize the difference between it and pemphigus vegetans of Hallopeau, it is preferable to refer to this disease as blastomycosislike pyoderma rather than as pyoderma vegetans (Williams and Stone).

Blastomycosislike pyoderma shows one or multiple large, verrucous, vegetating plaques with scattered pustules and elevated borders (Su et al). The plaques show considerable resemblance to those seen in blastomycosis (see p. 336). The location of the plaques varies considerably from case to case. In some instances, the face and legs are affected (Williams and Stone; Su et al); in others it is the intertriginous areas (Brunsting and Underwood). Some authors have observed an association with ulcerative colitis (Brunsting and Underwood; Forman).

Histopathology. The two major features of blastomycosislike pyoderma are pseudocarcinomatous hyperplasia and multiple abscesses in the dermis as well as in the hyperplastic epidermis. The abscesses are composed of neutrophils in some cases (Williams and Stone; Su et al) and of eosinophils in others (Brunsting and Underwood; Forman).

Histogenesis. Bacteria, most commonly *S. aureus*, can be regularly found in blastomycosislike pyoderma; however, the presence of several different strains and the variable response of patients to antibiotic therapy suggest that the bacteria are secondary invaders (Williams and Stone), although they may be responsible for the vegetating tissue reaction (Su et al). A deficiency in cellular immunity (Getlik et al) and a decrease in the chemotactic activity of the neutrophils have also been observed (Djawari and Hornstein).

Differential Diagnosis. In cases with largely eosinophils in the abscesses, pemphigus vegetans must be excluded by direct immunofluorescence (Ruzicka and Goerz). When there is marked pseudocarcinomatous hyperplasia, multiple biopsies may be necessary for differentiation from true squamous cell carcinoma (see p. 505).

ACUTE SEPTICEMIA

Two types of acute fulminating septicemia have cutaneous manifestations that are diagnostically significant. They are those caused by *Neisseria meningitidis* and *Pseudomonas*.

Acute Meningococcemia

In fulminating septicemic infections with *N. meningitidis*, extensive purpura is seen consisting of both petechiae and ecchymoses. The center of the petechiae may show a small pustule. In addition, shock, cyanosis, and severe consumption coagulopathy occur (Dalldorf and Jennette). Without treatment, death may occur within 12 hr to 24 hr. On autopsy, extensive hemorrhage is found in many internal organs, especially the lungs, kidneys, and adrenals.

On rare occasions, acute septicemia with purpura can be produced by other organisms, such as *Diplococcus pneumoniae*, *Streptococcus*, or *Staphylococcus aureus* (Plaut).

Histopathology. The cutaneous petechiae and ecchymoses show in many dermal vessels thrombi composed of neutrophils, platelets, and fibrin. In addition, there is an acute vasculitis with considerable damage to the vascular walls resulting in large and small areas of hemorrhage into the tissue. Also, neutrophils and nuclear dust are seen within and around the damaged vessels (Hill and Kinney). In most instances, many meningococci can be demonstrated in the luminal thrombi, within vessel walls, and around vessels as gram-negative diplococci. They are present not only in the cytoplasm of endothelial cells and neutrophils but also extracellularly (Hill and Kinney; Shapiro et al). Intraepidermal and subepidermal pustules filled with neutrophils may also be seen (Shapiro et al).

Histogenesis. In the past, vascular collapse and death were attributed to massive bilateral hemorrhage into the adrenal glands and were known as the Waterhouse–Friderichsen syndrome. However, it was then learned that death can occur without significant damage to the adrenals (Ferguson and Chapman). Therefore, it was assumed that the generalized hemorrhagic diathesis was caused by the consumptive depletion of plasma clotting factors and the resulting disseminated intravascular coagulation (Winkelstein et al). It seems likely, however, that there are two distinct pathogenic mechanisms operating in acute meningococcemia (Dalldorf and Jennette). First, a shocklike terminal phase is associated with the development of widerspread thrombosis of the pulmonary microcirculation. These thrombi, which are caused by meningococcal toxins, are composed of leukocytes as well as of fibrin and often also contain meningococci. They produce severe cor pulmonale, which cannot be prevented by treatment with heparin. Similar microthrombi are found also in the skin, spleen, heart, and liver. Second, a meningococcal endotoxin produces disseminated intravascular coagulation resulting in thrombi composed of fibrin only. These thrombi are found in the capillaries of the adrenal cortex and the kidney and may cause hemorrhagic infarction of the adrenal glands and renal cortical necrosis. This secondary phase of the disease can be modified with heparin therapy, but its control does not improve survival, because the adrenal and renal lesions are not immediately life-threatening, in contrast to the pulmonary lesions, which result in shock and death.

Pseudomonas Septicemia

The classic and diagnostic cutaneous lesions of *P. aeruginosa* or *P. cepacia* septicemia are referred to as *ecthyma gangrenosum*. *Pseudomonas* septicemia usually occurs in debilitated, leukemic, or severely burned patients, particularly after they have received treatment with several antibiotics. The cutaneous lesions may be single but usually are multiple. They consist of punched-out ulcers about 1 cm in diameter possessing a hemorrhagic border. They usually are preceded by a hemorrhagic bulla (Hall et al). In Tzanck smears prepared from the base of the lesions, gram-negative rods can be identified, confirming the diagnosis. Because of the rapid fatality of *Pseudomonas* septicemia, early institution of intravenous treatment with gentamicin sulfate is indicated.

In rare instances of *Pseudomonas* septicemia, multiple large, indurated, subcutaneous nodules develop (Schlossberg).

Histopathology. The ulcers show at their base a necrotizing vasculitis with only scant neutrophilic infiltration and little nuclear dust. There is, however, extensive bacillary infiltration of the perivascular region and of the adventitia and media of blood vessels. Nevertheless, the intima and the lumen usually are spared (Mandell et al). *Pseudomonas* bacilli first invade the walls of the deep subcutaneous vessels and then spread along the surfaces of the vessels to the dermis (Dorff et al). By causing perivascular and vascular necrosis, the bacilli cause extravasation of erythrocytes and the formation of ulcers.

The subcutaneous nodules are the result of cellulitis caused by the presence of large numbers of *Pseudomonas* bacilli (Schlossberg).

CHRONIC SEPTICEMIA

Meningococcemia and gonococcemia can occur in association with a chronic intermittent, benign eruption.

Chronic Meningococcemia

In persons with partial immunity to *N. meningitidis,* an infection with this organism produces chronic meningococcemia. This is characterized by recurrent attacks of fever, each lasting about 12 hr, associated with migratory joint pains and a papular and petechial eruption. Positive blood cultures are obtained during the febrile attacks.

Histopathology. The cutaneous lesions of chronic meningococcemia, in contrast to those of acute meningococcemia, show no bacteria and no vascular thrombosis or necrosis. Instead, one observes in papular lesions a perivascular infiltrate composed largely of lymphoid cells and only a few neutrophils (Ognibene and Ditto; Nielsen). In petechial lesions, one may find, in addition to a limited area of perivascular hemorrhage, a fairly high percentage of neutrophils and fibrinoid material in the walls of the vessels, so that the histologic picture resembles that of a leukocytoclastic vasculitis (Nielsen). The presence of meningococci cannot be demonstrated, not even through direct immunofluorescence testing (Ognibene and Ditto).

Chronic Gonococcemia

Patients with chronic gonococcemia, also referred to as disseminated gonococcal infection (Schoolnik et al), like those with chronic meningococcemia, have intermittent attacks of fever and polyarthralgia. The cutaneous lesions of the two diseases are also similar, except that those of chronic gonococcemia are only few in number and have a predominantly acral distribution. Also, in contrast to chronic meningococcemia, there are often, in addition to papules and petechiae, vesicopustules with a hemorrhagic halo, and, rarely, hemorrhagic bullae. Blood cultures often are positive for *N. gonorrhoeae,* but only during attacks of fever. A search for gonococci should also be made in possible sites of primary infection.

Histopathology. The capillaries in the upper dermis and middermis are surrounded by an infiltrate of neutrophils and a variable admixture of mononuclear cells and red cells. There often is nuclear dust, as in leukocytoclastic vasculitis. Fibrinoid material may be seen in the walls of some vessels, and fibrin thrombi in some lumina (Shapiro et al). Pustular lesions are usually seen in an intraepidermal location with neutrophils both within them and in the underlying dermis (Björnberg). Bullae are subepidermal in location (Ackerman).

Gram-negative diplococci are seen in tissue sections only on rare occasions in the walls of blood vessels (Ackerman et al). They are found more readily in direct smears of pus from freshly opened pustules. It is of interest that direct smears reveal gonococci more commonly than cultures (Abu-Nassar et al). However, *N. gonorrhoeae* can frequently be identified in tissue sections by use of fluorescent-antibody techniques (Kahn and Danielsson). For this purpose, fluorescein-labeled antigonococcus globulin is used. Diplococci, as well as single cocci and disintegrated antigenic material, are then seen, largely in a perivascular location. The reason that direct smears are more apt to show diplococci than cultures and that the fluorescent-antibody technique is particularly effective in demonstrating gonococci lies in the fact that smears and the fluorescent-antibody technique are not dependent on living organisms, as are cultures.

Histogenesis. Whereas most strains of gonococci are susceptible to the bactericidal action of normal serum, those causing disseminated gonococcal infection are resistant (Schoolnik et al).

MALAKOPLAKIA

Malakoplakia may affect various organs, most commonly the urinary tract and gastrointestinal tract. In rare instances, it involves an area of the skin. The lesions are the result of an inability of macrophages to phagocytize bacteria adequately. The most common organism grown in cultures of tissue material is *Escherichia coli* (Arul and Emmerson; Abdou et al; Nieland et al), but, in some instances, other bacteria such as *Staphylococcus aureus* (Sencer et al) are cultured. Some patients with lesions of malakoplakia have altered immune responsiveness as a result of immunosuppressive therapy for lymphoma (Almagro et al) or for renal transplantation (Sian et al; Nieland et al). The appearance of the cutaneous lesions is nonspecific and variable. Most commonly, one observes a fluctuant area (Sencer et al), a draining abscess (Abdou et al), draining sinuses (Sian et al), or an ulcer (Arul and Emmerson; Moore et al); however, in some patients, a solitary, tender nodule (Almagro et al) or a cluster of tender papules (Nieland et al) is seen. In cases involving the skin, the disease is benign and self-limited (Moore et al).

Histopathology. There are sheets of large, round or ovoid histiocytes containing fine, eosinophilic granules in their cytoplasm. These cells are referred to as von Hansemann cells (Arul and Emmerson; Almagro et al). Many of them contain, in addition to the granules, ovoid or round basophilic inclusions, referred to as Michaelis–Gutmann bodies, that vary in size from 5 μm to 15 μm (Moore et al). These bodies either are homogeneous or have a "target" appearance by showing concentric laminations (Arul and Emmerson; Nieland et al). In addition, the infiltrate may contain lymphocytes and plasma cells.

The Michaelis–Gutmann inclusion bodies, as well as the cytoplasmic granules, are periodic acid-Schiff (PAS)-positive and diastase-resistant. In addition, the Michaelis–Gutmann bodies stain with the von Kossa stain for calcium and contain small amounts of iron that may be demonstrated by Perls' stain. With the Gram stain, gram-negative bacteria may be seen in some of the histiocytes (Nieland et al).

Histogenesis. On *electron microscopic examination,* one observes within the cytoplasm of the von Hansemann cells numerous phagolysosomes corresponding to the PAS-positive granules. The phagolysosomes contain lamellae in a whorled or concentric arrangement (Chandra and Kapur). The Michaelis–Gutmann bodies develop within phagolysosomes by the progressive deposition of electron-dense calcific material on the whorled or concentric lamellae until they are ultimately completely calcified (Nieland et al). Bacteria may be seen in the cytoplasm of the von Hansemann cells and in various stages of digestion within phagolysosomes (Sencer et al).

Malakoplakia represents an acquired defect in the lysosomal digestion of phagocytized bacteria. In one reported case of malakoplakia caused by *E. coli*, the blood monocytes of the patient showed in vitro a decreased bactericidal activity toward *E. coli* after phagocytosis. This was associated with a poor release by the monocytes of beta-glucuronidase, a lysosomal enzyme (Abdou et al).

TUBERCULOSIS

When a normal, not previously infected guinea pig is inoculated intradermally with an adequate dose of *Mycobacterium tuberculosis*, a hard nodule develops at the site of the inoculation after 8 to 12 days. The nodule soon ulcerates, and the regional lymph nodes become enlarged and ultimately may drain pus. This represents the primary or Ghon complex. Histologic examination of the primary ulcer 10 to 14 days after inoculation reveals an acute inflammatory infiltrate with many neutrophils and many tubercle bacilli. Areas of tissue necrosis are also present. During the third and fourth weeks after inoculation, the histologic picture gradually changes. First monocytes and macrophages and then epithelioid cells appear and replace the neutrophils. During the fourth week after inoculation, distinct tubercles or tuberculoid structures appear both at the site of the inoculation and in the regional lymph nodes. Simultaneous with the formation of tuberculoid structures, the number of tubercle bacilli decreases rapidly (Sulzberger).

A typical tubercle consists of an accumulation of epithelioid cells surrounded by a wall of mononuclear cells. Usually, a few giant cells are present among the epithelioid cells. The epithelioid cells in the center of the tubercle may show various degrees of necrosis. If such typical tubercles are present, one speaks of a *tuberculous infiltrate*. In tuberculosis, however, one frequently does not find typical tubercles but only irregular accumulations of epithelioid cells within an inflammatory infiltrate, with or without necrosis and with or without giant cells. In that case, one speaks of a *tuberculoid infiltrate*.

The presence of a tuberculous or a tuberculoid infiltrate does not necessarily mean tuberculosis. Such an infiltrate may be seen in various other conditions as well. First, it can be produced by several infectious diseases, especially syphilis, lep-

rosy, atypical mycobacterial infections, and some deep fungus infections. In these diseases, as in tuberculosis, tubercles or tuberculoid structures form as the result of an immunologic response. Second, it can occur in instances of hypersensitivity to foreign substances, such as zirconium, beryllium, and certain dyes used in tattoos (see p. 224). Third, some foreign body reactions not associated with hypersensitivity show a tuberculoid structure, for instance, reactions to silk or nylon sutures, talc, starch, and cactus spines (see p. 222). Finally, well-developed tuberculoid structures are also seen in some cases of papular acne rosacea and in lupus miliaris disseminatus faciei, which is probably related to acne rosacea (see p. 199).

The establishment of a diagnosis of tuberculosis requires proof of the presence of tubercle bacilli. Their demonstration in the histologic sections of some forms of cutaneous tuberculosis, particularly lupus vulgaris, is very rarely possible with acid-fast staining; although fluorescent staining for mycobacteria with auramine or rhodamine is usually superior to acid-fast staining (Wilner et al), it is apt to give negative results in lupus vulgaris (Steigleder). Both guinea pig inoculation and bacterial cultures should be carried out. Cultures on special media at 37° C grow within 3 to 4 weeks, whereas guinea pig inoculations require 6 to 7 weeks for a positive result (Slany). Cultures are required also for isolating atypical mycobacteria, some of which cause lesions that both clinically and histologically resemble those caused by *M. tuberculosis* (see p. 303) (Weed and Macy).

Tuberculosis of the skin may be divided into primary and secondary tuberculosis. The latter develops in previously infected and sensitized persons owing to reactivation or reinfection. In secondary tuberculosis, the regional lymph nodes are not involved. Diagnosis of the various types of cutaneous tuberculosis is dependent on correlation of a number of factors, such as the presence or absence of bacteria in the histologic sections, the amount of bacteria in the histologic sections, the amount of necrosis, the amount of inflammatory infiltrate, the depth of the tuberculous or tuberculoid infiltrate, and the type of epidermal response.

Areas of necrosis, on histologic examination, show a loss of cellular outline. One observes eosinophilic granular material in which, unless the necrosis is advanced, some nuclei are still present. However, most of the nuclei show pyknosis (shrinkage) or karyorrhexis (fragmentation). The amount of necrosis, often referred to as caseation necrosis, usually is proportional to the number of bacteria present (see Histogenesis).

Before enzyme histochemical methods became available, the mononuclear cells present at the periphery of epithelioid cell granulomas, as seen in tuberculosis and sarcoidosis, were thought to be lymphocytes. It has since become generally recognized that the high content of lysosomal enzymes in most of these cells establishes them as monocytes. As such, they are derived from the bone marrow and are carried to the sites of granulomas through the blood stream (see p. 52). Within the granulomas, the monocytes develop into macrophages, which, in turn, give rise to both epithelioid cells and giant cells (Adams).

Electron microscopic studies have shown that tubercle bacilli are phagocytized by macrophages through the formation of membrane-lined phagosomes. Through interaction with primary lysosomes containing hydrolytic enzymes, such as acid phosphatase, the phagosomes develop into digestive vacuoles or secondary lysosomes (Dumont and Sheldon). Whether the disease progresses or is contained depends on whether the macrophages are able to kill all or nearly all tubercle bacilli within them before disintegrating, or whether they disintegrate first and thus release many viable bacilli. In the latter case, however, the bacilli may be phagocytized by a new series of macrophages. With each new series, the bactericidal ability of the macrophages may increase (Shima et al).

Disintegrating macrophages form areas of necrosis (caseation). In contrast, macrophages capable of digesting bacilli within them assume the appearance of epithelioid cells during the process of digestion. Such epithelioid cells may contain large, dense phagolysosomes containing digested bacterial organisms (Miller et al). In addition, since, in many infections, more macrophages enter the area than are needed to engulf the organisms present, macrophages that never have ingested bacilli can also develop into epithelioid cells (Papadimitriou and Spector).

Multinucleated giant cells usually form by the fusion of nonproliferating, that is, tritiated-thymidine-negative, macrophages or epithelioid cells. As macrophages mature into epithelioid cells and lose their ability to divide, they show a greater tendency to fuse into multinucleated giant cells (Carter and Roberts).

Delayed Hypersensitivity. Infection with tubercle bacilli in previously uninfected persons results in a delayed hypersensitivity reaction that is elicited by proteins present in the bacilli. In nonsensitized persons, an infection with tubercle bacilli at first attracts neutrophils; however, as soon as thymus-derived lymphocytes have become specifically sensitized to *M. tuberculosis*, they attract monocytes by means of their lymphokines and stimulate them to develop into macrophages. Macrophages are much more capable of digesting and destroy-

ing tubercle bacilli than are neutrophils. The antibodies in sensitized persons are carried by T lymphocytes, as is typical in delayed hypersensitivity reactions, also referred to as cellular immunity, since the antibodies do not freely circulate in the blood serum, as do the immunoglobulins.

When, for the purpose of testing, purified protein derivative (PPD) of tuberculin containing tuberculoproteins is applied to or injected into the skin of sensitized persons, it causes an influx of relatively few antibody-carrying lymphocytes, resulting in an antigen–antibody reaction. This reaction, through the release of lymphokines by the specifically sensitized T lymphocytes, leads not only to tissue destruction but also to the accumulation of monocytes, which, by developing into macrophages, remove the local damage produced by the antigen–antibody reaction. The predominantly perivascular accumulation of monocytes produces the positive tuberculin reaction within 24 hr to 48 hr of its application or injection. Thus, the response to tuberculin is similar to the response to patch tests observed in contact dermatitis, which is also a delayed hypersensitivity reaction (see p. 96).

Primary Tuberculosis

Primary infection with tuberculosis occurs only very rarely on the skin. In the great majority of cases, it presents itself in the lung as the so-called Ghon complex or primary complex. This consists of a small necrotic lesion at the periphery of one lung associated with a necrotic lesion in the hilar lymph nodes. The Ghon complex in the lung usually heals with scarring, although a few bacilli may persist for many years and then may reactivate. In rare instances, no healing takes place, and the primary lesion extends rapidly. Extension may be limited to the lungs or, through hematogenous dissemination, reach other organs. Widespread dissemination results in generalized miliary tuberculosis.

Primary infection of the skin with tuberculosis has always been a rare event. In the past, when tuberculosis was common, it was reported mainly in children (O'Leary and Harrison); nowadays, it is reported sporadically in adults, as a result, for instance, of mouth-to-mouth artificial respiration (Heilman and Muschenheim) or of inoculation during an autopsy (Goette et al). Usually, the cutaneous lesion arises within 2 to 4 weeks after the inoculation. It consists of an asymptomatic crust-covered ulcer referred to as tuberculous chancre. The regional lymph nodes are enlarged and may suppurate and produce draining sinuses.

Histopathology. The histologic development of the lesion is very much like that observed in experimental cutaneous inoculation of the guinea pig (see p. 297) (O'Leary and Harrison). In the earliest phase, the histologic picture is that of an acute neutrophilic reaction, with areas of necrosis resulting in ulceration. Numerous tubercle bacilli are present, particularly in the areas of necrosis (Goette et al). After 2 weeks, monocytes and macrophages predominate, but necrosis within the infiltrate remains a prominent feature. Three to 6 weeks after onset, epithelioid cells and giant cells begin to appear, while caseation necrosis is still prominent (Montgomery). As the proportion of epithelioid cells and giant cells gradually increases, caseation lessens, and the number of tubercle bacilli decreases until it is so greatly reduced that the bacilli may be impossible to demonstrate in histologic sections, and the only proof of their presence may be through animal inoculations and positive cultures. Simultaneous with the decrease in the number of tubercle bacilli in the lesion, the tuberculin test with PPD, previously negative, becomes positive (see Histogenesis above.)

Miliary Tuberculosis of the Skin

Involvement of the skin with miliary tuberculosis is rare, occurring mostly in infants and only exceptionally in adults. Usually, internal involvement is widespread as a result of hematogenous dissemination, and the cutaneous eruption is generalized, consisting of erythematous papules and pustules 2 mm to 5 mm in diameter. The tuberculin test generally is negative. The disease is usually fatal (Schermer et al).

There exists, however, a milder form of hematogenous dissemination of tubercle bacilli in neonates born of tuberculous mothers. This form shows limited visceral involvement and only a few scattered erythematous papules with central crusted dells. Antituberculous treatment is effective (McGray and Esterly).

Histopathology. In severe cases, the center of the papules shows a microabscess containing neutrophils, cellular debris, and numerous tubercle bacilli. This is surrounded by a zone of macrophages (Schermer at al).

In the milder form, the histologic picture in the skin is similar to that seen in the severe form, except that the Ziehl–Neelsen stain is negative for acid-fast organisms. A biopsy of the liver, however, shows focal caseating granulomas containing numerous acid-fast bacteria (McKay and Esterly).

Lupus Vulgaris

The lesions of lupus vulgaris are found on the head or neck in over 90% of the cases (Horwitz). The skin of and around the nose is frequently involved (Warin and Wilson Jones). The lesions consist of one or a few well-demarcated, reddish brown patches containing deep-seated nodules, each about 1 mm in size. If the blood is pressed out of the skin with a glass slide (diascopy), these nodules stand out clearly as yellowish brown macules, referred to because of their color as apple-jelly nodules. The disease is very chronic, with slow peripheral extension of the lesions. In the course of time, the affected areas become atrophic, with contraction of the tissue. It is a characteristic feature of lupus vulgaris that new lesions may appear in areas of atrophy. Superficial ulceration or verrucous thickening of the skin occurs occasionally. Squamous cell carcinoma develops at the margin of ulcers in rare instances.

Histopathology. Tubercles or tuberculoid structures composed of epithelioid cells and giant cells are present. Caseation necrosis within the tubercles is slight and may be absent (Fig. 17-2) (Montgomery). Although the giant cells usually are of the Langhans type, with peripheral arrangement of the nuclei, some can be of the foreign body type,

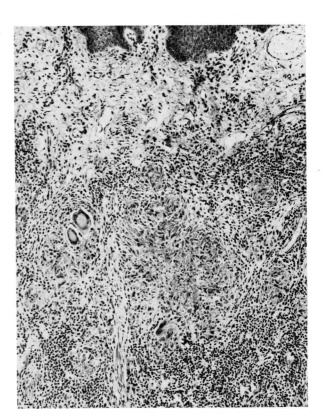

Fig. 17-2. Lupus vulgaris
Low magnification. There are several tubercles. The large tubercle in the center shows slight caseation necrosis. (×100)

with irregular arrangement of the nuclei (Fig. 17-3). In addition, there is an infiltrate of mononuclear cells. On staining for lysosomal enzymes, many of the mononuclear cells in the vicinity of the tubercles or tuberculoid structures show positive staining, indicating that they are monocytes, whereas those farther away do not stain and thus can be interpreted as lymphocytes (see also Histogenesis, p. 298) (Shima et al).

The extent and density of the mononuclear infiltrate are variable. In some instances, especially in cases showing ulceration, the inflammatory infiltrate dominates the histologic picture, so that one has to search for occasional tuberculoid structures; in other cases, the inflammatory infiltrate is slight.

Both the tubercles or tuberculoid structures and the mononuclear infiltrate usually are most pronounced in the upper dermis, but, in some areas, they may extend into the subcutaneous layer. They cause destruction of the cutaneous appendages. In areas of healing, extensive fibrosis may be present.

Secondary changes in the epidermis are common. The epidermis may undergo atrophy and subsequently destruction, causing ulceration, or it may become hyperplastic, showing acanthosis, hyperkeratosis, and papillomatosis. At the margin of ulcers, pseudocarcinomatous hyperplasia often exists. Unless a deep biopsy is done in such cases, one may see only the epithelial hyperplasia and a nonspecific inflammation, and the diagnosis may be missed (Warin and Wilson Jones). In rare instances, squamous cell carcinoma supervenes.

Tubercle bacilli are present in such small numbers that they can only very rarely be demonstrated by staining methods. Even cultures and guinea pig inoculations are not always successful. Thus, in one series of 31 cases, there were 7 patients in whom both cultures and guinea pig inoculations gave negative results (van der Lugt).

Histogenesis. Lupus vulgaris is a form of secondary tuberculosis developing in previously infected and sensitized persons. Hypersensitivity to PPD tuberculin is high. Although the mode of infection is often not apparent, the disease only rarely seems to be the result of an exogenous infection of the skin; usually it is due to hematogenous spread from an old, reactivated focus in the lung or due to lymphatic extension from a tuberculous cervical lymphadenitis (Montgomery; Horwitz).

Differential Diagnosis. For a discussion of differentiation of lupus vulgaris from sarcoidosis, see p. 233; for differentiation from atypical mycobacterial diseases, see p. 303.

Tuberculosis Verrucosa Cutis

Tuberculosis verrucosa cutis and its variant verruca necrogenica represent virulent exogenous infections of

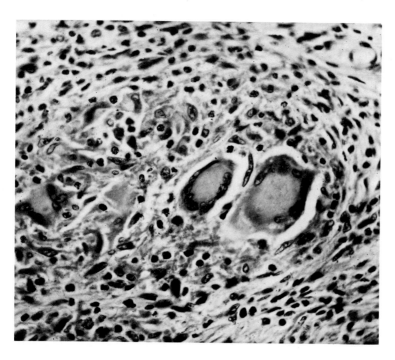

Fig. 17-3. Lupus vulgaris
High magnification of Figure 17-2. A tubercle contains several giant cells of the Langhans type with peripheral arrangement of the nuclei. (×400)

the skin in persons with a rather high degree of immunity. In tuberculosis verrucosa cutis, one usually observes a single lesion presenting as a verrucous plaque with an inflammatory border and showing gradual peripheral extension. The verrucous surface shows fissures from which pus often can be expressed. The most common sites are the hands and, in children, the knees, buttocks, and thighs (Wong et al). Verruca necrogenica differs from tuberculosis verrucosa cutis only in the mode by which it is contracted, namely from handling cadavers, and by its small size (Minkowitz et al).

Histopathology. The histologic picture shows hyperkeratosis, papillomatosis, and acanthosis. Beneath the epidermis, one observes an acute inflammatory infiltrate. Abscess formation may be seen in the upper dermis or within downward extensions of the epidermis. In the middermis, tuberculoid structures with a moderate amount of necrosis are usually present. Tubercle bacilli are more numerous in this disease than in lupus vulgaris and occasionally can be demonstrated histologically (Montgomery).

Scrofuloderma

Scrofuloderma, also called tuberculosis colliquativa cutis, represents a direct extension to the skin of an underlying tuberculous infection present most commonly in a lymph node or a bone. The lesion first manifests itself as a bluish red, painless swelling that breaks open and then forms an ulcer with irregular, undermined, bluish borders.

Histopathology. The center of the lesion usually shows nonspecific changes, such as abscess formation or ulceration. In the deeper portions and at the periphery of the lesion, however, if the biopsy specimen is adequate, one usually sees tuberculoid structures with a considerable amount of necrosis together with a pronounced inflammatory reaction (Fig. 17-4) (Montgomery). Usually, the number of tubercle bacilli is sufficient for them to be found in histologic sections.

Differential Diagnosis. For a discussion of differentiation of scrofuloderma from erythema induratum, see p. 250; for differentiation from gummatous syphilis, see p. 324.

Tuberculosis Cutis Orificialis

The lesions of tuberculosis cutis orificialis are shallow ulcers with a granulating base occurring singly or in small numbers on or near the mucosal orifices of patients with advanced internal tuberculosis. Most patients have a low degree of immunity. The ulcers, which are often very tender, may occur inside the mouth, on the lips, around the anus, or on the perineum (Regan and Harley) and, in the case of genitourinary tuberculosis, on the vulva (Fisher).

Histopathology. The histologic picture may show merely an ulcer surrounded by a nonspecific inflammatory infiltrate. Yet, in most instances, tu-

Fig. 17-4.   Scrofuloderma
Margin of an ulcer. On the right side of the photograph, one observes necrosis of epidermis and dermis. In the center are tuberculoid structures. On the left, the infiltrate is composed of lymphocytes and plasma cells. (×200)

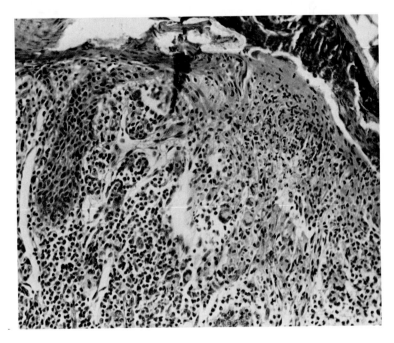

berculoid formations with pronounced necrosis are found deep in the dermis (Regan and Harley). Tubercle bacilli are easily demonstrated in the sections, even when the histologic appearance is nonspecific.

TUBERCULIDS

The *tuberculids*, a term first proposed in 1896 (Darier), according to some authors comprise two dermatoses, the papulonecrotic tuberculid, and lichen scrofulosorum (Morrison and Furie; Iden et al; Smith et al; Hudson; Ehring). Other authors also include some instances of erythema induratum (Braun-Falco et al).

Histogenesis. The concept of tuberculids has suffered in the past from two misconceptions. First, several diseases were called tuberculids because the skin lesions had a tuberculoid appearance on histologic examination, even though there was no clinical evidence of a coexisting tuberculosis. They are no longer considered tuberculids. These diseases include the "rosacealike tuberculid" or "micropapular tuberculid," now regarded as a granulomatous form of papular acne rosacea (see p. 199), and lupus miliaris disseminatus faciei, or "macropapular tuberculoid," now regarded as a dermatosis of unknown etiology possibly related to acne rosacea (see p. 200). Second, some cases were regarded as papulonecrotic tuberculid or as lichen scrofulosorum in spite of the absence of adequate evidence for a coexisting tuberculosis, only because they resembled one of these two diseases clinically and histologically. Thus, retrospectively, one may classify cases diagnosed as papulonecrotic tuberculid as instances of pityriasis lichenoides et varioliformis acuta of Mucha and Habermann (see p. 171), since both diseases are characterized by a largely lymphocytic vasculitis (Krüger and Weise); furthermore, some cases described as lichen scrofulosorum (Ockuly and Montgomery) may be regarded as instances of lichenoid or micropapular sarcoidosis (see p. 229) (Brunner and Robin; Thal; Kanaar), whereas others may be reclassified as cases of generalized papular granuloma annulare (see p. 234) (van der Lugt; Schumachers).

Since, until recently, no acceptable cases of either papulonecrotic tuberculid or lichen scrofulosorum had appeared in the literature for several decades (Smith et al; Iden et al), doubts as to the existence of these two entities have been expressed (Flegel; Lever and Schaumburg-Lever; Wolff). However, several recent publications suggest that they do exist, although rarely and then usually in persons who either live in developing countries or have recently emigrated from them (see below). The following prerequisites are necessary for a diagnosis of tuberculid to be acceptable: (1) tuberculin sensitivity must exist, (2) a simultaneous tuberculosis must be present, and (3) there must be a good response to tuberculostatica (Ehring).

The histogenesis of tuberculids is not fully understood. Tubercle bacilli are absent in tuberculids, probably having been destroyed at the site of the tuberculids by some immunologic mechanism. This mechanism in the papulonecrotic tuberculid consists of an Arthus reaction with vasculitis followed by a delayed hypersensitivity response with granuloma formation (Morrison and Furie). In the case of lichen scrofulosorum, there is only a delayed hypersensitivity reaction resulting in granuloma formation (Smith et al).

In regard to erythema induratum, evidence in favor of a tuberculous genesis is insufficient (see p. 249).

Papulonecrotic Tuberculid

A series of 91 cases of papulonecrotic tuberculid published in 1974 (Morrison and Furie) consisted largely of South African blacks, in whom the incidence of tuberculosis is high. Papulonecrotic lesions were present, more or less widely distributed. In four patients, lupus vulgaris developed from the lesions. Only in about one third of the cases was a focus of tuberculosis demonstrable, most commonly in lymph nodes or the lungs, but, irrespective of whether a deep tuberculous focus was known to exist, the response of the eruption to treatment with streptomycin and isoniazid was rapid and complete. Since then, an additional case has been reported in the United States in a patient with tuberculosis of cervical lymph nodes (Iden et al).

Histopathology. Early lesions show a leukocytoclastic vasculitis followed by a perivascular infiltrate of mononuclear cells (Morrison and Furie). Subsequently, a wedge-shaped area of necrosis forms, its broad base toward the epidermis (Iden et al). As this wedge is gradually cast off, epithelioid and giant cells gather around its periphery (Morrison and Furie).

Lichen Scrofulosorum

Seven cases of lichen scrofulosorum have been reported from London since 1976. Five of the seven cases concerned patients from overseas. Five had tuberculosis of lymph nodes (Smith et al; Breathnach and Black), and two had osseous tuberculosis (Hudson; Graham-Brown and Sarkany). Lichenoid papules were observed mainly on the trunk. They were skin-colored and often follicular in distribution, measuring from 0.5 mm to 3 mm in diameter. The papules in some cases showed grouping or an annular arrangement. Response to antituberculous treatment was excellent in all seven patients.

Histopathology. Superficial dermal granulomas are usually seen surrounding hair follicles or sweat ducts. The granulomas are composed of epithelioid cells, with some Langhans giant cells and a narrow margin of lymphoid cells at the periphery. Generally, caseation necrosis is absent (Smith et al). In one reported case, however, central caseation was observed (Hudson).

Differential Diagnosis. Distinction of lichen scrofulosorum from sarcoidosis may be impossible on histologic grounds alone (Smith et al).

INFECTIONS WITH ATYPICAL MYCOBACTERIA

Among the so-called atypical mycobacterial infections of the skin, those caused by *M. marinum* are by far the most common. However, there are several other mycobacteria that in rare instances may affect the skin.

The atypical mycobacteria are divided into four groups (Runyan). Group I is composed of the *photochromogens*, which develop a yellow color only when exposed to light. In this group are *M. marinum* and *M. kansasii*. Group II includes the *scotochromogens*, which develop a yellow pigment even when growing in the dark. The main species is *M. scrofulaceum*. Group III consists of the *nonchromogens*. In this group is *M. intercellulare*. In group IV are the *rapid growers*, which form colonies in culture at room temperature within 3 to 5 days, instead of the 2 to 3 weeks required by the other mycobacteria. In this group are *M. fortuitum* and *M. chelonei* (Dore et al).

Infection with *Mycobacterium Marinum*

Infections with *M. marinum*, formerly referred to also as *M. balnei*, can take place through minor abrasions incurred while bathing in swimming pools (Hellerström) or in ocean or lake water (Zeligman; Even-Paz et al; Izumi et al) or while cleaning home aquariums (Adams et al; Mansson et al; Marsch et al). Infected swimming pools have caused epidemics, the largest of which affected 290 persons (Philpott et al). The period of incubation usually is about 3 weeks but may be longer.

Clinically, most of the lesions caused by *M. marinum* are solitary and consist of indolent, dusky red, hyperkeratotic, papillomatous papules, nodules, or plaques. Superficial ulceration is seen occasionally. The fingers, knees, elbows, and feet are most commonly affected. In some instances, satellite papules arise (Even-Paz et al), or multiple intracutaneous or subcutaneous nodules arise in linear arrangement, as seen in sporotrichosis, several weeks after the appearance of the primary lesion at the periphery of an extremity (Dickey; Adams et al; Marsch et al). Lesions may form at different sites in the case of multiple injuries (Jolly and Seabury). Although spontaneous healing usually takes place within a year, the lesions persist in some patients for many years (Zeligman; Izumi et al).

Histopathology. Early lesions no more than 2 or 3 months old show a nonspecific inflammatory infiltrate composed of neutrophils, monocytes, and macrophages. In lesions about 4 months old, a few multinucleated giant cells and a few small epithelioid cell granulomas usually are present, and in lesions 6 months old or older, typical tubercles or tuberculoid structures may be seen (Mansson et al). Areas of necrosis are only occasionally present in the center of the granulomas. The epidermis often shows papillomatosis and hyperkeratosis, and there may be central ulceration.

Acid-fast organisms usually can be identified in histologic sections of early lesions that show a nonspecific inflammatory infiltrate (Adams et al). In contrast, tuberculoid granulomas generally no longer show acid-fast organisms, unless areas of central necrosis are present (Scholz-Jordan et al).

In histologic sections, the atypical mycobacteria appear slightly larger than *M. tuberculosis* and show transverse striation (Philpott et al). If acid-fast bacilli cannot be detected in histologic sections, they can be identified by culture or by animal inoculation, except in healing lesions.

Whereas primary lesions usually require a few months for the formation of tuberculoid granulomas, the sporotrichoid nodules that arise later show tuberculoid granulomas and a lack of acid-fast bacilli even when they have been present for only a few weeks (Dickey; Marsch et al).

Histogenesis. In some instances in which *M. marinum* is not demonstrable in biopsy specimens, it may be seen in smears of exudates (Even-Paz et al). When tissue homogenates are cultured on standard mycobacterial culture media, *M. marinum* shows optimal growth at 30°C to 33°C, rather than at 37°C, as do most other atypical mycobacteria and *M. tuberculosis*. *M. marinum* is not pathogenic to guinea pigs, but it is pathogenic to mice if inoculated into their footpads (Cott et al).

Differential Diagnosis. The granulomatous reaction produced by *M. marinum* often is very similar to that seen in tuberculosis verrucosa cutis or lupus vulgaris, so that cultures and animal inoculations are necessary for their differentiation.

Infection with Other Atypical Mycobacteria

Cutaneous infections with atypical mycobacteria other than *M. marinum* are rare. Although the infections may clinically resemble those caused by *M. marinum*, they generally do not occur through exposure in water.

Infection with *M. kansasii* in some patients has caused a verrucous nodular lesion on the hand with sporotrichoid nodules extending along the arm (Owens and McBride; Dore et al); in others, it has caused extensive verrucous granulomas (Maberry et al), a crusted ulcer (Hirsh and Saffold), or an abscess (Bolivar et al).

Reports of infections with atypical mycobacteria of groups II to IV are very few, but these infections follow the pattern of group I. The lesions in group II may be verrucous (Knox et al) or may consist of abscesses (Cott et al). In group III, one reported case showed a draining sinus (Schmidt et al). The lesions of group IV have been described either as crusted nodules (Yip et al) or as subcutaneous abscesses (Brock et al; Greer et al). The abscesses may result in ulcerations (Fenske and Millns).

Histopathology. In cases of infections caused by *M. kansasii*, a tuberculoid infiltrate has been found in most patients without the presence of acid-fast bacilli in the histologic sections (Maberry et al; Owens and McBride; Hirsh and Saffold; Dore et al). One patient, however, who clinically had abscesses showed on histologic examination numerous acid-fast bacilli in an infiltrate of acute and chronic inflammation (Bolivar et al).

In cases of infections caused by atypical mycobacteria of groups II to IV, histologic sections showed acid-fast bacilli in the patients with abscesses (Cott et al; Brock et al; Greer et al; Fenske and Millns). Also, in one case with a crusted nodule, numerous bacilli were found in the necrotic centers of granulomas (Yip et al). In contrast, cases with a nonspecific or granulomatous infiltrate without necrosis showed no acid-fast bacilli (Knox et al).

BURULI ULCERATION

Buruli ulceration, an infection caused by an atypical mycobacterium, *M. ulcerans,* is common in some parts of Central Africa. The infection consists of usually a solitary, large, deep, painless ulcer located in most instances on an extremity. Contagion is not a factor in transmission, but penetrating trauma is a recognized antecedent factor.

Histopathology. The infection begins as a subcutaneous nodule that ulcerates. At the base of the ulcer, one observes extensive areas of necrosis characterized by a "ghost" outline of tissue structure (Connor and Lunn). The fat cells are enlarged,

without nuclei, and are separated by fibrin (Ziefer et al). Acid-fast organisms are found in large quantities in the necrotic tissue without any associated inflammatory reaction in the adjacent viable tissue.

Histogenesis. The widespread necrosis of skin and subcutaneous tissue is caused by an exotoxin elaborated by *M. ulcerans*. This toxin, which is present in cultures of *M. ulcerans*, causes necrosis when inoculated into guinea pig skin (Krieg et al). Like *M. marinum, M. ulcerans* shows optimal cultural growth at 30°C to 33°C. It is pathogenic to mice when inoculated into their footpads (Cott et al).

LEPROSY

Leprosy, caused by *M. leprae*, predominantly affects the skin and peripheral nerves. Aside from the occasional initial manifestation of leprosy referred to as the indeterminate form, the disease can be divided into six types forming a spectrum (Ridley and Jopling; Ridley, 1974). The form of disease arising in an individual patient depends on his degree of resistance or immunity against *M. leprae*. On the one end of the spectrum is tuberculoid leprosy (TT), which occurs only in persons with a very high degree of immunity and which is characterized by only one or very few asymmetrically arranged lesions and, rarely, shows a few bacilli. This is followed by the borderline tuberculoid form (BT), the true borderline form (BB), the borderline lepromatous form (BL), and lepromatous leprosy (LL). Lepromatous leprosy has been subdivided into subpolar (LLs) and polar (LLp) leprosy (Ridley, 1974; Jolliffe). The number of lesions and the number of bacilli within the lesions increase with diminishing immunity. Thus, lepromatous leprosy shows widespread lesions with many bacilli. Only the two polar forms, TT, which affects only persons with a very high degree of immunity, and LLp, which arises in persons with a complete lack of immunity, are fairly stable, all the other forms being unstable. The disease may move spontaneously from BT to BL and ultimately to LLs; in contrast, under treatment with mycobactericidal drugs, the disease may move in the opposite direction (Pettit).

Clinical Appearance. In *indeterminate leprosy*, which may occur in the beginning of the disease, either a single hypochromic or erythematous macule or several such macules are present. In some instances, the lesions are hypoesthetic (Kwittken and Peck). Indeterminate leprosy may heal spontaneously or under treatment, or it may go on to any of the other forms of the disease (Convit and Ulrich).

Tuberculoid leprosy often shows only a single cutaneous lesion or, at most, very few asymmetrically arranged lesions. They are large, well-defined macules showing an active, often slightly raised border with clearing in the center (Rea and Levan, 1977). They are characterized by hypoesthesia, hypopigmentation, hair loss, and impairment of sweating. A superficial nerve in the vicinity of the lesion may be palpable.

Lepromatous leprosy, representing the completely anergic type, initially has cutaneous and mucosal lesions, with neural changes occurring later. The lesions usually are numerous and are symmetrically arranged. There are three clinical types: macular, nodular, and diffuse (Arnold and Fasal). In the macular type, numerous ill-defined, confluent, either hypopigmented or erythematous macules are seen. They are frequently slightly infiltrated. The nodular type, the classic and most common variety, may develop from the macular type or arise as such. It is characterized by papules, nodules, and diffuse infiltrates that are often dull red in color. Involvement of the eyebrows and forehead often results in a leonine facies, with a loss of eyebrows and eyelashes. The lesions themselves are not hypoesthetic, although, through involvement of the large peripheral nerves, disturbances of sensation develop, as well as trophic disturbances and nerve paralyses. The diffuse type of leprosy, common in Central America, especially in Mexico, shows diffuse infiltration of the skin without nodules. This infiltration may be quite inconspicuous except for the alopecia of the eyebrows and eyelashes it produces. Acral, symmetric anesthesia is generally present in the diffuse type (Rea and Levan, 1978).

Borderline leprosy exhibits clinical features of both tuberculoid and lepromatous leprosy, often with a prevalence of either one or the other, so that the patient may have borderline tuberculoid, true borderline, or borderline lepromatous leprosy. In the borderline tuberculoid form, the individual large macules resemble those of tuberculoid leprosy, but they are more numerous, often symmetrically distributed, and less sharply demarcated than in tuberculoid leprosy (Kwittken and Peck). In the borderline lepromatous form, a very characteristic feature is the presence of red, raised plaques with central clearing, resulting in an annular appearance (Arnold and Fasal).

Reactional leprosy may be classified as one of three types (Jolliffe). The most common form of reaction is known as the type 1 or lepra reaction, and patients in nonpolar categories of leprosy may have it, whether treated or untreated. Under treatment, there may be a shift toward the tuberculoid pole of the spectrum; this is called a reversal reaction. In untreated patients, the shift may be toward the lepromatous pole of the spectrum; this represents a downgrading reaction. The reaction in either case consists of swelling of the existing skin and nerve lesions associated with constitutional symptoms.

The type 2 reaction, referred to as erythema nodosum leprosum, occurs most commonly in lepromatous leprosy and rarely in borderline lepromatous leprosy. It may be seen not only in patients under treatment but also in untreated patients (Rea and Levan, 1975). Clinically, the reaction has a greater resemblance to erythema multiforme than to erythema nodosum. On normal skin between existing lepromatous lesions, one observes tender, red plaques and nodules together with areas of erythema and occasionally also purpura and vesicles. Ulceration, however, is rare. The eruption is widespread and is accompanied by fever, malaise, arthralgia, and leukocytosis. New lesions appear for only a few days in some cases but for weeks and even years in others (Jolliffe). This is the only type of reactional leprosy that responds to treatment with thalidomide (Jolliffe; Rea and Levan, 1978).

The type 3 reaction, called Lucio's phenomenon, occurs exclusively in diffuse lepromatous leprosy, in which it is a fairly common complication. It is usually seen in patients who have received either no or inadequate treatment (Rea and Levan, 1978). In contrast to erythema nodosum leprosum, fever, tenderness, and leukocytosis are absent, and the lesions are limited to the lower extremities, buttocks, and forearms. They consist of barely palpable, hemorrhagic, sharply marginated, irregular plaques. They develop into crusted lesions and, particularly on the legs, into ulcers (Rea and Levan, 1978). There may be repeated attacks or a continuous appearance of new lesions for years (Pursley et al).

Histopathology. Histologic examination in leprosy serves two purposes: establishment of the diagnosis and assignment of the disease to one of the seven recognized types. Assignment to one of the seven types requires clinical and histologic correlation. Since there may be variation in the histologic picture among different lesions of patients with borderline reactions (BT, BB, BL), the taking of multiple biopsy specimens is recommended in such patients (Ridley, 1977). It is probably advisable to assign priority to the clinical presentation over the histologic picture when the two are at variance, a situation that is not uncommon (Sehgal et al).

Indeterminate leprosy may be interpreted as a lesion in which a granuloma has not yet developed or in which the granuloma consists of only a few cells (Ridley, 1977). The dermis shows a nonspecific chronic inflammatory infiltrate around some of the blood vessels and skin appendages and perineurally. If nerves are infiltrated, it is usually possible to find a few acid-fast bacilli (Arnold and Fasal). Occasionally, the histologic picture of indeterminate leprosy is found in biopsies from patients with clinically well-established tuberculoid, borderline tuberculoid, or even borderline leprosy (Ridley, 1977; Sehgal et al). Since indeterminate leprosy usually represents a transitional stage, one may find fairly numerous lepra bacilli and occasional foamy macrophages in cases developing toward lepromatous leprosy and a few epithelioid cell granulomas in cases developing toward tuberculoid leprosy (Case Records, Massachusetts General Hospital, Case 21-1970).

Tuberculoid leprosy shows epithelioid cell granulomas that often are indistinguishable from those seen in sarcoidosis (Wiersema and Binford). The presence of a tuberculoid infiltrate and the scarcity or absence of bacilli are the result of an adequate immune response of the host to the lepra bacillus. A mild to moderate mononuclear cell infiltrate and, occasionally, giant cells, as in sarcoidosis, are present (Fig. 17-5). Since the epithelioid cell granulomas of tuberculoid leprosy form around dermal

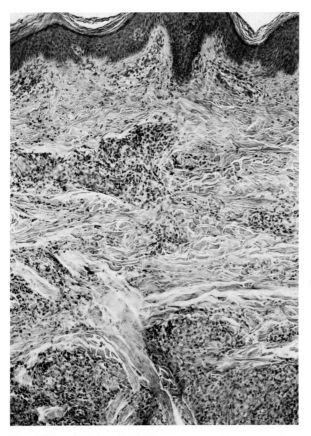

Fig. 17-5. Tuberculoid leprosy
The infiltrate shows epithelioid cell granulomas showing a slight admixture of monocytes, particularly at their margins. The histologic picture thus resembles that of sarcoidosis. (×100)

nerves undergoing necrosis, the granulomas of tuberculoid leprosy, like those of sarcoidosis, may show slight central necrosis. If present in the upper dermis, the infiltrate in tuberculoid leprosy, unlike that in lepromatous leprosy, does not necessarily remain separated from the epidermis by a free grenz zone but may touch the epidermis (Arnold and Fasal). Lepra bacilli usually are absent in quiescent lesions, but they may be found in small numbers if the specimen for biopsy is taken from the active margin of an extending lesion (Wiersema and Binford).

The following features aid in the differentiation of tuberculoid leprosy from sarcoidosis (see p. 233). First, in tuberculoid leprosy, if the biopsy specimen has been taken from the active margin of the lesion, bacilli may occasionally be found in the necrotic center of some of the granulomas on staining with the Fite stain. Second, in sections impregnated with silver, remnants of nerve tissue may be found in the necrotic center of some of the granulomas of tuberculoid leprosy. Third, since the granulomas of tuberculoid leprosy, in contrast to those of sarcoidosis, follow nerves, they often appear elongated (Wiersema and Binford).

Lepromatous leprosy as a rule shows an extensive cellular infiltrate that is almost invariably separated from the flattened epidermis by a narrow grenz zone of normal collagen. The infiltrate causes the destruction of the cutaneous appendages and extends into the subcutaneous fat. Macrophages with abundant foamy or vacuolated cytoplasm, so-called lepra cells or Virchow cells, predominate (Fig. 17-6). They resemble xanthoma cells and, on staining with fat stains, are shown to contain lipid, largely neutral fat and phospholipids rather than cholesterol. Because of the absence of cholesterol, the lipid is not doubly refractile, unlike the lipid in xanthoma. With the Fite stain, innumerable acid-fast, red-staining bacilli are seen measuring about 0.5 μm by 5 μm in size. They are found particularly within the lepra cells, where they often lie in bundles like packs of cigars or, if degenerated, in large clumps called globi (Fig. 17-7). In lepromatous leprosy, in contrast with tuberculoid leprosy, the nerves in the skin, although they may show considerable numbers of lepra bacilli, remain well preserved for a long time, and there is thus much less anesthesia in the cutaneous lesions of lepromatous leprosy than in those of tuberculoid leprosy (Wiersema and Binford).

In nonnodular diffuse lepromatous leprosy, one finds everywhere in the skin extensive infiltrates of foam cells containing many bacilli. Although

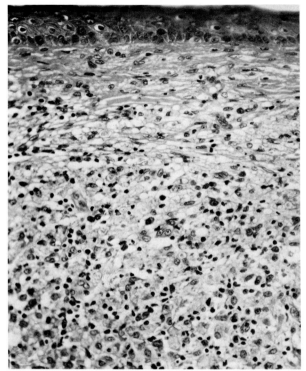

Fig. 17-6.   Lepromatous leprosy
The infiltrate is separated from the flattened epidermis by a narrow zone of normal collagen. Macrophages with abundant, foamy cytoplasm, so-called lepra cells, predominate. (×200)

Fig. 17-7.   Lepromatous leprosy
Fite stain. Numerous acid-fast lepra bacilli are present. They are found particularly within the lepra cells, where they tend to lie in bundles. (×800)

nodular lepromatous leprosy in the vast majority of cases also shows acid-fast bacilli in apparently normal skin, these bacilli are found only in small numbers in a perivascular distribution, often without foam cells. The perivascular distribution in the apparently normal skin of patients with nodular lepromatous leprosy suggests a hematogenous dissemination (Rea et al, 1975).

The large peripheral nerves in lepromatous leprosy contain large numbers of lepra bacilli, as many as are seen in the cutaneous infiltrate, with a minimal amount of inflammation. The Schwann cells are invaded, resulting in their destruction and subsequent fibrosis. Demyelinization ultimately is followed by axonal degeneration (Job and Desikan).

Autopsy reveals even in clinically quiescent cases bacilli in many organs, especially the liver and lymph nodes, including the visceral lymph nodes, as well as in the spleen, the adrenals, and the testes (Desikan and Job). The presence of bacillary depositions in the viscera explains the tendency toward relapse.

Borderline leprosy shows a wide range of histologic changes, depending on whether a case is one of borderline tuberculoid, true borderline, or borderline lepromatous leprosy. Generally, the cutaneous lesions show granulomatous aggregates containing both foamy macrophages and epithelioid cells. Usually, acid-fast bacilli can be found with ease, especially within macrophages (Kwittken and

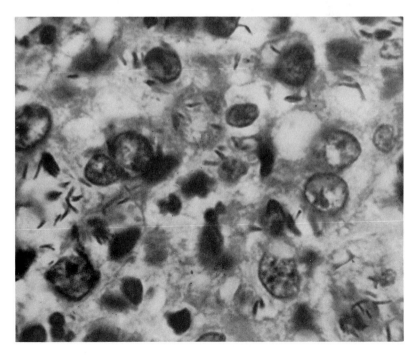

Peck). In contrast with lepromatous leprosy, lepra bacilli are not found in normal-appearing skin in borderline leprosy, not even in the borderline lepromatous form (Rea et al, 1975).

Reactional leprosy of type 1, referred to as the lepra reaction, shows a shift in the histologic picture toward the tuberculoid pole in patients with a "reversal reaction" and a shift toward the lepromatous pole in patients with a "downgrading reaction." The change in the type of leprosy usually is reflected also in changes in lepromin reactivity and lymphocyte transformation (see Histogenesis) (Jolliffe).

In *erythema nodosum leprosum*, or the type 2 reaction, the "erythema nodosum" lesions reveal the presence of a neutrophilic, leukocytoclastic vasculitis occasionally intermingled with eosinophils (Kramarsky et al). Scanty, fragmented bacilli are present around the vessels (Jolliffe). Small, foamy, histiocytic granulomas containing bacilli are scattered through the dermis and subcutis (Rea and Levan, 1975). Extravasated erythrocytes are often seen.

In *Lucio's phenomenon*, or the type 3 reaction, vascular changes are also prominent, but they differ from those seen in the type 2 reaction (Rea and Levan, 1978; Pursley et al). Endothelial proliferation leading to luminal obliteration is seen in association with thrombosis in the medium-sized vessels of the dermis and subcutis. There is a sparse, largely mononuclear infiltrate. Dense aggregates of acid-fast bacilli are found in the walls and the endothelium of normal-appearing vessels, as well as in vessels with proliferative changes. Ischemic necrosis, brought on by the vascular occlusion, leads to hemorrhagic infarcts and results in crusted erosions or frank ulcers.

Histogenesis. With respect to *immunologic reactivity*, patients with leprosy, particularly those with lepromatous leprosy, have a specific defect in cell-mediated immune responses to the lepra bacillus, which therefore cannot be eradicated from the body (Convit and Ulrich). The primary defect lies in the T lymphocytes, which can be stimulated only slightly or not at all to react against the lepra bacillus and thus do not adequately "instruct" macrophages to destroy phagocytized bacilli (Rea and Levan, 1977). This defect is specific for *M. leprae*, since, in the early phase of their disease, even patients with lepromatous leprosy show normal immunologic responses to antigens other than lepromin in both in vivo and in vitro testing (Rea et al, 1976). Generalized deficiencies in cell-mediated immune responses or excessive autoantibody production, as reported in many patients with lepromatous leprosy (Bullock), are remote sequelae of the disease. The specific

inability of T lymphocytes obtained from patients with lepromatous leprosy to react against lepromin is shown by the fact that, when these lymphocytes are incubated with lepromin, they show little or no production of macrophage migration inhibiting factor (MIF). In contrast, the lymphocytes of patients with tuberculoid leprosy produce significant amounts of MIF on exposure to lepromin (Katz et al). The lepromin-induced in vitro transformation of lymphocytes to lymphoblasts also varies with the type of leprosy. There is a progressively decreasing response by lymphocytes to lepromin as one descends from tuberculoid leprosy to lepromatous leprosy, with virtually no response at all by lymphocytes obtained from borderline lepromatous and lepromatous patients (Myrvang et al). In reversal reactions, there is a definite increase in the lymphocyte response to lepromin during the reaction and a decrease during the postreaction phase (Barnetson et al).

In advanced stages of lepromatous leprosy, there is apt to be hypergammaglobulinemia together with the presence of various antibodies, such as cryoglobulins of the mixed type, rheumatoid factor, or syphilis reagin (Rea and Levan, 1977).

In patients with either erythema nodosum leprosum or the Lucio phenomenon, deposits of immunoglobulin G (IgG) and the third component of complement (C3), as well as circulating immune complexes, have been found in the vessel walls of the dermal lesions. This suggests that both reactions are mediated by immune complexes (Wemambu et al; Sanchez et al; Quismorio et al).

The *lepromin skin test*, or Mitsuda test, consists of the intradermal injection of a crude preparation of *M. leprae* derived from autoclaved infected human tissue. A positive reaction consists of the formation of a nodule measuring 5 mm or more in diameter after 2 to 4 weeks. On histologic examination, the nodule shows an epithelioid cell granuloma. The reaction is positive only in the high resistance (tuberculoid and borderline tuberculoid) forms of the disease (Turk). In indeterminate leprosy, it may be positive or negative. The test detects the inability of patients at the lepromatous end of the spectrum to react to the injection of *M. leprae* with an epithelioid cell granuloma, and its main value is therefore as a marker of a specific absence of cell-mediated immunity to this organism. Because lepromin responsiveness is the rule in normal adults, it is of no diagnostic value (Rea and Levan, 1977).

M. leprae has not been grown on any culture media. However, like *M. marinum*, *M. leprae* can multiply if injected into the footpads of mice (Shepard). The nine-banded armadillo is much more susceptible than the mouse because of its low body temperature (32–35°C) and thus has become a useful research model for leprosy. When inoculated intradermally, subcutaneously, or intravenously with a suspension of *M. leprae*, 40% or more of nine-banded armadillos develop a disseminated infection after 15 to 34 months that histopathologically closely resembles lepromatous leprosy in humans (Storrs et al).

ELECTRON MICROSCOPY. On electron microscopy, *M. leprae* consists of an electron-dense cytoplasm lined by a trilaminal plasma membrane. Outside of this lies the bacterial cell wall surrounded by a radiolucent area, the waxy coating typical of mycobacteria (Kramarsky et al). Lepra bacilli are found in the skin predominantly in macrophages and in Schwann cells.

In *tuberculoid leprosy*, the Schwann cells of the cutaneous nerves at first contain lepra bacilli that possess an intact waxy coat. During the cell-mediated immune response against *M. leprae*, macrophages digest both the bacilli and the Schwann cells that contain them. After digestion, only macrophages with the appearance of epithelioid cells remain. The epithelioid cells in tuberculoid leprosy are free of mycobacteria and contain no lipid. On electron microscopy, they show a strongly positive reaction for acid phosphatase within numerous, well-preserved primary lysosomes (Job).

In *lepromatous leprosy*, in contrast, it is evident that the macrophages are incapable of digesting the lepra bacilli adequately. Initially, the bacilli are engulfed by phagocytic vacuoles into which primary lysosomes discharge their contents, causing partial lysis of the mycobacteria (Kramarsky et al). However, the multiplication of the mycobacteria is so rapid that the phagocytic vacuoles suffer damage as they become filled with lipid derived from the waxy coat of the mycobacteria (Imaeda). Thus, the foamy appearance of the macrophages that is evident by light microscopy is revealed by electron microscopy to be due to the presence of greatly enlarged, lipid-laden phagocytic vacuoles (Job). These lipid-laden vacuoles no longer are accessible to lysosomal enzymes, which are found in considerable concentration in the cytoplasm of the macrophages but outside of the phagocytic vacuoles (Job).

In *borderline leprosy*, bacterial growth activity and the cellular response are balanced, so that the mycobacteria do not multiply uninhibitedly, as they do in lepromatous leprosy. On electron microscopy, many of the cells containing bacilli have a cytologic appearance similar to that of epithelioid cells, and the phagolysosomes within them contain rather well preserved mycobacteria (Imaeda).

Differential Diagnosis.   The resemblance of and the consequent need to differentiate between lepromatous leprosy and xanthoma and between tuberculoid leprosy and sarcoidosis require re-emphasis, even though the differences have already been stressed in the histologic description.

ANTHRAX

Anthrax, caused by *Bacillus anthracis*, is enzootic in many countries. In the United States, anthrax occurs occasionally among workers in tanneries and wool-scouring mills through the handling of infected hides, wool, or hair imported from Asia (Matz and Brugsch). The lesion starts as a papule. The papule enlarges, and a hemorrhagic pustule forms. After the pustule has ruptured, a thick, black eschar covers the area. Marked erythema and edema surround the lesion. Characteristically, pain is slight or absent (Gold).

Histopathology.   At the site of the eschar, the epidermis is destroyed, and the ulcerated surface is covered with necrotic tissue. There is marked edema of the dermis. Numerous erythrocytes but only few inflammatory cells are present. The blood vessels are dilated, and their walls show diffuse degenerative changes.

Anthrax bacilli are present in large numbers and can be recognized in sections stained with routine stains, but they are best seen in sections stained with the Gram stain. The anthrax bacillus is a large, rod-shaped, encapsulated, gram-positive bacillus 6 μm to 10 μm long and 1 μm to 2 μm thick. Anthrax bacilli are found particularly in the necrotic tissue at the surface of the ulcer but also in the dermis. It is worth noting that phagocytosis of the bacilli by either neutrophils or histiocytes is absent (Lebowich et al).

TULAREMIA

Tularemia is caused by *Francisella (Pasteurella) tularensis*, a very small, gram-negative, pleomorphic coccobacillus. It is usually acquired by humans through direct contact with rodents (Young et al), but it may be transmitted from rodents to humans by insects, such as mosquitoes, ticks, or deerflies. The disease often occurs in small epidemics. It occurs in four types: (1) ulceroglandular, by far the most common, (2) oculoglandular, (3) pulmonary, and (4) typhoidal. Specific cutaneous lesions occur only in the ulceroglandular type.

In the ulceroglandular type, one or several painful ulcers occur as primary lesions at the site of infection, usually on the hands. Tender subcutaneous nodes may form along the lymph vessels that drain the primary lesion or lesions. There is considerable swelling of the regional lymph nodes, and the infection is associated with marked constitutional symptoms. Healing of the lesions takes place in 2 to 5 weeks.

Histopathology.   The primary ulcer shows at its base a nonspecific inflammatory infiltrate associated with a granulomatous reaction. In some cases, only a moderate number of epithelioid cells and a few giant cells are observed (Hitch and Smith). In others, however, large, well-developed tuberculoid granulomas are apparent (Lawless). These granulomas may show central necrosis with the presence of nuclear dust, so that there are, as in sporotrichosis (see p. 346), three zones: a central zone of necrosis, a "tuberculoid" zone surrounding it, and a peripheral "round cell" zone (Schuermann and Reich). Late lesions may show epithelioid cell tubercles that have no central necrosis and are surrounded by only a slightly inflammatory reaction, and they may thus have an appearance resembling that of sarcoidosis (Schuermann and Reich).

The tender nodes that may be found along lymph vessels show deep in the dermis and extending into the subcutaneous tissue multiple granulomas with a "sporotrichoid" arrangement into three zones. The central zone of necrosis in the granulomas may attain a much greater size than in the primary ulcer (Lawless). Similarly, the regional lymph nodes show multiple granulomas with irregularly shaped foci of necrosis (Reich).

F. tularensis, although present, does not stain in tissue sections. It can be demonstrated, however, in the exudate from cutaneous lesions or in tissue sections by the direct fluorescence-antibody technic with fluorescein-conjugated antiserum. In addition, specific agglutinins are present in the serum (Young et al).

Differential Diagnosis.   The histologic picture differs clearly from that of tuberculosis whenever the arrangement in three zones is present. Differentiation from sporotrichosis (see p. 346) and lymphogranuloma venereum (see p. 314), however, may be impossible.

ROCKY MOUNTAIN SPOTTED FEVER

Rocky Mountain spotted fever is caused by *Rickettsia rickettsii,* a very small, pleomorphic coccobacillus that is an obligate intracellular parasite. It is transmitted by ticks from infected animals. Contrary to its name, the disease is encountered most commonly in the Southeast of the United States.

After an incubation period of 1 to 2 weeks, chills and fever develop, and, a few days later, a rash appears that begins on the extremities and spreads to the trunk. The lesions at first are macular to papular but become purpuric within 2 to 3 days. There may be only petechiae but, in fatal cases, widespread ecchymoses are common. Because the diagnosis may not be made in the beginning and the course may be rapid, mortality exceeds 10%, despite the effectiveness of antibiotics such as tetracycline and chloramphenicol if given in time (Bradford and Hawkins). Whenever a diagnosis of Rocky Mountain spotted fever is suspected, a search should be made for an eschar indicating the site of a tick bite. One may find a hemorrhagic crust 8 mm by 10 mm in diameter surrounded by an erythematous ring (Walker et al, 1981).

Histopathology.   The small vessels of the dermis and of the subcutaneous fat show a necrotizing vasculitis with a perivascular infiltrate consisting mostly of lymphocytes and macrophages (Woodward et al). There is extravasation of erythrocytes. As a result of injury to the endothelial cells, luminal thrombosis and microinfarcts occur (Case Records, Massachusetts General Hospital, Case 18-1978). The causative organism, which is 0.3 μm by 1 μm in size, is too small to be visible by light microscopy, but it can be visualized by direct immunofluorescence, which thus is of considerable diagnostic value (see Histogenesis).

In addition to the cutaneous and subcutaneous vessels, the small vessels of the central nervous system are frequently involved. The vessels in many other organs may also be affected, leading, for instance, to focal necroses in the myocardium and liver and to acute interstitial pneumonitis (Case Records, Massachusetts General Hospital, Case 18-1978).

Histogenesis.   Since serologic tests such as the Weil–Felix complement fixation test may not become positive until 1 or 2 weeks after the onset of symptoms, *direct immunofluorescence testing* with fluorescein-labeled guinea pig antiserum to *R. rickettsii* is of great diagnostic value. *R. rickettsii* can be identified in monocytes from the buffy coat of the patient's blood or in cryostat sections of the patient's skin lesions (Woodward et al). Both substrates should be tested, since, in a series of 17 patients with Rocky Mountain spotted fever, examination of the skin alone gave a positive result in only 7 cases (Walker et al, 1978). In cases with a positive result, fluorescent coccal and bacillary forms are seen in endothelial cells and vascular walls of the dermis.

In patients with an eschar from a tick bite, a diagnosis of Rocky Mountain spotted fever may be possible already during the febrile period preceding the appearance of the skin lesions. Direct immunofluorescence testing of frozen sections of skin from the edge of the eschar with fluorescein-labeled antiserum to *R. rickettsii* reveals numerous immunofluorescent organisms of *R. rickettsii* within the dermal blood vessels (Walker et al, 1981).

Differential Diagnosis.   It is characteristic of the necrotizing vasculitis of Rocky Mountain spotted fever to show a predominantly mononuclear infiltrate (Walker et al, 1981).

CHANCROID

Chancroid, or "soft chancre," caused by *Hemophilus ducreyi,* is a venereal disease leading to one or several ulcers, chiefly in the genital region. The ulcers possess little if any induration and often have an undermined border. They are usually tender. Inguinal lymphadenitis, either unilateral or bilateral, is common and, unless treated, often results in an inguinal abscess called *bubo*.

Histopathology. The histologic changes observed beneath the ulcer are sufficiently distinct to permit a presumptive diagnosis of chancroid in many instances. The lesion consists of three vertically arranged zones and shows characteristic vascular changes (Margolis and Hood). The surface zone at the floor of the ulcer is rather narrow and consists of neutrophils, fibrin, erythrocytes, and necrotic tissue. The next zone is fairly wide and contains many newly formed blood vessels showing marked proliferation of their endothelial cells (Sheldon and Heyman). As a result of the endothelial proliferation, the lumina of the vessels are often occluded, leading to thrombosis. In addition, there are degenerative changes in the walls of the vessels. The deep zone is composed of a dense infiltrate of plasma cells and lymphoid cells.

Demonstration of Ducrey bacilli in tissue sections stained with the Giemsa stain, the Gram stain, or polychrome methylene blue is only rarely possible. The bacilli are most apt to be found between the cells of the surface zone (Sheldon and Heyman). In smears of serous exudate obtained from the undermined edge of the ulcer, Ducrey bacilli usually can be fairly easily seen on staining with the Giemsa or Gram stain. *H. ducreyi* is a fine, short, gram-negative coccobacillus, about 1.5 μm in length and 0.2 μm in width, often arranged in parallel chains, giving the appearance of a school of fish (Gaisin and Heaton). Fluorescent-antibody examination of smears is a very reliable method of establishing the diagnosis.

Histogenesis. On *electron microscopic examination* of tissue sections, coccobacilli are seen aggregated in groups in the interstitial space. They appear as rods about 1.3 μm long and 0.5 μm broad with rounded ends. Only rarely are bacilli seen in phagosomes of macrophages (Marsch et al).

GRANULOMA INGUINALE (DONOVANOSIS)

Granuloma inguinale, also called donovanosis, is a venereal disease caused by *Calymmatobacterium granulomatis,* which is found in the lesions as intracytoplasmic inclusion bodies called *Donovan bodies. C. granulomatis* is a gram-negative bacterium that grows only in a medium containing yolk of fertilized chicken eggs (Goldberg et al).

Granuloma inguinale occurs in the genital or perianal region either as a single lesion or as several lesions. The lesions consist of asymptomatic ulcers filled with exuberant granulation tissue that bleeds easily. The border of the ulcers is elevated and often has a serpiginous outline. Because the lesions spread by peripheral extension, they may attain a large size. In some instances, ulceration leads to mutilation owing to destruction of tissue (Fritz et al). In others, excessive granulation tissue causes vegetating lesions (Davis). Occasionally, squamous cell carcinoma supervenes (Beerman and Sonck; Davis).

Histopathology. In the center of the lesion, the epidermis is absent, whereas at the border, it shows acanthosis, which may reach the proportions of pseudocarcinomatous hyperplasia (Beerman and Sonck; Fritz et al). A dense infiltrate is present in the dermis that is composed predominantly of histiocytes and plasma cells. Scattered throughout this infiltrate are small abscesses composed of neutrophils. The number of lymphoid cells is conspicuously small.

Intracytoplasmic inclusion bodies, the Donovan bodies, are present within a variable number of histiocytes. The parasitized histiocytes, or macrophages, possess abundant cytoplasm and may measure 20 μm or more in diameter. Their cytoplasm has a multivacuolated appearance. Within each vacuole, also referred to as capsule, a small, ovoid Donovan body measuring 1 μm to 2 μm in diameter is seen (Fig. 17-8). In the cross sections of large histiocytes, several dozen such bodies may be observed (Davis and Collins).

The Donovan bodies are difficult to recognize in sections stained with hematoxylin-eosin. In sections stained with the Giemsa stain, they may be seen as ovoid bodies with intense bipolar staining surrounded by a lighter-staining vacuole or capsule. They are better visualized when a silver stain is used. The vacuole or capsule surrounding the Donovan bodies does not stain with silver stains (Davis).

Since the diagnosis of granuloma inguinale rests on the demonstration of the Donovan bodies, it may be pointed out that it is often easier to find them in smears made from crushed, fresh biopsy material and stained with the Wright or Giemsa stain than in routinely fixed tissue sections (Davis).

By far the best method for visualizing the Donovan bodies in tissue sections consists of cutting semithin sections 0.5 μm to 1 μm thick from plastic-embedded tissue blocks processed for electron microscopy and staining these sections with toluidine blue. The Donovan bodies then appear as dark, ovoid structures surrounded by a wide, clear vac-

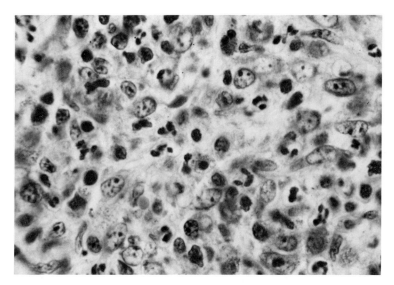

Fig. 17-8.   Granuloma inguinale (donovanosis)
The dense infiltrate is composed predominantly of histiocytes and plasma cells. There is a diffuse sprinkling of neutrophils. Several of the histiocytes contain within their cytoplasms aggregates of Donovan bodies. (×400)

uole or capsule (Davis and Collins). In some instances, several Donovan bodies are seen within the same vacuole (Dodson et al).

Histogenesis. Analogous to the findings in semithin sections, *electron microscopic examination* of Donovan bodies has shown that the bacteria are surrounded by a vacuole. By coalescence, larger vacuoles containing several Donovan bodies may form. Some vacuoles appear electron-lucent throughout, whereas others contain small amounts of amorphous granular material (Dodson et al). Each microorganism is limited on its outer surface by a corrugated bacterial cell wall, medial to which is a trilaminar plasma membrane. The corrugated appearance of the cell wall and the fact that division takes place by invagination of both the cell wall and the plasma membrane are features typical of gram-negative bacteria (Davis and Collins). The vacuoles surrounding the Donovan bodies are lined by a trilaminar limiting membrane (Dodson et al). This suggests that the vacuoles represent phagosomes, rather than capsules as originally assumed. An analogous situation exists in histoplasmosis, in which *Histoplasma capsulatum* also lies in phagosomes and possesses no capsule, contrary to what was once thought (see p. 345) (Davis and Collins).

Differential Diagnosis. The parasitism of histiocytes is strikingly similar to that observed in rhinoscleroma, histoplasmosis, and leishmaniasis. However, the small size of the Donovan bodies and the presence of small abscesses in the infiltrate usually make differentiation of granuloma inguinale from these three diseases possible (see Table 20-1, p. 358).

A difficult problem may be posed by the marked epidermal proliferation that is present occasionally in granuloma inguinale (Beerman and Sonck; Fritz et al). Several biopsies may be necessary to determine whether this represents merely pseudocarcinomatous hyperplasia (see p. 505) or squamous cell carcinoma.

RHINOSCLEROMA

Rhinoscleroma is a chronic infectious but only mildly contagious disease in which the nose, the pharynx, the larynx, the trachea, and occasionally also the skin of the upper lip are infiltrated with hard, granulomatous masses. The disorder always begins in the nose.

Histopathology. The cellular infiltrate is very rich in plasma cells and contains two striking structures: Mikulicz cells and Russell bodies. Because of their presence, the histologic picture of rhinoscleroma is diagnostic (Convit et al).

The Mikulicz cell is a large histiocyte measuring from 10 μm to 100 μm in diameter. It has a pale, vacuolated cytoplasm. Within the cytoplasm of the Mikulicz cells, one finds many bacilli, called *Klebsiella rhinoscleromatis* or Frisch bacilli (Fig. 17-9). They can be seen in sections stained with hematoxylin-eosin but are better visualized with the Giemsa stain or a silver stain. They also stain vividly red with the PAS technique (Fisher and Dimling). They are gram-negative rods that measure 2 μm to 3 μm in length and appear round or ovoid in cross sections. Although it is likely, it has not been proved that rhinoscleroma is caused by Frisch bacilli, since the disease has not been reproduced by cultures of this organism.

Russell bodies are round to ovoid formations measuring up to 40 μm in diameter. They thus can be twice as large as normal plasma cells. They have a homogeneous, bright red appearance and are light-refractile (Fig. 17-10). They are also PAS-positive. They arise within plasma cells as a result of excessive synthesis of immunoglobulins (see Histogenesis).

In long-standing lesions, marked fibrosis is present (Hoffmann et al). The mucosal epithelium overlying the cellular infiltrate often shows hyperplasia, which may be so pronounced as to give rise to a mistaken diagnosis of squamous cell carcinoma (Fisher and Dimling).

Histogenesis. *Electron microscopy* reveals numerous vacuoles of varying size within the Mikulicz cells. Some vacuoles contain one or a few bacilli up to 4 μm in length. They are surrounded by a characteristic coat of finely granular, filamentous material arranged in a radial fashion. This coating material contains mucopolysaccharides and is responsible for the positive PAS-reaction of the bacteria (Fukuhara and Klingmüller). Other vacuoles, however, contain no bacteria but merely small amounts of finely granular material similar to that coating the bacteria (Hoffmann et al). Since the vacuoles are lined by a limiting membrane, they can be regarded as phagosomes (Hoffmann et al).

The Russell bodies form within plasma cells through enlargement of the rough endoplasmic reticulum and the accumulation of amorphous or granular electron-dense material within the cisternae. When the plasma cell is overloaded with this material, the nucleus and cytoplasmic organelles degenerate. The material involved in the morphogenesis of the Russell bodies represents immunoglobulin, as shown by immunofluorescence (Erlach et al). (See also p. 51.)

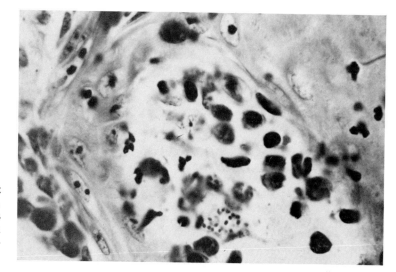

Fig. 17-9.   Rhinoscleroma
Giemsa stain. There are several Mikulicz cells, the cytoplasm of which is pale, foamy, and vacuolated. One Mikulicz cell contains in its cytoplasm many Frisch bacilli, which appear here as small, round, deeply staining bodies. (×900)

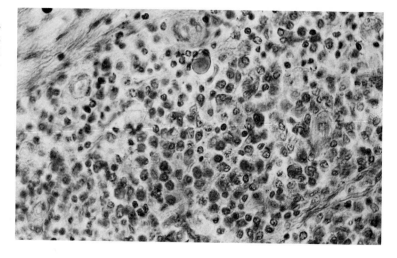

Fig. 17-10.   Rhinoscleroma
The infiltrate contains many plasma cells and one Russell body. The Russell body is larger than the cells in the infiltrate and has a homogeneous, brilliant red, light-refractile cytoplasm. (×400)

Differential Diagnosis. Parasitized histiocytes are also observed in granuloma inguinale, histoplasmosis, and leishmaniasis. For their differentiation, see Oriental Leishmaniasis (p. 357; see also Table 20-1, p. 358). Rhinoscleroma differs from the other three diseases by the abundance of plasma cells and the presence of Russell bodies, which are therefore of considerable diagnostic value. However, Russell bodies are not specific for rhinoscleroma; they may occur in other diseases when an infiltrate rich in plasma cells is present—for instance, in syphilis, lupus vulgaris, and squamous cell carcinoma.

LYMPHOGRANULOMA VENEREUM

Lymphogranuloma venereum is a venereal disease. The organism causing it is a member of the species *Chlamydia trachomatis* (see Histogenesis). Chlamydiae are bacterialike and definitely are not viruses (Schachter). They are related to rickettsiae in structure, metabolism, and mode of reproduction and by containing two nucleic acids, both deoxyribonucleic acid (DNA) and ribonucleic acid (RNA).

The incubation period of lymphogranuloma venereum varies from 3 to 30 days but on the average is 7 days. The primary lesion is a small erosion or papule 5 mm to 8 mm in size. This heals within a few days and may pass unnoticed. Within 1 to 2 weeks after the appearance of the primary lesion, enlargement of the inguinal lymph nodes begins, usually on one side only but occasionally bilaterally. Inguinal lymphadenopathy occurs in all heterosexual men infected with this disease but in only some women. The involved inguinal lymph nodes at first are firm but subsequently develop multiple areas of suppuration, resulting in draining sinuses. The lymphadenopathy usually subsides within 2 to 3 months. Rarely, elephantiasis of the penis and scrotum or chronic penile ulcerations arise as a late complication (Hopsu-Havu and Sonck).

In women in whom the infection begins in the lower portion of the vagina, drainage is to the iliac and anorectal lymph nodes rather than to the inguinal lymph nodes, causing a proctitis. Rectal stricture and perineal ulcerations are fairly common late complications in these women (Sonck). Proctitis and rectal strictures also occur in homosexual men (Becker).

Histopathology. The changes in the initial papule are nonspecific. In the lymph nodes, so-called stellate abscesses represent the characteristic lesion and, although not specific for lymphogranuloma venereum, are highly suggestive.

The earliest change in the lymph nodes consists of the formation of small, scattered islands of epithelioid cells. Often, a few giant cells are found among the epithelioid cells. As these islands increase in size, they become embedded in a chronic granulation tissue containing many plasma cells. With a further increase in size, the centers of the epithelioid cell islands undergo necrosis and become filled with numerous neutrophils, as well as some macrophages (Sheldon and Heyman). These central abscesses tend to have a triangular or a quadrangular shape with elongated corners, resulting in a stellate appearance (Fig. 17-11). The epithelioid cells surrounding the abscesses show a palisading arrangement. As the abscesses enlarge gradually, they coalesce and lose their stellate appearance. No organisms can be identified in histologic sections (Sheldon and Heyman).

Histogenesis. There are several strains of *Chlamydia trachomatis* that are related antigenically. They include the organisms responsible for trachoma, inclusion conjunctivitis, nongonococcal urethritis, and lymphogranuloma venereum (Schachter). Chlamydiae are bacterialike and differ from viruses in that they have two nucleic acids and a discrete cell wall similar to that found in gram-negative bacteria. Furthermore, they contain certain enzymes, multiply within the host cell by binary fission, and undergo no eclipse phase. The sole feature that chlamydiae share with viruses is the obligatory intracellular nature of their parasitism. For this reason, they grow well in the yolk sac and in cell cultures (Schachter).

Chlamydiae undergo a developmental cycle and, as can be seen by *electron microscopy*, occur in two forms: elementary body and initial body (Filipp and Metz). The elementary body is adapted to an extracellular environment and is infective for other cells. It measures about 0.3 μm in diameter and consists of a round, electron-dense inner body surrounded by an electron-lucid halo and a membrane. After entering a host cell by means of phagocytosis, it develops into a metabolically active initial body 0.5 μm to 1 μm in diameter. Multiplication takes place by division of the nucleus. This division results in two elementary bodies, which, on leaving the host cell, can infect other cells (Schachter).

CAT-SCRATCH DISEASE

Two to three weeks after a person has been scratched by a cat, a large, tender swelling of a group of lymph nodes may develop in the drainage area of the scratch. In some patients, the cat scratch heals in a normal fashion; in others, one or several papules appear 2 to 4 days after the scratch has occurred (Daniels and MacMurray). In some instances, the affected lymph nodes become fluctuant as a result of suppuration. The average duration of lymph node enlargement is 2 months.

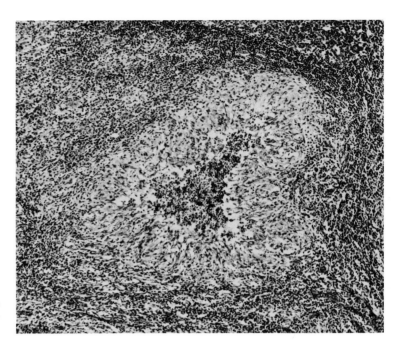

Fig. 17-11. Lymphogranuloma venereum
In the lymph node is a stellate abscess surrounded by epithelioid cells in a palisade formation. (×100)

Histopathology. The primary papules at the site of the scratch show one or several acellular areas of necrosis in the dermis. These areas are of various shapes, including round, triangular, and stellate. Surrounding them are several layers of histiocytic and epithelioid cells, with the innermost layer showing a palisading arrangement. A few giant cells may be present. The periphery of the epithelioid cell reaction is surrounded by a zone of lymphoid cells (Johnson and Helwig).

The reaction in the lymph nodes is similar to that observed in the skin, except that the central areas of necrosis in the epithelioid cell granulomas undergo abscess formation through the accumulation of numerous neutrophils (Daniels and MacMurray). As the abscesses enlarge, they become confluent.

Histogenesis. The agent that causes cat-scratch disease has not been identified. However, the great resemblance of the changes in the lymph nodes to those observed in lymphogranuloma venereum (see p. 314) makes it likely that cat-scratch disease is caused by a chlamydialike organism.

BIBLIOGRAPHY

Impetigo

AMON RB, DIMOND RL: Toxic epidermal necrolysis. Rapid differentiation between staphylococcal- and drug-induced disease. Arch Dermatol 111:1433–1437, 1975

DIMOND RL, WOLFF HH, BRAUN-FALCO O: The staphylococcal scalded skin syndrome. Br J Dermatol 96:483–492, 1977

DIMOND RL, WUEPPER KD: Das staphylogene Lyell-Syndrom. Hautarzt 28:447–455, 1977

ELIAS PM, FRITSCH P, EPSTEIN EH JR: Staphylococcal scalded skin syndrome. (Review) Arch Dermatol 113:207–219, 1977

ELIAS PM, LEVY SW: Bullous impetigo. Occurrence of localized scalded skin syndrome in an adult. Arch Dermatol 112:856–858, 1976

ELLIS FA: Subcorneal pustular dermatosis. Arch Dermatol 78:580–588, 1958

FRITSCH P, ELIAS P, VARGA J: The fate of staphylococcal exfoliatin in newborn and adult mice. Br J Dermatol 95:275–284, 1976

KAPLAN EL, ANTHONY BF, CHAPMANN SS et al: Epidemic acute glomerulonephritis associated with type 49 streptococcal pyoderma. Am J Med 48:9–27, 1970

KELLY C, TAPLIN D, ALLEN AM: Streptococcal ecthyma. Arch Dermatol 103:306–310, 1971

LEVINE J, NORDEN CW: Staphylococcal scalded-skin syndrome in an adult. N Engl J Med 287:1339–1340, 1972

MELISH ME, GLASGOW LA: The staphylococcal scalded-skin syndrome. N Engl J Med 282:1114–1119, 1970

MELISH ME, GLASGOW LA, TURNER MD: The staphylococcal scalded-skin syndrome: Isolation and partial characterization of the exfoliative toxin. J Infect Dis 125:129–140, 1972

NOBLE WC, PRESBURY D, CONNOR BL: Prevalence of streptococci and staphylococci in lesions of impetigo. Br J Dermatol 91:115–116, 1974

PACHINGER W: Staphylogenes Lyell-Syndrome bei einer Erwachsenen mit Agranulocytose. Z Hautkr 55:57–67, 1980

PETER G, SMITH AL: Group A streptococcal infections of the skin and pharynx. N Engl J Med 297:311–317, 1977

REID LH, WESTON WL, HUMBERT JR: Staphlococcal scalded skin syndrome. Arch Dermatol 109:239–241, 1974

RIDGWAY HB, LOWE NJ: Staphylococcal syndrome in an adult with Hodgkin's disease. Arch Dermatol 115:589–590, 1979

RITTER VON RITTERSHAIN G: Die exfoliative Dermatitis jüngerer Säuglinge. Centralzeitschrift für Kinderheilkunde 2:3–23, 1878

STEIGLEDER GK: Zur Differentialdiagnose des Pemphigus vulgaris aus dem Blasengrundausstrich. Arch Klin Exp Dermatol 202:1–9, 1955

WUEPPER KD, DIMOND RL, KNUTSON DD: Studies of the mechanism of epidermal injury by a staphylococcal epidermolytic toxin. J Invest Dermatol 65:191–200, 1975

Erysipelas

TAPPEINER J, PFLEGER L: Zur Histopathologie cutaner Lymphgefässe beim chronisch-rezidivierenden Erysipel der unteren Extremitäten. Hautarzt 15:517–518, 1970

Acute Deep Folliculitis (Furuncle)

PINKUS H: Furuncle. J Cutan Pathol 6:517–518, 1979

Chronic Superficial Folliculitis

MONTGOMERY H: Acne necrotica miliaris of the scalp. Arch Dermatol Syph 36:40–44, 1937

STRITZLER C, FRIEDMAN R, LOVEMAN AB: Acne necrotica. Arch Dermatol Syph 64:464–469, 1951

Chronic Deep Folliculitis

BOGG A: Folliculitis decalvans. Acta Derm Venereol (Stockh) 43:14–24, 1963

LAYMON CW, MURPHY RJ: The cicatrial alopecias. J Invest Dermatol 8:99–122, 1947

MEINHOF W, BRAUN-FALCO O: Über die Folliculitis sycosiformis atrophicans barbae Hoffmann (Sycosis lupoides Milton-Brocq, Ulerythema sycosiforme Unna). Dermatol Wochenschr 152:153–167, 1966

MOYER DG, WILLIAMS RM: Perifolliculitis capitis abscedens et suffodiens. Arch Dermatol 85:378–384, 1962

SUTER L: Folliculitis decalvans. Hautarzt 32:429–431, 1981

Pseudofolliculitis of the Beard

STRAUSS JS, KLIGMAN AM: Pseudofolliculitis of the beard. Arch Dermatol 74:533–542, 1956

Follicular Occlusion Triad

BRUNSTING HA: Hidradenitis suppurativa: Abscess of the apocrine sweat glands. Arch Dermatol Syph 39:108–120, 1939

CURRY SS, GAITHER DH, KING LE JR: Squamous cell carcinoma arising in dissecting perifolliculitis of the scalp. J Am Acad Dermatol 4:673–678, 1981.

DJAWARI D, HORNSTEIN OP: Recurrent chronic pyoderma with cellular immunodeficiency. Dermatologica 161:116–123, 1980

DVORAK VC, ROOT RK, MACGREGOR RR: Host-defensive mechanisms in hidradenitis suppurative. Arch Dermatol 113:450–453, 1977

HYLAND CH, KHEIR SM: Follicular occlusion disease with elimination of abnormal elastic tissue. Arch Dermatol 116:925–928, 1980

MCMULLAN FH, ZELIGMAN I: Perifolliculitis capitis abscedens et suffodiens. Arch Dermatol 73:256–263, 1956

MOSCHELLA SL, KLEIN MH, MILLER RJ: Perifolliculitis capitis abscedens et suffodiens. Arch Dermatol 96:195–197, 1967

MOYER DG, WILLIAMS RM: Perifolliculitis capitis abscedens et suffodiens. Arch Dermatol 85:378–384, 1962

PILLSBURY DM, SHELLEY WB, KLIGMAN AM: Dermatology, p 481. Philadelphia, WB Saunders, 1956

STRAUSS JS: Acne conglobata. In Fitzpatrick TB, Eisen AZ, Wolff K et al (eds): Dermatology in General Medicine, 2nd ed, pp 452–453. New York, McGraw-Hill, 1979

Blastomycosislike Pyoderma (Pyoderma Vegetans)

BRUNSTING LA, UNDERWOOD LJ: Pyoderma vegetans in association with chronic ulcerative colitis. Arch Dermatol Syph 60:161–172, 1949

DJAWARI D, HORNSTEIN OP: In vitro studies on microphage functions in chronic pyoderma vegetans. Arch Dermatol Res 263:97–104, 1978

FORMAN L: Pemphigus vegetans of Hallopeau. Arch Dermatol 114:627–628, 1978

GETLIK A, FARKAS J, PALENIKOVA O et al: Pyoderma vegetans bei zellulärer Immunitätsdefizienz. Dermatol Monatsschr 166:645–648, 1980

RUZICKA T, GOERZ G: Beobachtungen bei der Pyodermite végétante Hallopeau. Z Hautkr 54:24–32, 1979

SU WPD, DUNCAN SC, PERRY HO: Blastomycosis-like pyoderma. Arch Dermatol 115:170–173, 1979

WILLIAMS HM JR, STONE OJ: Blastomycosis-like pyoderma. Arch Dermatol 93:226–228, 1966

Acute Septicemia

DALLDORF FG, JENNETTE JC: Fatal meningococcal septicemia. Arch Pathol 101:6–9, 1977

DORFF, GI, GEIMER NF, ROSENTHAL DR et al: Pseudomonas septicemia. Illustrated evolution of its skin lesion. Arch Intern Med 128:591–595, 1971

FERGUSON JH, CHAPMAN OD: Fulminating meningococcic infections and the so-called Waterhouse-Friderichsen syndrome. Am J Pathol 24:763–795, 1948

HALL JH, CALLAWAY JL, TINDALL JP et al: *Pseudomonas aeruginosa* in dermatology. Arch Dermatol 97:312–324, 1968

HILL WR, KINNEY TD: The cutaneous lesions in acute meningococcemia. JAMA 134:513–518, 1947

MANDELL JN, FEINER HP, PRICE NM et al: *Pseudomonas cepacia* endocarditis and ecthyma gangrenosum. Arch Dermatol 113:199–202, 1977

PLAUT ME: Staphylococcal septicemia and pustular purpura. Arch Dermatol 99:82–85, 1969

SCHLOSSBERG D: Multiple erythematous nodules as a manifestation of *Pseudomonas aeruginosa* septicemia. Arch Dermatol 116:446–447, 1980

SHAPIRO L, TEISCH JA, BROWNSTEIN MH: Dermatohistopathology of chronic gonococcal sepsis. Arch Dermatol 107:403–406, 1973

WINKELSTEIN A, SONGSTER CL, CARAS TS et al: Fulminant meningococcemia and disseminated intravascular coagulation. Arch Intern Med 124:55–59, 1969

Chronic Septicemia

ABU-NASSAR H, FRED HL, YOW EM: Cutaneous manifestations of gonococcemia. Arch Intern Med 112:731–737, 1963

ACKERMAN AB: Hemorrhagic bullae in gonococcemia. N Engl J Med 282:793–794, 1970

ACKERMAN AB, MILLER RC, SHAPIRO L: Gonococcemia and its cutaneous manifestations. Arch Dermatol 91:227–232, 1965

BJÖRNBERG A: Benign gonococcal sepsis. Acta Derm Venereol (Stockh) 50:313–316, 1970

KAHN G, DANIELSSON D: Septic gonococcal dermatitis. Arch Dermatol 99:421–425, 1969

NIELSEN LT: Chronic meningococcemia. Arch Dermatol 102:97–101, 1970

OGNIBENE AJ, DITTO MR: Chronic meningococcemia. Arch Intern Med 114:29–32, 1964

SCHOOLNIK GK, BUCHANAN TM, HOLMES KK et al: Gonococci causing disseminated gonococcal infection are resistant to the bactericidal action of normal human sera. J Clin Invest 58:163–1173, 1976

and histopathological classification of leprosy. Dermatologica 161:93–96, 1980

SHEPARD CC: The experimental disease that follows the injection of human leprosy bacilli into foot-pads of mice. J Exp Med 112:445–454, 1960

STORRS EE, BINFORD CH, MIGAKI G: Experimental lepromatous leprosy in nine-banded armadillos (*Dasypus novemcinctus* Linn). Am J Pathol 92:813–816, 1978

TURK JL: Leprosy as a model of subacute and chronic immunologic disease. J Invest Dermatol 67:457–463, 1976

WEMAMBU SNC, TURK JL, WATERS MFR et al: Erythema nodosum leprosum: A clinical manifestation of the Arthus phenomenon. Lancet 2:933–935, 1969

WIERSEMA JP, BINFORD CH: The identification of leprosy among epithelioid cell granulomas of the skin. Int J Lepr 40:10–32, 1972

Anthrax

GOLD H: Anthrax. Arch Intern Med 96:387–396, 1955

LEBOWICH RJ, MCKILLIP BG, CONBOY JR: Cutaneous anthrax. Am J Clin Pathol 13:505–515, 1943

MATZ MH, BRUGSH HG: Anthrax in Massachusetts, 1943 to 1962. JAMA 188:635–638, 1964

Tularemia

HITCH JM, SMITH DC: Cutaneous manifestations of tularemia. Arch Dermatol Syph 38:859–876, 1938

LAWLESS TK: Tularemia. (Review) Arch Dermatol Syph 44:147–160, 1941

REICH H: Zur Kenntnis der Tularämie hautnaher (regionaler) Lymphknoten. Arch Dermatol Syph (Berlin) 192:175–188, 1950

SCHUERMANN H, REICH H: Zur Klinik und Histologie des cutan lokalisierten tularämischen Primäraffekts. Arch Dermatol Syph (Berlin) 190:579–604, 1950

YOUNG LS, BICKNELL DS, ARCHER BG et al: Tularemia epidemic: Vermont, 1968. N Engl J Med 280:1253–1260, 1969

Rocky Mountain Spotted Fever

BRADFORD WD, HAWKINS HK: Rocky Mountain spotted fever in childhood. Am J Dis Child 131:1228–1232, 1977

Case Records of the Massachusetts General Hospital, Case 18-1978. Rocky Mountain spotted fever. N Engl J Med 298:1071–1078, 1978

WALKER DH, CAIN BG, OLMSTEAD M: Laboratory diagnosis demonstration of *Rickettsia rickettsii* in cutaneous lesions. Am J Clin Pathol 69:619–623, 1978

WALKER DH, GAY RM, VALDES-DAPENA M: The occurrence of eschars in Rocky Mountain spotted fever. J Am Acad Dermatol 4:571–576, 1981

WOODWARD TE, PEDERSEN CE JR, OSTER CN et al: Prompt confirmation of Rocky Mountain spotted fever: Identification of rickettsia in skin tissues. J Infect Dis 134:297–301, 1976

Chancroid

GAISIN A, HEATON CL: Chancroid: Alias the soft chancre. Int J Dermatol 14:188–197, 1975

MARGOLIS RJ, HOOD AF: Chancroid: Diagnosis and treatment. J Am Acad Dermatol 6:493–499, 1982

MARSCH WC, HAAS N, STÜTTGEN G: Ultrastructural detection of *Haemophilus ducreyi* in biopsies of chancroid. Arch Dermatol Res 263:153–157, 1978

SHELDON WH, HEYMAN A: Studies on chancroid. Am J Pathol 22:415–425, 1946

Granuloma Inguinale

BEERMAN H, SONCK CE: The epithelial changes in granuloma inguinale. Am J Syph 36:501–510, 1952

DAVIS CM: Granuloma inguinale. JAMA 211:632–636, 1970

DAVIS CM, COLLINS C: Granuloma inguinale: An ultrastructural study of *Calymmatobacterium granulomatis*. J Invest Dermatol 53:315–321, 1969

DODSON RF, FRITZ GS, HUBLER WR JR et al: Donovanosis: A morphologic study. J Invest Dermatol 62:611–614, 1974

FRITZ GS, HUBLER WR, DODSON RF et al: Mutilating granuloma inguinale. Arch Dermatol 111:1464–1465, 1975

GOLDBERG J, WEAVER RH, PACKER H: Studies on granuloma inguinale. I. Bacteriologic behavior of *Donovania granulomatis*. Am J Syph 37:60–70, 1953

Rhinoscleroma

CONVIT J, KERDEL-VEGAS F, GORDON B: Rhinoscleroma. Arch Dermatol 84:55–62, 1961

ERLACH E, GEBHART W, NIEBAUER G: Ultrastructural investigations on the morphogenesis of Russell bodies. (Abstr) J Cutan Pathol 3:145, 1976

FISHER ER, DIMLING C: Rhinoscleroma. Arch Pathol 78:501–512, 1964

FUKUHARA S, KLINGMÜLLER G: Elektronenmikroskopische Untersuchungen des Rhinoscleroms. Arch Dermatol Res 254:263–274, 1975

HOFFMANN E, LOOSE LD, HARKIN JC: The Mikulicz cell in rhinoscleroma. Am J Pathol 73:47–58, 1973

Lymphogranuloma Venereum

BECKER LE: Lymphogranuloma venereum. Int J Dermatol 15:26–33, 1976

FILIPP N, METZ J: Erregernachweis bei Lymphogranulomatosis inguinalis. Eine elektronenmikroskopische Untersuchung. Hautarzt 26:411–415, 1975

HOPSU-HAVU VK, SONCK CE: Infiltrative, ulcerative, and fistular lesions of the penis due to lymphogranuloma venereum. Br J Vener Dis 49:193–202, 1973

SCHACHTER J: Chlamydial infections. N Engl J Med 298:428–435, 490–495, 1978

SHELDON WH, HEYMAN A: Lymphogranuloma venereum. Am J Pathol 23:653–671, 1947

SONCK CE: Lymphogranuloma inguinale. Hautarzt 23:280–286, 1972

Cat-Scratch Disease

DANIELS WB, MACMURRAY FG: Cat-scratch disease. Arch Intern Med 88:736–751, 1951

JOHNSON WT, HELWIG EB: Cat-scratch disease. Histopathologic changes in the skin. Arch Dermatol 100:148–154, 1969

18 Treponemal Diseases

SYPHILIS

Acquired syphilis occurs on the skin in two stages: early and late. The early stage comprises primary and secondary syphilis; the late stage, tertiary syphilis. During the early stage, the causative organism, *Treponema pallidum* (*Spirochaeta pallida*), can often be demonstrated in the cutaneous lesions either by dark-field examination of tissue fluid or by silver staining or fluorescent-antibody staining of tissue sections (see p. 322). During the late stage, no spirochetes can be demonstrated in the cutaneous lesions.

Primary syphilis is characterized by the syphilitic, or hard, chancre, which usually is a single lesion but may be multiple. The typical, or hunterian, chancre is represented by a brownish red, indurated, round papule or plaque with an eroded surface, usually measuring from 1 cm to 2 cm in diameter. Occasionally, the chancre shows ulceration. The regional lymph nodes are enlarged.

Secondary syphilis is characterized by a more or less generalized eruption composed usually of macules or papules brownish red in color. In some instances, there are papulosquamous lesions that resemble guttate psoriasis. In the anogenital region, the papules may become large, verrucous, and moist; then they are called condylomata lata. (They must be differentiated from condylomata acuminata, a variety of verruca; see p. 376.) On the palms and the soles, discrete, hyperkeratotic, centrally pitted papules may be present (syphilis cornée). Ulcerating lesions in secondary syphilis are very rare and occur only in severe cases, so-called lues maligna. In secondary syphilis, there may be recurrent attacks, with later attacks usually having fewer but larger lesions that may be grouped, annular, or serpiginous.

Occasionally, a benign, self-limited hepatitis occurs during secondary syphilis with tenderness and enlargement of the liver and, in some cases, jaundice. In rare instances, an acute nephrosis or glomerulonephritis occurs in secondary syphilis.

Tertiary syphilis often shows only a single lesion, but there are occasionally several lesions. A superficial nodular type and a deep gummatous type occur. Lesions of the nodular type show a smooth, atrophic center and an active serpiginous border composed of nodules that may be superficially ulcerated. Lesions of the gummatous type begin as a soft cutaneous or subcutaneous swelling that breaks down to form one or several ulcers with a punched-out appearance. In rare instances, juxta-articular nodes occur. They are painless, subcutaneous, fibrous nodules, often symmetrically situated in the vicinity of joints. The elbows and knees are the sites of predilection.

Histopathology. The two fundamental pathologic changes in syphilis are swelling and proliferation of endothelial cells, and a predominantly perivascular infiltrate composed of lymphoid cells and many plasma cells. In late secondary and in tertiary syphilis, one usually also finds a granulomatous infiltrate of epithelioid and giant cells.

Primary Syphilis. In a typical hard chancre, the epidermis shows slight acanthosis at the margin of the lesion. Toward the center, the epidermis gradually becomes thinner and appears edematous and permeated by inflammatory cells. In the center, the epidermis may be absent (Fig. 18-1). An infiltrate composed of lymphoid cells and many plasma cells is present in the dermis. It is compact in the center and consists of individual perivascular islands at the margin. The capillaries show considerable proliferation of their endothelial cells (Fig. 18-2), and their walls may be invaded by the cellular infiltrate.

On staining with a silver stain, such as the Levaditi stain or the Warthin–Starry stain, spirochetes usually can be found in the epidermis and in the dermis around the walls of capillaries. If seen in their full length, which is rare, spirochetes generally show 8 to 12 spiral convolutions, each measuring from 1 μm to 1.2 μm in length. When spirochetes are stained with silver, it must be remembered that silver also stains melanin and reticulum fibers. Differentiation may cause some difficulties but should be possible on the basis of the fact that the melanin in the dendritic processes of melanocytes has a granular appearance, the granules being thicker and more heavily stained than *T. pallidum*. It has therefore been suggested that a silver stain be performed routinely on all specimens in which early syphilis is suspected (Jeerapaet and Ackerman).

Histologic examination of swollen regional lymph nodes in primary syphilis most commonly reveals

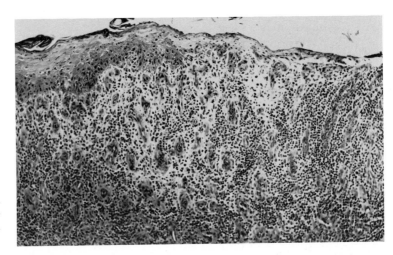

Fig. 18-1.   Primary syphilis
Low magnification. The margin of an erosion is shown. The epidermis gradually becomes thinner as it approaches the erosion. (×100)

Fig. 18-2.   Primary syphilis
High magnification of Figure 18-1. The capillaries show proliferation of their endothelial cells. Many plasma cells are present in the dense infiltrate. (×400)

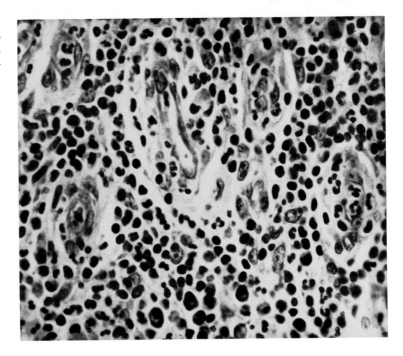

a chronic inflammatory infiltrate containing many plasma cells. In addition, there are endothelial proliferation and follicular hyperplasia. Spirochetes are numerous and can nearly always be identified with the Warthin–Starry stain. In some instances, noncaseating granulomas resembling those of sarcoidosis are found in the lymph nodes (Hartsock et al).

Histogenesis. There are *immunologic methods* for the demonstration of *T. pallidum* in tissue sections. For direct immunofluorescence testing, fluorescein-labeled syphilitic rabbit serum may be applied to tissue sections. However, frozen sections are required for this method (Yobs et al). In contrast, immunoperoxidase localization of *T. pallidum* can be carried out with formaldehyde-fixed and paraffin-embedded tissue sections (Beckett and Bigbee). This method utilizes rabbit anti-*T. pallidum* antiserum and a goat antirabbit immunoglobulin G (IgG)-horseradish peroxidase conjugate.

Electron microscopic examination of lesions of early syphilis has revealed the presence of *T. pallidum* in the epidermis as well as in the dermis, largely extracellularly but also intracellularly (Metz and Metz). In the epidermis, *T. pallidum* has been seen even within nuclei (Sykes et al). In the dermis, *T. pallidum* is occasionally found in the endothelial cells of capillaries but not in the lumen; however, it is frequently observed in lymphatic channels (Sykes et al). In addition, some spirochetes are found within phagocytic vacuoles and phagolysosomes of macrophages, neutrophils, and plasma cells (Azar et al). It is evident that not all spirochetes found intracellularly in the dermis have been phagocytized, since they are seen occasionally either entering or leaving a fibroblast (Sykes et al; Wecke et al).

T. pallidum shows three or four basal nodules at each end. From each of these nodules, a long axial filament extends to the other end of the cytoplasmic body. These filaments are located between the plasma membrane and the outer cell wall. Being contractile, they are responsible for the contractile and spiral motions of the spirochete (Klingmüller et al). The diameter of the organism is about 170 nm, and that of the axial filaments about 25 nm (Sykes et al).

Secondary Syphilis. The histologic picture in secondary syphilis, like the clinical picture, is quite variable. Often, the findings are nonspecific, since, in about one quarter of the biopsy specimens, plasma cell infiltration is either absent or very sparse, and vascular changes are seen in only about half of the cases (Abell et al). The histologic picture actually may be misleading in that it may be suggestive of other diseases, such as lichen planus, psoriasis, erythema annulare contrifugum, and, particularly, pityriasis lichenoides et varioliformis acuta (Jeerapaet and Ackerman). In occasional cases, when the infiltrate is heavy, atypical-appearing nuclei may be present and may then suggest the possibility of mycosis fungiodes (Cochran et al) or of non-Hodgkin's lymphoma (Gartmann and Klein). Still, a biopsy examination can be helpful in suggesting the possibility of secondary syphilis in unsuspected cases. A silver stain is recommended in all cases that are suspected of being secondary syphilis; it shows the presence of spirochetes in about one third of the cases of secondary syphilis, mainly within the epidermis and less commonly around the blood vessels of the superficial plexus. In some instances, the silver

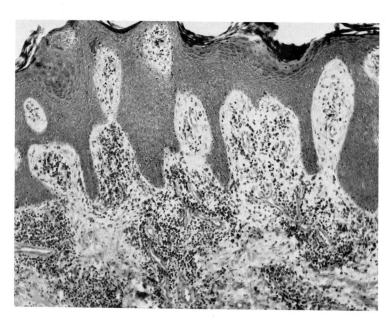

Fig. 18-3. Secondary syphilis
Low magnification. The vessels throughout the dermis show endothelial proliferation. The cellular infiltrate is located around the vessels in coat-sleeve-like arrangement. (×100)

stain is positive even when dark-field examination of the patient's lesions is negative (Jeerapaet and Ackerman).

As in primary syphilis, the most common histologic changes in secondary syphilis are those affecting the blood vessels, which may show dilatation, thickening, and an increased number of large endothelial cells (Fig. 18-3) and the presence of a perivascular infiltrate containing plasma cells (Fig. 18-4). The perivascular infiltrate may be seen around superficial as well as deeper dermal blood vessels. In addition, it may obscure the dermal–epidermal interface. Frequently, there is also epidermal hyperplasia (Jeerapaet and Ackerman). There is considerable histologic overlap among the various clinical forms of secondary syphilis, such as the macular, papular, and papulosquamous types (Abell et al; Paterou et al). Nevertheless, epidermal changes are least in the macular type and most pronounced in the papulosquamous type of lesion. In papulosquamous lesions, the epidermal changes may greatly resemble psoriasis and, as a result of the exocytosis of neutrophils, show microabscesses resembling spongiform pustules (Jeerapaet and Ackerman; Abell et al). Small, well-circumscribed epithelioid cell granulomas, some of them with giant cells, are present in the infiltrate, at times even in early secondary syphilis (Kahn and Gordon). In lesions more than 2 to 3 months old, such granulomas are a regular finding (Paterou et al).

Condylomata lata show the same changes in the dermis as papular lesions. Thus, an infiltrate usually containing a significant admixture of plasma cells is present around the blood vessels throughout the dermis. The overlying epithelium is hyperplastic, shows edema, and contains many neutrophils. At a later stage, the epithelium may be absent in the center, but there is still epithelial hyperplasia at the periphery of the lesion, as well as marked exocytosis (Jeerapaet and Ackerman).

Syphilis cornée shows a central keratotic, in part parakeratotic, plug invaginating the epidermis (Kerdel-Vegas et al). The dermis shows the usual changes of secondary syphilis.

Ulcerating lesions occur in the very rare lues maligna. They may show, in addition to pronounced endothelial swelling and proliferation, accumulation of fibrinoid material within many vessels. This causes partial to complete occlusion of lumina and thus results in infarction necrosis of the dermis and epidermis (Fisher et al; Degos et al). Spirochetes are characteristically absent in the ulcers. In some cases, vascular changes are absent, so that it is possible that defective cell-mediated

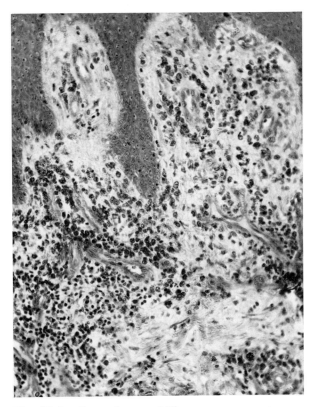

Fig. 18-4. Secondary syphilis
High magnification of Figure 18-3. The perivascular infiltrate contains many plasma cells. (×200)

immunity plays an important role in the pathogenesis (Adam and Korting; Petrozzi et al). Other cases may represent precocious nodulo-ulcerative syphilis, even though they lack a granulomatous infiltrate (Pariser).

In addition to finding small, sarcoidlike granulomas in papular lesions of early secondary syphilis, one may find in lesions of late secondary syphilis extensive aggregates of epithelioid cells and giant cells intermingled with many lymphoid and plasma cells, as seen typically in tertiary syphilis (Lantis et al). Conversely, lesions of early tertiary syphilis may show vascular changes and many plasma cells without any epithelioid and giant cell reaction. Thus, it is not always possible on the basis of histologic examination to assign cutaneous lesions of syphilis to either secondary or tertiary syphilis.

The *hepatitis* that may occur in secondary syphilis most commonly shows a nonspecific hepatitis on biopsy of the liver, but, in some instances, one may find a granulomatous or a cholestatic hepatitis.

The hepatitis is sometimes associated with areas of hepatic necrosis (Longstreth et al).

The *nephrosis* or *glomerulonephritis* of secondary syphilis shows proliferative changes in the glomeruli (Tourville et al).

Histogenesis. It has been shown that the renal changes occurring in secondary syphilis are an immune complex disease involving treponemal antigen. Not only has *direct immunofluorescence* shown granular deposits of immunoglobulins and complement along the glomerular basement membrane (Tourville et al; Bansal et al), but, in addition, *indirect immunofluorescence* antibody studies employing rabbit treponemal antibody and sheep anti-rabbit globulin conjugate have demonstrated the presence of treponemal antigen in the glomerular deposits (Tourville et al).

Tertiary Syphilis. In tertiary syphilis, granulomas are the characteristic lesion.

In *nodular tertiary syphilis*, the granulomas are small, but they are absent in only exceptional cases. The granulomatous process is limited to the dermis. Scattered islands of epithelioid cells, which usually are intermingled with a few multinucleated giant cells, are embedded in an infiltrate of lymphoid and plasma cells (Fig. 18-5). As a rule, caseation necrosis is not extensive, and it may be absent. The blood vessels often show endothelial swelling (Pembroke et al).

In *gummatous tertiary syphilis*, the granulomatous process is more extensive than it is in the nodular form, and it involves the subcutaneous tissue in addition to the dermis. Epithelioid and giant cells are numerous, and massive caseation necrosis occurs in the center of the lesion (Fig. 18-6). The epithelioid and giant cells are located mainly in the vicinity of the areas of caseation. Because of the deep extension of the process, not only the vessels of the dermis, as in nodular tertiary syphilis, but also the large vessels of the subcutaneous layer are markedly involved (Holtzmann and Hassenpflug).

Histogenesis. Vascular changes are prominent in gummatous tertiary syphilis; however, it is unlikely that vascular changes are the cause of the caseation necrosis, since they are as severe in areas without caseation as in those with caseation. Rather, the caseation is part of the immune phenomenon occurring in tertiary syphilis. The granulomas of tertiary syphilis basically are a reaction of cellular immunity, and their occurrence is due to renewed activity of *T. pallidum*, probably resulting from a decrease in circulating humoral antibodies against the organism (Wigfield).

Differentiation of nodular tertiary syphilis from lupus vulgaris may be difficult if caseation is slight or absent. The only difference then lies in the sparsity of plasma cells in lupus vulgaris. The gummatous type of tertiary syphilis greatly resembles scrofuloderma and erythema induratum. Scrofuloderma differs by not showing vascular changes, but erythema induratum, in which obliterative vascular changes similar to those of gummatous tertiary syphilis may be found, often cannot be excluded without clinical data.

In *juxta-articular nodes*, the histologic picture varies with the age of the lesion. Early lesions are fairly cellular and show within a dense fibrous

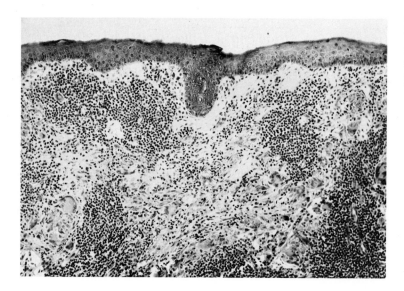

Fig. 18-5. Nodular tertiary syphilis
There are several islands of epithelioid and multinucleated giant cells. They are surrounded by an infiltrate containing a large proportion of plasma cells. (×100)

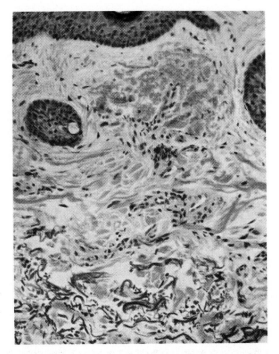

Solar degeneration. Basophilic degeneration is present in the upper dermis. The collagen bundles there have been replaced by amorphous material staining faintly basophilic with hematoxylin-eosin. (See p. 271.) (×100)

Molluscum contagiosum. In the horny layer, numerous large basophilic molluscum bodies lie enmeshed in a network of eosinophilic horny fibers. (See p. 370.) (×350)

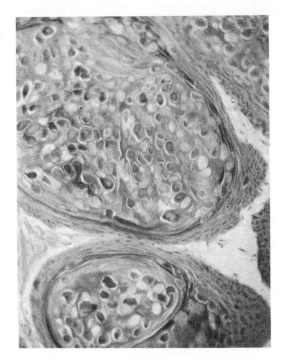

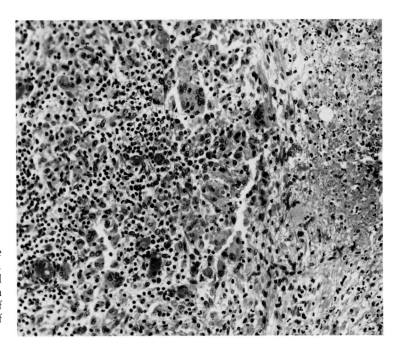

Fig. 18-6. Gummatous tertiary syphilis
On the left side of the field, the infiltrate consists of lymphoid cells and plasma cells. In the center, numerous epithelioid and multinucleated giant cells are present. On the right side is part of the large area of caseation necrosis that forms the center of the gumma. ($\times 200$)

tissue granulomatous areas that are composed of epithelioid cells, lymphocytes, and plasma cells, with an occasional multinucleated giant cell (Tuta and Coombs). Older lesions show an increasing amount of fibrosis and hyalinization. In the late stage, the node is composed of hyalinized collagen with little or no cellular infiltrate (Freeman). The center may contain amorphous material and occasionally also cholesterol clefts (Kalz and Newton).

SYPHILIS OF INTERNAL ORGANS. Without going into details about the histologic appearance of lesions of syphilis in the internal organs, it may be pointed out that late syphilis may cause two types of reactions in the internal organs: gumma and diffuse interstitial inflammation. The latter reaction is more common.

The gummata in internal organs show the same histologic changes as those observed in the skin.

Diffuse interstitial syphilitic inflammation manifests itself as accumulations of lymphoid and plasma cells around the small blood vessels. As a result of the long-continued inflammation, there is gradual degeneration of the parenchymatous structures and their replacement by fibrous tissue. This type of reaction produces, for instance, syphilitic hepatic cirrhosis. Syphilis of the aorta is also of the diffuse type. It predominantly affects the thoracic portion of the aorta, in which one observes (1) fragmentation and loss of the elastic tissue of the media; (2) an inflammatory infiltrate with a predominance of plasma cells around the blood vessels, including the vasa vasorum; and (3) formation of fibrous scar tissue (Sohn and Levine).

In general paresis, examination of the brain reveals that the gyri are shrunken, while the sulci and ventricles are widened. The meninges are usually thickened. The ganglion cells of the cerebral cortex are reduced in number, and those remaining appear degenerated. There is proliferation of the astrocytes in both the cortex and the white matter. *T. pallidum* can be demonstrated in the cortex in approximately 50% of the cases. In tabes dorsalis, there is atrophy of the posterior columns of the spinal cord together with atrophy of the posterior spinal roots. Microscopically, an infiltrate of lymphocytes and plasma cells is found to be present in the leptomeninges and in the intraspinal portion of the posterior roots (Luxon).

YAWS (FRAMBESIA TROPICA)

Yaws is caused by *T. pertenue*, which is morphologically indistinguishable from *T. pallidum*. Yaws is endemic in humid regions of the tropical belt around the globe. It is not a venereal disease but is transmitted by direct contact among children, usually with the hands (Guthe). Three stages are recognized. However, they may overlap.

The *primary lesion* starts in childhood as a papule, which often enlarges and becomes papillomatous and crusted.

Secondary yaws, which develops subsequently, consists of crops of infectious, relapsing skin lesions consisting of frambesiform (raspberrylike) papillomata that resemble the primary lesion. Healing takes place with atrophic scarring (Lanigan-O'Keeffe et al). Hyperkeratotic, tender lesions can develop on the palms and soles.

Late or tertiary yaws develops after a long latent period in adolescence or in later life. It consists of ulcerating lesions comparable to gummas. Ulcerations at the mucocutaneous borders of the mouth and the nose may progress to considerable destruction in the mouth and the upper respiratory tract; these destructive lesions are referred to as rhinopharyngitis mutilans or gangosa. In addition, the bones may show extensive destructive lesions. However, the central nervous system and the cardiovascular system show no clinical involvement.

Histopathology. The *primary lesion* shows considerable acanthosis and papillomatosis. There is pronounced edema of the epidermis, and numerous neutrophils are seen migrating into the epidermis, leading to the formation of intraepidermal microabscesses. The dermis shows a dense infiltrate composed predominantly of plasma cells but also containing neutrophils, lymphoid cells, histiocytes, fibroblasts, and a few eosinophils. In contrast with syphilis, the blood vessels show little or no endothelial proliferation (Williams; Hasselmann, 1957).

The *secondary lesions* show the same histologic appearance as the primary lesion. Although the secondary lesions of yaws resemble condylomata lata in their epidermal changes, they differ from condylomata lata in that their infiltrate has a diffuse rather than a perivascular arrangement.

In *late yaws,* the ulcerative lesions greatly resemble those seen in late syphilis in histologic appearance (Williams). Vascular changes are slight or absent (Hasselmann, 1957).

The causative organism, *T. pertenue,* can be demonstrated in the lesions during the first two stages of the disease by dark-field examination. Also, large numbers of organisms can be seen between the epidermal cells on silver impregnation. Thus, an important biologic difference exists between *T. pertinue,* which is almost entirely epidermotropic, and *T. pallidum,* which is found also in the dermis (see p. 322) (Hasselmann, 1952).

PINTA

Pinta, like yaws, is caused by a treponema that is morphologically indistinguishable from *T. pallidum.* It is called *T. carateum.* Pinta is endemic in Central America. It is not a venereal disease but is transmitted by personal skin-to-skin contact. Three stages exist.

The *primary lesion* starts as a red papule, which by peripheral extension grows into an oval or rounded patch 10 cm or more in diameter. Often, small papules surround the extending primary lesion and gradually merge with it. The lesion shows scaling but no oozing.

In the *secondary stage,* disseminated lesions appear. These are called pintids. They, too, show peripheral enlargement and may coalesce. They are often covered with scales and thus may resemble psoriasis. At first, the lesions are red, but, later, they assume a purple or a slate color, depending on the amount of melanin present in them.

The *tertiary stage* is characterized by the presence of dyschromic lesions that consist of alternating areas of hyperpigmentation and depigmentation resembling vitiligo.

Pinta is a benign but, especially in the tertiary stage, a disfiguring disease because of the presence of dyschromic lesions. No lesions of the bones, the central nervous system, or the cardiovascular system occur.

Histopathology. The *primary lesion* shows mild acanthosis. There is edema of the epidermis with migration of lymphoid cells into the epidermis. The basal layer shows liquefaction degeneration and loss of melanin. The upper dermis contains numerous melanophages. Thus, even in this early stage, the pigment mechanism is greatly disturbed. In addition to the melanophages, the upper dermis contains a fairly heavy cellular infiltrate composed of plasma cells, lymphoid cells, and occasional histiocytes and neutrophils (Pardo-Castello and Ferrer). Swelling of the endothelium of the dermal blood vessels is either mild or absent (Hasselmann). The causative organism, *T. carateum,* can be demonstrated in great numbers by dark-field examination and by silver impregnation between the cells of the epidermis.

In the *secondary stage,* the lesions show essentially the same histologic changes as the primary lesions, including the presence of many treponemata.

In the *tertiary stage,* the hyperpigmented areas show atrophy of the epidermis with absence of melanin in the basal cell layer. The upper dermis, however, contains accumulations of melanophages intermingled with a moderate number of lymphoid cells. Treponemata still are present in considerable numbers among the cells of the epidermis. The depigmented lesions, which represent the final stage of the disease, show atrophy of the epidermis, complete absence of melanin, even in the dermis, no inflammatory infiltrate, and no treponemata. However, some early depigmented lesions still may show a mild inflammatory infiltrate in the dermis and treponemata in the epidermis (Pardo-Castello and Ferrer).

Histogenesis. *Electron microscopic examination* has revealed in the depigmented areas of tertiary or late pinta the absence of basal epidermal melanocytes (Rodriguez et al). However, Langerhans cells, are present, and some of them contain a few melanosomes enclosed within lysosomes.

BIBLIOGRAPHY

Syphilis

ABELL E, MARKS R, WILSON JONES E: Secondary syphilis: A clinicopathological review. Br J Dermatol 93:53–61, 1975

ADAM W, KORTING GW: Lues maligna. Arch Klin Exp Dermatol 210:14–26, 1960

AZAR HH, PHAM TD, KURBAN AK: An electron microscopic study of a syphilitic chancre. Arch Pathol 90:143–150, 1970

BANSAL RC, COHN H, FANI K et al: Nephrotic syndrome and granulomatous hepatitis. Arch Dermatol 114:1228–1229, 1978

BECKETT JH, BIGBEE JW: Immunoperoxidase localization of *Treponema pallidum*. Arch Pathol 103:135–138, 1979

COCHRAN RIE, THOMSON J, FLEMING KA et al: Histology simulating reticulosis in secondary syphilis. Br J Dermatol 95:251–254, 1976

DEGOS R, TOURAINE R, COLLART P et al: Syphilis maligne précoce d'évolution mortelle (avec examen anatomique). Bull Soc Fr Dermatol Syph 77:10–15, 1970

FISHER DA, CHANG LW, TUFFANELLI DL: Lues maligna. Arch Dermatol 99:70–73, 1979

FREEMAN HE: Juxta-articular nodules. Arch Dermatol Syph 43:206–207, 1941

GARTMANN H, KLEIN R: Syphilis: Klinisch und histologisch ein malignes Lymphom vortäuschend. Z Hautkr 53:846–856, 1978

HARTSOCK RJ, HALLING LW, KING FM: Luetic lymphadenitis. Am J Clin Pathol 53:304–314, 1970

HOLTZMANN H, HASSENPFLUG K: Tertiärsyphilitische Lymphknotenbeteiligung vom granulierenden Typ bei einem Kranken mit plattenartigen Gummen der Haut. Arch Klin Exp Dermatol 215:230–245, 1962

JEERAPAET P, ACKERMAN AB: Histologic patterns of secondary syphilis. Arch Dermatol 107:373–377, 1973

KAHN LB, GORDON W: Sarcoid-like granulomas in secondary syphilis. Arch Pathol 92:334–337, 1971

KALZ F, NEWTON BL: Syphilitic juxtaarticular nodules. Arch Dermatol Syph 48:626–634, 1943

KERDEL-VEGAS F, KOPF AW, TOLMACH JA: Keratoderma punctatum syphiliticum: Report of a case. Br J Dermatol 66:449–454, 1954

KLINGMÜLLER G, ISHIBASHI Y, RADKE K: Der elektronenmikroskopische Aufbau des *Treponema pallidum*. Arch Klin Exp Dermatol 233:197–205, 1968

LANTIS LR, PETROZZI JW, HURLEY HJ: Sarcoid granuloma in secondary syphilis. Arch Dermatol 99:748–752, 1969

LONGSTRETH P, HOKE AQ, MCELROY C: Hepatitis and bone destruction as uncommon manifestation of early syphilis. Arch Dermatol 112:1451–1454, 1976

LUXON LM: Neurosyphilis. (Review) Int J Dermatol 19:310–317, 1980

METZ J, METZ G: Elektronenmikroskopischer Nachweis von *Treponema pallidum* in Hauteffloreszenzen der unbehandelten Lues I und II. Arch Dermatol Forsch 243:241–254, 1972

PARISER H: Precocious noduloulcerative cutaneous syphilis. Arch Dermatol 111:76–77, 1975

PATEROU M, STAVRIANEAS N, CIVATTE J et al: Histologie de la syphilis secondaire. Ann Dermatol Venereol 106:923–925, 1979

PEMBROKE AC, MICHELL PA, MCKEE PH: Nodulo-squamous tertiary syphilide. Clin Exp Dermatol 5:361–364, 1980

PETROZZI JW, LOCKSHIN NA, BERGER BJ: Malignant syphilis. Arch Dermatol 109:387–389, 1974

SOHN D, LEVINE S: Luetic aneurysms of the aortic valve, sinus of Valsalva, and aorta. Am J Clin Pathol 46:99–102, 1966

SYKES JA, MILLER JN, KALAN AJ: *Treponema pallidum* within cells of a primary chancre from a human female. Br J Vener Dis 50:40–44, 1974

TOURVILLE DR, BYRD LH, KIM DU et al: Treponemal antigen in immunopathogenesis of syphilitic glomerulonephritis. Am J Pathol 82:479–492, 1976

TUTA JA, COOMBS RA: Symmetric syphilitic granulomas of the elbow. Arch Dermatol Syph 46:375–378, 1942

WECKE J, BARTUNEK J, STÜTTGEN G: *Treponema pallidum* in early syphilitic lesions in humans during high-dosage penicillin therapy. An electron microscopical study. Arch Dermatol Res 257:1–15, 1976

WIGFIELD AS: Immunological phenomena in syphilis. Br J Vener Dis 41:275–285, 1965

YOBS AR, BROWN L, HUNTER EF: Fluorescent antibody technique in early syphilis. Arch Pathol 77:220–225, 1964

Yaws (Frambesia Tropica)

GUTHE T: Clinical, serological and epidemiological features of framboesia tropica (yaws) and its control in rural communities. Acta Derm Venereol (Stockh) 49:343–368, 1969

HASSELMANN CM: Experimental evidence and clinical studies as basis for nomenclature in frambesia tropica (yaws). Arch Dermatol 66:107–122, 1952

HASSELMANN CM: Comparative studies on the histopathology of syphilis, yaws and pinta. Br J Vener Dis 33:5–23, 1957

LANIGAN-O'KEEFE FM, HOLMES JG, HILL D: Infections and active yaws in a midland city. Br J Dermatol 79:325–330, 1967

WILLIAMS HU: Pathology of yaws. Arch Pathol 20:596–630, 1935

Pinta

HASSELMANN CM: Studien über die Histopathologie von Pinta, Frambösie und Syphilis. Arch Klin Exp Dermatol 201:1–8, 1955

HASSELMANN CM: Comparative studies on the histopathology of syphilis, yaws and pinta. Br J Vener Dis 33:5, 1957

PARDO-CASTELLO V, FERRER I: Pinta. Arch Dermatol Syph 45:843–864, 1942

RODRIGUEZ HA, ALBORES-SAAVEDRA J, LOZANO MM et al: Langerhans' cells in late pinta. Arch Pathol 91:302–306, 1971

19 Fungal Diseases

TINEA (DERMATOPHYTOSIS)

Among the dermatophytes causing superficial infections, two, *Trichophyton rubrum* and *Pityrosporum,* are by far the most common. Still, the following fungi should also be listed as potential causes of superficial fungus infections:

Microsporum audouini, M. canis

Trichophyton mentagrophytes, T. schoenleinii, T. tonsurans, T. verrucosum, T. violaceum

Epidermophyton floccosum

Clinically, nine regional types of fungal infections can be recognized: tinea capitis, tinea barbae, tinea faciei, tinea corporis, tinea cruris, tinea of the hands and feet, onychomycosis, favus of the scalp, and tinea versicolor and pityrosporum folliculitis of the upper trunk.

Tinea capitis is caused in the United States mainly by *T. tonsurans* (Rasmussen and Ahmed). Until about 1960, *M. audouini* and *M. canis* were the most common causes of tinea capitis. *T. violaceum* has been the cause in only exceptional cases. In contrast with the two types of *Microsporum,* which show fluorescence in Wood's light and cause scalp infections in children only, the two types of *Trichophyton* do not fluoresce in Wood's light and occasionally affect the scalp of adults. In all four types of tinea capitis, the affected hairs tend to break off either at the level of the scalp or slightly above it. Whereas *M. audouini* and *T. violaceum* usually produce only a slight inflammatory reaction, *M. canis* often produces pronounced inflammation of the affected areas of the scalp, so-called kerion celsi. Infection with *T. tonsurans* produces a marked inflammatory reaction (kerion celsi) in some patients, whereas in others one observes only slight scaling and broken-off hairs (black dot ringworm) (Rasmussen and Ahmed).

Tinea barbae, rare in the United States, may be caused by *T. mentagrophytes* but usually is due to *T. verrucosum (faviforme).* Infection of the bearded region with *T. verrucosum* is referred to also as cattle ringworm, since it is usually contracted from cattle. Both *T. mentagrophytes* and *T. verrucosum* cause a kerionlike, soft, nodular inflammatory infiltration in the bearded region of men (Birt and Wilt). *T. verrucosum* infections may also affect the scalp.

Tinea faciei consists of a persistent eruption of red macules, papules, and patches, with some of the latter showing an arcuate border. It is caused usually by *T. rubrum* and occasionally by *T. mentagrophytes* (Pravda and Pugliese).

Tinea corporis may be caused by *M. canis, T. mentagrophytes, T. rubrum,* or *T. verrucosum (faviforme),* with *T. rubrum* being by far the most common cause in the United States. If caused by *M. canis,* tinea corporis manifests itself as several annular lesions with a raised papulovesicular border and central clearing. If the disease is caused by *T. mentagrophytes,* one finds one or at the most a few annular lesions showing little or no central clearing. If it is caused by *T. rubrum,* there are large patches showing central clearing and a polycyclic scaling border, which may be quite narrow and thread-like. Occasionally, *T. rubrum* causes an asymptomatic nodular perifolliculitis in circumscribed areas. It is seen most commonly on the legs in association with an infection of the soles by *T. rubrum,* particularly in women who shave their legs (Cremer; Wilson et al), but it may also occur in other areas (Mikhail). If caused by *T. verrucosum,* tinea corporis manifests itself as grouped follicular pustules referred to as agminate folliculitis (Birt and Wilt).

Tinea cruris, usually caused by *T. rubrum* and occasionally by *T. mentagrophytes* or *E. floccosum*, produces sharply demarcated areas, often with a raised border, on the upper and inner surfaces of the thighs. From there, the eruption can extend to the perineal and perianal regions and, in men, to the scrotum.

Tinea of the feet and hands is caused usually by *T. rubrum* and occasionally by *T. mentagrophytes*. In cases of infection with *T. rubrum*, the soles and sometimes also the palms show diffuse erythema and superficial scaling; in cases of infection with *T. mentagrophytes*, the lesions consist of maceration between the toes and an erythematous, vesicular eruption on the soles and palms.

Onychomycosis, caused usually by *T. rubrum*, shows disintegration of the nail substance.

Favus, rare in the United States, is caused by *T. schoenleinii*. It affects mainly the scalp, where it produces inflammation with formation of perifollicular hyperkeratotic crusts, called scutula. Destruction of the hair ensues. Healing takes place with scarring.

Two dermatoses, tinea vesicolor and *Pityrosporum* folliculitis, are caused by the genus *Pityrosporum*. Tinea versicolor generally affects the upper trunk, where one finds areas of brownish discoloration that may lighten in color to appear hypopigmented. On gentle scraping, the surface of the discolored areas shows fine, branny scaling. *Pityrosporum* folliculitis shows red follicular papules or follicular pustules, predominantly on the upper back and anterior chest, measuring 2 mm to 4 mm in size (Potter et al).

Histopathology. For the demonstration of fungi in histologic sections, two stains can be used: the periodic acid-Schiff (PAS) reaction (see p. 43), which stains fungi deeply red, and the methenamine silver nitrate method, which stains fungi black. Fungi stain positively with the PAS reaction because of the presence of cellulose and chitin in their cell walls, two substances that are rich in polysaccharides (Kligman et al). The PAS reaction of fungi, being caused by polysaccharides, is diastase-resistant, unlike the PAS reaction of glycogen. Whenever this stain is used for the demonstration of fungi in the dermis, it is advisable first to clear the tissue sections of glycogen by exposing them to diastase, since glycogen granules in the dermis may resemble fungal spores (Fetter).

In histologic sections, fungi may present two structures: hyphae (or mycelia) and spores. Hyphae are threadlike structures that may be septate or nonseptate; they grow by extending and branching. Spores appear as round or ovoid bodies; they grow by budding.

Tinea of the Glabrous Skin. In tinea of the glabrous skin, which includes tinea faciei, tinea corporis, tinea cruris, and tinea of the feet and hands, fungi occur only in the horny layers of the epidermis and, with two exceptions, *T. rubrum* and *T. verrucosum* (see below), do not invade hairs and hair follicles. In histologic sections, even on staining with the PAS reaction or with methenamine silver nitrate, the number of fungi seen in the horny layer usually is small, so that they may be easily missed. In occasional instances, however, they are present in sufficient numbers that, even in sections stained with hematoxylin–eosin, they can be recognized as faintly basophilic structures. In infections with *Microsporum* or *Trichophyton*, only hyphae are seen, and, in infections with *E. floccosum*, chains of spores are present.

In the absence of demonstrable fungi, the histologic picture of fungal infections of the glabrous skin is not diagnostic. Depending on the degree of reaction of the skin to the presence of fungi, one sees the histologic features of an acute, a subacute, or a chronic dermatitis (see p. 94). If blisters are present, as they may be in tinea of the feet or hands due to *T. mentagrophytes*, they present the histologic picture of intraepidermal "spongiotic" vesicles like those seen in acute or subacute dermatitis.

Two fungal infections of the glabrous skin, those with *T. rubrum* and with *T. verrucosum*, occasionally are associated with an invasion of hairs and hair follicles and a subsequent perifolliculitis.

The nodular perifolliculitis caused by *T. rubrum* shows, on staining with the PAS reaction or with methenamine silver nitrate, numerous mycelia and spores not only within hairs and hair follicles but also in the inflammatory infiltrate of the dermis. Whereas the spores present within hairs or hair follicles measure about 2 μm in diameter, those located in the dermis, especially within multinucleated giant cells, may be larger, measuring up to 6 μm in size (Mikhail). The fungal elements reach the dermis through a break in the follicular wall. The dermal infiltrate shows, besides central necrosis and occasionally also suppuration, lymphoid cells, histiocytes, epithelioid cells, and scattered multinucleated giant cells (Wilson et al).

The agminate folliculitis caused by *T. verrucosum* (*faviforme*) shows, on staining with the PAS reaction, mycelia and spores within hairs and hair follicles (Birt and Wilt). The dermis around the hair follicles, however, contains no fungi. Depending on the severity and on the stage of the inflammatory reaction, either an acute or a chronic inflammatory infiltrate is predominant around the hair follicles in the dermis. In well-established lesions, the inflammatory infiltrate contains many plasma cells, as well as microabscesses and small aggregates of foreign body giant cells (Birt and Wilt).

Tinea Versicolor.   In contrast to other fungal infections of the glabrous skin, the horny layer in lesions of tinea versicolor contains abundant amounts of fungal elements, which can often be visualized in sections stained with hematoxylin-eosin as faintly basophilic structures. *Pityrosporum* is present as a combination of both hyphae and spores (Fig. 19-1), often referred to as spaghetti and meatballs.

Histogenesis. At one time, two yeast forms of *Pityrosporum* were recognized: *P. orbiculare* and *P. ovale,* with the former present predominantly on the trunk, and the latter found mainly in the scalp. It was then thought that *P. orbiculare* was the causative fungus of tinea versicolor (Roberts). However, recent investigations on the metabolism of both *P. ovale* and *P. orbiculare,* as well as the observation of transitional forms in the same strain of *Pityrosporum* in culture, support the concept that the two fungi are one and the same (Porro et al). In addition to the widespread presence of the yeast phase of *Pityrosporum,* a few short rods resembling hyphae are seen in 8% of normal subjects (Roberts). In patients with tinea versicolor, *Pityrosporum* becomes dimorphous by forming, in addition to spores, numerous septate hyphae. The organism then becomes pathogenic (McGinley et al). The factors that set off this yeast-to-hypha transformation are unknown.

On *electron microscopy,* the thick-walled hyphae of *Pityrosporum* are seen to be oval in cross sections and from 1 μm to 3 μm thick. They are thus much thicker than the horny cells, which measure only about 0.3 μm in diameter. Nevertheless, hyphae are seen not only outside of horny cells but quite frequently also inside them (Keddie).

The difference in the degree of pigmentation among lesions of tinea versicolor is due to the fact that *Pityrosporum* can produce a substance that directly inhibits the normal mechanism of epidermal pigmentation (Jung and Bohnert). Electron microscopic study of hypopigmented lesions has shown that, in such areas, melanocytes produce abnormally small melanosomes, which are not transferred to keratinocytes (Charles et al). In areas of hyperpigmentation, in contrast, the melanosomes are large, unpackaged, and heavily melanized (Allen et al). It is unknown how the fungus can initiate the production of either small or large melanosomes.

Pityrosporum *Folliculitis.*   The involved pilosebaceous follicles show dilatation of their infundibulum as a result of plugging with keratinous material. Inflammatory cells are present both within and around the infundibulum (Berretty et al). In some instances, the follicular epithelium is disrupted, and an abscess is seen in the peri-infundibular dermis (Potter et al; Heid et al). In every instance, PAS-stained sections show PAS-positive, diastase-resistant, spheric to oval, singly budding yeast organisms 2 μm to 4 μm in size. They are located predominantly within the infundibulum and at the dilated orifice of the follicular lumen but are occasionally observed also in the perifollicular dermis. No mycelial elements are seen.

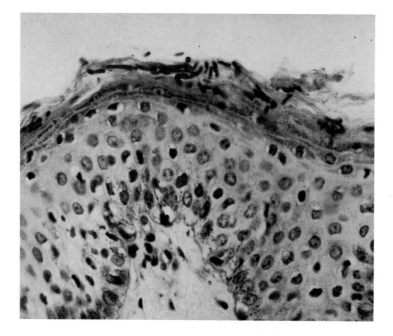

Fig. 19-1.   Tinea versicolor
Periodic acid-Schiff stain. The horny layer contains hyphae and spores. (× 400)

Histogenesis. It may be assumed that *Pityrosporum* organisms, through causing hyperkeratosis in the follicular ostium, prevent the normal flow of sebum, thus causing the follicular, acnelike lesions (Berretty et al).

Tinea Capitis and Tinea Barbae.

In tinea capitis and tinea barbae, fungi are usually demonstrable in the hair follicles, with the occasional exception of infections due to *T. tonsurans* or *T. verrucosum (faviforme),* in which fungi may no longer be found (see below). In tinea capitis and tinea barbae, the fungi generally are found both within and around the hair, and they descend in the hair to a line about 30 μm above the zone of beginning keratinization (Graham et al). The dermis, which contains no fungi, shows a perifollicular infiltrate of varying intensity, depending on the degree of reaction of the patient. The infiltrate is most pronounced in patients with kerion celsi. In addition to a chronic inflammatory infiltrate, multinucleated giant cells may be present in the vicinity of disrupted or degenerated hair follicles (Graham et al).

Tinea capitis due to *T. tonsurans* and tinea capitis or barbae due to *T. verrucosum (faviforme)* often show a clinically pronounced kerion celsi reaction and follicular pustules. Histologically, they show a marked inflammatory reaction consisting largely of neutrophils within the hair follicles and a chronic inflammatory infiltrate surrounding the hair follicles. Not infrequently, in cases with a severe inflammatory reaction, fungi can no longer be demonstrated either by microscopic examination or by culture (Birt and Wilt; Zaslow and Derbes). However, direct immunofluorescence staining using fluorescein-labeled *T. mentagrophytes* antiserum, discloses the presence of fungal antigens, even in the absence of demonstrable fungal structures not only within hair shafts but also in the dermal inflammatory infiltrate (Imamura et al). As a result of cross sensitivity, an anti-*T. mentagrophytes* conjugate demonstrates the localization of all dermatophyte antigens.

Histogenesis. The formation of kerion celsi in the scalp or the bearded region in response to certain fungi, especially *M. canis, T. tonsurans,* and *T. verrucosum (faviforme),* can be regarded as an immunologic reaction. In favor of this view are (1) the tendency of lesions of the kerion celsi type to heal by themselves; (2) the occasional absence of fungi in markedly reactive lesions caused either by *T. verrucosum (faviforme)* (Birt and Wilt) or by *T. tonsurans* (Zaslow and Derbes); and (3) the strongly positive intradermal trichophytin reaction in patients with a kerion type of *T. tonsurans* infection, as compared with a negative trichophytin reaction in patients with a noninflammatory type of *T. tonsurans* infection (Rasmussen and Ahmed).

Favus.

Mainly hyphae and only a few spores of *T. schoenleinii* are present in the stratum corneum of the epidermis around and within hairs (Fig. 19-2). The scutula consist of keratinized as well as parakeratotic cells, exudate, and inflammatory cells intermingled with segmented hyphae and spores that are well preserved at the periphery but appear

Fig. 19-2. Favus
Periodic acid-Schiff stain. A diagonal section of a hair follicle is shown. The fungus *Trichophyton schoenleinii* is present as segmented hyphae within and around the hair. (×400)

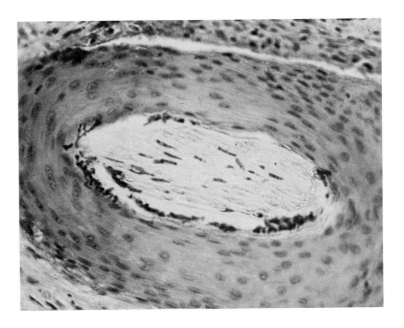

degenerated and granular in the center of the scutula (Dvoretzky et al). In active areas, the dermis shows a pronounced inflammatory infiltrate containing multinucleated giant cells and many plasma cells in association with degenerating hair follicles. In old areas, there is fibrosis and an absence of pilosebaceous structures (Graham et al).

Erythrasma

Erythrasma is caused by *Corynebacterium minutissimum*, a diphtheroid bacterium rather than a fungus as formerly thought (Sarkany et al).

Erythrasma shows well-demarcated, reddish brown, slightly scaling patches in intertriginous areas, especially in the groins, in the axillae, and between the toes. The affected areas show a coral red fluorescence in Wood's light.

Histopathology.   The causative organism is present in the horny layer in small amounts as gram-positive rods and filaments.

CANDIDIASIS

Candida albicans is a dimorphous fungus exhibiting both yeast and filamentous growth on the skin. It exists in a commensal relationship with man. The spectrum of infection may be divided into three groups (Maize and Lynch): acute mucocutaneous candidiasis, chronic mucocutaneous candidiasis, and disseminated candidiasis.

Acute Mucocutaneous Candidiasis

Acute mucocutaneous candidiasis, the usually encountered, benign, self-limited form of candidiasis, is caused by environmental changes that act either locally, like heat and sweating, or systemically, like antibiotic or corticosteroid therapy. It results in a localized infection of intertriginous areas, either alone or in association with oral, vulvar, or paronychial lesions. Intertriginous lesions show areas of erythema lined by an epidermal fringe. Small, superficial pustules may be seen either along the fringe or peripheral to it as satellite lesions.

Histopathology.   The primary lesion is a subcorneal pustule resembling that of impetigo (Maibach and Kligman). In some instances, the pustules have a spongiform appearance, so that they are indistinguishable from the spongiform pustules of Kogoj seen in pustular psoriasis (see p. 141) (Degos et al).

The fungal organisms are present, usually in small amounts only, in the stratum corneum. They consist of mycelia, which predominate by far, and ovoid spores, some of the latter in the budding stage. The mycelia, which are septate and show branching, measure from 2 μm to 4 μm in diameter, and the size of the ovoid spores varies from 3 μm to 5 μm (Table 19-1). They stain well with both the PAS and the Gram stains (Louria et al).

Histogenesis. On *electron microscopy,* the majority of the mycelia and spores are found to be situated inside the cells of the stratum corneum, many of which are parakeratotic (Scherwitz).

Chronic Mucocutaneous Candidiasis

In chronic mucocutaneous candidiasis, a defect in cell-mediated immunity leads to more or less widely disseminated lesions of candidiasis on the skin and mucous membranes. Systemic lesions, however, do not occur (Kirkpatrick et al). Three major types are recognized.

One type is associated with one of the lethal immune deficiencies. This includes the Nezelof syndrome, with hypoplasia of the thymus, DiGeorge's syndrome, which is associated with congenital absence of the thymus and parathyroids, and the "Swiss" type of agammaglobulinemia, in which there is hypoplasia not only of the thymus but also of all lymphoid tissue, resulting in both defective cell-mediated immunity and hypogammaglobulinemia (Higgs and Wells). The candidiasis is generally mild and is often limited to the oral cavity. Death usually occurs before the age of 2 from severe infections such as viral pneumonia.

The second type, which also starts in early life, is associated with usually nonlethal immune deficiencies. In some instances, it affects only the oral mucosa, but there is usually also more or less widespread involvement of the skin and nails (Shama and Kirkpatrick). There are two special variants. One is candidiasis with endocrinopathy, often showing autosomal recessive inheritance. The most frequent endocrinopathies are hypoadrenalism, hypoparathyroidism, and hypothyroidism; they may be multiple and their onset may precede or follow the onset of the candidiasis (Kirkpatrick and Montes; Richman et al). The other variant is candidal granuloma, in which numerous hyperkeratotic, crusted lesions are present, mainly on the face and scalp but also elsewhere (Hauser and Rothman; Kugelman et al).

The third type is chronic mucocutaneous candidiasis of late onset. It is associated with a thymoma that may be benign or malignant and that in some instances is accompanied by myasthenia gravis (Schoch; Maize and Lynch).

TABLE 19-1. Histologic Appearance of the Tissue and the Fungi in Fungal Diseases

Disease	Histologic Appearance of Tissue	Average Size of Spores (μm)	Appearance of Fungus in Dermis
Candidiasis	When invasive, nonspecific chronic inflammatory infiltrate	4	Hyphae and a few spores
North American blastomycosis	Epithelial hyperplasia; giant cells and inflammatory infiltrate with formation of small abscesses	10	Thick-walled spores in giant cells and tissue; budding forms *Double Contour*
Paracoccidioidomycosis	Like North American blastomycosis	30	Spores with multiple budding resembling a marine pilot's wheel
Lobomycosis	Macrophages; large giant cells	10	Spores with single budding, often in chains
Chromoblastomycosis	Like North American blastomycosis	10	Thick-walled, dark-brown spores, often in clusters; some cells possess cross walls
Coccidioidomycosis	Verrucous nodules: like blastomycosis, except that caseation may occur; subcutaneous abscesses: central necrosis surrounded by a granulomatous infiltrate	40	Thick-walled spores with granular cytoplasm; the larger spores contain endospores
Cryptococcosis	Gelatinous reaction: many spores; granulomatous reaction: fewer spores	7	Spores with wide gelatinous capsule
Histoplasmosis	Chronic inflammatory infiltrate with foci of necrosis	3	Numerous spores surrounded by a clear halo in the cytoplasm of large histiocytes
Sporotrichosis	Primary lesion: nonspecific inflammatory infiltrate; subcutaneous nodules: three zones—suppurative, tuberculoid, and round cell	5	Usually, spores can be seen only if diastase is used before PAS. Occasionally, asteroid forms of spores are present.
Actinomycosis	Nonspecific inflammatory infiltrate with abscess formation	150	Large, irregularly lobulated granules with radiating, branching filaments

Histopathology. The histologic findings are identical with those of acute mucocutaneous candidiasis, except in cases of candidal granuloma.

Candidal granuloma shows pronounced papillomatosis and hyperkeratosis and a dense infiltrate in the dermis composed of lymphoid cells, neutrophils, plasma cells, and multinucleated giant cells. The infiltrate may extend into the subcutis (Hauser and Rothman). *Candida albicans* usually is present only in the stratum corneum (Hauser and Rothman; Degos et al; Kugelman et al). In some instances, however, fungal elements are found also within hairs (Hellier et al), in the viable epidermis (Engel), and in the dermis (Papazian and Koch; Ezold and Schönborn).

Histogenesis. In some patients with chronic mucocutaneous candidiasis, the defect in cell-mediated immunity is selective for *Candida albicans*. In such cases, there is specific anergy to *Candida albicans* in skin tests, lack of *Candida*-induced lymphocyte transformation, and lack of migration inhibition factor to *Candida;* however, the lymphocyte proliferative responses are normal to the mitogens phytohemagglutinin, concanavalin A, and pokeweed mitogen. Also, the response to antigens such as mumps antigen, streptokinase–streptodornase, and dinitrochlorobenzene (DNCB) is normal (Horsmanheimo et al; Rockoff). In other patients, however, the defect in cell-mediated immunity is not limited to *Candida albicans* but rather affects many aspects of T-cell function (Kirkpatrick et al). Chemotactic and phagocytic functions of the neutrophils may be deficient, in addition to the impaired functioning of T lymphocytes (Djawari et al).

Disseminated Candidiasis

Disseminated, or systemic, candidiasis is a not uncommon serious complication among patients with impaired host-defense mechanisms, particularly among those with hematologic malignancies. The diagnosis is often difficult to establish, since *Candida* organisms can be cultured from blood specimens in only 25% of the patients (Bodey and Luna). Unless treated, the disease is rapidly fatal. It has been emphasized that the triad of fever, papular rash, and diffuse muscle tenderness must be regarded as presumptive evidence of disseminated candidiasis (Jarowski et al; Grossman et al). Unfortunately, the characteristic skin lesions are seen in only 13% of the patients (Bodey and Luna).

The characteristic cutaneous lesions of disseminated candidiasis consist of single or, more commonly, multiple red or purpuric papulonodules 0.5 cm to 1 cm in diameter. They frequently have a pale center. These papulonodules are seen most commonly on the trunk and the proximal portions of the extremities (Grossman et al).

Histopathology. Histologic examination reveals focally within the dermis, at the site of vascular damage, one or several aggregates of hyphae and spores, generally visible only in sections stained with the PAS reaction or with methenamine silver. Some of the spores, which are 3 µm to 6 µm in diameter, show budding (Bodey and Luna). The aggregates of hyphae and spores may lie in an area of leukocytoclastic vasculitis (Grossman et al), within a microabscess (Jacobs et al), or in an area of only mild inflammation (Bodey and Luna). The aggregates of *Candida* often are small, and step

sections through the biopsy specimen may thus be necessary to find them.

Since the diffuse muscle tenderness is caused by infiltration of muscle tissue by yeast organisms, biopsy of a tender muscle area may also aid in establishing the diagnosis of disseminate candidiasis (Kressel et al).

Histogenesis. Only about half of the infections in disseminated candidiasis are caused by *Candida albicans*, with *Candida tropicalis* and *Candida krusei* causing the remainder (Bodey and Luna).

ASPERGILLOSIS

Three major forms of cutaneous aspergillosis exist: (1) primary cutaneous aspergillosis caused by *Aspergillus flavus*, (2) primary cutaneous aspergillosis caused by *A. fumigatus* or *A. niger*, and (3) secondary cutaneous aspergillosis occurring in disseminated aspergillosis caused by *A. fumigatus*.

Primary cutaneous aspergillosis caused by *A. flavus* is the most common form and is very serious. It occurs largely in patients under immunosuppressive treatment for hematologic malignancies. One observes either one or several papules or plaques, which rapidly progress into necrotic ulcers that are often covered by a heavy black eschar (Prystowski et al; Carlile et al; Estes et al). Usually, the lesions appear at sites at which an intravenous administration unit had been secured to an arm or hand. Death often results from secondary systemic dissemination of the *A. flavus* infection (Prystowski et al; Estes et al).

Primary cutaneous or subcutaneous aspergillosis due to *A. fumigatus* or *A. niger* occurs on rare occasions in patients in apparently good health and without systemic involvement (Caro and Dogliotti; Cahill et al; Paldrok). In addition, *A. niger* may colonize burn wounds and subsequently invade viable tissue (Panke et al).

Secondary cutaneous aspergillosis caused by *A. fumigatus* and associated with systemic involvement, especially of the lungs, shows multiple scattered lesions as a result of an embolic hematogenous spread (Young et al; Findley et al). In most patients, the host defenses are altered by severe primary disease such as leukemia or immunosuppressive therapy. Death results from widespread systemic lesions of *A. fumigatus*.

Histopathology. In the two serious forms of cutaneous aspergillosis, the primary form due to *A. flavus* and the secondary form due to *A. fumigatus*, numerous aspergillus hyphae are seen in the dermis when sections are stained with the PAS reaction or with the silver methenamine stain. The hyphae, which measure 2 µm to 4 µm in diameter (Carlile et al), are septate and show branching at an acute angle. Spores are absent. In the primary form due to *A. flavus,* many hyphae may be seen invading blood vessels (Prystowski et al). Very little inflammation is seen in some instances (Estes et al), whereas an inflammatory reaction with some giant cells may be present in others (Carlile et al).

In patients with primary cutaneous or subcutaneous aspergillosis due to *A. fumigatus* or *A. niger,* the number of hyphae present is relatively small, and there may be a well-developed granulomatous reaction (Caro and Dogliotti; Cahill et al).

PHYCOMYCOSIS (MUCORMYCOSIS)

Infection of the skin with fungi of the two genera *Rhizopus* and *Mucor* is rare. Nevertheless, four types of infection may occur.

(1) Primary cutaneous phycomycosis may cause ulcers in debilitated patients with diabetes or uremia or in patients receiving immunosuppression. Such ulcers may heal (Roberts) or may lead to fatal systemic spreading of the infection (Veliath et al). Also, patients with extensive burns may suffer a severe superimposed infection with phycomycosis (Rabin et al).

(2) Secondary cutaneous phycomycosis may develop in debilitated patients with systemic phycomycosis. It may manifest itself as indurated nodules (Meyer et al) or as an area of infarction (Kramer et al).

(3) Contaminated adhesive tape may cause formation of pustules progressing to areas of deep ulceration in patients who are not debilitated or immunosuppressed (Hammond and Winkelmann; Gartenberg et al).

(4) Chronic subcutaneous phycomycosis may occur in tropical and subtropical areas in persons who are otherwise healthy, leading to slowly enlarging, painless, firm swelling, most commonly on the face (Herstoff et al).

Histopathology.   Within areas of nonspecific necrosis or granulation tissue, one observes very large, long, nonseptate hyphae with right-angled branching (Veliath et al). In cross or tangential sections, the hyphae appear ring-shaped or oval (Fig. 19-3) (Hammond and Winkelmann). They are easily located even in routinely stained sections because of their very large size, up to 30 μm in diameter (Rabin et al). Nevertheless, on staining with PAS or silver methenamine, the hyphae are visualized much better. No spores are seen. In patients with invasive primary infection of the skin or with systemic infection extending to the skin, the walls and lumina of the blood vessels contain many hyphae (Veliath et al). In some instances, numerous entangled hyphae may be present as thrombi within dermal blood vessels (Meyer et al).

CUTANEOUS ALTERNARIOSIS

The fungus *alternaria* generally is nonpathogenic for humans; however, on rare occasions, in persons who otherwise are healthy, it can cause lesions on the face that show either large, sharply demarcated, slightly infiltrated, reddish plaques with scaling and crusting (Mikoshiba et al) or scattered crusted ulcers (Higashi and Asada). More commonly, cutaneous lesions occur

Fig. 19-3. Phycomycosis (Mucormycosis)
Periodic acid-Schiff stain. Very large, long, nonseptate hyphae are seen within an area of necrotic tissue. The ring-shaped structures represent cross sections of hyphae. (×200)

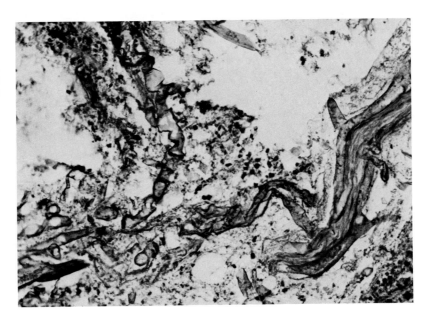

in patients who either have a debilitating disease (Pedersen et al) or are receiving immunosuppressive therapy (Chevrant-Breton et al). The lesions then usually consist of crusted ulcers but may be papulonodular or vegetating, with location on the limbs or the head (Chevrant-Breton et al).

Histopathology. Brownish, broad, septate hyphae 3 μm to 15 μm in diameter may be seen either only in the stratum corneum (Higashi and Asada) or extending also into the stratum spinosum (Pedersen et al) and into the dermis (Chevrant-Breton et al). Large, round spores 10 μm to 15 μm in diameter may be seen either free in the dermal inflammatory infiltrate (Pedersen et al) or within giant cells (Mikoshiba et al). Both the hyphae and spores stain deeply with PAS.

CUTANEOUS PROTOTHECOSIS

A rare type of infection, cutaneous protothecosis usually occurs in otherwise healthy persons either as a single lesion (Nabai and Mehregan; Mayhall et al) or as a few scattered lesions (Wolfe et al). The clinical appearance is quite variable. There may be raised papillomatous plaques (Tindall and Fetter; Mars et al), superficially ulcerated plaques (Nabai and Mehregan), or superficial ulcers (Wolfe et al). Spontaneous healing may occur (Dogliotti et al).

Histopathology. The histologic appearance, like the clinical appearance, is not characteristic, so that the diagnosis depends on the finding of the organisms. Usually, there is a mixed inflammatory infiltrate with areas of necrosis and fairly numerous giant cells. In sections stained with hematoxylineosin, the organisms stain faintly or not at all. On staining with PAS or silver methenamine, however, the spores stain well and are seen both within giant cells and free in the tissue (Wolfe et al).

Individual spores are spheric and measure 6 μm to 10 μm in diameter (Mars et al). However, as the result of septation, many spores contain endospores and then are considerably larger. Further subdivision of daughter cells within the parent cell leads to the formation of "sporangia" containing as many as 50 spores lying clustered together as morulalike structures (Nabai and Mehregan). Ultimately, such a sporangium breaks down into individual spores.

Histogenesis. *Prototheca* is a genus of saprophytic, achloric (nonpigmented) algae. These organisms reproduce asexually by way of internal septation, producing autospores identical to the parent cell. *Prototheca* forms

creamy, yeastlike colonies on Sabouraud's medium between 25°C and 37°C. These colonies become visible within 48 hr (Wolfe et al).

NORTH AMERICAN BLASTOMYCOSIS

North American blastomycosis, caused by *Blastomyces dermatitidis*, occurs in three forms: primary cutaneous inoculation blastomycosis, pulmonary blastomycosis, and systemic blastomycosis (Harrell and Curtis).

Primary cutaneous inoculation blastomycosis is very rare and seems to occur only as a laboratory or autopsy room infection (Table 19-2). It starts at the site of injury on a hand or wrist as an indurated, ulcerated, solitary lesion that has been called chancriform. It is followed by lymphangitis and lymphadenitis of the affected arm. Small nodules may be present along the involved lymph vessel. Spontaneous healing takes place within a few weeks or months (Wilson et al).

Pulmonary blastomycosis, the usual route of acquisition of the infection, may be asymptomatic or may produce mild to moderately severe, acute pulmonary signs, such as fever, chest pain, cough, and hemoptysis. In rare instances, acute pulmonary blastomycosis is accompanied by erythema nodosum (Smith et al). The pulmonary lesions either resolve or progress to chronic pulmonary blastomycosis with cavity formation. Immunosuppressants only very rarely activate pulmonary blastomycosis (Table 19-2) (Berger and Kraman).

In systemic blastomycosis, the lungs are the primary site of infection. Granulomatous and suppurative lesions may occur in many different organs, but they are most commonly found, aside from the lungs, in the skin, the bones, the male genital system, and the central nervous system. The mortality rate of systemic blastomycosis, in excess of 80% prior to the advent of amphotericin B, has decreased to about 10% (Witorsch and Utz). It has long been recognized, however, that there is a benign systemic form of blastomycosis in which cutaneous lesions are the only clinical manifestation (Wilson et al; Macauley; Klapman et al). It may be pointed out that the same phenomenon of a benign systemic form with only cutaneous lesions occurs, though rarely, subsequent to pulmonary infection in several other deep mycoses, for instance, in coccidioidomycosis, cryptococcosis, histoplasmosis, and sporotrichosis (Table 19-2) (Procknow and Loosli).

Cutaneous lesions are very common in systemic blastomycosis, occurring in about 70% of the patients (Witorsch and Utz). They may be solitary or numerous. They occur in two types, either as verrucous lesions, the more common type, or as ulcerative lesions. Verrucous lesions show central healing with scarring and slowly advancing, raised, verrucous border that is beset by a large number of pustules or small, crusted abscesses. Ulcerative lesions begin as pustules and rapidly develop into ulcers with a granulating base. In addition, subcutaneous abscesses may occur; they usually develop as

TABLE 19-2.   Some Clinical Data Concerning the "Deep" Fungal Infections

Disease	Occurrence of Primary Cutaneous Inoculation	Existence of a Benign Systemic Form with Only Cutaneous Lesions	Progression to Generalized Systemic Disease Possible	Activation of the Disease by Lymphoma or Medication with Corticosteroids
North American blastomycosis	Very rare	Rare	No	Very rare
Paracoccidioidomycosis	No	No		
Chromomycosis	Very common	Questionable	No	
Coccidioidomycosis	Very rare	Very rare	No	Common
Cryptococcosis	No	Rare	Yes	Common
Histoplasmosis	Very rare	Rare	No	Occasional
Sporotrichosis	Very common	Rare	Yes	Rare

an extension of bone lesions. A most unusual early cutaneous manifestation of systemic blastomycosis is a widespread pustular eruption (Hashimoto et al).

In the benign systemic form of blastomycosis with only cutaneous lesions, the lesions usually are of the verrucous type. There are often only one or two lesions, the face being the most common site of involvement (Klapman et al).

Lesions of the oral or nasal mucosa are seen in about one fourth of the patients with systemic blastomycosis. They present either as ulcers or as heaped-up masses of friable tissue. In some instances, they are contiguous with cutaneous lesions (Witorsch and Utz).

Histopathology.   In primary cutaneous inoculation blastomycosis, the primary lesion shows a nonspecific inflammatory infiltrate without epithelioid or giant cells. Numerous organisms, many in a budding state, are present. The nodules that may be found along the lymphatic vessel show an identical histologic picture. The regional lymph nodes, however, already show a granulomatous reaction with numerous giant cells, in which the organisms are predominantly located (Wilson et al).

For an examination of the verrucous lesions of systemic blastomycosis, it is important that the specimen for biopsy be taken from the active border. One then observes considerable downward proliferation of the epidermis often amounting to pseudocarcinomatous hyperplasia. Intraepidermal abscesses often are present. Occasionally, multi-nucleated giant cells are completely enclosed by the proliferating epidermis (Fig. 19-4). The dermis is permeated by a polymorphous infiltrate. Neutrophils usually are present in large numbers and form small abscesses. Multinucleated giant cells are scattered throughout the dermis. Usually, they lie alone and not within groups of epithelioid cells; occasionally, however, one observes tuberculoid formations, although without evidence of caseation necrosis (Moore). In the ulcerative lesions, the dermal changes are the same as in the verrucous lesions, but the epidermis is absent (Littman et al).

The spores of *B. dermatitidis* are found in histologic sections often only after a diligent search. Occasionally, they are found lying free in the tissue, particularly in the abscesses and in pustules. However, they are most apt to be found within the giant cells. One or several spores may lie within a giant cell (Fig. 19-5). When in this location, the spores are easily spotted, even in sections stained with routine stains. Unstained, the spores resemble small, round holes punched out of the cytoplasm of the giant cells. On high magnification, the spores are seen to have a thick wall, which gives them a double-contoured appearance. They measure 8 μm to 15 μm in diameter (average, 10 μm). Occasionally, spores showing a single broad-based bud are seen. As in most fungal infections, many more spores are visualized in sections stained with the

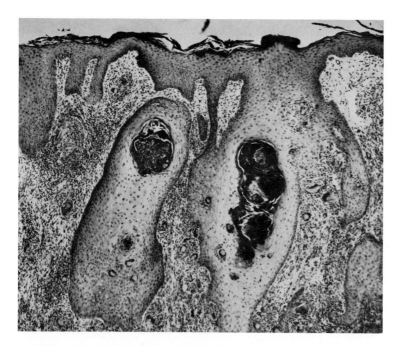

Fig. 19-4. North American blastomycosis
Low magnification. There is marked epidermal hyperplasia. Many multinucleated giant cells are present in the dermis and are also enclosed in the downward proliferations of the epidermis. (×50)

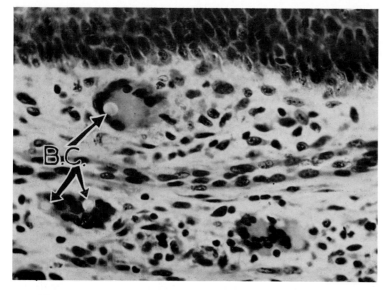

Fig. 19-5. North American blastomycosis
High magnification of Figure 19-4. Three blastomyces cells (*B.C.*), or spores, are shown lying in the cytoplasm of giant cells. (×400)

PAS reaction or with methenamine silver than in routinely stained sections.

The histologic appearance of the visceral lesions in North American blastomycosis is analogous to that of the cutaneous lesions. The number of neutrophils is often great, and numerous abscesses may be present (Littman et al).

Histogenesis. Of great value is the demonstration of the spores of *B. dermatitidis* in tissue sections either by direct immunofluorescence (Kaplan and Kraft) or by immunoperoxidase (Russell et al). The required antiserum is prepared in rabbits with pure cultures of fungi and is conjugated either with fluorescein isothiocyonate or with horseradish peroxide. The antiserum can be applied to fresh as well as to formalin-fixed, paraffin-embedded tissue sections. Prior staining with hematoxylin-eosin does not interfere with the procedure.

Corresponding antisera are valuable also for the demonstration of the spores of *Coccidioides immitis, Cryptococcus neoformans, Histoplasma capsulatum,* and *Sporotrichum schenckii.*

Differential Diagnosis.   The verrucous lesions of systemic blastomycosis must be differentiated from tuberculosis verrucosa cutis, chromoblastomycosis, and cryptococcosis. Tuberculosis verrucosa cutis shows no spores in the tissue. In addition, the number of neutrophils is smaller, and areas of caseation necrosis usually are present. The distinctive features of chromoblastomycosis and cryptococcosis are discussed under those headings (see below).

PARACOCCIDIOIDOMYCOSIS

Paracoccidioidomycosis, also called *South American blastomycosis,* is a chronic granulomatous disease caused by *Paracoccidioides brasiliensis.* Unless treated, it is almost invariably fatal in its usual systemic form. Whereas the treatment used to include sulfonamides and amphotericin B (Wilson), the present treatment of choice is the oral administration of ketoconazole (Cucé et al). The disease occurs exclusively in South and Central America, mainly in Brazil.

Paracoccidioides brasiliensis gains entrance into the human body through inhalation. The lungs are the site of the primary infection, which often is asymptomatic and then can be recognized only through a positive paracoccidioidin skin test (Londero and Ramos). Most commonly, the first clinical manifestation of the disease is the appearance of lesions in the oropharynx and on the gingivae. The lesions in the mouth begin as papules and nodules that then ulcerate. Subsequently, extensive granulomatous, ulcerated lesions develop in the mouth, nose, larynx, and pharynx. Extensive cervical lymphadenopathy develops, with suppuration of some of the lymph nodes. The oral lesions may extend to the neighboring skin, with formation of similar granulomatous, ulcerated lesions around the mouth and nose (Londero and Ramos).

Through both lymphatic and hematogenous spread, the disease may subsequently involve many lymph nodes, both subcutaneous and visceral, as well as the lower gastrointestinal tract. In cases with wide dissemination, the lungs are often involved, presenting a clinical picture greatly resembling chronic pulmonary tuberculosis (Salfelder et al). Adrenal insufficiency due to destruction of the adrenal glands, uncommon in other systemic mycoses except histoplasmosis, is seen not infrequently (Murray et al).

Rarely, widely scattered cutaneous lesions resulting from hematogenous spread are observed during the stage of dissemination. The lesions may be papular, pustular, nodular, papillomatous, or ulcerated (Furtado).

Histopathology.   Examination of cutaneous or mucosal lesions reveals in some areas a granulomatous infiltrate showing epithelioid and giant cells in association with an acute inflammatory infiltrate and abscess formation (Götz). The fungus spores may lie within giant cells or free in the infiltrate, especially in the abscesses. They are best demonstrated with the PAS reaction or with methenamine silver.

Many of the fungus spores present in the tissue show only single buds or no buds at all; for detection of the diagnostic multiple budding, many sections often have to be searched (Salfelder et al). In spores with multiple budding, peripheral buds are distributed over the whole surface of the ball-shaped fungus cell. Because of protrusion of the peripheral buds, such yeast cells in cross sections have the appearance of a marine pilot's wheel. Whereas nonbudding or singly budding spores measure from 6 μm to 20 μm in diameter, spores with multiple budding may measure up to 60 μm in size.

Occasionally, histologic examination does not reveal spores with multiple budding. The resemblance to North American blastomycosis then is such that cultural studies are necessary for differentiation (Perry et al).

LOBOMYCOSIS

Lobomycosis is characterized by asymptomatic, keloidal, nodular lesions that may coalesce to plaques. The lesions generally are limited to one area. There is no tendency toward healing. Except for the occasional involvement of a regional lymph node, the condition is limited to the skin (Azulay et al). The infection, which is probably caused by a minor local injury, occurs sporadically in the South American tropics and in Panama (Tapia et al). The causative fungus is designated *Loboa loboi.*

Histopathology.   The dermis shows an extensive infiltrate of macrophages and large giant cells. Numerous fungus spores lie both within these cells and outside of them, and, since the fungus does not stain with hematoxylin-eosin, there may be so many unstained areas that the section may have a sievelike appearance (Tapia et al).

On staining with the PAS reaction or with methenamine silver, the fungus spores are seen to measure from 6 μm to 12 μm in size, averaging 10 μm. They possess a thick capsule about 1 μm in diameter. They form single chains in some areas, the fungal elements being joined together by small, tubular bridges (Jaramillo et al). The spores occasionally show single budding (Bhawan et al).

Histogenesis. The macrophages contain abundant PAS-positive granular material that appears to consist of fragments of fungal capsules, indicating that the host macrophages are unable to digest the glycoproteins in the capsules (Bhawan et al).

CHROMOMYCOSIS

Chromomycosis is a cutaneous mycosis in which the primary lesion is thought to develop as a result of traumatic implantation of the fungus into the skin (Carrion; Vollum; Greer et al). In addition to the usual cutaneous type of chromomycosis, there are two rare forms, subcutaneous and cerebral.

The cutaneous type of chromomycosis is caused by one of five closely related species of pigmented fungi that appear alike in tissue sections: *Phialophora verrucosa, Fonsecaea pedrosoi, F. compactum, F. (Wangiella) dermatitidis,* and *Cladosporium carrionii* (Vollum). These fungi are saprophytes that can be found growing in soil, decaying vegetation, or rotten wood in subtropical and tropical countries. The occasional occurrence of chromomycosis in Finland and northern Russia is attributed to decaying wood in hot saunas (Putkonen; Ariewitsch).

The cutaneous lesions are most commonly located on the lower extremities and consist of verrucous nodules and plaques. While some of the lesions heal with scarring, new ones may appear in the vicinity as a result of spreading of the fungus along superficial lymphatic vessels (Derbes and Friedman). In rare instances, hematogenous dissemination may cause extensive cutaneous lesions (Ariewitsch; Azulay and Serruya; Caplan).

The subcutaneous cystic type of chromomycosis is usually caused by *Phialophora gougerotii* (formerly called *Sporotrichum gougerotii*) (Young and Ulrich; Kempson and Sternberg). In rare instances, it is due to *F. (Wangiella) dermatitidis* (Greer et al). It consists of a solitary, asymptomatic, subcutaneous cyst located most commonly on the hands and ankles.

Cerebral chromomycosis is caused by a fungus different from those causing cutaneous chromomycosis and is not associated with lesions of the skin. This fungus, called *Cladosporium trichoides,* in contrast to the organisms causing cutaneous chromomycosis, shows not only spores but also mycelia (Symmers; Watson).

Histopathology. The cutaneous type of chromomycosis resembles North American blastomycosis in histologic appearance. There is considerable hyperplasia of the epidermis. The dermis shows extensive infiltration with a polymorphous granulation tissue containing many multinucleated giant cells and small abscesses composed of neutrophils. Tuberculoid formations may be present, but caseation necrosis is absent, as in North American blastomycosis (Moore et al; French and Russell). In some cases, there are numerous aggregates of epithelioid cells, each aggregate having a small abscess in its center (Nödl).

In the subcutaneous type of chromomycosis, the abscess is lined by a fibrous wall that, on its inner side, shows a granulomatous reaction composed of histiocytes, epithelioid cells, and usually also giant cells. The center of the abscess consists of necrotic debris and numerous neutrophils (Kempson and Sternberg; Greer et al).

The causative organisms in both the cutaneous and the subcutaneous types are found within giant cells as well as free in the tissue, especially in the abscesses. They appear as conspicuous, dark brown, thick-walled, ovoid or spheric spores varying in size from 6 μm to 12 μm (French and Russell) and lying either singly or in chains or clusters (Fig. 19-6). Reproduction is by intracellular wall formation and septation, not by budding, and, in some of the spores, cross walls can be seen. Inasmuch as budding is absent, the designation *chromoblastomycosis,* even though it is still occasionally used, is inappropriate. Because of their brown pigmentation, the spores can be easily seen without the use of special staining. In cases with marked hyperplasia of the epidermis, fungus spores can be seen, as in North American blastomycosis, within microabscesses or giant cells surrounded by epidermal proliferation; even transepidermal elimination of fungal spores may be observed (Batres et al).

Histogenesis. Although percutaneous inoculation of the fungus is widely accepted as the mode of infection, the fact that the cutaneous manifestations show no chancriform syndrome but rather a granulomatous infiltrate resembling that of North American blastomycosis suggests that the cutaneous lesions of chromomycosis may arise by hematogenous dissemination from a silent primary pulmonary focus (Wilson). Though this view is supported by occasional reports of hematogenous dissemination (see above) and by the observation of multiple areas of calcification in the chest x-ray film of a patient with chromomycosis (Caplan), convincing evidence is lacking.

COCCIDIOIDOMYCOSIS

Coccidioidomycosis is caused by *Coccidioides immitis.* Like blastomycosis, it occurs in three forms: primary cutaneous inoculation coccidioidomycosis, pulmonary coccidiodomycosis, and systemic coccidioidomycosis. The disease is endemic in certain regions of the Southwestern United States, especially in the San Joaquin and Sacramento valleys in southern California, in southern Arizona, and in the northwest of Mexico (Schwartz and Lamberts). The fungus is resident in the soil of these areas, which have an arid or semiarid climate, and is inhaled with dust particles.

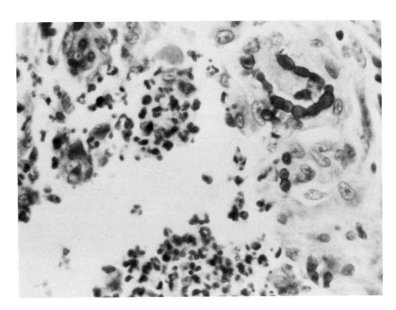

Fig. 19-6. Chromomycosis
Epithelioid cells and multinucleated giant cells form the wall of an abscess. Two chains of pigmented fungal spores are located in the right upper corner. In addition, three fungal spores lie in the right center. (×400)

Primary cutaneous inoculation coccidioidomycosis is very rare. In a few instances, like primary cutaneous inoculation blastomycosis, it has occurred as a laboratory or an autopsy room infection (Trimble and Doucette; Overholt and Hornick; Carroll et al); but, unlike primary cutaneous inoculation blastomycosis, it has also been found as a naturally occurring infection through injuries by thorns or splinters (Harrell and Honeycutt; Levan and Huntington; Winn). A tender, ulcerated nodule forms within 1 to 3 weeks at the site of inoculation and may enlarge into a granulomatous, ulcerated plaque. This is followed, as in the case of accidental inoculation with *B. dermatitidis*, by regional lymphangitis and lymphadenitis. Healing usually takes place within a few months, but, in one reported patient, meningitis developed, requiring prolonged intrathecal treatment with amphotericin B (Winn).

Pulmonary coccidioidomycosis, the usual route of acquiring the infection, is very common in endemic areas; on the basis of positive skin tests with coccidioidin, it has been established that 85% to 90% of the population in the Southwestern United States have been infected with coccidioidomycosis (Medoff and Kobayashi). The infection may be asymptomatic; however, in about 40% of those infected, symptoms of an acute respiratory infection develop and usually subside without sequelae. Development of erythema nodosum is not uncommon. In 2% to 8% of the cases, the pulmonary lesions progress into chronic pulmonary disease with cavity formation before finally healing (Harrell and Honeycutt).

Systemic coccidioidomycosis follows the primary pulmonary infection in only about 1 of each 10,000 cases in light-skinned persons. However, Mexicans are about 5 times, blacks 25 times, and Filipinos 175 times more likely to acquire systemic disease (Deresinski and Stevens). Before amphotericin B and ketoconazole became available, systemic coccidioidomycosis had a mortality rate of about 50%.

In systemic coccidioidomycosis, many organs, especially the meninges, the lungs, the bones, and the lymph nodes, may be involved. Cutaneous lesions occur in 15% to 20% of the cases (Levan and Huntington). They consist either of verrucous nodules and plaques or of subcutaneous abscesses, which may break through the skin. A rare manifestation is the sudden widespread appearance of small pustules on an erythematous base (Bayer et al), just as has been described in North American blastomycosis (see p. 337). In rare instances, the only clinical manifestation of systemic coccidioidomycosis consists of one or a few cutaneous nodules or plaques; in this case, the prognosis is good (Table 19-2) (Levan and Kwong; Schwartz and Lamberts).

Immunosuppressive therapy may cause activation of a latent pulmonary infection of coccidioidomycosis. Dissemination of the infection is frequently explosive and may be fatal (Table 19-2) (Deresinski and Stevens; Lynch et al). Therefore, all patients with a history of travel or residence in endemic areas should receive a coccidioidin skin test and have a chest roentgenogram before immunosuppressive therapy is initiated (Schwartz and Lamberts).

Histopathology. In primary cutaneous inoculation coccidioidomycosis, one observes a dense inflammatory infiltrate of neutrophils, eosinophils, lymphoid cells, and plasma cells with an occasional giant cell. Small abscesses may be seen (Trimble and Doucette). Spores, and in some cases also hyphae, are present (Levan and Huntington). The regional lymph nodes show a well-developed granulomatous reaction consisting of epithelioid and giant cells, within and outside of the latter of which spores are found.

The nodose skin lesions occurring in primary pulmonary coccidioidomycosis have the same histologic appearance as those in idiopathic erythema nodosum (Winer).

The verrucous nodules and plaques of the skin in systemic coccidioidomycosis histologically resemble blastomycosis. However, they show less of a tendency toward abscess formation, and caseation necrosis may occur (Moore). The causative organisms are found as spores free in the tissue as well as within multinucleated giant cells. As a rule, they are present in large numbers.

The subcutaneous abscesses of systemic coccidioidomycosis resemble scrofuloderma in histologic appearance. Surrounding a central area of necrosis is a granulomatous infiltrate that is tuberculoid in type and composed of lymphoid cells, plasma cells, epithelioid cells, and some giant cells. Numerous spores are present extracellularly as well as intracellularly in the giant cells (Moore). The pustules seen in a few cases show the presence of spores within them (Bayer et al).

The spores of *Coccidioides immitis* vary in size from 10 μm to 80 μm (Fig. 19-7), the average size being about 40 μm. Thus, the fungi of *Coccidioides* are much larger than those of *Blastomyces*, *Cryptococcus*, or *Phialophora*. The spores are round and thick-walled and have a granular cytoplasm. Multiplication takes place by the formation of endospores, which may be seen lying inside the larger spores (Fig. 19-8). The endospores are released into the tissue by rupture of the spore wall. Endospores may measure up to 10 μm in diameter.

Histogenesis. The coccidioidin skin test, which consists of the intradermal injection of 0.1 ml of a 1:100 dilution of coccidioidin, is of value in distinguishing between primary pulmonary infection and systemic infection. The test converts from negative to positive within a few weeks of the primary pulmonary infection and remains positive in patients with adequate immunity. In contrast, patients with disseminated disease tend to have a persistently negative skin test (Carroll et al).

CRYPTOCOCCOSIS

Cryptococcosis, though quite rare, occurs throughout the world. The causative fungus, *Cryptococcus neoformans*, is found in avian excreta and in the soil. The respiratory tract is the only established portal of entry into the body. The resulting pulmonary cryptococcosis may be symp-

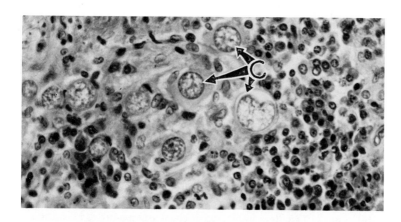

Fig. 19-7. Coccidioidomycosis
The *Coccidioides* spores (C) are large—larger than those of other fungi—and show considerable variation in size. Their cytoplasm is granular. (×400)

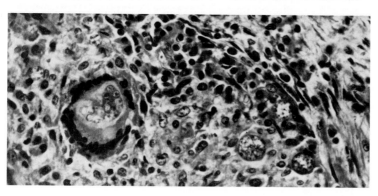

Fig. 19-8. Coccidioidomycosis
A large *Coccidioides* spore, which contains numerous endospores, lies within a giant cell. (×400)

tomatic or asymptomatic. In the latter case, the fact that an infection with *Cryptococcus* has taken place can be established, as in the case of histoplasmosis, either by the indirect immunofluorescence technique for the presence of circulating antibodies or by the complement fixation test for antigen (Warr et al). At least 90% of symptomatic cryptococcal infections of the lungs either resolve spontaneously or are cured by amphotericin B therapy or surgery (Schupbach et al).

In patients with active disease, cryptococcosis often manifests itself as a widespread systemic disease with predominant involvement of the brain and meninges and presence of the fungus in the spinal fluid. In addition, there may be osseous lesions and involvement of the kidneys and prostate. The systemic form is fatal without therapy in 70% to 80% of the cases, and, in cases with involvement of the central nervous system, it is almost invariably fatal, unless amphotericin B is administered. Cutaneous lesions are found in 10% to 15% of the cases of systemic cryptococcosis. In rare instances, lesions of the oral mucosa also occur (Cawley et al).

In some instances, systemic cryptococcosis, rather than being widespread after the primary asymptomatic or symptomatic pulmonary infection, shows only one or a few lesions without central nervous system involvement, for instance, in the skin, the lymph nodes, the bones, or the eyes (Littman and Walter). In cases in which only cutaneous lesions are present, the disease usually takes a benign course, ending with healing of the lesions, even without treatment (Gandy; Brier et al; Rook and Woods; Blanc and Bazex), although, in some cases, amphotericin B has been administered (Miura et al; Saúl et al). Occasionally, however, systemic cryptococcosis with lesions initially limited to the skin is followed by wide dissemination of the disease with a fatal ending (Table 19-2) (Sarosi et al).

The appearance of the cutaneous lesions is not diagnostic and is quite variable. The lesions may consist of papules, pustules, nodules, infiltrated plaques (Miura et al), subcutaneous swellings or abscesses (Brier et al; Rook and Woods), or ulcers (Crounse and Lerner; Blanc and Bazex). In infections limited to the skin, generally only one or possibly two lesions are present, whereas, in cases with widespread systemic infection, there are often multiple cutaneous lesions (Cawley et al; Crounse and Lerner; Schupbach et al; Chu et al).

Many patients with systemic cryptococcosis are "compromised hosts," having diseases leading to a depression of their immunologic status, particularly Hodgkin's disease (Noble and Fajardo) and leukemia (Cawley et al). Through the same mechanism of depression of the immunologic status, the prolonged administration of corticosteroids or immunosuppressants may cause cryptococcosis to become systemic (Table 19-2) (Sarosi et al; Schupbach et al; Chu et al).

Histopathology. Two types of histologic reactions to infection with *Cryptococcus neoformans* may occur in the skin as well as elsewhere: gelatinous and granulomatous. Both types may be seen in the same skin lesion (Moore; Chu et al). Gelatinous lesions show numerous organisms in aggregates and only very little tissue reaction (Fig. 19-9). In contrast, granulomatous lesions show a pronounced tissue reaction consisting of histiocytes, giant cells, lymphoid cells, and fibroblasts; areas of necrosis may also be seen. The organisms are present in a much smaller number than in gelatinous lesions. They are found mainly within giant cells and histiocytes but are encountered also free in the tissue (Gutierrez et al).

Cryptococcus neoformans, a round to ovoid spore, measures from 4 μm to 12 μm in diameter in the gelatinous reaction but often only 2 μm to 4 μm in the granulomatous reaction (Gutierrez et al). Like *Blastomyces dermatitidis,* it multiplies by budding. Usually, it is surrounded by a capsule. The capsule does not stain with hematoxylin-eosin or

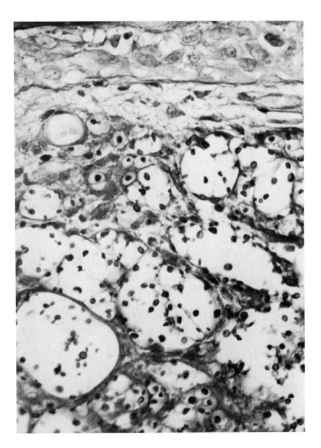

Fig. 19-9. Cryptococcosis
A large mass of spores is located directly beneath the epidermis. Each spore is surrounded by a wide gelatinous capsule. (×400) (Courtesy of S. William Becker, M.D.)

with the PAS reaction, but, because of the presence of acid mucopolysaccharides, it stains metachromatically purple with methylene blue (Linell et al), blue with alcian blue (Ruiter and Ensink), and red with mucicarmine (Littman and Walter). When the alcian blue stain and the PAS reaction are combined, the yeast cell stains red and the surrounding capsule blue. In areas in which *Cryptococcus neoformans* has a wide, gelatinous capsule, the inflammatory infiltrate is minimal, leading to the so-called gelatinous reaction. However, yeast cells located within a granulomatous infiltrate show only a narrow capsule and in some instances no capsule at all (Gutierrez et al).

Histogenesis. *Cryptococcus neoformans* is inhaled as a relatively small, nonencapsulated organism measuring approximately 3 μm in diameter. Under favorable nutrient conditions in the human host, the size of the organism increases up to 12 μm, and a wide gelatinous capsule forms. The lack of a tissue reaction to encapsulated *Cryptococcus neoformans* is best explained by the fact that the thick capsule prevents contact of the organism with the host tissue and thus inhibits phagocytosis of the organism (Gutierrez et al). The factors that lead to loss of the capsule and the subsequent development of a granulomatous reaction are not entirely clear, but aging of the organism may be a factor.

On *electron microscopy*, the mucinous capsule of *Cryptococcus neoformans* is seen to consist of radially arranged fibrillary material, with the fibrils having a beaded appearance and showing intertwining (Collins et al).

Ever since cases of cryptococcosis with only one or a few cutaneous lesions have been described, some authors have assumed that a purely cutaneous form of cryptococcosis produced by cutaneous inoculation exists (Gandy; Brier et al; Miura et al). However, the fact that purely cutaneous lesions show no chancriform syndrome characterized by regional lymphadenopathy speaks against the theory of primary inoculation of the skin (Schupbach et al). It has been recommended that all cases that seem to be purely cutaneous cryptococcosis should be considered potentially disseminated (Noble and Fajardo). Cultural studies should include the spinal fluid, sputum, prostatic fluid, and urine to rule out disseminated disease (Sarosi et al).

Differential Diagnosis. In the granulomatous type of reaction, *Cryptococcus neoformans* may have no capsule, may be small, with an average diameter of only 3 μm, and is found largely within macrophages and giant cells. Histologic differentiation from *Histoplasma capsulatum* may then be impossible and may require culture or staining by the fluorescent-antibody technic (Gutierrez et al).

HISTOPLASMOSIS

Histoplasmosis is caused by the fungus *Histoplasma capsulatum*, which exists in the soil of endemic areas and enters the body by inhalation. Although scattered areas of low endemicity exist in many parts of the world, there is only one large endemic area located in the central eastern states of the United States. On the basis of positive histoplasmin skin tests, it has been estimated that 30 million persons in this area have undergone pulmonary infection with *H. capsulatum*. In the geographic area bounded by the Mississippi and Ohio river valleys, 85% to 90% of the population have positive skin tests for histoplasmin (Goodwin and Des Prez), and, in heavily endemic areas of this region, the entire population reacts positively (Goodwin et al, 1976).

Histoplasmosis, like blastomycosis and coccidioidomycosis, occurs in three forms: primary cutaneous inoculation histoplasmosis, pulmonary histoplasmosis, and disseminated histoplasmosis.

Primary cutaneous inoculation histoplasmosis, a very rare event, is benign and self-limited in duration. It generally occurs as a laboratory infection and presents as a chancriform syndrome, with a nodule or ulcer at the site of inoculation and associated lymphangitis and axillary lymphadenitis (Tosh et al; Tesh and Schneidau).

Primary pulmonary histoplasmosis, representing the usual way of acquiring the infection, is entirely asymptomatic in the great majority of cases; however, in some infected persons, the primary infection produces acute pulmonary histoplasmosis with symptoms resembling those of influenza. Chronic pulmonary histoplasmosis with formation of cavities develops in 1 of 2000 infections (Goodwin et al, 1976). It resembles pulmonary tuberculosis in its symptoms and, unless treated, may end fatally. Disseminated histoplasmosis develops in only 1 of 50,000 infections, with a somewhat greater frequency in infants (Goodwin et al, 1976). Whereas chronic pulmonary histoplasmosis generally occurs in patients with pre-existing pulmonary disease, disseminated histoplasmosis arises on the basis of an inborn defect in the cellular immune mechanisms. The occasional occurrence of disseminated histoplasmosis in patients with lymphoma (Cawley and Curtis; Ende et al) and in patients receiving immunosuppressive treatment (Kauffman et al) is due to the depression of the immune response in such patients (Table 19-2).

Disseminated histoplasmosis presents a variable clinical picture, depending on the degree of parasitization. Cases with severe degrees of parasitization (acute disseminated disease) occur principally in infants and are often fatal even when treated. One observes high, persistent fever, hepatosplenomegaly and anemia, leukocytopenia, and thrombocytopenia. Cases with moderate degrees of parasitization (subacute disseminated disease) occur in both adults and infants, who, if adequately treated, may survive. Fever, hepatosplenomegaly, and bone marrow depression are mild to moderate. Adrenal involvement leading to adrenal insufficiency, as well as gastrointestinal ulceration, meningitis, and endocarditis, are common. Cases with mild degrees of parasitization (chronic disseminated disease) are associated with destructive focal lesions and occur almost exclusively in adults. There may or may not be fever, hepatosplenomegaly, bone marrow depression, adrenal insufficiency, meningitis, or endocarditis. In the chronic form, the response to treatment generally is good (Goodwin et al, 1980). If no cutaneous or oral lesions are present, the most useful diagnostic method is a bone marrow biopsy and occasionally also biopsy of the liver or of a palpable lymph node (Kauffman et al).

Cutaneous lesions occur in only 6% of patients with disseminated histoplasmosis (Studdard et al; Goodwin et al, 1980). In contrast, lesions of the oral mucosa occur in about half of all cases and are especially common in chronic disseminated histoplasmosis, so that they have been called a hallmark of chronic disseminated histoplasmosis (Hay). The cutaneous lesions most commonly consist of either papules or nodules that undergo ulceration (Chanda and Callen), large plaquelike lesions (Goodwin et al, 1980), or primary ulcers (Studdard et al). In some instances, purpuric or crusted lesions with a tendency to ulcerate are seen (Miller et al). Lesions of the oral mucosa generally consist of ulcers. A rare cutaneous manifestation is a generalized pruritic erythroderma (Samovitz and Dillon; Cramer).

In rare instances, systemic histoplasmosis, instead of disseminating widely, causes only localized lesions either in the oral cavity (Curtis and Grekin; Nejedly and Baker) or in one area of the skin (Symmers) and ultimately heals (Table 19-2). Even widespread mucocutaneous histoplasmosis with papular or nodular lesions on the skin has been observed without internal lesions and has shown clearing of all lesions under treatment with amphotericin B (Soo-Hoo et al). Also, one reported patient with generalized erythroderma due to histoplasmosis had no internal lesions (Cramer).

Histopathology. Histologic examination of a lesion of primary cutaneous inoculation histoplasmosis stained with methenamine silver shows numerous yeast cells within the cytoplasm of histiocytes (Tesh and Schneidau).

The cutaneous and mucosal lesions of either localized or widely disseminated systemic histoplasmosis often show ulceration and foci of necrosis in a chronic inflammatory infiltrate. A few giant cells may also be present (Miller et al; Nejedly and Baker). The diagnostic feature in all types of cutaneous lesions is the presence of numerous spores of *H. capsulatum* within the abundant cytoplasm of macrophages and occasionally also within giant cells (Dumont and Piché; Chanda and Callen).

The spores of *H. capsulatum* usually can be recognized in sections stained with hematoxylin-eosin. They appear as round or oval bodies surrounded by a clear space that was originally interpreted as a capsule. The spores, not including the clear space surrounding them, measure from 2 μm to 4 μm in diameter. A similar clear space is seen even more distinctly on staining with the Gram stain or Giemsa stain, since the spores are then deeply basophilic. On staining with methenamine silver, it becomes apparent that *H. capsulatum* does not possess a capsule. Instead, the inner portion of the clear space stains more intensely than the center of the spore and is thus shown to represent the cell wall of the fungus, whereas the outer part of the clear space forms a halo separating the cell wall of the fungus from the cytoplasm of the macrophage (Dumont and Piché).

On *electron microscopy*, it can be seen that each spore of *H. capsulatum*, including its halo, is located within a phagosome that is lined by a trilaminar membrane. The halo is partly filled with granular, cytoplasmic material (Dumont and Piché).

H. capsulatum is a dimorphous fungus that grows in culture at temperatures below 35°C and on natural substrates as a mycelial fungus elaborating macroaleuriospores (8–16 μm) and microaleuriospores (2–5 μm). When inhaled, the latter sprout and transform into small budding yeasts that are 2 μm to 5 μm in diameter. In cultures at a temperature of 37°C, the organism also grows in the yeastlike form (Rippon).

Differential Diagnosis. The histologic appearance of histoplasmosis, characterized by the presence of parasitized macrophages within a chronic inflammatory infiltrate, is much like that of rhinoscleroma, granuloma inguinale, and cutaneous leishmaniasis. For their differential diagnosis, see Table 20-1, p. 358. It may be pointed out that, in addition, only in histoplasmosis is the causative organism stained by the usual fungal stains, such as the PAS reaction and methenamine silver. For a discussion of differential diagnosis from cryptococcosis, see p. 344.

African Histoplasmosis

The cause of African histoplasmosis is *H. duboisii*. The disease occurs almost exclusively in Central Africa. It almost always involves the skin and often also the subcutaneous tissue, bones, and lymph nodes. The patient's general health is not affected (Lucas; Nethercott et al). However, there is a relatively rare disseminated form that involves many internal organs in addition to the skin, the bones, and lymph nodes and is fatal (Williams et al).

The cutaneous lesions may be one, a few, or many. They consist of papules, nodules, and plaques that often ulcerate (Flegel et al). In addition, there may be large, subcutaneous granulomas that develop into fluctuant, nontender abscesses (Lucas). Furthermore, purulent bone lesions may result in draining sinus tracts extending through the skin (Nethercott et al).

Histopathology.   The cutaneous lesions show a dense, polymorphous cellular infiltrate containing numerous giant cells and scattered histiocytes, lymphocytes, and plasma cells. There are focal aggregates of neutrophils forming small abscesses (Flegel et al). Numerous yeast cells, 8 μm to 15 μm in diameter, are present mainly in the giant cells but also in histiocytes and extracellularly (Nethercott et al).

Histogenesis. In spite of the fact that African histoplasmosis differs in its clinical character and in the size of the organism from classic histoplasmosis, it is clear that *H. capsulatum* and *H. duboisii* are variants of the same species, since, after prolonged in vitro growth at 37°C, the small yeast cells of *H. capsulatum* can assume the same size as those of *H. duboisii* (Nethercott et al). The primary portal of entry for African histoplasmosis is not known.

SPOROTRICHOSIS

Sporotrichosis, caused by *Sporothrix schenckii,* occurs in four forms: (1) primary cutaneous inoculation sporotrichosis, (2) asymptomatic pulmonary sporotrichosis, (3) unifocal systemic sporotrichosis, and (4) multifocal systemic sporotrichosis. Primary cutaneous inoculation sporotrichosis is by far the most common of the clinically apparent forms. However, the use of the sporotrichin skin test has revealed that, in certain areas, such as Louisiana and Arizona, up to 10% of the population have had an asymptomatic pulmonary infection with sporotrichosis (Lynch et al). Development of either unifocal or multifocal systemic sporotrichosis from an asymptomatic pulmonary infection, although rare, occurs particularly in persons with a depressed immune response, such as patients with lymphoma or persons receiving corticosteroids for a prolonged period of time (Lynch et al).

Primary cutaneous inoculation sporotrichosis most commonly manifests itself as lymphocutaneous sporotrichosis but may occur as fixed cutaneous sporotrichosis. The lymphocutaneous form starts with a painless papule located most commonly on a finger or hand. This papule grows into an ulcer. Subsequently, a chain of asymptomatic nodules appears along the lymph vessel draining the area. These lymphatic nodules may undergo suppuration with subsequent ulceration. Systemic sporotrichosis very rarely develops from primary cutaneous inoculation sporotrichosis, with only one proved instance (Seabury and Dascomb). However, in some cases, primary cutaneous inoculation sporotrichosis can spread widely in the skin and the subcutaneous tissues, thus extending from an arm to the trunk (Smith et al).

In the fixed cutaneous form, usually a solitary plaque is seen, most commonly on an arm or the face. It may show superficial crusting (Dellatorre et al) or a verrucous surface (Lurie; Carr et al; Itani; Dolezal). There is no tendency toward lymphatic spread.

Unifocal systemic sporotrichosis subsequent to asymptomatic pulmonary infection may affect the lungs, a single joint or symmetric joints, the genitourinary tract, or, rarely, the brain (Wilson et al). Chronic pulmonary sporotrichosis greatly resembles pulmonary tuberculosis (Baum et al).

Multifocal systemic sporotrichosis nearly always shows widely scattered cutaneous lesions, which start as nodules or as subcutaneous abscesses and undergo ulceration (Stroud). Whereas some patients have only cutaneous lesions (Krause), others show either from the beginning or later in the course of the disease involvement of several joints (Stroud) or of the lungs (Smith et al). Such patients can be improved or cured with potassium iodide given alone or in combination with amphotericin B (Cawley; Parker et al). However, some patients with involvement of many visceral organs or of the brain have died (Collins; Geraci et al).

Histopathology.   Primary lesions of sporotrichosis that are only a few weeks old and are ulcerated usually show a nonspecific inflammatory infiltrate composed of neutrophils, lymphoid cells, plasma cells, and histiocytes (Fetter). If the primary lesion is older and possesses an elevated border or appears verrucous, small, intraepidermal abscesses are often found in the hyperplastic epidermis, and the dermis shows, scattered through an inflammatory infiltrate, not only small abscesses but also giant cells and small granulomas (Fetter; Lurie; Itani).

The lymphatic nodules of primary cutaneous inoculation sporotrichosis, as well as the cutaneous nodules of multifocal systemic sporotrichosis, at first show scattered granulomas within an inflammatory infiltrate (Male). At a later stage, through coalescence, the nodules may show the characteristic arrangement of the infiltrate in three zones: a central "suppurative" zone composed of neutrophils; surrounding it, a "tuberculoid" zone; and peripheral to it, a "round cell" zone of lymphoid cells and plasma cells (Lurie; Stroud).

In the plaques of fixed cutaneous sporotrichosis, one observes a granulomatous infiltrate containing fairly numerous giant cells (Lurie; Itani; Dellatorre et al). In plaques with a verrucous surface, one finds, in addition, epidermal hyperplasia (Lurie; Itani; Dolezal).

In many instances, it is not possible to recognize the causative organisms of *S. schenckii* in tissue sections. This seems to be true especially in cases of sporotrichosis reported from the United States (Segal and Jacobs) and from Europe (Male). In these areas, negative findings are common even if, prior to staining with the PAS reaction, the sections are cleared of glycogen granules either with amylase or with a 1:1000 solution of malt diastase at 37°C for 1 hr (Fetter). Nor has staining with methenamine silver, rather than with the PAS reaction, increased the frequency of positive findings (Male). Even in cases with positive findings, numerous sections often have to be examined before one or a few organisms are visualized (Fetter and Tindall). Apparently, there are significant geographic differences, since, in a series of cutaneous sporotrichosis reported from Japan, 98% of the cases showed spores in tissue sections on staining with the PAS reaction (Kariya and Iwatsu). If present, the spores of *S. schenckii* appear as round to oval bodies 4 μm to 6 μm in diameter that stain more strongly at the periphery than in the center (Fig. 19-10) (Fetter and Tindall). Single or, occasionally, multiple buds are present. In some instances, small, cigar-shaped bodies up to 8 μm in length are also present (Stroud). In only very few cases can clumps of branching, nonseptate hyphae be demonstrated with the PAS reaction or the methenamine silver stain (Maberry et al; Stroud).

Asteroid bodies have been observed in only a few cases of sporotrichosis occurring in the United States (Moore and Ackerman; Pinkus and Grekin). However, they are found frequently in cases of sporotrichosis from South Africa (Lurie), Japan (Kariya and Iwatsu), and Australia (Auld and Beardsmore), with an incidence varying from 39% to 65%. Asteroid bodies, visible even in sections stained with hematoxylin-eosin, show a central spore 5 μm to 10 μm in diameter. Surrounding the spore are radiating elongations of a homogeneous eosinophilic material (Fig. 19-11). Measurements of the greatest diameter vary from 7 μm to 25 μm, with a mean of 20 μm (Lurie).

Histogenesis. In nearly all cases of sporotrichosis, even in those without demonstrable fungi in the tissue, *S. schenkii* can be grown easily on Sabouraud's medium. At room temperature, it grows in a mycelial form with conidiophores bearing conidia as a "bouquet" at the tip; at 37°C, it grows in a yeast form (Segal and Jacobs). At 39°C, there is no growth, a fact that has led to the use of local thermotherapy (Male; Kariya and Iwatsu).

Differential Diagnosis.   If the fungus is not found in sections, a diagnosis of sporotrichosis can only be suspected; however, it can be excluded in dubious cases by a negative cutaneous sporotrichin test (Male). The subcutaneous abscesses of tularemia and of infections with *Mycobacterium marinum* may have the same histologic appearance as the cutaneous and subcutaneous nodules and abscesses of sporotrichosis.

Fig. 19-10.   Sporotrichosis
Periodic acid-Schiff stain. Several round to oval spores of *Sporothrix schenckii* are present. They stain more strongly at the periphery than in the center. One spore, located in the center, shows single budding. (×400)

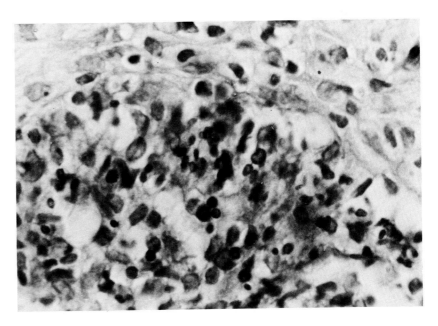

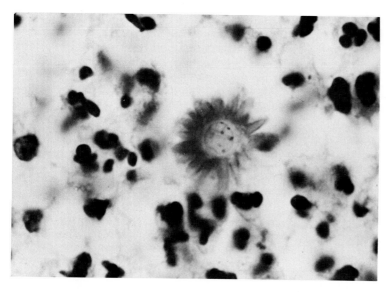

Fig. 19-11. Sporotrichosis
A large spore with radiating "asteroid" elongations is shown. (×1350) (Courtesy of Hermann Pinkus, M.D.)

ACTINOMYCOSIS

Actinomycosis is caused by *Actinomyces israelii,* an anaerobic or microaerophilic, gram-positive bacterium formerly thought to be a fungus. *Actinomyces israelii* is frequently found as a saprophyte in tonsillar crypts or carious teeth. Actinomycosis occurs in three major clinical forms: cervicofacial, thoracic, and abdominal. Very rarely, *Actinomyces israelii* is one of the organisms causing mycetoma (see p. 350).

Cervicofacial actinomycosis produces an area of "wooden" hardness of the skin over the mandible or maxilla, with multiple draining sinuses discharging purulent material that often contains characteristic yellowish "sulfur granules."

Thoracic actinomycosis produces areas of infiltration of the lungs with or without abscess formation. The infection may extend to the thoracic wall, which becomes indurated and shows multiple draining sinuses often containing "sulfur granules."

Intestinal actinomycosis primarily affects a portion of the intestinal tract, especially the appendix or colon, resulting in an indurated mass with formation of an abscess. The process may extend to adjacent loops of bowel and to the anterior abdominal wall, with formation of multiple draining sinuses. Rarely, when the rectum is primarily affected, multiple perianal and perineal sinuses result (Fry et al).

Occasionally hematogenous dissemination leads to multiple abscesses in the skin, the subcutaneous tissue, and muscle. Usually, thoracic actinomycosis is the primary site. There is intermittent draining, and "sulfur granules" may be present in the drainage (Varkey et al).

Histopathology. Histologic examination of the indurated skin shows extensive granulation tissue containing abscesses that may lead into sinuses. The granulation tissue is nonspecific in appearance. In the early phase of the disease, the tissue surrounding the abscesses is composed of lymphoid cells, plasma cells, histiocytes, and fibroblasts, whereas, in the late phase, fibroblasts may predominate. Thus, the diagnosis can be established only by the finding of the "sulfur granules." Because they occur almost exclusively in abscesses or sinuses, an area containing purulent material should be chosen as the site for biopsy.

The "sulfur granules," representing colonies of filamentous bacteria, range in size from 25 μm to 3700 μm, averaging 290 μm (Brown). Many granules thus are large enough to be visible macroscopically. In histologic sections, the "sulfur granules" appear irregularly lobulated (Fig. 19-12). On staining with hematoxylin-eosin, they are homogeneous and basophilic, although many granules show central degeneration and loss of basophilia. At their periphery, they show a radiating fringe of eosinophilic clubs 1 μm to 7 μm wide and 5 μm to 25 μm long (Brown). The granules are surrounded by neutrophils that are attached to the peripheral clubs and often lie in parallel rows. On staining with the Gram stain or methenamine silver, the granules show a dense, central mass of tangled filaments surrounded by radiating, branching filaments, some of which terminate in a club. The filamentous bacteria average 1 μm in width and 13 μm in length.

Differential Diagnosis. The filaments of *Actinomyces israelii* have the same diameter as those of

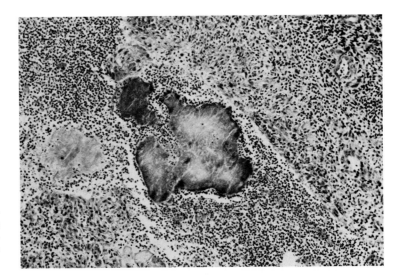

Fig. 19-12. Actinomycosis
A large, basophilic, lobulated "sulfur gran-ule" of *Actinomyces israelii* is present. The granule measures several hundred micro-meters in diameter and is surrounded by closely attached neutrophils. (×50)

Nocardia but differ from *Nocardia* by not being acid-fast. The filaments or hyphae of the fungi causing eumycetoma (see p. 350) are thicker than those of *Actinomyces israelii*, measuring from 2 μm to 5 μm in diameter (Zaias et al).

NOCARDIOSIS

The genus *Nocardia* is characterized by aerobic, gram-positive, filamentous bacteria that fragment into bacillary forms and frequently are acid-fast (Frazier et al). Two species are known: *N. asteroides* and *N. brasiliensis*.

N. asteroides is an opportunist and thus is usually found in "compromised hosts," persons receiving either immunosuppressants or corticosteroids. Nocardiosis due to *N. asteroides* most commonly affects primarily the lungs and less commonly the brain. There is a tendency toward fatal hematogenous dissemination (Welsh et al). Subcutaneous abscesses may occur as part of the hem-atogenous dissemination; however, in some instances, they present the only clinical manifestation (Frazier et al). Very rarely, *N. asteroides* is one of the organisms causing mycetoma, a purely cutaneous infection (see below).

N. brasiliensis usually acts as a primary pathogen. It may cause a primary infection of the lungs, common in Mexico (Rippon). In contrast to infection with N. aster-oides draining sinuses resembling those of thoracic actinomycosis occasionally extend to the chest wall. In rare instances, multiple subcutaneous abscesses are found in association either with pulmonary or urinary tract infection (Karassik et al; Diamond and Bennett) or with widespread fatal hematogenous dissemination (Mahvi). A benign, self-limited form of infection with *N. brasiliensis* is lymphocutaneous nocardiosis, also referred to as sporotrichoid nocardiosis. It shows a primary chancri-form ulcer on a finger and multiple subcutaneous nod-ules along the lymphatics (Moore and Conrad; Zecler et al). In addition, *N. brasiliensis* is a fairly common cause of mycetoma (see below).

Histopathology.   In the subcutaneous tissue, as well as in other organs, one finds abscesses com-posed of neutrophils and surrounded by only slight fibroblastic proliferation (Welsh et al).

The organisms of *N. asteroides* and *N. brasiliensis* present in the areas of suppuration do not differ morphologically from each other and can be dif-ferentiated only by culture. They do not stain with hematoxylin-eosin. Being gram-positive, however, they appear in sections stained with a Gram stain as basophilic, branching filaments about 1 μm in diameter. These filaments, rather than aggregating into "sulfur granules" like *Actinomyces israelii*, have a tendency to break up into short bacillary seg-ments like *Mycobacterium tuberculosis*. The possibil-ity of confusion with *M. tuberculosis* is increased by the fact that *Nocardia* nearly always is acid-fast, although not as strongly as *M. tuberculosis*. How-ever, the fact that even the bacillary segments stain well with methenamine silver aids in their differ-entiation from *M. tuberculosis* (Robboy and Vickery; Karassik et al).

MYCETOMA

Actinomycetoma and eumycetoma look alike clinically. Both represent an indolent local infection characterized by induration associated with draining sinuses. This infection occurs most frequently on a foot, which explains the synonym "Madura foot."

Actinomycetoma is caused by a group of filamentous bacteria, among which *N. brasiliensis* and *Streptomyces madurae* are the most common. In rare instances, *N. asteroides*, commonly the cause of pulmonary nocardiosis, and *Actinomyces israelii*, commonly the cause of actinomycosis, produce a mycetoma on the feet or hands (Zaias et al; Barnetson and Milne).

Eumycetoma is caused by a group of true fungi with thick, septate hyphae, including *Allescheria boydii, Madurella grisea*, and *Madurella mycetomi* (Barnetson and Milne).

Differentiation between actinomycetoma and eumycetoma is important because of the different responses to treatment. On the one hand, the filamentous bacteria producing actinomycetoma often respond to treatment with antibiotics such as sulfones (Zaias et al), sulfadiazine plus tetracycline (Kamalam et al), or trimethoprim plus sulfamethoxazole (Nitidandhaprabhas and Sittapairochana). Only in cases of infection with *Actinomyces israelii* is penicillin the treatment of choice (Zaias et al). On the other hand, the fungi causing eumycetoma are resistant to all forms of drug therapy.

Although much more common in tropical regions, both actinomycetoma and eumycetoma are seen occasionally in the United States (Montes et al; Zaias et al; Butz and Ajello). Both show subcutaneous nodules, usually on a foot but occasionally on a hand, that eventuate in abscesses and draining sinuses. Gradually, the muscles and tendons are damaged, and osteomyelitis develops. Granules are discharged from the draining sinuses. These granules are black in cases of eumycetoma caused by *Madurella grisea* and *Madurella mycetomi* (Butz and Ajello; Taralakshmi et al), whereas they are colorless in eumycetoma caused by *Allescheria boydii* and in all cases of actinomycetoma (Zaias et al; Barnetson and Milne). Both actinomycetoma and eumycetoma are local infections without a tendency toward systematic spreading.

Histopathology. The histologic picture in actinomycetoma and eumycetoma is essentially the same as that described for actinomycosis (Khandari et al; Zaias et al). Granules are found within abscesses. Most granules measure between 0.5 mm and 2 mm in diameter (Butz and Ajello). The black granules that are seen in eumycetoma caused by *Madurella grisea* and *Madurella mycetomi* show the hyphae embedded in an interstitial brownish cement substance (Taralakshmi et al).

A Gram stain is of considerable value in distinguishing between actinomycetoma and eumycetoma; the fine, branching filaments, only about 1 μm thick, within the grains of actinomycetoma are gram-positive, whereas the grains of actinomycetoma are gram-negative (Zaias et al). Both the filaments of actinomycetoma and the hyphae of eumycetoma stain with the PAS reaction and with methenamine silver. It can then be seen that the granules of actinomycetoma consist of fine, branching filaments only about 1 μm thick, whereas the granules of eumycetoma are composed of septate hyphae 4 μm to 5 μm thick (Taralakshmi et al). The study of discharged granules crushed on a slide and stained with lactophenol blue particularly allows differentiation between the thin filaments of actinomycetoma and the thicker hyphae of eumycetoma (Zaias et al).

BOTRYOMYCOSIS

In botryomycosis, there may be one, several, or even many areas of swelling and induration that usually discharge pus intermittently through sinus tracts. The grains that are characteristic of botryomycosis are seen only rarely in the discharge (Picou et al), although they may be obtained by curettage of the sinus tracts (Leibowitz et al). In some instances, areas of induration are present that do not discharge (Bishop et al). Although the condition is apt to be chronic and suppuration may extend into underlying muscles and bones, the patient's general health is not affected, and the prognosis is good, even without antibiotic treatment (Waisman; Picou et al).

Histopathology. Histologic examination reveals nonspecific granulation tissue with foci of suppuration. Within some of the suppurative foci, one finds grains that appear basophilic on staining with hematoxylin-eosin (Picou et al). The number and size of the grains varies greatly; whereas, in some instances, only a few small grains measuring 7 μm to 40 μm in size are found (Kansky), in others, grains are quite numerous and measure up to 2 mm in size (Bishop et al; Picou et al). On staining with the Gram stain, one usually finds gram-positive cocci within and on the surface of the grains embedded in a homogeneous pink material (Waisman; Harman et al; Picou et al). In a few instances, however, gram-negative rods are seen (Bishop et al). Acid-fast and methenamine silver stains are negative. On culture, the gram-positive cocci, usually are found to be *Staphylococcus aureus*, and the gram-negative rods *Pseudomonas aeruginosa*. Only very rarely have other organisms, such as *Proteus*, been identified (Bishop et al).

Histogenesis. Whereas the grains of actinomycetoma and eumycetoma are microcolonies, the grains of botryomycosis consist largely of amorphous material in which the bacteria appear to be trapped (Picou et al). This amorphous material represents a formidable barrier to penetration of the granules with antibiotics, making prolonged treatment necessary (Bishop et al).

BIBLIOGRAPHY

Tinea (Dermatophytosis)

ALLEN HB, CHARLES CR, JOHNSON BL: Hyperpigmented tinea versicolor. Arch Dermatol 112:1110–1112, 1976

BERRETTY P, NEUMANN M, HAUSMANN R et al: Follikulitis, verursacht durch Pityrosporum. Hautarzt 31:613–615, 1980

BIRT AR, WILT JC: Mycology, bacteriology, and histopathology of suppurative ring-worm. Arch Dermatol 69:441–448, 1954

CHARLES CR, SIRE DJ, JOHNSON BL et al: Hypopigmentation in tinea versicolor: A histochemical and electron microscopic study. Int J Dermatol 12:48–58, 1973

CREMER G: A special granulomatous form of mycosis on the lower legs caused by *Trichophyton rubrum Castellani*. Dermatologica 107:28–37, 1953

DVORETZKY I, FISHER BK, MOVSHOVITZ M et al: Favus. Int J Dermatol 19:89–92, 1980

FETTER BF: Human cutaneous sporotrichosis due to *Sporotrichum schenckii*; Technique for demonstration of organisms in tissue. Arch Pathol 71:416–419, 1961

GRAHAM JH, JOHNSON WC, BURGOON CF et al: Tinea capitis. Arch Dermatol 89:528–543, 1964

HEID E, GOSSHANS E, PROVENCHER D et al: Folliculites pityrosporiques. Ann Dermatol Venereol 105:133–138, 1978

IMAMURA S, TANAKA M, WATANABE S: Use of immunofluorescence staining in kerion. Arch Dermatol 111:906–909, 1975

JUNG EG, BOHNERT E: Mechanism of depigmentation in pityriasis versicolor alba. Arch Dermatol Res 256:333–334, 1976

KEDDIE FM: A novel cellular reaction caused by tinea versicolor: Extracellular glycogen deposits. J Invest Dermatol 53:363–372, 1969

KLIGMAN AM, MESCON H, DELAMATER ED: The Hotchkiss-McManus stain for the histopathologic diagnosis of fungus diseases. Am J Clin Pathol 21:86–91, 1951

MCGINLEY KJ, LANTIS LR, MARPLES RR: Microbiology of tinea versicolor. Arch Dermatol 109:168–171, 1970

MIKHAIL GR: Trichophyton rubrum granuloma. Int J Dermatol 9:41–46, 1970

PORRO MN, PASSAI S, CAPRILLI F et al: Induction of hyphae in cultures of *Pityrosporum* by cholesterol and cholesterol esters. J Invest Dermatol 69:531–534, 1977

POTTER BS, BURGOON CF JR, JOHNSON WC: Pityrosporon folliculitis. Arch Dermatol 107:388–391, 1973

PRAVDA DJ, PUGLIESE MM: Tinea faciei. Arch Dermatol 114:250–252, 1978

RASMUSSEN JE, AHMED AR: Trichophytin reactions in children with tinea capitis. Arch Dermatol 114:371–372, 1978

ROBERTS SOB: *Pityrosporum orbiculare*: Incidence and distribution on clinically normal skin. Br J Dermatol 81:264–269, 1969

SARKANY I, TAPLIN D, BLANK H: Incidence and bacteriology of erythrasma. Arch Dermatol 85:578–582, 1962

WILSON JW, PLUNKETT OA, GREGERSEN A: Nodular granulomatous perifolliculitis of the legs caused by *Trichophyton rubrum*. Arch Dermatol 69:258–277, 1954

ZASLOW L, DERBES VJ: The immunologic nature of kerion celsi formation. Dermatol Int 8:1–4, 1971

Candidiasis

BODEY GP, LUNA M: Skin lesions associated with disseminated candidiasis. JAMA 229:1466–1468, 1974

DEGOS R, GARNIER G, CIVATTE J: Pustulose par *Candida albicans* avec lésions psoriasiformes rappelant le psoriasis pustuleux. Bull Soc Fr Dermatol Syph 69:231–233, 1962

DJAWARI D, HORNSTEIN OP, GROSS J et al: Defect of phagocytosis and intracellular killing of *Candida albicans* by granulocytes in patients with familiar and non-familiar chronic mucocutaneous candidosis. Arch Dermatol Res 260:159–161, 1977

ENGEL MF: Monilial granuloma with hypergammaglobulinemia. Arch Dermatol 84:192–198, 1961

EZOLD M, SCHÖNBORN C: Über ein Granuloma candidamyceticum des Erwachsenen. Z Hautkr 37:379–392, 1964

GROSSMAN ME, SILVERS DN, WALTHER RR: Cutaneous manifestations of disseminated candidiasis. J Am Acad Dermatol 2:111–116, 1980

HAUSER FV, ROTHMAN S: Monilial granuloma. Arch Dermatol Syph 61:297–310, 1950

HELLIER FF, LA TOUCHE CJ, ROWELL NR: Monilial granuloma treated by amphotericin B. Br J Dermatol 75:375–381, 1963

HIGGS JM, WELLS RS: Klassifizierung der chronischen mucocutanen Candidiasis mit Betrachtungen zum klinischen Bild und zur Therapie. Hautarzt 25:159–165, 1974

HORSMANHEIMO M, KROHN K, VIROLAINEN M et al: Immunologic features of chronic granulomatous mucocutaneous candidiasis before and after treatment with transfer factor. Arch Dermatol 115:180–184, 1979

JACOBS MI, MAGID MS, JAROWSKI CI: Disseminated candidiasis. Arch Dermatol 116:1277–1279, 1980

JAROWSKI CI, FIALK MA, MURRAY HW et al: Fever, rash and muscle tenderness. A distinctive clinical presentation of disseminated candidiasis. Arch Intern Med 138:544–546, 1978

KIRKPATRICK CH, MONTES LF: Chronic mucocutaneous candidiasis. J Cutan Pathol 1:211–229, 1974

KIRKPATRICK CH, RICH RR, BENNETT JE: Chronic mucocutaneous candidiasis: Model-building in cellular immunity. Ann Intern Med 74:955–978, 1971

KRESSEL B, SZEWCZYK C, TUAZON CU: Early clinical recognition of disseminated candidiasis by muscle and skin biopsy. Arch Intern Med 138:429–433, 1978

KUGELMAN TP, CRIPPS DJ, HARRELL ER JR: *Candida* granuloma with epidermophytosis. Arch Dermatol 88:150–157, 1963

LOURIA DB, STIFF DP, BENNETT B: Disseminated moniliasis in the adult. Medicine (Baltimore) 41:307–337, 1962

MAIBACH HI, KLIGMAN AM: The biology of experimental human cutaneous moniliasis (*Candida albicans*). Arch Dermatol 85:233–257, 1962

MAIZE JC, LYNCH PJ: Chronic mucocutaneous candidiasis of the adult. Arch Dermatol 105:96–98, 1972

PAPAZIAN CE, KOCH R: Monilial granuloma with hypothyroidism. N Engl J Med 262:16–18, 1960

RICHMAN RA, ROSENTHAL IM, SOLOMON LM et al: Candidiasis and multiple endocrinopathy. Arch Dermatol 111:625–627, 1975

ROCKOFF AS: Chronic mucocutaneous candidiasis. Arch Dermatol 115:322–323, 1979

SCHERWITZ C: Ultrastructure of human cutaneous candidosis. J Invest Dermatol 78:200–205, 1982

SCHOCH EP JR: Thymic conversion of *Candida albicans* from commensalism to pathogenism. Arch Dermatol 103:311–319, 1971

SHAMA SK, KIRKPATRICK CH: Dermatophytosis in patients with chronic mucocutaneous candidiasis. J Am Acad Dermatol 2:285–294, 1980

Aspergillosis

CAHILL KM, EL MOFTY AM, KAWAGUCHI TP: Primary cutaneous aspergillosis. Arch Dermatol 96:545–547, 1967

CARLILE JR, MILLET RE, CHO CT et al: Primary cutaneous aspergillosis in a leukemic child. Arch Dermatol 114:78–80, 1978

CARO I, DOGLIOTTI M: Aspergillosis of the skin. Dermatologica 146:244–248, 1973

ESTES SA, HENDRICKS AA, MERZ WG et al: Primary cutaneous aspergillosis. J Am Acad Dermatol 3:397–400, 1980

FINDLEY GH, ROUX HF, SIMSON JW: Skin manifestations in disseminated aspergillosis. Br J Dermatol 85, Suppl 7:94–97, 1971

PALDROCK H: Report on a case of subcutaneous dissemination of *Aspergillus niger*, type Awamori. Acta Derm Venereol (Stockh) 45:275–282, 1965

PANKE TW, MCMANUS AT, SPEBAR MJ: Infection of a burn wound by *Aspergillus niger*. Am J Clin Pathol 72:230–232, 1979

PRYSTOWSKY SD, VOGELSTEIN, B, ETTINGER DS et al: Invasive aspergillosis. (Review) N Engl J Med 295:655–658, 1976

YOUNG RC, BENNETT JE, VOGEL CL et al: Aspergillosis: The spectrum of the disease in 98 patients. Medicine (Baltimore) 49:147–173, 1970

Phycomycosis (Mucormycosis)

GARTENBERG G, BOTTONE EJ, KEUSCH GT et al: Hospital-acquired mucormycosis (*Rhizopus rhizopodiformis*) of skin and subcutaneous tissue. N Engl J Med 299:1115–1118, 1978

HAMMOND DE, WINKELMANN RK: Cutaneous phycomycosis. Arch Dermatol 115:990–992, 1979

HERSTOFF JK, BOGAARS H, MCDONALD CJ: Rhinophycomycosis entomopthorae. Arch Dermatol 114:1674–1678, 1978

KRAMER BS, HERNANDEZ AD, REDDICK RL et al: Cutaneous infarction. Manifestation of disseminated mucormycosis. Arch Dermatol 113:1075–1076, 1977

MEYER RD, KAPLAN MH, ONG M et al: Cutaneous lesions in disseminated mucormycosis. JAMA 225:737–738, 1973

RABIN ER, LUNDBERG GD, MITCHELL ET: Mucormycosis in severely burned patients. N Engl J Med 264:1286–1289, 1961

ROBERTS HJ: Cutaneous mucormycosis. Arch Intern Med 110:108–112, 1962

VELIATH AJ, RAO R, PRABHU R et al: Cutaneous phycomycosis (mucormycosis) with fatal pulmonary dissemination. Arch Dermatol 112:509–512, 1976

Cutaneous Alternariosis

CHEVRANT-BRETON J, BOISSEAU-LEBREUIL M, FRÉOUR E et al: Les alternarioses cutanées humaines. A propos de trois cas. Revue de la littérature. Ann Dermatol Venereol 108:653–662, 1981

HIGASHI N, ASADA Y: Cutaneous alternariosis with mixed infection of *Candida albicans*. Arch Dermatol 108:558–560, 1973

MIKOSHIBA H, OKUBO S, WAKAMATSU K et al: Cutaneous alternariosis. J Dermatol (Tokyo) 6:67–73, 1979

PEDERSEN NB, MARDH PA, HALLBERG T et al: Cutaneous alternariosis. Br J Dermatol 94:201–209, 1976

Cutaneous Protothecosis

DOGLIOTTI M, MARS PW, RABSON AR et al: Cutaneous protothecosis. Br J Dermatol 93:473–474, 1975

MARS PW, RABSON AR, RIPPEY JJ et al: Cutaneous protothecosis. Br J Dermatol 85, Suppl 7:76–84, 1971

MAYHALL CG, MILLER CW, EISEN AZ et al: Cutaneous protothecosis. Arch Dermatol 112:1749–1752, 1976

NABAI H, MEHREGAN AH: Cutaneous protothecosis. Report of a case from Iran. J Cutan Pathol 1:180–185, 1974

TINDALL JP, FETTER BF: Infections caused by achloric algae (protothecosis). Arch Dermatol 104:490–500, 1971

WOLFE ID, SACKS HG, SAMORODIN CS et al: Cutaneous protothecosis in a patient receiving immunosuppressive therapy. Arch Dermatol 112:829–832, 1976

North American Blastomycosis

BERGER R, KRAMAN S: Acute miliary blastomycosis after "short-course" corticosteroid treatment. Arch Intern Med 141:1223–1225, 1981

HARRELL ER, CURTIS AC: North American blastomycosis. Am J Med 27:750–766, 1959

HASHIMOTO K, KAPLAN RJ, DAMAN LA et al: Pustular blastomycosis. Int J Dermatol 16:277–280, 1977

KAPLAN W, KRAFT DE: Demonstration of pathogenic fungi in formalin-fixed tissues by immunofluorescence. Am J Clin Pathol 52:420–432, 1969

KLAPMAN MH, SUPERFON NP, SOLOMON LM: North American blastomycosis. Arch Dermatol 101:653–658, 1970

LITTMAN ML, WICKER EH, WARREN AS: Systemic North American blastomycosis. Am J Pathol 24:339–365, 1948

MACAULAY WL: Is cutaneous blastomycosis a systemic disease? Arch Dermatol 73:560–563, 1956

MOORE M: Mycotic granulomata and cutaneous tuberculosis: A comparison of the histopathologic response. J Invest Dermatol 6:149–181, 1945

PROCKNOW JJ, LOOSLI CG: Treatment of the deep mycoses. Arch Intern Med 101:765–781, 1958

RUSSELL B, BECKETT JH, JACOBS PH: Immunoperoxidase localization of *Sporothrix schenckii* and *Cryptococcus neoformans*. Arch Dermatol 115:433–435, 1979

SMITH JG JR, HARRIS JS, CONANT NF et al: An epidemic of North American blastomycosis. JAMA 158:641–646, 1955

WILSON JW, CAWLEY EP, WEIDMAN FD et al: Primary cutaneous North American blastomycosis. Arch Dermatol 71:39–45, 1955

WITORSCH P, UTZ JP: North American blastomycosis: A study of 40 patients. (Review) Medicine (Baltimore) 47:169–200, 1968

Paracoccidioidomycosis

CUCÉ LC, WROCLAWSKI E, SAMPAIO SAP: Treatment of paracoccidioidomycosis, candidiasis, chromomycosis, lobomycosis, and mycetoma with ketoconazole. Int J Dermatol 19:405–408, 1980

FURTADO TA: Mechanism of infection in South American blastomycosis. Dermatol Tropica 2:27–32, 1963

GÖTZ H: Klinische und experimentelle Studien über das Granuloma paracoccidioides. Arch Dermatol Syph (Berlin) 198:507–528, 1954

LONDERO AT, RAMOS CD: Paracoccidioidomycosis. Am J Med 52:771–775, 1972

MURRAY HW, LITTMAN ML, ROBERTS RB: Disseminated paracoccidioidomycosis (South American blastomycosis). Am J Med 56:209–220, 1974

PERRY HO, WEED LA, KIERLAND RR: South American blastomycosis. Arch Dermatol Syph 70:477–482, 1954

SALFELDER K, DOEHNERT G, DOEHNERT HR: Paracoccidioidomycosis. Anatomic study with complete autopsies. Virchows Arch (Pathol Anat) 348:51–76, 1969

WILSON JW: Therapy of systemic fungus infections in 1961. Arch Intern Med 108:292–316, 1961

Lobomycosis

AZULAY RD, CARNEIRO JA, CUNHA DGS et al: Keloidal blastomycosis (Lobo's disease) with lymphatic involvement. Int J Dermatol 15:40–42, 1976

BHAWAN J, BAIN RW, PURTILO DT et al: Lobomycosis. J Cutan Pathol 3:5–16, 1976

JARAMILLO D, CORTÉZ A, RESTREPO A et al: Lobomycosis. J Cutan Pathol 3:180–189, 1976

TAPIA A, TORRES-CALCINDO A, AROSEMENA R: Keloidal blastomycosis (Lobo's disease) in Panama. Int J Dermatol 17:572–574, 1978

Chromomycosis

ARIEWITSCH AM: Über die Metastasierung der Chromomykose-Infektion. Dermatol Wochenschr 153:685–689, 1967

AZULAY RD, SERRUYA J: Hematogenous dissemination in chromoblastomycosis. Arch Dermatol 95:57–60, 1967

BATRES E, WOLF JE JR, RUDOLPH AH et al: Transepithelial elimination of cutaneous chromomycosis. Arch Dermatol 114:1231–1232, 1978

CAPLAN RM: Epidermoid carcinoma arising in extensive chromoblastomycosis. Arch Dermatol 97:38–41, 1968

CARRION AL: Chromoblastomycosis and related infections. Int J Dermatol 14:27–32, 1975

DERBES VJ, FRIEDMAN L: Chromoblastomycosis. Dermatol Tropica 3:201–206, 1964

FRENCH AJ, RUSSELL SR: Chromoblastomycosis. Arch Dermatol Syph 67:129–134, 1953

GREER KE, GROSS GP, COOPER PH et al: Cystic chromomycosis due to *Wangiella dermatitidis*. Arch Dermatol 115:1433–1434, 1979

KEMPSON RL, STERNBERG WH: Chronic subcutaneous abscess caused by pigmented fungi, a lesion distinguishable from cutaneous chromoblastomycosis. Am J Clin Pathol 39:598–606, 1963

MOORE M, COOPER ZK, WEISS RS: Chromomycosis (chromoblastomycosis). JAMA 122:1237–1243, 1943

NÖDL F: Zur Histologie der Chromomykose. Z Hautkr 35:305–309, 1963

PUTKONEN T: Die Chromomykose in Finnland. Hautarzt 17:507–509, 1966

SYMMERS WSC: A case of chromoblastomycosis (cladosporiosis) occurring in Britain as a complication of polyarteritis treated with cortisone. Brain 83:37–51, 1962

VOLLUM DI: Chromomycosis: A review. Br J Dermatol 96:454–458, 1977

WATSON KC: Cerebral chromoblastomycosis. J Pathol Bacteriol 84:233–237; 1962

WILSON JW: Therapy of systemic fungous infections in 1961. Arch Intern Med 108:292–316, 1961

YOUNG JM, ULRICH E: Sporotrichosis produced by *Sporotrichum gougeroti*. Arch Dermatol 67:44–52, 1953

Coccidioidomycosis

BAYER AS, YOSHIKAWA TT, GALPIN JE et al: Unusual syndromes of coccidioidomycosis. Medicine (Baltimore) 55:131–152, 1976

CARROLL GF, HALEY LD, BROWN JM: Primary cutaneous coccidioidomycosis. Arch Dermatol 113:933–936, 1977

DERESINSKI SC, STEVENS DA: Coccidioidomycosis in compromised hosts. Medicine (Baltimore) 54:377–395, 1975

HARRELL ER, HONEYCUTT WM: Coccidioidomycosis, a traveling fungus disease. Arch Dermatol 87:188–196, 1963

LEVAN NE, HUNTINGTON, RW JR: Primary cutaneous coccidioidomycosis in agricultural workers. Arch Dermatol 92:215–220, 1965

LEVAN NE, KWONG MQ: Coccidioidomycosis: Persistent pulmonary lesion, solitary "disseminated" lesion of face. Arch Dermatol 87:511–513, 1963

LYNCH PJ, RATHER EP, RUTALA PJ: Pemphigus and coccidioidomycosis. Cutis 22:581–583, 1978

MEDOFF G, KOBAYASHI GS: Strategy in the treatment of systemic fungus infections. N Engl J Med 302:145–155, 1980

MOORE M: Mycotic granulomata and cutaneous tuberculosis: A comparison of the histopathologic response. J Invest Dermatol 6:149–181, 1945

OVERHOLT EL, HORNICK RB: Primary cutaneous coccidioidomycosis. Arch Intern Med 114:149–153, 1964

SCHWARTZ RA, LAMBERTS RJ: Isolated nodular cutaneous coccidioidomycosis. J Am Acad Dermatol 4:38–46, 1981

TRIMBLE JR, DOUCETTE J: Primary cutaneous coccidioidomycosis. Arch Dermatol 74:405–410, 1956

WINER LH: Histopathology of the nodose lesion of acute coccidioidomycosis. Arch Dermatol Syph 61:1010–1024, 1950

WINN WA: Primary cutaneous coccidioidomycosis. Arch Dermatol 92:221–228, 1965

Cryptococcosis

BLANC C, BAZEX J: Un cas de cryptococcose cutanée primitive chez un sujet sain. Ann Dermatol Venereol 106:807–811, 1979

BRIER RL, MOPPER C, STONE J: Cutaneous cryptococcosis. Arch Dermatol 75:262–263, 1957

CAWLEY EP, GREKIN RH, CURTIS AC: Torulosis. J Invest Dermatol 14:327–344, 1950

CHU AC, HAY RJ, MACDONALD DM: Cutaneous cryptococcosis. Br J Dermatol 103:95–100, 1980

COLLINS DN, OPPENHEIM JA, EDWARDS MR: Cryptococcosis associated with systemic lupus erythematosus. Arch Pathol 91:78–88, 1971

CROUNSE RG, LERNER AB: Cryptococcosis. Arch Dermatol 77:210–215, 1958

GANDY WM: Primary cutaneous cryptococcosis. Arch Dermatol Syph 62:97–104, 1950

GUTIERREZ F, FU YS, LAURIE HI: Cryptococcosis histologically resembling histoplasmosis. Arch Pathol 99:347–352, 1975

LINELL F, MAGNUSSON B, NORDEN A: Cryptococcosis. Acta Derm Venereol (Stockh) 33:103–122, 1953

LITTMAN ML, WALTER JE: Cryptococcosis: Current status. (Review) Am J Med 45:922–933, 1968

MIURA T, AKIBA H, SAITO N et al: Primary cutaneous cryptococcosis. Dermatologica 142:374–379, 1971

MOORE M: Cryptococcosis with cutaneous manifestations. J Invest Dermatol 28:159–182, 1957

NOBLE RC, FAJARDO LF: Primary cutaneous cryptococcosis. Review and morphologic study. Am J Clin Pathol 57:13–22, 1972

ROOK A, WOODS B: Cutaneous cryptococcosis. Br J Dermatol 74:43–49, 1962

RUITER M, ENSINK GJ: Acute primary cutaneous cryptococcosis. Dermatologica 128:185–201, 1964

SAROSI GA, SILBERFARB PM, TOSH FE: Cutaneous cryptococcosis, a sentinel of disseminated disease. Arch Dermatol 104:1–3, 1971

SAÚL A, LAVALLE P, RODRÍGUEZ G: Cutaneous cryptococcosis. Int J Dermatol 19:457–458, 1980

SCHUPBACH CW, WHEELER CE JR, BRIGGAMAN RA et al: Cutaneous manifestations of disseminated cryptococcosis. Arch Dermatol 112:1734–1740, 1976

WARR W, BATES JH, STONE A: The spectrum of pulmonary cryptococcosis. Ann Intern Med 69:1109–1116, 1968

Histoplasmosis

CAWLEY EP, CURTIS AC: Histoplasmosis and lymphoblastoma. J Invest Dermatol 11:443–453, 1948

CHANDA JJ, CALLEN JP: Isolated nodular cutaneous histoplasmosis. Arch Dermatol 114:1197–1198, 1978

CRAMER HJ: Erythrodermatische Hauthistoplasmose. Dermatologica 146:249–255, 1973

CURTIS, AC, GREKIN JN: Histoplasmosis. JAMA 134:1217–1224, 1947

DUMONT A, PICHÉ C: Electron microscopic study of human histoplasmosis. Arch Pathol 87:168–178, 1969

ENDE N, PIZZOLATO P, ZISKIND J: Hodgkin's disease associated with histoplasmosis. Cancer 5:763–769, 1952

FLEGEL H, KNABEN U, WESTPHAL HJ: Afrikanische Histoplasmose. Hautarzt 31:50–52, 1980

GOODWIN RA JR, DES PREZ RM: Histoplasmosis. Am Rev Respir Dis 117:929–956, 1978

GOODWIN RA JR, OWENS FT, SNELL JD et al: Chronic pulmonary histoplasmosis. Medicine (Baltimore) 55:413–452, 1976

GOODWIN RA JR, SHAPIRO JL, THURMAN GA et al: Disseminated histoplasmosis: Clinical and pathologic correlations. (Review) Medicine (Baltimore) 59:1–33, 1980

HAY RJ: The skin and systemic fungal infection. Clin Exp Dermatol 4:365–371, 1979

KAUFFMAN CA, ISRAEL KS, SMITH JW et al: Histoplasmosis in immunosuppressed patients. Am J Med 64:923–932, 1978

LUCAS AO: Cutaneous manifestations of African histoplasmosis. Br J Dermatol 82:435–447, 1970

MILLER HE, KEDDIE FM, JOHNSTONE HG et al: Histoplasmosis. Arch Dermatol Syph 56:715–739, 1947

NEJEDLY RF, BAKER LA: Treatment of localized histoplasmosis with 2-hydroxystilbamidine. Arch Intern Med 95:37–40, 1955

NETHERCOTT JR, SCHACHTER RK, GIVAN KF et al: Histoplasmosis due to *Histoplasma capsulatum var* duboisii in a Canadian immigrant. Arch Dermatol 114:595–598, 1978

RIPPON JW: Medical Mycology, p 323. Philadelphia, WB Saunders, 1974

SAMOVITZ M, DILLON TK: Disseminated histoplasmosis presenting as exfoliative erythroderma. Arch Dermatol 101:216–219, 1970

SOO-HOO TS, ADAMS BA, YUSOF D: Disseminated primary cutaneous histoplasmosis. Aust J Dermatol 21:105–107, 1980

STUDDARD J, SNEED WF, TAYLOR MR JR et al: Cutaneous histoplasmosis. (Review of cutaneous lesions) Am Rev Respir Dis 113:689–693, 1976

SYMMERS WSC: Localized cutaneous histoplasmosis. Br Med J 2: 790–792, 1956

TESH RB, SCHNEIDAU JD JR: Primary cutaneous histoplasmosis. N Engl J Med 275:597–599, 1966

TOSH FE, BALHUIZEN J, YATES JL et al: Primary cutaneous histoplasmosis. Arch Intern Med 114:118–119, 1964

WILLIAMS AO, LAWSON EA, LUCAS AO: African histoplasmosis due to *Histoplasma duboisii*. Arch Pathol 92:306–318, 1971

Sporotrichosis

AULD JC, BEARDSMORE GL: Sporotrichosis in Queensland: A review of 37 cases at the Royal Brisbane Hospital. Aust J Dermatol 20:14–22, 1979

BAUM GL, DONNERBERG RL, STEWART D et al: Pulmonary sporotrichosis. N Engl J Med 280:410–413, 1969

CARR RD, STORKAN MA, WILSON JW et al: Extensive verrucous sporotrichosis of long duration. Arch Dermatol 89:124–130, 1964

CAWLEY EP: Sporotrichosis, a protean disease, with report of a disseminated subcutaneous gummatous case of the disease. Ann Intern Med 30:1287–1292, 1949

COLLINS WT: Disseminated ulcerating sporotrichosis with widespread visceral involvement. Arch Dermatol Syph 56:523–528, 1947

DELLATORRE DL, LATTERAND A, BUCKLEY HR et al: Fixed cutaneous sporotrichosis of the face. J Am Acad Dermatol 6:97–100, 1982

DOLEZAL JF: Blastomycoid sporotrichosis. J Am Acad Dermatol 4:523–527, 1981

FETTER BF: Human cutaneous sporotrichosis. Arch Pathol 71:416–419, 1961

FETTER BF, TINDALL JF: Cutaneous sporotrichosis. Arch Pathol 78:613–617, 1964

GERACI JE, DRY TJ, ULRICH JA et al: Experiences with 2-hydroxystilbamadine in systemic sporotrichosis. Arch Intern Med 96:478–489, 1955

ITANI Z: Die Sporotrichose. Hautarzt 22:110–113, 1971

KARIYA H, IWATSU T: Statistical survey of 100 cases of sporotrichosis. J Dermatol 6:211–217, 1979

KRAUSE H: Kasuistischer Beitrag zur Sporotrichose. Hautarzt 19:428–432, 1968

LURIE HI: Histopathology of sporotrichosis. Arch Pathol 75:421–437, 1963

LYNCH PJ, VOORHEES JJ, HARRELL ER: Systemic sporotrichosis. (Review) Ann Intern Med 73:23–30, 1970

MABERRY JD, MULLINS JF, STONE OJ: Sporotrichosis with demonstration of hyphae in human tissue. Arch Dermatol 93:65–67, 1966

MALE O: Diagnostische und therapeutische Probleme bei der kutanen Sporotrichose. Z Hautkr 49:505–515, 1974

MOORE M, ACKERMAN LV: Sporotrichosis with radiate formation in tissue. Arch Dermatol 53:253–264, 1946

PARKER JD, SAROSI GA, TOSH FE: Treatment of extracutaneous sporotrichosis. Arch Intern Med 125:858–863, 1970

PINKUS H, GREKIN JN: Sporotrichosis with asteroid tissue forms. Arch Dermatol Syph 61:813–819, 1950

SEABURY JH, DASCOMB HE: Experience with amphotericin B for the treatment of systemic mycoses. Arch Intern Med 102: 960–964, 1958

SEGAL RJ, JACOBS PH: Sporotrichosis. Int J Dermatol 18:639–644, 1979

SMITH PW, LOOMIS GW, LUCKASEN JL et al: Disseminated cutaneous sporotrichosis. Arch Dermatol 117:143–144, 1981

STROUD JD: Sporotrichosis presenting as pyoderma gangrenosum. Arch Dermatol 97:667–670, 1968

WILSON DE, MANN JJ, BEANETT JE et al: Clinical features of extracutaneous sporotrichosis. Medicine (Baltimore) 46:265–279, 1967

Actinomycosis

BROWN JR: Human actinomycosis. A study of 181 subjects. Hum Pathol 4:319–330, 1973

FRY GR, MARTIN, WJ, DEARING WH et al: Primary actinomycosis of the rectum. Proc Mayo Clin 40:296–299, 1965

VARKEY B, LANDIS FJ, TANG TT et al: Thoracic actinomycosis. Dissemination to skin, subcutaneous tissue, and muscle. Arch Intern Med 134:689–693, 1974

ZAIAS N, TAPLIN D, REBELL G: Mycetoma. Arch Dermatol 99:215–225, 1969

Nocardiosis

DIAMOND RD, BENNETT JE: Disseminated *Nocardia brasiliensis* infection. Arch Intern Med 131:735–736, 1973

FRAZIER AR, ROSENOW EC III, ROBERTS GD: Nocardiosis. Mayo Clin Proc 50:657–663, 1975

KARASSIK SL, SUBRAMANYAM L, GREEN RE et al: Disseminated *Nocardia brasiliensis* infection. Arch Dermatol 112:370–372, 1976

MAHVI TA: Disseminated nocardiosis caused by *Nocardia brasiliensis*. Arch Dermatol 89:426–431, 1964

MOORE M, CONRAD AH: Sporotrichoid nocardiosis caused by *Nocardia brasiliensis*. Arch Dermatol 95:390–393, 1967

RIPPON JW: *Nocardia*: A geographic prevalence. Arch Dermatol 113:237, 1977

ROBBOY SJ, VICKERY AL JR: Tinctorial and morphologic properties distinguishing actinomycosis and nocardiosis. N Engl J Med 282:593–596, 1970

WELSH JD, RHOADES ER, JAQUES W: Disseminated nocardiosis involving spinal cord. Arch Intern Med 108:73–79, 1961

ZECLER E, GILBOA Y, ELKINA L et al: Lymphocutaneous nocardiosis due to *Nocardia brasiliensis*. Arch Dermatol 113:642–643, 1977

Mycetoma

BARNETSON R ST C, MILNE LJR: Mycetoma. (Review) Br J Dermatol 99:227–230, 1978

BUTZ WC, AJELLO L: Black grain mycetoma. Arch Dermatol 104:197–201, 1971

KAMALAM A, SUBRAMANYAM R, AUGUSTINE SM et al: Restoration of bones in mycetoma. Arch Dermatol 111:1178–1180, 1975

KHANDARI KC, MOHAPATRA LN, SEHGAL VN et al: Black grain mycetoma of foot. Arch Dermatol 89:867–870, 1964

MONTES LF, FREEMAN RG, MCCLARIN W: Maduromycosis due to *Madurella grisea*. Arch Dermatol 99:74–79, 1969

NITIDANDHAPRABHAS P, SITTAPAIROCHANA D: Treatment of nocardial mycetoma with trimethoprim and sulfamethoxazole. Arch Dermatol 111:1345–1348, 1975

TARALAKSHMI VV, PANKAJALAKSHMI VV, ARUMUGAM S et al: Mycetoma caused by *Madurella mycetomii* in Madras. Aust J Dermatol 19:125–129, 1978

ZAIAS N, TAPLIN D, REBELL G: Mycetoma. Arch Dermatol 99:215–225, 1969

Botryomycosis

BISHOP GF, GREER KE, HORWITZ DA: *Pseudomonas* botryomycosis. Arch Dermatol 112:1568–1570, 1976

HARMAN RRM, ENGLISH MP, HALFORD M et al: Botryomycosis. Br J Dermatol 102:215–222, 1980

KANSKY A: Botryomycosis. Acta Derm Venereol (Stockh) 44:369–376, 1964

LEIBOWITZ MR, ASVAT MS, KALLA AA et al: Extensive botryomycosis in a patient with diabetes and chronic active hepatitis. Arch Dermatol 117:739–742, 1981

PICOU K, BATRES E, JARRATT M: Botryomycosis. A bacterial cause for mycetoma. Arch Dermatol 115:609–610, 1979

WAISMAN M: Staphylococcic actinophytosis (botryomycosis). Arch Dermatol 86:525–529, 1962

20 Diseases Caused by Protozoa

Three different diseases are caused by *Leishmania:* oriental leishmaniasis, caused by *L. tropica;* American leishmaniasis, caused by *L. brasiliensis;* and kala-azar, caused by *L. donovani*. These three types of organisms cannot be differentiated morphologically. However, they do differ immunologically (Koerber et al).

ORIENTAL LEISHMANIASIS

Oriental leishmaniasis, also called cutaneous leishmaniasis, is endemic to countries of the Middle East and Central Asia, as well as to India, North Africa, and the European countries bordering the eastern Mediterranean Sea (Barsky et al). It is a benign, though often disfiguring, disease that remains limited to the skin. It is transmitted by sandflies of the genus *Phlebotomus*. The incubation period varies with the size of the inoculum and ranges from weeks to months (Rau et al).

The clinical manifestations of oriental leishmaniasis can be divided into acute leishmaniasis, chronic leishmaniasis, leishmaniasis recidivans, and disseminated anergic cutaneous leishmaniasis (Farah and Malak). Leishmaniasis, similar to leprosy, is a spectral disease in which the clinical features depend on the response of the host to the parasite.

Acute leishmaniasis designates primary lesions lasting 1 to 2 years or less. Ordinarily, a single lesion is seen. Multiple lesions occur occasionally and are the result of multiple infective bites by the sandfly (Farah and Malak). The lesions, which are asymptomatic, start as papules, grow into nodules that usually ulcerate, and ultimately heal with a depressed scar.

Chronic leishmaniasis refers to primary lesions lasting longer than 1 to 2 years, possibly several years. This occurs in 3% to 10% of the cases (Hart et al). One or, occasionally, several red raised plaques are present. Ulceration is uncommon. In some instances, the presence of "apple-jelly" nodules causes a considerable resemblance to lupus vulgaris (Hart et al).

Leishmaniasis recidivans indicates a reactivation process occurring many years after the primary infection. It shows circinate papules at or near the periphery of scars of previously healed lesions.

Disseminated anergic cutaneous leishmaniasis, a very rare event in oriental leishmaniasis, consists of widespread nodular or plaquelike lesions (Cohen).

Histopathology. In acute leishmaniasis, during the first few months, the dermal infiltrate consists predominantly of large macrophages filled with great numbers of leishmania organisms (Fig.20-1). In addition, lymphoid cells and a few plasma cells are present. When ulceration sets in, secondary infiltration with neutrophils occurs. The leishmania organisms are present exclusively within macrophages (Bourlond-Reinert and Nicolay). The parasitized macrophages measure 20 μm to 30 μm in diameter. After several months' duration, primary lesions show a gradual reduction in the number of organisms, so that it may be difficult to find them. At the same time, the number of macrophages decreases, and a granulomatous infiltrate develops that contains epithelioid cells and multinucleated giant cells (Lagerholm et al). In the stage of healing, no organisms may be detectable, so that the diagnosis can be made only by means of culture or skin testing.

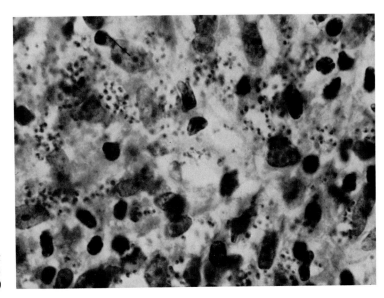

Fig. 20-1.   Oriental leishmaniasis
Numerous leishmania organisms are present
within macrophages. They possess a nucleus
and a small paranucleus or kinetoplast. (×600)

In chronic leishmaniasis, one finds a granulomatous infiltrate intermingled with lymphocytes and histiocytes. It is often indistinguishable from that of lupus vulgaris. However, the lack of caseation necrosis and the sparsity of plasma cells in the infiltrate may help in the distinction (Kurban et al). A few leishmania organisms can be found occasionally on careful searching (Kurban et al; Farah and Malak).

In leishmaniasis recidivans, the histologic changes combine features of both the acute and the chronic forms. The dermis shows an infiltrate of macrophages, lymphoid cells, and some plasma cells as well as tuberculoid granulomas. The number of leishmania organisms is variable. They are difficult to find in some cases (Farah and Malak) but are numerous in others (Schewach-Millet et al).

In disseminated anergic cutaneous leishmaniasis, numerous macrophages full of leishmania organisms are seen (Cohen).

The leishmania organisms, which represent protozoa, appear in sections as round to oval bodies from 2 μm to 4 μm in size. They have no capsule. Within each body is a relatively large, deeply basophilic, round nucleus about 1 μm in diameter and, in addition, a small rodlike paranucleus, or kinetoplast. Although visible in routine stains, leishmania organisms are seen best when a Giemsa stain is used. With this stain, the nucleus and the kinetoplast appear bright red.

Histogenesis. Since in the late stage of acute leishmaniasis and in the chronic and recidivans forms the histologic sections may show no organisms, it is advisable that material obtained by scraping either the edge of an ulcer or a biopsy specimen be inoculated on Novy-MacNeal-Nicolle (N-N-N) medium. The leishmanin skin test, which uses an extract of cultured promastigotes, is a useful diagnostic aid only in persons not living in an endemic area (Bryceson). The test is positive in all persons having or having had leishmaniasis, with the exception of those with the disseminated anergic form.

On *electron microscopy,* as many as 20 leishmania organisms may be seen in one macrophage. Some of them are seen lying free in the cytoplasm, whereas others lie within phagosomes (Sandbank). Each leishmania organism possesses a plasma membrane. Aside from the nucleus, the most conspicuous structures are the flagellum with its basal body and the kinetoplast. The rod-shaped kinetoplast is located within a large mitochondrion (Fukuhara and Klingmüller). It is so rich in deoxyribonucleic acid (DNA) that it was at one time regarded as a second nucleus, or paranucleus. The flagellum and its basal body lie at a right angle to the kinetoplast. The flagellum is surrounded by a large, pear-shaped pocket representing an invagination of the plasma membrane of the parasite (Bourlond-Reinert and Nicolay). Within this invagination, the flagellum lies outside the parasite, extending slightly beyond the confines of the parasite (Sandbank). Its basal body is attached to the kinetoplast (Nicolay and Bourlond-Reinert). When the parasite changes from its promastigote to its flagellar form outside the human body, either in the animal host or in the culture medium, the flagellum increases in length up to 25 μm.

Differential Diagnosis.   A leishmania organism can easily be differentiated from other parasites by the presence of a nucleus and a kinetoplast.

TABLE 20-1.   Points of Differentiation of Four Cutaneous Diseases Showing Parasitized Macrophages

Disease	Distinctive Features in the Histologic Appearance of the Infiltrate	Size of the Organism (μm)	Appearance of the Organism in the Tissue
Rhinoscleroma	Mikulicz cells, on the average, are larger than the parasitized macrophages in the other three diseases. There are more plasma cells than in the other three diseases. Russell bodies are present.	2–3	Round or oval bodies
Granuloma inguinale	Small abscesses composed of neutrophils are scattered through the infiltrate.	1–2 (smaller than in the other three diseases)	Encapsulated round or oval bodies
Histoplasmosis	Foci of necrosis are common.	2–4	Round or oval bodies surrounded by a clear halo
Leishmaniasis		2–4	Not encapsulated round or oval bodies containing a nucleus and a paranucleus, or kinetoplast

In addition to leishmaniasis, three other cutaneous diseases are characterized by an infiltrate containing large parasitized macrophages. They are rhinoscleroma and granuloma inguinale, caused by bacteria, and histoplasmosis, caused by a fungus. In spite of great similarities, these four diseases have points of differentiation that in most instances make a histologic diagnosis possible (Table 20-1).

AMERICAN LEISHMANIASIS

American leishmaniasis, also called mucocutaneous leishmaniasis, is caused by *L. brasiliensis*. It occurs in South America, especially Brazil and Peru, and, less frequently, in Central America and Mexico. It is transmitted by flies of the genus *Phlebotomus*.

The initial lesion or lesions have the same appearance as in oriental leishmaniasis. However, in a significant number of cases, this is followed several years later, as many as 15 to 25 years after the healing of the primary cutaneous ulcer, by severely destructive mucocutaneous lesions, which affect especially the nasopharynx and are caused by hematogenous and lymphatic dissemination of the parasite (Walton et al). This secondary involvement, known as espundia, indicates a decrease in the immunologic competence of the host, as shown by the fact that it may be induced by immunosuppressive therapy (Moriearty).

Disseminated anergic cutaneous leishmaniasis, a very uncommon event in oriental leishmaniasis, occurs somewhat more commonly in American leishmaniasis, but it is still rare. Widely scattered nodules, plaques, and ulcerated lesions are seen. However, involvement of mucous membranes either is absent (Convit et al) or consists of minimal lesions of the nasal mucosa (Convit and Kerdel-Vegas; Simpson et al).

Histopathology. In early lesions of American leishmaniasis, as in oriental leishmaniasis, one observes macrophages containing leishmania organisms. However, the number of organisms is as a rule smaller than in oriental leishmaniasis, so that, occasionally, no organisms can be seen even in early lesions (Price and Silvers). Usually, a few tuberculoid granulomas are also present (Snow et al). The ulcerative mucosal lesions of espundia show predominantly a nonspecific inflammatory infiltrate. There are only a few leishmania organisms within macrophages and few or no tuberculoid formations (Fasal). If only a few organisms are present, the diagnosis can be established by culture of tissue homogenate or aspirate on N-N-N medium, by the leishmanin skin test, or by indirect immunofluorescence testing of the patient's serum (Walton et al).

In the disseminated anergic form of American leishmaniasis, the lesions contain numerous macrophages with abundant cytoplasm that is filled with many leishmania organisms. The presence of such large numbers of leishmania organisms is the result of an anergic state, as shown by a negative intradermal test with leishmanin (Convit et al; Simpson et al).

POST-KALA-AZAR DERMAL LEISHMANIASIS

Kala-azar, caused by *L. donovani*, is characterized by chronic, irregular fever, anemia, weight loss, and marked enlargement of the spleen and often also of the liver. Cutaneous lesions may occur, especially in India, 1 to 5 years after apparent recovery. These lesions may be one of three types: (1) hypopigmented or hyperpigmented macular lesions, (2) erythematous macular lesions, or (3) nodular lesions (Gupta and Bhattacharjee). The pigmentary macules are found predominantly on the trunk, and the erythematous macules on the face, often in a butterfly distribution (Yesudian and Thambiah). The nodules, which are asymptomatic and rarely larger than 1 cm in diameter, occur predominantly on the face, especially around the mouth and nose, and to a lesser extent also on the trunk and extremities. Patients may have macules or nodules or both (Girgla et al).

Histopathology. The pigmentary macules show in the upper dermis an infiltrate of lymphocytes, plasma cells, and histiocytes. A few intracellular leishmania bodies are found after a prolonged search in some cases, but none are found in others (Girgla et al).

The erythematous lesions generally contain a more pronounced cellular infiltrate than the pigmentary macules and a larger proportion of plasma cells. Leishmania organisms are somewhat more numerous in the erythematous than in the pigmentary lesions (Gupta and Bhattacharjee).

The nodular lesions show, separated from the epidermis by a narrow zone of normal collagen and extending into the subcutaneous fat, a compact cellular infiltrate composed largely of histiocytes and epithelioid cells intermingled with lymphoid cells (Yesudian and Thambiah). In addition, there may be numerous plasma cells, and, occasionally, a few giant cells. The number of leishmania organisms present within the histiocytes is fairly small in some cases (Gupta and Bhattacharjee); in others, however, large numbers are found (Yesudian and Thambiah; Girgla et al).

BIBLIOGRAPHY

Oriental Leishmaniasis

BARSKY S, STORINO W, SALGEA K et al: Cutaneous leishmaniasis. Arch Dermatol 114:1354–1355, 1978

BOURLOND-REINERT L, NICOLAY M: Leishmaniose cutanée: Étude ultrastructurale. Dermatologica 151:113–124, 1975

BRYCESON A: Cutaneous leishmaniasis. Br J Dermatol 94:223–226, 1976

COHEN HA: Induction of delayed-type sensitivity to leishmania parasite in a case of leishmaniasis cutanea diffusa with BCG and cord-factor (trehalose-6-6'-dimycolate). Acta Derm Venereol (Stockh) 59:547–549, 1979

FARAH FS, MALAK JA: Cutaneous leishmaniasis. Arch Dermatol 103:467–474, 1971

FUKUHARA S, KLINGMÜLLER G: Elektronenmikroskopische Untersuchungen der Leishmaniasis cutanea. Arch Dermatol Res 255:305–316, 1976

HART M, LIVINGOOD CS, GOLTZ RW et al: Late cutaneous leishmaniasis. Arch Dermatol 99:455–458, 1969

KOERBER WA JR, KOEHN MC, JACOBS PH et al: Treatment of cutaneous leishmaniasis with antimony sodium gluconate. Arch Dermatol 114:1226, 1978

KURBAN AK, MALAK JA, FARAH F et al: Histopathology of cutaneous leishmaniasis. Arch Dermatol 93:396–401, 1966

LAGERHOLM B, GIP L, LODIN A: The histopathological and cytological diagnosis of cutaneous leishmaniasis in two cases of *Leishmania tropica*. Acta Derm Venereol (Stockh) 48:600–607, 1968

NICOLAY M, BOURLOND-REINERT L: Une leishmaniose cutanée. Arch Belges Dermatol 29:327–331, 1973

RAU RC, DUBIN HV, TAYLOR WB: *Leishmania tropica* infections in travellers. Arch Dermatol 112:197–201, 1976

SANDBANK M: Cutaneous leishmaniasis. Ultrastructural study of three cases. Arch Dermatol Res 257:195–201, 1976

SCHEWACH-MILLET M, FISHER BK, SEMAH D: Leishmaniasis recidivans treated with sodium stibogluconate. Cutis 28:67–89, 1981

American Leishmaniasis

CONVIT J, KERDEL-VEGAS F: Disseminated cutaneous leishmaniasis. Arch Dermatol 91:439–447, 1965

CONVIT J, REYES O, KERDEL-VEGAS F: Disseminated anergic cutaneous leishmaniasis. Arch Dermatol 76:213–217, 1957

FASAL P: American leishmaniasis or leishmaniasis mucocutanea. In Simons RDGP (ed): Handbook of Tropical Dermatology and Medical Mycology, Vol 1, p 375. Amsterdam, Elsevier, 1952

MORIEARTY PL: Diagnosis and prognosis of New World leishmaniasis. Arch Dermatol 114:962–963, 1978

PRICE SM, SILVERS DN: New World leishmaniasis. Arch Dermatol 113:1415–1416, 1977

SIMPSON MH, MULLINS JF, STONE OF: Disseminated anergic cutaneous leishmaniasis. Arch Dermatol 97:301–303, 1968

SNOW JH, SATULSKY EM, KEAN BH: American cutaneous leishmaniasis. Arch Dermatol Syph 57:90–101, 1948

WALTON BC, PAULSON JE, ARJONA MA et al: American cutaneous leishmaniasis. JAMA 228:1256–1258, 1974

Post-Kala-Azar Dermal Leishmaniasis

GIRGLA HS, MARSDEN RA, SINGH GM et al: Post-kala-azar dermal leishmaniasis. Br J Dermatol 97:307–311, 1977

GUPTA PC, BHATTACHARJEE B: Histopathology of post-kala-azar dermal leishmaniasis. J Trop Med Hyg 56:110–117, 1953

YESUDIAN P, THAMBIAH AS: Amphotericin B therapy in dermal leishmanoid. Arch Dermatol 109:720–722, 1974

21 Diseases Caused by Viruses

INTRODUCTION

Viruses are obligatory intracellular parasites that differ from the larger microorganisms, such as bacteria, in that they are not cells (White). They lack organelles, such as ribosomes and mitochondria, hence have no metabolism of their own, and consequently must use the organelles, the energy, and many of the enzymes of the host cell for their replication. In doing so, viruses disturb the metabolism of the host cell irreversibly and thus act as pathogens (Luger).

Viruses are composed of a central core of nucleoprotein called the *nucleoid*, which contains either deoxyribonucleic acid (DNA) or ribonucleic acid (RNA). The core is surrounded by the capsid, the subunits of which, called *capsomers*, contain the major antigenic components of the virus. The core and the capsid form the essential part of the virus or virion. Viruses that replicate in the nucleus, on leaving the nucleus, may acquire an outer coat derived from the nuclear membrane, whereas virions that replicate in the cytoplasm may derive an outer coat from the plasma membrane (EM 31).

Before viruses can enter a cell, they must be able to attach themselves to specific receptors of the plasma membrane; thus, they are species-specific. Viruses enter the cytoplasm of a cell by a process akin to phagocytosis, that is, by becoming enveloped by the plasma membrane of the cell as an outer coat. Once inside the cell, the viruses induce the synthesis of an "uncoating" protein. As their outer coat and their capsid are being digested by the "uncoating" protein, the uncoated nucleoids lose their characteristic structure. The viruses now are in "eclipse" and are not apparent until replication has taken place and new virions or viruses, each composed of a core and a capsid, have been formed. During the process of replication, the proteins of the cell follow the genetic code of the specific virus nucleic acid, and the proteins that are formed are characteristic of the virus rather than of the cell. The first proteins formed after the "uncoating" are specific enzymes needed for replication of the virus nucleic acids. The proteins constituting the capsid are also synthesized (Luger). Thousands of viruses may be released from an infected cell.

The diameter of viruses infecting the skin varies from 20 nm for the echoviruses to 300 nm for the poxviruses. Under favorable conditions, the latter group of viruses may be recognizable with the light microscope—for example, variola viruses as Paschen bodies. As a rule, however, viruses can be seen with the light microscope only when aggregated into inclusion bodies.

Inclusion bodies usually are roughly spherical. Their average size is about 7 µm, analogous to the size of an erythrocyte. They tend to be eosinophilic with most staining methods. Electron microscopy has shown that inclusion bodies represent sites in which virus replication is occurring or has occurred. In some viral infections, such as molluscum contagiosum, they contain masses of virions and are Feulgen-positive; in contrast, in other viral infections, such as herpesvirus infections, the viruses have left the inclusion bodies, except for a few residual nucleoids, and the inclusion bodies are then Feulgen-negative (Southam et al). Since inclusion bodies are found in locations in which the respective viruses either are replicating or have replicated, they are seen in the cytoplasm in the case of poxvirus infections, and in the nucleus in the case of herpesvirus infections. When located in the nucleus, they are surrounded by a clear halo as a result of margination of the nuclear chromatin (Pinkerton).

Aside from the recognition of inclusion bodies, the

inoculation of laboratory animals or of cell cultures can often prove the existence of a specific virus infection. Also, in some instances, direct immunofluorescence staining of viral antigen is used, employing specific antibody conjugates (Liu and Llanes-Rodas). Serologic tests may also be of value, particularly if an increase in antibody titer has occurred in the course of a disease. The titer of antibodies may be determined either by complement fixation or by neutralization (Artenstein and Demis).

Electron microscopy has been of great value in the study of the anatomy of various viruses and of the replication of viruses in tissue; it is also occasionally useful for the purpose of diagnosing viral diseases. Most cutaneous viruses remain well preserved in formalin-fixed, paraffin-embedded tissue blocks, and even sections stained for light microscopy can be reprocessed for electron microscopy with good results (Blank et al).

Four groups of viruses can affect the skin or the adjoining mucous surfaces: (1) the herpesvirus group, including herpes simplex types 1 and 2 and the varicella-zoster virus, DNA-containing organisms that multiply within the nucleus of the host cell; (2) the poxvirus group, including smallpox, milkers' nodules, orf, and molluscum contagiosum, DNA-containing agents that multiply within the cytoplasm; (3) the papovavirus group, including the various types of verrucae and focal epithelial hyperplasia; they contain DNA and replicate in the nucleus; and (4) the picornavirus group, including coxsackievirus group A, causing hand-foot-and-mouth disease; these viruses contain RNA rather than DNA in their nucleoid.

HERPES SIMPLEX

Two viruses that show no cross immunity can cause herpes simplex: herpes simplex virus type 1 (orofacial type) and type 2 (genital type), often referred to as HSV-1 and HSV-2, respectively. The primary infection with HSV-1 takes place subclinically in childhood in 85% to 90% of the cases (Blank and Haines). In approximately 10% of the population, an acute gingivostomatitis occurs, usually in childhood and rarely in early adult life (Southam et al). Primary infection may also occur in rare instances as a respiratory infection, as infected eczema (Kaposi's varicelliform eruption, see p. 368), or as keratoconjunctivitis. Primary infection with HSV-2 generally occurs on the genitalia after puberty by venereal contact. Occasionally, an infant contracts HSV-2 as an intrauterine infection or by direct contact with the infected birth canal (see p. 362).

Primary infections are always caused by infection from another person. The incubation period in the case of genital herpes simplex varies between 3 and 14 days and on the average is 5 days (Chang et al). Recurrent infections of the oral cavity, the skin, or the genitals can be due either to reactivation of a latent infection or to a new infection.

Recurrent infections of HSV-1 occur most commonly as herpes labialis on or near the vermilion border of the lips. Recurrences may be triggered by excess exposure to sunlight or by febrile illnesses, but they also occur spontaneously. Instead of the lips, however, any part of the skin or oral mucosa can be affected by HSV-1. Even though most infections of the genitalia and adjoining skin are caused by HSV-2, some infections in this area are caused by HSV-1, probably as a result of orogenital contact (Chang et al). However, genital infections with HSV-1 are less apt to recur than those with HSV-2; the rate of recurrence in one series was 14% for HSV-1 infections as compared with 60% for HSV-2 infections (Reeves et al).

Both primary and recurrent herpes simplex, in their earliest stage, show one or several groups of vesicles on an inflamed base. If located on a mucous surface, the vesicles quickly change into erosions, whereas, on the skin, they may become pustular before becoming covered by crusts.

The following are special forms of cutaneous herpes simplex: *Kaposi's varicelliform eruption* (eczema herpeticum), which is discussed on p. 368; *herpetic folliculitis of the bearded region*, a benign eruption of grouped vesiculofollicular lesions that heals within a few weeks (Izumi et al); and *herpetic whitlow*, which consists of painful, deep-seated vesicles limited to the paronychial or volar aspects of the distal phalanx of a finger. Herpetic whitlow occurs largely in medical personnel following minor injuries and may be caused by either HSV-1 or HSV-2. In the latter case, it may be a primary infection (Giacobetti). There may be periodically recurring attacks (Haburchak).

Herpes simplex pneumonia usually is fatal. Though rare, it may occur in children as well as in adults and is thought to be an aspiration infection, since it usually follows a herpes simplex infection of the mouth, the esophagus, or the trachea (Herout et al; Nash and Foley).

Herpes simplex encephalitis is the most frequent and devastating of acute viral infections of the brain in the United States today (Nolan et al). It has a fairly high mortality rate, and some of those who survive have severe residual cerebral damage. Infants and children as well as adults may be affected. Only a few patients have a history of recurrent herpes labialis before the onset of the encephalitis (Leider et al).

Herpes Simplex in Compromised Hosts. Three forms of herpes simplex are characteristically found in children or adults with impairment of the cellular immune system. Such impairment may be caused (a) by congenital diseases such as the Wiskott–Aldrich syndrome or dysplasia of the thymus (Sutton et al; Joseph and Vogt), (b) by lymphoma or leukemia (Solomon), (c) by severe burns (Foley et al), and, most commonly, (d) by prolonged immunosuppressive therapy (Orenstein et al; Keane et al). There may be three manifestations: (1) chronic ulcerative herpes simplex, (2) generalized acute mucocutaneous herpes simplex, and (3) systemic herpes simplex.

Chronic ulcerative herpes simplex shows persistent ulcers and erosions, usually starting on the face (Logan et al) or in the perineal region (Vonderheid et al). There may be gradual, widespread extension (Vonderheid et al), and the infection may progress into systemic herpes simplex (Shneidman et al). The occurrence of chronic perianal ulcerative herpes simplex lesions has recently been described in young male homosexuals as the result of severe acquired immunodeficiency (Siegel et al). (See also Kaposi's sarcoma, p. 637).

Generalized acute mucocutaneous herpes simplex starts with a localized vesicular eruption, which is located in the genital region in cases of HSV-2 infection (Rendtorf and Fowinkel; Long et al; Lopyan et al) but has been observed in various areas in cases of HSV-1 infection (Solomon). Rapid dissemination associated with fever takes place, suggestive of smallpox (Rendtorf and Fowinkel) or varicella (Long et al). In some instances, death results without the presence of visceral lesions (Sutton et al; Lopyan et al).

Systemic herpes simplex usually follows oral or genital lesions of herpes simplex. It causes areas of necrosis, particularly in the liver, adrenals, and pancreas, and leads rapidly to death (Lee and Fortuny; Keane et al; Elliott et al). In some patients, a few cutaneous lesions of herpes simplex are also present (Orenstein et al). In patients without cutaneous or mucosal lesions of herpes simplex, the virus may be cultured in vivo from the throat or buffy coat (Taylor et al).

Congenital Herpes Simplex. Since up to 1% of patients in prenatal clinics have HSV-2 infections by culture of the vagina and one third of these have lesions, the potential of congenital herpes simplex infection is considerable (Honig et al). Early intrauterine infection secondary to maternal viremia and transplacental spread may result in disturbed embryogenesis. Late intrauterine infections and neonatal infections occurring during passage of the fetus through the birth canal may result in encephalitis, hepatoadrenal necrosis, and pneumonia (Komorous et al). In over 50% of all babies with congenital HSV-2 infection, localized cutaneous lesions of herpes simplex are an initial manifestation facilitating the diagnosis. In vertex deliveries, the scalp is a common site for the development of initial herpetic vesicles. Conversely, infants delivered by breech often have lesions of the buttocks and perianal area (Honig et al). It is very rare, however, for this localized herpes simplex to remain the only manifestation (Tasaki et al). Since at least half of the babies die of systemic herpes simplex infection and neurologic and ocular sequelae occur in at least one third of the survivors, a cesarean section is recommended as a prophylactic measure in parturient women with lesions of genital herpes simplex (Nahmias et al).

Histopathology. The characteristic lesion in herpes simplex of the skin is an intraepidermal vesicle produced by profound degeneration of epidermal cells, resulting in marked acantholysis. The degen-

eration of the epidermal cells occurs in two forms: ballooning degeneration and reticular degeneration. These degenerative changes are typical of viral vesicles, making them histologically distinct from the vesicles seen in other vesiculobullous diseases (see Classification of Bullae, p. 92). However, as in all vesiculobullous diseases, it is important that an early lesion be selected for biopsy; otherwise, secondary changes, especially invasion of inflammatory cells, may obscure the diagnostic features.

Ballooning degeneration causes marked swelling of epidermal cells. Such swollen balloon cells have a homogeneous, eosinophilic cytoplasm (Figs. 21-1, 21-2). They may have one nucleus or may be multinucleated. Because the balloon cells lose their intercellular bridges, acantholysis occurs: the cells become separated from one another, and unilocular vesicles result. The processes of ballooning degeneration occurs mainly at the base of viral vesicles, leading to a dissolution of the lower epidermis, so that the vesicle that formed intraepidermally ultimately has a subepidermal location in many places. Ballooning degeneration can also affect the epithelial cells of hair follicles and sebaceous glands.

Reticular degeneration represents a process in which the epidermal cells become greatly distended by intracellular edema, so that many of the cell walls burst. Through coalescence of neighboring, similarly affected cells, a multilocular vesicle results, the septa of which are formed by resistant cellular walls (Fig. 21-3). Reticular degeneration occurs mainly in the upper portion and at the periphery of viral vesicles. In old vesicles, the cellular walls no longer are resistant and disappear. In this way, the originally multilocular portions of the vesicle may become unilocular. It should be pointed out that, in contrast to ballooning degeneration, reticular degeneration is not specific for viral vesicles, since it also occurs in the vesicles of dermatitis (see p. 95).

The upper dermis of viral vesicles shows an inflammatory infiltrate, the density of which depends on the severity of the reaction. In severe reactions, as seen especially in primary infections with herpes simplex virus, the dermis may show a severe vasculitis characterized by the presence of fibrinoid deposits and a dense inflammatory infiltrate with many neutrophils both within and around the capillary walls. In addition, there may be extravasation of erythrocytes, fragmentation of the nuclei of neutrophils, and, occasionally, necrosis of vascular walls (Cheatham et al).

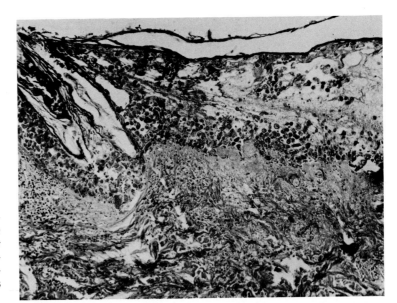

Fig. 21-1.   Herpes simplex
Low magnification. There is marked ballooning degeneration of the cells at the floor of the vesicle. The cells of a hair follicle shown at the left also show ballooning degeneration. Reticular degeneration, observed at the top of the vesicle, is only slight. (×100)

Fig. 21-2.   Herpes simplex
High magnification of Figure 21-1. Balloon cells at the floor of a vesicle are shown. On the right, an eosinophilic inclusion body surrounded by a halo lies in the nucleus of a balloon cell (L). (×400)

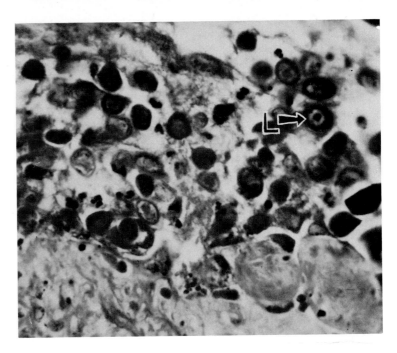

Inclusion bodies are seen quite frequently in the center of enlarged, round nuclei of balloon cells. The inclusion bodies are eosinophilic and usually are surrounded by a clear space or halo (see Fig. 21-2). They measure from 3 μm to 8 μm in diameter. (Concerning the nature of the inclusion bodies, see p. 360.)

Herpetic folliculitis of the bearded region shows pronounced changes in the outer root sheath of the affected hair follicles with ballooning degeneration and formation of multinucleated epithelial giant cells. The heavy inflammatory perifollicular infiltrate can cause destruction of some of the hair follicles (Izumi et al).

Chronic ulcerative herpes simplex may be impossible to diagnose as being of viral genesis in specimens that are devoid of epidermis. However, viral changes may be seen in the epidermis at the margin of the ulcer, including epithelial giant cells with intranuclear inclusions (Logan et al; Vonder-

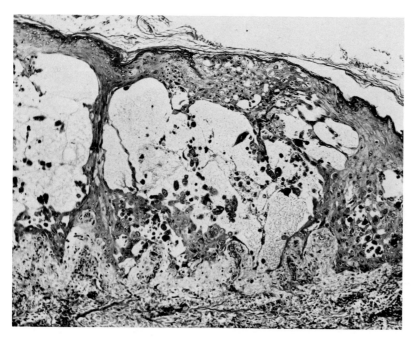

Fig. 21-3.   Herpes simplex
Reticular degeneration is present, especially at the top of the vesicle, resulting in a multilocular vesicle. In addition, ballooning degeneration is present at the floor of the vesicle. (×200)

heid et al). Viral cultures may be the best way to prove the diagnosis.

Visceral Lesions.   In *herpes simplex pneumonia*, the alveolar lining cells show eosinophilic inclusion bodies in their nuclei as the most characteristic feature (Herout et al; Nash and Foley).

In *herpes simplex encephalitis,* the brain shows extensive areas of necrosis, particularly of the medial surfaces of the temporal lobes. Eosinophilic intranuclear inclusion bodies may be present in the cerebral cortex (Leider et al). In addition, the herpes simplex virus can be recovered on cultures of necrotic brain tissue (Jewett).

In *systemic herpes simplex of compromised hosts and of the newborn*, autopsy reveals characteristic foci of necrosis in the liver and the adrenals and, in some instances, also in the lungs and the brain with the presence of intranuclear eosinophilic inclusion bodies (Catalano et al; Patrizi et al).

Tzanck Smear.   For a rapid, though preliminary diagnosis, cytologic examination is often useful. It is carried out on a smear taken from the floor of an early, freshly opened vesicle and stained with the Giemsa stain (Honig et al). As a rule, many acantholytic balloon cells with either one or several nuclei are seen (Graham et al). The presence of so many balloon cells is due to the fact that the smear is taken from the floor of the blister, where ballooning degeneration is most pronounced.

Viral Identification. The herpes simplex virus can be directly identified either by culture or by direct immu-

nofluorescence testing. For the culture, material from the floor of a blister or other infected material is inoculated on cell cultures consisting of HeLa cells or human amnion cells or fibroblasts. The virus has a cytopathogenic effect on the cells of the culture. This effect is specifically inhibited, or neutralized, by prior addition to the cell culture of a serum containing herpes simplex antibodies (Luger). Direct immunofluorescence examination for the presence of the viral antigen in cells infected with herpes simplex virus is carried out by the preparation of smears of such cells to which is added, first, rabbit serum containing herpes simplex antibody and then fluorescein-conjugated antirabbit serum globulin of mice (Liu and Llanes-Rodas). For determination of the antibody titer in the patient's serum, the complement fixation reaction is usually used.

Histogenesis. On *electron microscopy*, the herpes simplex virus is found to be spheric. Its DNA-containing core measures approximately 40 nm in diameter. The virion has a diameter of about 100 nm and together with its outer coat measures around 135 nm (Morecki and Becker). Ultrastructurally, the virion of herpes simplex is indistinguishable from that of varicella (see p. 367) (Bastian et al).

HSV-1 and HSV-2 differ not only in their antigenicity, since each type is preferentially neutralized by its own specific antiserum, but also in their effects on tissue cultures and in their growth characteristics on the chorioallantoic membrane of chick embryos (Nahmias and Dowdle).

Primary infection with either HSV-1 or HSV-2, which may be subclinical (and very often is, particularly in the case of HSV-1), is followed by the emergence of specific circulating antibodies and latency of the infection. In a proportion of persons infected with either HSV-1 or HSV-2, the virus can become activated intermittently and give rise to recurrent lesions. The first few recurrences usually are accompanied by a rise in the antibody titer; thereafter, however, the appearance of lesions is unrelated to the antibody titer (Higgins). With few exceptions, patients with recurrent herpes simplex have higher levels of circulating antibody to herpes simplex virus than control subjects (Gange et al).

Although recurrences, particularly in the case of HSV-2, can be based on reinfection, they are often based on reactivation of a latent infection. It is now generally accepted that, after the primary infection of the skin or mucosa, the virus makes its way to the nuclei of the cells of the regional sensory ganglia, where it resides in a latent, nonreplicative state (Bierman). Thus, the herpes simplex virus was recovered from trigeminal ganglia obtained at autopsy in six of seven unselected patients. This suggests the trigeminal ganglia as a likely site of latent virus causing recurrent herpes labialis (Baringer and Swoveland).

Two possible mechanisms have been proposed for the production of endogeneous recurrences. One suggests that trigger factors cause activation of the virus in the ganglia and that the virus then travels down nerves to the epithelium. The other theory proposes that infectious viruses are frequently or continuously released to distal epithelial sites and that, when local conditions are appropriate, the virus can induce a recurrent lesion (Blank).

Differential Diagnosis.   Although the viral vesicles produced by the herpes simplex virus and by the varicella-zoster virus have the same histologic appearance, and although the two viruses are indistinguishable by electron microscopy, herpes simplex and varicella-zoster differ in their antigenicity and in their growth in culture (see p. 367).

Herpes simplex vesicles must be differentiated from vesicles of pemphigus vulgaris. Even though the blisters of pemphigus vulgaris, like viral vesicles, show acantholysis and degeneration of epidermal cells, differentiation usually is quite easy, because the ballooning degeneration in viral vesicles represents a far more profound degeneration than that occurring in the blisters of pemphigus vulgaris. Furthermore, viral vesicles are never seen in a suprabasal location, since viral degeneration causes lysis of the basal layer from the dermis. The presence of eosinophilic nuclear inclusion bodies in the viral vesicles further aids in the differentiation.

VARICELLA AND HERPES ZOSTER

Varicella and herpes zoster are produced by the same virus, the varicella-zoster virus. Varicella results from contact of the nonimmune host with this virus, whereas herpes zoster occurs in persons who are partially immune as a result of having previously had varicella either clinically or subclinically. Although varicella occasionally develops in children exposed to herpes zoster, exogenous infection causes herpes zoster only very rarely. In most instances in which herpes zoster has been acquired through exposure to varicella or herpes zoster, the patients had a defect of cellular immunity (Rado et al; Sokal and Firat; Rogers and Tindall). As a rule, herpes zoster is caused by reactivation of a latent virus infection that originally took place in either a spinal or a cranial sensory ganglion as a result of hematogenous dissemination during the initial varicella infection. On reactivation, the virus spreads from the ganglion along the corresponding sensory nerve or nerves to the skin (Cheatham; Blank and Haines).

Varicella.   In varicella, a generalized eruption develops after an incubation period of about 2 weeks, usually as the result of a respiratory tract infection. About 95% of the patients are children. Serious complications are very rare in normal children. The lesions of varicella begin as small papules, which develop into vesicles. In mild cases, most vesicles become crusted without changing into pustules. A slightly hemorrhagic base to the vesicles may be seen in severe cases. New lesions continue to develop for several days so that, in varicella, in contrast to variola, lesions in different stages of development can be observed.

Three systemic complications can occur in varicella without the existence of immunosuppression: *primary varicella pneumonia*, which occurs in approximately 14% of adults with varicella and carries a mortality of at least 10% (Triebwasser et al); *Reye's syndrome*, a rare, fatal encephalopathy occurring in infants or children in association with varicella or other viral infections (Takashima and Becker); and *neonatal varicella*, which results in severe, usually fatal disseminated varicella in the infant if the mother has developed varicella less than 5 days before delivery (Takashima and Becker).

VARICELLA IN COMPROMISED HOSTS.   In patients with impairment of the cellular immune system, as seen in lymphoma and as a result of treatment with immunosuppressants, continued viral replication may lead not only to a prolonged course but also to dissemination to various organs. Thus, varicella pneumonia is not uncommon, even in children, and death may result from dissemination (Cheatham et al; Takashima and Becker).

Herpes Zoster.   Although herpes zoster occurs largely in adults, particularly in those of advanced age, about 5% of patients with herpes zoster are children under 15 years of age. The course in children without immune defects usually is mild (Rogers and Tindall). The eruption in herpes zoster consists of groups of vesicles situated on an inflammatory base and arranged along the course of a sensory nerve. The base of the lesions frequently appears hemorrhagic, and some of the lesions may become necrotic and ulcerate. Not infrequently, in addition to the localized eruption, there are a few scattered lesions elsewhere and, rarely, a generalized eruption, including mucosal lesions, indistinguishable from that of varicella (Merselis et al).

HERPES ZOSTER IN COMPROMISED HOSTS. Both the incidence and the severity of herpes zoster are greatly increased in patients with impaired cellular immunity. The incidence of herpes zoster is particularly high in patients with advanced Hodgkin's disease receiving chemotherapy or radiation (Sokal and Firat). In children, as in adults, the incidence of herpes zoster in this high-risk group is about 50%. The eruption is either localized or disseminated, and some patients may even have two separate episodes (Reboul et al). Rarely, varicella develops in place of a disseminated herpes zoster (Nasemann et al).

Whereas patients with disseminated herpes zoster but without associated serious illness have a good prognosis, patients with impaired cellular immunity may develop widespread, fatal systemic manifestations, such as pneumonia (Kain et al), gastroenteritis (Cheatham), or encephalitis (Appelbaum et al).

Histopathology. The cutaneous lesions of varicella and herpes zoster are histologically indistinguishable from those seen in herpes simplex (see p. 362). Also, the same type of intranuclear eosinophilic inclusion bodies are seen in the epithelial cells in and about the vesicles in all three diseases. Frequently, however, the degree of leukocytoclastic vasculitis and hemorrhage are more pronounced in varicella and, particularly, in herpes zoster than in herpes simplex. In severe cases of varicella and in disseminated herpes zoster, eosinophilic inclusion bodies have also been observed in the dermis within the nuclei of capillary endothelial cells and of fibroblasts bordering the affected vessels (Cheatham et al). In contrast, in localized herpes zoster, in which the virus reaches the epidermis by way of the cutaneous nerves rather than the capillaries, inclusion bodies have been demonstrated within neurilemmal cells of the small nerves in the dermis underlying the vesicles (Cheatham).

Visceral Lesions. The visceral lesions caused by hematogenous dissemination in varicella and herpes zoster are indistinguishable from one another and from those produced by herpes simplex. However, the neural lesions in herpes zoster are quite specific for that disease (see below).

In fatal cases of *pneumonia due to varicella or herpes zoster*, the autopsy reveals intranuclear eosinophilic inclusion bodies in bronchiolar epithelial cells and alveolar cells (Frank; Merselis et al).

Fatal *systemic varicella* or *herpes zoster* usually occurs in children or adults with an inherited,

acquired, or induced defect in cellular immunity (Blank). One finds areas of focal necrosis containing intranuclear eosinophilic inclusion bodies in various organs, especially the liver, the kidneys, the adrenals, and the lungs (Cheatham et al). However, in varicella, even in the case of widespread lesions with inclusion bodies in many internal organs, invasion of the central nervous system is rare except in neonates (Takashima and Becker).

In fatal cases of *neonatal varicella*, widespread lesions are the rule. These lesions may even involve the brain. In contrast, in Reye's syndrome occurring in infants or children in conjunction with varicella as acute and severe encephalopathy and fatty degeneration of the viscera, particularly of the liver, no inclusion bodies are found, and no virus can be isolated from either the brain or the viscera (Takashima and Becker).

The *neural lesions in herpes zoster* begin either in a dorsal root ganglion or in a cranial nerve ganglion with a severe inflammatory infiltrate that is associated with necrosis of ganglion cells and nerve fibers and with hemorrhage (Cheatham). The affected ganglia in herpes zoster have been shown on light microscopy to contain intranuclear eosinophilic inclusion bodies (Cheatham). Furthermore, the presence of the varicella-zoster virus in the ganglia has been demonstrated by electron microscopy (Ghatak and Zimmerman) and by culture with monkey kidney cells (Bastian et al). Inflammatory and degenerative changes extend from the involved ganglia along the sensory nerves to the skin. In addition, inflammatory and degenerative changes extend proximally from the ganglion to the posterior nerve root and into the spinal cord, producing a unilateral, segmental myelitis in the posterior columns (Denny-Brown et al).

Asymptomatic upward extension of the virus along the spinal cord from the dorsal root ganglion to the brain apparently is not uncommon, in view of the facts that about one fourth of the patients with herpes zoster have pleocytosis of the spinal fluid (Appelbaum et al; Gold) and that the varicella-zoster virus occasionally can be isolated from the spinal fluid of such patients (Gold). However, fatal cases of encephalomyelitis (Rose et al) or encephalitis (Appelbaum et al) are rare in herpes zoster and occur only in compromised hosts.

Tzanck Smear. Cytologic examination of the contents of vesicles, useful as a preliminary diagnostic test, is carried out in varicella and herpes zoster in the same way as in herpes simplex (see p. 364).

Viral Identification. The herpes simplex virus and the varicella-zoster virus are indistinguishable by electron microscopy (Bastian et al). However, in contrast with herpes simplex, the varicella-zoster virus does not grow in ordinary tissue cultures, although it does grow in tissue cultures containing human fetal diploid kidney cells or monkey kidney cells (Weller et al). Also, whereas the herpes simplex virus is a pathogen for several laboratory animals such as the rabbit, the varicella-zoster virus is not pathogenic for any animal (Gold). Furthermore, the herpes simplex and varicella-zoster viruses differ in their antigenicity, so that, on serologic testing for varicella-zoster virus antibodies, an increase in antibody titer in the course of the disease is found to occur only in varicella (see p. 365).

Histogenesis. On *electron microscopic examination* of the cutaneous lesions of varicella and herpes zoster, virus particles are found in the capillary endothelium in varicella and in the axons of dermal nerves in herpes zoster in some cases (Hasegawa) but not in others (Orfanos and Runne). The reason for the sparsity or absence of virions in the dermis is the fact that replication of the virus in the skin takes place almost exclusively in the keratinocytes of the involved epidermis. If present in sufficient numbers, the virions within the epidermal nuclei may lie partially in crystalloid aggregates (Nasemann et al). Some virus particles consist only of a hollow coat, or capsid, whereas others show within the capsid a DNA-containing core, or nucleoid (Bastian et al). The nucleoid averages 40 nm in diameter, and the capsid 100 nm (Morecki and Becker). On leaving the nucleus for the cytoplasm, most virions are enveloped by an outer coat derived from the nuclear membrane, increasing the size of the virus particle from about 100 nm to about 150 nm. When many virions are present, they may be seen in a crystalloid arrangement in the cytoplasm as well as in the nuclei (Nasemann et al). Subsequently, the virions are extruded into the intercellular space (EM 31), where they are phagocytized by macrophages. As a result of this phagocytosis, the phagolysosomes of the macrophages may contain numerous virions (Orfanos and Runne). It is worth noting that both the herpes simplex virus and the varicella-zoster virus can often be identified by electron microscopy even in tissue that has not been specifically prepared for electron microscopy but has been routinely fixed in formalin and embedded in paraffin (Morecki and Becker).

VARIOLA

The global eradication of variola, or smallpox, has apparently been achieved. The last case observed in a formerly endemic area occurred in Somalia in 1977 (Breman and Arita).

Variola, caused by one of the poxviruses, poxvirus variolae, has an incubation period of 12 to 13 days. It usually begins with a generalized eruption that at first consists of papules. After 2 or 3 days, the papules are transformed into vesicles that are characteristically umbilicated. After 3 more days, the vesicles change into pustules. In severe cases, the lesions may have a hemorrhagic base. It is typical of variola that all lesions are at the same stage of development.

Histopathology. Reticular degeneration is prominent in variola, especially in the early stage of vesiculation. Therefore, early vesicles are multilocular. Balloon cells are few in number and small in size, and they are not multinucleated (Michelson and Ikeda).

The demonstration of eosinophilic, intracytoplasmic inclusion bodies is of great diagnostic value, since it characterizes the infection as one caused by the poxvirus group and excludes infection by the herpesvirus group (Nasemann).

Visceral Lesions. Visceral lesions are rarely prominent in variola. However, vesicles occur not only on the palate and in the pharynx but also in the trachea and the esophagus. The pulmonary lesions usually are bacterial in type by the time they are observed, but they probably have a viral basis (Blank and Rake). A decrease in the number of platelets is commonly seen in severe cases. The hemorrhagic form of variola bears some similarity to disseminated intravascular coagulation, in which, as a result of extensive thrombosis of small blood vessels, there is depletion of platelets, fibrinogen, prothrombin, and various coagulation factors, causing extensive hemorrhage in many organs followed by death (Fulginiti).

Histogenesis. Variola is caused by one of the poxviruses, which, on the basis of their morphology, can be divided into two classes. One class comprises viruses that are rectangular ("brick-shaped"), have DNA cores in the shape of biconcave disks, and measure approximately 250 nm by 310 nm in diameter. In this class are the viruses of variola, vaccinia, cowpox, and molluscum contagiosum. The second class comprises viruses that are cylindrical and measure approximately 140 nm by 310 nm. In this class are the virus of paravaccinia, which causes milkers' nodules, and the virus that causes orf (Davis and Musil).

Differential Diagnosis. In herpex simplex, varicella, and herpes zoster, in contrast with variola, ballooning degeneration usually predominates, and multinucleated balloon cells are commonly seen; however, the histologic structure of the vesicles is not a reliable criterion for the differentiation of variola from the other three diseases, since old vesicles of variola that are in the suppurative stage often become unilocular through rupture of the septa, and, in occasional instances, reticular degeneration in the other three diseases is more pronounced than usual. The demonstration of intracytoplasmic inclusion bodies differentiates variola from herpes simplex, varicella, and herpes zoster. However, vaccinia and milkers' nodules also show eosinophilic, intracytoplasmic inclusion bodies. Thus, a definitive diagnosis of variola can be made only by virologic methods. Among these methods are (1) isolation of the virus in tissue culture followed by identification of the virus by neutralization with variola or vaccinia antiserum; (2) fluorescent-antibody staining of the virus; and (3) electron microscopic identification of the virus in vesicular fluid or scrapings (Fulginiti).

ECZEMA HERPETICUM AND ECZEMA VACCINATUM (KAPOSI'S VARICELLIFORM ERUPTION)

Eczema herpeticum and eczema vaccinatum, both of which often are referred to as Kaposi's varicelliform eruption, occur only in patients with a pre-existing dermatosis, usually atopic dermatitis (Barton and Brunsting). Occasionally, however, other forms of dermatitis, such as seborrheic dermatitis, or other dermatoses, such as Darier's disease (Loeffel and Meyer), benign familial pemphigus (Otsuka et al), pemphigus foliaceus (Silverstein and Burnett), mycosis fungoides (Segal and Watson; Taulbee and Johnson), Sézary's syndrome (Case Records, Massachusetts General Hospital), and ichthyosis vulgaris (Verbov et al) may provide the "soil" on which Kaposi's varicelliform eruption develops.

Eczema herpeticum is usually caused by HSV-1; however, in rare instances, it is caused by HSV-2 (Hazen and Eppes). Eczema herpeticum can occur either as a primary or as a recurrent type of infection (Wheeler and Abele). A primary type of infection with HSV-1 takes place in persons without circulating HSV-1 antibodies. Since primary infection with HSV-1 occurs, usually subclinically, in nearly all children (Blank and Haines), the great majority of patients with the primary type of eczema herpeticum are infants and children. The recurrent type of eczema herpeticum occurs in patients with circulating HSV-1 antibodies. The first attack of eczema herpeticum, whether of the primary or recurrent type, is the result of exogenous infection, whereas subsequent attacks may be due either to reinfection or to reactivation (see p. 361). The primary type of eczema herpeticum can be expected to be a serious disease with viremia and potential internal organ involvement resulting in death (Wheeler and Abele). In contrast, the recurrent type of eczema herpeticum generally shows no viremia and internal organ involvement except in immunologically compromised patients (Case Records, Massachusetts General Hospital). Occasionally, in both the primary

and the recurrent types of eczema herpeticum, bacterial infection of the skin with subsequent septicemia may cause death (Wheeler and Abele; Taulbee and Johnson).

Eczema vaccinatum results from the accidental inoculation of the vaccinia virus. As a consequence of the global eradication of variola, vaccination against variola is no longer necessary, and eczema vaccinatum is thus no longer seen.

Clinically, eczema herpeticum and eczema vaccinatum look alike. Primary and recurrent eczema herpeticum also cannot be differentiated clinically but only through the herpes simplex virus antibody titer of the serum (see below) (Wheeler and Abele). They all show a more or less extensive eruption composed of vesicles and pustules that may be umbilicated. These vesicles and pustules are situated chiefly on the areas of the pre-existing dermatosis but also on normal skin. The face is usually the site of severest involvement and may show marked edema. There are fever and prostration. The mortality of eczema herpeticum lies around 10%, with most of the fatalities occurring in infants and children with a primary type of herpetic infection (Nasemann) and in adults with inadequate cellular immunity (Taulbee and Johnson).

Histopathology.   On histologic examination, both eczema herpeticum and eczema vaccinatum show vesicles and pustules of the viral type. Even though the pustules show only necrotic epidermis in their center, one may still see reticular and ballooning degeneration at their periphery (Lynch; Lausecker). In instances of eczema herpeticum, but not in eczema vaccinatum, multinucleated epithelial giant cells often are present (Lausecker; von Weiss et al). Because of the presence of innumerable inflammatory cells, especially neutrophils, the demonstration of inclusion bodies is often difficult. If they are found, they are located exclusively in the cytoplasm in eczema vaccinatum and exclusively in the nucleus in eczema herpeticum.

Differential Diagnosis.   Since eczema herpeticum and eczema vaccinatum look alike clinically, and since the histologic similarity is great in the absence of inclusion bodies and of multinucleated epithelial cells, differentiation of the two diseases may have to depend on nonhistologic means, such as a history of possible exposure to the vaccinia virus and a number of laboratory tests.

Among the tests are (1) inoculation of HeLa cell or human amnion cell cultures, without and with the addition of sera containing antibodies to the herpes simplex virus and to the vaccinia virus, respectively, for the purpose of neutralization; (2) direct immunofluorescence examination for the presence of viral antigen (see p. 364); and (3) the complement fixation reaction, or the viral neutralization reaction. If carried out during the course of the disease, this last test reveals an increase in the antibody titer with herpes simplex antigen in the sera of patients with the primary type of eczema herpeticum (von Weiss et al; Wheeler and Abele). Patients with eczema vaccinatum show an increase in the antibody titer with the use of vaccinia antigen (Marchionini and Nasemann). In patients with eczema herpeticum of the recurrent type who already have a high antibody titer, no significant increase in the titer occurs (Wheeler and Abele).

MILKERS' NODULES

Milkers' nodules are acquired from cows the udders of which are infected with pseudocowpox or paravaccinia, a disease that, in contrast to cowpox or vaccinia, does not provide cross immunity to variola.

Clinically, infected persons show, after an incubation period of 4 to 7 days, usually on their fingers, one to three or, rarely, more lesions measuring 1 cm to 2 cm in diameter. The lesions usually are painless. During a period of approximately 6 weeks, they pass through six clinical stages, each lasting about 1 week (Leavell and Phillips): (1) the maculopapular stage; (2) the target stage, during which the lesions have a red center, a white ring, and a red halo; (3) the acute weeping stage; (4) the nodular stage, which shows hard, nontender nodules; (5) the papillomatous stage, in which the nodules have an irregular surface; and (6) the regressive stage, during which the lesions involute without scarring.

Histopathology. During the maculopapular and target stages, that is, during the first 2 weeks, the histologic picture is consistent with a viral infection. During the maculopapular stage, one observes vacuolization of cells in the upper third of the stratum malpighii, leading in some areas to multilocular vesicles. Fairly numerous eosinophilic inclusion bodies are seen in the cytoplasm of the vacuolated epidermal cells (Katzenellenbogen; Marchionini and Nasemann; Evins et al; Leavell and Phillips). In addition, intranuclear eosinophilic inclusion bodies are present in some cases (Evins et al; Leavell and Phillips). During the target stage, vacuolated epidermal cells with inclusion bodies are no longer seen in the red center, in which the cells have been destroyed by the virus, but only in the surrounding white ring (Leavell and Phillips). The epidermis in stages 1 and 2 shows elongation of the rete ridges, and the dermis contains many newly formed, dilated capillaries and a mononuclear infiltrate.

In stage 3, the acute weeping stage, the histologic picture is no longer diagnostic, since the epidermis is necrotic throughout. A massive infiltrate of mononuclear cells extends throughout the dermis.

In stages 4 and 5, the epidermis shows acanthosis with fingerlike downward projections, and the dermis shows vasodilatation and chronic inflammation. In the final, sixth stage, there is resolution of the histologic changes.

Histogenesis. On *electron microscopy*, the paravaccinia virus is found to be cylindrical in shape and to have convex ends. It consists of a dense DNA core surrounded by a less dense, wide capsid and by two narrow, electron-dense outer layers. On the average, the virion measures 140 nm by 310 nm. Mature virus particles are present not only in the upper stratum malpighii but also within keratin fibrils of keratinocytes (Davis and Musil). In tissue cultures, the paravaccinia virus produces a cytopathic effect on human skin fibroblasts and bovine kidney cells (Leavell and Phillips).

ECTHYMA CONTAGIOSUM (ORF)

Ecthyma contagiosum, or orf, is a benign, self-limited viral infection contracted by the handling of infected sheep. The incubation time varies from 3 to 6 days (Johannessen et al). Clinically, the lesions in infected humans appear on exposed surfaces and vary in number from one to several. They show considerable clinical resemblance to the lesions of milkers' nodules and pass through the same six stages as described for milkers' nodules, healing usually within 5 to 6 weeks (Leavell).

Histopathology. The histologic picture of orf during the six stages is identical to that seen during the corresponding stages in milkers' nodules (Leavell). Vacuolization of cells in the upper stratum malpighii, resulting in multilocular vesicles, is seen in the first two stages. Only in this early phase, particularly in the white ring of target lesions, are eosinophilic inclusion bodies found within vacuolated cells. They are usually located within the cytoplasm but occasionally also within the nucleus (Leavell; Tarnick et al). The presence of inclusion bodies only in early lesions may explain why some authors have been unable to find them (Seifert and Saito) and others have failed to discuss their presence or absence in histologic sections (Wheeler et al; Yeh and Soltani; Johannessen et al).

Histogenesis. *Electron microscopic examination* in orf reveals in the cytoplasm of keratinocytes viral particles of similar size and shape to those seen in milkers' nodules (Leavell and Phillips; Johannessen et al). The two viruses also produce similar cytopathic changes in tissue cultures of various cell types, including bovine and rhesus monkey kidney cells and human amnion cells (Leavell and Phillips; Naggington and Whittle). Only the fact that one type of virus is transmitted by cows and the other by sheep suggests that they are different viruses.

MOLLUSCUM CONTAGIOSUM

Molluscum contagiosum consists of a variable number of small, discrete, waxy, skin-colored, dome-shaped papules usually 2 mm to 4 mm in size and having an umbilicated center. When the lesion is fully developed, a small amount of a curdlike substance can be expressed from its center. In occasional instances, a papule of molluscum contagiosum appears markedly inflamed (Henao and Freeman). Ultimately, the lesions involute spontaneously. During involution, there may be mild inflammation and tenderness (Steffen and Markman).

Histopathology.   In molluscum contagiosum, the epidermis grows down into the dermis as multiple, often closely packed lobules. Many epidermal cells contain large, intracytoplasmic inclusion bodies, the so-called molluscum bodies (Fig. 21-4). These first appear as single, minute, ovoid eosinophilic structures in the lower cells of the stratum malpighii at a level one or two layers above the basal cell layer. The basal cell layer itself does not contain molluscum bodies (Lutzner). The molluscum bodies increase considerably in size as the infected cells move toward the surface; at the level of the midepidermis, their size already exceeds the original size of the invaded cells. The molluscum bodies in the upper layers of the epidermis displace and compress the nucleus of each invaded cell, so that the nucleus appears as a thin crescent at the periphery of the cell. At the level of the wide, but poorly defined, granular layer, the staining reaction

of the molluscum bodies changes from eosinophilic to basophilic (Mescon et al). In the horny layer, numerous large, basophilic molluscum bodies measuring up to 35 μm in diameter lie enmeshed in a network of eosinophilic horny fibers (see Plate 2, facing p. 324). In the center of the lesion, the stratum corneum ultimately disintegrates, releasing the molluscum bodies. Thus, a central crater forms.

The surrounding dermis usually shows little or no inflammatory reaction, except in rare instances in which the lesion of molluscum contagiosum ruptures and discharges molluscum bodies and horny material into the dermis. This results in a pronounced inflammatory infiltrate containing lymphoid cells, neutrophils, macrophages, and often also a few foreign body giant cells (Henao and Freeman).

During the period of spontaneous involution, a mononuclear infiltrate may be seen in close apposition to the lesion infiltrating between the infected epidermal cells (Steffen and Markman).

Histogenesis. On *electron microscopic examination,* the molluscum inclusion bodies are found to contain, embedded in a protein matrix, large numbers of molluscum contagiosum viruses (EM 32). The virus of molluscum contagiosum belongs to the poxvirus group (see p. 367). Like the viruses of variola, vaccinia, and cowpox, it is "brick-shaped" and measures approximately 300 nm by 240 nm. It consists of an electron-dense nucleoid approximately 230 nm in length that appears rectangular

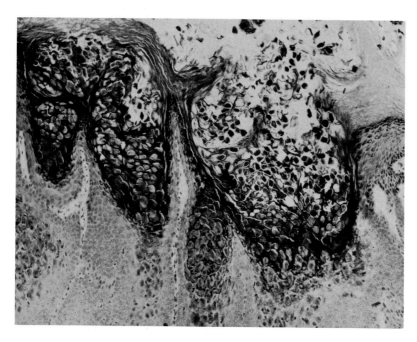

Fig. 21-4. Molluscum contagiosum
Numerous intracytoplasmic inclusion bodies, so-called molluscum bodies, are seen forming in the lower epidermis. They grow in size as they move toward the surface. (× 100)

in front view and dumbbell-shaped in profile (EM 32, inset). As seen in front view, the nucleoid is composed of interwoven filaments measuring approximately 6 nm in diameter and representing fibrous DNA. The nucleoid is surrounded by a medium electron-dense amorphous coat representing the capsid (EM 32, inset). Peripheral to this is a thin trilaminar outer membrane (Robinson et al; Hasegawa et al).

The virus of molluscum contagiosum has not been grown in tissue culture. In an attempt to explain this failure to replicate, one group of investigators inoculated tissue cultures of chick embryo cells with extracts from skin lesions of patients with molluscum contagiosum (Robinson et al). Although the viral particles were quickly adsorbed to the cell surface and phagocytized by these cells and the outer membrane of the viral particles was lysed, the viral coat or capsid failed to rupture. Thus, the viral DNA was not extruded into the cytoplasm, and replication of the virus was blocked. It could be postulated that the viral coat remained present around the nucleoid because the virus of molluscum contagiosum fails to induce the synthesis of "uncoating" protein in the host cells (see p. 360).

The spontaneous disappearance of molluscum contagiosum may well represent a cell-mediated immune rejection of the lesion by the host, since the involution is accompanied by a mononuclear cell infiltrate (Steffen and Markman). A similar dense mononuclear cell infiltrate has been observed in spontaneously regressing verrucae planae (Tagami et al), verrucae vulgares (Berman and Winkelmann), and deep palmoplantar warts (Berman et al) and has been interpreted as a cellular immune response (see pp. 372 and 375).

VERRUCA

Three classifications of verrucae exist. First is the traditional classification, which is based on clinical appearance and location and which includes (1) verruca vulgaris or common wart, including filiform wart; (2) deep, hyperkeratotic palmoplantar wart; (3) superficial, mosaic-type palmoplantar wart; (4) verruca plana; (5) epidermodysplasia verruciformis; and (6) condyloma acuminatum. Second is a histologic classification, which recognizes (1) inclusion warts (myrmecia) seen in deep, hyperkeratotic palmoplantar warts; (2) papillomatous warts with foci of vacuolization and parakeratosis, seen in common warts, in superficial, mosaic-type palmoplantar warts, and in condylomata acuminata; (3) warts with diffuse vacuolization in the upper epidermis, seen in verrucae planae and in some instances of epidermodysplasia verruciformis; and (4) warts with "dysplastic" vacuolization, seen in some cases of epidermodysplasia verruciformis. Third is a new classification based on the fact that there are several types of human papillomaviruses, each with a distinct DNA genome and type-specific antigen. The various types can be recognized by radiolabeling the human papillomavirus DNA and

using it for molecular hybridization with free viral DNA (Orth et al, 1978). Four serotypes have thus been definitely characterized: human papillomavirus type 1 (HPV-1) is specifically associated with deep, hyperkeratotic palmoplantar warts (myrmecia warts); HPV-2 with superficial, mosaic-type palmoplantar warts, as well as with common and filiform warts; HPV-3 with verrucae planae and the benign variant of epidermodysplasia verruciformis; and HPV-5 (at first called HPV-4) with the dysplastic type of epidermodysplasia verruciformis (Kienzler et al, 1979). The specificity of these four serotypes has been confirmed by direct immunofluorescence testing on various types of warts using anti-HPV-1, anti-HPV-2, anti-HPV-3, and anti-HPV-5 fluorescein-labeled guinea pig immunoglobulin G (IgG) (Kienzler et al, 1981). Two other serotypes have been found, but they show less specificity, although HPV-4 is associated largely with superficial, mosaic-type palmoplantar warts and common warts (Gross et al), and HPV-6 largely with condylomata acuminata (Grussendorf; Gross et al). In addition, a new type with distinct antigenic properties, HPV-7, was detected in warts on the hands of nine butchers (Orth et al, 1981).

Verruca Vulgaris

Verrucae vulgares are circumscribed, firm, elevated papules with a papillomatous ("verrucous"), hyperkeratotic surface. They may occur singly or in groups. Generally, they are associated with little or no tenderness. Verrucae vulgares may occur anywhere on the skin but are seen most commonly on the dorsal aspects of the fingers and hands. They often occur on the soles of the feet as superficial clusters referred to as mosaic warts. Rarely, verrucae vulgares occur on the oral mucosa. Filiform warts, variants of verruca vulgaris, show a threadlike, horny projection arising from a horny base. They are seen most commonly on the face and scalp.

Development of a squamous cell carcinoma in a verruca vulgaris is very rare but may occur (Grussendorf and Gahlen; Goette; Shelley and Wood).

Histopathology. Verrucae vulgares show acanthosis, papillomatosis, and hyperkeratosis. The rete ridges are elongated and, at the periphery of the verruca, are often bent inward so that they appear to point radially toward the center (Fig. 21-5). The characteristic features that distinguish verruca vulgaris from other papillomas (see p. 474) are foci of vacuolated cells, vertical tiers of parakeratotic cells, and foci of clumped keratohyaline granules (Fig. 21-6). These three changes are quite pronounced in young verrucae vulgares but are slight and even absent in old ones. The foci of vacuolated cells are located in the upper stratum malpighii and in the granular layer (Fig. 21-6). The vacuolated

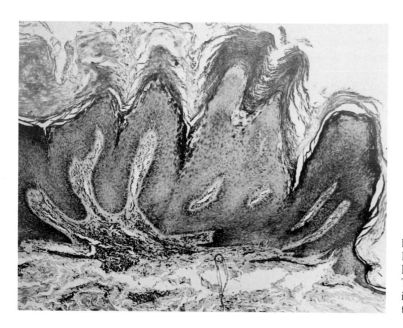

Fig. 21-5. Verruca vulgaris
Low magnification. One observes hyper-keratosis, acanthosis, and papillomatosis. The rete ridges are elongated and bent inward at both margins and thereby appear to point radially to the center. (×100)

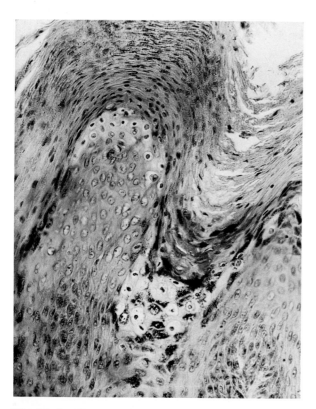

Fig. 21-6. Verruca vulgaris
High magnification of Figure 21-5. Groups of large, vacuolated cells lie in the upper stratum malpighii and in the granular layer. A tier of parakeratotic cells lies over the crest of a papillomatous elevation. (×400)

cells possess small, round, deeply basophilic nuclei that are surrounded by a narrow clear halo and by pale-staining cytoplasm. These cells contain few or no keratohyaline granules, even when they are located in the granular layer. The vertical tiers of parakeratotic cells are often located at the crests of papillomatous elevations of the rete malpighii overlying a focus of vacuolated cells. In comparison with ordinary parakeratotic nuclei, the nuclei of the parakeratotic cells in verrucae vulgares are larger and more deeply basophilic, and many of them appear rounded rather than elongated (Blank et al). Whereas no granular cells are generally seen overlying the papillomatous crests, they are increased in number and size in the intervening valleys and contain heavy, irregular clumps of keratohyaline granules (Fig. 21-6).

In filiform warts, the papillae are much more elongated than in verrucae vulgares. They contain dilated capillaries, and small areas of hemorrhage may be seen in the thickened horny layer at the tip of the filiform wart.

Involution of verrucae vulgares is associated with a mononuclear cell infiltration, exocytosis, and degenerative epidermal changes. These findings suggest that regression represents a cell-mediated immune rejection of the wart (Berman and Winkelmann, 1980). Similar findings have been made in involuting verrucae planae (see p. 375), in involuting deep palmoplantar warts (see p. 373), and in involving lesions of molluscum contagiosum (see p. 371).

Histogenesis. The wart virus, or human papillomavirus, is a DNA virus belonging to the papova group. No difference has been noted in *electron microscopic* appearance among the virus particles in the seven types of HPV. Only the quantity varies in the different types, being sparse in HPV-2 (verruca vulgaris) and HPV-6 (condyloma acuminatum) and profuse in HPV-1 (myrmecia wart), HPV-3 (verruca plana), and HPV-5 (dysplastic epidermodysplasia verruciformis (Laurent et al, 1975, 1978). Not infrequently, no virus particles can be found in verrucae vulgares on electron microscopic examination (Rowsen and Mahy; Almeida et al).

The virus particles are spheric bodies with a diameter of about 50 nm. Each particle consists of an electron-dense nucleoid with a stippled appearance surrounded by a less dense capsid (Gianotti et al; Rajagopalan et al). The wart virus replicates in the nucleus, where the viral particles, when present in large numbers, are located as dense aggregates in a crystalloid arrangement (EM 33) (Cornelius et al). The wart virus does not grow in tissue cultures and is not pathogenic for any animal.

Although warts are very common, especially in children and adolescents, defective cell-mediated immunity predisposes to the development of some types of warts. It has been stated that cell-mediated immunity, measured by the percentage of circulating T-cells, sensitization to dinitrochlorobenzene (DNCB), and lymphocyte response to phytohemagglutinin, is on the average near to normal in patients with plantar or genital warts; in contrast, a statistically significant defect exists in patients with verrucae vulgares, and an even greater defect is found in patients with verrucae planae or epidermodysplasia verruciformis (Obalek et al). The frequency of warts in children with renal transplants receiving immunosuppressive therapy is 3 times that of the general childhood population (Ingelfinger et al).

Differential Diagnosis. For a discussion of differentiation of verruca vulgaris from other papillomas, see p. 474.

Deep Palmoplantar Warts (Myrmecia)

Deep palmoplantar warts are usually associated with considerable tenderness and occasionally with swelling and redness. Although they may be multiple, they do not coalesce as do mosaic warts, which are verrucae vulgares. Deep palmoplantar warts occur not only on the palms and soles but also on the lateral aspects and tips of the fingers and toes. Unlike superficial, mosaic-type palmoplantar warts, deep palmoplantar warts usually are covered with a thick callus. When the callus is removed with a scalpel, the wart proper becomes apparent as soft, granular, white or brownish tissue. Even

though there exists a plantar verrucous carcinoma that may initially show a clinical resemblance to plantar warts, it is uncertain that plantar warts can change into carcinoma (see p. 505) (Swanson and Taylor).

Histopathology. Whereas superficial, mosaic-type palmoplantar warts have a histologic appearance analogous to that of verruca vulgaris and represent serotype HPV-2 or HPV-4, deep palmoplantar warts were first described in 1950 as inclusion warts (Strauss et al) and again in 1951 as myrmecia—meaning anthill—warts (Lyell and Miles). They represent serotype HPV-1.

Myrmecia or inclusion warts are characterized by the presence of an abundance of keratohyalin, which differs from normal keratohyalin by being eosinophilic. Starting already in the lower epidermis, one observes within the cytoplasm of many cells numerous eosinophilic granules, which enlarge in the upper stratum malpighii and coalesce to form large, irregularly shaped, homogeneous "inclusion bodies." They either encase the vacuolated nucleus or are separated from it by perinuclear vacuolization (Kaufmann et al). It has been pointed out that these homogeneous eosinophilic bodies resemble molluscum bodies, except that they do not displace the nucleus laterally (Lyell and Miles). An actual granular layer does not exist. The homogeneous, eosinophilic intracytoplasmic material seems to merge with the keratin formed by less altered cells. The nuclei in the stratum corneum persist, appearing as deeply basophilic round bodies surrounded by a wide, clear zone (Fig. 21-7). Aside from showing the large intracytoplasmic eosinophilic inclusions, some of the cells in the upper stratum malpighii with vacuolated nuclei also show a small intranuclear eosinophilic "inclusion body." It is round and of about the same size as the nucleolus, which, however, is basophilic (Fig. 21-8). Both disappear as the vacuolated nucleus changes into a smaller, deeply basophilic structure.

On regressing, deep palmoplantar warts show a mononuclear cell infiltrate as evidence of a cell-mediated immune response and, subsequently, thrombosis of the dermal blood vessels. Thrombosis results in hemorrhage and in degeneration and necrosis of epidermal cells (Berman et al).

Histogenesis. On *electron microscopic examination*, both the large, irregular cytoplasmic inclusions and the small, round intranuclear inclusions are seen as sharply demarcated, very electron-dense bodies showing no recognizable internal structure owing to their intense electron density (Almeida et al). Because of their relationship

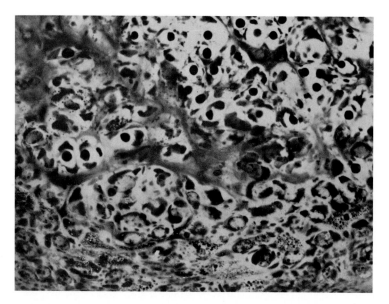

Fig. 21-7.   Deep palmoplantar wart (myrmecia)
In the lower portion of the illustration, the nuclei of the epidermal cells are vacuolated. In the upper portion, many of the nuclei are round and deeply basophilic and are surrounded by a clear zone. The deeply basophilic nuclei have been shown by electron microscopy to contain numerous virus particles. The cytoplasm of many cells contains large, irregularly shaped, homogeneous, eosinophilic ''inclusions'' representing keratohyalin. (×200)

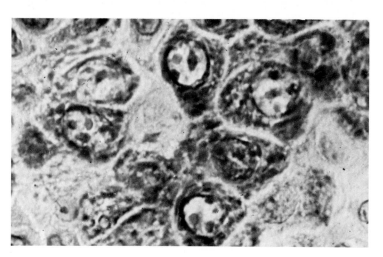

Fig. 21-8.   Deep palmoplantar wart (myrmecia)
The epidermal cells have large, vacuolated nuclei. Five of the nuclei each contain a round eosinophilic body, formerly thought to represent an inclusion body but actually representing keratohyalin. The darker, basophilic particles in the nuclei are nucleoli. (×600)

to tonofilaments, the cytoplasmic inclusions are readily identifiable as keratohyaline granules, and so are the intranuclear inclusions, because of their identity in density and texture to the cytoplasmic inclusions (Chapman et al; Kaufmann et al).

Viral particles are first seen in the upper portion of the stratum malpighii within and around the nucleolus. Their number increases, and, in cells just beneath the stratum corneum, nucleoli are no longer detected. In many instances, the material of the nucleus appears to be entirely replaced by virus particles except for a thin rim of chromatin closely applied to the nuclear membrane. The particles tend to be arranged in regular or crystalline formations (EM 33). In the stratum corneum, no normal cell structures are recognizable, but there remain large, compact aggregates of virus particles surrounded by keratinous matter (Almeida et al).

Verruca Plana

Verrucae planae are slightly elevated, flat, smooth papules. They may be the color of normal skin, but they usually have a brownish hue. The face and the dorsa of the hands are affected most commonly. In rare instances, there is more extensive involvement, with lesions also on the extremities and neck.

Histopathology.   Verrucae planae show hyperkeratosis and acanthosis but, unlike verrucae vulgares, have no papillomatosis, only slight elongation of the rete ridges, and no areas of parakeratosis.

In the upper stratum malpighii, including the granular layer, there is diffuse vacuolization of the cells (Fig. 21-9). Some of the vacuolated cells are

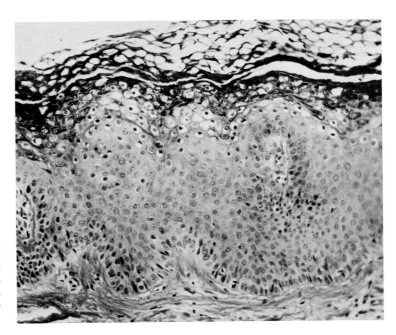

Fig. 21-9.   Verruca plana
One observes hyperkeratosis and acanthosis but no papillomatosis or parakeratosis. Numerous vacuolated cells lie in the upper stratum malpighii, including the granular layer. The horny layer has a pronounced basket-weave appearance resulting from the vacuolization of the horny cells. (×200)

enlarged to about twice their normal size. The nuclei of the vacuolated cells lie in the center of the cells, and some of them appear deeply basophilic. The granular layer is uniformly thickened, and the stratum corneum has a pronounced basket-weave appearance resulting from vacuolization of the horny cells. The dermis appears normal.

When verrucae planae regress spontaneously, a mononuclear cell infiltration is seen in the upper dermis, with exocytosis of mononuclear cells into the epidermis and degenerative epidermal changes (Tagami et al; Berman and Winkelmann, 1977). These findings suggests that the involution is mediated by cellular immunity, as in verruca vulgaris (see p. 372), deep palmoplantar warts (see p. 373), and molluscum contagiosum (see p. 370).

Histogenesis. Verrucae planae are induced by HPV-3. On *electron microscopic examination,* they reveal marked cytoplasmic edema. The tonofilaments are dislodged to the periphery of the cell. The keratohyaline granules appear normal (Laurent et al, 1978). Viral particles are numerous in the nuclei of the vacuolated cells (Laurent et al, 1975).

Epidermodysplasia Verruciformis

Two variants of epidermodysplasia verruciformis (EV) exist: one caused by HPV-3, the same type that causes verrucae planae, and the other caused by HPV-5 (formerly referred to as HPV-4). In rare instances, both HPV-3 and HPV-5 are found in the same patient (Jablonska et al, 1979).

In EV due to HPV-3, the clinical picture resembles that of extensive verrucae planae except for familial occurrence, onset in childhood, and, in some instances, the presence of confluent pigmented plaques, particularly on the legs. Malignant degeneration of the warts does not occur (Jablonska et al, 1979).

In EV due to HPV-5, the eruption shows, in addition to flat, wartlike lesions, red and brownish red patches and characteristic hypopigmented, scaling patches resembling lesions of tinea versicolor. Like EV due to HPV-3, the disorder starts in early life and often is familial, probably with autosomal recessive inheritance (Jablonska et al, 1979). In contrast to EV due to HPV-3, malignant changes within lesions in exposed areas is a common occurrence, manifesting itself usually as Bowen's disease but occasionally as squamous cell carcinoma (Prawer et al; Yabe et al).

Histopathology. In EV due to HPV-3, the histologic changes are identical to those of verruca plana and consist of marked diffuse vacuolization of the cells in the upper epidermis (see above) (Jablonska et al, 1979).

In EV due to HPV-5, the epidermal changes are apt to be uneven, extending deep into the epidermis in some areas and being quite superficial in others. The affected cells are swollen and irregularly shaped. Rather than being clear, their cytoplasm stains a pale blue and may have a foamy appearance (Johnson et al). Whereas some nuclei appear pyknotic, others appear large, round, and empty owing to marginal distribution of the chromatin (Kaufmann et al; Feuerman et al; Guilhou et al). The irregular shape of the cells and the emptiness of the nuclei gives the swollen cells a "dysplastic" appearance (Kienzler et al, 1979).

Histogenesis. The *electron microscopic findings* in EV due to HPV-3 are identical to those seen in verrucae planae (see p. 375). In EV due to HPV-5, the swollen, dysplastic cells are filled with ribosomes, whereas the tonofilaments appear greatly reduced (Laurent et al, 1978). Viral particles are seen, often in a crystalline array, within nuclei located in the stratum granulosum. In contrast, the swollen cells in the stratum malpighii show virions in their nuclei in some cases (Guilhou et al) but not in others (Prawer et al; Feuerman et al).

Viral particles are absent in lesions of Bowen's disease or squamous cell carcinoma arising within lesions of EV (Jablonska et al, 1970). However, viral particles have been observed in the upper layers of the epidermis overlying malignant lesions (Yabe et al).

Most patients with EV have a significant depression of their cell-mediated immune function (Glinski et al; Prawer et al). However, in some patients, no such abnormality is found (Kienzler et al, 1979). Cell-mediated

immunity has been found to be impaired to the same extent in patients with EV induced by HPV-3 and HPV-5, although lesions of Bowen's disease have been observed only in patients infected with HPV-5. Thus, the development of Bowen's carcinoma appears to be related to the oncogenic potential of the HPV-5 type rather than to the extent of the T-cell defect (Glinski et al).

Condyloma Acuminatum

Condylomata acuminata, or anogenital warts, can occur on the penis, on the female genitals, and around as well as within the anus. They consist of fairly soft, verrucous papules that occasionally coalesce into cauliflowerlike masses.

Malignant degeneration has been observed in rare instances of condylomata acuminata. This degeneration may manifest itself as a solitary lesion of Bowen's disease, which may either remain as such (Oriel and Whimster; Grussendorf and Bär) or progress into squamous cell carcinoma (Boxer and Skinner). In other cases, an invasive squamous cell carcinoma develops (Bauer and Friederich; Kerl and Pickel). This may result in metastases (Sonck). (Concerning the development of bowenoid papulosis in patients with condylomata acuminata, see p. 377.)

Giant condylomata acuminata of Buschke and Loewenstein is an erroneous designation, since this condition represents a verrucous carcinoma (see p. 505) (Kraus and Perez-Mesa). Clinically, the resemblance to a large aggregate of condylomata acuminata is very great, especially in the early stage. The most frequent location is the glans penis and foreskin of uncircumcised males. A large verrucous tumor develops. The diagnosis of verrucous carcinoma becomes evident by the deep penetration that results in multiple fistulas extending into the urethra, through which pus and urine are discharged (Becker et al). In spite of the aggressive local behavior of these tumors, regional lymph node metastases have been observed only rarely (Dawson et al).

In rare instances, verrucous carcinoma can occur also on the vulva (Doutre et al) and in the anal region, where it may cause a rectal stricture (Judge).

Histopathology. In condyloma acuminatum, the stratum corneum is only slightly thickened. Lesions located on mucosal surfaces show parakeratosis. The stratum malpighii shows papillomatosis and considerable acanthosis, with thickening and elongation of the rete ridges. The rete ridges branch to such a degree that the picture of pseudocarcinomatous hyperplasia may result. A considerable number of mitotic figures may be present. Usually, squamous cell carcinoma can be ruled out because the epithelial cells show an orderly arrangement and the border between the epithelial proliferations and the dermis is sharp (Fig. 21-10). The most

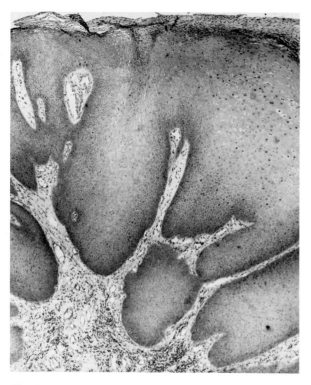

Fig. 21-10.   Condyloma acuminatum
There is pronounced acanthosis. Many cells of the stratum malpighii appear vacuolated and have a round, hyperchromatic nucleus. (×50)

characteristic feature, important for the diagnosis, is the presence of areas in which the epithelial cells show distinct perinuclear vacuolization. These vacuolated epithelial cells are relatively large and possess a hyperchromatic, round nucleus resembling the nuclei seen in the upper portion of the epidermis in verrucae vulgares. It must be kept in mind, however, that vacuolization is a normal occurrence in the upper portion of all mucosal surfaces, so that vacuolization in condylomata acuminata can be regarded as being possibly of viral genesis only if it extends into the deeper portions of the stratum malpighii. The dermis in condylomata acuminata usually appears edematous and shows dilated capillaries and a moderately dense, chronic inflammatory infiltrate.

Giant Condylomata Acuminata of Buschke and Loewenstein.   Although, in general, histologic differentiation between condyloma acuminatum and squamous cell carcinoma is easy, differentiation between condyloma acuminatum and the verrucous carcinoma of Buschke and Loewenstein can be very difficult. In fact, it was the histologic resemblance to condyloma acuminatum that led to the erroneous interpretation of this tumor as giant condyloma acuminatum. Only the deep penetration of verrucous carcinoma with displacement of the underlying tissue is analogous to the invasion of tissue seen in squamous cell carcinoma (Machacek and Weakley). In contrast to other types of squamous cell carcinoma, the ratio of nucleus to cytoplasm is low in verrucous carcinoma, and the invasive strands of tumor usually possess a well-developed basal cell layer (Kraus and Perez-Mesa). (For a further discussion of verrucous carcinoma, see p. 505.)

Histogenesis. Condylomata acuminata are associated largely with the serotype HPV-6 (Grussendorf; Gross et al). The concentration of virions in condylomata lata is low. Thus, on electron microscopic examination of nine condylomata acuminata, virions were found in only one case; some questionable virions were found in another case, and none was found in the remainder (Nasemann and Schaeg).

BOWENOID PAPULOSIS OF THE GENITALIA

Only in the last few years has bowenoid papulosis of the genitalia been recognized as a frequently occurring entity. Multiple small, reddish brown papules are seen varying from 2 mm to 10 mm in size, with an average diameter of 4 mm (Wade et al). Some lesions are distinctly verrucous in appearance. They are seen in young adults,

almost all under the age of 40. The lesions are located in men on the glans and shaft of the penis and in women in the perineal and vulvar areas. Generally, the lesions are diagnosed clinically as genital warts, and the histologic finding of "Bowen's disease" appears incongruous.

The lesions have a definite tendency toward spontaneous resolution; however, whereas some lesions regress, others may appear that in turn may also regress (Berger and Hori). Still, in some patients, lesions have persisted for more than 10 years (Wade et al). Usually, more than a dozen lesions are present, although, in exceptional cases, only one or two are found (Lupulescu et al). So far, only one patient with bowenoid papulosis has shown development of a plaque of true Bowen's disease, located on the scrotum and 10 cm in size; however, the lesions of bowenoid papulosis did not begin to appear until the patient had reached the age of 42 (De Villez and Stevens). It is of interest that approximately one third of the patients with bowenoid papulosis have a history of genital warts. Others have had previous genital infections with herpes simplex (Wade et al; Kaufman et al).

Histopathology.   On many occasions, multiple biopsy specimens of bowenoid papulosis have been obtained. In one instance, as many as seven specimens were obtained (Wade et al). In nearly all cases, each specimen showed the typical features of Bowen's disease (Berger and Hori; Katz et al; Wade et al; Bhawan; Faber and Hagedorn). These features consist of crowding and an irregular, "windblown" arrangement of the nuclei, many of which are large, hyperchromatic, and pleomorphic. Dyskeratotic and multinucleated keratinocytes are also present, as are atypical mitoses (for a detailed description of Bowen's disease, see p. 496). In a few instances, the coexistence of bowenoid papulosis and condylomata acuminata has been observed in the same patient (Kimura et al; Hödl) and even within the same lesion (Grussendorf and Gahlen; Steffen).

Histogenesis. It seems likely that bowenoid papulosis of the genitalia is related to genital warts, even though proof is inadequate. Most authors have been unable to find viruslike particles in the nuclei (Lupulescu et al; Berger and Hori; Wade et al; Bhawan; Faber and Hagedorn; Hödl). After a long search, some investigators found viruslike particles in a few nuclei (Kimura et al; Katz et al; Zelickson and Prawer); however, in one case, the size of the particles was only 35 nm to 50 nm, rather than 46 nm to 52 nm as seen in human papillomavirus (Zelickson and Prawer), and, in another case, the size of the particles varied greatly from 30 nm to 70 nm (Kimura et al). Nevertheless, it should be remembered, that, first, viral particles are rarely demonstrable in condylomata acuminata (see above) and, secondly, no viruses can be demonstrated in the lesions of Bowen's disease arising in epidermodysplasia verruciformis (see p. 376).

In some instances, the atypicality of the lesions of bowenoid papulosis is not as pronounced as is often the case in true Bowen's disease. It has therefore been suggested that the presence of atypical-appearing cells is the result of either irritation or resolution (Indianer). It is possible that the bowenoid papules represent atypical but biologically benign condylomata acuminata (Hödl).

A possible relationship between bowenoid papulosis of the vulva and herpes simplex virus type 2 (HSV-2) has been postulated because of the frequent finding of HSV-2-induced antigens in the cells of the carcinoma in situ (Kaufman et al).

Differential Diagnosis.   Bowenoid papulosis of the genitalia is easily differentiated from Bowen's disease on the basis of clinical data, such as onset at an earlier average age, multiplicity of lesions, smaller size of lesions, verrucoid appearance of some lesions, and tendency toward spontaneous regression.

It is recommended that, in cases of bowenoid papulosis, any recent application of podophyllum resin as a therapeutic measure be excluded. The changes induced by podophyllum resin consist of clumping, pyknosis, and distortion of the epidermal nuclei, with formation of epithelial giant cells as a result of aborted mitoses (Sullivan and King). These histologic changes may persist for as long as 2 weeks after application of the agent (Connors and Ackerman).

ORAL FOCAL EPITHELIAL HYPERPLASIA

A rare condition first described in American Indians (Archard et al), oral focal epithelial hyperplasia has since been found to occur in many countries and races. It is seen mainly in children, often in small endemic foci (van Wyk). Although the disease is chronic, spontaneous remissions occur.

The lesions are limited to the oral mucosa, the mucosa of the lower lip being most commonly involved (Stiefler et al). One observes numerous soft, white papules 2 mm to 4 mm in diameter. Most of them are discrete, but some are confluent. The lesions are asymptomatic.

Histopathology.   The oral epithelium shows acanthosis with thickening and elongation of the rete ridges. Throughout the epithelium, one observes scattered areas in which the cells show marked vacuolization and stain only faintly (Kuhlwein et al). The vacuolization usually is most pronounced in the upper portion of the epithelium, but it may extend into the broadened rete ridges.

The basal cell layer, however, does not become vacuolated. Some of the vacuolated cells have been found to be binuclear (Lutzner et al).

Histogenesis.   Some authors have found no viral particles on *electron microscopic examination* (Orfanos et al; Stiefler et al). Others, however, have found intranuclear particles consistent in appearance and size with the human papillomavirus as seen in the various types of verrucae (see p. 373) (van Wyk; Goodfellow and Calvert; Kuhlwein et al; Petzoldt and Pfister; Lutzner et al). Whereas, in one case, the virus was identified as HPV-1 (Petzoldt and Pfister), in two other cases, the virus showed no cross reaction with HPV-1, -2, -3, or -5 (Lutzner et al).

Differential Diagnosis.   The histologic appearance of the affected oral epithelium in focal epithelial hyperplasia is identical to that seen in oral epithelial nevus, or white sponge nevus (see p. 475) (Kuhlwein et al).

HAND-FOOT-AND-MOUTH DISEASE

Hand-foot-and-mouth disease occurs in small epidemics affecting mainly children. It nearly always takes a mild course and lasts less than a week. Small vesicles occur that may be confined to the mouth, where they result in small ulcers. If present on the skin, only a few vesicles are generally seen on the palms of the hands, soles of the feet, and ventral surface and sides of the fingers and toes (Fields et al). They are surrounded by an erythematous halo.

The disease is caused by a coxsackievirus, an enterovirus and member of the picornavirus group that contains RNA. In most instances, coxsackievirus type A16 has been isolated; only rarely have other types, such as A5 or A9 been found (Miller and Tindall).

Histopathology.   Early vesicles are intraepidermal, whereas old vesicles may be subepidermal in location. There is pronounced reticular degeneration of the epidermis resulting in multilocular vesiculation (Miller and Tindall). In the deep layers of the epidermis, some ballooning degeneration may be found (Evans and Waddington). Neither inclusion bodies nor multinucleated giant cells are present. A nonspecific inflammatory infiltrate is present in the vesicles as well as in the underlying dermis.

Histogenesis.   The coxsackievirus can be cultured from the stool and occasionally also from the vesicles. The virus grows well on human epithelial cell cultures and on monkey kidney tissue cultures. On inoculation, it is pathogenic to suckling mice (Miller and Tindall).

BIBLIOGRAPHY

Introduction

ARTENSTEIN MS, DEMIS DJ: Recent advances in the diagnosis and treatment of viral diseases of the skin. (Review) N Engl J Med 270:1101–1111, 1964

BLANK H, DAVIS C, COLLINS D: Electron microscopy for the diagnosis of cutaneous viral infections. Br J Dermatol 83:69–80, 1970

LIU C, LLANES-RODAS R: Application of the immunofluorescent technic to the study of pathogenesis and rapid diagnosis of viral infections. Am J Clin Pathol 57:829–834, 1972

LUGER A: Verlauf und Behandlung der Infektionen mit dem Herpesvirus hominis. II. Therapie. Z Hautkr 46:399–408, 1971

PINKERTON H: Rickettsial, chlamydial, and viral diseases. In Anderson WAD, Kissane JM (eds): Pathology, 7th ed, Vol. 1, pp 452–496. St Louis, CV Mosby, 1977

SOUTHAM JC, COLLEY IT, CLARKE NG: Oral herpetic infection in adults. Br J Dermatol 80:248–256, 1968

WHITE DO: Viral infections of the skin. (Review) Aust J Dermatol 11:5–13, 1970

Herpes Simplex

BARINGER JR, SWOVELAND P: Recovery of herpes simplex virus from human trigeminal ganglions. N Engl J Med 288:648–650, 1973

BASTIAN FO, RABSON AS, YEE CL et al: Herpesvirus varicellae. Arch Pathol 97:331–333, 1974

BIERMAN SM: The mechanism of recurrent infection by Herpesvirus hominis. Arch Dermatol 112:1459–1461, 1976

BLANK H: Herpetism. Arch Dermatol 115:1440–1441, 1979

BLANK H, HAINES H: Viral diseases of the skin, 1975. A 25-year perspective. J Invest Dermatol 67:169–176, 1976

CATALANO LW JR, SAFLEY GH, MUSCLES M et al: Disseminated herpes virus infection in a newborn infant: Virologic, serologic, coagulation and interferon studies. J Pediatr 79:393–400, 1971

CHANG TW, FIUMARA NJ, WEINSTEIN L: Genital herpes. JAMA 229:544–545, 1974

CHEATHAM WJ, WELLER TH, DOLAN TF et al: Varicella: Report of two fatal cases with necropsy, virus isolation, and serologic studies. Am J Pathol 32:1015–1035, 1956

ELLIOT WC, HOUGHTON DC, BRYANT RE et al: Herpes simplex type 1 hepatitis in renal transplantation. Arch Intern Med 140:1656–1660, 1980

FOLEY FD, GREENAWALD KA, NASH G et al: Herpesvirus infection in burned patients. N Engl J Med 282:652–656, 1970

GANGE RW, DE BATS A, PARK JR et al: Cellular immunity and circulating antibody to herpes simplex virus in subjects with recurrent herpes simplex lesions and controls. Br J Dermatol 93:539–544, 1975

GIACOBETTI R: Herpetic whitlow. Int J Dermatol 18:55–58, 1979

GRAHAM JG, BINGUL O, BURGOON CB JR: Cytodiagnosis of inflammatory dermatoses. Arch Dermatol 87:118–127, 1963

HABURCHAK DR: Recurrent herpetic whitlow due to herpes simplex virus type 2. Arch Intern Med 138:1418–1419, 1978

HEROUT V, VORTEL V, VONDRACKOVA A: Herpes simplex involvement of the lower respiratory tract. Am J Clin Pathol 46:411–419, 1966

HIGGINS PG: Recurrent herpes simplex virus infections. Br J Dermatol 91:111–113, 1974

HONIG PJ, HOLZWANGER J, LEYDEN JJ: Congenital herpes simplex virus infections. Arch Dermatol 115:1329–1333, 1979

IZUMI AK, KIM R, ARNOLD H JR: Herpes sycosis. Arch Dermatol 106:372–374, 1972

JEWETT JJ: Herpes simplex encephalitis. N Engl J Med 292:531, 1975

JOSEPH TJ, VOGT PJ: Disseminated herpes with hepatoadrenal necrosis in an adult. Am J Med 56:735–739, 1974

KEANE JT, MALKINSON FD, BRYANT J et al: Herpesvirus hominis hepatitis and disseminated intravascular coagulation. Occurrence in an adult with pemphigus vulgaris. Arch Intern Med 136:1312–1317, 1976

KOMOROUS JM, WHEELER CE, BRIGGAMAN RA et al: Intrauterine herpes simplex infections. Arch Dermatol 113:918–922, 1977

LEE JC, FORTUNY IE: Adult herpes simplex hepatitis. Hum Pathol 3:277–281, 1972

LEIDER W, MAGOFFIN RL, LENNETTE EH et al: Herpes-simplex-virus encephalitis. N Engl J Med 273:341–347, 1965

LIU C, LLANES-RHODAS C: Application of the immunofluorescent technic to the study of pathogenesis and rapid diagnosis of viral infections. Am J Clin Pathol 57:829–834, 1972

LOGAN WS, TINDALL JP, ELSON ML: Chronic cutaneous herpes simplex. Arch Dermatol 103:606–614, 1971

LONG JC, WHEELER CE JR, BRIGGAMAN RA: Varicella-like infection due to herpes simplex. Arch Dermatol 114:406–409, 1978

LOPYAN L, YOUNG AW JR, MENEGUS M: Generalized acute mucocutaneous herpes simplex type 2 with fatal outcome. Arch Dermatol 113:816–818, 1977

LUGER A: Verlauf und Behandlung der Infektionen mit dem Herpesvirus hominis. I. Epidemiologie, Klinik und Serologie. (Review) Z Hautkr 46:387–394, 399–408, 1971

MORECKI R, BECKER NH: Human herpesvirus infection. Its fine structure identification in paraffin-embedded tissue. Arch Pathol 86:292–296, 1968

NAHMIAS AJ, DOWDLE WR: Antigenic and biologic differences in Herpesvirus hominis. Prog Med Virol 10:110–159, 1968

NAHMIAS AJ, VISENTINE AM, JOSEY WE: Cesarean section and genital herpes. N Engl J Med 296:1359, 1977

NASH G, FOLEY FD: Herpetic infection of the middle and lower respiratory tract. Am J Clin Pathol 54:857–863, 1970

NOLAN DC, CARRUTHERS MM, LERNER M: Herpesvirus hominis encephalitis in Michigan. N Engl J Med 282:10–13, 1970

ORENSTEIN JM, CASTADOT MJ, WILENS SL: Fatal herpes hepatitis associated with pemphigus vulgaris and steroids in an adult. Hum Pathol 5:489–493, 1974

PATRIZI G, MIDDLEKAMP JN, REED CA: Fine structure of herpes simplex virus in hepatoadrenal necrosis in the newborn. Am J Clin Pathol 49:325–341, 1968

REEVES WC, COREY L, ADAMS HG et al: Risk of recurrence after first episodes of genital herpes. N Engl J Med 305:315–319, 1981

RENDTORF CF, FOWINKEL EW: Herpes simplex skin lesions simulating smallpox. JAMA 192:998–1000, 1965

SHNEIDMAN DW, BARR RJ, GRAHAM JH: Chronic cutaneous herpes simplex. JAMA 241:592–594, 1979

SIEGEL FP, LOPEZ C, HAMMER GS et al: Severe acquired immunodeficiency in male homosexuals, manifested by chronic perianal ulcerative herpes simplex lesions. N Engl J Med 305:1439–1444, 1981

SOLOMON M: Herpes simplex virus from skin lesions of myelogenous leukemia. Arch Intern Med 107:100–104, 1961

SOUTHAM JC, COLLEY IT, CLARKE NG: Oral herpetic infection in adults. Br J Dermatol 80:248–256, 1968

SUTTON AL, SMITHWICK EM, KIM D: Fatal disseminated Herpesvirus hominis type 2 infection in an adult with associated thymic dysplasia. Am J Med 56:545–553, 1974

TASAKI T, MORI R, MINAMISHIMA Y et al: Rezidivierende neonatale herpetische Infektion. Z Hautkr 50:69–71, 1975

TAYLOR RJ, SAUL SH, DOWLING JN et al: Primary disseminated

herpes simplex infection with fulminant hepatitis following renal transplantation. Arch Intern Med 141:1519–1521, 1981

VONDERHEID EC, MILSTEIN, HJ, THOMPSON KD et al: Chronic herpes simplex: Infection in cutaneous T-cell lymphoma. Arch Dermatol 116:1018–1022, 1980

Varicella and Herpes Zoster

APPELBAUM E, KREPS SI, SUNSHINE A: Herpes zoster encephalitis. Am J Med 32:25–31, 1962

BASTIAN FO, RABSON AS, YEE CL et al: *Herpesvirus varicellae.* Arch Pathol 97:331–333, 1974

BLANK H, HAINES H: Viral diseases of the skin, 1975: A 25-year perspective. J Invest Dermatol 67:169–176, 1976

CHEATHAM WJ: The relation of heretofore unreported lesions to pathogenesis of herpes zoster. Am J Pathol 29:401–411, 1953

CHEATHAM WJ, WELLER TH, DOLAN TF et al: Varicella: Report of two fatal cases with necropsy, virus isolation, and serologic studies. Am J Pathol 32:1015–1035, 1956

DENNY-BROWN D, ADAMS RD, FITZGERALD PJ: Pathologic features of herpes zoster. Arch Neurol Psychiatr 51:216–231, 1944

FRANK L: Varicella pneumonitis. Arch Pathol 50:450–456, 1950

GHATAK NR, ZIMMERMAN HM: Spinal ganglion in herpes zoster. A light and electron microscopic study. Arch Pathol 95:411–415, 1973

GOLD E: Serologic and virus-isolation studies of patients with varicella or herpes-zoster infection. N Engl J Med 274:181–185, 1966

HASEGAWA T: Further electron microscopic observations of herpes zoster virus. Arch Dermatol 103:45–49, 1971

KAIN HK, FELDMAN CA, COHN LH: Herpes zoster generalisatus pneumonia. Arch Intern Med 110:98–101, 1962

MERSELIS JG JR, KAYE D, HOOK EW: Disseminated herpes zoster. Arch Intern Med 113:679–686, 1964

MORECKI R, BECKER NH: Human herpes-virus infection. Its fine structure identification in paraffin-embedded tissue. Arch Pathol 86:292–307, 1968

NASEMANN T, MENZEL I, SCHAEG G: Generalisierte Varicellen bei Morbus Hodgkin. Licht- und elektronenoptische Beobachtungen. Hautarzt 24:530–535, 1973

ORFANOS CE, RUNNE U: Virus-Ausbreitung, Virus-Replikation und Virus-Elimination in der menschlichen Haut beim Zoster. Hautarzt 26:181–190, 1975

RADO JP, TAKO J, GEDER L et al: Herpes zoster house epidemic in steroid-treated patients. Arch Intern Med 116:329–335, 1965

REBOUL F, DONALDSON SS, KAPLAN HS: Herpes zoster and varicella infections in children with Hodgkin's disease. Cancer 41:95–99, 1978

ROGERS RS III, TINDALL JP: Herpes zoster in children. Arch Dermatol 106:204–207, 1972

ROSE FC, BRETT EM, BURSTON J: Zoster encephalomyelitis. Arch Neurol 11:155–172, 1964

SOKAL JE, FIRAT D: Varicella-zoster infection in Hodgkin's disease. Am J Med 39:452–463, 1965

TAKASHIMA S, BECKER LE: Neuropathology of fatal varicella. Arch Pathol 103:209–213, 1979

TRIEBWASSER JH, HARRIS RE, BRYANT RE et al: Varicella pneumonia in adults. Medicine (Baltimore) 46:409–423, 1967

WELLER TH, WITTON HM, BELL EJ: The etiologic agents of varicella and herpes zoster. Isolation, propagation, and cultural characteristics in vitro. J Exp Med 108:843–868, 1958

Variola

BLANK H, RAKE G: Viral and Rickettsial Diseases of the Skin, Eye, and Mucous Membranes of Men, pp 9, 105. Boston, Little, Brown & Co, 1955

BREMAN JG, ARITA I: The confirmation and maintenance of smallpox eradication. N Engl J Med 303:1263–1273, 1980

DAVIS CM, MUSIL G: Milker's nodule. Arch Dermatol 101:305–311, 1970

FULGINITI VA: Smallpox and complications of smallpox vaccination. In Fitzpatrick TB, Eisen AZ, Wolff K et al (eds): Dermatology in General Practice, 2nd ed, pp 1616–1623. New York, McGraw-Hill, 1979

MICHELSON HE, IKEDA K: Microscopic changes in variola. Arch Dermatol Syph 15:138–164, 1927

NASEMANN T: Viruskrankheiten der Haut, der Schleimhäute und des Genitales, pp 51–54. Stuttgart, Georg Thieme Verlag, 1974

Eczema Herpeticum and Eczema Vaccinatum (Kaposi's Varicelliform Eruption)

BARTON RL, BRUNSTING LA: Kaposi's varicelliform eruption. Arch Dermatol Syph 50:99–104, 1944

BLANK H, HAINES H: Viral diseases of the skin, 1975. A 25-year perspective. J Invest Dermatol 67:169–176, 1976

Case Records of the Massachusetts General Hospital, Case 37-1975. Kaposi's varicelliform eruption. N Engl J Med 293:598–603, 1975

HAZEN PG, EPPES RB: Eczema herpeticum caused by herpesvirus type 2. Arch Dermatol 113:1085–1086, 1977

LAUSECKER H: Kaposis varicelliforme Eruption—Ekzema herpetiforme. Arch Dermatol Syph (Berlin) 196:183–222, 1953

LOEFFEL ED, MEYER JS: Eczema vaccinatum in Darier's disease. Arch Dermatol 102:451–456, 1970

LYNCH FW: Kaposi's varicelliform eruption. Arch Dermatol Syph 51:129–137, 1945

MARCHIONINI A, NASEMANN T: Zur Diagnostik der durch Viren der Pockengruppe hervorgerufenen Erkrankungen des Menschen. Arch Klin Exp Dermatol 202:69–102, 1955

NASEMANN T: Viruskrankheiten der Haut, der Schleimhäute und des Genitales, p 144. Stuttgart, Georg Thieme Verlag, 1974

OTSUKA F, NIIMURA N, HARADA S et al: Generalized herpes simplex complicating Hailey-Hailey's disease. J Dermatol (Tokyo) 8:63–68, 1981

SEGAL RJ, WATSON W: Kaposi's varicelliform eruption in mycosis fungoides. Arch Dermatol 114:1067–1069, 1978

SILVERSTEIN EA, BURNETT JW: Kaposi's varicelliform eruption complicating pemphigus foliaceus. Arch Dermatol 95:214–216, 1967

TAULBEE KS, JOHNSON SC: Disseminated cutaneous herpes simplex infection in cutaneous T-cell lymphoma. Arch Dermatol 117:114–115, 1981

VERBOV J, MUNRO DD, MILLER A: Recurrent eczema herpeticum associated with ichthyosis vulgaris. Br J Dermatol 86:638–640, 1972

VON WEISS JF, KIBRICK S, LEVER WF: Eczema herpeticum as complication of Darier's disease. Ann Intern Med 62:1293–1296, 1965

WHEELER CE JR, ABELE DC: Eczema herpeticum, primary and recurrent. Arch Dermatol 93:162–173, 1966

Milkers' Nodules

DAVIS CM, MUSIL G: Milker's nodule. Arch Dermatol 101:305–311, 1970

EVINS S, LEAVELL UW JR, PHILLIPS IA: Intranuclear inclusions in milker's nodules. Arch Dermatol 103:91–93, 1971

KATZENELLENBOGEN I: Studies on milker's nodules. Dermatologica 105:69–78, 1952

LEAVELL UW JR, PHILLIPS IA: Milker's nodules. Arch Dermatol 111:1307–1311, 1975

MARCHIONINI A, NASEMANN T: Zur Diagnostik der durch Viren der Pockengruppe hervorgerufenen Erkrankungen des Menschen. Arch Klin Exp Dermatol 202:69–102, 1959

Ecthyma Contagiosum (Orf)

JOHANNESSEN JV, KROGH KH, SOLBERG J et al: Human orf. J Cutan Pathol 2:256–283, 1975

LEAVELL UW JR: Orf. In Fitzpatrick TB, Eisen AZ, Wolff K et al (eds): Dermatology in General Practice, 2nd ed, pp 1623–1625. New York, McGraw-Hill, 1979

LEAVELL UW JR, PHILLIPS IA: Milker's nodules. Arch Dermatol 111:1307–1311, 1975

NAGGINGTON J, WHITTLE CH: Human orf: Isolation of virus by tissue culture. Br Med J 2:1324–1327, 1961

SEIFERT HW, SAITO Y: Ecthyma contagiosum mit Virusnachweis im Negative-Staining-Verfahren. Hautarzt 28:188–191, 1977

TARNICK M, SEBASTIAN G, HORN K et al: Vorkommen von Ekthyma contagiosum (Orf) beim Menschen. Dermatol Wochenschr 162:402–407, 1976

WHEELER CE, CAWLEY EP, JOHNSON J: Ecthyma contagiosum (orf). Arch Dermatol 71:481–485, 1955

YEH HP, SOLTANI K: Ultrastructural studies in human orf. Arch Dermatol 109:390–392, 1974

Molluscum Contagiosum

BERMAN A, WINKELMANN RK: Involuting common warts. J Am Acad Dermatol 3:356–362, 1980

HASEGAWA H, FUJIWARA E, AMETANI T et al: Further electron microscopic observation of molluscum contagiosum virus. Arch Klin Exp Dermatol 235:319–328, 1969

HENAO M, FREEMAN RG: Inflammatory molluscum contagiosum. Arch Dermatol 90:479–482, 1964

LUTZNER MA: Molluscum contagiosum, verruca and zoster viruses. Arch Dermatol 87:436–444, 1963

MESCON H, GRAY M, MORETTI G: Molluscum contagiosum. J Invest Dermatol 23:293–308, 1954

ROBINSON HJ JR, PROSE PH, FRIEDMAN-KIEN AE et al: The molluscum contagiosum virus in chick embryo cell cultures: An electron microscopic study. J Invest Dermatol 52:51–56, 1969

STEFFEN C, MARKMAN JA: Spontaneous disappearance of molluscum contagiosum. Arch Dermatol 116:923–924, 1980

TAGAMI H, TAKIGAWA M, OGINO A et al: Spontaneous regression of plane warts after inflammation. Arch Dermatol 113:1209–1213, 1977

Verruca

ALMEIDA JD, HOWATSON AF, WILLIAMS MG: Electron microscope study of human warts: Sites of virus production and nature of the inclusion bodies. J Invest Dermatol 38:337–345, 1962

BAUER KM, FRIEDERICH HC: Peniscarcinoma auf dem Boden vorbehandelter Condylomata acuminata. Z Hautkr 39:150–163, 1965

BECKER FT, WALDER HJ, LARSON DM: Giant condylomata acuminata. Arch Dermatol 100:184–186, 1969

BERMAN A, DOMNITZ JM, WINKELMANN RK: Plantar warts recently turned black. Arch Dermatol 118:47–51, 1982

BERMAN A, WINKELMANN RK: Flat warts undergoing involution. Histologic findings. Arch Dermatol 113:1219–1221, 1977

BERMAN A, WINKELMANN RK: Involuting common warts. J Am Acad Dermatol 3:356–362, 1980

BLANK H, BUERK M, WEIDMAN F: The nature of the inclusion body of verruca vulgaris: A histochemical study of the nucleotids. J Invest Dermatol 16:19–30, 1951

BOXER RJ, SKINNER DG: Condylomata acuminata and squamous cell carcinoma. Urology 9:72–78, 1977

CHAPMAN GB, DRUSIN LM, TODD JE: Fine structure of the human wart. Am J Pathol 42:619–642, 1963

CORNELIUS CE, WITKOWSKI JA, WOOD MG: Viral verruca, human papova virus infection. Arch Dermatol 98:377–384, 1968

DAWSON DF, DUCKWORTH JK, BERNHARDT H et al: Giant condyloma and verrucous carcinoma of the genital area. Arch Pathol 79:225–231, 1965

DOUTRE MS, BEYLOT C, BIOULAC P et al: Tumeur de Buschke-Löwenstein: Deux case féminins. Ann Dermatol Venereol 106:1031–1034, 1979

FEUERMAN EJ, SANDBANK M, DAVID M: Two siblings with epidermodysplasia verruciformis with large clear cells in the epidermis. Acta Derm Venereol (Stockh) 59:513–520, 1979

GIANOTTI F, CAPUTO R, CALIFANO A: Ultrastructural study of epidermodysplasia verruciformis Lewandowsky and Lutz. Arch Klin Exp Dermatol 235:161–172, 1969

GLINSKI W, OBALEK S, JABLONSKA S et al: T cell defect in patients with epidermodysplasia verruciformis due to human papillomavirus type 3 and 5. Dermatologica 162:141–147, 1981

GOETTE DK: Carcinoma in situ in verruca vulgaris. Int J Dermatol 19:98–101, 1980

GROSS G, PFISTER H, HAGEDORN M et al: Correlation between human papillomavirus (HPV) type and histology of warts. J Invest Dermatol 78:160–164, 1982

GRUSSENDORF EI: Lichtmikroskopische Untersuchungen an typisierten Viruswarzen. Arch Dermatol Res 268:141–148, 1980

GRUSSENDORF EI, BÄR T: Condylomata acuminata associated with Morbus Bowen (carcinoma in situ). Dermatologica 155:50–58, 1977

GRUSSENDORF EI, GAHLEN W: Metaplasia of a verruca vulgaris into spinocellular carcinoma. Dermatologica 150:295–299, 1975

GUILHOU JJ, MALBOS S, BARNÉON S et al: Epidermodysplasie verruciforme (deux observations). Étude immunologique. Ann Dermatol Venereol 107:611–619, 1980

INGELFINGER JR, GRUPE WE, TOPOR M et al: Warts in a pediatric renal transplant population. Dermatologica 155:7–12, 1977

JABLONSKA S, BICZYSKO W, JAKUBOWICZ K et al: The ultrastructure of transitional states in Bowen's disease and invasive Bowen's carcinoma in epidermodysplasia verruciformis. Dermatologica 140:186–194, 1970

JABLONSKA S, ORTH G, JARZABEK-CHORZELSKA M et al: Epidermodysplasia verruciformis versus disseminate verrucae planae. J Invest Dermatol 72:114–119, 1979

JOHNSON SAM, MONTGOMERY H, TUURA JL et al: Two cases of unusual vacuolar degeneration of the epidermis. Epidermodysplasia verruciformis? Arch Dermatol 85:53–64, 1962

JUDGE JR: Giant condyloma acuminatum involving vulva and rectum. Arch Pathol 88:46–48, 1969

KAUFMANN J, MEVES C, OTT F: Die Epidermodysplasia verruciformis Lewandowsky-Lutz in licht- und elektronenoptischem Vergleich mit den übrigen Papova-Virus Akanthomen. Arch Dermatol Res 261:39–54, 1978

KERL H, PICKEL H: Maligne Umwandlung von Condylomata acuminata der Vulva. Z Hautkr 46:155–162, 1971

KIENZLER JL, LAURENT R, COPPEY J et al: Épidermodysplasie verruciforme. Ann Dermatol Venereol 106:549–563, 1979

KIENZLER JL, ORTH G, LAURENT R: Human papillomavirus specific association with different types of warts. (Abstr) J Cutan Pathol 8:142, 1981

KRAUS FT, PEREZ-MESA C: Verrucous carcinoma. Cancer 19:26–38, 1966

LAURENT R, AGACHE P, COUME-MARQUET J: Ultrastructure of clear cells in human viral warts. J Cutan Pathol 2:140–148, 1975

LAURENT R, COUME-MARQUET S, KIENZLER JL et al: Comparative electron microscopic study of clear cells in epidermodysplasia

verruciformis and flat warts. Arch Dermatol Res 263:1–12, 1978

LYELL A, MILES JAR: The myrmecia. A study of inclusion bodies in warts. Br Med J 1:912–915, 1951

MACHACEK GF, WEAKLEY DR: Giant condylomata acuminata of Buschke and Lowenstein. Arch Dermatol 82:41–47, 1960

NASEMANN T, SCHAEG G: Electron microscopic examination of condylomata acuminata. J Cutan Pathol 3:147, 1976

OBALEK S, GLINSKI W, HAFTEK M et al: Comparative studies on cell-mediated immunity in patients with different warts. Dermatologica 161:73–83, 1980

ORIEL JD, WHIMSTER IW: Carcinoma in situ associated with virus containing anal warts. Br J Dermatol 84:71–73, 1971

ORTH G, JABLONSKA S, BREITBARD F et al: The human papilloma viruses. Bull Cancer 65:151–154, 1978

ORTH G, JABLONSKA S, FAVRE M et al: Identification of papillomavirus in butchers' warts. J Invest Dermatol 76:97–102, 1981

PRAWER SE, PASS F, VANCE JC et al: Depressed immune function in epidermodysplasia verruciformis. Arch Dermatol 113:495–499, 1977

RAJAGOPALAN K, BAHRU J, LOO DSC et al: Familial epidermodysplasia verruciformis of Lewandowsky and Lutz. Arch Dermatol 105:73–78, 1972

ROWSON KEK, MAHY BWJ: Human papova (wart) virus. Bacteriol Rev 31:110–131, 1967

SHELLEY WB, WOOD MG: Transformation of the common wart into squamous cell carcinoma in a patient with primary lymphedema. Cancer 48:820–824, 1981

SONCK CE: Condylomata acuminata mit Übergang in Karzinom. Z Hautkr 46:273–278, 1971

STRAUSS MJ, BUNTING H, MELNICK JL: Virus-like particles and inclusion bodies in skin papillomas. J Invest Dermatol 15:433–444, 1950

SWANSON NA, TAYLOR WB: Plantar verrucous carcinoma. Arch Dermatol 116:794–797, 1980

TAGAMI H, TAKIGAWA M, OGINO A et al: Spontaneous regression of plane warts after inflammation. Arch Dermatol 113:1209–1213, 1977

YABE, Y, YASUE M, YOSHINO N et al: Viral particles in early malignant lesions. J Invest Dermatol 71:225–228, 1978

Bowenoid Papulosis of the Genitalia

BERGER BW, HORI Y: Multicentric Bowen's disease of the genitalia. Spontaneous regression of lesions. Arch Dermatol 114:1698–1699, 1978

BHAWAN J: Multicentric pigmented Bowen's disease: A clinically benign squamous cell carcinoma in situ. Gynecol Oncol 10:201–205, 1980

CONNORS RC, ACKERMAN AB: Histologic pseudomalignancies of the skin. Arch Dermatol 112:1767–1780, 1976

DE VILLEZ RL, STEVENS CS: Bowenoid papules of the genitalia. A case progressing to Bowen's disease. J Am Acad Dermatol 3:149–152, 1980

FABER M, HAGEDORN M: A light and electron microscopic study of bowenoid papulosis. Acta Derm Venereol (Stockh) 61:397–403, 1981

GRUSSENDORF EI, GAHLEN W: Morbus Bowen bei Condylomata acuminata. Hautarzt 25:443–447, 1974

HÖDL S: Genitale bowenoide Papulose. Z Hautkr 56:368–377, 1981

INDIANER L: Controversies in dermatopathology. J Dermatol Surg Oncol 5:321–328, 1979

KATZ HI, POSALAKY Z, MCGINLEY D: Pigmented penile papules with carcinoma in situ changes. Br J Dermatol 99:155–162, 1978

KAUFMAN RH, DREESMAN GR, BUREK J et al: Herpesvirus-induced antigens in squamous-cell carcinoma in situ of the vulva. N Engl J Med 305:483–488, 1981

KIMURA S, HIRAI A, HARADA R et al: So-called multicentric pigmented Bowen's disease. Dermatologica 157:229–237, 1978

LUPULESCU A, MEHREGAN AH, RAHBARI H et al: Venereal warts vs. Bowen's disease. JAMA 237:2520–2522, 1977

STEFFEN C: Concurrence of condylomata acuminata and bowenoid papulosis. Am J Dermatopathol 4:5–8, 1982

SULLIVAN M, KING LS: Effects of resin of podophyllum on normal skin, condylomata acuminata and verrucae vulgares. Arch Dermatol 56:30–47, 1947

WADE TR, KOPF AW, ACKERMAN AB: Bowenoid papulosis of the genitalia. Arch Dermatol 115:306–308, 1979

ZELICKSON AS, PRAWER SE: Bowenoid papulosis of the penis. Demonstration of intranuclear viral-like particles. Am J Dermatopathol 2:305–308, 1980

Oral Focal Epithelial Hyperplasia

ARCHARD HO, HECK, JW, STANLEY HR: Focal epithelial hyperplasia. Oral Surg 20:201–212, 1965

GOODFELLOW A, CALVERT H: Focal epithelial hyperplasia of the oral mucosa. Br J Dermatol 101:341–344, 1979

KUHLWEIN A, NASEMANN T, JÄNNER M et al: Nachweis von Papillomviren bei fokaler epithelialer Hyperplasie Heck. Hautarzt 32:617–621, 1981

LUTZNER M, KUFFER R, BLANCHET-BARDON C et al: Different papillomaviruses as the causes of oral warts. Arch Dermatol 118:393–399, 1982

ORFANOS CE, STRUNK V, GARTMANN H: Fokale epitheliale Hyperplasie der Mundschleimhaut: Hecksche Krankheit. Dermatologica 149:163–175, 1974

PETZOLDT D, PFISTER H: HPV-1 DNA in lesions of focal epithelial hyperplasia Heck. Arch Dermatol Res 268:313–314, 1980

STIEFLER RE, SOLOMON MP, SHALITA AR: Heck's disease (focal epithelial hyperplasia). J Am Acad Dermatol 1:499–502, 1979

VAN WYK CW: Focal epithelial hyperplasia: Recently discovered in South America. Br J Dermatol 96:381–388, 1977

Hand-Foot-and-Mouth Disease

EVANS AD, WADDINGTON E: Hand, foot and mouth disease in South Wales, 1964. Br J Dermatol 79:309–317, 1967

FIELDS JP, MIHM MC JR, HELLREICH PD et al: Hand, foot, and mouth disease. Arch Dermatol 99:243–246, 1969

MILLER GD, TINDALL JP: Hand-foot-and-mouth disease. JAMA 203:827–830, 1968

Lipidoses

22

The term *lipidoses* may be applied to a group of diseases in which, owing to a generalized or local disturbance of the lipid metabolism, the lesions contain lipid substances.

The lipidoses can be divided into the following four groups:

1. *Systemic Lipidoses with Altered Serum Lipoprotein Values*
    Hyperlipoproteinemia, types I to V
    Tangier disease
2. *Tissue Storage Lipidoses*
    Niemann–Pick disease
    Gaucher's disease
    Angiokeratoma corporis diffusum (Fabry's disease), fucosidosis
    Lipogranulatomatosis (Farber's disease)
3. *Histiocytosis X*
    Xanthoma disseminatum
4. *Predominantly Cutaneous Lipidoses*
    Diffuse normolipemic plane xanthoma
    Verruciform xanthoma
    Juvenile xanthogranuloma
    Necrobiotic xanthogranuloma with paraproteinemia
    Reticulohistiocytosis
    Congenital self-healing reticulohistiocytosis
    Progressive nodular histiocytoma
    Generalized eruptive histiocytoma

HYPERLIPOPROTEINEMIA

The division of hyperlipoproteinemia into five types, as proposed in 1967 (Fredrickson et al), is based on the paper electrophoretic separation of the plasma lipoproteins in barbital buffer, pH 8.6, containing 1% albumin (Lees and Hatch). Four fractions are thus obtained; they are, in order of increasing electrophoretic mobility, chylomicrons, beta-lipoproteins, pre-beta-lipoproteins, and alpha-lipoproteins. These four fractions correlate well with those obtained by fractionation of lipoproteins by means of analytic ultracentrifugation, whereby the ultracentrifugal flotation rate is expressed in Svedberg flotation units (S_f). The chylomicrons, having an ultra-centrifugal flotation rate in excess of S_f 400, contain about 81% triglycerides and 9% cholesterol; the pre-beta-lipoproteins or very-low-density (VLD) lipoproteins, with an S_f of from 20 to 400, contain approximately 52% triglycerides and 22% cholesterol; and the beta-lipoproteins or low-density (LD) lipoproteins, with an S_f of 0 to 20, have only about 9% triglycerides but 47% cholesterol (Fleischmajer, 1971). The beta-lipoprotein molecules, in contrast to the pre-beta-lipoprotein molecules and chylomicrons, are of such small size that they cause no turbidity of the plasma. Presently, six, rather than five, types of hyperlipoproteinemia are recognized owing to the fact that type II has been subdivided into types IIA and IIB (Table 22-1). Types I, III, and V are rare, whereas types IIA, IIB, and IV are quite common (Fisher and Truitt).

Type I: *Hyperchylomicronemia*. First described in 1932 (Bürger and Grütz), this very rare condition has an autosomal recessive inheritance and begins in infancy. It is always associated with hepatosplenomegaly and abdominal cramps (Holt et al). There is a deficiency in lipoprotein lipase activity in the plasma as well as in the tissue (Ferrans et al).

Type IIA: *Hyperbetalipoproteinemia*. This condition, also referred to as familial hypercholesterolemia, has an autosomal dominant mode of inheritance. In the homozygote, the disease is apt to be severe, with development of xanthomas in childhood and death from coronary

383

TABLE 22-1. Biochemical and Clinical Data in Hyperlipoproteinemia

	I	IIA	IIB	III	IV	V
	Hyperchylo-micron	Hyperbeta	Combined	Broad-Beta	Pre-Beta	Mixed Pre-Beta Chylomicron
Chylomicrons	↑					↑
Pre-Beta (VLD)			↑	↑	↑	↑
Beta (LD)		↑	↑	↑		
Cholesterol	(+)	+ +	+	+ +	+	+
Triglycerides	+ + +		+	+ +	+ +	+ + +
Supernatant	Creamy	Clear	Slightly turbid	Turbid	Milky	Creamy
Infranatant	Clear					Turbid
Eruptive Xan-thoma	+		(+)	+	+ +	+
Tuberous Xan-thoma		+	(+)	+	(+)	
Tendon Xan-thoma		+ +	(+)	+		
Xanthelasma		+ +		+		
Plane Xanthoma		(+)		+		
Cardiovascular		+ +	+	+ +	+	
Diabetes			+	+	+ +	+
Hepatomegaly ⎫ Pancreatitis ⎭	+				(+)	+

VLD = very low density; LD = low density.

occlusion at a rather early age (Lever et al; Maher et al). In the heterozygote, however, symptoms usually do not develop until the third to sixth decade of life (Brown and Goldstein).

Type IIB: *Combined Hyperlipoproteinemia.* This newly recognized type, which has autosomal dominant inheritance, shows a usually moderate elevation in both LD (beta) and VLD (pre-beta) lipoproteins. Subjects with familial combined hyperlipoproteinemia generally do not manifest their disease until adulthood. It is of interest that, within families with type IIB, instances of hyperbetalipoproteinemia (type IIA) and hyperprebetalipoproteinemia (type IV) may also be found (Fisher and Truitt).

Type III: *Broad-Beta Lipoproteinemia.* There is a usually marked increase in both LD (beta) and VLD (pre-beta) lipoproteins so that, on paper electrophoresis, the beta and pre-beta bands merge. The disease is recessively transmitted (Fleischmajer, 1969) and usually does not start until adult life (Holimon and Wasserman).

Type IV: *Hyperprebetalipoproteinemia.* This type shows an autosomal dominant inheritance (Fleischmajer, 1971). Although elevation of triglycerides may be present already in childhood, clinical symptoms do not arise until adult life (Schreibman et al).

Type V: *Mixed Pre-Beta and Chylomicronemia.* Biochemically, this type is a combination of types I and IV. There occasionally is a deficiency of lipoprotein lipase activity in plasma and tissue that is similar to that seen in type I (Schreiber and Shapiro; Fleischmajer, 1971).

As a rule, the six types of hyperlipoproteinemia are well-defined entities. However, there are instances in which the type IV electrophoretic pattern can be converted into type V by minor dietary measures, and, in families of type V probands, relatives can be found with the type IV pattern; therefore, it is evident that some relationship exists between types IV and V (Borrie and Slack).

The hyperlipoproteinemias in their idiopathic form can evoke several other diseases, such as atherosclerosis, diabetes, or pancreatitis (see Systemic Lesions and Table 22-1). In addition, rather than occurring as a primary disorder, several types of hyperlipoproteinemia may occur secondary to other diseases. Thus, hyperlipoproteinemia of type IIA may be induced by myxedema, biliary cirrhosis, or nephrosis; hyperlipoproteinemia of type IV may be brought on by diabetes or by von Gierke's disease (also called Cori type I glycogenosis); and hyperlipoproteinemia of type V may develop in myxedema, nephrosis, or pancreatitis (Roberts et al;

Fleischmajer, 1971). Occasionally, the hyperlipoprotein-emia in diabetes mellitus or in Cori type I glycogenesis is of type V rather than of type IV (Roberts et al).

Cutaneous lesions may occur in all six types of hyper-lipoproteinemia (Table 22-1). They may be divided into eruptive xanthomas, tuberous xanthomas, tendon xan-thomas, xanthelasmata, and plane xanthomas.

Eruptive xanthomas are typical of triglyceridemia or hyperlipemia and therefore may occur in all five types of hyperlipoproteinemia that are associated with an increase in the concentration of either chylomicrons or pre-beta-lipoproteins in the plasma (types I, IIB, III, IV, V). Eruptive xanthomas consist of small, soft, yellowish papules with a predilection for the buttocks and the posterior aspects of the thighs. They come and go with fluctuations in the concentration of triglycerides in the plasma (Lever et al; Cornelius).

Tuberous xanthomas are found predominantly in cases with an increase in beta-lipoproteins, that is, in types IIA and III and, rarely, in types IIB and IV. They are large nodes or plaques located most commonly on the elbows, knees, fingers, and buttocks.

Tendon xanthomas occur in patients with excessive plasma levels of beta-lipoproteins, that is, in types IIA and III and, rarely, in type IIB. The Achilles tendons and the extensor tendons of the fingers are most fre-quently affected.

Xanthelasmata consist of slightly raised, yellowish, soft plaques on the eyelids. Although xanthelasmata are the commonest of the cutaneous xanthomas in type IIA and may occur in type III hyperlipoproteinemia, they also occur frequently in persons with normal lipoprotein levels. It is estimated that two thirds of all persons with xanthelasma palpebrarum have normal serum lipid levels (Polano; Pedace and Winkelmann).

Plane xanthomas develop in skin folds and especially in the palmar creases. They occur in type III hyperlipo-proteinemia and in biliary cirrhosis producing type IIA.

Systemic lesions that can be evoked by the idiopathic hyperlipoproteinemias include atherosclerosis, diabetes, and hepatosplenomegaly with pancreatitis (Table 22-1). Atherosclerosis is associated mainly with elevated beta-lipoprotein values and, to a lesser degree, with elevated pre-beta-lipoprotein values. Whereas atherosclerotic cor-onary heart disease occurs mainly in types IIA and III and occasionally in types IIB and IV, occlusive peripheral vascular disease, particularly of the lower extremities, is a common occurrence in type III. Diabetes occurs most commonly with elevated pre-beta-lipoprotein values in types IIB, III, IV, and V. Hepatosplenomegaly and pancreatitis causing severe abdominal cramps are found mainly in association with chylomicronemia (types I and V) and less commonly with elevated pre-beta-lipoprotein values (type IV) (Roberts et al).

Histopathology. The histologic appearance of xanthomas of the skin and the tendons is charac-terized by the presence of xanthoma or foam cells. Foam cells are macrophages that, because of their ability to phagocytize, have become filled with lipid droplets. In routine sections, xanthoma cells are seen to have a reticulated or foamy cytoplasm (Fig. 22-1), because the lipid droplets have dis-solved and have been extracted from the cytoplasm during the automatic processing carried out on routine specimens. However, the lipid droplets can be seen when frozen or formalin-fixed sections are stained with fat stains such as scarlet red or Sudan red (Fig. 22-2).

Xanthoma cells usually have only one nucleus, although they may have several. The nuclei of multinucleated xanthoma cells either are irregularly distributed, as in foreign body giant cells, or lie near the center of the cell, grouped in a wreathlike arrangement around a small island of nonfoamy cytoplasm and surrounded by foamy cytoplasm. A cell with the latter type of nuclear arrangement is called a Touton giant cell (Fig. 22-3). Some differ-ences exist in the histologic appearance and chem-ical composition of the various types of xanthoma.

Eruptive xanthomas, when of recent origin, often show a considerable admixture of nonfoamy cells, among them lymphoid cells, histiocytes, and neu-trophils, whereas the number of well-developed foam cells may still be small (Fig. 22-4). Fully

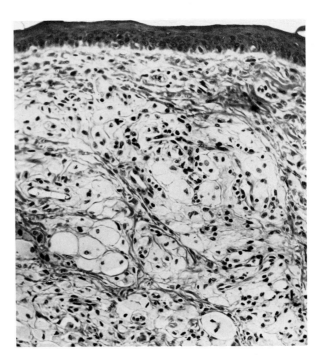

Fig. 22-1. Xanthoma tuberosum, early lesion
Numerous xanthoma cells (foam cells) are present. Fi-brosis is slight. (× 200)

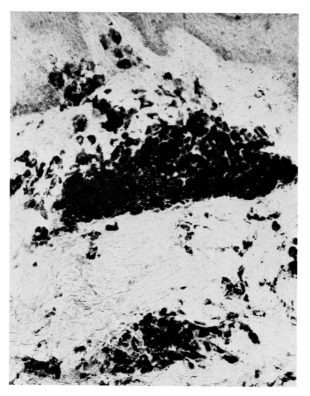

Fig. 22-2. Xanthoma tuberosum, early lesion
Scarlet red stain for fat. The xanthoma cells are filled with lipid material. (×100)

developed eruptive xanthomas contain more triglycerides and fewer cholesteryl esters than the other types of xanthoma (Baes et al). Thus, like the subcutaneous fat and lipid in the sebaceous glands, eruptive xanthomas stain orange red with scarlet red, and the lipid within them is usually not doubly refractile on polariscopic examination of frozen sections. With a decrease in serum triglycerides, the xanthoma triglycerides are mobilized more rapidly than cholesterol, so that resolving eruptive xanthomas are rich in cholesterol (Parker et al).

Tuberous xanthomas consist of large and small aggregates of xanthoma or foam cells. In early lesions, there usually is a slight admixture of nonfoamy cells, among them lymphoid cells, histiocytes, and neutrophils. In well-developed lesions, the infiltrate is composed almost entirely of foam cells (see Fig. 22-1), and, in aging lesions, fibroblasts appear (see Fig. 22-3). Ultimately, collagen bundles replace many of the foam cells. Tuberous xanthomas contain more cholesteryl esters than eruptive xanthomas (Baes et al). The foam cells of tuberous xanthomas therefore stain brownish red rather than orange red with Sudan red or scarlet red and are doubly refractile on polariscopic examination.

Tendon xanthomas are identical to tuberous xanthomas in histologic appearance and chemical composition.

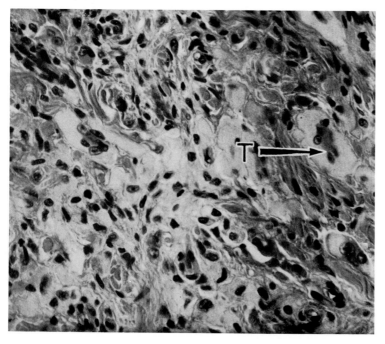

Fig. 22-3. Xanthoma tuberosum, late lesion
In addition to xanthoma cells, many fibroblasts are present. On the right side is a typical Touton giant cell (*T*). The nuclei lie near the center of the Touton cell, grouped around a small island of nonfoamy cytoplasm and surrounded by foamy cytoplasm. (×400)

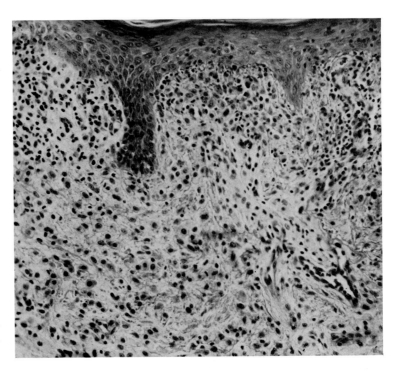

Fig. 22-4.   Eruptive xanthoma
In this early lesion, the foam cells are fairly small. There is an admixture of inflammatory cells. (×200)

Xanthelasmata located on the eyelids differ from tuberous xanthomas by the fairly superficial location of the foam cells and the nearly complete absence of fibrosis.

Plane xanthomas, located usually in the palmar creases, also lack fibrosis. Similar to tuberous and tendon xanthomas and to xanthelasmata, plane xanthomas stain brownish red with Sudan red or scarlet red and show double refraction on polariscopic examination.

Systemic Lesions.   Atherosclerosis of the coronary arteries is accelerated and extensive in patients with hyperlipoproteinemia of types IIA, IIB, III, and IV. The peripheral arteries often are excessively atheromatous in type III (Amatruda et al). The bone marrow, lymph nodes, liver, and spleen often contain foam cells in types I, IV, and V, their number generally being dependent on the degree of hypertriglyceridemia (Roberts et al). The number of foam cells in the liver and spleen is particularly high in patients with hepatosplenomegaly and pancreatitis, as seen especially in types I and V; in addition, the liver shows extensive fatty degeneration, and the pancreas fibrosis (Bruton and Kanter).

The type IV or type V hyperlipoproteinemia observed secondary to von Gierke's disease, or Cori type I glycogenosis, is a result of a deficiency in hepatic glucose-6-phosphatase. The inability of the patient to dephosphorylate glucose-6-phosphate to glucose leads to hepatomegaly as a result of glycogen storage and to hyperlipoproteinemia as a result of increased fat synthesis (Cuttino et al). On histologic examination, the hepatic cells appear vacuolated like plant cells because of the accumulation of glycogen.

Also of interest are the findings in the liver of patients having hyperlipoproteinemia type IIA secondary to biliary cirrhosis. Such patients have pronounced jaundice, which precedes the appearance of xanthomatous lesions often by several years. The blood serum is clear but, owing to its high content of bilirubin, intensely green. The cutaneous lesions consist of xanthelasmata and often also of plane xanthomas in the palmar creases. The biliary cirrhosis, which is responsible for the hyperbetalipoproteinemia, is produced in the great majority of cases by a pericholangiolitis that leads to obliteration of the interlobular bile ducts (Ahrens et al). In rare instances, the biliary cirrhosis is produced by an obstruction of the extrahepatic bile ducts (Ahrens et al), or, in infants, by a congenital hypoplasia of the interlobular bile ducts (Ito et al).

Histogenesis. *Electron microscopic examination* of the foam cells in tuberous xanthomas shows that all of the lipid is located within histiocytic foam cells. No lipid is seen in interstitial regions or in the walls of blood vessels.

The lipid within the foam cells is present predominantly as large lipid droplets of low electron density that are not membrane-bound and measure from 0.3 μm to 1.8 μm in diameter. Small amounts of lipid are membrane-bound either as elongated, electron-lucid cholesterol crystals or as electron-dense "ceroid" granules, or they are seen within residual myelin figures (Bulkley et al). The paucity of membrane-bound lipid indicates that lysosomal digestion is a minor metabolic pathway and that nonlysosomal lipid storage in foam cells is the characteristic tissue response in tuberous xanthoma.

In patients with eruptive xanthomas due to hypertriglyceridemia, electron microscopy reveals accumulations of lipid droplets in the intercellular spaces of the dermal capillary walls, indicating that lipoproteins cross the vascular wall. The lipid particles are phagocytized by capillary pericytes and by pericapillary macrophages, which constitute the major component of tissue foam cells. The macrophages contain, in addition to lipid droplets without a limiting membrane, numerous lysosomes, including myelin figures, indicating attempts at lysosomal digestion (Parker and Odland). In resolving eruptive xanthomas that are largely depleted of triglycerides, the foam cells show a cholesterol-rich lipid pattern, as seen in the foam cells of tuberous xanthomas, that includes cholesterol crystals and ceroid granules (Bulkley et al).

TANGIER DISEASE

In Tangier disease, a rare disorder with autosomal recessive inheritance, the plasma alpha-lipoproteins are greatly decreased. This is associated with reduced concentrations of cholesterol and phospholipids in the plasma. In contrast to the low plasma cholesterol level, the cholesteryl ester concentration is increased in many tissues, including the skin.

Clinically, patients with hypoalphalipoproteinemia have markedly enlarged tonsils that show orange yellow striations. The spleen is moderately enlarged, and there are intermittent sensory and motor neuropathies (Herbert et al). The skin usually is free of lesions (Ferrans and Fredrickson). In one reported patient, however, numerous scattered papules were noted, mainly on the trunk (Waldorf et al).

Histopathology. In routinely stained sections of the skin, no abnormality is noted. However, on staining with scarlet red or oil red O, irrespective of whether the skin has papular lesions or appears normal, the dermis shows deposits of lipids both within macrophages and extracellularly (Waldorf et al; Krebs and Kuske). The lipid material stains positively with the Schultz stain, indicating the presence of cholesterol or cholesteryl esters. It is markedly birefringent under the polarizing microscope, as seen when cholesteryl esters are present.

Lipid deposits, usually recognizable even in routinely stained sections as foam cells, are found in the tonsils as well as in the liver, spleen, lymph nodes, bone marrow, and peripheral nerves (Ferrans and Fredrickson).

Histogenesis. Normal high-density lipoproteins or alpha-lipoproteins are absent from the plasma in patients with Tangier disease. Electron microscopy of the abnormal high-density lipoproteins in the plasma has revealed the presence of abnormal particles resulting from an abnormal chylomicron metabolism. These particles may be targets for phagocytosis and may be at least one source of the cholesteryl esters that accumulate in the tissues of patients with Tangier disease (Herbert et al).

NIEMANN–PICK DISEASE

Niemann–Pick disease, like Gaucher's disease and Fabry's disease, represents a sphingolipidosis. It is an intralysosomal storage disease in which, as a result of a deficiency of sphingomyelinase, sphingomyelin accumulates in the cells of the mononuclear phagocytic system in the spleen, liver, lymph nodes, and bone marrow, as well as in the central nervous system and in other tissues (Brady). Cholesterol accumulates secondarily. In spite of this widespread involvement, the skin is spared. Niemann–Pick disease is transmitted as an autosomal recessive trait.

Four types of Niemann–Pick disease are recognized (Crocker). Hepatosplenomegaly is found in all four types.

Type A, by far the most common type, represents the rather rapidly progressive, infantile form. It shows severe involvement of the central nervous system, with death occurring at 1 to 3 years of age. In association with cachexia, a diffuse yellow brown pigmentation of the skin occurs (Thannhauser). Rarely, papular eruptive xanthomas are seen in association with a secondary hyperlipemia (Crocker and Farber).

Type B, the adult type, has been given this designation because, even though it starts in early life, patients usually reach adulthood in reasonably good health. This is due to the fact that the central nervous system is spared (Lynn and Terry).

Type C, the juvenile type, and Type D, the Nova Scotia type, start in childhood. In both types, there is progressive central nervous system involvement leading to death in adolescence (Crocker and Farber).

Histopathology. The brownish discoloration of the skin is due to the presence of increased amounts of melanin in the basal cell layer of the epidermis. The eruptive xanthomas show the histologic features already described (see p. 385).

The characteristic cell of Niemann–Pick disease is a large foam cell 20 μm to 90 μm in diameter.

Because of the presence of fairly uniform vacuoles, these cells have a mulberry appearance. The lipids within these cells stain with scarlet red and Sudan black B (Crocker and Farber).

Histogenesis. The diagnosis of Niemann–Pick disease is established through assays for sphingomyelinase activity on sonicated leukocyte preparations or on cultured skin fibroblasts. Leukocytes or skin fibroblasts from patients with the classic type A Niemann–Pick disease do not hydrolyze sphingomyelin at all (Gal et al), whereas leukocytes and skin fibroblasts from patients with the other types possess a moderate amount of hydrolytic activity (Wenger et al).

On *electron microscopic examination*, the foam cells are found to contain, as a result of the enzymatic defect, numerous lipid-filled secondary lysosomes as well as concentrically laminated residual bodies, so-called myelin bodies (Lynn and Terry). Ultimately, the lysosomes lose their enclosing membrane and appear as large, lipid-filled vacuoles (Miller and Reimann).

GAUCHER'S DISEASE

Gaucher's disease represents an intralysosomal storage disease in which, as a result of a deficiency of glucocerebrosidase (beta-glucosidase), glucocerebroside accumulates mainly in cells of the mononuclear phagocytic system in the spleen, liver, bone marrow, and lymph nodes and sometimes in other tissues (Brady et al). The skin, however, is spared. The serum lipids are normal. Gaucher's disease is transmitted as an autosomal recessive trait.

The most common form of Gaucher's disease by far is type I, the adult, or nonneuropathic form. It is characterized by splenomegaly and aggregates of Gaucher cells in the bone marrow of the long bones and pelvis causing pain. There is thinning of the cortex of the affected bones that is readily recognizable on x-ray examination. Pathologic fractures may result. Many patients with type I Gaucher's disease have a normal life span. The other two types are very rare. They are type II, the infantile or acute neuropathic form, and type III, the juvenile or subacute neuropathic form. Both are fatal (Peters et al).

In type I, brownish tan pigmentation of the skin often becomes apparent in adult life. It may be diffuse or patchy and is seen on exposed parts of the body. In addition, diffuse or striped pigmentation may be seen on the shins (Thannhauser). Wedge-shaped, brownish thickenings, so-called pingueculae, are often seen on the bulbar conjunctiva of each eye.

Histopathology. The hyperpigmented skin shows increased amounts of melanin in the basal cell layer of the epidermis.

Gaucher cells have a characteristic appearance.

They are large, 20 μm to 100 μm in diameter. They possess one or several small nuclei and a pale, striated, wrinkled cytoplasm. The cytoplasm is periodic acid-Schiff (PAS)-positive but stains only faintly with fat stains.

Histogenesis. The diagnosis of Gaucher's disease can be established by an assay for glucocerebrosidase on the sonicated leukocytes of the patient. This assay shows greatly reduced activity (Lee et al). In addition, the tartrate-resistant (i.e., nonprostatic) serum acid phosphatase level is greatly elevated. These two determinations may make a search for Gaucher cells in the bone marrow unnecessary (Lee et al).

Electron microscopic examination of Gaucher cells shows numerous membrane-bound secondary lysosomes filled with tubular structures 20 nm to 30 nm in diameter. These tubular structures represent aggregated glucocerebroside molecules and correspond to the cytoplasmic striations seen in Gaucher cells by light microscopy (Hibbs et al).

ANGIOKERATOMA CORPORIS DIFFUSUM (FABRY'S DISEASE)

Fabry's disease, like Niemann–Pick disease and Gaucher's disease, represents a sphingolipidosis. As a result of a deficiency in the lysosomal hydrolase alpha-galactosidase, formerly called ceramide trihexosidase, the sphingoglycolipid ceramide trihexoside (galactosyl–galactosyl–glucosyl–ceramide) cannot be cleaved (Kint). As a consequence, there is progressive accumulation of ceramide trihexoside in many types of cells and in many organs, including the endothelial cells and pericytes of blood vessels throughout the body. In addition, smooth muscle cells, ganglion cells, nerves, the epithelial cells of the cornea, the kidney, the skin, and many other organs may be affected (Sagebiel and Parker).

The cutaneous eruption in most instances of Fabry's disease consists of innumerable small "angiomas," which are usually only 1 mm to 2 mm in size. The greatest number of lesions is located on the lower trunk. The first lesions, as a rule, begin to appear in late childhood. In occasional instances, cutaneous lesions are absent (Clarke et al). A few angiomas may be present in the mouth.

Systemic manifestations include the gradual development of renal insufficiency and, often, hypertension as a result of lipid deposits in the glomeruli. Death usually occurs in the fourth or fifth decade of life and is most commonly caused by renal failure (Ruiter, 1957). In some patients, death may occur as the result of myocardial infarction or of a cerebrovascular accident (Wise et al). Early symptoms of the disease that may precede the development of the cutaneous lesions are paresthesias of the hands and feet subsequent to changes in temperature.

Rt in Alcohol or Frozen Section (1st choice)

Histopathology. In routine sections, one observes only slight hyperkeratosis and a somewhat hyperplastic epidermis. The subepidermal capillaries are dilated and may be enclosed by the hyperplastic epidermis (Fig. 22-5). There often is

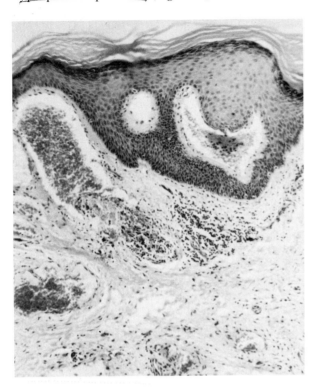

Fig. 22-5. Angiokeratoma corporis diffusum (Fabry's disease)
Superficial capillaries, some of them completely enclosed by the hyperplastic epidermis, are dilated, as are some of the more deeply situated vessels. One of them, in the left lower corner, is thrombosed. (×100)

also moderate dilatation of the more deeply situated vessels of the skin. Occasionally, one observes within some of the dilated capillaries fibrinous thrombi showing partial organization (Nakamura et al). Whereas the presence of glycolipid deposits in the heart muscle, the kidneys, and the macrophages of the bone marrow generally can be suspected even on routine fixation and staining because of swelling and vacuolization of the affected cells, the amount of glycolipid in the skin is small and therefore can be detected only by the use of special stains on unfixed or formalin-fixed frozen sections. Staining with Sudan black B demonstrates the lipids particularly well and is therefore preferable to staining with scarlet red (Frost et al). The PAS reaction is strongly positive and diastase-resistant, since it stains the carbohydrate component of the glycolipid (Hashimoto et al, 1965). Because the lipid material is doubly refractile, it can be demonstrated by means of polariscopic examination of unfixed or formalin-fixed frozen sections. Lipid deposits are not restricted to the cutaneous areas showing lesions but are present also in normal-appearing skin (de Groot).

Lipid deposits in the skin are seen particularly in the endothelial cells and pericytes of the cutaneous capillaries (Fig. 22-6) but also in many fibroblasts and in the arrector pilorum muscles (Ruiter, 1954; Pittelkow et al; Tarnowski and Hashimoto, 1969).

Systemic Lesions. On routine fixation and staining, the aorta and the large blood vessels show considerable thickening of their media as a result of marked vacuolization in their muscle bundles. Similar changes are seen in the heart muscle (Ruiter, 1957). In the kidneys, marked foamy vacuolization is seen not only in the walls

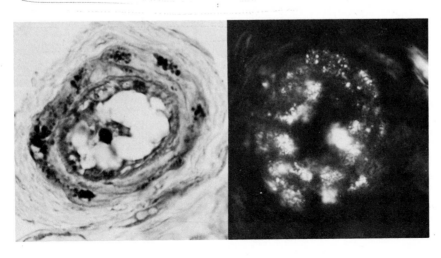

Fig. 22-6. Angiokeratoma corporis diffusum (Fabry's disease)
Cutaneous capillary. (*Left*) Staining with sudan black B reveals lipid granules in the endothelial cells and pericytes. (*Right*) Frozen section in polarized light shows the lipid granules to be doubly refractile. (×800) (Courtesy of M. Ruiter, M.D.)

of the large blood vessels but especially also in the glomerular endothelium, the epithelium of Bowman's capsule, the loops of Henle, and the distal tubules. In patients who have died of uremia, there is marked fibrosis of the kidney, particularly of the glomeruli. The glomerular changes have been shown by means of renal biopsies to be present even in patients with still normal renal function (Wallace; Burkholder et al). However, there generally is proteinuria in such instances, and the urinary sediment shows both intra- and extracellular lipid globules that are birefringent and thus show Maltese crosses under polarized light. A bone marrow biopsy also shows varying numbers of lipid-filled macrophages (von Gemmingen et al).

Histogenesis. The disease is inherited as an X-linked recessive trait, since the locus of the responsible gene is on the X chromosome (Wallace). There is complete penetrance in the hemizygous male and only occasional and usually mild penetrance in the heterozygous female (Burda and Winder). The affected male transmits the defective gene to all his daughters, and, in the heterozygous female, each conception carries a 50% probability of transmittal of the defective gene—to a male child as disease, or to a female child as a trait or mild disease (von Gemmingen et al). Patients with this disease as well as female carriers of the disease show a usually asymptomatic corneal opacity referred to as cornea verticillata. This condition represents a dystrophy of the corneal epithelium that is visible only by slit-lamp examination (von Gemmingen et al; Wallace).

Dilatation of the dermal blood vessels is the result of damage brought on by lipid deposits in the vascular walls (Ruiter, 1957). Thus, the vascular lesions represent not true angiomas but angiectases. Damage to endothelial cells is also responsible for the occasional formation of thrombi (Nakamura et al).

On *electron microscopic examination* of the skin, large, electron-dense lipid deposits are seen to be present in endothelial cells, pericytes, and fibroblasts (EM 34). They may be seen also in arrector pilorum muscles and in the secretory, ductal, and myoepithelial cells of eccrine glands (Nakamura et al). On high magnification, these deposits show a lamellar structure with a periodicity of 5 nm that is diagnostic for the intracytoplasmic inclusions of Fabry's disease (Hashimoto et al, 1976; Luderschmidt and Wolff). Many of the inclusions are surrounded by a membrane, but others are not. The smaller, membrane-bound inclusions show acid phosphatase activity when stained for acid phosphatase prior to staining for electron microscopy. Inclusions that are membrane-bound and contain acid phosphatase activity represent phagolysosomes that are engorged with lipid material. In contrast, the acid-phosphatase-negative, non-membrane-bound lamellar structures represent glycolipid aggregates. As "foreign bodies" to the cell, however, they may become surrounded by a membrane and fuse with primary

lysosomes, thus being transformed into secondary phagolysosomes. The presence of numerous large lysosomes filled with lipid material, including large residual bodies (EM 34), suggests that a genetic deficiency of a lysosomal enzyme prevents the lysosomes from adequately digesting the glycolipid material within them (Hashimoto et al, 1965, 1976; Tarnowski and Hashimoto, 1968). Alpha-galactosidase, in which patients with Fabry's disease are deficient, represents one of the lysosomal enzymes (Hashimoto et al, 1976).

Hemizygous patients with Fabry's disease show a marked reduction in alpha-galactosidase activity in the serum, in circulating neutrophils, and in cultures of their fibroblasts (Kint). This is associated with increased levels of ceramide trihexoside in the serum. In addition, these patients excrete large amounts of ceramide trihexoside in their urine (Brady et al). Heterozygous patients with Fabry's disease may show only a slightly reduced or even normal alpha-galactosidase activity. Nevertheless, they show corneal opacities and, on electron microscopy, intracytoplasmic lamellar lipid deposits in endothelial cells and pericytes of the skin (Hashimoto et al, 1976; Luderschmidt and Wolff). The prenatal diagnosis of Fabry's disease can be made by the demonstration of deficient alpha-galactosidase activity in cultured amniotic fluid cells obtained by amniocentesis in the 15th to 16th weeks of gestation (Brady; Michaelsson).

Fucosidosis

Fucosidosis, the result of a deficiency of the lysosomal enzyme alpha-L-fucosidase, leads to an accumulation of fucose-containing glycolipids in many locations. Three variants of fucosidosis are recognized, but only type III is associated with cutaneous lesions, which consist of angiokeratomas indistinguishable from those seen in angiokeratoma corporis diffusum of Fabry (Dvoretzky and Fisher).

In contrast to Fabry's disease, fucosidosis is transmitted as an autosomal recessive, rather than as an X-linked recessive, condition. In the typical patient, psychomotor regression is first noticed at the age of 12 to 18 months and is associated with spasticity and seizures. Ectasia of cutaneous vessels develops earlier than in Fabry's disease, between 6 months and 8 years of age (Dvoretzky and Fisher; Epinette et al).

Histopathology. Markedly dilated capillary spaces are present in the papillary dermis (Epinette et al). The endothelial cells lining these spaces appear swollen and vacuolated. In addition, the secretory coils of the sweat glands consist of swollen, finely vacuolated cells (Kornfeld et al). Dermal macrophages contain lipid material staining positively with oil red O and Sudan black (Epinette et al).

Histogenesis. On *electron microscopy,* numerous greatly distended, vacuolated lysosomes with finely granular content are seen not only in endothelial cells, fibroblasts, and histiocytes but also in keratinocytes and in the secretory cells of the eccrine glands (Epinette et al; Kornfeld et al).

Alpha-L-fucosidase activity in leukocytes is reduced to less than 10% of the level seen in normal controls (Epinette et al; Kornfeld et al).

LIPOGRANULOMATOSIS (FARBER'S DISEASE)

A rare autosomal recessive disease first described in 1952 (Farber), lipogranulomatosis represents a sphingolipidosis in which, as a result of low ceramidase activity, ceramide is found in an excessive concentration in various organs, including the skin (Schmoeckel and Hohlfed).

The disease starts in early infancy with hoarseness, painful periarticular and tendinous swellings leading to flexion contractures, and cutaneous–subcutaneous nodules that are most pronounced over the wrists and ankles. Involvement of cranial nerves and of the spinal cord leads to death, usually during the first year of life (Battin et al). Occasionally, however, patients survive for a longer period of time (Zetterström).

Histopathology.   Aggregates of histiocytes and fibroblasts are found in the cutaneous–subcutaneous nodules and in the tendinous and synovial swellings. Foamy histiocytes are only rarely found in the skin but are generally present in visceral and neural lesions (Zetterström; Battin et al). However, staining of frozen sections of cutaneous lesions shows the presence of lipid and PAS-positive material in histiocytes and fibroblasts, a result indicative of the presence of glycolipids.

Histogenesis. On *electron microscopy,* histiocytes and fibroblasts show within their cytoplasm lipid vacuoles as well as vacuoles filled with commalike curved rods called curvilinear bodies that are regarded as specific for the disease and referred to also as Farber bodies (Schmoeckel and Hohlfed). In addition, lipid vacuoles with transverse membranes, referred to as zebra bodies, are seen in endothelial cells (Battin et al; Schmoeckel and Hohlfed).

HISTIOCYTOSIS X

Histiocytosis X is a disease of unknown cause characterized by a proliferation of histiocytes. Three clinical forms are recognized: Letterer–Siwe disease, Hand–Schüller–Christian disease, and eosinophilic granuloma.

The three conditions are not sharply demarcated from each other, and transitional cases among them are common. In general, if the histiocytosis occurs during the first year of life, it is characterized by major and often fatal visceral involvement (Letterer–Siwe disease). If it develops during early childhood, the disease is expressed predominantly in osseous lesions and is associated with usually minor visceral involvement (Hand–Schüller–Christian disease). In older children and adults, histiocytosis X is as a rule localized and appears most commonly as one or several lesions of a bone (eosinophilic granuloma). Cutaneous lesions are very commonly encountered in Letterer–Siwe disease and occur occasionally in the two other forms.

Transformation of some of the histiocytes into lipid-laden foam cells occurs in some cases. It may be seen in all three forms of histiocytosis X and is not related to the duration of the disease. The formation of foam cells, if it occurs, is usually limited to a few organs, especially the meninges, bones, and spleen, whereas the histiocytic infiltrations located in the skin, liver, lungs, and lymph nodes show only little tendency toward lipidization. It appears likely that the presence of lipids within histiocytes is the result of inadequate digestion of phagocytized lipids (see Histogenesis). The values for serum lipids are within normal limits in histiocytosis X.

Letterer–Siwe disease, or acute disseminated histiocytosis X, usually occurs in infants. Rarely, it is seen in older children or adults. The prognosis generally is serious, particularly if the disease is extensive (Nezelof et al, 1979). However, in some cases, the degree of dysfunction of an organ may be more significant than the number of organs involved (Lahey). The most common manifestations are fever, anemia, thrombocytopenia, enlargement of the liver and spleen, lymphadenopathy, and pulmonary infiltrations. Osteolytic lesions are uncommon except in the pars mastoidea of the temporal bone, resulting in a clinical picture of otitis media. In about 80% of the cases, cutaneous lesions are present. They often are the first sign of the disease and are therefore of considerable diagnostic importance.

The cutaneous lesions usually consist of petechiae and papules. In some cases, one observes numerous closely set, brownish papules covered with scales or crusts. This type of eruption may be extensive, involving particularly the scalp, face, and trunk. The resemblance of this eruption to seborrheic dermatitis or Darier's disease often is striking (Laymon and Sevenants; Cancilla et al). In rare instances, a widespread cutaneous eruption indistinguishable from that seen in Letterer–Siwe disease is the only clinical manifestation in infants (Zachariae; Metz et al; Wolfson et al) and also the elderly (Benisch et al; Chevrant-Breton; Berman et al). The prognosis in such cases is very good. In infants, the eruption may consist of only a few scattered papules appearing intermittently (Eng).

In *Hand–Schüller–Christian disease,* or chronic disseminated histiocytosis X, diabetes insipidus, exophthalmos, and multiple defects of the bones, especially of the cranium, represent the classic triad. However, any one or even all three of the cardinal symptoms may be absent, and involvement may occur in entirely different organs. For example, enlargement of the liver, spleen, or lymph nodes may be found. Pulmonary involvement is rare and, if present, usually is mild. Osteolytic lesions of the long bones may result in a spontaneous fracture. Also, as in Letterer–Siwe disease, involvement of the temporal bone may manifest itself as otitis media. Hand–Schüller–Christian disease takes a chronic course, usually extending over years. The mortality rate without treatment is about 30%.

Cutaneous lesions occur in about one third of the cases (Curtis and Cawley). In rare instances, cutaneous lesions represent the only manifestation of the disease (Feuerman and Sandbank). Three types of skin lesions may occur. Most common are infiltrated plaques undergoing ulceration, especially in the axillae, the anogenital region, and the mouth, as seen also in eosinophilic granuloma (Curtis and Cawley; Malzoon and Wood). Next in frequency is an extensive eruption of coalescing, scaling, or crusted papules, as seen also in Letterer–Siwe disease (Altman and Winkelmann, 1963; Freeman). Finally, in rare instances only, one observes scattered, soft, yellowish, papular xanthomata. When they are the only manifestation of Hand–Schüller–Christian disease, they are both clinically and histologically indistinguishable from the cutaneous lesions seen in juvenile xanthogranuloma except for the presence of Langerhans granules on electron microscopy (see p. 398) (Hu and Winkelmann). Diabetes insipidus is present in some instances in association with the papular xanthomata (Jausion et al; Altman and Winkelmann, 1963) and lytic bone lesions or diffuse lymphadenopathy in others (Thannhauser). In most of these cases, the course is benign, but a fatal outcome has been observed (Thelander; Crocker, 1951). An additional type of eruption, *xanthoma disseminatum,* is discussed separately, because its relationship to Hand–Schüller–Christian disease is not generally accepted (see p. 396).

Eosinophilic granuloma, or chronic localized histiocytosis X, represents the third and least severe disease in this group. The lesions are either solitary or few in number. Most common are lesions of the bones, but the skin or the oral mucosa is occasionally involved, either with or without osseous lesions (Kierland et al). In some cases, diabetes insipidus is also present (Kierland et al; Koch and Panscherewski; Cohen and Ehrenfeld). Even though the disease is chronic, there is a tendency toward spontaneous healing. In rare instances, however, cases originally diagnosed as eosinophilic granuloma have progressed into typical Hand–Schüller–Christian disease (Engelbreth-Holm et al).

The cutaneous lesions may be of two types: they may consist of an extensive eruption of crusted papules, as seen also in Letterer–Siwe and Hand–Schüller–Christian disease (Lever and Leeper), or they may consist of one or several erythematous infiltrated plaques with a tendency to ulcerate, as seen also in Hand–Schüller–Chris-

tian disease (Curtis and Cawley; McCreary). The two types of cutaneous lesions may be present simultaneously.

Histopathology.   Not only clinically but also histologically, a close relationship exists among the three forms of histiocytosis. Generally, three kinds of histologic reactions can occur in histiocytosis: proliferative, granulomatous, and xanthomatous. In all three types, the histiocyte is the basic cell type. Several authors have pointed out that these three types of reaction may occur as consecutive stages, the proliferative reaction being the first, followed by the granulomatous and then by the xanthomatous reactions (Engelbreth-Holm et al). However, each of the three reactions may arise as such, and healing can occur during any one of them. In addition, the three histologic reactions are not sharply demarcated and may overlap or occur together in different organs of the same patient and even in different areas of the same organ (Laymon and Sevenants).

A definite relationship exists, nevertheless, between the type of histologic reaction and the clinical type of disease. In general, the proliferative reaction with its almost purely histiocytic infiltrate is typical of Letterer–Siwe disease, the granulomatous reaction of eosinophilic granuloma, and the xanthomatous reaction of Hand–Schüller–Christian disease; however, in Hand–Schüller–Christian disease, the xanthomatous reaction often is present in only a few organs, especially the meninges, bones, and spleen, whereas other involved organs, including the skin, may instead show the proliferative or granulomatous type of reaction (Laymon and Sevenants; Altman and Winkelmann, 1963). Thus, lipid-containing cells need not be and often are not present in the skin lesions of Hand–Schüller–Christian disease.

The histologic reaction present in the skin depends on the type of skin lesion. Since more than one type of skin lesion is occasionally present, different types of histologic reactions may be found in the same patient.

The *proliferative reaction* is encountered in the skin in petechiae, in hemorrhagic and nonhemorrhagic papules, in the eruption resembling seborrheic dermatitis, and, occasionally, in the often extensive eruption of scaling and crusting papules resembling Darier's disease, entirely independent of whether the lesions occur in Letterer–Siwe disease, Hand–Schüller–Christian disease, or eosinophilic granuloma.

Histologically, the proliferative reaction is characterized in the skin by the presence of an extensive infiltrate of histiocytes. The infiltrate usually lies close to the epidermis and invades it (Fig. 22-7). It may even destroy the epidermis, resulting in ulceration. The histiocytes composing the infiltrate appear as large, rounded cells with abundant, slightly eosinophilic cytoplasm. The nucleus is usually eccentric in location and indented or kidney-shaped (Fig. 22-8). In some patients, especially in infants with a rapidly fatal course, the nuclei may appear pleomorphic and even atypical, being large, irregularly shaped, and hyperchromatic (Altman and Winkelmann, 1963). In some areas, these cells are outlined distinctly and even separated by edema whereas in other areas, their cytoplasm is confluent (Sweitzer and Laymon; Wells). A few scattered lymphoid cells and varying numbers of eosinophils may be present. Extravasated erythrocytes frequently lie within the aggregates of histiocytes. Occasionally, some of the histiocytes have a foamy cytoplasm and stain positive with fat stains. In persistent lesions, one may find within the histiocytic infiltrate a few multinucleated histiocytes, indicating a transition to the granulomatous reaction (Eberhartinger and Santler).

The granulomatous reaction is found in the skin most commonly in infiltrated plaques in the genital area, in the axillary region, or on the scalp, but it

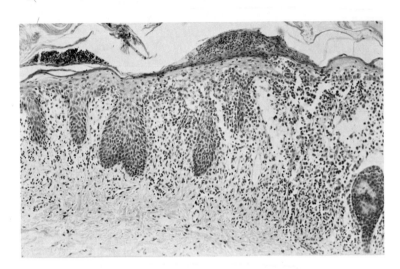

Fig. 22-7. Histiocytosis X, proliferative reaction
Low magnification. This reaction, typical of Letterer–Siwe disease, shows in the upper portion of the dermis an infiltrate composed almost entirely of loosely aggregated histiocytes. The infiltrate has invaded the epidermis in many areas. (×100)

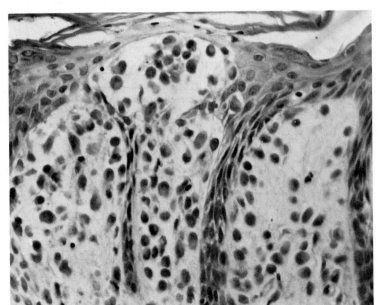

Fig. 22-8. Histiocytosis X, proliferative reaction
High magnification. The histiocytes of the infiltrate possess irregularly shaped nuclei and abundant, well-demarcated cytoplasm. In the center, the infiltrate has invaded the epidermis. (×400)

is occasionally seen also in the extensive eruption of scaling or crusted papules that may occur in Hand–Schüller–Christian disease and eosinophilic granuloma.

Histologically, the granulomatous reaction shows extensive aggregates of histiocytes often extending deep into the dermis. Eosinophils are present in various quantities. Generally, they lie in clusters instead of being diffusely scattered (Fig. 22-9). Irregularly shaped, multinucleated giant cells are seen frequently (Fig. 22-10). In addition, some neutrophils, lymphoid cells, and plasma cells may be present. Frequently, extravasations of erythrocytes are found. True foam cells are usually absent. Occasionally, however, some of the histiocytes possess a vacuolated cytoplasm and, on staining for fat, reveal small amounts of lipids (Farber; Curtis and Cawley; McCreary; Lever and Leeper).

The *xanthomatous reaction* is encountered in the skin only in the rarely occurring yellow, papular

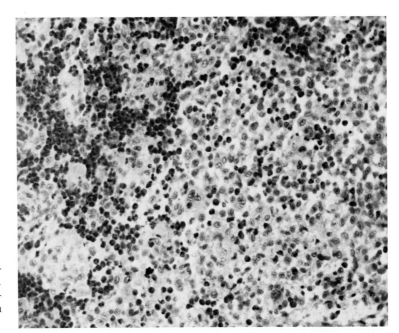

Fig. 22-9. Histiocytosis X, granulomatous reaction
This biopsy specimen, taken from an infiltrated plaque of eosinophilic granuloma, contains rather large histiocytes and eosinophils. Many of the eosinophilis lie in clusters. (×200)

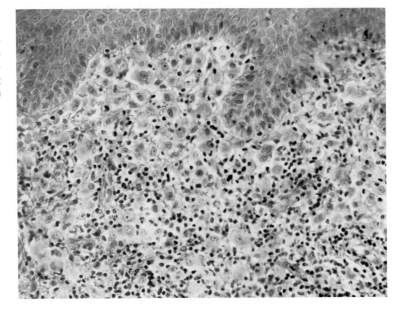

Fig. 22-10. Histiocytosis X, granulomatous reaction
This biopsy specimen, taken from an infiltrated, partially ulcerated plaque of Hand–Schüller–Christian disease, shows, in addition to large histiocytes, several giant cells and an inflammatory infiltrate. (×200)

xanthoma lesions of Hand–Schüller–Christian disease.

Histologically, the xanthomatous reaction reveals in the dermis numerous foam cells, as well as varying numbers of histiocytes and some eosinophils (Fig. 22-11). Multinucleated giant cells are frequently present. They are mainly of the foreign body type but occasionally have the appearance of Touton giant cells (lipid-containing giant cells). Thus, the histologic picture usually is more polymorphous than that seen in the tuberous xanthomas associated with the various types of hyperlipoproteinemia and represents a xanthogranuloma rather than a true xanthoma (Thannhauser; Altman and Winkelmann, 1963). The lipid is birefringent on polariscopic examination.

Visceral Lesions. The visceral lesions seen in histiocytosis X show the same three types of reactions just described for the skin. The organs most commonly affected are the spleen, liver, lungs, lymph nodes, and bones (Engelbreth-Holm et al; Sweitzer and Laymon; Thannhauser). In the triad occasionally seen in Hand–Schüller–Christian dis-

ease, the diabetes insipidus is caused by granulomatous infiltration of the posterior pituitary gland, the tuber cinereum, or the hypothalamus; the exophthalmos, by retro-orbital accumulations of granulomatous tissue; and the multiple defects in the skull, by the osteolytic effect of granulomatous infiltrations (Avioli et al).

Histogenesis. On *electron microscopic examination,* one third to one half of the histiocytes present in the cutaneous and visceral lesions of all three forms of histiocytosis are found to contain in their cytoplasm so-called Langerhans granules (Basset and Turiaf; Tarnowski and Hashimoto; Gianotti and Caputo; Wolff and Braun-Falco; Nezelof et al, 1979; Eady). In some cells, they are found in great numbers (Wolff and Braun-Falco). Langerhans granules are most abundant in lesions composed of nonlipidized histiocytes and are scanty or absent in xanthogranulomatous lesions (Nezelof et al, 1979). These granules, absent in normal histiocytes, are morphologically indistinguishable from the Langerhans granules present in normal epidermal Langerhans cells (see p. 18) both by transmission electron microscopy (Wolff; Nezelof et al, 1973) and in freeze-fracture replicas (Caputo et al). In addition, epidermal Langerhans cells and histiocytosis X cells are practically indistinguishable from each other in shape and structure of the nucleus, and both possess a well-developed Golgi zone and irregular cell borders (Elema and Poppema). In addition, enzymes known to be present in Langerhans cells, such as adenosine-triphosphatase and leucyl-beta-naphthylamidase, can be demonstrated also in histiocytosis X cells (Elema and Poppema). Both types of cells have surface receptors for the third component of complement (C3) and immunoglobulin (Ig), and both can phagocytize erythrocytes in cultures (Nezelof et al, 1977). In view of so many similarities, it appears quite likely that histiocytosis X is a proliferative disorder of the Langerhans histiocyte (Nezelof et al, 1973).

The lipid vacuoles that may accumulate in the cells of histiocytosis X on electron microscopy are of varying sizes and have no limiting membrane. Surrounding the lipid vacuoles are numerous primary lysosomes. It is possible that the lipid accumulates in the histiocytosis X cells as a result of impaired lysosomal degradation (Zemel et al).

Differential Diagnosis. For differentiation of the xanthomatous reaction of histiocytosis X from juvenile xanthogranuloma, see p. 398.

Xanthoma Disseminatum

Xanthoma disseminatum differs sufficiently from histiocytosis X that it warrants separate consideration, although it may represent merely a variant of Hand–Schüller–Christian disease.

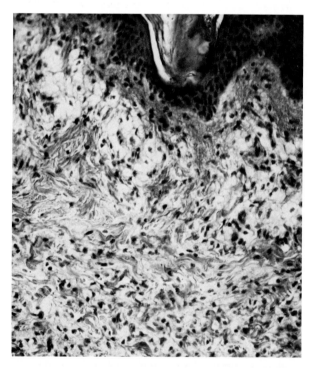

Fig. 22-11.   Histiocytosis X, xanthomatous reaction
This biopsy specimen, taken from a yellow nodule of Hand–Schüller–Christian disease, shows groups of foam cells in the upper dermis. The lower dermis contains histiocytes. (×200)

In this rare condition, of which fewer than 30 cases have been reported (Crocker, 1979), numerous widely disseminated but often closely set and even coalescing, round to oval, orange or yellow brown papules and nodules are found mainly on the flexor surfaces, such as the neck, axillae, antecubital fossae, groins, and perianal region. Often, there are lesions around the eyes. The mucous membranes are commonly affected. In addition to oral lesions, there may be extensive yellowish nodules in the pharynx and larynx occasionally leading to dyspnea and requiring tracheotomy (Altman and Winkelmann, 1962). Diabetes insipidus is encountered fairly often but usually is mild. Characteristically, internal lesions other than diabetes insipidus are absent. Occasionally, cutaneous lesions are the only manifestation (Altman and Winkelmann, 1962). Although xanthoma disseminatum usually is observed in adults, it may occur in children (Crocker, 1951; Sonnex et al).

Histopathology. In early lesions, large histiocytes dominate the histologic picture. With aging of the lesions, lipidization of histiocytes increases with formation of foam cells. Mature lesions show a histologic picture that is regarded as typical for xanthoma disseminatum, namely, a mixture of histiocytes, xanthoma cells, inflammatory cells, and numerous Touton giant cells (Altman and Winkelmann, 1962; Kumakiri et al). Occasionally, however, only few Touton giant cells are present (Mishkel et al). Some lesions consist almost exclusively of foam cells (Kalz et al; Kumakiri et al). The lipid present in the foam cells is doubly refractile (Mishkel et al).

Histogenesis. Proponents of the view that xanthoma disseminatum is an independent syndrome, rather than a variant of Hand–Schüller–Christian disease, have pointed out the predominant occurrence in adults; the common involvement of the pharynx and larynx, not seen in Hand–Schüller–Christian disease; the absence of bone lesions and of exophthalmos; and the prevalence of foam cells, uncommon in the cutaneous lesions of histiocytosis X (Altman and Winkelmann, 1962; Crocker, 1979). However, except for their predominant distribution on the flexural surfaces, where they often coalesce, the cutaneous lesions are similar in both diseases, and both diseases share the fairly common occurrence of diabetes insipidus. A case of xanthoma disseminatum with multiple osseous lesions has even been described (Mishkel et al).

Decisive for the question of whether xanthoma disseminatum represents a variant of histiocytosis X is the presence or absence of Langerhans granules. They were found in one reported case (Perrot et al) but were absent in four other cases (Ferrando and Bombi; Kumakiri et al; Sonnex et al). It is possible that, in the one case in which Langerhans granules were seen, the actual diagnosis was histiocytosis X. The possibility that Langer-

hans granules were not seen in the other four cases because of pronounced lipidization appears less likely but cannot be entirely excluded.

DIFFUSE NORMOLIPEMIC PLANE XANTHOMA

In diffuse normolipemic plane xanthoma, a rather rare disorder, one observes patches or, more commonly, diffuse areas of orange yellow discoloration of the skin. Whereas patchy areas have a recognizable border and, often, a slight degree of palpable infiltration, the diffuse areas have a poorly defined border. The face, particularly the periorbital areas, and the upper trunk are sites of predilection. The lesions usually persist indefinitely.

Some cases of diffuse normolipemic plane xanthoma can be regarded as idiopathic, not being associated with any other illness (Altman and Winkelmann). In other instances, diffuse normolipemic plane xanthoma has developed in areas of erythroderma (Walker and Sneddon) or secondary to leukemia (Lynch and Winkelmann) or paraproteinemia, particularly cryoglobulinemia (Feiwel; Kodama et al). The most common association, however, is with multiple myeloma (Levin et al; Moschella; Marien and Smeenk). The plane xanthomatosis often antedates the multiple myeloma by many years (Levin et al). In patients with this association, hyperlipoproteinemia of type IIA, III, or IV is not uncommon (Moschella; Marien and Smeenk).

Histopathology. Histologic examination reveals large sheets and clusters of foam cells, as well as foam cells singly and in small groups, diffusely scattered throughout the dermis. In some areas, the foam cells lie in thin streaks between collagen bundles (Fleischmajer et al), and, occasionally, a perivascular arrangement of foam cells is noted (Altman and Winkelmann). There may be an admixture of histiocytes and lymphoid cells; rarely, Touton giant cells are also seen (Walker and Sneddon). There is no fibrosis. Staining with Sudan IV reveals droplets of lipid in the foam cells (Altman and Winkelmann). Scattered foam cells have been observed even in the normal-appearing skin (Marien and Smeenk).

VERRUCIFORM XANTHOMA

Verruciform xanthoma, a rare condition, occurs as a solitary verrucous lesion most commonly in the oral cavity (Shafer; Buchner et al) but occasionally also on the vulva (Santa Cruz and Martin) or the penis (Kraemer et al). Verruciform xanthoma also occurs as a secondary development in lesions with prominent epidermal hyperplasia, such as epidermal nevus (Barr and Plank) and inflammatory linear verrucous epidermal nevus, or ILVEN (Grosshans and Laplanche).

Histopathology.   There is marked elongation of the rete ridges extending to a uniform level in the dermis. An infiltrate of foam cells is confined to the elongated dermal papillae located between the rete ridges (Barr and Plank).

JUVENILE XANTHOGRANULOMA

Juvenile xanthogranuloma, a designation that has gradually replaced the old term nevoxanthoendothelioma, generally is a benign disorder in which one or several and occasionally numerous red to yellow nodules are present. Their usual size is from 0.5 cm to 1 cm in diameter, but there is also a ''macronodular'' variant in which the nodules measure several centimeters in diameter (Nödl; Gartmann and Tritsch; Schmid and Usener). The lesions may be present at birth (Helwig and Hackney) but usually arise in early infancy. However, development in childhood or in adult life is by no means uncommon (Gartmann and Tritsch; Rodriguez and Ackerman). Although the lesions usually involute spontaneously within a year, they may persist for several years (Gartmann and Tritsch; Rodriguez and Ackerman).

In occasional instances, nodular lesions of the iris (Blank et al) or of the epibulbar area (Cogan et al) are found in association with juvenile xanthogranuloma. Lesions of the iris may lead to hemorrhages into the anterior chamber of the eye and to glaucoma. In several reported cases of juvenile xanthogranuloma, there were pulmonary infiltrations (Lamb and Lain; Nödl; Lottsfeldt

and Good; Schmid and Usener), hepatosplenomegaly (Lamb and Lain; Nödl), swelling of a testis (Helwig and Hackney; Nödl), or pericardial infiltration (Webster et al).

Histopathology.   Early lesions may show large accumulations of histiocytes without any lipid infiltration intermingled with only a few lymphoid cells and eosinophils (Fig. 22-12) (Nödl; Gartmann and Tritsch). Usually, however, some degree of lipidization is present, even in very early lesions. One finds then in some of the histiocytes a pale, vacuolated cytoplasm staining positive with fat stains (Esterly et al). In mature lesions, a granulomatous infiltrate is usually present containing foam cells, foreign body giant cells, and Touton giant cells as well as histiocytes, lymphocytes, and eosinophils. The presence of giant cells, most of them Touton giant cells, showing a perfect ''wreath'' of nuclei is quite typical for juvenile xanthogranuloma (Fig. 22-13) (Gartmann and Tritsch; Webster et al). Older, regressing lesions show proliferation of fibroblasts and fibrosis replacing part of the infiltrate.

Histogenesis. *Electron microscopy* has revealed that the lesion is composed of macrophages with complex pseudopodia. In mature lesions, one finds in the macrophages varying numbers of lysosomal structures containing lipid, but most lipid material is found as vacuoles not bound by a trilaminar membrane (EM 35) (Gonzalez-Crussi and Campbell; Esterly et al; Wolff et al).

Juvenile xanthogranuloma is generally regarded as an

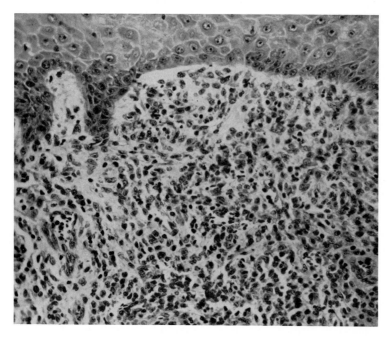

Fig. 22-12.   Juvenile xanthogranuloma, early lesion
There is a uniform infiltrate of histiocytes or macrophages without lipid infiltration. ($\times 200$)

independent entity, a reactive granuloma of unknown cause (Helwig and Hackney; Nödl; Gartmann and Tritsch). In the past, the view that juvenile xanthogranuloma represents an abortive, monosymptomatic, purely cutaneous form of Hand–Schüller–Christian disease was considered by several authors (Crocker; Nilsby; Thannhauser). As points in favor of a relationship between juvenile xanthogranuloma and Hand–Schüller–Christian disease, the following resemblances were cited. First, clinically, both diseases usually have their onset early in life and tend to involute spontaneously. Second, histologically, both have histiocytes as the basic cell type and, with aging of the lesions, show progressive lipidization and formation of giant cells. Third, internal lesions of the same type as seen in Hand–Schüller–Christian disease occur occasionally in cases of juvenile xanthogranuloma (see above). Finally, in rare instances, even fatal cases of Hand–Schüller–Christian disease have at their onset cutaneous lesions indistinguishable from those seen in juvenile xanthogranuloma (Thelander; Crocker). However, a strong argument against any relationship between juvenile xanthogranuloma and Hand–Schüller–Christian disease is the absence of Langerhans granules in the histiocytes of juvenile xanthogranuloma on electron microscopic examination (Gonzalez-Crussi and Campbell; Esterly et al; Wolff et al), whereas all three forms of histiocytosis, from one third to one half of the histiocytes these characteristic organelles (see p. 396).

Differential Diagnosis. In spite of their close histologic resemblance, juvenile xanthogranuloma differs from Hand–Schüller–Christian disease in certain aspects. In its early stage, it differs by the monomorphous appearance of massively aggregated histiocytes, and in its granulomatous stage by a milder inflammatory reaction with fewer eosinophils than in Hand–Schüller–Christian disease and by the prevalence of wreath-shaped Touton giant cells. These Touton giant cells are rarely seen in significant numbers in the xanthomatous lesions of Hand–Schüller–Christian disease, in which irregularly shaped giant cells of the foreign body type predominate. Differentiation of juvenile xanthogranuloma from dermatofibroma with lipidization can be difficult. However, dermatofibromas with lipidization only rarely show wreath-shaped Touton giant cells, may show areas of hemosiderin deposits, and often have a hyperplastic epidermis.

NECROBIOTIC XANTHOGRANULOMA WITH PARAPROTEINEMIA

A rare disorder, necrobiotic xanthogranuloma with paraproteinemia can be recognized clinically and histologically and thus represents a well-defined entity (Kossard and Winkelmann). Large, indurated plaques showing

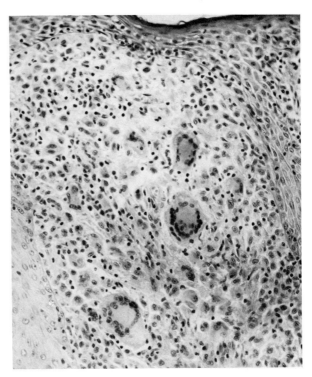

Fig. 22-13.   Juvenile xanthogranuloma, mature lesion
Many histiocytes or macrophages show a vacuolated cytoplasm and thus have the appearance of foam cells. Several giant cells possess a perfect "wreath" of nuclei, a feature that is quite typical for juvenile xanthogranuloma. Most wreath-shaped giant cells are Touton giant cells. ($\times 200$)

atrophy, telangiectasia, and occasionally also ulceration are present on the trunk, often together with subcutaneous nodules (Frank and Weidman; Kossard and Winkelmann). The skin of the thorax may show diffuse induration (Rupec et al). In many patients, papules, nodules, and plaques are present also on the face, especially in the periorbital region (Rendall et al). The facial plaques may also undergo ulceration (Kossard and Winkelmann).

Histopathology. Granulomatous masses are present either as focal aggregates or as large, intersecting bands occupying the dermis and subcutis. The intervening tissue separating the granulomas shows extensive hyaline necrobiosis (Kossard and Winkelmann). The granulomas show histiocytes, foam cells, and often also an admixture of inflammatory cells. A distinctive feature is the presence of numerous large giant cells, both of the Touton type with a peripheral rim of foamy cytoplasm and of the foreign body type (Rendall et al).

Histogenesis. In all patients tested for it, serum protein electrophoresis showed an IgG monoclonal paraprotein, which, on immunoelectrophoresis, had kappa light chains in some cases and lambda light chains in others (Rendall et al; Kossard and Winkelmann; Rupec et al). In two patients, bone marrow examination revealed multiple myeloma (Kossard and Winkelmann).

RETICULOHISTIOCYTOSIS

Two types of reticulohistiocytosis are recognized: reticulohistiocytic granuloma and multicentric reticulohistiocytosis. Both types occur almost exclusively in adults. The histologic picture is the same in the two types.

In *reticulohistiocytic granuloma,* one observes usually a single nodule and occasionally a few nodules, most commonly on the head and neck. The nodules are smooth and measure from 0.5 cm to 2 cm in diameter (Zak; Purvis and Helwig; Davies and Wood; Nödl). They usually involute spontaneously.

In *multicentric reticulohistiocytosis,* one finds, in addition to numerous nodules, a polyarthritis that may either precede or follow the cutaneous lesions. The nodules are present in many areas of the skin, with a predilection for the face and hands. In about half of the patients, nodules are present also on the oral or nasal mucosa (Barrow and Holubar). The size of the nodules ranges from a few millimeters to several centimeters, and they may become confluent. The polyarthritis may be mild or severe, but it has been found to be absent so far in only one case (Goette et al). If severe, it may be mutilating, especially on the hands, through destruction of articular cartilage and subarticular bone (Orkin et al). In most instances, the disease gradually loses its activity after several years (Barrow and Holubar).

Histopathology. The characteristic histologic feature in both reticulohistiocytic granuloma and multicentric reticulohistiocytosis is the presence of numerous large histiocytes showing abundant eosinophilic, finely granular cytoplasm with a "ground-glass" appearance. The histiocytes either have one nucleus or are multinucleated (Purvis and Helwig; Orkin et al). Early lesions show numerous mononuclear histiocytes and only a few multinucleated histiocytes with relatively few nuclei (Fig. 22-14) (Albert et al; Coode et al). As the lesions age, the number as well as the size of the giant cells increase, and fully matured lesions consist predominantly of strikingly large, round to oval or polygonal, multinucleated histiocytic giant cells showing an irregular distribution of nuclei. These giant cells may measure up to 50 μm in diameter (Coode et al). They often seem to lie within an empty space due to shrinkage of their cytoplasm (Fig. 22-15) (Nödl).

In early lesions, the large, predominantly mononuclear histiocytes lie intermingled with a rather pronounced inflammatory infiltrate composed largely of lymphoid cells but often also containing neutrophils and eosinophils (see Fig. 22-14) (Ikezawa and Nakajima). In older lesions, the inflammatory reaction is replaced more or less by fibrous tissue surrounding almost every large histiocyte (see Fig. 22-15) (Davies and Wood).

The contents of the large mononucleated or multinucleated histiocytes with "ground-glass" cytoplasm is somewhat variable; however, in all cases, the cytoplasm is strongly PAS-positive and

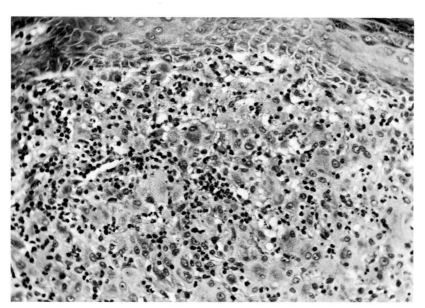

Fig. 22-14. Reticulohistiocytosis, early lesion
The large histiocytes with "ground-glass" cytoplasm are predominantly mononuclear, in contrast with those shown in Figure 22-15, which are largely multinuclear. A rather pronounced inflammatory infiltrate is present. (×200)

diastase-resistant. In some cases, the PAS-positive material is extractable by lipid solvents such as chloroform or acetone, indicating that the PAS-positive polysaccharide is attached to a lipid and represents a glycolipid (Albert et al). In other cases, the PAS reactivity is not abolished after extraction with lipid solvents, indicating the presence of a glycoprotein rather than a glycolipid (Davies et al; Ikezawa and Nakajima). Nevertheless, in most cases, lipids are present in small amounts in the "ground-glass" cytoplasm of the large histiocytes (Barrow and Holubar). The presence of phospholipids is indicated by a positive reaction with Baker's acid hematin (Davies et al), and the presence of neutral fat by positive staining with scarlet red (Albert et al; Orkin et al). Cholesterol is regularly absent, as demonstrated by a negative Schultz reaction, and so are cholesterol esters, since there is no birefringence (Anderson et al).

The polyarthritis present in nearly all instances of multicentric reticulohistiocytosis is caused by the same type of infiltrate as found in the cutaneous lesions. In early or mild cases, the granulomatous infiltrate is confined to the synovial membrane (Albert et al; Orkin et al). In patients with mutilating arthritis, the granulomatous infiltrate is found also in the subarticular cartilage and bone, leading to fragmentation and degeneration of bone (Montgomery et al).

Systemic lesions usually are absent in patients who have died of unrelated diseases. In a few instances, aggregates of histiocytes were found either in the pleura on biopsy (Fast) or on autopsy in bone, lymph nodes, and endocardium (Warin et al) or in muscle, perineural fat, and stomach (Ehrlich et al); however, there is inadequate evidence for the assumption that multicentric reticulohistiocytosis causes clinically significant lesions in locations other than the skin and joints (Chevrant-Breton; Coode et al).

Histogenesis. Enzyme histochemical staining has demonstrated in the large cells of reticulohistiocytosis the typical enzyme pattern of histiocytes, such as the presence of acid phosphatase and adenosine triphosphatase (Dammert and Niemi) as well as of nonspecific esterase (Coode et al).

Electron microscopic examination has revealed within the large histiocytes numerous electron-dense lysosomes (Ebner and Gebhart). However, only few secondary lysosomal vacuoles are present. Thus, these cells do not show evidence of active phagocytosis (Coode et al). Lipid vacuoles within the histiocytes are present in some cases (Ebner and Gebhart; Flam et al) but absent in others (Coode et al; Tani et al). This suggests that lipid

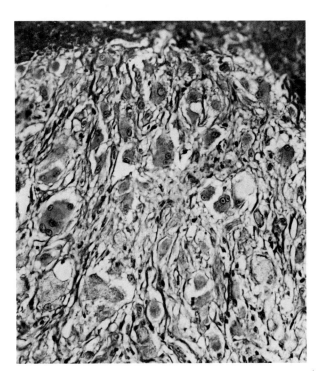

Fig. 22-15.   Reticulohistiocytosis, late lesion
Numerous large, multinucleated giant cells with a pale, finely granular, "ground-glass" cytoplasm are present. (×200) (Courtesy of Joseph Albert, M.D.)

accumulation does not play a major role in the pathogenesis of multicentric reticulohistiocytosis and may merely represent a degenerative process within the histiocytes (Tani et al). Ultracytochemical studies have shown that the PAS-positive reaction within the histiocytes is related to the presence of numerous lysosomes (Tani et al). No Langerhans granules are observed in the histiocytes (Ebner and Gebhart; Flam et al; Coode et al; Tani et al).

Differential Diagnosis.   Juvenile xanthogranuloma, which occurs rarely in adults, differs from reticulohistiocytosis in the appearance of its histiocytes. In juvenile xanthogranuloma, the cytoplasm of the histiocytes does not have a "ground-glass" appearance, and, except in very early lesions, abundant lipids are present in many histiocytes, giving them a foamy appearance. If giant cells are present in juvenile xanthogranuloma, at least some of them are Touton giant cells, which show a regular arrangement of nuclei in a wreathlike fashion and, peripheral to them, foamy cytoplasm. This contrasts with the irregular arrangement of nuclei in the giant cells of reticulohistiocytosis.

CONGENITAL SELF-HEALING RETICULOHISTIOCYTOSIS

The first case of congenital self-healing reticulohistiocytosis, a rare condition, was reported in 1973 (Hashimoto and Pritzker). Five additional cases have been reported since. In five of the six reported cases, scattered papules and small nodules were present at birth; in one case, they began to appear 17 days after birth (Hashimoto et al). The number of lesions varies from a dozen (Mascaro et al) to many more widely disseminated over the entire skin (Rufli and Fricker). The nodules may show central crusting. Spontaneous involution of all lesions takes place within 1 to 3½ months.

Histopathology.   The lesions show densely aggregated histiocytes with abundant eosinophilic cytoplasm. In some cells, the cytoplasm has a "ground-glass" appearance (Hashimoto and Pritzker). Multinucleated cells are present in some cases (Laugier et al), whereas only a few binucleated cells are seen in others (Rufli and Fricker). The histiocytes may invade and damage the epidermis (Mascaro et al). An admixture of inflammatory cells, including eosinophils, may be present (Rufli and Fricker). In many cells, portions of the cytoplasm are PAS-positive and diastase-resistant (Hashimoto and Pritzker). The histologic picture resembles that of reticulohistiocytosis of the adult type except for the prevalence of mitotic figures (Hashimoto et al).

Histogenesis. *Electron microscopic examination* carried out in four cases revealed within the histiocytes numerous lysosomal dense bodies, many of which contained myelinlike concentric laminations (Hashimoto and Pritzker; Laugier et al). Langerhans granules were observed in three of the four cases. They were present in varying proportions in the histiocytes: from a few cells (Hashimoto et al), to 10% of the cells (Hashimoto and Pritzker), to as many as 25% of the cells (Bonifazi et al).

Differential Diagnosis.   Histologic differentiation from Letterer–Siwe disease may be impossible on a purely cytologic basis (Mascaro et al). However, large cellular aggregates as seen in congenital self-healing reticulohistiocytosis are exceptional in Letterer–Siwe disease.

PROGRESSIVE NODULAR HISTIOCYTOMA

Only two cases of progressive nodular histiocytoma, a clinically distinct histiocytic proliferation, have been described (Taunton et al; Burgdorf et al). One observes a widespread eruption of hundreds of lesions consisting of papules varying from 2 mm to 10 mm in size and raised nodules measuring from 1 cm to 3 cm in diameter. Conjunctival, oral, or laryngeal lesions may occur. New lesions arise without involution of any of the lesions.

Histopathology.   The histologic picture, in contrast to the clinical picture, is not diagnostic. Two patterns can be recognized that may be found side by side: a cellular and a fibrous pattern (Burgdorf et al). In the cellular areas, numerous histiocytes and foam cells are seen together with an occasional Touton giant cell; in the fibrous areas, fibroblasts and collagen predominate, with the collagen bundles occasionally arranged in a storiform ("matted") pattern. Sudan black B and oil red O stains done on frozen tissue confirm the presence of lipid in areas of foam cells.

Differential Diagnosis.   The two patterns seen in progressive nodular histiocytoma resemble those seen in dermatofibroma: a fibrous pattern (dermatofibroma) and a cellular pattern (histiocytoma) (see p. 597).

GENERALIZED ERUPTIVE HISTIOCYTOMA

A rare dermatosis, generalized eruptive histiocytoma is characterized by the presence of innumerable flesh-colored to reddish papules that develop in crops and involute spontaneously. However, as a result of the continuous development of new lesions, the disorder may persist indefinitely (Herzberg; Winkelmann and Muller). Ultimately, after several years' duration, the eruption may subside (Winkelmann and Muller; Caputo et al). Yet even after complete regression, the eruption may recur (Sohi et al). Although most patients are adults, the condition may arise already in infancy (Winkelmann et al). In rare instances, oral lesions have been observed (Winkelmann and Muller).

Histopathology.   Histologic examination reveals a monomorphous infiltrate composed of histiocytes with a large, pale nucleus and abundant pale cytoplasm (Winkelmann and Muller). Multinucleated giant cells are absent (Winkelmann et al). In some lesions, an inflammatory infiltrate is present consisting predominantly of lymphocytes (Winkelmann et al), neutrophils (Cramer), or eosinophils (Herzberg). Lipid stains are negative (Herzberg; Sohi et al).

Histogenesis. On *electron microscopic examination*, the histiocytes show a large number of lysosomal structures but no significant phagocytosis (Muller et al; Caputo et al). Small aggregates of lipid are seen in only a few cells (Muller et al), and no Langerhans cell granules are present (Winkelmann et al).

Differential Diagnosis.   Even though the histologic picture of this condition is indistinguishable from the earliest stage of juvenile xanthogranuloma (see p. 398) or xanthoma disseminatum (see p. 397), the failure of the lesions to progress to lipidization is characteristic of generalized eruptive histiocytoma. The absence of "ground-glass" cytoplasm and of giant cells distinguishes this disorder from reticulohistiocytosis.

BIBLIOGRAPHY

Hyperlipoproteinemia

AHRENS EH JR, PAYNE MA, KUNKEL HG et al: Primary biliary cirrhosis. Medicine (Baltimore) 29:299–364, 1950

AMATRUDA JM, MARGOLIS S, HUTCHINS GM: Type III hyperlipoproteinemia. Arch Pathol 98:51–54, 1974

BAES H, VAN GENT CM, PRIES C: Lipid composition of various types of xanthoma. J Invest Dermatol 51:286–293, 1968

BORRIE P, SLACK J: A clinical syndrome characteristic of primary type IV-V hyperlipoproteinemia. Br J Dermatol 90:245–253, 1974

BROWN MS, GOLDSTEIN JL: Familial hypercholesterolemia: A genetic defect in the low-density lipoprotein receptor. N Engl J Med 294:1386–1390, 1976

BRUTON OC, KANTER AJ: Idiopathic familial hyperlipemia. Am J Dis Child 82:153–159, 1951

BÜRGER M GRÜTZ O: Über hepatosplenomegale Lipidose mit xanthomatösen Veränderungen. Arch Dermatol Syph (Berlin) 166:542–575, 1932

BULKLEY BH, BUJA M, FERRANS VJ et al: Tuberous xanthoma in homozygous Type II hyperlipoproteinemia. Arch Pathol 99:293–300, 1975

CORNELIUS CE: Disappearance of eruptive xanthoma following carbohydrate restriction. Arch Dermatol 96:45–50, 1967

CUTTINO JT JR, SUMMER GK, HILL HD: Treatment of eruptive xanthomas in Cori type I glycogenosis. Arch Dermatol 101:469–471, 1970

FERRANS VJ, BUJA LM, ROBERTS WC et al: The spleen in type I hyperlipoproteinemia. Am J Pathol 64:67–96, 1971

FISHER WR, TRUITT DH: The common hyperlipoproteinemias. (Review) Ann Intern Med 85:497–508, 1976

FLEISCHMAJER R: Familial hyperlipoproteinemia type III. Arch Dermatol 100:401–406, 1969

FLEISCHMAJER R: Diagnosis and treatment of familial lipoproteinemias. (Review) Int J Dermatol 10:251–258, 1971

FREDRICKSON DS, LEVY RI, LEES RS: Fat transport in lipoproteins: An integrated approach to mechanisms and disorders. N Engl J Med 276:34–44, 94–103, 148–156, 215–225, 273–281, 1967

HOLIMON JL, WASSERMAN AJ: Autopsy findings in type 3 hyperlipoproteinemia. Arch Pathol 92:415–417, 1971

HOLT LE, AYLWARD FX, TIMBRES HG: Idiopathic familial lipemia. Johns Hopkins Hosp Bull 64:279–314, 1939

ITO J, SUGAI T, SAITO T: Atresia of the intrahepatic bile ducts with xanthomatosis. Arch Dermatol 96:53–58, 1967

LEES RS, HATCH FT: Sharper separation of lipoprotein species by paper electrophoresis in albumin-containing buffer. J Lab Clin Med 61:518–528, 1963

LEVER WF, SMITH PAJ, HURLEY NA: Idiopathic hyperlipemia and primary hypercholesteremic xanthomatosis. I. Clinical data and analysis of the plasma lipids. J Invest Dermatol 22:33–69, 1954

MAHER JA, EPSTEIN FH, HAND EA: Xanthomatosis and coronary heart disease. Arch Intern Med 102:437–454, 1958

PARKER F, BAGDADE JD, ODLAND GF et al: Evidence for the chylomicron origin of lipids accumulating in diabetic eruptive xanthoma. J Clin Invest 49:2172–2187, 1970

PARKER F, ODLAND GF: Electron microscopic similarities between experimental xanthoma and human eruptive xanthomas. J Invest Dermatol 52:136–147, 1969

PEDACE FJ, WINKELMANN RK: Xanthelasma palpebrarum. JAMA 193:893–894, 1965

POLANO MK: Die Xanthelasmatosen der Haut. Arch Dermatol Syph (Berlin) 181:139–172, 1940

ROBERTS WC, LEVY RI, FREDRICKSON DS: Hyperlipoproteinemia. (Review) Arch Pathol 90:46–56, 1970

SCHREIBER MM, SHAPIRO SI: Secondary eruptive xanthoma. Type V hyperlipoproteinemia. Arch Dermatol 100:601–603, 1969

SCHREIBMAN PH, WILSON DE, ARKY RA: Familial type IV hyperlipoproteinemia. N Engl J Med 281:981–985, 1969

Tangier Disease

FERRANS VJ, FREDRICKSON DS: The pathology of Tangier disease. Am J Pathol 78:101–158, 1975

HERBERT PN, FORTE T, HEINEN RJ et al: Tangier disease. One explanation of lipid storage. N Engl J Med 299:519–521, 1978

KREBS A, KUSKE H: Familiäre Analphalipoproteinämie ("Tangier disease"). Dermatologica 138:196–198, 1969

WALDORF DS, LEVY RI, FREDRICKSON DS: Cutaneous cholesterol ester deposition in Tangier disease. Arch Dermatol 95:161–165, 1967

Niemann–Pick Disease

BRADY RO: The sphingolipidoses. N Engl J Med 275:312–318, 1966

CROCKER AC: The cerebral defect in Tay-Sachs disease and Niemann-Pick disease. J Neurochem 7:69–80, 1961

CROCKER AC, FARBER S: Niemann-Pick disease: A review of 18 patients. Medicine (Baltimore) 37:1–95, 1958

GAL AE, BRADY RO, HIBBERT SR et al: A practical chromogenic procedure for the detection of homozygotes and heterozygous carriers of Niemann-Pick disease. N Engl J Med 293:632–636, 1975

LYNN R, TERRY RDL: Lipid histochemistry and electron microscopy in adult Niemann-Pick disease. Am J Med 37:987–994, 1964

MILLER WL, REIMANN BEF: Childhood variant of Niemann-Pick disease. Am J Pathol 58:450–457, 1972

THANNHAUSER S: Lipidoses, 3rd ed, p 551. New York, Grune & Stratton, 1958

WENGER DA, BARTH G, GITHENS JA: Nine cases of spingomyelin lipidoses, a new variant in Spanish-American children. Am J Dis Child 131:955–961, 1977

Gaucher's Disease

BRADY RO, KANFER JW, BRADLEY RM et al: Demonstration of a deficiency of glucose-cerebroside-cleaving enzyme in Gaucher's disease. J Clin Invest 45:1112–1115, 1966

HIBBS RG, FERRANS VJ, CIPRIANO PR et al: A histochemical and electron microscopic study of Gaucher cells. Arch Pathol 89:137–153, 1970

LEE RE, ROBINSON DB, GLEW RH: Gaucher's disease. I. Modern enzymatic and anatomic methods of diagnosis. Arch Pathol 105:102–104, 1981

PETERS SP, LEE RE, GLEW RH: Gaucher's disease. A review. Medicine (Baltimore) 56:425–442, 1977

THANNHAUSER S: Lipidoses, 3rd ed, pp 494–495. New York, Grune & Stratton, 1958

Angiokeratoma Corporis Diffusum (Fabry's Disease), Fucosidosis

BRADY RO: Fabry's disease: Antenatal detection. Science 172:174–175, 1971

BRADY RO, GAL AE, BRADLEY RM et al: Enzymatic defect in Fabry's disease. N Engl J Med 276:1163–1167, 1967

BURDA CD, WINDER PR: Angiokeratoma corporis diffusum universale (Fabry's disease) in female subjects. Am J Med 42:293–301, 1967

BURKHOLDER PM, UPDIKE SJ, WARE RA et al: Clinicopathologic, enzymatic, and genetic features in a case of Fabry's disease. Arch Pathol 104:17–25, 1980

CLARKE JTR, KNAACK J, CRAWHALL JC et al: Ceramide trihexidosis (Fabry's disease) without skin lesions. N Engl J Med 284:233–235, 1971

DE GROOT WP: Angiokeratoma corporis diffusum Fabry. Dermatologica 128:321–349, 1964

DVORETZKY I, FISHER BK: Fucosidosis. Int J Dermatol 18:213–216, 1979

EPINETTE WW, NORINS AL, DREW AL et al: Angiokeratoma corporis diffusum with alpha-L-fucosidase deficiency. Arch Dermatol 107:754–757, 1973

FROST P, SPAETH GL, TANAKA Y: Fabry's disease: Glycolipid lipidosis. Arch Intern Med 117:440–446, 1966

HASHIMOTO K, GROSS BG, LEVER WF: Angiokeratoma corporis diffusum (Fabry). Histochemical and electron microscopic studies of the skin. J Invest Dermatol 44:119–128, 1965

HASHIMOTO K, LIEBERMAN P, LAMKIN N JR: Angiokeratoma corporis diffusum (Fabry's disease): A lysosomal disease. Arch Dermatol 112:1416–1423, 1976

KINT JA: Fabry's disease: Alpha-galactosidase deficiency. Science 167:1268–1269, 1970

KORNFELD M, SNYDER RD, WENGER DA: Fucosidosis with angiokeratoma. Arch Pathol 101:478–485, 1977

LUDERSCHMIDT C, WOLFF HH: Intracytoplasmic granules with lamellae as signs of heterozygous Fabry's disease. Am J Dermatopathol 2:57–61, 1980

MICHAELSSON G: Prenatal diagnosis of skin disorders. Acta Derm Venereol (Stockh) Suppl 95:64–66, 1981

NAKAMURA T, KANEKO H, NISHINO I: Angiokeratoma corporis diffusum (Fabry disease): Ultrastructural studies of the skin. Acta Derm Venereol (Stockh) 61:37–41, 1981

PITTELKOW RB, KIERLAND RR, MONTGOMERY H: Polariscopic and histochemical studies in angiokeratoma corporis diffusum. Arch Dermatol 76:59–64, 1957

RUITER M: Histologic investigation of the skin in angiokeratoma corporis diffusum in particular with regard to the associated disturbance of phosphatid metabolism. Dermatologica 109:273–286, 1954

RUITER M: Some further observations on angiokeratoma corporis diffusum. Br J Dermatol 69:137–144, 1957

SAGEBIEL RW, PARKER F: Cutaneous lesions of Fabry's disease: Glycolipid lipidosis. J Invest Dermatol 50:208–213, 1968

TARNOWSKI WM, HASHIMOTO K: Lysosomes in Fabry's disease. Acta Derm Venereol (Stockh) 48:143–151, 1968

TARNOWSKI WM, HASHIMOTO K: New light microscopic findings in Fabry's disease. Acta Derm Venereol (Stockh) 49:386–389, 1969

VON GEMMINGEN G, KIERLAND RR, OPITZ JM: Angiokeratoma diffusum (Fabry's disease). Arch Dermatol 91:206–218, 1965

WALLACE HJ: Anderson-Fabry disease. (Review) Br J Dermatol 88:1–23, 1973

WISE D, WALLACE HJ, JELLINEK EH: Angiokeratoma corporis diffusum. Q J Med 31:177–206, 1962

Lipogranulomatosis (Farber's Disease)

BATTIN J, VITAL C, AZANZA X: Une neurolipidose rare avec lésions nodulaires souscutanées et articulaires: La lipogranulomatose disseminée de Farber. Ann Dermatol Syph 97:241–248, 1970

FARBER S: A lipid metabolic disorder: Disseminated "lipogranulomatosis." A syndrome with similarity to, and important difference from, Niemann-Pick and Hand-Schüller-Christian disease. Am J Dis Child 84:499–500, 1952

SCHMOECKEL C, HOHLFED M: A specific ultrastructural marker for disseminated lipogranulomatosis (Farber). Arch Dermatol Res 266:187–196, 1979

ZETTERSTRÖM R: Disseminated lipogranulomatosis (Farber's disease). Acta Paediatr 47:501–510, 1958

Histiocytosis X, Xanthoma Disseminatum

ALTMAN J, WINKELMANN RK: Xanthoma disseminatum. Arch Dermatol 86:582–596, 1962

ALTMAN J, WINKELMANN RK: Xanthomatous cutaneous lesions of histiocytosis X. Arch Dermatol 87:164–170, 1963

AVIOLI LV, LASERSOHN JT, LOPRESTI JM: Histiocytosis X (Schüller-Christian disease): A clinicopathologic survey. Medicine (Baltimore) 42:119–147, 1963

BASSET F, TURIAF J: Identification par le microscope électronique de particles de nature probablement virale dans les laisions granulomateuses d'une histiocytose "X" pulmonaire. C R Acad Sci [D] (Paris) 261:3701–3703, 1965

BENISCH B, PEISON B, CARTER H: Histiocytosis of the skin in an elderly man. Am J Clin Pathol 67:36–40, 1977

BERMAN B, CHANG DL, SHUPACK JL: Histiocytosis: Treatment with topical nitrogen mustard. J Am Acad Dermatol 3:23–29, 1980

CANCILLA PA, LAHEY ME, CARNES WH: Cutaneous lesions of Letterer-Siwe disease. Cancer 20:1986–1991, 1967

CAPUTO R, PELUCHETTI D, MONTI M: Freeze-fracture of Langerhans granules. A comparative study. J Invest Dermatol 66:297–301, 1976

CHEVRANT-BRETON J: La maladie de Letterer-Siwe de l'adulte. Revue de la littérature. Ann Dermatol Venereol 105:301–305, 1978

COHEN HA, EHRENFELD EN: Granulome éosinophile de la peau et des muqueuses associé au diabète insipide. Ann Dermatol Syph 89:602–610, 1962

CROCKER AC: Skin xanthomas in childhood. Pediatrics 8:573–597, 1951

CROCKER AC: Xanthoma disseminatum. In Fitzpatrick TB, Eisen AZ, Wolff K et al (eds): Dermatology in General Practice, 2nd ed, pp 1173–1174. New York, McGraw-Hill, 1979

CURTIS AC, CAWLEY EP: Eosinophilic granuloma of bone with cutaneous manifestations. Arch Dermatol 55:810–818, 1947

EADY RAJ: Letterer-Siwe disease in an elderly patient: Histological and ultrastructural findings. Clin Exp Dermatol 4:413–420, 1979

EBERHARTINGER C, SANTLER R: Reticulose vom Typ der Abt-Letterer-Siweschen Erkrankung. Arch Klin Exp Dermatol 208:367–379, 1959

ELEMA JD, POPPEMA S: Infantile histiocytosis X (Letterer-Siwe disease). Cancer 42:555–565, 1978

ENG AM: Papular histiocytosis X. Am J Dermatopathol 3:205–206, 1981

ENGLEBRETH-HOLM J, TEILUM G, CHRISTENSEN E: Eosinophil granuloma of bone: Schüller-Christian's disease. Acta Med Scand 118:292–312, 1944

FARBER S: The nature of "solitary or eosinophilic granuloma" of bone. Am J Pathol 17:625–631, 1941

FERRANDO J, BOMBI JA: Ultrastructural aspects of normolipidemic xanthomatosis. Arch Dermatol Res 266:143–159, 1979

FEUERMAN EJ, SANDBANK M: Histiocytosis X with skin lesions as the sole clinical expression. Acta Derm Venereol (Stockh) 56:269–277, 1976

FREEMAN SA: A benign form of Letterer-Siwe disease. Aust J Dermatol 12:165–171, 1971

GIANOTTI F, CAPUTO R: Skin ultrastructure in Hand-Schüller-Christian disease. Arch Dermatol 100:342–349, 1969

HU CH, WINKELMANN RK: Unusual normolipidemic cutaneous xanthomatosis: A comparison of two cases illustrating the differential diagnosis. Acta Derm Venereol (Stockh) 57:421–429, 1977

JAUSION H, ROUSSEL A, BELLALUNE A: Curieuse évolution d'une xanthomatose éruptive, avec diabète insipide. Bull Soc Fr Dermatol Syph 61:469–471, 1954

KALZ F, HOFFMAN M, LAFRANCE A: Xanthoma disseminatum. Dermatologica 140:129–141, 1970

KIERLAND RB, EPSTEIN JG, WEBER WE: Eosinophilic granuloma of skin and mucous membranes. Arch Dermatol 75:45–54, 1957

KOCH H, PANSCHEREWSKI D: Das eosinophile Granulom im Bereich der Mundschleimhaut. Hautarzt 14:173–177, 1963

KUMAKIRI M, SUDOH M, MIURA Y: Xanthoma disseminatum. J Am Acad Dermatol 4:291–299, 1981

LAHEY ME: Prognosis in reticuloendotheliosis in children. J Pediatr 51:664–671, 1962

LAYMON CW, SEVENANTS JJ: Systemic reticuloendothelial granuloma. Arch Dermatol Syph 57:873–890, 1948

LEVER WF, LEEPER RW: Eosinophilic granuloma of the skin. Arch Dermatol Syph 57:85–96, 1950

MALZOON S, WOOD MG: Multifocal eosinophilic granuloma with skin ulceration. Histiocytosis X of the Hand-Schüller-Christian type. Arch Dermatol 116:218–220, 1980

MCCREARY JH: Eosinophilic granuloma of the skin. Arch Dermatol Syph 58:372–380, 1948

METZ J, METZ G, LECHNER W: Kutane Histiozytose X. Hautarzt 31:486–490, 1980

MISHKEL MA, COCKSHOTT WP, NAZIR DJ et al: Xanthoma disseminatum. Arch Dermatol 113:1094–1100, 1977

NEZELOF C, BASSET F, ROUSSEAU MF: Histiocytosis X: Histogenetic arguments for a Langerhans cell origin. Biomedicine 18:365–371, 1973

NEZELOF C, DIEBOLD D, ROUSSEAU-MERCK MF: Ig surface receptors and erythrophagocytic activity of histiocytosis X cells in vitro. J Pathol 122:105–113, 1977

NEZELOF C, FRILEUX-HERBET F, CRONIER-SACHOT J: Disseminated histiocytosis X. Analysis of prognostic factors based on a retrospective study of 50 cases. Cancer 44:1824–1838, 1979

PERROT H, THIVOLET J, HERMIER C et al: Xanthoma disseminatum. Aspect ultrastructural d'histiocytose X. Bull Soc Fr Dermatol Syph 79:674–675, 1972

SONNEX TS, RYAN TJ, DAWBER RPR: Progressive xanthoma disseminatum. Br J Dermatol 105, Suppl 19:79–81, 1981

SWEITZER SE, LAYMON CW: Letterer-Siwe disease. Arch Dermatol Syph 59:549–559, 1949

TARNOWSKI WM, HASHIMOTO K: Langerhans' cell granules in histiocytosis X. Arch Dermatol 96:298–304, 1967

THANNHAUSER SJ: Lipidoses, 3rd ed, pp 345–424. New York, Grune & Stratton, 1958

THELANDER HE: Xanthomatosis. J Pediatr 34:490–501, 1949

WELLS GC: The pathology of adult type Letterer-Siwe disease. Clin Exp Dermatol 4:407–412, 1979

WOLFF HH, BRAUN-FALCO O: Zur Diagnostik und Therapie des Morbus Hand-Schüller-Christian. Hautarzt 23:163–169, 1972

WOLFF K: The Langerhans cell. In Current Problems in Dermatology, Vol 4, pp 79–145. Basel, S Karger, AG, 1972

WOLFSON SL, BOTERO F, HURWITZ S et al: "Pure" cutaneous histiocytosis X. Cancer 48:2236–2238, 1981

ZACHARIAE H: Histiocytosis X in two infants. Br J Dermatol 100:433–438, 1979

ZEMEL H, DEEKEN J, ASEL N et al: The ultrastructural features of normolipemic plane zanthoma. Arch Pathol 89:111–117, 1970

Diffuse Normolipemic Plane Xanthoma

ALTMAN J, WINKELMANN RK: Diffuse normolipemic plane xanthoma. Arch Dermatol 85:633–640, 1962

FEIWEL M: Xanthomatosis in cryoglobulinaemia and other paraproteinaemias with report of a case. Br J Dermatol 80:719–729, 1968

FLEISCHMAJER R, HYMAN AB, WEIDMAN AI: Normolipemic plane xanthomas. Arch Dermatol 89:319–323, 1964

KODAMA H, NAKAGAWA S, TANIOKU K: Plane xanthomatosis with antilipoprotein antibody. Arch Dermatol 105:722–727, 1972

LEVIN WC, ABOUMRAD MH, RITZMANN SE et al: Gamma-type I myeloma and xanthomatosis. Arch Intern Med 114:688–693, 1964

LYNCH PJ, WINKELMANN RK: Generalized plane xanthoma and systemic disease. Arch Dermatol 93:639–646, 1966

MARIEN KJC, SMEENK G: Plane xanthomata associated with multiple myeloma and hyperlipoproteinemia. Br J Dermatol 93:407–415, 1975

MOSCHELLA SL: Plane xanthomatosis associated with myelomatosis. Arch Dermatol 101:683–687, 1970

WALKER AE, SNEDDON IB: Skin xanthoma following erythroderma. Br J Dermatol 80:580–587, 1968

Verruciform Xanthoma

BARR RJ, PLANK CJ: Verruciform xanthoma of the skin. J Cutan Pathol 7:422–428, 1980

BUCHNER A, HANSEN LS, MERRILL PW: Verruciform xanthoma of the oral mucosa. Arch Dermatol 117:563–565, 1981

GROSSHANS E, LAPLANCHE G: Verruciform xanthoma or xanthomatous transformation of inflammatory epidermal nevus. J Cutan Pathol 8:382–384, 1981

KRAEMER BB, SCHMIDT WA, FOUCAR E et al: Verruciform xanthoma of the penis. Arch Dermatol 117:516–518, 1981

SANTA CRUZ DJ, MARTIN SA: Verruciform xanthoma of the vulva. Am J Clin Pathol 71:224–228, 1979

SHAFER WB: Verruciform xanthoma. Oral Surg 31:784–789, 1971

Juvenile Xanthogranuloma

BLANK H, EGLICK PG, BEERMAN H: Nevoxanthoendothelioma with ocular involvement. Pediatrics 4:349–354, 1949

COGAN DG, KUWABARA T, PARKE D: Epibulbar nevoxanthoendothelioma. Arch Ophthalmol 59:717–725, 1958

CROCKER AC: Skin xanthomas in childhood. Pediatrics 8:573–597, 1951

ESTERLY NB, SAHIHI T, MEDENICA M: Juvenile xanthogranuloma. An atypical case with study of ultrastructure. Arch Dermatol 105:99–102, 1972

GARTMANN H, TRITSCH H: Klein- und grossknotiges Naevoxanthoendotheliom. Arch Klin Exp Dermatol 215:409–421, 1963

GONZALES-CRUSSI F, CAMPBELL R: Juvenile xanthogranuloma. Ultrastructural study. Arch Pathol 89:65–72, 1970

HELWIG EB, HACKNEY VC: Juvenile xanthogranuloma (nevoxanthoendothelioma). Am J Pathol 30:625–626, 1954

LAMB JH, LAIN ES: Nevo-xanthoendothelioma. Its relation to juvenile xanthoma. South Med J 30:585–594, 1937

LOTTSFELDT FJ, GOOD RA: Juvenile xanthogranuloma with pulmonary lesions. Pediatrics 33:233–238, 1964

NILSBY J: Juvenile xanthoma. Acta Paediatr 41:373–380, 1952

NÖDL F: Systematisierte grossknotige Naevoxanthoendotheliome. Arch Klin Exp Dermatol 208:601–615, 1959

RODRIGUEZ J, ACKERMAN AB: Xanthogranuloma in adults. Arch Dermatol 112:43–44, 1976

SANDERS TE: Intraocular juvenile xanthogranuloma (Nevoxantho-endothelioma). Am J Ophthalmol 53:455–462, 1962

SCHMID AH, USENER M: Grossknotiges Naevoxanthoendotheliom mit Lungenbeteiligung. Arch Klin Exp Dermatol 228:239–248, 1967

THANNHAUSER SJ: Juvenile xanthoma. Its relation to, and variation from, the skin lesions of eosinophilic xanthomatous granuloma. In Lipidoses, 3rd ed, pp 362–364. New York, Grune & Stratton, 1958

THELANDER HE: Xanthomatosis. J Pediatr 34:490–501, 1949

WEBSTER SB, REISTER HC, HARMAN LE JR: Juvenile xanthogranuloma with extracutaneous lesions. Arch Dermatol 93:71–76, 1966

WOLFF HH, VIGL E, BRAUN-FALCO O: Juveniles Xanthogranulom und Organmanifestationen. Hautarzt 26:268–272, 1975

Necrobiotic Xanthogranuloma with Paraproteinemia

FRANK SB, WEIDMAN AI: Xanthoma disseminatum. Arch Dermatol Syph 65:88–94, 1952

KOSSARD S, WINKELMANN RK: Necrobiotic xanthogranuloma with paraproteinemia. J Am Acad Dermatol 3:257–270, 1980

RENDALL JR, VANHEGAN RI, ROBB-SMITH AHT et al: Atypical multicentric reticulohistiocytosis with paraproteinemia. Arch Dermatol 113:1576–1582, 1977

RUPEC M, HAVEMANN K, AUST W et al: Zur Frage der Hautveränderungen bei einer Doppelparaproteinämie. Arch Dermatol Res 268:191–206, 1980

Reticulohistiocytosis

ALBERT J, BRUCE W, ALLEN AC et al: Lipoid dermato-arthritis. Reticulohistiocytoma of the skin and joints. Am J Med 28:661–667, 1960

ANDERSON TE, CARR AJ, CHAPMAN RS et al: Myositis and myotonia in a case of multicentric reticulohistiocytosis. Br J Dermatol 80:39–45, 1968

BARROW MV, HOLUBAR K: Multiple reticulohistiocytosis. A review of 33 patients. Medicine (Baltimore) 48:287–305, 1969

CHEVRANT-BRETON J: La réticulo-histiocytose multicentrique. Revue de la littérature récente (depuis 1969). Ann Dermatol Venereol 104:745–753, 1977

COODE PE, RIDGWAY H, JONES DB: Multicentric reticulohistiocytosis: Report of two cases with ultrastructure, tissue culture and immunology studies. Clin Exp Dermatol 5:281–293, 1980

DAMMERT K, NIEMI K: Reticulohistiocytosis (lipoid dermatoarthritis) of the skin and joints. Acta Derm Venereol (Stockh) 46:210–216, 1966

DAVIES NEJ, ROENIGK HH JR, HAWK WA et al: Multicentric reticulohistiocytoma of the skin. Arch Dermatol 97:543–547, 1968

DAVIES BT, WOOD SR: The so-called reticulohistiocytoma of the skin. A comparison of two distinct types. Br J Dermatol 67:205–211, 1955

EBNER H, GEBHART W: Zur Ultrastruktur der multizentrischen Reticulohistiocytose. Arch Dermatol Forsch 240:259–270, 1971

EHRLICH GE, YOUNG I, NOSHENY SZ et al: Multicentric reticulohistiocytosis: A multisystem disorder. Am J Med 52:830–840, 1972

FAST A: Cardiopulmonary complications in multicentric reticulohistiocytosis. Arch Dermatol 112:1139–1141, 1976

FLAM M, RYAN SC, MAH-POY GL et al: Multicentric reticulohistiocytosis. Am J Med 52:841–848, 1972

GOETTE DK, ODOM RB, FITZWATER JE: Diffuse cutaneous reticulohistiocytosis. Arch Dermatol 118:173–176, 1982

IKEZAWA Z, NAKAJIMA H: A study of multicentric reticulohistiocytosis (lipoid dermatoarthritis). J Dermatol (Tokyo) 3:289–302, 1976

MONTGOMERY H, POLLEY HF, PUGH DG: Reticulohistiocytoma (reticulohistiocytic granuloma). Arch Dermatol 77:61–71, 1958

NÖDL F: Zur Histogenese der riesenzelligen Reticulohistiocytome. Arch Klin Exp Dermatol 207:275–290, 1958

ORKIN M, GOLTZ RW, GOOD RA et al: A study of multicentric reticulohistiocytosis. Arch Dermatol 89:640–654, 1964

PURVIS WE, HELWIG EB: Reticulohistiocytic granuloma ("reticulohistiocytoma") of the skin. Am J Clin Pathol 24:1005–1015, 1954

TANI M, HORI K, NAKANISHI T et al: Multicentric reticulohistiocytosis. Arch Dermatol 117:485–499, 1981

WARIN RP, EVANS CD, HEWITT M et al: Reticulohistiocytosis (lipoid dermatoarthritis). Br Med J 1:1387–1391, 1957

ZAK FG: Reticulohistiocytoma ("ganglioneuroma") of the skin. Br J Dermatol 62:351–355, 1950

Congenital Self-Healing Reticulohistiocytosis

BONIFAZI E, CAPUTO R, CECI A et al: Congenital self-healing histiocytosis. Arch Dermatol 118:267–272, 1982

HASHIMOTO K, GRIFFIN D, KOHSBAKI M: Self-healing reticulohistiocytosis. Cancer 49:331–337, 1982

HASHIMOTO K, PRITZKER MS: Electron microscopic study of reticulohistiocytoma. An unusual case of congenital self-healing reticulohistiocytosis. Arch Dermatol 107:263–270, 1973

LAUGIER P, HUNZIKER N, LAUT J et al: Réticulo-histiocytose d'évolution bénigne (type Hashimoto-Pritzker). Ann Dermatol Syph 102:21–35, 1975

MASCARO JM, ALAGIA A, MASCARO-GALY C: Réticulose congénitale auto-involutive (type Hashimoto-Pritzker). Ann Dermatol Venereol 105:223–227, 1978

RUFLI T, FRICKER HS: Kongenitale, selbstheilende Retikulohistiozytose. Z Hautkr 54:554–558, 1979

Progressive Nodular Histiocytoma

BURGDORF WHC, KUSCH SL, NIX TE JR et al: Progressive nodular histiocytoma. Arch Dermatol 117:644–649, 1981

TAUNTON OD, YESHURUN D, JARRATT M: Progressive nodular histiocytoma. Arch Dermatol 114:1505–1508, 1978

Generalized Eruptive Histiocytoma

CAPUTO R, ALESSI E, ALLEGRA F: Generalized eruptive histiocytoma. Arch Dermatol 117:216–221, 1981

CRAMER HJ: Multiple Reticulohistiocytome der Haut ohne nachweisbare Zweiterkrankung. Hautarzt 14:297–302, 1963

HERZBERG JJ: Eruptive, symmetrisch angeordnete eosinophile Granulome der Haut. Arch Klin Exp Dermatol 212:282–297, 1961

MULLER SA, WOLFF, K, WINKELMANN RK: Generalized eruptive histiocytoma. Arch Dermatol 96:11–17, 1967

SOHI AS, TIWARI VD, SUBRAMANIAN DSV et al: Generalized eruptive histiocytoma. Dermatologica 159:471–475, 1979

WINKELMANN RK, KOSSARD S, FRAGA S: Eruptive histiocytoma of childhood. Arch Dermatol 116:565–570, 1980

WINKELMANN RK, MULLER SA: Generalized eruptive histiocytoma. Arch Dermatol 88:586–596, 1963

Metabolic Diseases

23

AMYLOIDOSIS

Three forms of amyloidosis occur: primary systemic amyloidosis, secondary systemic amyloidosis, and localized amyloidosis. Primary systemic amyloidosis, which involves mainly mesenchymal tissue, is associated with cutaneous lesions in about 30% of the cases (Rubinow and Cohen). In contradistinction, secondary systemic amyloidosis, which occurs secondary to chronic inflammatory diseases and shows amyloid deposits mainly in the parenchymal organs, shows no cutaneous lesions. Localized amyloidosis may occur in the skin in three variants: lichenoid amyloidosis, macular amyloidosis, and nodular amyloidosis. In addition, amyloid is deposited occasionally in the stroma or the adjacent connective tissue of certain epithelial tumors. Such depositions may be found, for instance, in basal cell epithelioma and in Bowen's disease (Brownstein and Helwig, 1970b).

Amyloid can often be recognized in histologic sections stained with hematoxylin-eosin, provided that it is present in sufficiently large amounts. It then appears as homogeneous, faintly eosinophilic aggregates that contain clefts as the result of shrinkage of the amyloid during the process of fixation and dehydration. Three staining methods are mainly used for the demonstration of amyloid: crystal violet, Congo red, and thioflavine T. Better results are obtained when crystal violet, which causes reddish metachromasia, is used on unfixed, frozen sections rather than on paraffin-embedded sections (Hashimoto et al; Black and Wilson Jones). The method regarded as most reliable for the demonstration of amyloid consists of staining paraffin-embedded sections with alkaline Congo red and studying the sections in polarized light. The amyloid then shows greenish birefringence (Shapiro et al). This method is superior to staining paraffin-embedded sections with thioflavine T and examining them with a fluorescence microscope, because greenish fluorescence after staining with thioflavine T is seen occasionally as a false-positive reaction in a variety of conditions (Brownstein and Helwig, 1970b). Even greenish birefringence following staining with alkaline Congo red is not specific for amyloid, as shown by the fact that it is frequently found also in colloid milium, hyalinosis cutis et mucosae, and porphyria. Fortunately, clinical differentiation of these three diseases from amyloidosis only rarely causes difficulties.

Even though the amyloid in primary, secondary, and localized amyloidosis is of different origin (see Histogenesis for the various types), it stains alike with the above-mentioned staining methods. However, a distinction of primary from secondary amyloidosis is possible by the treatment of sections with potassium permanganate prior to staining with Congo red. Primary amyloid is resistant to this treatment, retaining its affinity to Congo red and its green birefringence on polarization, whereas secondary amyloid loses its Congo red affinity and polarization characteristics (Sweet et al).

Primary Systemic Amyloidosis

In primary systemic amyloidosis, mesenchymal tissues rather than parenchymal organs are mainly involved.

407

Amyloid deposits are often found in the smooth and striated musculature, in the connective tissue, in the walls of blood vessels, and in peripheral nerves. Myocardial insufficiency and gastrointestinal bleeding are common and may result in death. Some involvement of parenchymatous organs, especially of the kidneys and liver, usually occurs. Renal failure is a late development but may be the cause of death (Kyle).

Among cutaneous lesions, petechiae and ecchymoses are most common (Kyle). They are the result of involvement of cutaneous blood vessels and are seen mainly on the face, especially on the eyelids and in the periorbital region. Minor trauma may precipitate these lesions, referred to by some as pinch purpura. In addition, there may be discrete or coalescing papules or plaques. They usually have a waxy color but may be bluish red as the result of hemorrhage into them (Natelson et al; Beacham et al). In rare instances, one observes firm cutaneous or subcutaneous nodules or plaques or areas of induration of the skin resembling morphea (Brownstein and Helwig, 1970c). Bullae that may be induced by minor trauma and may be hemorrhagic occur occasionally (Bluhm et al; Beacham et al; Westermark et al). Among oral lesions, macroglossia is common, occurring in 17% of the patients (Kyle and Bayrd).

Histopathology. Examination of cutaneous lesions reveals faintly eosinophilic, amorphous, often fissured masses of amyloid deposited in the dermis as well as in the subcutaneous tissue. Quite frequently, accumulations of amyloid are deposited close to the epidermis. They may or may not be separated from the overlying epidermis by a narrow zone of collagen (Fig. 23-1). In addition, deposits of amyloid may be seen in the membrana propria surrounding the sweat glands as well as around and within the walls of blood vessels (Fig. 23-2). The involvement of the walls of blood vessels is responsible for the frequent presence of extravasated erythrocytes. Inflammatory cells are absent or scarce (Westermark, 1979). Bullae arise by cleavage in extensive dermal amyloid deposits and thus form intradermally, rather than at the epidermal-dermal junction (Bluhm et al; Westermark et al).

In the subcutaneous tissue, one may find large aggregates of amyloid and amyloid infiltration of the walls of the blood vessels as well as so-called amyloid rings, which are formed by the deposition of amyloid around individual fat cells (Fig. 23-2) (Westermark, 1979). The fat cells may then appear as if cemented together by the amyloid substance.

If there are no skin lesions or macroglossia, biopsy of the rectal mucosa, including submucosa, is the recommended procedure for the demonstration of amyloid. Positive results are obtained in more than 60% of the patients (Kyle). Other tissues from which specimens for biopsy may be obtained are the gingiva and the small intestine. Biopsy of normal-appearing skin in patients without skin lesions is also worthwhile; positive findings are obtained in about 40% of the patients (Brownstein and Helwig, 1970c; Rubinow and Cohen). Small deposits are found most commonly in the walls of small blood vessels of the dermis or the subcutaneous tissue but occasionally also around eccrine glands and around fat cells. The forearm is the area recommended for biopsy (Rubinow and Cohen).

Systemic Lesions. Not only in the skin and in the subcutaneous tissue, but also throughout the body, the small arteries and veins may show amyloid deposits (Brunsting and MacDonald; Rukawina et al). The tongue, the heart muscle, the smooth musculature of the gastrointestinal and

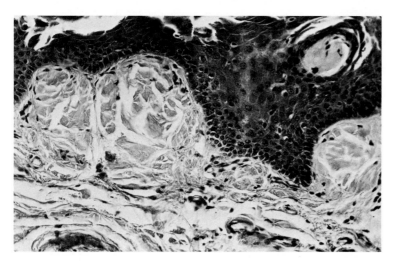

Fig. 23-1.   Primary systemic amyloidosis
Amorphous, fissured masses of amyloid are present in the upper dermis. The amyloid material greatly resembles that seen in colloid milium (see Fig. 23-4). (×200)

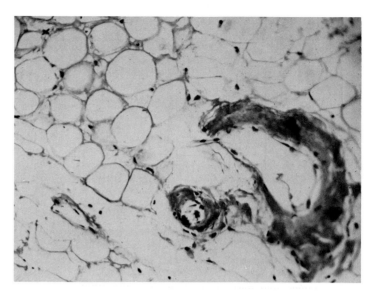

Fig. 23-2.   Primary systemic amyloidosis
Subcutaneous fat. Amyloid is deposited in the walls of two blood vessels and around fat cells, forming so-called amyloid rings. (× 400)

urinary tracts, and, in some instances, the skeletal muscles are infiltrated by amyloid (Rukawina et al). Not infrequently, deposits of amyloid are found in renal glomeruli (Kyle). Also, in many cases, as the result of vascular involvement, the liver and the spleen show some degree of parenchymatous damage (Rukawina et al).

Relationship to Multiple Myeloma. Primary systemic amyloidosis, like multiple myeloma, represents a plasma cell dyscrasia (Buxbaum et al). Even though the two diseases can occur together, the clinical features of one disease generally predominate. Thus, pronounced osteolytic lesions and pathologic fractures are rare in patients with primary systemic amyloidosis.

It is customary to distinguish between primary systemic amyloidosis and amyloidosis with myeloma (Kyle and Bayrd). The differences between these two groups lie (1) in the appearance and number of plasma cells in the bone marrow, (2) in the amount of monoclonal protein in the serum and urine, and (3) in the presence or absence of radiologically apparent skeletal lesions. However, differentiation is sometimes difficult, because the two groups constitute different aspects of the same disease process (Kyle). As many as 88% of the patients with primary systemic amyloidosis have been found on immunoelectrophoretic examination to have a monoclonal paraprotein in the serum or urine, compared to 100% of the patients who have amyloidosis with myeloma (Kyle). Thus, it can be assumed that, if carefully studied by immunoelectrophoresis and if followed long enough, all patients with primary systemic amyloidosis will ultimately show paraproteinemia as evidence of a plasma cell dyscrasia (Franklin).

Histogenesis. It has become apparent that the amyloid in different forms of amyloidosis has different origins,

even though no difference can be observed by electron microscopy in its structure. In primary systemic amyloidosis, including "myeloma-associated amyloidosis," the amyloid originates from monoclonal immunoglobulin light chains (L chains) produced by plasma cells in the bone marrow and is therefore referred to as *amyloid light chain (AL) protein*. In secondary systemic amyloidosis, the amyloid is derived from a serum protein that is not an immunoglobulin and is deposited as amyloid A (AA) protein (see p. 410). In lichenoid and in macular amyloidosis, tonofilaments of keratinocytes are the basic material that is transformed into amyloid (see p. 411). Finally, in nodular amyloidosis, plasma cells produce the amyloid locally (see p. 411).

The amyloid in primary systemic amyloidosis is derived from L chains secreted by bone marrow plasma cells into the serum. In contrast to the L chains that are produced under normal conditions and in patients with the usual form of multiple myeloma, the L chains produced in primary systemic amyloidosis are, for reasons yet unknown, "amyloidogenic." At sites at which the amyloid is deposited, the amyloidogenic L chains undergo partial proteolysis within lysosomes of macrophages and then are deposited extracellularly, in association with a polysaccharide, as insoluble amyloid filaments. Chemical studies have demonstrated that the amyloid filaments have as their major protein component either an intact L chain or the amino-terminal fragment of an L chain, or both an intact L chain and its amino-terminal fragment (Glenner and Page).

On *electron microscopy,* amyloid deposits consist of straight, nonbranching, nonanastomosing, often irregularly arranged filaments usually 6 nm to 7 nm in diameter (Hashimoto and Kumakiri). On high magnification, these filaments are seen to possess a higher degree of electron density at their periphery than in their center and thus have the appearance of hollow cylinders (Glenner and Page; Goerttler et al). The length of the filaments has not been determined, because a single filament cannot be seen in its entirety, but it has been estimated to be of the order of 800 nm (Kyle and Bayrd).

Secondary Systemic Amyloidosis

Secondary systemic amyloidosis occurs secondary to chronic inflammatory diseases, among which rheumatoid arthritis and osteomyelitis are the most common (Kyle and Bayrd). Lepromatous leprosy may also cause secondary systemic amyloidosis. Tuberculosis used to be the most common cause. Certain chronic cutaneous diseases, such as stasis ulcer, hidradenitis suppurativa, and dystrophic epidermolysis bullosa, can also lead to secondary systemic amyloidosis (Brownstein and Helwig, 1970a).

Clinically, hepatomegaly and proteinuria are the initial manifestations, followed by nephrosis and uremia. The skin is free of lesions.

Histopathology. The parenchymatous organs, such as the kidneys, liver, spleen, and adrenals, are predominantly involved, beginning with deposits of amyloid in the interstitial tissue and in the walls of blood vessels. Progressive accumulation leads to replacement of the parenchymal cells by amyloid. In the kidneys, glomerular deposits are the most serious event, although deposits are found also in the peritubular tissue. Involvement of the follicles in the spleen leads to a gross appearance known as sago spleen.

The preferred procedure for the diagnosis of secondary systemic amyloidosis is biopsy of the rectal mucosa, since biopsy of the kidney or liver may result in uncontrollable hemorrhage. However, biopsy of normal skin, including subcutaneous fat, has also been found to be worthwhile; in about half of the patients, deposits are found with the alkaline Congo red method, particularly as amyloid rings in the subcutaneous fat, but occasionally also within the walls of blood vessels, around eccrine glands, or free in the dermis (Rubinow and Cohen). An even higher number of positive findings may be obtained by the examination of abdominal subcutaneous fat (Westermark, 1972).

Histogenesis. The filaments of secondary systemic amyloidosis are composed of *AA (amyloid A) protein,* which is unrelated to any immunoglobulin. Its precursor, referred to as *serum amyloid A-related (SAA) protein,* is an alpha-globulin that is present in small quantities in normal serum and in increased amounts in the sera of elderly persons, pregnant women, and patients with many unrelated diseases. AA protein constitutes the amino-terminal portion of SAA protein, from which it may be derived by proteolysis (Franklin). This enzymatic process takes place within lysosomes of macrophages that are receiving antigenic stimulation by a variety of chronic diseases (Breathnach and Black). The AA is then excreted by the macrophages and deposited extracellularly.

Lichenoid and Macular Amyloidosis

In lichenoid amyloidosis, also called lichen amyloidosus, closely set, discrete, brownish red papules often showing some scaling are seen most commonly on the legs, especially the shins, although they may occur elsewhere. Through the coalescence of papules, plaques may form on the legs that often possess a verrucous surface and then resemble hypertrophic lichen planus or lichen simplex chronicus. Usually, the lesions of lichenoid amyloidosis itch severely.

Macular amyloidosis is characterized by moderately pruritic macules showing pigmentation with a reticulated or rippled pattern. Although macular amyloidosis may occur anywhere on the trunk or extremities, the upper back is a fairly common site (Shanon and Sagher). The eruption may be easily passed off as postinflammatory hyperpigmentation by physicians unfamiliar with the condition (Brownstein and Hashimoto).

The existence of a close relationship between lichenoid and macular amyloidosis is borne out not only by the fact that the two conditions not infrequently occur together (Kurban et al; Brownstein and Hashimoto; Toribio et al) but also by the fact that they can change from one into the other: from macular to lichenoid amyloidosis as a result of chronic irritation of the skin from scratching (Bedi and Datta), and from lichenoid to macular amyloidosis under treatment with intralesional injections of corticosteroids (Brownstein et al). In addition, the histologic findings are similar, and the histogenesis is identical.

Histopathology. Lichenoid and macular amyloidosis show deposits of amyloid that are limited to the papillary dermis and thus do not extend beyond the subpapillary plexus. Most of the amyloid is situated within the dermal papillae. Although the deposits usually are smaller in macular amyloidosis than in lichenoid amyloidosis, differentiation of the two on the basis of the amount of amyloid is not possible, since the amount is variable in both conditions in different papillae (Brownstein and Hashimoto). The two conditions actually differ only in the appearance of the epidermis, which shows acanthosis and hyperkeratosis in lichenoid amyloidosis but not in macular amyloidosis. Occasionally, the amount of amyloid in macular amyloidosis is so small that it is missed, even when special stains are used on frozen sections. In such in-

[handwritten margin note: Frozen section best for Congo Red]

stances, more than one biopsy may be necessary to confirm the diagnosis (Black and Wilson Jones).

In areas in which the entire dermal papilla is filled with amyloid, the amyloid appears homogeneous in both lichenoid and macular amyloidosis. In lesions in which the dermal papillae are only partially filled, as seen more often in macular than in lichenoid amyloidosis, the amyloid has a globular appearance, resembling the colloid bodies found in lichen planus. These amyloid bodies in some areas lie in direct contact with the overlying basal cells of the epidermis. Similar colloid bodies are also found in some sections within the epidermis, but, in contrast with those located at the epidermal-dermal junction, they do not stain as amyloid. In addition, there often is a striking degree of pigmentary incontinence (Black and Wilson Jones).

Histogenesis. The light microscopic findings in lichenoid and macular amyloidosis indicate that degenerating epidermal cells are discharged into the dermis, where they are converted into amyloid. The epidermal origin of the amyloid in lichenoid and macular amyloidosis has been confirmed by *electron microscopy* (Kumakiri and Hashimoto; Hashimoto and Kobayashi). Also on electron microscopy, the degenerating epidermal cells resemble the colloid bodies seen in lichen planus (see p. 155). They contain the following components: (1) tonofilaments; (2) degenerated, wavy tonofilaments that are thicker but less electron-dense than normal tonofilaments; (3) lysosomes; and (4) typical filaments of amyloid, 6 nm to 10 nm thick, that are straight and nonbranching (Hashimoto and Kobayashi). It may be assumed that the degenerated, wavy tonofilaments are recognized as foreign and are digested by the cell's own lysosomes. Such digestion produces amyloid filaments. A conversion of tonofilaments into amyloid filaments requires that the alpha-pleated sheet configuration of the tonofilaments change into the beta configuration of amyloid (Glenner). Although colloid bodies form amyloid in lichenoid and macular amyloidosis, they are unable to do so in lichen planus, because they are destroyed by the inflammatory reaction accompanying lichen planus (Hashimoto and Kobayashi).

On *direct immunofluorescence,* all specimens of lichenoid or macular amyloidosis fluoresce positively for immunoglobulins or complement, particularly immunoglobulin M (IgM) and the third component of complement (C3). Also, staining for kappa and lambda light chains is positive. The immunofluorescent pattern is globular and thus is similar to that of lichen planus, except for the absence of fibrin. It suggests that the globular aggregates of lichenoid or macular amyloidosis, like the colloid bodies of lichen planus, act as a filamentous sponge on which immunoglobulins and complement are absorbed (MacDonald et al).

The epidermal derivation of the amyloid in lichenoid and macular amyloidosis is also supported by histochemical and immunologic findings. In contrast to the amyloid of systemic amyloidosis, the amyloid of lichenoid and macular amyloidosis shows fluorescence for disulfide bonds as normally seen in the stratum corneum, suggesting that cross-linking of sulfhydryl groups occurs in amyloidogenesis (Danno and Horio). Furthermore, immunofluorescence studies with an antikeratin antiserum have shown intense staining of the amyloid for the antikeratin antibody (Masu et al).

The amyloid that may be found in the stroma or in the adjacent connective tissue of *basal cell epithelioma* and other epithelial tumors has a similar appearance on electron microscopy and direct immunofluorescence to that seen in lichenoid and macular amyloidosis, suggesting that it too is derived from tonofilaments (Weedon and Shand; Weedon; Hashimoto and Kobayashi). This amyloid also shows positive staining with antikeratin antiserum (Masu et al).

Nodular Amyloidosis

In nodular amyloidosis, a rare condition of which only 29 cases had been reported by 1976 (Goerttler et al), one or several nodules are encountered, usually on the legs (Potter and Johnson) or face (Goerttler et al) but occasionally elsewhere. The nodules commonly measure from 1 cm to 3 cm in diameter. In their center, the skin may appear atrophic as a result of involution of the amyloid (Rodermund). In exceptional instances, plaques rather than nodules are seen (Lindemayr and Partsch).

Histopathology. Beneath an atrophic epidermis are large masses of amyloid, which extend through the entire dermis into the subcutaneous fat. Amyloid deposits are also found within the walls of blood vessels, in the membrana propria of the sweat glands, and around fat cells (Lindemayr and Partsch). A chronic inflammatory infiltrate containing a significant admixture of plasma cells is present in most cases at the periphery of the masses of amyloid (Rodermund; Brownstein and Helwig, 1970b; Goerttler et al).

Histogenesis. On *electron microscopic examination,* mature plasma cells located at the periphery of the amyloid deposits show a well-developed ergastoplasma and numerous mitochondria, making it likely that amyloid is formed within them (Goerttler et al). Fibroblasts are seen completely encased by the amyloid masses. The fibroblasts contain ample amorphous material in their greatly dilated rough endoplasmic reticulum. This finding has been interpreted as an indication that the fibroblasts are highly active and produce amyloid (Runne and Orfanos). It seems more likely, however, that the material in the rough endoplasmic reticulum is retained there as a result of a disturbance in excretion into the extracellular space (Goerttler et al). The histogenesis of the amyloid in localized nodular cutaneous amyloidosis seems to be similar to that in localized nodular pulmonary amyloidosis; the amyloid in the latter is derived from light polypeptide chains of an immunoglobulin that is produced by plasma cells present in the lesion (Page et al).

Although amyloid was found in a rectal biopsy in one patient with nodular amyloidosis, neither this patient nor any other patient with nodular amyloidosis reported in the literature has developed evidence of primary systemic amyloidosis (Goerttler et al).

Differential Diagnosis.   On a histologic basis, differentiation of nodular amyloidosis from primary systemic amyloidosis is not possible.

COLLOID MILIUM AND NODULAR COLLOID DEGENERATION

Three types of colloid degeneration of the skin occur: (1) juvenile colloid milium, (2) adult colloid milium, and (3) nodular colloid degeneration. Types 1 and 3 are very rare.

Juvenile colloid milium has its onset before puberty and shows numerous round or angular, brownish, waxy papules located mainly on the face (Ebner and Gebhart, 1978) but in some instances also on the sides of the neck (Wooldridge and Frerichs) or in the nuchal region (Percival and Duthie).

Adult colloid milium, which starts in adult life, in some instances involves the dorsa of the hands in addition to the face and neck (Holzberger; Hashimoto et al, 1975).

Sun exposure often seems to be a precipitating factor (Ebner and Gebhart, 1978).

Nodular colloid degeneration shows either a single large nodule on the face (Dupre et al) or multiple nodules on the face (Sullivan and Ellis) or the chin and scalp (Kawashima et al). Sun exposure does not seem to play a role, since, in some instances, the lesions are limited to the trunk (Reuter and Becker).

Histopathology.   The histologic findings differ in the three types of colloid degeneration, since the colloid in the juvenile form is of epidermal origin, whereas that in the other two forms is of dermal origin (Ebner and Gebhart, 1977, 1978).

In *juvenile colloid milium*, basal cells are transformed into colloid bodies (Wooldridge and Frerichs; Ebner and Gebhart, 1977). In some areas, colloid islands can also be seen within the epidermis (Percival and Duthie; Ebner and Gebhart, 1977). In areas in which the colloid masses fill the papillary dermis, the overlying epidermis appears flattened but still shows transformation of some basal cells into colloid bodies (Percival and Duthie). The colloid material within the papillary dermis appears homogeneous and faintly eosinophilic and contains dilated capillaries, scattered fibroblasts, and, often, melanophages.

In *adult colloid milium*, a narrow zone of connective tissue usually separates the homogeneous masses of colloid located in the papillary dermis from the overlying epidermis (Fig. 23-3). Elastic tissue staining shows some elastic fibers in this

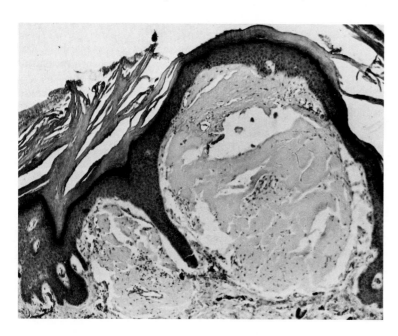

Fig. 23-3.   Colloid milium, adult type
Two round, homogeneous, fissured masses of colloid are present in the uppermost dermis. The colloid material greatly resembles the amyloid material seen in primary systemic amyloidosis (see Fig. 23-1). (×100)

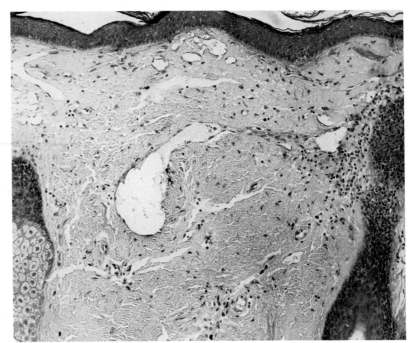

Fig. 23-4. Nodular colloid degeneration
Large masses of colloid are present throughout the dermis. Scattered nuclei of fibroblasts are present within the colloid. The cutaneous appendages are well preserved. (×100)

narrow zone of connective tissue (Ebner and Gebhart, 1978). In addition, solar elastotic fibers are usually seen at the base of the colloid deposits (Graham and Marques).

In *nodular colloid degeneration*, the epidermis is flattened. The upper three fourths of the dermis are occupied with pale pink, homogeneous material; in some lesions, even the entire dermis is filled with this material (Fig. 23-4) (Kawashima et al). Scattered nuclei of fibroblasts are present within the colloid (Dupre et al). There are scattered clefts or fissures. Some dilated capillaries are seen. The hair follicles and sebaceous glands appear well preserved (Sullivan and Ellis).

Histogenesis. The colloid in all three types shows considerable resemblance to amyloid not only in its histologic appearance but also in its histochemical reactions (Graham and Marques). However, colloid differs from amyloid in its electron microscopic appearance (see below).

Histochemical staining shows that colloid, like amyloid, is periodic-acid Schiff (PAS)-positive and diastase-resistant. It shows affinity for Congo red and stains metachromatically purplish to red with methyl violet and crystal violet (Graham and Marques). As in the case of amyloid, these reactions are more pronounced when frozen sections are used in place of formalin-fixed, paraffin-embedded material (Hashimoto et al, 1972). In addition, both substances show greenish birefringence after staining with alkaline Congo red, and both show

greenish fluorescence after staining with thioflavine T (Graham and Marques). The greenish birefringence in the Congo-red-stained frozen sections is very weak in some instances of adult colloid milium (Hashimoto et al, 1972; Ebner and Gebhart, 1978), in contrast to the distinct birefringence in juvenile colloid milium (Ebner and Gebhart, 1978).

Electron microscopy in a case of *juvenile colloid milium* has shown that the colloid consists of tightly packed bundles of filaments, 8 nm to 10 nm thick, in a weavy or whorled arrangement (Ebner and Gebhart, 1977). This is quite in contrast with the straight appearance of amyloid filaments. The predominantly filamentous composition of the colloid material explains the distinct greenish birefringence seen in Congo-red-stained sections (Ebner and Gebhart, 1978). The epidermal derivation of the colloid in juvenile colloid milium is borne out by the presence within the bundles of filaments of cellular organelles, such as mitochondria and melanosomes, and particularly of desmosomes. Because the colloid is derived from colloid bodies, direct immunofluorescence shows the presence of "trapped" immunoglobulins and complement, just as in the colloid bodies of lichen planus (see p. 156) and in the amyloid of lichenoid and macular amyloidosis (see p. 411).

In *adult colloid milium*, the colloid masses are seen on electron microscopic examination to consist primarily of a structureless, amorphous substance (Hashimoto et al, 1975). On high magnification, very fine filaments, only 2 nm in width, may be seen embedded in the amorphous substance (Ebner and Gebhart, 1978). This colloid material is not related to collagen, because it does not contain hydroxyproline or hydroxylysine (Hashimoto et al, 1975). It is assumed that adult colloid is synthesized in fibroblasts (Hashimoto et al, 1972; Ebner and Gebhart, 1978).

The colloid in *nodular colloid degeneration*, similar to that in adult colloid milium, consists of an amorphous substance and short, wavy, irregularly arranged filaments (Kawashima et al). The diameter of these filaments is 3 nm to 4 nm (Dupre et al). These electron microscopic findings exclude nodular amyloidosis as the diagnosis, since in this condition the filaments have a diameter of about 6 nm to 7 nm and are long and straight.

HYALINOSIS CUTIS ET MUCOSAE (LIPOID PROTEINOSIS)

In hyalinosis cutis et mucosae, a disorder inherited as an autosomal recessive trait, there are rather widespread depositions of a hyaline material. The skin, the oral mucosa, and the larynx show the most pronounced involvement. Not infrequently, the hyaline material, largely a glycoprotein, also has a lipid component, and the term *lipoid proteinosis* is therefore also used for this

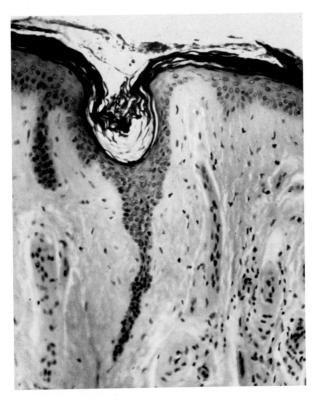

Fig. 23-5.   Hyalinosis cutis et mucosae
The hyaline material consists of thick, homogeneous bundles that extend perpendicular to the skin surface. In addition, thick hyaline mantles surround the blood vessels. (×200)

disease. Basically, however, the hyalin consists of basement membrane collagen, that is, type IV collagen (see Histogenesis).

Clinically, one observes papular and nodular lesions on the face. Areas of diffuse infiltration associated with hyperkeratosis are seen on the elbows, knees, hands, and occasionally elsewhere. The papules and nodules on the face cause pitted scars, giving the skin a pigskin-leather appearance. Beads of small nodules may be present along the free margin of the eyelids. The tongue is firm because of diffuse infiltration. Extension of the infiltration to the frenulum of the tongue restricts normal movement of the tongue, and infiltration of the vocal cords causes hoarseness, which may be present already at birth. The occurrence of convulsive seizures is not uncommon (Holtz and Schulze; Caplan).

Histopathology. The earliest change consists of thickening of the capillary walls due to the deposition of hyaline material within and around the basement membrane (van der Walt and Heyl). In well-developed lesions, the skin presents a striking and diagnostic picture. Beneath a hyperkeratotic and occasionally papillomatous epidermis, a homogeneous, eosinophilic hyalin mantle surrounds the vessels throughout the dermis and also the sweat glands, the epithelium of which becomes atrophic. The dermis, which usually is thickened considerably, consists in its upper portion also of hyaline material arranged in homogeneous bundles and staining a pale pink with hematoxylin-eosin. In areas of papillomatosis, these bundles often run perpendicular to the skin surface (Fig. 23-5). In the lower dermis, the hyalin deposits are focal and not as diffuse as in the upper dermis. In the areas of hyalin, the nuclei of the fibroblasts and the vascular walls are well preserved. Mantles of hyalin similar to those seen around the vessels and sweat glands often surround the hair follicles (Fleischmajer et al, 1969). In addition, the arrectores pilorum show marked infiltration with hyaline material (Caplan).

The hyaline material is strongly PAS-positive and diastase-resistant, indicating the presence of neutral mucopolysaccharides. Elastic fibers are absent in the hyaline material. However, reticulum fibers are present (Ungar and Katzenellenbogen; Eberhartinger and Niebauer). They may be seen as concentric rings within the hyalin surrounding the sweat glands (Fleischmajer et al, 1969), as well as in the intercellular spaces of smooth muscle bundles and around blood vessels (Ishibashi). Staining for acid mucopolysaccharides with alcian blue is negative at pH 0.9 but slightly positive at pH 2.9. The fact that staining with alcian blue at *p*H 2.9 is negative after prior exposure to hyaluronidase indicates that the acid mucopolysaccharides are largely hyaluronic acid (Fleischmajer et al, 1969). Staining with Congo red and crystal violet may give slightly positive results (Fleischmajer et al, 1969).

Lipid stains have given varying results. Although lipids are present in most instances, there is occasionally no reaction to lipid stains (Grosfeld et al; Rasiewicz et al). Also, one lesion may contain lipids while another lesion in the same patient contains none (Fleischmajer et al, 1969). Of the various lipids, neutral fat is present most commonly, as shown by a positive reaction to staining with Sudan III or IV or oil red O (Wood et al: Ungar and Katzenellenbogen; Eberhartinger and Niebauer; McCusker and Caplan). The neutral fat is distributed as numerous small droplets throughout the hyaline material, particularly around the blood vessels (Fig. 23-6). The fact that staining with Sudan is in most instances dark orange rather than bright orange red indicates that neutral fat is not the only lipid present (Wood et al). As shown by a positive Schultz reaction, cholesterol is often present (Wood et al; Eberhartinger and Niebauer; McCusker and Caplan), but only as free cholesterol and not as cholesterol ester, since the lipid material in frozen sections is not birefringent (Ramos e Silva; Wood et al). Phospholipids are absent or present in only small amounts, as shown by the test most specific for phospholipids, Baker's acid hematein test, which is either negative (Wood et al; McCusker and Caplan) or weakly positive (Eberhartinger and Niebauer).

Systemic Lesions. Intracranial calcification has been noted quite frequently by x-ray examination in patients with hyalinosis cutis et mucosae and has been held responsible for the occurrence of convulsive seizures in these patients (Holtz and Schulze; Laymon and Hill). Autopsy findings have established that the calcium is deposited within the walls of capillaries located in the hippocampal gyri of the temporal lobes (Holtz). The fact that, after decalcification, a mantle of PAS-positive material is seen around the endothelium of these vessels indicates that hyalinization preceded calcification of the capillary walls (Holtz).

The very widespread distribution of the pericapillary hyalin deposits has been established by biopsies and autopsies. Deposits have been found not only in the submucosa of the upper respiratory and digestive tracts, but also in the submucosa of the stomach, jejunum, rectum, and vagina, in the retina between the vitreous membrane and the

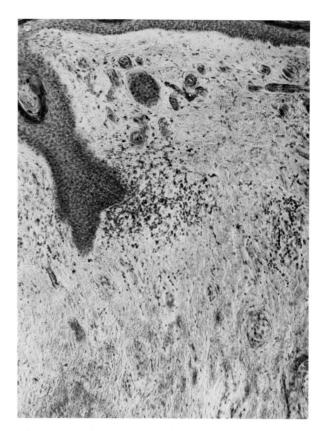

Fig. 23-6.   Hyalinosis cutis et mucosae
Scarlet red stain for neutral fat. Numerous small lipid droplets are seen throughout the hyaline material, particularly around the blood vessels. (×100)

pigment epithelium, and in the testes, pancreas, lungs, kidneys, and elsewhere (Holtz; Caplan).

Histogenesis. PAS-positive neutral mucopolysaccharides are a characteristic component of the hyaline material. Since this PAS-positive material disappears following digestion with pepsin, it can be concluded that it is bound to a protein and thus represents a glycoprotein (Fleischmajer et al, 1969). Lipids are not an essential feature of the disease. If present, they can be removed with lipid solvents without damage to the protein–carbohydrate complex. This suggests that the lipids are either free or loosely bound to the hyaline material (McCusker and Caplan).

On *electron microscopic examination*, the hyaline material is seen to be composed of small filaments 1 nm to 2 nm wide, larger filaments 5 nm to 10 nm wide, and amorphous material (Hashimoto et al). Interspersed in this hyaline material are fibrils with cross striation characteristic of collagen fibrils (Ishibashi). Most of these fibrils measure only 30 nm to 35 nm in diameter and thus are thinner than mature collagen fibrils (Kint), the diameter

TABLE 23-1. Classification of the Porphyrias

	Type; Heredity; Onset	Cutaneous Manifestations	Extra-cutaneous Manifestations	Urine	Feces	Erythrocytes	Enzymatic Defect
Erythropoietic Porphyria	Ery; Rec; Infancy	Blisters; Severe scarring	Red teeth; Hemolytic anemia	Uro I	Copro I	Uro I; Stable fluorescence	Uroporphyrinogen III cosynthetase
Erythropoietic Protoporphyria	Ery; Dom; Childhood	Burning; Edema; Thickening; Rarely, blisters	Rarely, fatal liver disease	Negative	Protoporphyrin continuously	Protoporphyrin; Transient fluorescence	Ferrochelatase; (Heme synthetase)
Hepatoerythrocytic Porphyria	Ery and Hep; Rec; Childhood	Blisters; Severe scarring; Thickening	Decreased liver function	Uro I; Uro III	Copro I; Copro III	Protoporphyrin	?Ferrochelatase and uroporphyrinogen decarboxylase
Acute Intermittent Porphyria (AIP)	Hep; Dom; Young adulthood	Negative	Abdominal pain; Neuropathy; Psychoses	ALA, PBG continuously	Negative	Negative	Uroporphyrinogen I synthetase
Porphyria Variegata	Hep; Dom; Young adulthood	Same as PCT	Same as AIP	ALA, PBG during attacks	Protoporphyrin continuously	Negative	Protoporphyrinogen oxidase
Porphyria Cutanea Tarda (PCT)	Hep; Dom; Middle age	Blisters; Scarring; Thickening	Decreased liver function; Siderosis	Uro III; Continuous fluorescence		Negative	Uroporphyrinogen III decarboxylase
Hereditary Coproporphyria	Hep; Dom; Young adulthood	Same as PCT	Same as AIP	Copro, ALA, PBG during attacks	Copro continuously	Negative	Coproporphyrinogen oxidase

AIP = acute intermittent porphyria
Ery = erythropoietic
Hep = hepatic
Dom = autosomal dominant
Rec = autosomal recessive

Uro = uroporphyrin
Copro = coproporphyrin
ALA = delta-aminolevulinic acid
PBG = porphobilinogen
PCT = porphyria cutanea tarda

of which varies between 70 nm and 140 nm (see p. 31). The epidermal basement membrane may appear intact, the hyaline material being present beneath it (Ishibashi), but, in some areas, the basement membrane is obscured as the result of hyalin infiltration (Hashimoto et al).

Perivascular basement membranes show multiplication and are often masked by infiltrating hyalin (Hashimoto et al). Around many vessels, a multilayered basement membrane is seen that gradually loses its layered appearance farther away from the vessel, becoming a homogeneous, dense collection of partially filamentous and partially amorphous material representing hyalin. This suggests that the layered basement membrane and the hyalin are basically the same material (Ishibashi).

The smooth musculature of the tunica dartos shows widening of the intercellular spaces owing to the presence of ample filamentous and amorphous material. This material forms multiple layers of basement membrane adjacent to the muscle cells, as in the case of the dermal blood vessels, and peripheral to it appears as a wide, homogeneous zone (Ishibashi).

Since endothelial cells, pericytes, and smooth muscle cells show a dilated, rough-surfaced endoplasmic reticulum filled with filamentous and amorphous material, it can be assumed that the accumulation of hyalin in these cells is due to an abnormality in the synthetic process of the basement membrane (Ishibashi). The hyalin surrounding the sweat glands also represents abnormal and excessive production of basement membrane material by myoepithelial cells. The collagen present in basement membranes is type IV collagen (see p. 31). It is synthesized by epithelial or endothelial cells (see p. 13), and, in contrast to the usual collagen, consisting of type I collagen, it is composed of procollagen molecules, which, instead of undergoing conversion to collagen molecules, interact with glycoprotein (see p. 13) (Kefalides). The presence of glycoprotein in type IV collagen and in hyalin causes their strongly positive PAS reaction. In addition, it is evident that the hyalin contains type III collagen, since light microscopic examination reveals the presence of reticulum fibers and electron microscopic examination shows interspersed, small collagen fibrils analogous to reticulum fibrils (see p. 31). Type III collagen is produced by fibroblasts.

The conclusion that the hyalin in hyalinosis cutis et mucosae consists essentially of type IV collagen has been confirmed by indirect immunofluorescence performed with antibodies against types I, III, and IV collagens. Immunofluorescence in a lesion of hyalinosis cutis et mucosae revealed a reduction in type I collagen, normal distribution of type III collagen, and a marked increase in type IV collagen around small blood vessels (Fleischmajer et al, 1981).

A close analogy exists between the hyalin of hyalinosis cutis et mucosae and the hyalin sheath surrounding the tumor islands of cylindroma, since this sheath, on electron microscopy, is seen to contain similar fine filaments and amorphous material and is located adjoining epithelial–dermal junctions (see p. 550) (Hashimoto et al).

Differential Diagnosis. Porphyria shows deposits of hyalin around the superficial dermal capillaries indistinguishable from the deposits of hyalin seen in hyalinosis cutis et mucosae. There is, however, no involvement in the deeper dermis. Also, involvement of the membrana propria of the sweat glands is rare. In addition, the cutaneous lesions in porphyria are limited to sun-exposed areas. *Amyloid, Colloid Millium*

PORPHYRIA *Genetic*

Seven types of porphyria are recognized (Table 23-1). The light sensitivity in the six types with cutaneous lesions is caused by wavelengths that are absorbed by the porphyrin molecule. These wavelengths lie in the 400-nm range, representing longwave ultraviolet light (UVA) and visible light (Konrad et al).

In *erythropoietic porphyria,* a very rare disease, recurrent vesiculobullous eruptions in sun-exposed areas of the skin gradually result in mutilating ulcerations and scarring (Haining et al; Stretcher).

In *erythropoietic protoporphyria,* the usual reaction to light is erythema and edema followed by thickening and superficial scarring of the skin (Gschnait et al). In rare instances, vesicles are present that may resemble those seen in hydroa vacciniforme (see p. 212) (Ryan; Horkay et al; DeLeo et al). The protoporphyrin is formed in reticulocytes in the bone marrow and is then carried in circulating erythrocytes and in the plasma. When a smear of blood from a patient is examined under the fluorescence microscope, large numbers of red-fluorescing erythrocytes are seen. The protoporphyrin is cleared from the plasma by the liver and excreted into the bile and feces (Mathews-Roth). It is not found in the urine. In rare instances, fatal liver disease develops quite suddenly, usually in persons of middle age (MacDonald et al) but occasionally in patients only in the second decade of life (Cripps and Goldfarb; Wells et al). (See also Histogenesis).

Hepatoerythrocytic porphyria, a very rare form first recognized in 1975 (Piñol Aguadé et al), shows clinical resemblance to erythropoietic porphyria in severe cases and to erythropoietic protoporphyria in less severe cases (Czarnecki). Vesicular eruptions lead to ulceration, severe scarring, and sclerosis (Simon et al). Liver damage develops with increasing age (Hönigsmann and Reichel).

In *porphyria variegata,* different members of the same family may have either cutaneous manifestations identical to those of porphyria cutanea tarda or systemic involvement analogous to acute intermittent porphyria or both, or the condition may remain latent (Fromke et al; Hunter). The presence of protoporphyrin in the feces distinguishes porphyria variegata from porphyria cutanea tarda (Table 23-1) (Mustajoki). Also, a sharp fluorescence emission peak at 626 nm is specific for the plasma of porphyria variegata (Poh-Fitzpatrick; Corey et al).

In *porphyria cutanea tarda*, the most common form of porphyria, blisters occur through a combination of sun exposure and minor trauma mainly on the dorsa of the hands but sometimes also on the face. Mild scarring may result. The skin of the face and the dorsa of the hands often is thickened and sclerotic. Hypertrichosis of the face is common. Evidence of hepatic cirrhosis with siderosis is regularly present but generally is mild (Elder et al). In rare instances, a malignant hepatoma or a carcinoma metastatic to the liver induces porphyria cutanea tarda (Keczkes and Barker), or a malignant hepatoma develops in a patient with porphyria cutanea tarda (Waddington).

In *hereditary coproporphyria*, a very rare disorder, there are episodic attacks of abdominal pain and a variety of neurologic and psychiatric disturbances analogous to those seen in acute intermittent porphyria and porphyria variegata (Roberts et al). In some cases, there are also cutaneous manifestations indistinguishable from those of porphyria cutanea tarda and porphyria variegata (Roberts et al; Poh-Fitzpatrick).

Histopathology. The histologic changes seen in the skin lesions are the same in all six types of porphyria with cutaneous lesions. Differences are based on the severity rather than on the type of porphyria. Deposits of hyalin are regularly seen, and bullae are seen in some instances. In addition, sclerosis of the collagen is present in old lesions (Kint et al; Epstein et al).

In mild cases, homogeneous, pale, eosinophilic deposits of hyalin are limited to the immediate vicinity of the blood vessels in the papillary dermis (Epstein et al). These deposits are best visualized with a PAS stain, since they are PAS-positive and diastase resistent (Fig. 23-7).

In severely involved areas, seen most commonly in erythropoietic protoporphyria, the perivascular mantles of hyalin are wide enough in the papillary dermis to coalesce with those of adjoining capillaries. In addition, deeper blood vessels may show homogeneous hyaline material around them, and similar homogeneous material may be found throughout the dermis and occasionally even around eccrine glands (Ozasa et al). PAS staining demonstrates this material particularly well. In some instances, it also contains acid mucopolysaccharides, shown with alcian blue or the colloidal iron stain (Epstein et al), or lipids, demonstrable with Sudan IV or Sudan black B (Peterka et al; Ryan; Ozasa et al). In addition, the PAS-positive epidermal-dermal basement membrane zone may be thickened (Epstein et al).

In areas of sclerosis, as seen especially in porphyria cutanea tarda, the collagen bundles are thickened. In contrast to scleroderma, PAS-positive, diastase-resistant material is often present throughout the dermis even in the late stage (Epstein et al).

The bullae, most commonly seen in porphyria cutanea tarda and least commonly in erythropoietic protoporphyria, arise subepidermally above the PAS-positive basement membrane zone (Fig. 23-7). It is quite characteristic of the bullae of porphyria cutanea tarda that the dermal papillae often extend irregularly from the floor of the bulla into the bulla cavity (Feldaker et al; Corey et al). This phenomenon, referred to as festooning, is explained by the rigidity of the upper dermis induced by the presence of hyalin around the capillaries in the papillae and the papillary dermis.

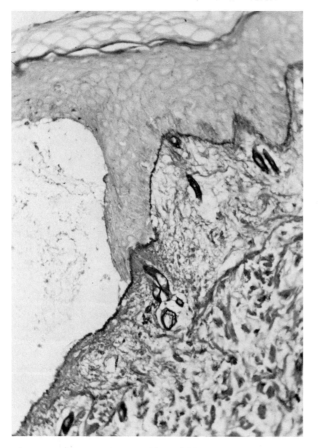

Fig. 23-7. Porphyria cutanea tarda
On staining with the PAS reaction after diastase digestion, the PAS-positive basement membrane zone is seen at the floor of the blister. PAS-positive hyalin is present in the walls of capillaries in the upper dermis. (×200)

Histogenesis. On *electron microscopic examination*, the hyaline material observed in the skin lesions of porphyria appears indistinguishable from the hyalin of hyalinosis cutis and mucosae (Kint et al). Concentric multiplication of the basement membrane is seen around the dermal blood vessels. Peripheral to this multilayered basement membrane, one observes a thick mantle of unlayered material with the same filamentous and amorphous composition as the basement membrane. Often, a gradual transition from the layered to the unlayered zone can be observed (Ryan and Madill; Anton-Lamprecht and Meyer). Scattered through the thick, unlayered zone are solitary collagen fibrils with an average diameter of only 35 nm, in contrast to the 100 nm of mature collagen (Kint; Anton-Lamprecht and Meyer). In cases with severe involvement, intermingled filamentous and amorphous material is seen throughout the upper dermis and even in the middermis, giving the impression of being independent of the blood vessels (Epstein et al).

The hyaline material appears to be excessively synthesized basement membrane material produced by hypertrophic endothelial cells (Anton-Lamprecht and Meyer). Thus, just as in hyalinosis cutis et mucosae, it represents type IV collagen, which is rich in glycoprotein (see p. 13). The presence of small collagen fibrils analogous to reticulum fibrils suggests the presence also of some type III collagen (see p. 31).

Direct immunofluorescence testing has revealed in the majority of patients the presence of immunoglobulins, particularly IgG (Epstein et al), and occasionally also of complement (Cormane et al) in the walls of blood vessels and at the epidermal-dermal junction of light-exposed skin. It is unlikely that these deposits indicate an immunologic phenomenon; rather, they are the result of "trapping" of immunoglobulins and complement in the filamentous material (see p. 156).

The *enzymatic defect* causing each form of porphyria is known with the exception of hepatoerythropoietic porphyria, in which the deficiency is assumed but not yet proved because of the only recent recognition of the disease and the scarcity of cases (Table 23-1). Enzyme determinations may be carried out on cultured skin fibroblasts, erythrocytes, or liver tissue.

Of special significance is the recognition of porphyria cutanea tarda as a disorder inherited as an autosomal dominant trait. The great rarity of its familial occurrence had led to the assumption that it was an acquired disease caused by liver damage induced usually by alcohol but occasionally by other agents such as estrogen (Roenigk and Gottlob). The inherited defect is a decrease in the tissue uroporphyrinogen decarboxylase activity, usually measured on the erythrocytes (Kushner et al). Although it occurs occasionally in early life and without an eliciting factor (Cruces Prado et al), porphyria cutanea tarda in most instances has its onset in middle age. This is because full expression of the disease generally requires concordance of the inherited enzymatic defect and an acquired factor, usually hepatic siderosis. Porphyria cutanea tarda in the same family can be overt, subclinical (in which case there is excessive excretion of uroporphyrins), or latent (in which case there is decreased uroporphyrinogen decarboxylase activity only) (Benedetto et al). The enzyme defect persists during phlebotomy-induced remissions (Felsher et al).

Liver damage is generally mild and chronic in porphyria cutanea tarda. In erythropoietic protoporphyria, however, liver function tests are usually normal, even though microscopic deposits of protoporphyrin in the liver are frequently found (DeLeo et al). Yet, in rare instances, death occurs from liver failure developing swiftly after the initial detection of hepatic dysfunction (MacDonald et al). Patients with such liver failure have very high levels of protoporphyrin in the erythrocytes and, at the time of death, show extensive deposits of protoporphyrin in a cirrhotic liver. The protoporphyrin in hepatocytes and Kupffer cells appears as dark brown granules (Wells et al). This pigment exhibits birefringence on polariscopic examination and, in unstained sections viewed with ultraviolet light, shows red autofluorescence (MacDonald et al). In patients with normal liver function tests, biopsy of the liver may or may not show portal and periportal fibrosis (Cripps and Goldfarb). Even in the absence of fibrosis, some biopsy specimens show protoporphyrin deposits (Cripps and Goldfarb), and, in some instances, biopsy specimens showing no protoporphyrin when examined by light microscopy, by polarization microscopy, or under ultraviolet light, nevertheless show protoporphyrin crystals on electron microscopy (MacDonald et al).

Pseudoporphyria Cutanea Tarda

In patients with chronic renal failure receiving maintenance hemodialysis, an eruption indistinguishable from that of porphyria cutanea tarda may develop on the dorsa of the hands and fingers during the summer months (Gilchrest et al). Rarely, blisters are seen also on the face, and atrophic scarring develops (Thivolet et al). In a large series of 180 patients receiving hemodialysis, 28, or 16%, showed this type of eruption (Perrot et al). Although normal porphyrin levels in urine, stool, and plasma are the rule in hemodialyzed patients developing clinical signs of porphyria cutanea tarda, the clinical manifestations in some patients are accompanied by markedly elevated plasma, urinary, and fecal porphyrin levels (Poh-Fitzpatrick et al, 1978, 1980). In others, plasma porphyrin levels are markedly elevated, whereas the urinary porphyrin concentration is not increased as the result of chronic renal failure (Lichtenstein et al; Topi et al). In one patient from the latter group, the level of red cell uroporphyrinogen decarboxylase was determined and found to be reduced (Lichtenstein et al).

A similar eruption limited to the dorsa of the hands and fingers may appear in patients with chronic renal failure receiving furosemide. In some of these patients, however, a more extensive eruption of large bullae is seen involving also the feet, shins, and trunk (Burry and Lawrence; Keczkes and Farr). The possibility has been suggested that such cases represent instances of furosemide-induced bullous pemphigoid (see p. 13) (Castel et al).

Histopathology. In patients with normal porphyrin levels and with blisters limited to the dorsa of the hands and fingers, the histologic picture is indistinguishable from that seen in mild cases of porphyria (see p. 418). The superficial blood vessels show thickened walls, and the PAS-positive basement membrane zone is often also thickened. Blisters are subepidermal, with festooned dermal papillae. The blisters are situated above the PAS-positive basement membrane zone (Thivolet et al).

Histogenesis. *Electron microscopic findings* are identical to those of porphyria (see p. 419) (Perrot et al). As in porphyria, immunoglobulins are often seen in vessel walls and at the epidermal-dermal junction. Complement is also occasionally seen (Gilchrest et al; Perrot et al).

CALCINOSIS CUTIS

Four forms of calcinosis cutis exist: metastatic calcinosis, dystrophic calcinosis, idiopathic calcinosis, and subepidermal calcified nodule.

Metastatic Calcinosis Cutis

Metastatic calcification develops as the result of either hypercalcemia or hyperphosphatemia. Hypercalcemia may result from (1) primary hyperparathyroidism, (2) excessive intake of vitamin D (Wilson et al), (3) excessive intake of milk and alkali (Wermer et al), or (4) extensive destruction of bone through osteomyelitis or metastases of a carcinoma (Mulligan). Hyperphosphatemia occurs in chronic renal failure as the result of a decrease in renal clearance of phosphorus and is associated with a compensatory drop in the serum calcium level. The low level of ionized calcium in the serum stimulates parathyroid secretion, leading to secondary hyperparathyroidism and to resorption of calcium and phosphorus from bone. The demineralization of bone causes both osteodystrophy and metastatic calcification (Katz et al; Kolton and Pedersen).

Metastatic calcification most commonly affects the media of blood vessels and the kidneys. In addition, other visceral organs may be involved, such as the myocardium, the stomach, and the lungs (Katz et al; Kuzela et al).

Metastatic calcification in the subcutaneous tissue is seen occasionally in association with renal hyperparathyroidism (Katz et al), in uremia (Parfitt), in hypervitaminosis D (Wilson et al), and as the result of excessive intake of milk and alkali (Wermer et al), but hardly ever in primary hyperparathyroidism (Mulligan). Palpable, hard nodules, occasionally of considerable size, are located mainly in the vicinity of the large joints (Katz et al). With an increase in size, the nodules may become fluctuant (Putkonen and Wangel).

Instances of *cutaneous metastatic calcinosis* are rare. Most reports have concerned patients with renal hyperparathyroidism and osteodystrophy. The cutaneous lesions may consist of firm, white papules (Posey and Ritchie), papules in a linear arrangement (Putkonen and Wangel), symmetric, nodular plaques (Kolton and Pedersen), or papules and nodules from which a granular, whitish substance can be expressed (Eisenberg and Bartholow).

Calcification in and around muscular vessels in the deep dermis or in the subcutaneous tissue may occur in primary or secondary hyperparathyroidism and lead to occlusion of these vessels and to infarctive ulcerations, especially on the legs (Winkelmann and Keating).

Histopathology. Calcium deposits are recognized easily in histologic sections, since they stain deep blue with hematoxylin-eosin. They stain black with the von Kossa stain for calcium. The calcium occurs as a rule as massive deposits when located in the subcutaneous fat (Fig. 23-8) and usually as granules and small deposits when located in the dermis. Large deposits of calcium often evoke a foreign body reaction, so that giant cells, an inflammatory infiltrate, and fibrosis may be present around them (Kolton and Pedersen).

In areas of infarctive necrosis, as a result of calcification of dermal or subcutaneous vessels, the involved vessels show calcification of their walls and intravascular fibrosis with attempts at recanalization of the obstructed lumina (Winkelmann and Keating).

Dystrophic Calcinosis Cutis

In dystrophic calcinosis cutis, the calcium is deposited in previously damaged tissue. The values for serum calcium and phosphorus are normal, and the internal organs are spared. There may be numerous large deposits of calcium (calcinosis universalis) or only a few deposits (calcinosis circumscripta).

Calcinosis universalis occurs as a rule in patients with dermatomyositis, but, exceptionally, it has also been seen in patients with systemic scleroderma (Velayos et al). Large deposits of calcium are found in the skin and subcutaneous tissue and often also in muscles and tendons (see p. 458) (Wheeler et al; Muller et al, 1959b). In dermatomyositis, if the patient survives, the nodules of dystrophic calcinosis gradually resolve.

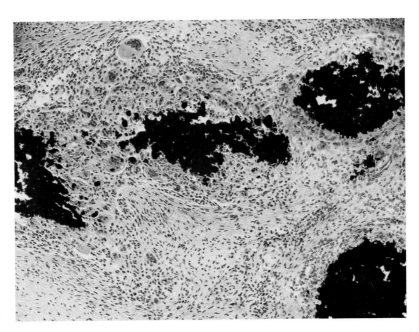

Fig. 23-8. Metastatic calcinosis cutis
The condition was caused by hypercalcemia produced by prolonged and excessive intake of vitamin D. The von Kossa stain for calcium demonstrates irregular masses of calcium surrounded by a foreign body giant cell reaction in the subcutaneous fat. (×100)

Calcinosis circumscripta occurs as a rule in patients with systemic scleroderma; however, rarely, it may be observed in patients with widespread morphea (Muller et al, 1959a; Holmes). Generally, in the presence of calcinosis, systemic scleroderma manifests itself as acrosclerosis. The association of acrosclerosis and calcinosis is often referred to as the Thibierge–Weissenbach syndrome or as the CRST or CREST syndrome, since the manifestations usually consist of **c**alcinosis cutis, **R**aynaud's phenomenon, **s**clerodactyly, and **t**elangiectasia, and often also **e**sophageal dysfunction (Muller et al, 1959a; Carr et al; Velayos et al). Patients with this syndrome often, but not always, have a better prognosis than those with generalized scleroderma or systemic sclerosis (see p. 464).

Lupus erythematosus is only rarely associated with dystrophic calcinosis cutis (Kabir and Malkinson).

Aside from occurring in the connective tissue diseases, dystrophic calcinosis is often seen in subcutaneous fat necrosis of the newborn (see p. 255) and, rarely, in the subcutaneous nodules occurring in Ehlers–Danlos disease (see p. 78).

Histopathology.   As in metastatic calcinosis cutis, the calcium in dystrophic calcinosis cutis usually is present as granules or small deposits in the dermis and as massive deposits in the subcutaneous tissue (Holmes). A foreign body giant cell reaction is often found around large deposits of calcium (Reich). The calcium deposits usually are located in areas in which the collagen or fatty tissue appears degenerated as a result of the disease preceding the calcinosis.

Idiopathic Calcinosis Cutis

Even though the underlying connective tissue disease in some instances of dystrophic calcinosis cutis may be mild and can be overlooked unless specifically searched for, there remain cases of idiopathic calcinosis cutis that resemble dystrophic calcinosis cutis but show no underlying disease (Paegle; Cornelius et al; Haim and Friedman-Birnbaum).

There are two entities that are generally regarded as special manifestations of idiopathic calcinosis cutis: tumoral calcinosis and idiopathic calcinosis of the scrotum.

Tumoral calcinosis consists of numerous large, subcutaneous, calcified masses that may be associated with papular and nodular skin lesions of calcinosis (Whiting et al; Pursley et al). The disease usually is familial and is associated with hyperphosphatemia (Mozaffarian et al; Pursley et al). Otherwise, the resemblance of tumoral calcinosis to the dystrophic calcinosis universalis seen with dermatomyositis is great.

Idiopathic calcinosis of the scrotum consists of multiple asymptomatic nodules of the scrotal skin. The nodules begin to appear in childhood or in early adult life, increase in size and number, and sometimes break down to discharge chalky contents (Shapiro et al).

Histopathology.   *Tumoral calcinosis* shows in the subcutaneous tissue large masses of calcium surrounded by a foreign body reaction (Reich). In addition, intradermal aggregates are present in some cases. Discharge of calcium may take place either through areas of ulceration or by means of transepidermal elimination (Pursley et al).

Idiopathic calcinosis of the scrotum is characterized by variously sized calcific masses, some showing a pronounced surrounding granulomatous foreign body reaction, and others showing none (Shapiro et al; Fisher and Dvoretzky).

Histogenesis. Two authors have studied lesions of idiopathic calcinosis cutis by electron microscopy (Paegle; Cornelius et al). They agree that the deposits consist of pleomorphic calcium phosphate (apatite) crystals. However, according to one opinion, the earliest deposits of calcium are situated extracellularly in the ground substance (Paegle), whereas, according to the other opinion, the earliest calcium deposits lie within collagen fibrils and subsequently extend into the ground substance as the apatite crystals grow (Cornelius et al).

Subepidermal Calcified Nodule

In subepidermal calcified nodules, also referred to as cutaneous calculi, usually a single small, raised, hard nodule is present. Occasionally, however, there are two or three nodules (Woods and Kellaway; Tezuka), and, in some instances, there are numerous (Shmunes and Wood) or even innumerable nodules (Eng and Mandrea). Most patients are children, but, in some patients, a nodule is present already at birth (Winer) or does not appear until adult life (Steigleder and Elschner). In most instances, the surface of the nodule is verrucous, but it may be smooth. The most common location of the nodule is the face.

Histopathology. The calcified material is located predominantly in the uppermost dermis, although, in large nodules, it may extend into the deep layers of the dermis. The calcium is present largely as closely aggregated globules (Fig. 23-9). In some instances, however, there are also one or several large, homogeneous masses of calcified material (Woods and Kellaway; Tezuka). Both the globules and the homogeneous masses occasionally contain well-preserved nuclei (Woods and Kellaway). Macrophages and foreign body giant cells may be seen arranged around the large, homogeneous masses (Woods and Kellaway). The epidermis is often hypertrophic. Calcium granules may be seen within the epidermis, indicative of transepidermal elimination (Duperrat and Goetschel; Eng and Mandrea).

Histogenesis. The primary event seems to be the formation of large, homogeneous masses that undergo calcification and break up into numerous calcified globules (Tezuka). The origin of the homogeneous masses is obscure. It is not likely that they originate from a specific pre-existing structure, such as sweat ducts (Winer) or nevus cells (Steigleder and Elschner), as has been assumed.

GOUT

In the early stage of gout, there usually are irregularly recurring attacks of acute arthritis. In the late stage,

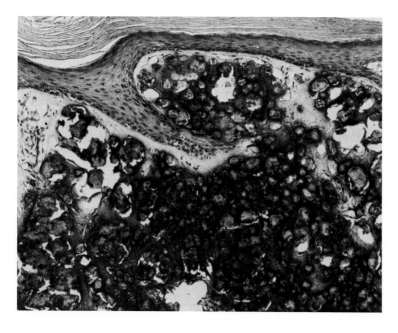

Fig. 23-9.   Subepidermal calcified nodule
Granules and globules of calcium are located beneath the epidermis.

deposits of monosodium urate form within and around various joints, leading to chronic arthritis with destruction in the joints and the adjoining bone. During this late stage, urate deposits, called tophi, may occur in the subcutaneous tissue. The incidence of tophaceous lesions in gout has significantly decreased since 1950, from 14% to 3%, even though the incidence of gout has remained unchanged. Improved methods of treatment account for this decrease (O'Duffy et al).

Tophi are seen most commonly on the helix of the ears, over the bursae of the elbows, and on the fingers and toes (Lichtenstein et al). They may attain a diameter of several centimeters. When large, tophi may discharge a chalky material. In rare instances, intracutaneous tophi are seen on the fingers as firm, yellowish nodules usually only 3 mm to 5 mm in size (Gottron and Korting).

Histopathology. For the histologic examination of tophi, fixation in alcohol is preferable to fixation in formalin; formalin destroys the characteristic urate crystals and merely leaves amorphous material (Lichtenstein et al).

On fixation in alcohol, tophi are seen to consist of variously sized, sharply demarcated aggregates of needle-shaped urate crystals lying closely packed in the form of bundles or sheaves. The crystals often have a brownish color and are doubly refractile on polariscopic examination. The aggregates of urate crystals are surrounded by a granulomatous infiltrate containing many foreign body giant cells (Gottron and Korting). As a secondary phenomenon, calcification, and occasionally also

ossification, may take place in the sodium urate aggregates (Lichtenstein et al).

Even when the specimen has been fixed in formalin, the diagnosis of gout can be made without difficulty because of the characteristic rim of foreign body giant cells and macrophages surrounding the aggregates of amorphous material (Fig. 23-10).

Histogenesis. Gout, a dominantly inherited disorder, is characterized by hyperuricemia. An asymptomatic stage of hyperuricemia precedes the development of gouty arthritis by many years. In the opinion of some authors, the hyperuricemia is solely the result of excessive production of uric acid through increased synthesis of purines (Yü et al). Other authors regard patients with gout as a heterogeneous group, with some patients showing diminished renal excretion of uric acid, others excessive synthesis of uric acid, and still others both overproduction and hypoexcretion of urate (Seegmiller; Reif et al).

OCHRONOSIS

In ochronosis, which is inherited as an autosomal recessive trait, homogentisic acid accumulates over the course of years in many tissues, especially in the cartilage of the joints, of the ears, and of the nose, in ligaments and tendons, and in the sclerae. This results in osteoarthritis, in blackening of cartilages, ligaments, and tendons, and in patchy pigmentation of the sclerae. In the

Fig. 23-10. Gout
Deposits of urate are surrounded by a granulomatous reaction containing many foreign body giant cells. On the left, part of the urate is present as needle-shaped crystals. (×100)

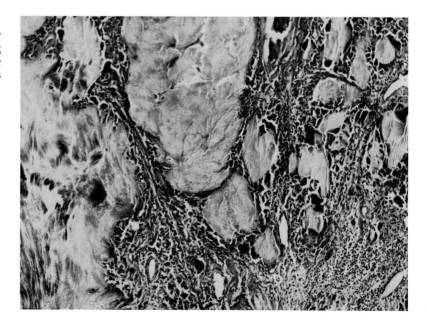

course of time, homogentisic acid accumulates also in the dermis in sufficient amounts to cause patchy brownish pigmentation of the skin.

Histopathology. The ochronotic pigment, as seen in sections of the dermis stained with hematoxylin-eosin, has a yellow brown color. It does not stain with silver nitrate as melanin does but becomes black when stained with cresyl violet or methylene blue (Laymon). The skin shows ochronotic pigment as fine granules free in the tissue as well as in the endothelial cells of blood vessels, in the basement membrane and the secretory cells of sweat glands, and within scattered macrophages (Lichtenstein and Kaplan). The most striking finding, however, is the presence of the ochronotic pigment within collagen bundles causing homogenization and swelling of the bundles. Some collagen bundles assume a bizarre shape; they appear rigid and tend to fracture transversely with jagged or pointed ends (Findlay et al). As the result of the breaking up of degenerated collagen bundles, irregular, homogeneous, light brown clumps lie free in the tissue (Fig. 23-11) (Friderich and Nikolowski; Laymon). There may be scattered foreign body giant cells in the vicinity of the ochronotic clumps (Kutty et al). In addition, ochronotic pigment can be found within elastic fibers (Teller and Winkler).

Histogenesis. In ochronosis, because of an inborn lack of homogentisic acid oxidase, the two amino acids

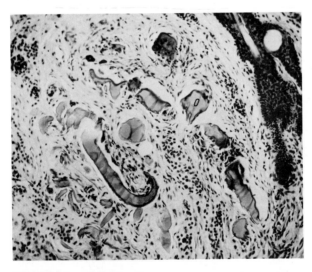

Fig. 23-11.   Ochronosis
The ochronotic pigment is present within degenerated and swollen collagen bundles, most of which appear broken up into irregularly shaped clumps. (× 160) (Friderich H, Nikolowski W: Arch Dermatol Syph (Berlin) 192:273–289, 1951)

tyrosine and phenylalanine cannot be catabolized beyond homogentisic acid. Most of the homogentisic acid is excreted in the urine. The urine, on standing or after the addition of sodium hydroxide, turns black (alkaptonuria), since, through oxidation and polymerization, homogentisic acid is converted into a dark-colored insoluble product. However, some of the homogentisic acid gradually accumulates in certain tissues. It is bound irreversibly to collagen fibers as a polymer after oxidation to benzoquinone-acetic acid (Zannoni et al).

On *electron microscopic examination* of early lesions, one observes deposition of amorphous, electron-dense ochronotic pigment around individual collagen fibrils within collagen fibers (Atwood et al). This causes the collagen fibrils to lose their periodicity and to degenerate (Kutty et al). Gradually, the collagen fibrils disappear as they are replaced by ochronotic pigment. Ultimately, the ochronotic pigment occupies entire collagen fibers and, by fusion, entire collagen bundles (Atwood et al; Kutty et al). Cross sections of such bundles then reveal a large, homogeneous, electron-dense aggregate that in some instances shows remnants of collagen fibrils at its periphery (Teller and Winkler). Particles of ochronotic pigment can also be found in elastic fibers (Teller and Winkler) and within macrophages (Kutty et al).

MUCINOSES

Five types of cutaneous mucinosis occur: (1) generalized myxedema; (2) pretibial myxedema; (3) lichen myxedematosus or papular mucinosis; (4) reticular erythematous mucinosis or plaquelike mucinosis; and (5) scleredema.

Regular demonstration of the presence of mucin in the dermis is possible only in pretibial myxedema and in lichen myxedematosus. In reticular erythematous mucinosis, it is possible in most cases. In generalized myxedema, the amount of mucin usually is too small to be demonstrable, and, in scleredema, mucin may be present only in the early stage.

The mucin found in these five diseases represents an increase in the mucin that is normally present in the ground substance of the dermis. It consists of proteins bound to hyaluronic acid, an acid mucopolysaccharide or glycosaminoglycan. As a result of the great water-binding capacity of hyaluronic acid, dermal mucin contains a considerable amount of water. This water is largely removed during the process of dehydration of the specimen; consequently, in routine sections, the mucin, because of its marked shrinkage, appears largely as threads and granules.

The mucin present in the five types of mucinosis stains a light blue in sections stained with hematoxylin-eosin. It also stains with colloidal iron. It is alcian-blue-positive at *p*H 2.5 but negative at *p*H 0.5 and shows metachromasia with toluidine blue at *p*H 7.0 and 4.0 but no metachromasia below *p*H 2.0 (Holubar and Mach; Cohn et al). It is PAS-negative (indicating the absence of neutral mucopolysaccharides) and aldehyde-fuchsin-negative (indicating the absence of sulfated acid mucopolysaccharides). The mucin is completely removed on incubation of histologic sections with testicular hyaluronidase for 1 hr at 37°C (Johnson and Helwig).

Generalized Myxedema

In generalized myxedema, caused by hypothyroidism, the entire skin appears swollen, dry, pale, and waxy. It is firm to the touch. In spite of its edematous appearance, the skin does not pit on pressure. There is often a characteristic facial appearance: the nose is broad, the lips are swollen, and the eyelids are puffy.

Histopathology. Usually, routinely stained sections show no abnormality, except in severe cases, in which one may observe swelling of the collagen bundles with splitting up of the bundles into individual fibers with some bluish threads and granules of mucin interspersed (Reuter). However, with histochemical stains, such as colloidal iron, alcian blue, or toluidine blue, it is possible, at least in severe cases, to demonstrate small amounts of mucin, mainly in the vicinity of the blood vessels and hair follicles (Gabrilove and Ludwig; Cawley et al).

Pretibial Myxedema

Usually, the lesions are limited to the anterior aspects of the legs, but they may extend to the dorsa of the feet. They consist of raised, nodular, yellow, waxy plaques with prominent hair follicles.

Pretibial myxedema usually occurs in association with thyrotoxicosis and not infrequently becomes more pronounced after treatment of the thyrotoxicosis. It nearly always occurs in association with exophthalmos. Rarely, pretibial myxedema, with or without exophthalmos, occurs in nonthyrotoxic thyroid disease such as chronic lymphocytic thyroiditis, the patient being either euthyroid or hypothyroid (Lynch et al).

Histopathology. Mucin in large amounts is present in the dermis, particularly in the middle and lower thirds. As a result, the dermis is greatly thickened. The mucin occurs not only as individual

threads and granules but also as extensive deposits resulting in the splitting up of collagen bundles into fibers and wide separation of the fibers. As a result of shrinkage of the mucin during the process of fixation and dehydration, empty spaces are seen within the mucin deposits (Fig. 23-12). The number of fibroblasts is as a rule not increased, but, in areas in which there is much mucin, some fibroblasts have a stellate shape and are then referred to as mucoblasts (Cawley et al; Konrad et al).

Histogenesis. On *electron microscopic examination*, two types of cells can be recognized: stellate mucoblasts and fibroblasts (Korting et al). The mucoblasts have numerous long, branching, intertwining processes. The cisternae of their rough endoplasmic reticulum are greatly dilated and filled with amorphous, moderately electron-dense material. This material also coats the surface of the mucoblasts and collagen fibers and is present as small, irregular clumps within otherwise empty-appearing spaces (Konrad et al). The fibroblasts also appear as actively synthesizing cells; they contain and are surrounded by filamentous material (Korting et al).

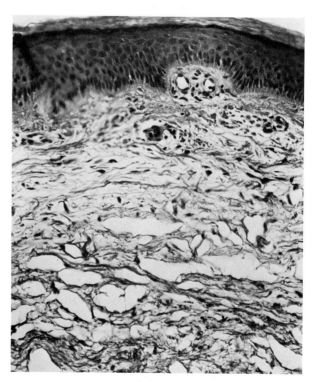

Fig. 23-12.   Pretibial myxedema
Considerable amounts of mucin are present, especially in the middle portion of the dermis, separating the llagen bundles as well as individual collagen fibers. The empty spaces are caused by shrinkage of the mucin during the process of fixation and dehydration. (× 200)

Of interest is the almost invariable presence of long-acting thyroid stimulator (LATS) in the serum of patients with pretibial myxedema. There is, however, a rather poor correlation between the severity of the skin lesions and the level of serum LATS; furthermore, LATS is detected in 40% to 60% of patients with an active exophthalmic goiter but without pretibial myxedema. Thus, LATS cannot be regarded as the cause of pretibial myxedema (Schermer et al). It appears likely that the IgG LATS represents an autoantibody that is produced by lymphocytes in thyroid disease, especially in thyrotoxicosis, and is a reflection, rather than a cause, of the underlying disease (Lynch et al).

The restriction of the myxedema largely to the pretibial area may be explained by the finding that fibroblasts from the pretibial area synthesize 2 to 3 times more hyaluronic acid than fibroblasts from other areas when incubated with serum from patients with pretibial myxedema (Cheung et al).

Lichen Myxedematosus

Lichen myxedematosus, or papular mucinosis, is characterized by a more or less extensive eruption of asymptomatic, soft papules generally 2 mm to 3 mm in diameter. Though densely grouped, they usually do not coalesce. The face and arms are most commonly affected. In some instances, in addition to papules, large nodules may be present, especially on the face (Hill et al). Although the disease is very chronic, spontaneous resolution has been reported (Hardie et al).

A variant of lichen myxedematosus is *scleromyxedema*, in which one observes, in addition to a generalized eruption of papules as in lichen myxedematosus, diffuse thickening of the skin associated with erythema. There is marked accentuation of the skin folds, particularly on the face. In contrast with scleroderma, the thickened skin in scleromyxedema is freely movable.

Histopathology.   In lichen myxedematosus, fairly large amounts of mucin are present (Fig. 23-13). In contrast with pretibial myxedema, however, the mucinous infiltration is found only in circumscribed areas, is most pronounced in the upper dermis, and is associated with an increase in fibroblasts and collagen (Dalton and Seidell; Montgomery and Underwood). The collagen bundles may show a rather irregular arrangement.

Scleromyxedema.   The histologic picture found in the papules in scleromyxedema resembles that seen in lichen myxedematosus. In the diffusely thickened skin, one finds extensive proliferation of fibroblasts throughout the dermis associated with irregularly arranged bundles of collagen. In many areas, the collagen bundles are split up into individual fibers by mucin. As a rule, the amount of mucin is greater in the upper half than in the lower half of the dermis (Rudner et al).

Autopsy examination of patients with scleromyxedema has not shown mucinous deposits in any internal organs (Montgomery and Underwood;

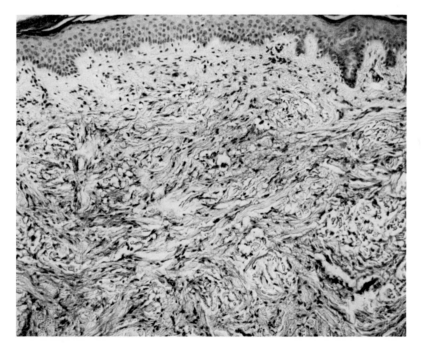

Fig. 23-13.   Lichen myxedematosus (scleromyxedema) In addition to fairly large amounts of mucin, there is extensive proliferation of fibroblasts associated with irregularly arranged bundles of collagen. (×100)

Rudner et al; Braun-Falco and Weidner). In one reported patient, the autopsy was thought to reveal the coexistence of scleromyxedema and multiple myeloma (see Histogenesis below) (Proppe et al).

Histogenesis. *Electron microscopic examination* of scleromyxedema reveals an increase in the number of fibroblasts. They show considerable activity, as indicated by the presence of a markedly dilated rough endoplasmic reticulum and long cytoplasmic processes. These fibroblasts produce both collagen and ground substance. The presence of many collagen fibrils with reduced diameter, similar to those seen in scleroderma, indicates that it is young collagen. In many areas, one observes rather small bundles of young collagen fibrils, with each fibril richly coated with ground substance (Hardmeier and Vogel).

The presence of a *monoclonal component* (M component) or paraprotein in the sera of patients with lichen myxedematosus and scleromyxedema has been noted in nearly all cases that have been adequately tested. Its absence has been noted in one case (Howsden et al); in another case, it was absent at first but present later on (Carli-Basset et al).

In nearly all instances, the paraprotein is an IgG, although, in one reported instance, it was an IgM (Braun-Falco and Weidner). The IgG paraprotein is a very basic protein because of an increased lysine content in its light chains (Lawrence et al). Thus, in most instances, it migrates more slowly than gamma-globulin on serum electrophoresis and may even migrate toward the cathode rather than toward the anode (Shapiro et al). In instances in which it migrates with the same speed as gamma-globulin, immunoelectrophoresis is required for its recognition (Piper et al). The IgG of lichen myxematosus differs from the IgG of multiple myeloma not only by usually showing slower electrophoretic migration but also by the fact that its IgG molecules nearly always possess light chains of the lambda type, although light chains of the kappa type have occasionally been found (Lai A Fat et al; Danby et al; Archibald and Calvert). In contrast, in multiple myeloma with elevated values for IgG, only about one third of the reported cases with IgG molecules have lambda light chains, and two thirds have kappa light chains (James et al). In addition to showing a monoclonal IgG, many cases of lichen myxedematosus show hyperplasia of plasma cells in the bone marrow (Perry et al, 1960b; Piper et al; Feldman et al; Braun-Falco and Weidner). These plasma cells have been shown to synthesize the monoclonal IgG (Suurmond and van Furth; Lai A Fat et al). In some cases, the plasma cells in the bone marrow have been regarded as atypical in appearance (McCarthy et al; Krebs and Müller).

The role of the monoclonal IgG in lichen myxedematosus is not clear. Since its presence in the dermal mucin has been demonstrated by direct immunofluorescence (McCarthy et al; Rowell et al; Sawada and Ohashi), it has been speculated that it might stimulate fibroblasts

to increased activity (Piper et al); however, it seems more likely that it represents an autoantibody and, like the IgG LATS in pretibial myxedema, is a consequence rather than the cause of lichen myxedematosus (Lawrence et al).

The coexistence of *multiple myeloma* and lichen myxedematosus has been assumed in three cases. In one case, a diagnosis of multiple myeloma appears unlikely, because the autopsy revealed no atypical plasma cells in the bone marrow (Proppe et al). In the second case, the presence of atypical plasma cells in the bone marrow was regarded as evidence of multiple myeloma; however, the remission of both the cutaneous manifestations and the abnormalities of the bone marrow under treatment with cytostatica and prednisone makes the diagnosis of multiple myeloma uncertain (Krebs and Müller). In a third case, reported only as a case demonstration, not only were atypical plasma cells seen in the bone marrow, but also numerous foci of osteolysis were found in the skull, so that multiple myeloma cannot be excluded (Schnyder and Kaufmann).

Reticular Erythematous Mucinosis

Erythematous, reticulated areas with irregular but well-defined margins are present, usually in the center of the chest and of the upper back. First described in 1960 as being composed of confluent papules and called plaque-like mucinosis (Perry et al, 1960a), similar cases showing coalescent macules, rather than papules, were designated reticular erythematous mucinosis in 1974 (Steigleder et al). It has since become apparent that macular and papular lesions can coexist (Steigleder; Kocsard and Munro; Stevanović). In rare instances, lesions spare the trunk and are present on the arms and face (Morison et al). The eruption is asymptomatic. It is chronic but usually responds well to rather small doses of antimalarial drugs of the 4-aminoquinoline group, such as chloroquin.

Histopathology. Two histologic features are usually present: small amounts of dermal mucin, and a mild to moderately pronounced mononuclear infiltrate situated predominantly around blood vessels and hair follicles (Perry et al, 1960a; Steigleder).

In papular lesions, the amounts of mucin usually are fairly conspicuous. As a rule, mucin can be recognized even in routinely stained sections (Fig. 23-14). The mucin stains with alcian blue and usually also with mucicarmine. In addition, there often is metachromasia on staining with toluidine blue or with the Giemsa stain (Perry et al, 1960a; Steigleder; Stevanović). Fibroblasts with bipolar processes are located in the mucinous deposits (Herzberg).

In macular lesions, the mucin may be missed in routinely stained sections and become apparent

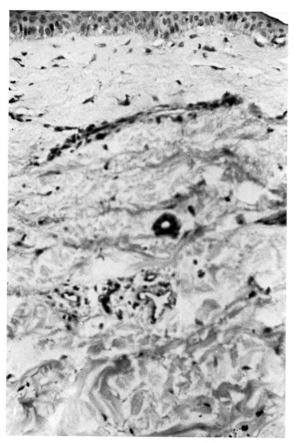

Fig. 23-14.   Reticular erythematous mucinosis
Mucinous deposits are visible as threads and streaks between collagen bundles even in this routinely stained section. Fibroblasts with bipolar processes are located in the vicinity of the mucin. (× 100)

only on staining with alcian blue. However, it usually does not stain with mucicarmine and shows no metachromasia with toluidine blue or with the Giemsa stain (Steigleder et al; Kocsard and Munro). In some instances, no mucin is found even on staining with alcian blue (Smith et al; Rufli); the diagnosis then depends on the presence of the mononuclear infiltrate, the clinical appearance, and the response of the patient to treatment with antimalarial drugs.

Scleredema

Scleredema, occasionally also called scleredema adultorum even though it may occur in children (Greenberg et al), is characterized by diffuse, nonpitting swelling and induration of the skin. Its cause is unknown, but it

frequently follows an infectious disease such as influenza or tonsillitis. Usually, it begins on the face and extends from there to the neck and upper trunk. In about three quarters of the patients, complete resolution takes place within a few months; in the remaining fourth, the disease may persist for as many as 40 years (Fleischmajer et al). Although visceral lesions may occur, only one instance of death from scleredema has been recorded (see below).

Diabetes is commonly associated with persistent scleredema and, in most of these instances, is quite resistant to antidiabetic therapy (Fleischmajer et al; Cohn et al). It has been suggested that the association of persistent scleredema with maturity-onset diabetes be recognized as a special form of scleredema (Krakowski et al).

Histopathology. The dermis in scleredema is about 3 times thicker than normal. The collagen bundles are thickened and separated by clear spaces, causing "fenestration" of the collagen. The secretory coils of the sweat glands, surrounded by fat tissue, are located in the upper dermis or the middermis, rather than, as normally, in the lower dermis or at the junction of the dermis and the subcutaneous fat. Since the distance between the epidermis and the sweat glands is unchanged, it can be concluded that much of the subcutaneous fat in scleredema has been replaced by dense collagenous bundles (Fleischmajer et al). No increase in the number of fibroblasts is noted in association with the hyperplasia of the collagen; in fact, their number may be strikingly decreased (Kövary et al).

In most instances, especially in early cases, histochemical staining reveals the presence of hyaluronic acid between the bundles of collagen, particularly in the areas of fenestration. The hyaluronic acid can best be demonstrated with the colloidal iron stain (Cohn et al). Staining with toluidine blue usually reveals metachromasia, which is most evident at pH 7.0, weaker at pH 5.0, and absent at pH 1.5, indicating the presence of only nonsulfated acid mucopolysaccharides (Holubar and Mach).

In some instances, staining with toluidine blue at pH 7.0 is more intense if unfixed cryostat sections are used in place of formalin-fixed material (Niebauer and Ebner). However, in some cases, even frozen sections fail to stain with alcian blue or toluidine blue (Curtis and Shulak). It may be postulated that, in cases of long standing in which the disease has reached a steady stage of collagen turnover, staining for hyaluronic acid may give negative results (Fleischmajer et al).

Systemic Lesions. Occasionally, the tongue and some skeletal muscles are involved (Curtis and Shulak), and, on histologic examination, the muscle bundles show edema and loss of striation (Reichenberger). In a few reported cases, pleural and pericardial effusions were present (Vallee; Curtis and Shulak). In one such case, the disease terminated in death, and autopsy revealed, in addition to pleural and pericardial effusions, diffuse edema of the heart, the liver, and the spleen (Leinwand).

Histogenesis. In some but not all patients with long-standing and widespread scleredema, a monoclonal gammopathy is found in the serum with either Ig-kappa or IgG-lambda. No immunoglobulin deposits have been found in involved skin sites (Kövary et al).

Differential Diagnosis. It can be difficult to differentiate between scleroderma and scleredema. As a rule, however, in scleroderma, the collagen in the subcutaneous tissue appears homogenized and hyalinized and stains only lightly with eosin and with the Masson trichrome stain, whereas, in scleredema, the collagen bundles in the subcutaneous tissue are thickened without being hyalinized and stain normally with eosin and the trichrome stain (see p. 463) (Fleischmajer and Perlish).

MUCOPOLYSACCHARIDOSES Genetic

The mucopolysaccharidoses (MPS) comprise a group of diseases in which, as the result of a deficiency of specific lysosomal enzymes, there is inadequate degradation of mucopolysaccharides, or glycosaminoglycans. Consequently, this material accumulates within lysosomes of various cells in many organs, including the skin. Greatly elevated levels of mucopolysaccharides are present in the blood serum and in the urine.

So far, seven types of mucopolysaccharidoses have been recognized. There is marked variation in the manifestations not only from type to type but also within the same type. The most common features, any or all of which may be present or absent, include dwarfism, skeletal deformities, hepatosplenomegaly, corneal clouding, and progressive mental deterioration with premature death from cardiorespiratory complications. In many instances, there is a characteristic facial appearance with thick lips, flattened nose, and hirsutism referred to as gargoylism. The mode of transmission is autosomal recessive in all types of MPS except type II, the Hunter syndrome, in which it is X-linked recessive.

Of the seven types of MPS, only types I to III will be discussed here. MPS I presents as three distinctive variants, even though they are all caused by a deficiency of the same enzyme. MPS I H, Hurler's syndrome, causes severe mental retardation and death, usually within the first decade of life (Hambrick a contrast, persons with MPS I S, Scheie's sy normal intelligence, no dwarfism, and a expectancy (Horiuchi et al). MPS I H/S, Scheie syndrome, is intermediate between th variants. MPS II, Hunter's syndrome, occurs form, with mental retardation and early death, and in a mild form, in which mental function is normal and survival to adult life is the rule (Prystowsky et al). MPS III, Sanfilippo's syndrome, has mild somatic changes but severe mental retardation (Lasser et al).

The skin in all seven types of MPS usually appears thickened and inelastic. However, the only type in which distinctive cutaneous lesions are found frequently, though not invariably, is MPS II, Hunter's syndrome. They consist of ivory white papules or small nodules, usually 3 mm to 4 mm in size, that may coalesce to form ridges in a reticular pattern on the upper trunk, especially in the scapular region (Prystowsky et al). This has been referred to as pebbling of the skin.

Histopathology. In all seven types of MPS, the normal-appearing or slightly thickened skin, on staining with the Giemsa stain or toluidine blue, shows metachromatic granules within fibroblasts, so that the fibroblasts resemble mast cells (Hambrick and Scheie). The granules also stain with alcian blue and with colloidal iron (Horiuchi et al). Fixation in absolute alcohol in some instances demonstrates the metachromasia better than fixation in formalin (Freeman). In addition, metachromatic granules are occasionally present in some epidermal cells (Hambrick and Scheie; Belcher, 1972b) and in the secretory and ductal cells of eccrine glands (Belcher, 1973).

The cutaneous papules seen only in Hunter's syndrome show not only metachromatic granules within dermal fibroblasts but also extracellular deposits of metachromatic material between collagen bundles and fibers (Freeman).

In all types of mucopolysaccharidosis, metachromatic granules are seen also in the cytoplasm of circulating lymphocytes when smears of them are stained with toluidine blue after fixation in absolute methanol, a finding that aids in the rapid diagnosis of mucopolysaccharidosis (Belcher, 1972a).

Histogenesis. Biochemical studies have shown that, in MPS I, as a result of a deficiency in alpha-L-iduronidase, there is an increased urinary excretion of heparan sulfate and dermatan sulfate (chondroitin sulfate). In MPS II, the same two substances are excessively excreted owing to a deficiency in iduronate sulfatase. In MPS III, there is excessive excretion of heparan sulfate. In MPS IV, the Morquio syndrome, one finds increased urinary excretion of keratan sulfate; in MPS VI, the Maroteau–Lamy syndrome, increased excretion of dermatan sulfate; in

MPS VII, the Sly syndrome, increased excretion of heparan sulfate and dermatan sulfate, as in MPS I and II, but as a result of a deficiency in beta-glucuronidase; and, in MPS VIII, the Di Ferrante syndrome, increased excretion of heparan sulfate and keratan sulfate (Pinnell and McKusick).

By staining for acid phosphatase and by electron microscopy, the metachromatic granules in the skin and in the lymphocytes have been identified as lysosomes that contain acid mucopolysaccharides, which they are incapable of degrading (Belcher 1972a; 1973).

Electron microscopic examination of the skin reveals in most fibroblasts numerous electron-lucent, greatly dilated, membrane-bound vacuoles representing lysosomes. Some of the vacuoles contain granular material or, less commonly, myelinlike structures representing residual bodies (DeCloux and Friederici; Horiuchi et al). Lysosomes are present also in macrophages, showing the same characteristics as in fibroblasts (Lasser et al). In addition, from 5% to 20% of the epidermal cells contain lysosomal vacuoles, with acid phosphatase activity, varying from a solitary vacuole to 20 or 30 vacuoles per cell (Belcher, 1972b).

The dermal Schwann cells also contain electron-lucent lysosomes. In addition, some Schwann cells occasionally show laminated membranous structures ("zebra bodies"). These structures resemble those found in the brain of some patients with mucopolysaccharidosis. In the brain, they contain gangliosides as the result of a deficiency in the lysosomal hydrolase beta-d-galactosidase (Belcher 1972b). The deposition of gangliosides in the brain leads to mental deterioration through the degeneration and loss of neurons (McKusick).

ACANTHOSIS NIGRICANS

Four types of acanthosis nigricans exist: malignant, inherited, endocrine, and idiopathic (Brown and Winkelmann). The malignant type as a rule differs from the three benign types by showing more extensive and more pronounced lesions. The histologic picture is essentially the same in all four types.

The *malignant* type is associated with a malignant tumor, most commonly an abdominal, particularly a gastric, carcinoma (Mikhail et al). However, in rare instances, the tumor may be a lymphoma, such as Hodgkin's disease (Ackerman and Lantis), or an osteogenic sarcoma (Garrott). The sign of Leser–Trélat, which is characterized by the sudden appearance of numerous seborrheic keratoses in association with a malignant tumor, is regarded by some as an early stage (Curth, 1976) or incomplete form (Jacobs and Rigel) of the malignant type of acanthosis nigricans. The seborrheic keratoses seen in this sign may be accompanied (Schwartz and Burgess; Jacobs and Rigel) or followed (Ronchese) by lesions of acanthosis nigricans (see p. 480).

The *inherited* type may have its onset during infancy, childhood, or adulthood.

The *endocrine* type is associated most commonly with a pituitary tumor, usually manifesting itself as acromegaly. In other instances, the endocrine disorder consists of diabetes, Addison's disease, or the Stein–Leventhal syndrome (Brown and Winkelmann). Obesity may or may not be present (Hollingsworth and Amatruda).

In the *idiopathic* type, the most common type, there is no associated malignancy, endocrine disorder, or genetic predisposition. Obesity is often present, but without clear-cut evidence for its being of endocrine genesis (Hollingsworth and Amatruda).

Clinically, all four types of acanthosis nigricans present papillomatous brownish patches, predominantly in the intertriginous areas such as the axillae, the neck, and the genital and submammary regions. In extensive cases of acanthosis nigricans of the malignant type, mucosal surfaces, such as the mouth, the vulva, and the palpebral conjunctivae, may be involved (Mikhail et al).

Histopathology. Histologic examination reveals hyperkeratosis and papillomatosis but only slight, irregular acanthosis and usually no hyperpigmentation. Thus, the term *acanthosis nigricans* has little histologic justification.

In a typical lesion, the dermal papillae project upward as fingerlike projections. The valleys between the papillae show mild to moderate acanthosis and are filled with keratotic material (Fig. 23-15). In contrast, the stratum malpighii at the tips of the papillae and often also on the sides of the protruding papillae appears thinned. The rete ridges as a rule are poorly developed.

Slight hyperpigmentation of the basal layer is demonstrable with silver nitrate staining in some cases but not in others (Brown and Winkelmann). The brownish color of the lesions thus is caused by hyperkeratosis rather than by melanin.

Histogenesis. The relationship of the malignant type of acanthosis nigricans to the coexisting malignant tumor is obscure. Although, in one case of malignant acanthosis nigricans, many cells of the malignant tumor were identified by means of histochemistry and electron microscopy as enterochromaffinlike cells belonging to the APUD series of endocrine cells (Hage and Hage), this finding has not been confirmed (Curth, 1979).

Differential Diagnosis. Differentiation of acanthosis nigricans from other benign papillomas, particularly from epidermal nevi and from the hyperkeratotic type of seborrheic keratosis, often is impossible. As a rule, however, epidermal nevi show more marked acanthosis than acanthosis nigricans and considerable elongation of the rete ridges.

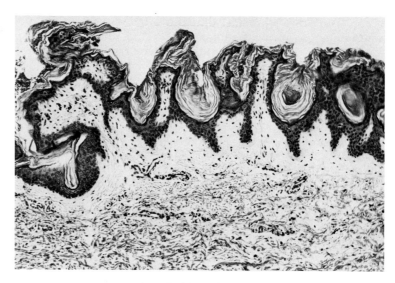

Fig. 23-15.   Acanthosis nigricans
One observes hyperkeratosis and papillomatosis. Some of the dermal papillae project upward as fingerlike projections. As is usually the case, acanthosis and hyperpigmentation are slight. (× 100)

Confluent and Reticulated Papillomatosis

First described in 1927 (Gougerot and Carteaud), confluent and reticulated papillomatosis shows slightly hyperkeratotic and papillomatous pigmented papules that are confluent in the center and reticulated at the periphery. The site of predilection is the sternal region. In the view of some authors, this disorder represents a variant of acanthosis nigricans either of the inherited or of the idiopathic type (Kesten and James). Other authors, however, regard it as a disease entity because of its location and reticulated pattern (Hamilton et al).

Histopathology.   Mild hyperkeratosis and papillomatosis are present, as is focal acanthosis limited largely to the valleys between elongated papillae (Kesten and James). Thus, the histologic changes are similar to but milder than those of acanthosis nigricans.

Histogenesis.   Heavy colonization with *Pityrosporum orbiculare* has been observed in patients with confluent and reticulated papillomatosis, so that this disorder has been regarded as a peculiar host reaction to *P. orbiculare* (Roberts and Lachapelle; Yesudian et al). However, in some cases, mycologic examination has shown absence of this organism (Thomsen; Hamilton et al).

IDIOPATHIC HEMOCHROMATOSIS

In idiopathic hemochromatosis, large amounts of iron are deposited in various organs of the body, especially in the parenchymal cells of the liver and pancreas and in the myocardial fibers. The classic tetrad of idiopathic hemochromatosis consists of hepatic cirrhosis, diabetes, hyperpigmentation of the skin, and cardiac failure.

Pigmentation of the skin is present in 80% to 90% of the patients with idiopathic hemochromatosis at the time the diagnosis is made, but it is often so mild as to attract little attention (Cawley et al; Milder et al). The pigmentation is most pronounced in exposed areas, especially on the face. Its color usually is brown or bronze but may be bluish. The pigmentation is caused largely, if not entirely, by melanin and not by iron.

Histopathology.   Histologic examination of pigmented skin, especially from exposed areas, shows melanin to be present in increased amounts in the basal layer of the epidermis (Cawley et al; Perdrup and Poulsen). Hemosiderin can be demonstrated in the skin of most patients with the aid of an iron stain, such as Perls' stain. It is found as blue-staining granules mainly around blood vessels, both extracellularly and within macrophages, and in the basement membrane zone of the sweat glands and within cells of the connective tissue surrounding these glands (Cawley et al; Perdrup and Poulsen). In rare instances, some iron is present in the epidermis, particularly in the basal cell layer, and in the epithelial cells of the sweat glands (Weintraub et al).

In selecting a site for biopsy, it is not necessary to choose a pigmented area, because, if deposits of iron are present in the skin, they are not limited to the areas of pigmentation. It is important, however, not to take a specimen from the legs, where deposits of iron are frequently found in association with even minor venous stasis or as a consequence of a preceding inflammation that may no longer be evident.

A skin biopsy no longer represents an important test for establishing the diagnosis of idiopathic hemochromatosis; it is merely of confirmatory value. Determinations in the serum of the level of iron, the iron-binding capacity, and the degree of saturation of transferrin with iron and, above all, biopsy of the liver have replaced the skin biopsy in importance (Milder et al).

Liver biopsy is of value in determining the quantity of iron present in the liver, the distribution of the iron, and the degree of fibrosis. In idiopathic hemochromatosis, the iron is deposited largely in the parenchymal cells of the liver. Usually, it is possible to distinguish the findings in an alcoholic patient with iron overload from those in a patient with idiopathic hemochromatosis. In the alcoholic patient, iron deposits are less heavy and are located predominantly in the Kupffer cells rather than in the parenchymal cells. Fatty degeneration of the hepatocytes and portal inflammatory infiltrates are common features of alcoholic liver disease that are rarely seen in idiopathic hemochromatosis (Milder et al). However, it must be realized that alcohol intake has a strong influence on the development of hepatic fibrosis in persons with excess hepatic parenchymal iron as the result of clinically silent hemochromatosis (Rowe et al). If alcoholic liver damage is superimposed, recognition of liver damage brought on by hemochromatosis can be very difficult, and family studies are needed to establish the genetic nature of the disorder (Milder et al).

Histogenesis. It is generally accepted that idiopathic hemochromatosis is an inherited disease, since one or more abnormalities in iron metabolism can be recognized in 25% to 75% of first-degree relatives of patients with the disease (Edwards et al). However, the mode of inheritance is a matter of dispute. Whereas some authors have proposed that idiopathic hemochromatosis is inherited as an autosomal dominant disorder (Feller et al; Rowe et al), others have suggested an autosomal recessive mode of inheritance (Scheinberg; Cartwright et al). It is probable, therefore, that idiopathic hemochromatosis is a genetically heterogeneous syndrome (Crosby).

The exact nature of the defect leading to excessive iron storage is not known. It is possible that the primary defect lies in the intestinal mucosal cells, since it has been shown through the oral administration of radioactive iron that there is an increased rate of intestinal absorption of iron in idiopathic hemochromatosis (Heilmeyer). Through this increased rate of absorption, the degree of saturation of transferrin with iron is very high. Consequently, not all of the iron passing from the intestinal tract can be bound to transferrin, and it is therefore deposited in a variety of organs (Heilmeyer). Iron accumulates particularly in the parenchyma of the liver and pancreas and in the myocardium, and by damaging the cells in which it accumulates, it causes hepatic cirrhosis, diabetes, and cardiac insufficiency.

Two observations indicate that the cutaneous pigmentation in idiopathic hemochromatosis is caused by melanin and not by hemosiderin. The first observation concerns a patient who, in addition to having idiopathic hemochromatosis, had vitiligo. The areas of vitiligo were fully depigmented despite the finding on histologic examination that they contained just as much iron as deeply pigmented areas (Perdrup and Poulsen). The second observation was made in a black patient with idiopathic hemochromatosis who had three epidermal cysts. Although the patient had noticed no change in his skin color, he had observed progressive darkening of the cysts, and histologic examination revealed considerable amounts of melanin both in the walls of the cysts and in their keratinous contents (Leyden et al).

The increase in the amount of melanin found in the skin of patients with hemochromatosis is brought about by the presence of iron in the skin. The iron stimulates melanocytic activity either by increasing oxidative processes (Robert and Zürcher) or by reacting with epidermal sulfhydryl groups and reducing their inhibitory effect on the enzyme system governing melanin synthesis (Buckley). (See also Argyria, p. 265.)

VITAMIN A DEFICIENCY (PHRYNODERMA)

Deficiency of vitamin A is very rare in the United States, occurring mainly in Asia and Africa. It has been recently described, however, as occurring after small bowel bypass surgery for obesity (Wechsler). Vitamin A deficiency results in cutaneous changes to which the name *phrynoderma* has been given. These changes consist of dryness and roughness of the skin and the presence of conical, follicular keratotic lesions. In addition to causing cutaneous changes, deficiency of vitamin A may cause night-blindness, xerophthalmia, and keratomalacia.

Histopathology. The skin shows moderate hyperkeratosis with marked distention of the upper part of the hair follicles by large, horny plugs (Fasal; Wechsler). The sebaceous gland lobules are greatly reduced in size. In addition, one may find evidence of atrophy of the sweat glands, such as flattening of the secretory cells (Frazier and Hu). In severe cases, the sweat glands and sebaceous glands may undergo keratinizing metaplasia (Bessey and Wolbach).

Differential Diagnosis. Histologic differentiation of phrynoderma from ichthyosis vulgaris and keratosis pilaris is impossible, except in very severe cases of phrynoderma, in which the sweat glands and the sebaceous glands show keratinizing metaplasia. Pityriasis rubra pilaris differs from phrynoderma by showing, in addition to hyperkeratosis and follicular plugging, spotted parakeratosis, irregular acanthosis, and an inflammatory infiltrate in the upper dermis.

PELLAGRA

Pellagra is caused by a deficiency of nicotinic acid (niacin) or its precursor, the essential amino acid tryptophan. As a dietary deficiency disease, it may occur in chronic alcoholics. It may also occur in patients with the carcinoid syndrome; the tumor cells divert tryptophan towards serotonin, thus depressing endogenous niacin production (see p. 595) (Castiello and Lynch). In addition, pellagra is a well-recognized complication of isoniazid therapy for tuberculosis. Since isoniazid is a structural analogue of niacin, it can cause the suppression of endogenous niacin production (Cohen et al).

Besides showing cutaneous lesions, pellagra often presents gastrointestinal symptoms and mental changes, resulting in the triad of the three Ds: dermatitis, diarrhea, and dementia (Stratigos and Katsambas).

The cutaneous lesions are precipitated by sunlight. Thus, the dorsa of the hands, wrists, and forearms, the face, and the nape of the neck are predominantly involved. In the early stage, there is erythema, which usually is sharply demarcated; in severe cases, it may be accompanied by vesicles or bullae. Later, the skin becomes thickened, scaling, and pigmented.

Histopathology. The histologic changes of the skin are nonspecific. Early lesions present a chronic inflammatory infiltrate in the upper dermis. Vesicles, if present, arise as in erythema multiforme either subepidermally, owing to edema in the papillary dermis, or intraepidermally, owing to degenerative changes in the epidermis (Moore et al).

In older lesions, one observes hyperkeratosis with areas of parakeratosis. The amount of melanin in the basal layer of the epidermis is increased, and the dermis may show fibrosis in addition to chronic inflammation (Moore et al).

Hartnup Disease

First described in 1956 (Baron et al) and named in 1957 after the family in which it was first observed (Dent), Hartnup disease is transmitted as an autosomal recessive trait. It first manifests itself in early childhood and often improves with advancing age. A photosensitivity eruption is present that usually is indistinguishable from pellagra (Halvorsen and Halvorsen; Fazekas et al). However, in some cases, the cutaneous reaction to sun exposure resembles poikiloderma atrophicans vasculare (Clodi et al) or, because of the prominence of vesicles, hydroa vacciniforme (Ashurst). In addition, there may be cerebellar ataxia and mental retardation. Hartnup disease, in contrast to pellagra, does not respond to treatment with niacin (Ashurst).

Histopathology. The cutaneous eruption in Hartnup disease shows the same histologic changes as seen in pellagra (see above). In patients with poikilodermalike changes, one observes flattening of the epidermis and the presence of a chronic inflammatory infiltrate and of melanophages in the upper dermis (Clodi et al).

Histogenesis. The sun-sensitivity eruption with its resemblance to pellagra is caused by an enzymatic defect in the transport of tryptophan and a resultant decrease in the endogenous production of niacin. The defect in tryptophan transport consists of both an intestinal defect in tryptophan absorption and a renal tubular defect causing inadequate reabsorption of amino acids, including tryptophan. Thus, chromatographic study of the urine shows a constant aminoaciduria, particularly the presence of tryptophan and of indolic substances derived from tryptophan, a finding that establishes the diagnosis (Halvorsen and Halvorsen; Clodi et al; Fazekas et al).

OCULOCUTANEOUS TYROSINOSIS

Oculocutaneous tyrosinosis, also referred to as the Richner–Hanhart syndrome and tyrosinemia type II, is transmitted as an autosomal recessive trait. It is characterized by very tender hyperkeratotic papules and plaques on the palms and soles arising in infancy or childhood, bilateral keratitis, which may lead to corneal opacities, and mental retardation. In some families, however, ocular changes are absent (Rehák et al). A diet low in tyrosine and phenylalanine improves the disease manifestations.

Histopathology. In most instances, the histologic findings in the keratotic lesions are not diagnostic, merely showing hyperkeratosis, parakeratosis, and acanthosis (Larrègue et al). In one reported case, an intraepidermal bulla was seen (Zaleski et al) and, in another, there were homogeneous, refractile, eosinophilic inclusions 2 μm to 3 μm in diameter in the stratum corneum and stratum spinosum. These inclusions were regarded as lipidlike granules (Goldsmith et al).

Histogenesis. As a result of a genetic deficiency in hepatic tyrosine aminotransferase, the levels of tyrosine in the blood and urine are markedly elevated (Hunziker).

BIBLIOGRAPHY

Amyloidosis
BEACHAM BE, GREER KE, ANDREWS BS et al: Bullous amyloidosis. J Am Acad Dermatol 3:506–510, 1980

BEDI TR, DATTA BN: Diffuse biphasic cutaneous amyloidosis. Dermatologica 158:433–437, 1979

BLACK MM, WILSON JONES E: Macular amyloidosis. Br J Dermatol 84:199–209, 1971

BLUHM JF III, JOHNSON SC, NORBACK DH: Bullous amyloidosis. Arch Dermatol 116:1164–1168, 1980

BREATHNACH SM, BLACK MM: Systemic amyloidosis and the skin. Clin Exp Dermatol 4:517–536, 1979

BROWNSTEIN MH, HASHIMOTO K: Macular amyloidosis. Arch Dermatol 106:50–57, 1972

BROWNSTEIN MH, HASHIMOTO K, GREENWALD G: Biphasic amyloidosis: Link between macular and lichenoid forms. Br J Dermatol 88:25–29, 1973

BROWNSTEIN MH, HELWIG EB: Systemic amyloidosis complicating dermatoses. Arch Dermatol 102:1–7, 1970a

BROWNSTEIN MH, HELWIG EB: The cutaneous amyloidoses. I. Localized forms. Arch Dermatol 102:8–19, 1970b

BROWNSTEIN MH, HELWIG EB: The cutaneous amyloidoses. II. Systemic forms. Arch Dermatol 102:20–28, 1970c

BRUNSTING LA, MACDONALD ID: Primary systemic amyloidosis with macroglossia: A syndrome related to Bence Jones proteinuria and myeloma. J Invest Dermatol 8:145–165, 1947

BUXBAUM JN, HURLEY ME, CHUBA J et al: Amyloidosis of the AL type. Am J Med 67:867–878, 1979

DANNO K, HORIO T: Sulphhydryl and disulphide stainings of amyloid: A comparison with hyaline body. Acta Derm Venereol (Stockh) 61:285–289, 1981

FRANKLIN EC: Amyloid and amyloidosis of the skin. J Invest Dermatol 67:451–456, 1976

GLENNER GG: Amyloid deposits and amyloidosis. The beta-fibrilloses. N Engl J Med 302: 1283–1292, 1333–1343, 1980

GLENNER GG, PAGE DL: Amyloid, amyloidosis and amyloidogenesis. Int Rev Exp Pathol 15:2–92, 1976

GOERTTLER E, ANTON-LAMPRECHT I, KOTZUR B: Amyloidosis cutis nodularis. Hautarzt 27:16–25, 1976

HASHIMOTO K, GROSS BG, LEVER WF: Lichen amyloidosus. Histochemical and electron microscopic studies. J Invest Dermatol 45:204–219, 1965

HASHIMOTO K, KOBAYASHI H: Histogenesis of amyloid in the skin. Am J Dermatopathol 2:165–171, 1980

HASHIMOTO K, KUMAKIRI M: Colloid–amyloid bodies in PUVA-treated human psoriatic patients. J Invest Dermatol 72:70–80, 1979

KUMAKIRI M, HASHIMOTO K: Histogenesis of primary localized cutaneous amyloidosis: Sequential change of epidermal keratinocytes to amyloid via filamentous degeneration. J Invest Dermatol 73:150–162, 1979

KURBAN AK, MALAK JA, AFIFI AK et al: Primary localized macular cutaneous amyloidosis: Histochemistry and electron microscopy. Br J Dermatol 85:52–60, 1971

KYLE RA: Amyloidosis. Int J Dermatol 19:537–539, 1980; 20:20–25, 1981

KYLE RA, BAYRD ED: Amyloidosis: Review of 236 cases. Medicine (Baltimore) 54:271–299, 1975

LINDEMAYR W, PARTSCH H: Plattenartig infiltrierte lokalisierte Hautamyloidose. Hautarzt 21:104–107, 1970

MACDONALD DM, BLACK MM, RAMNARAIN N: Immunofluorescence studies in primay localized cutaneous amyloidosis. Br J Dermatol 96:635–641, 1977

MASU S, HOSOKAWA M, SEIJI M: Amyloid in localized cutaneous amyloidosis: Immunofluorescence studies with anti-keratin antiserum. Acta Derm Venereol (Stockh) 61:381–384, 1981

NATELSON EA, DUNCAN WC, MACOSSAY CR et al: Amyloidosis palpebrarum. Arch Intern Med 125:304–307, 1979

PAGE DL, ISERSKY, HARADA M et al: Immunoglobulin origin of localized nodular pulmonary amyloidosis. Res Exp Med (Berlin) 159:75–86, 1972

POTTER BA, JOHNSON WC: Primary localized amyloidosis cutis. Arch Dermatol 103:448–451, 1971

RODERMUND OE: Zur Amyloidosis cutis nodularis atrophicans (Gottron 1950). Arch Klin Exp Dermatol 230:153–171, 1967

RUBINOW A, COHEN AS: Skin involvement in generalized amyloidosis. Ann Intern Med 88:781–785, 1978

RUKAWINA JG, BLOCK WD, JACKSON CE et al: Primary systemic amyloidosis. (Review) Medicine (Baltimore) 35:239–334, 1956

RUNNE U, ORFANOS CE: Amyloid production by dermal fibroblasts. Br J Dermatol 97:155–166, 1977

SHANON J, SAGHER F: Interscapular cutaneous amyloidosis. Arch Dermatol 102:195–198, 1970

SHAPIRO L, KURBAN AK, AZAR HA: Lichen amyloidosus. A histochemical and electron microscopic study. Arch Pathol 90:499–508, 1970

SWEET J, BEAR RA, LANG AP: Amyloidosis and systemic lupus erythematosus. Hum Pathol 12:853–856, 1981

TORIBIO J, QUIÑONES PA, VIGIL TR et al: Mixed (lichenoid and macular) cutaneous amyloidoses. Acta Derm Venereol (Stockh) 55:221–226, 1975

WEEDON D: The composition of amyloid. Aust J Dermatol 20:133–134, 1979

WEEDON D, SHAND E: Amyloid in basal cell carcinomas. Br J Dermatol 101:141–146, 1979

WESTERMARK P: Occurrence of amyloid deposits in the skin in secondary systemic amyloidosis. Acta Pathol Microbiol Scand (A) 80:718–720, 1972

WESTERMARK P: Amyloidosis of the skin: A comparison between localized and systemic amyloidosis. Acta Derm Venereol (Stockh) 59:341–345, 1979

WESTERMARK P, ÖHMAN S, DOMAR M et al: Bullous amyloidosis. Arch Dermatol 117:782–784, 1981

Colloid Milium, Nodular Colloid Degeneration

DUPRE A, BONAFE JF, PIERAGGI MT et al: Paracolloid of the skin. J Cutan Pathol 6:304–309, 1979

EBNER H, GEBHART W: Colloid milium: Light and electron microscopic investigations. Clin Exp Dermatol 2:217–226, 1977

EBNER H, GEBHART W: Vergleichende Untersuchungen bei juvenilem und adultem Colloid Milium. Arch Dermatol Res 261:231–244, 1978

GRAHAM JH, MARQUES AS: Colloid milium: A histochemical study. J Invest Dermatol 49:497–507, 1967

HASHIMOTO K, KATZMAN RL, KANG AH et al: Electron microscopical and biochemical analysis of colloid milium. Arch Dermatol 111:49–59, 1975

HASHIMOTO K, MILLER F, BERESTON ES: Colloid milium. Histochemical and electron microscopic studies. Arch Dermatol 105:684–694, 1972

HOLZBERGER PC: Concerning adult colloid milium. Arch Dermatol 82:711–716, 1960

KAWASHIMA Y, MATSUBARA T, KINBARA T et al: Colloid degeneration of the skin. J Dermatol (Tokyo) 4:115–121, 1977

PERCIVAL BH, DUTHIE DA: Notes on a case of colloid pseudo-milium. Br J Dermatol 60:399–404, 1948

REUTER MJ, BECKER SW: Colloid degeneration (collagen degeneration) of the skin. Arch Dermatol Syph 46:695–704, 1942

SULLIVAN M, ELLIS FA: Facial colloid degeneration in plaques. Arch Dermatol 84:816–823, 1961

WOOLDRIDGE WE, FRERICHS JE: Amyloidosis. A new clinical type. Arch Dermatol 82:230–234, 1960

Hyalinosis Cutis et Mucosae (Lipoid Proteinosis)

CAPLAN RM: Visceral involvement in lipoid proteinosis. Arch Dermatol 95:149–155, 1967

EBERHARTINGER C, NIEBAUER G: Beitrag zur Kenntnis der Lipoidproteinose Urbach-Wiethe. Hautarzt 10:54–65, 1959

FLEISCHMAJER R, NEDWICH A, RAMOS E, SILVA J: Hyalinosis cutis et mucosae. J Invest Dermatol 52:495–503, 1969

FLEISCHMAJER R, TIMPL R, GRAVES P et al: Hyalinosis cutis et mucosae. A basal lamina disease. (Abstr) J Invest Dermatol 76:314–315, 1981

GROSFELD JCM, SPAAS J, VAN DE STAAK WJBM et al: Hyalinosis cutis et mucosae. Dermatologica 130:239–266, 1965

HASHIMOTO K, KLINGMÜLLER G, RODERMUND OE: Hyalinosis cutis et mucosae. Acta Derm Venereol (Stockh) 52:179–195, 1972

HOLTZ KH: Über Gehirn- und Augenveränderungen bei Hyalinosis cutis et mucosae (Lipoidproteinose) mit Autopsiebefund. Arch Klin Exp Dermatol 214:289–306, 1962

HOLTZ KH, SCHULZE W: Beitrag zur Klinik und Pathogenese der Hyalinosis cutis et mucosae (Lipoid-Proteinose Urbach–Wiethe). Arch Dermatol Syph (Berlin) 192:206–237, 1950

ISHIBASHI A: Histogenesis of hyalinosis cutis et mucosae. J Dermatol 5:265–278, 1978

KEFALIDES NA: Basement membranes: Structural and biosynthetic considerations. J Invest Dermatol 65:85–92, 1975

KINT A: A comparative electron microscopic study of the perivascular hyaline from porphyria cutanea tarda and from lipoid proteinosis. Arch Klin Exp Dermatol 239:203–212, 1970

LAYMON CW, HILL EM: An appraisal of hyalinosis cutis et mucosae. Arch Dermatol 75:55–65, 1957

MCCUSKER JJ, CAPLAN RM: Lipoid proteinosis (lipoglycoproteinosis). Am J Pathol 40:599–613, 1962

RAMOS E, SILVA S: Lipoid proteinosis. Arch Dermatol Syph 47:301–326, 1943

RASIEWICZ W, RUBISZ-BRZEZINSKA J, KONECKI J: Hyalinosis cutis et mucosae Urbach–Wiethe. Dermatologica 130:145–157, 1965

UNGAR H, KATZENELLENBOGEN I: Hyalinosis of skin and mucous membranes. Arch Pathol 63:65–74, 1957

VAN DER WALT JJ, HEYL T: Lipoid proteinosis and erythropoietic protoporphyria. Arch Dermatol 104:501–507, 1971

WOOD MG, URBACH F, BEERMAN H: Histochemical study of a case of lipoid proteinosis. J Invest Dermatol 26:263–274, 1956

Porphyria

ANTON-LAMPRECHT I, MEYER B: Zur Ultrastruktur der Haut bei Protoporphyrinämie. Dermatologica 141:76–83, 1970

BENEDETTO AV, KUSHNER JP, TAYLOR JS: Porphyria cutanea tarda in three generations of a single family. N Engl J Med 298:358–362, 1978

BURRY JN, LAWRENCE JR: Phototoxic blisters from high frusemide dosage. Br J Dermatol 94:495–499, 1976

CASTEL T, GRATACOS R, CASTRO J et al: Bullous pemphigoid induced by frusemide. Clin Exp Dermatol 6:635–638, 1981

COREY TJ, DE LEO VA, CHRISTIANSON H et al: Variegate porphyria. Clinical and laboratory features. J Am Acad Dermatol 2:36–43, 1980

CORMANE RH, SZABO E, TIO TY: Histopathology of the skin in acquired and hereditary porphyria cutanea tarda. Br J Dermatol 85:531–539, 1971

CRIPPS DJ, GOLDFARB SS: Erythropoietic protoporphyria: Hepatic cirrhosis. Br J Dermatol 98:349–354, 1978

CRUCES PRADO MJ, ENRIQUEZ DE SALAMANCA R, VEREA HERNANDO M et al: Two cases of infantile and familial porphyria cutanea tarda. Dermatologica 161:205–210, 1980

CZARNECKI DB: Hepatoerythropoietic porphyria. Arch Dermatol 116:307–311, 1980

DE LEO VA, MATHEWS-ROTH M, POH-FITZPATRICK M et al: Erythropoietic protoporphyria. Ten years' experience. Am J Med 60:8–22, 1976

ELDER GH, LEE GB, TOVEY JA: Decreased activity of hepatic uroporphyrinogen decarboxylase in sporadic porphyria cutanea tarda. N Engl J Med 299:274–278, 1978

EPSTEIN JH, TUFFANELLI DL, EPSTEIN WL: Cutaneous changes in the porphyrias. Arch Dermatol 107:689–698, 1973

FELDAKER M, MONTGOMERY H, BRUNSTING LA: Histopathology of porphyria cutanea tarda. J Invest Dermatol 24:131–137, 1955

FELSHER BF, NORRIS ME, SHIH JC: Red-cell uroporphyrinogen decarboxylase activity in porphyria cutanea tarda and in other forms of porphyria. N Engl J Med 299:1095–1098, 1978

FROMKE VL, BOSSENMAIR I, CARDINAL R et al: Porphyria variegata. Study of a large kindred in the United States. Am J Med 65:80–88, 1978

GILCHREST B, ROWE JW, MIHM MC JR: Bullous dermatosis in hemodialysis. Ann Intern Med 83:480–483, 1975

GSCHNAIT F, WOLFF K, KONRAD K: Erythropoietic protoporphyria: Submicroscopic events during the acute photosensitivity flare. Br J Dermatol 92:545–557, 1975

HAINING RG, COWGER ML, SHURTLEFF DB et al: Congenital erythropoietic porphyria. Am J Med 44:624–637, 1968

HÖNIGSMANN H, REICHEL K: Hepatoerythrozytäre Porphyrie. Hautarzt 30:95–97, 1979

HORKAY J, BALOGH E, VITALIS S: Protoporphyria erythropoietica. Z Hautkr 43:639–643, 1968

HUNTER GA: Clinical manifestations of the porphyrias: A review. Aust J Dermatol 20:120–122, 1979

KECZKES K, BARKER DJ: Malignant hepatoma associated with acquired cutaneous porphyria. Arch Dermatol 112:78–82, 1976

KECZKES K, FARR M: Bullous dermatosis of chronic renal failure. Br J Dermatol 95:541–546, 1976

KINT A: A comparative electron microscopic study of the perivascular hyaline from porphyria cutanea tarda and from lipoid proteinosis. Arch Klin Exp Dermatol 239:203–212, 1970

KINT A, GHEORGHIN G, DE BERSAQUES J: Étude comparative au microscope électronique de la substance hyaline dans divers types de porphyrie. Arch Belges Dermatol Syph 27:31–40, 1971

KONRAD K, HÖNIGSMANN H, GSCHNAIT F et al: Mouse model for protoporphyria. II. Cellular and subcellular events in the photosensitivity flare of the skin. J Invest Dermatol 65:300–310, 1975

KUSHNER JP, BARBUTO AJ, LEE GR: An inherited enzymatic defect in porphyria cutanea tarda. J Clin Invest 58:1089–1097, 1976

LICHTENSTEIN JR, BABB EJ, FELSHER BF: Porphyria cutanea tarda (PCT) in a patient with chronic renal failure on hemodialysis. Br J Dermatol 104:575–578, 1981

MACDONALD DM, GERMAIN D, PERROT H: The histopathology and ultrastructure of liver disease in erythropoietic protoporphyria. Br J Dermatol 104:7–17, 1981

MATHEWS-ROTH, MM: Erythropoietic protoporphyria: Diagnosis and treatment. N Engl J Med 297:98–100, 1977

MUSTAJOKI P: Variegate porphyria. Ann Intern Med 89:238–244, 1978

OZASA S, YAMAMOTO S, MAEDA M et al: Erythropoietic protoporphyria. J Dermatol (Tokyo) 4:85–89, 1977

PERROT H, GERMAIN D, EUVRARD S et al: Porphyria cutanea tarda-like dermatosis by hemodialysis. Arch Dermatol Res 259:177–185, 1977

PETERKA ES, FUSARO RM, GOLTZ RW: Erythropoietic protoporphyria. II. Histological and histochemical studies of cutaneous lesions. Arch Dermatol 92:357–361, 1965

PIÑOL-AGUADÉ J, HERRERO C, ALMEIDA J et al: Porphyrie hépatoérythrocytaire. Une nouvelle forme de porphyrie. Ann Dermatol Syph 102:129–136, 1975

POH-FITZPATRICK MB: A plasma porphyrin fluorescence marker for variegate porphyria. Arch Dermatol 116:543–547, 1980

POH-FITZPATRICK MB, BELLET N, DE LEO VA et al: Porphyria cutanea tarda in two patients treated with hemodialysis for chronic renal failure. N Engl J Med 299:292–294, 1978

POH-FITZPATRICK MB, MASULLO AS, GROSSMAN ME: Porphyria cutanea tarda associated with chronic renal failure and hemodialysis. Arch Dermatol 116:191–195, 1980

ROBERTS DT, BRODIE MJ, MOORE MR et al: Hereditary coproporphyria presenting with photosensitivity induced by the contraceptive pill. Br J Dermatol 96:549–553, 1977

ROENIGK HH, GOTTLOB ME: Estrogen-induced porphyria cutanea tarda. Arch Dermatol 102:260–266, 1970

RYAN EA: Histochemistry of the skin in erythropoietic proto-porphyria. Br J Dermatol 78:501–518, 1966

RYAN EA, MADILL GT: Electron microscopy of the skin in erythropoietic protoporphyria. Br J Dermatol 80:561–570, 1968

SIMON N, BERKÓ G, SCHNEIDER I: Hepato-erythropoietic porphyria presenting as scleroderma and acrosclerosis in a sibling pair. Br J Dermatol 663–668, 1977

STRETCHER GS: Erythropoietic porphyria. Arch Dermatol 113:1553–1557, 1977

THIVOLET J, EUVRARD S, PERROT H et al: La pseudo-porphyrie cutanée tardive des hémodialyses. Ann Dermatol Venereol 104:12–17, 1977

TOPI GC, D'ALESSANDRO GL, CANCARINI GC et al: Porphyria cutanea tarda in a haemodialysed patient. Br J Dermatol 104:579–580, 1981

WADDINGTON RT: A case of primary liver tumor associated with porphyria. Br J Surg 59:653–654, 1972

WELLS MM, GOLITZ LE, BENDER BJ: Erythropoietic protoporphyria with hepatic cirrhosis. Arch Dermatol 116:429–432, 1980

Calcinosis Cutis

CARR RD, HEISEL EB, STEVENSON TD: CRST syndrome. Arch Dermatol 92:519–525, 1965

CORNELIUS CE III, TENENHOUSE A, WEBER JC: Calcinosis cutis. Arch Dermatol 98:219–229, 1968

DUPERRAT B, GOETSCHEL G: Calcification nodulaire solitaire con-génitale de la peau (Winer, 1952). Ann Dermatol Syph 90:283–287, 1963

EISENBERG E, BARTHOLOW PV JR: Reversible calcinosis cutis. N Engl J Med 268:1216–1220, 1963

ENG AM, MANDREA E: Perforating calcinosis cutis presenting as milia. J Cutan Pathol 8:247–250, 1981

FISHER BK, DVORETZKY I: Idiopathic calcinosis of the scrotum. Arch Dermatol 114:957, 1978

HAIM S, FRIEDMAN-BIRNBAUM R: Two cases of circumscribed calcinosis. Dermatologica 143:111–114, 1971

HOLMES R: Morphoea with calcinosis. Clin Exp Dermatol 4:125–128, 1979

KABIR DJ, MALKINSON FD: Lupus erythematosus and calcinosis cutis. Arch Dermatol 100:17–22, 1969

KATZ AI, HAMPERS CL, MERRILL JP: Secondary hyperparathy-roidism and renal osteodystrophy in chronic renal failure. (Review) Medicine (Baltimore) 48:333–374, 1969

KOLTON B, PEDERSEN J: Calcinosis cutis and renal failure. Arch Dermatol 110:256–257, 1974

KUZELA DC, HUFFER WE, CONGER JD et al: Soft tissue calcification in chronic dialysis patients. Am J Pathol 86:403–424, 1977

MOZAFFARIAN G, LAFFERTY FW, PEARSON OH: Treatment of tu-moral calcinosis with phosphorus deprivation. Ann Intern Med 77:741–745, 1972

MULLER SA, BRUNSTING LA, WINKELMANN RK: Calcinosis cutis: Its relationship to scleroderma. Arch Dermatol 80:15–21, 1959a

MULLER SA, WINKELMANN RK, BRUNSTING LA: Calcinosis in dermatomyositis. Arch Dermatol 79:669–673, 1959b

MULLIGAN RM: Metastatic calcification. (Review) Arch Pathol 43:177–230, 1947

PAEGLE RD: Ultrastructure of mineral deposits in calcinosis cutis. Arch Pathol 82:474–482, 1966

PARFITT AM: Soft tissue calcification in uremia. Arch Intern Med 124:544–556, 1969

POSEY RE, RITCHIE EB: Metastatic calcinosis cutis with renal hyperparathyroidism. Arch Dermatol 95:505–508, 1967

PURSLEY TV, PRINCE MJ, CHAUSMER AB et al: Cutaneous mani-festations of tumoral calcinosis. Arch Dermatol 115:1100–1102, 1979

PUTKONEN T, WANGEL GA: Renal hyperparathyroidism with metastatic calcification of the skin. Dermatologica 118:127–144, 1959

REICH H: Das Teutschlaender-Syndrom. Hautarzt 14:462–468, 1963

SHAPIRO L, PLATT N, TORRES-RODRIGUEZ VM: Idiopathic calcinosis of the scrotum. Arch Dermatol 102:199–204, 1970

SHMUNES E, WOOD MG: Subepidermal calcified nodules. Arch Dermatol 105:593–597, 1972

STEIGLEDER GK, ELSCHNER H: Lokalisierte Calcinosis. Hautarzt 8:127–128, 1957

TEZUKA T: Cutaneous calculus: Its pathogenesis. Dermatologica 161:191–199, 1980

VELAYOS EE, MASI AT, STEVENS MB et al: The "CREST" syndrome. Comparison with systemic sclerosis (scleroderma). Arch Intern Med 139:1240–1249, 1979

WERMER P, KUSCHNER M, RILEY EA: Reversible metastatic calci-fication associated with excessive milk and alkali intake. Am J Med 14:108–115, 1953

WHEELER CE, CURTIS AC, CAWLEY EP et al: Soft tissue calcification with special reference to its occurrence in the collagen diseases. Ann Intern Med 36:1050–1075, 1952

WHITING DA, SIMSON IW, KALLMEYER JC et al: Unusual cutaneous lesions in tumoral calcinosis. Arch Dermatol 102:465–473, 1970

WILSON CW, WINGFIELD WL, TOONE EC JR: Vitamin D poisoning with metastatic calcification. Am J Med 14:116–123, 1953

WINER LH: Solitary congenital nodular calcification of the skin. Arch Dermatol Syph 66:204–211, 1952

WINKELMANN RK, KEATING FR JR: Cutaneous vascular calcifica-tion, gangrene and hyperparathyroidism. Br J Dermatol 83:263–268, 1970

WOODS B, KELLAWAY TD: Cutaneous calculi. Br J Dermatol 75:1–11, 1963

Gout

GOTTRON HA, KORTING GW: Chronische Hautgicht. Arch Klin Exp Dermatol 204:483–499, 1957

LICHTENSTEIN L, SCOTT HW, LEVIN MH: Pathologic changes in gout. Am J Pathol 32:871–895, 1956

O'DUFFY JD, HUNDER GG, KELLY PJ: Decreasing prevalence of tophaceous gout. Mayo Clin Proc 50:227–228, 1975

REIF MC, CONSTANTINER A, LEVITT MF: Chronic gouty nephrop-athy: A vanishing syndrome? N Engl J Med 304:535–536, 1981

SEEGMILLER JE: Skin manifestations of gout. In Fitzpatrick TB, Eisen AZ, Wolff K et al (eds): Dermatology in General Medicine, 2nd ed, pp 1106–1112. New York, McGraw-Hill, 1979

YÜ TF, BERGER L, DORPH DJ et al: Renal function in gout. V. Factors influencing the renal hemodynamics. Am J Med 67:766–771, 1979

Ochronosis

ATWOOD HD, CLIFTON S, MITCHELL RE: A histological, histochem-ical and ultrastructural study of dermal ochronosis. Pathology 3:115–121, 1971

FINDLAY GH, MORRISON JGL, SIMSON IW: Exogeneous ochronosis and pigmented colloid milium from hydroquinone bleaching creams. Br J Dermatol 93:613–622, 1975

FRIDERICH H, NIKOLOWSKI W: Endogene Ochronose. Arch Der-matol Syph (Berlin) 192:273–289, 1951

KUTTY MK, IGBAL QM, TEH EC: Ochronotic arthropathy. Arch Pathol 96:100–103, 1973

LAYMON CW: Ochronosis. Arch Dermatol 67:553–560, 1953

LICHTENSTEIN L, KAPLAN L: Hereditary ochronosis. Am J Pathol 30:99–125, 1954

TELLER H, WINKLER K: Zur Klinik und Histopathologie der endogenen Ochronose. Hautarzt 24:537–543, 1973

ZANNONI VG, MALAWISTA SE, LA DU BN: Studies on ochronosis. II. Studies on benzoquinone-acetic acid, a probable intermediate in the connective tissue pigmentation of alcaptonuria. Arthritis Rheum 5:547–556, 1962

Mucinoses

ARCHIBALD GC, CALVERT HT: Hypothyroidism and lichen myxoedematosus. Arch Dermatol 113:684–685, 1977

BRAUN-FALCO O, WEIDNER F: Skleromyxödem Arndt-Gottron mit Knochenmarks-Plasmocytose und Myositis. Arch Belges Dermatol Syph 26:193–217, 1970

CARLI-BASSET C, LORETTE G, ALISON Y et al: Apparition retardée d'une globuline monoclonale au cours d'une mucinose papuleuse. Ann Dermatol Venereol 106:175–179, 1979

CAWLEY EP, LUPTON CH JR, WHELLER CE et al: Examination of normal and myxedematous skin. Arch Dermatol 76:537–543, 1957

CHEUNG HS, NICOLOFF JT, KAMIEL MB et al: Stimulation of fibroblast biosynthetic activity by serum of patients with pretibial myxedema. J Invest Dermatol 71:12–17, 1978

COHN BA, WHEELER CE JR, BRIGGAMAN RA: Scleredema adultorum of Buschke and diabetes mellitus. Arch Dermatol 101:27–35, 1970

CURTIS AC, SHULAK BM: Scleredema adultorum. Arch Dermatol 92:526–541, 1965

DALTON JE, SEIDELL MA: Studies on lichen myxedematosus (papular mucinosis). Arch Dermatol 67:194–209, 1954

DANBY FW, DANBY CWE, PRUZANSKI W: Papular mucinosis with IgG (kappa) M component. Can Med Assoc J 114:920–922, 1976

FELDMAN P, SHAPIRO L, PICK AI et al: Scleromyxedema. Arch Dermatol 99:51–56, 1969

FLEISCHMAJER R, FALUDI G, KROL S: Scleredema and diabetes mellitus. Arch Dermatol 101:21–26, 1970

FLEISCHMAJER R, PERLISH JS: Glycosaminoglycans in scleroderma and scleredema. J Invest Dermatol 58:129–132, 1972

GABRILOVE JL, LUDWIG AW: The histogenesis of myxedema. J Clin Endocrinol 17:925–931, 1957

GREENBERG LM, GEPPERT C, WORTHEN HG et al: Scleredema "adultorum" in children. Pediatrics 32:1044–1054, 1963

HARDIE RA, HUNTER JAA, URBANIAK S et al: Spontaneous resolution of lichen myxedematosus. Br J Dermatol 100:727–730, 1979

HARDMEIER T, VOGEL A: Elektronenmikroskopische Befunde beim Skleromyxödem Arndt-Gottron. Arch Klin Exp Dermatol 237:722–736, 1970

HERZBERG J: Das REM-Syndrom. Z Hautkr 56:1317–1325, 1981

HILL TG, CRAWFORD JN, ROGERS CC: Successful management of lichen myxedematosus. Arch Dermatol 112:67–69, 1976

HOLUBAR K, MACH KW: Scleredema (Buschke). Acta Derm Venereol (Stockh) 47:102–110, 1967

HOWSDEN SM, HERNDON JH JR, FREEMAN RG: Lichen myxedematosus. Arch Dermatol 111:1325–1330, 1975

JAMES K, FUDENBERG H, EPSTEIN WL et al: Studies on a unique diagnostic serum globulin in papular mucinosis (lichen myxedematosus). Clin Exp Immunol 2:153–166, 1967

JOHNSON WC, HELWIG EB: Cutaneous focal mucinosis. Arch Dermatol 93:13–20, 1966

KOCSARD E, MUNRO VF: Reticular erythematous mucinosis (REM syndrome) of Steigleder. Aust J Dermatol 19:121–124, 1978

KONRAD K, BRENNER W, PEHAMBERGER H: Ultrastructural and immunological findings in Graves' disease with pretibial myxedema. J Cutan Pathol 7:99–108, 1980

KORTING GW, NÜRNBERGER F, MÜLLER G: Zur Ultrastruktur der Bindegewebszellen beim Myxoedema circumscriptum praetibiale. Arch Klin Exp Dermatol 229:381–389, 1967

KÖVARY PM, VAKILZADEH F, MACHER E et al: Monoclonal gammopathy in scleredema. Arch Dermatol 117:536–539, 1981

KRAKOWSKI A, COVO J, BERLIN C: Diabetic scleredema. Dermatologica 146:193–198, 1973

KREBS A, MÜLLER A: Lichen myxoedematosus und multiples Myelom vom Typ IgG/kappa. Hautarzt 31:649–653, 1980

LAI A FAT RFM, SUURMOND D, RADL J et al: Scleromyxedema (lichen myxedematosus) associated with a paraprotein, IgG₁ of the type kappa. Br J Dermatol 88:107–116, 1973

LAWRENCE DA, TYE MJ, LISS M: Immunochemical analysis of the basic immunoglobulin in papular mucinosis. Immunochemistry 9:41–49, 1972

LEINWAND I: Generalized scleredema. Report with autopsy findings. Ann Intern Med 34:226–238, 1951

LYNCH PJ, MAIZE JC, LISSON JC: Pretibial myxedema and nonthyrotoxic thyroid disease. Arch Dermatol 107:107–111, 1973

MCCARTHY JT, OSSERMAN E, LOMBARDO PC et al: An abnormal serum globulin in lichen myxedematosus. Arch Dermatol 89:446–450, 1964

MONTGOMERY H, UNDERWOOD LJ: Lichen myxedematosus (differentiation from cutaneous myxedemas or mucoid states). J Invest Dermatol 20:213–236, 1953

MORISON WL, SHEA CR, PARRISH JA: Reticular erythematous mucinosis syndrome. Arch Dermatol 115:1340–1342, 1979

NIEBAUER G, EBNER H: Skleroedema (Buschke). Dermatol Monatsschr 156:940–941, 1970

PERRY HO, KIERLAND RR, MONTGOMERY H: Plaque-like form of cutaneous mucinosis. Arch Dermatol 82:980–985, 1960a

PERRY HO, MONTGOMERY H, STICKNEY JM: Further observations on lichen myxedematosus. Ann Intern Med 53:955–969, 1960b

PIPER W, HARDMEIER T, SCHÄFER E: Das Skleromyxödem Arndt-Gottron: Eine paraproteinämische Erkrankung. Schweiz Med Wochenschr 97:829–838, 1967

PROPPE A, BECKER V, HARDMEIER T: Skleromyxödem Arndt-Gottron und Plasmocytom. Hautarzt 20:53–59, 1969

REICHENBERGER M: Betrachtungen zum Skleroedema adultorum Buschke. Hautarzt 15:339–345, 1964

REUTER MJ: Histopathology of the skin in myxedema. Arch Dermatol Syph 24:55–71, 1931

ROWELL NR, WAITE A, SCOTT DG: Multiple serum protein abnormalities in lichen myxedematosus. Br J Dermatol 81:753–758, 1969

RUDNER EJ, MEHREGAN A, PINKUS H: Scleromyxedema. Arch Dermatol 93:3–12, 1966

RUFLI T: REM-Syndrom. Dermatologica 159:413–415, 1979

SAWADA Y, OHASHI M: Scleromyxedema. J Dermatol (Tokyo) 7:207–212, 1980

SCHERMER DR, ROENIGK HH JR, SCHUMACHER OP et al: Relationship of long-acting thyroid stimulator to pretibial myxedema. Arch Dermatol 102:62–67, 1970

SCHNYDER UW, KAUFMANN J: Skleromyxoedema Arndt-Gottron, Plasmozytom (Ig-Kappa-Typ). Dermatologica 159:407–409, 1979

SHAPIRO CM, FRETZIN D, NORRIS S: Papular mucinosis. JAMA 214:2052–2054, 1970

SMITH NP, SANDERSON KV, CROW KD: Reticular erythematous mucinosis syndrome. Clin Exp Dermatol 1:99–103, 1976

STEIGLEDER GK: Plaque-artige Form der cutanen Mucinose (PCM) und retikuläre erythematöse Mucinosis (REM-Syndrom). Z Hautkr 50:25–32, 1975

STEIGLEDER GK, GARTMANN H, LINKER U: REM-syndrome: Reticular erythematous mucinosis (round-cell erythematosis), a new entity? Br J Dermatol 91:191–199, 1974

STEVANOVIĆ DV: Mucinosis in erythematous plaques of Steigleder and Perry. Dermatol Monatsschr 166:736–746, 1980

SUURMOND D, VAN FURTH R: Scleromyxedema (lichen myxedematosus) and paraproteinemia. Dermatologica 138:320–327, 1969

VALLEE BL: Scleredema: A systemic disease. N Engl J Med 235:207–213, 1946

Mucopolysaccharidoses

BELCHER RW: Ultrastructure and cytochemistry of lymphocytes in the genetic mucopolysaccharidoses. Arch Pathol 93:1–7, 1972a

BELCHER RW: Ultrastructure of the skin in the genetic mucopolysaccharidoses. Arch Pathol 94:511–518, 1972b

BELCHER RW: Ultrastructure and function of eccrine glands in the mucopolysaccharidoses. Arch Pathol 96:339–341, 1973

DE CLOUX RJ, FRIEDERICI HHR: Ultrastructural studies of the skin in Hurler's syndrome. Arch Pathol 88:350–358, 1969

FREEMAN RG: A pathological basis for the cutaneous papules of mucopolysaccharidosis II (the Hunter syndrome) J Cutan Pathol 4:318–328, 1977

HAMBRICK GW JR, SCHEIE HG: Studies of the skin in Hurler's syndrome. Arch Dermatol 85:455–471, 1962

HORIUCHI R, ISHIKAWA H, ISHII Y et al: Mucopolysaccharidosis with special reference to Scheie syndrome. J Dermatol (Tokyo) 3:171–178, 1976

LASSER A, CARTER DM, MAHONEY MJ: Ultrastructure of the skin in mucopolysaccharidoses. Arch Pathol 99:173–176, 1975

MCKUSICK VA: The nosology of the mucopolysaccharidoses. Am J Med 47:730–747, 1969

PINELL SR, MCKUSICK VA: The genetic mucopolysaccharides. In Fitzpatrick TB, Eisen AZ, Wolff K et al (eds): Dermatology in General Practice, 2nd ed, pp 1155–1159. New York, McGraw-Hill, 1979

PRYSTOWSKY SD, MAUMENEE IH, FREEMAN RG et al: A cutaneous marker in the Hunter syndrome. Arch Dermatol 113:602–605, 1977

Acanthosis Nigricans, Confluent and Reticulated Papillomatosis

ACKERMAN AB, LANTIS LR: Acanthosis nigricans associated with Hodgkin's disease. Arch Dermatol 95:202–205, 1967

BROWN J, WINKELMANN RK: Acanthosis nigricans: A study of 90 cases. (Review) Medicine (Baltimore) 47:33–51, 1968

CURTH HO: Classification of acanthosis nigricans. Int J Dermatol 15:592–593, 1976

CURTH HO: Does the cancer accompanying acanthosis nigricans contain endocrine cells of the APUD series? Acta Derm Venerol (Stockh) 59:261–263, 1979

GARROTT TC: Malignant acanthosis nigricans associated with osteogenic sarcoma. Arch Dermatol 106:384–385, 1972

GOUGEROT H, CARTEAUD A: Papillomatose pigmentée innominée. Bull Soc Fr Dermatol Syph 34:719–721, 1927

HAGE E, HAGE J: Malignant acanthosis nigricans: A para-endocrine syndrome. Acta Derm Venereol (Stockh) 57:169–172, 1977

HAMILTON D, TAVAFOGHI V, SHAFER JC et al: Confluent and reticulated papillomatosis of Gougerot and Carteaud. J Am Acad Dermatol 2:401–410, 1980

HOLLINGSWORTH DR, AMATRUDA TT JR: Acanthosis nigricans and obesity. An endocrine abnormality? Arch Intern Med 124:481–487, 1969

JACOBS MI, RIGEL DS: Acanthosis nigricans and the sign of Leser-Trélat associated with adenocarcinoma of the gallbladder. Cancer 48:325–328, 1981

KESTEN BM, JAMES HD: Pseudoatrophoderma colli, acanthosis nigricans, and confluent and reticular papillomatosis. Arch Dermatol 75:525–542, 1957

MIKHAIL GR, FACHNIE DM, DRUKKER BH et al: Generalized malignant acanthosis nigricans. Arch Dermatol 115:201–202, 1979

ROBERTS SDB, LACHAPELLE JM: Confluent and reticulate papillomatosis (Gougerot-Carteaud) and Pityrosporon orbiculare. Br J Dermatol 81:841–845, 1969

RONCHESE F: Keratoses, cancer and "the sign of Leser-Trélat." Cancer 18:1003–1006, 1965

SCHWARTZ RA, BURGESS GH: Florid cutaneous papillomatosis. Arch Dermatol 114:1803–1806, 1978

THOMSEN K: Confluent and reticulated papillomatosis (Gougerot-Carteaud). Acta Derm Venereol (Stockh) 59, Suppl 85:185–187, 1979

YESUDIAN P, KAMALAM S, RAZACK A: Confluent and reticulated papillomatosis (Gougerot-Carteaud). Acta Derm Venereol (Stockh) 53:381–384, 1973

Idiopathic Hemochromatosis

BUCKLEY WR: Localized argyria. Arch Dermatol 88:531–539, 1963

CARTWRIGHT GE, EDWARDS CQ, KRAVITZ K et al: Hereditary hemochromatosis. Phenotypic expression of the disease. N Engl J Med 301:175–179, 1979

CAWLEY EP, HSU YT, WOOD BT et al: Hemochromatosis of the skin. Arch Dermatol 100:1–6, 1969

CROSBY WH: Hemochromatosis. Arch Intern Med 133:1072, 1974

EDWARDS CQ, CARROLL M, BRAY P et al: Hereditary hemochromatosis. N Engl J Med 297:7–13, 1977

FELLER ER, PONT A, WANDS JR et al: Familial hemochromatosis. N Engl J Med 296:1422–1426, 1977

HEILMEYER L: Pathogenesis of hemochromatosis. Medicine (Baltimore) 46:209–215, 1967

LEYDEN JL, LOCKSHIN NA, KRIEBEL S: The black keratinous cyst. A sign of hemochromatosis. Arch Dermatol 106:379–381, 1972

MILDER MS, COOK JD, STRAY S et al: Idiopathic hemochromatosis, an interim report. Medicine (Baltimore) 59:34–49, 1980

PERDRUP A, POULSEN H: Hemochromatosis and vitiligo. Arch Dermatol 90:34–37, 1964

ROBERT P, ZÜRCHER H: Pigmentstudien. I. Mitteilung. Über den Einfluss von Schwermetallverbindungen, Hämin, Vitaminen, mikrobiellen Toxinen, Hormonen und weiteren Stoffen auf die Dopamelaninbildung in vitro und die Pigmentbildung in vivo. Dermatologica 100:217–241, 1950

ROWE JW, WANDS JR, MEZEY E et al: Familial hemochromatosis: Characteristics of the precirrhotic stage in a large kindred. Medicine (Baltimore) 56:197–211, 1977

SCHEINBERG IH: The genetics of hemochromatosis. Arch Intern Med 132:126–128, 1973

WEINTRAUB LR, DEMIS DJ, CONRAD ME et al: Iron excretion by the skin. Selective localization of iron[59] in epithelial cells. Am J Pathol 46:121–127, 1965

Vitamin A Deficiency (Phrynoderma)

BESSEY OA, WOLBACH SB: Vitamin A, physiology and pathology. JAMA 110:2072–2080, 1938

FASAL P: Clinical manifestations of vitamin deficiencies as observed in the Federated Malay States. Arch Dermatol Syph 50:160–166, 1944

FRAZIER CN, HU C: Nature and distribution according to age of cutaneous manifestations of vitamin A deficiency. Arch Dermatol Syph 33:825–852, 1936

WECHSLER HL: Vitamin A deficiency following small-bowel bypass surgery for obesity. Arch Dermatol 115:73–75, 1979

Pellagra, Hartnup Disease

ASHURST PJ: Hydroa vacciniforme occurring in association with Hartnup disease. Br J Dermatol 81:486–492, 1969

BARON DN, DENT CE, HARRIS H et al: Hereditary pellagralike skin rash with temporary cerebellar ataxia, constant renal aminoaciduria and other bizarre chemical features. Lancet 2:421–428, 1956

CASTIELLO RJ, LYNCH PJ: Pellagra and the carcinoid syndrome. Arch Dermatol 105:574–577, 1972

CLODI PH, DEUTSCH E, NIEBAUER G: Krankheitsbild mit poikilodermieartigen Hautveränderungen, Aminoacidurie und Indolaceturie. Arch Klin Exp Dermatol 218:165–176, 1964

COHEN LK, GEORGE W, SMITH R: Isoniazid-induced acne and pellagra. Arch Dermatol 109:377–381, 1974

DENT CE: Hartnup disease. An inborn error of metabolism. Arch Dis Child 32:363–372, 1957

FAZEKAS A, SZEGÖ L, MAACZ J: Beiträge zum Krankheitsbild des Hartnup-Syndroms. Dermatol Wochenschr 153:751–760, 1967

HALVORSEN L, HALVORSEN S: Hartnup disease. Pediatrics 31:29–34, 1963

MOORE RA, SPIES TD, COOPER ZK: Histopathology of the skin in pellagra. Arch Dermatol Syph 46:106–111, 1942

STRATIGOS JD, KATSAMBAS A: Pellagra: A still existing disease. Br J Dermatol 96:99–106, 1977

Oculocutaneous Tyrosinosis

GOLDSMITH LA, KANG E, BIENFANG DC et al: Tyrosinemia with plantar and palmar keratosis and keratitis. J Pediatr 83:798–805, 1973

HUNZIKER N: Richner-Hanhart syndrome and tyrosinemia type II. Dermatologica 160:180–189, 1980

LARRÈGUE M, DE GIACOMONI P, ODIÈVRE P et al: Modification des kératinocytes au cours de la tyrosinose oculo-cutanée: Syndrome de Richner-Hanhart. Ann Dermatol Venereol 107:1023–1030, 1980

REHÁK A, SELIM MM, YADAV G: Richner-Hanhart syndrome (tyrosinaemia-II) (report of four cases without ocular involvement). Br J Dermatol 104:469–475, 1981

ZALESKI WA, HILL A, KUSHNIRUK W: Skin lesions in tyrosinosis: Response to dietary treatment. Br J Dermatol 88:335–340, 1973

24 Pigmentary Disorders

ADDISON'S DISEASE

Addison's disease represents a hypofunction of the adrenal cortex and is characterized by weakness, hypotension, and hyperpigmentation of the skin and oral mucosa. In some cases, hyperpigmentation is the initial symptom (Clerkin and Sayegh).

The hyperpigmentation is most pronounced in areas of the skin exposed to the sun, at sites of pressure, and on the genitalia. Pigmentation of the oral mucosa usually is patchy.

Histopathology. The histologic picture is not diagnostic. The hyperpigmentation is the result of an increase in the activity of melanocytes without an increase in their number (Lerner). Increased amounts of melanin are present in the epidermis and occasionally also in the upper dermis. In the epidermis, the melanin is located chiefly in the basal cells but may be found also in the upper layers of the stratum malpighii. In the upper dermis, a moderate number of melanin-laden macrophages (melanophages) may be present (Montgomery and O'Leary).

Histogenesis. Most commonly, Addison's disease is the result of an idiopathic atrophy of the adrenal glands, probably on an autoimmune basis. This explains the occasional association of the disease with other autoimmune diseases. Other causes of adrenal hypofunction are damage to the adrenal glands by tuberculosis, metastatic carcinoma, and several deep fungus infections, particularly paracoccidioidomycosis and histoplasmosis (see pp. 339 and 344).

The diagnosis of Addison's disease is established by the failure of the adrenal cortex to respond adequately to stimulation by intravenously administered adrenocorticotropic hormone (ACTH). There is not only a subnormal increment in the plasma cortisol level but also an inadequate increase in the urinary output of 17-ketosteroids and 17-hydroxycorticosteroids (Clerkin and Sayegh).

The hyperpigmentation in Addison's disease is caused by an increased release of melanocyte-stimulating hormone (MSH) from the pituitary gland. Since the damaged adrenal glands in Addison's disease respond weakly to stimulation by ACTH, the pituitary gland, as a compensatory phenomenon, increases its output of ACTH. The overproduction of MSH is due to the fact that the synthesis and secretion of ACTH and MSH are controlled by a common mechanism (Abe et al).

Differential Diagnosis. A diagnosis of Addison's disease cannot be made from histologic sections, because the same histologic picture is observed in nonspecific hyperpigmentation of the skin and in persons with naturally dark skin.

ALBINISM

Albinism, also referred to as oculocutaneous albinism, shows a generalized lack of pigmentation of the skin and the hair from birth on. In addition, the eyes show lack of pigmentation of their fundi, translucent irides, and nystagmus. The condition is recessively inherited.

There are two types of albinism: a tyrosinase-positive type, in which the epidermal melanocytes are dopa-positive, and a tyrosinase-negative type, in which the melanocytes are dopa-negative. The two types are easily distinguished by the incubation of plucked anagen hair bulbs in a solution of tyrosine or dopa. In the tyrosinase-positive type, the hair bulbs darken on incubation (Kugelman and Van Scott; King et al). In the other type, the melanocytes do not darken (Witkop et al; Jung and Anton-Lamprecht). Patients with dopa-positive epidermal melanocytes may show melanin pigmentation in the form of ephelides in sun-exposed areas of the skin (Tsuji and Saito); in the course of their lives, these persons may acquire a slight capacity for pigmentation of the skin, hair, and eyes, whereas patients with dopa-negative melanocytes fail to form pigment throughout their lives (Jung and Anton-Lamprecht).

Histopathology. Histologic examination shows the presence of basal "clear cells" in both types of albinism; however, silver stains fail to show any melanin. In patients with the dopa-positive type of albinism, the epidermal melanocytes form pigment if sections of skin are incubated with dopa (Kugelman and Van Scott; Tsuji and Saito) or if epidermal scrapings are incubated with tyrosine solution (Kugelman and Van Scott); in contrast, in patients with the dopa-negative type of albinism, the epidermal melanocytes do not form pigment.

Histogenesis. *Electron microscopic examination* in albinism shows normally structured melanocytes in the epidermis. In tyrosinase-positive albinism, some melanosomes contain melanin, thus representing stage III and IV melanosomes (Tsuji and Saito). In contrast, in tyrosinase-negative albinism, the melanosomes contain no melanin and are present as stage I and II premelanosomes (Hishida); and, even though prolonged stimulation in vivo by ultraviolet light leads to an increase in the number of melanocytes in the epidermis as well as to an increase in the number of melanosomes within the melanocytes, the melanosomes remain devoid of melanin (Jung and Anton-Lamprecht).

The absence of tyrosinase activity in tyrosinase-negative albinism represents a deficiency in this enzyme. However, the defect in tyrosinase-positive albinism is not clear. Since the tyrosinase is kinetically normal, the defect must involve some other step in melanin synthesis, such as substrate transport or production of an inhibitor (King et al).

PIEBALDISM (PATTERNED LEUKODERMA)

In piebaldism, an autosomally dominant disorder, one finds irregularly shaped areas without pigmentation that are present from birth and are associated in about 85% of the cases with a white forelock arising from a depigmented area in the center of the forehead. The cutaneous areas lacking pigmentation have a predilection for the ventral skin, that is, the center of the face, the ventral chest, and the abdomen. Small islands of hyperpigmentation, 1 cm to 5 cm in diameter, are present, usually within the depigmented areas (Jimbow et al). The condition used to be called partial albinism, but this term is no longer used because of the difference in pathogenesis between oculocutaneous albinism and piebaldism.

A variant of piebaldism is the *Klein–Waardenburg syndrome*, also dominantly inherited, in which one observes lateral displacement of the inner canthi of the eyes, heterochromia of the irides, and congenital deafness. About half of the patients have a white forelock, and about 12% have patches of depigmentation from birth (Reed et al).

Histopathology. The depigmented skin and hair show absence of melanin and a negative dopa reaction. The islands of hyperpigmentation contain dopa-positive melanocytes in normal numbers (Jimbow et al). In epidermal sheets stained with adenosine triphosphatase, the number of Langerhans cells is the same in normal and depigmented skin (Bonerandi et al).

Histogenesis. *Electron microscopic examination* of the depigmented skin usually reveals a complete absence of melanocytes; in contrast, Langerhans cells are normal in appearance and distribution (Perrot et al). In some instances only, an occasional melanocyte is seen with unmelanized elipsoidal or spherical melanosomes (Breathnach et al; Jimbow et al).

The small islands of hyperpigmentation show within melanocytes and keratinocytes some normal ellipsoidal, lamellated melanosomes but largely abnormal, spherical, granular melanosomes (Jimbow et al).

VITILIGO

Vitiligo represents an acquired patchy loss of pigment of the skin. The patches are sharply though irregularly demarcated and are often surrounded by hyperpigmented skin. The areas may slowly increase in size. The scalp hair and eyelashes are only rarely affected.

In the *Vogt–Koyanagi–Harada syndrome*, an aseptic meningitis is often the initial symptom, followed by uveitis and dysacousia. In a high percentage of the patients, patches of vitiligo involving the skin and frequently also the eyelashes and scalp develop. Alopecia areata is often also present (Howsden et al).

Histopathology. The essential process in vitiligo is the destruction of melanocytes. With silver stains or the dopa reaction, long-standing lesions of vitiligo reveal no melanocytes. Early lesions and the peripheral zone of enlarging lesions that are hypopigmented rather than completely depigmented still show a few dopa-positive melanocytes and some melanin granules in the basal layer (Brown et al). At the border of the patches of vitiligo, the melanocytes often appear large and possess long dendritic processes filled with melanin granules. The presence of a dermal lymphocytic infiltrate at the border of the depigmented areas has been described by some authors (Bazex et al; Klaus and Moellmann; Nordlund et al, 1980).

Histogenesis. *Electron microscopic studies* have confirmed the absence of melanocytes in areas of long-standing vitiligo (Birbeck et al; Żelickson and Mottaz). In the hypopigmented peripheral zone, most melanocytes show signs of degeneration (Morohashi et al). No full agreement exists with regard to the number and distribution of Langerhans cells. Some observers have noted an increase in the number of Langerhans cells in the vitiliginous epidermis (Riley; Zelickson and Mottaz; Klaus and Moellmann). Others have noted no increase in the total number of Langerhans cells but a shift toward a location in the basal cell layer (Birbeck et al; Mishima et al). However, in a thorough study using adenosine triphosphatase activity for the demonstration of Langerhans cells in epidermal sheets, no increase in the concentration of Langerhans cells was found in areas of vitiligo (Brown et al). Furthermore, it was pointed out that, in regions of thin epidermis, Langerhans cells frequently occupy a position close to or even in apposition to the basement membrane zone both in normal and in vitiliginous skin.

It appears likely that vitiligo represents an autoimmune phenomenon. In favor of this view are the occasional coexistence of vitiligo and idiopathic uveitis (Nordlund et al, 1981) and the frequent presence of vitiligo in the Vogt–Koyanagi–Harada syndrome. The Vogt–Koyanagi–Harada syndrome represents an autoimmune reaction not only to uveal melanin but probably also to meningeal, cochleal, and epidermal melanin, resulting in the destruction of melanin-producing cells (Howsden et al; Nordlund et al, 1980). Also, the occasional presence of a lymphocytic infiltrate in which some of the lymphocytes are in contact either with melanocytes (Bazex et al) or with Langerhans cells (Klaus and Moellmann) suggests an immunologic phenomenon.

CHÉDIAK–HIGASHI SYNDROME

The Chédiak–Higashi syndrome is a rare disorder, inherited as an autosomal recessive trait, that is characterized by the presence of giant granules in the granulocytes and monocytes of the peripheral blood. Patients with this disorder have a greatly increased susceptibility to bacterial infections. In early childhood, an "accelerated phase" tends to develop that is associated with pancytopenia, lymphadenopathy, and splenomegaly (White and Clawson). In some patients, lymphomalike infiltra-

tions develop. Death usually occurs before the age of 10 as the result either of infection or of complications of the "accelerated phase."

The skin and hair of patients with this syndrome are very fair, and the eyes show translucency of the irides with photophobia and nystagmus, causing a considerable clinical resemblance to oculocutaneous albinism (Blume and Wolff).

Histopathology. In sections stained with silver, the epidermis shows sparse, irregularly shaped, large melanin granules (Moran and Estevez). The distribution of these granules is quite haphazard, with fairly numerous granules in some areas and no granules in others. Similar large, irregularly shaped melanin granules are scattered through the upper dermis within melanophages (Bedoya). The hairs also contain large, clumped, sparse melanin granules.

Blood smears, on staining with the Wright or Giemsa stain, reveal numerous coarse granules in the neutrophils and monocytes (Moran and Estevez).

Histogenesis. *Electron microscopic examination* reveals within melanocytes giant particles of irregular shape surrounded by a limiting membrane, representing giant melanosomes. They further increase in size by fusing with other giant particles (Zelickson et al). Within the giant particles, one observes a granular matrix and filaments showing periodicity and varying degrees of pigmentation indicative of melanosomes (Deprez et al). The largest particles show signs of degeneration leading to vacuolization and the formation of residual bodies (Zelickson et al). In addition, normal melanosomes are present in the melanocytes and are transferred to keratinocytes; however, there, they are packaged into abnormally large phagolysosomes (Zelickson et al). Similar abnormally large, membrane-bound phagolysosomes are found in the hair (Blume and Wolff). It is likely that the giant melanosomes in melanocytes and the giant phagolysosomes in keratinocytes form because of a defect in their membranes (Zelickson et al). The fact that, within the keratinocytes, the melanosomes, rather than being dispersed, lie within relatively few large phagolysosomes causes the hypopigmentation.

The giant granules present in neutrophils and monocytes also form as a result of a membrane defect. They develop by the fusion of primary lysosomes with one another and with cytoplasmic material, resulting in the formation of huge secondary lysosomes, or phagolysosomes (White and Clawson). Even though microorganisms are phagocytized into phagocytic vacuoles in a normal fashion, their inactivation is delayed or prevented because of the unavailability of primary lysosomes to discharge their bactericidal enzymes into the phagocytic vacuoles.

RETICULATE PIGMENTED DERMATOSIS OF THE FLEXURES

A dominantly inherited dermatosis also referred to as Dowling–Degos disease, reticulate pigmented dermatosis of the flexures usually does not start until adulthood. It then spreads slowly without causing any symptoms. The lesions consist of heavily pigmented macules arranged in a reticular pattern with a tendency to coalesce in the center of the lesions. Flexural areas are predominantly involved, particularly the axillae, the groins, and, in women, the inframammary regions (Wilson Jones and Grice; Howell and Freeman). In later life, wide areas of the skin can be affected.

Histopathology. The histologic findings are characteristic, consisting of thin, branching, heavily melanized epidermal downward proliferations arising from the lower border of the epidermis as well as from the infundibulum of follicles (Wilson Jones and Grice). In some instances, small horn cysts within the epidermal proliferations cause an appearance closely resembling that of an adenoid seborrheic wart (Smith et al). In general, epidermal involvement predominates in pigmented areas, and follicular involvement in nonpigmented areas (Bardach).

Histogenesis. On *electron microscopy*, the melanocytes show an increase in the number of melanosomes, the average size of which does not differ from those seen in normal Caucasoid skin. In the keratinocytes, however, the melanosomes are only rarely seen aggregated in membrane-bound spaces as seen in Caucasoid skin; instead, they appear largely dispersed as in black skin (Howell and Freeman; Grosshans et al).

BIBLIOGRAPHY

Addison's Disease
ABE K, NICHOLSON E, LIDDLE GW et al: Radioimmunoassay of beta-MSH in human plasma and tissues. J Clin Invest 46:1609–1616, 1967

CLERKIN EP, SAYEGH S: Melanosis as the initial symptom of Addison's disease. Lahey Clin Found Bull 15:173–176, 1966

LERNER AB: Melanin pigmentation. Am J Med 19:902–924, 1955

MONTGOMERY H, O'LEARY PA: Pigmentation of the skin in Addison's disease, acanthosis nigricans and hemochromatosis. Arch Dermatol Syph 21:970–984, 1930

Albinism
HISHIDA H: Electron microscopic studies of melanosomes in oculo-cutaneous albinism. Jpn J Dermatol (Series A) 83:119, 1973

JUNG EG, ANTON-LAMPRECHT I: Untersuchungen über Albinismus. Arch Dermatol Forsch 240:123–137, 1971

KING RA, OLDS DP, WITKOP CJ: Characterization of human hair bulb tyrosinase: Properties of normal and albino enzyme. J Invest Dermatol 71:136–139, 1978

KUGELMAN TP, VAN SCOTT EJ: Tyrosinase activity in melanocytes of human albinos. J Invest Dermatol 37:73–76, 1961

TSUJI T, SAITO T: Multiple naevocellular naevi in brothers with albinism. Br J Dermatol 98:685–692, 1978

WITKOP CJ JR, WHITE J, NANCE WE: Heterogeneity in human albinism. (Abstr) J Invest Dermatol 54:100, 1970

Piebaldism
BONERANDI JJ, BARAN R, BRETON A et al: Piebaldisme. Étude anatomo-clinique et ultrastructurale de trois cas. Ann Dermatol Venereol 105:67–72, 1978

BREATHNACH AS, FITZPATRICK TB, WYLLIS LMA: Electron microscopy of melanocytes in human piebaldism. J Invest Dermatol 45:28–37, 1965

JIMBOW K, FITZPATRICK TB, SZABO G et al: Congenital circumscribed hypomelanosis: A characterization based on electron microscopic study of tuberous sclerosis, nevus depigmentosus, and piebaldism. J Invest Dermatol 64:50–62, 1975

PERROT H, ORTONNE JP, THIVOLET J: Ultrastructural study of leukodermic skin in Waardenburg-Klein syndrome. Acta Derm Venereol (Stockh) 57:195–200, 1977

REED WB, STONE VM, BODER E et al: Pigmentary disorders in association with congenital deafness. Arch Dermatol 95:176–186, 1967

Vitiligo
BAZEX A, BALAS D, BAZEX J: Maladie de Vogt-Koyanagi-Harada. Ann Dermatol Venereol 104:849–853, 1977

BIRBECK MS, BREATHNACH AS, EVERALL JD: An electron microscope study of basal melanocytes and high-level clear cells (Langerhans cells) in vitiligo. J Invest Dermatol 37:51–64, 1961

BROWN J, WINKELMANN RK, WOLFF K: Langerhans cells in vitiligo. J Invest Dermatol 49:386–390, 1967

HOWSDEN SM, HERNDON JH JR, FREEMAN RG: Vogt-Koyanagi-Harada syndrome and psoriasis. Arch Dermatol 108:395–398, 1973

KLAUS S, MOELLMANN G: Vitiligo. In: Proceedings of the First International Workshop on Vitiligo. J Invest Dermatol 71:165, 1978

MISHIMA Y, KAWASAKI H, PINKUS H: Dendritic cell dynamics in progressive depigmentations. Arch Dermatol Forsch 247:67–87, 1972

MOROHASHI M, HASHIMOTO K, GOODMAN TF JR et al: Ultrastructural studies of vitiligo, Vogt-Koyanagi syndrome, and incontinentia pigmenti achromians. Arch Dermatol 113:755–766, 1977

NORDLUND JJ, ALBERT D, FORGET B et al: Halo nevi and the Vogt-Koyanagi-Harada syndrome. Arch Dermatol 116:690–692, 1980

NORDLUND JJ, TAYLOR NT, ALBERT DM et al: The prevalence of vitiligo and poliosis in patients with uveitis. J Am Acad Dermatol 4:528–536, 1981

RILEY RA: A study of the distribution of epidermal dendritic cells in pigmented and unpigmented skin. J Invest Dermatol 48:28–38, 1967

ZELICKSON AS, MOTTAZ JH: Epidermal dendritic cells. Arch Dermatol 98:652–659, 1968

Chédiak–Higashi Syndrome
BEDOYA V: Pigmentary changes in Chédiak-Higashi syndrome. Br J Dermatol 85:336–347, 1971

BLUME RS, WOLFF SM: The Chédiak-Higashi syndrome: Studies in four patients and a review of the literature. Medicine (Baltimore) 51:247–280, 1972

DEPREZ P, LAURENT R, GRISCELLI C et al: La maladie de Chédiak-Higashi. Ann Dermatol Venereol 105:841–849, 1978

MORAN TJ, ESTEVEZ JM: Chédiak-Higashi disease. Arch Pathol 88:329–339, 1969

WHITE JG, CLAWSON CC: The Chédiak-Higashi syndrome: The nature of the giant neutrophil granules and their interactions with cytoplasm and foreign particulates. Am J Pathol 98:151–196, 1980

ZELICKSON AS, WINDHORST DB, WHITE JG et al: The Chédiak-Higashi syndrome: Formation of giant melanosomes and the basis of hypopigmentation. J Invest Dermatol 49:575–581, 1967

Reticulate Pigmented Anomaly of the Flexures

BARDACH HG: Morbus Dowling-Degos mit Beteiligung des Kapillitiums. Hautarzt 32:182–186, 1981

GROSSHANS E, GEIGER JM, HANAU D et al: Ultrastructure of early pigmentary changes in Dowling-Degos disease. J Cutan Pathol 7:77–87, 1980

HOWELL JB, FREEMAN RG: Reticular pigmented anomaly of the flexures. Arch Dermatol 114:400–403, 1978

SMITH EL, DOWLING GB, WILSON JONES E: Acquired axillary and inguinal pigmentation: An epidermal naevoid abnormality not to be confused with acanthosis nigricans. Br J Dermatol 85:295–296, 1971

WILSON JONES E, GRICE K: Reticulate pigmented anomaly of the flexures. Arch Dermatol 114:1150–1157, 1978

Connective Tissue Diseases

25

LUPUS ERYTHEMATOSUS

Two types of lupus erythematosus are generally recognized: discoid lupus erythematosus (DLE), and systemic lupus erythematosus (SLE). It is widely realized, however, that a division of lupus erythematosus into only two types represents an oversimplification. Yet subdivision into additional intermediate types has met with difficulties, since, like leprosy, lupus erythematosus represents a spectrum of clinical forms in which DLE and SLE can be regarded as polar expressions of disease activity (Provost, 1979a). One can recognize at least two intermediate types, disseminated DLE, which shows widespread discoid lesions and usually mild systemic involvement (Prystowsky and Gilliam; O'Loughlin et al, 1978a), and subacute cutaneous lupus erythematosus, which shows widespread erythematous, confluent, often annular or polycyclic, nonscarring cutaneous lesions in association with severe photosensitivity and mild systemic illness (Sontheimer et al; Maciejewski). Since the systemic lesions in these two types generally are mild, such cases almost always carry a good prognosis. The importance of adequate laboratory data for an evaluation of the seriousness of the illness and its prognosis has long been recognized. A combination of clinical and laboratory data was used in the "Criteria for the Classification of Systemic Lupus Erythematosus" set forth by the American Rheumatism Association (ARA) in 1972 (Cohen and Canoso). These criteria are still widely employed, even though they do not include important data, such as those relative to the antinuclear-antibody (ANA) titer, the concentration of serum anti-native deoxyribonucleic acid (DNA), the serum complement levels, renal biopsy changes, and cutaneous immuno-fluorescence findings (O'Loughlin et al, 1978a). The proposed criteria are based on 14 manifestations that include 21 items. A person is said to have SLE if any four or more of the following 14 manifestations are present serially or simultaneously (Cohen and Canoso):

1. Facial erythema
2. Discoid lupus
3. Raynaud's phenomen
4. Alopecia
5. Photosensitivity
6. Oral or nasopharyngeal ulcerations
7. Arthritis without deformity
8. Lupus erythematosus cells
9. Chronic false-positive serologic tests for syphilis
10. Profuse proteinuria exceeding 3.5 g/day
11. Cellular casts
12. One or both of the following: pleuritis, pericarditis
13. One or both of the following: psychosis, convulsions
14. One or more of the following: hemolytic anemia, white blood cell count of less than 4,000/mm^3, thrombocytopenia of less than 100,000/mm^3

Since only four manifestations are required for a diagnosis of SLE in this rather liberal interpretation, many cases of the two intermediate types qualify as instances of SLE.

On a histologic basis, differentiation between DLE and SLE generally is not possible, since early lesions of DLE may resemble those of SLE, and lesions with the histologic appearance of DLE can occur in SLE.

445

Discoid Lupus Erythematosus

Characteristically, the cutaneous lesions of DLE consist of well-defined, erythematous, slightly infiltrated, "discoid" patches that often show adherent thick scales and follicular plugging. In old lesions, one often sees atrophic scarring associated occasionally with verrucous hyperkeratosis, especially at the periphery of the lesions (Uitto et al). However, involution of the lesions without scarring can also occur (Bielicky and Trapl).

In many instances, the discoid cutaneous lesions are limited to the face, where the malar areas and the nose are affected predominantly. In addition, the scalp, ears, oral mucosa, and vermilion border of the lips may be involved.

In patients with *disseminated discoid lupus erythematosus,* discoid lesions are seen predominantly on the upper trunk and upper limbs, usually but not always in association with lesions on the head (O'Loughlin et al). SLE may eventually develop in some of these patients (Millard and Rowell). Although discoid cutaneous lesions are typical of DLE, they are also seen in as many as 14% of the patients with SLE (Estes and Christian).

In the so-called *subacute cutaneous lupus erythematosus,* which represents about 9% of all cases of lupus erythematosus, extensive erythematous, nonscarring lesions are present usually on the face, neck, upper trunk, extensor part of the arms, and dorsa of the hands and fingers (Sontheimer et al). The lesions may be annular or polycyclic. In addition, maculopapular lesions and, rarely, vesicles may be present (Maciejewski). Patients with this form of lupus erythematosus frequently have mild systemic manifestations, and half of them have four or more of the ARA criteria for SLE. However, renal disease is rare (Sontheimer et al).

Histopathology.   In most instances of *discoid lesions,* a diagnosis of lupus erythematosus is possible on the basis of a combination of histologic findings. The five important changes in the skin are (1) hyperkeratosis with keratotic plugging; (2) thinning and flattening of the stratum malpighii; (3) hydropic degeneration of basal cells; (4) a patchy, chiefly lymphoid cell infiltrate with a tendency toward arrangement about the cutaneous appendages (Fig. 25-1); and (5) edema, vasodilatation, and a slight extravasation of erythrocytes in the upper dermis. However, not all five changes are present in every case.

The epidermal changes consist of mild to moderate hyperkeratosis. As a rule, parakeratosis is not conspicuous, and it may be absent. Keratotic plugs are found mainly in the follicular openings, but they may also occur in the openings of eccrine ducts. The follicles inside the dermis may contain concentric layers of keratin instead of hairs (Fig. 25-1). Focal hydropic degeneration of the basal layer, also referred to as liquefaction degeneration, represents the most significant histologic change in lupus erythematosus (Fig. 25-2). In its absence, a histologic diagnosis of lupus erythematosus is difficult and often impossible (see below).

The epidermal changes encountered in discoid

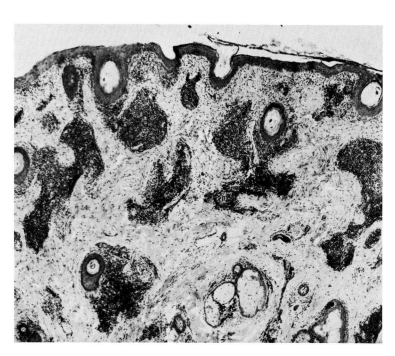

Fig. 25-1.   Discoid lupus erythematosus
Low magnification. There is keratotic plugging, and the follicles inside the dermis contain concentric layers of keratin instead of hairs. The epidermis is atrophic and devoid of rete ridges. The inflammatory infiltrate is patchy and largely located in the vicinity of hair follicles. (×50)

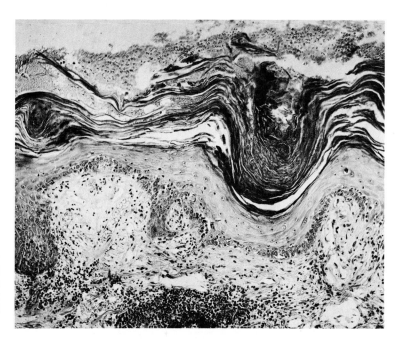

Fig. 25-2. Discoid lupus erythematosus
High magnification. There are hyperkeratosis and keratotic plugging, atrophy of the stratum malpighii, hydropic degeneration of the basal layer, edema of the upper dermis, and a patchy infiltrate composed of lymphoid cells. (× 100)

lesions vary in different types of lesions, so that thinning and flattening of the stratum malpighii do not always predominate. In cases showing clinically verrucous hyperkeratosis, the epidermis appears hyperplastic, papillomatous, and hyperkeratotic, causing considerable resemblance to a hypertrophic solar keratosis (von Eickstedt and Hassenpflug). In lesions of DLE that clinically do not show adherent scaling or keratotic plugging, the epidermis may show few if any changes and, in particular, no hydropic changes in the basal layer (Bielicky and Trapl).

The dermis shows edema in its upper portion. As a result of the subepidermal edema, the thickened basement membrane zone may be apparent even in routinely stained sections, so that one need not resort to a periodic acid-Schiff (PAS) stain (Clark et al). Frequently, small foci of extravasated erythrocytes are seen in the edematous upper dermis. In dark-skinned persons, melanin often is seen within melanophages in the upper dermis, since the hydropic degeneration in the basal cells causes these cells to lose their melanin (pigmentary incontinence). The capillaries and, in the lower dermis, the larger vessels are dilated, and their walls may show edema; however, proliferative or obliterative changes are absent. An increase in the ground substance, that is, in hyaluronic acid, is common in the middle and lower dermis but is generally mild, so that it is often not clearly evident in sections stained with hematoxylin-eosin and is

best demonstrated with the colloidal iron technique (Panet-Raymond and Johnson). Large amounts of mucin leading to the separation of collagen bundles is seen only rarely (Weigand et al). Fibrinoid deposits in the dermis are also encountered only rarely in discoid lesions, and even then only in early discoid lesions. (For a description of the fibrinoid changes, see Systemic Lupus Erythematosus, p. 450.)

The inflammatory infiltrate in the dermis usually is distinctly patchy. In areas such as the face or scalp, where there are many pilosebaceous structures, the infiltrate is located mainly in the vicinity of the hair follicles and the sebaceous glands. Frequently, one can observe hydropic changes in the basal layer of the hair follicles. In the absence of hydropic changes in the epidermis, this finding has considerable diagnostic value. The infiltrate, by impinging upon the pilosebaceous structures, causes their gradual atrophy and disappearance. Occasionally, a mild inflammatory infiltrate is also present in the upper dermis, invading the epidermis. Not infrequently, the infiltrate extends into the subcutaneous fat (Clark et al). The infiltrate in DLE is composed predominantly of lymphoid cells but also contains a small number of plasma cells and histiocytes.

Colloid bodies, referred to also as Civatte bodies, are occasionally seen in sections of DLE (Copeman et al). They are round to ovoid, have an eosinophilic, homogeneous appearance, and measure approximately 10 μm in diameter. They form as the result of dyskeratosis of individual epidermal cells and are present in the lower epidermis or in the papillary dermis. Colloid bodies are not specific for any one disease. Although found most commonly in lichen planus (see p. 153), they may be seen in several other diseases with damage to the basal cells, such as lupus erythematosus, poikiloderma, and benign lichenoid keratosis (Sümegi). When located in the dermis, colloid bodies are PAS-positive and diastase-resistant and, on direct immunofluorescence staining, often are found to contain immunoglobulins (IgG, IgM, IgA), complement, and fibrin. This staining does not represent an immunologic phenomenon but is the result of passive absorption (see p. 156).

Staining with the PAS reaction often shows broadening of the PAS-positive, diastase-resistant subepidermal basement membrane zone. Also, the capillary walls show thickening, homogenization, and an increase in the intensity of the PAS reaction (Stoughton and Wells; Beljaewa et al). Thickening of the basement membrane zone is also often seen around hair follicles. However, in areas of pronounced hydropic degeneration of the basal cells, the PAS-positive subepidermal basement zone may be fragmented and even absent (Ueki).

The histologic changes in *subacute cutaneous lupus erythematosus* differ only in degree from those seen in the discoid lesions. The hydropic degeneration of the basal cell layer and the edema of the dermis are more pronounced than in the discoid lesions,

whereas the hyperkeratosis and the inflammatory infiltrate are less prominent (Sontheimer et al). Colloid bodies in the lower epidermis are quite common (Kennedy and Gold). Occasionally, the edema in the upper dermis and, with it, the hydropic degeneration of the basal cell layer are severe enough to cause the formation of clefts and even vesicles between the epidermis and the dermis (Fig. 25-3) (McCreight and Montgomery; Maciejewski). Focal extravasations of erythrocytes are quite common. Also, there may be fibrinoid deposits in the dermis. (For a description of the fibrinoid deposits, see Systemic Lupus Erythematosus.)

Differential Diagnosis.   The epidermal changes seen in the discoid lesions of lupus erythematosus must be differentiated from those of lichen planus, since both diseases may show hydropic degeneration of the basal cell layer (see p. 152). Yet, whereas, in DLE, hydropic degeneration persists, in lichen planus, it is followed by dissolution of the basal cell layer and by replacement of the basal cells by squamous cells. Also, the triangular elongation of the rete ridges seen as "saw-toothing" in lichen planus is not observed in DLE; instead, the epidermis as a rule appears flattened. (For a discussion of the overlap syndrome lichen planus/lupus erythematosus, see pp. 152 and 155.)

The dermal changes in DLE consisting of a patchy infiltrate must be differentiated from four other diseases in which the dermal infiltrate may

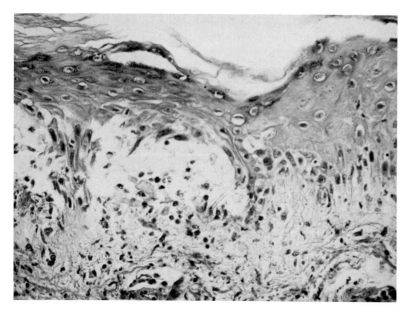

Fig. 25-3.   Subacute cutaneous lupus erythematosus
Edema of the upper dermis and pronounced hydropic degeneration of the basal layer have led to the formation of a subepidermal bulla. (×200)

also be patchy. The five diseases with a patchy dermal infiltrate, called the *five* Ls because they all begin with the letter L, are **L**upus erythematosus, lymphocytic **L**ymphoma, **L**ymphocytoma cutis, polymorphous **L**ight eruption of the plaque type, and **L**ymphocytic infiltration of the skin of Jessner. Lupus erythematosus can easily be differentiated from the four other diseases if a signficant degree of hydropic degeneration of the basal cell layer is present. However, since this degeneration is occasionally absent in lupus erythematosus, the following additional points of differentiation may be important. In lymphocytic lymphoma (see p. 732) and in lymphocytoma cutis, also referred to as pseudolymphoma of Spiegler–Fendt (see p. 753), the infiltrate usually is heavier than in lupus erythematosus and shows no tendency to arrange itself around pilosebaceous structures. Furthermore, in lymphocytic lymphoma, atypical lymphocytes often are present, and the cells of the infiltrate are more tightly packed than in an inflammatory infiltrate. In lymphocytoma cutis, there usually are, in addition to lymphocytes, cells with the appearance of histiocytes, and the infiltrate is often arranged in lymphoid follicles, the light-staining nuclei of the histiocytes suggesting germinal centers. Also, single rows of cells extending between collagen bundles, so-called Indian filing, is commonly seen in both lymphocytic lymphoma and lymphocytoma cutis but not in lupus erythematosus.

In the other two diseases, the plaque type of polymorphous light eruption and Jessner's lymphocytic infiltration of the skin, the dermal infiltrate is indistinguishable from that seen in early, non-scarring lesions of lupus erythematosus. In the plaque type of polymorphous light eruption, which, like lupus erythematosus, as a rule responds well to therapy with antimalarial drugs of the 4-amino-quinoline group, such as chloroquine, differentiation from DLE is best accomplished by direct immunofluorescence testing of a skin biopsy specimen, since deposits of immunoglobulins and complement are usually found at the dermal-epidermal junction in lesions of DLE but not in those of polymorphous light eruption (see p. 211) (Pohle and Tuffanelli; Chorzelski et al). In addition, phototesting with wavelengths shorter than 320 nm may be carried out, although it is not always reliable, as shown by the fact that not only all patients with polymorphous light eruption but also about one third of the patients with DLE show a positive phototest (Fisher et al). Testing for circulating antinuclear antibodies similarly is of limited usefulness; although nearly always negative in polymorphous light eruption, it is negative also in almost half of all patients with DLE (see p. 211) (Peterson and Fusaro; Fisher et al). (For a discussion of differentiation between DLE and Jessner's lymphocytic infiltration of the skin, see p. 457.)

Systemic Lupus Erythematosus

SLE is associated with systemic symptoms and leads to death within 10 years in about half of the patients (Kellum and Haserick; Estes and Christian). The demarcation of SLE from DLE and other connective tissue diseases is not always easy. A diagnosis of SLE is justified in the presence of four or more of the 14 manifestations listed by the ARA (see p. 445) (Cohen and Canoso). Furthermore, a diagnosis of SLE is indicated in any patient who has at least three of the following four symptoms: (1) a cutaneous eruption consistent with lupus erythematosus, (2) renal involvement, (3) serositis, and (4) joint involvement. The diagnosis is also very likely if the first two of these four manifestations are present (Ropes). It should be pointed out, however, that a diagnosis of SLE requires confirmation by laboratory tests (see Histogenesis).

Cutaneous lesions often are lacking at first in SLE. Only about 20% of SLE patients demonstrate prominent cutaneous features at the onset of their disease (Provost, 1979a), and, in about 20% of the cases, cutaneous lesions are absent throughout the course of the disease (Dubois and Tuffanelli; Estes and Christian). Usually, the cutaneous eruption consists of erythematous, slightly edematous patches without a significant degree of scaling and without atrophy. As a rule, the patches are not sharply demarcated. The most common site of involvement is the malar region, but any area of the skin may be involved, particularly the palms and fingers. Occasionally, the lesions show a petechial, vesicular, or ulcerative component. Rarely, in the late stage, some of the lesions may assume the appearance of poikiloderma atrophicans vasculare (see p. 460). Well-defined "discoid" lesions with atrophic scarring, as seen typically in DLE, occur in about 15% of the patients with SLE (Estes and Christian). They may precede all other clinical manifestations of SLE and, if they do, are convincing evidence that a transition from DLE to SLE is possible (Scott and Rees). A relatively benign course characterizes SLE in most patients with preceding DLE (Callen).

It has been established, however, that patients in whom the disease changes from DLE to SLE have persistent multiple abnormal laboratory findings from the beginning. This is in contrast to cases of simple DLE, in which most abnormal laboratory findings, if present at all, are transient (Millard and Rowell).

The systemic manifestations of SLE include arthralgia, the most common symptom. Renal involvement, referred to as lupus nephritis, may produce a nephrotic syndrome and, ultimately, uremia (Baldwin et al, 1970).

In addition, there may be pleurisy and pericarditis as manifestations of serositis, and seizures and psychoses as evidence of central nervous system involvement. Raynaud's phenomenon may occur, although it is more commonly seen in mixed connective tissue disease (MCTD) (see p. 457). Irregular fever, malaise, and weakness are common. The laboratory findings include leukopenia and an elevated erythrocyte sedimentation rate in many cases and thrombocytopenia in occasional instances. Proteinuria, hematuria, and the presence of cellular casts in the urine sediment indicate renal involvement. (For a discussion of immunologic abnormalities, see Histogenesis.)

The coexistence of SLE and systemic scleroderma or dermatomyositis has been repeatedly described (Dubois et al). It is known as overlap syndrome and refers to the coexistence of related but nevertheless separate diseases (Sharp and Anderson). This is in contrast to mixed connective tissue disease, which has become recognized as a disease entity (see p. 457).

For a discussion of the induction of SLE by various drugs, see Drug-Induced Lupus Erythematosus, p. 263.

Histopathology. Early lesions of SLE of the erythematous, edematous type may show only slight and nonspecific changes (Pruniéras and Montgomery). However, in well-developed lesions, the histologic changes correspond to those described for subacute cutaneous lupus erythematosus (see p. 448). One observes hydropic degeneration of the basal cell layer in association with edema of the upper dermis and extravasation of erythrocytes (Pruniéras and Montgomery). The findings in well-defined "discoid" lesions of SLE are similar to those described for the discoid lesions in DLE (see

p. 446). Hyperkeratosis and inflammatory changes may be quite pronounced in lesions of this type.

Fibrinoid deposits in the connective tissue of the skin are often seen in the erythematous, edematous lesions, especially in patients with SLE. Such fibrinoid deposits consist of the precipitation of fibrin in the ground substance. As a rule, the fibrinoid deposits are not as pronounced in the dermis as in the connective tissue of visceral organs, where they were first described in 1941 (Klemperer et al). Furthermore, fibrinoid deposits in the dermis are not specific for lupus erythematosus but occur also in several other dermatoses, especially in leukocytoclastic vasculitis. As a result of the precipitation of fibrin, which is characterized by strong eosinophilia, homogeneous, strongly eosinophilic, "fibrinoid" material is seen between and within the collagen bundles, so that the collagen fibers and bundles appear thickened and more deeply eosinophilic than normal (Fig. 25-4). The fibrinoid deposits may be seen occasionally also in the walls of dermal capillaries. Thus, vascular changes, if present, are part of the connective tissue changes. In addition, fibrinoid deposits may be seen in the subepidermal basement membrane zone and, in some cases, within areas of edema in the upper dermis (Fig. 25-5).

Because of the homogenizing effect of the fibrinoid deposits on the collagen and vascular walls, the presence of these deposits was originally interpreted as a process of collagen degeneration; however, electron microscopic studies have revealed no damage to the collagen fibrils, and direct

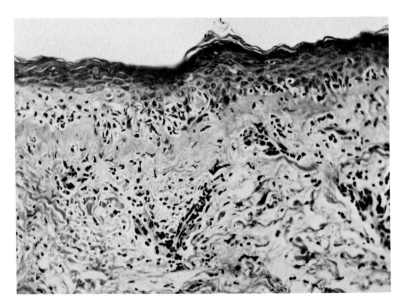

Fig. 25-4. Systemic lupus erythematosus
The epidermis is atrophic and shows marked liquefaction degeneration of the basal layer. Some of the collagen bundles appear thickened as a result of the precipitation of fibrinoid material on them. Only a mild perivascular inflammatory infiltrate is present. (×100)

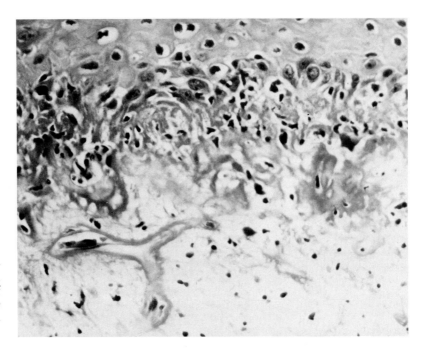

Fig. 25-5. Systemic lupus erythematosus
There are marked liquefaction degeneration of the basal layer and edema of the upper dermis. Precipitation of fibrinoid material can be seen in the zone of subepidermal edema and around a capillary. (× 200)

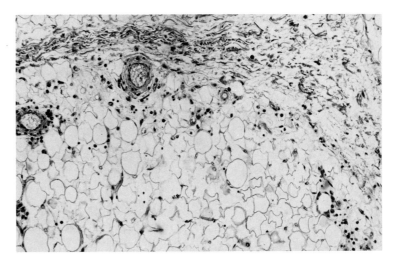

Fig. 25-6. Systemic lupus erythematosus, subcutaneous layer
The fat cells show mucoid degeneration. A scattered lymphocytic infiltrate is present. The collagen is increased in amount and shows precipitation of fibrinoid material. (× 100)

immunofluorescence studies carried out with fluorescein-labeled rabbit antisera against human fibrin have shown that the fibrinoid deposits consist, at least in part, of fibrin (Gitlin et al).

The fibrinoid deposits are strongly PAS-positive and diastase-resistant. In addition, one often finds in areas of fibrinoid deposits an increase in the amount of ground substance, particularly of hyaluronic acid, so that areas in which there are fibrinoid deposits stain positive with alcian blue (Cawley et al) and often show metachromasia on staining with toluidine blue (Pruniéras and Montgomery).

The subcutaneous fat is often involved in SLE. It may show focal mucoid degeneration with a reactive lymphocytic infiltrate. The trabeculae of collagen separating the fat lobules may be increased in thickness and show edema and fibrinoid deposits similar to those seen in the collagen bundles of the dermis (Fig. 25-6). These histologic changes in the subcutaneous fat produce no clinically apparent lesions. Still, except for being much milder, they resemble the histologic changes that occur in lupus erythematosus profundus, also referred to as lupus erythematosus panniculitis (see p. 455).

It deserves mention that, in occasional instances of SLE, pruritic, nonpurpuric urticarialike lesions are present that, on histologic examination, in most instances show a leukocytoclastic vasculitis (O'Loughlin et al, 1978b). Also, whitish atrophic lesions may occur in SLE that both clinically and histologically resemble those of malignant atrophic papulosis of Degos (Dubin and Stawiski; Black and Hudson).

Systemic Lesions.   Visceral involvement usually is widespread in patients who have died of SLE. However, some of the lesions are small, so that they may be overlooked on gross inspection and are found only on histologic examination. The renal glomeruli, endocardium, serous membranes, spleen, lungs, cardiac and skeletal muscle, and visceral fat deposits are commonly affected.

The renal changes are by far the most important, because they are the most common cause of death in SLE. They can be assessed by percutaneous renal biopsy. Most authors recommend a renal biopsy as part of the initial evaluation of all patients with SLE, with the exception of those with inadequate platelet function (Kant et al). The view has been expressed, however, that the prognostic information obtained from renal biopsies is generally less than that of even the simplest clinical classification, so that a renal biopsy in SLE provides mainly redundant information (Fries et al). However, this view is not generally held, since, in the view of most investigators, determination of the type and degree of histologic changes in the kidneys is of prognostic value regardless of the absence or severity of clinical renal disease (Appel et al).

The renal findings in SLE have been divided on a histologic basis into five classes (Kant et al):

1. Normal.
2. Predominantly mesangial lupus nephritis. The glomerular hypercellularity is confined to the mesangium.
3. Predominantly membranous lupus nephritis. There is fairly diffuse, uniform thickening of the glomerular capillary wall.
4. Predominantly proliferative lupus nephritis. One observes mainly intracapillary but often also extracapillary cellular proliferation and abundant mesangial and subendothelial deposits of fibrinoid material. These changes are referred to as *focal* if less than 50% of the glomeruli are affected and as *diffuse* when most of the glomeruli are abnormal.
5. Sclerosis. This is a terminal stage, with extensive glomerular sclerosis.

Whereas predominantly mesangial lupus nephritis generally has a good prognosis, diffuse proliferative lupus nephritis is the most serious renal lesion in SLE. Although some investigators have found that focal proliferative lupus nephritis generally follows a benign course (Baldwin et al, 1977), others have noted that most patients who at first show only focal proliferative changes ultimately develop diffuse proliferative lupus nephritis with its poor prognosis (Appel et al).

The characteristic "wire-loop" lesion of lupus nephritis is the result of subendothelial deposits of fibrinoid material, a common occurrence in lupus nephritis. Since the deposits contain fibrinoid material, they are PAS-positive and diastase-resistant (Muehrcke et al).

Whereas only about two thirds of the patients with SLE show renal changes by light microscopy, all patients show changes on *electron microscopy* and *direct immunofluorescence* (Appel et al). Subendothelial deposits of electron-dense material are found in all biopsy specimens of SLE, whereas mesangial and subepithelial deposits are not always present (Ben Bassat et al). Immunofluorescence studies show that these deposits contain immune complexes in addition to fibrin, particularly anti-DNA immune complexes, as demonstrated by elution studies (Provost, 1979a). The amount of subendothelial electron-dense deposits present is regarded as important to the prognosis (Appel et al). Unlike patients with small subendothelial deposits, patients with extensive deposits show considerable proteinuria and often a decrease in renal function (Ben Bassat et al).

The verrucous endocarditis of SLE, the so-called Libman–Sacks syndrome, occurs mainly on the mitral and tricuspid valves. In the subendothelial connective tissue, one finds a chronic inflammatory infiltrate together with fibrinoid deposits followed by fibrosis and the formation of small vegetations on the valve leaflets (Klemperer et al).

The serous membranes, such as the pleura, epicardium, and peritoneum, may show in their submucosa a chronic inflammatory infiltrate associated with fibrinoid deposits (Klemperer et al).

In the spleen, periarterial fibrosis around the follicular arteries is a common lesion in SLE and is highly characteristic of this disease. Thick, concentrically layered rings of sclerotic collagen fibers surround the arteries.

Noninfectious involvement of the lungs in SLE may occur either with acute symptoms of pneumonitis or with chronic pulmonary infiltrates (Matthay et al).

The myocardium and the skeletal muscles may

show small foci of degeneration in the muscle bundles, usually associated with mild to moderately severe reactive inflammation in the interfascicular connective tissue. These changes are identical to those of dermatomyositis, although they are much milder (Klemperer et al; Erbslöh and Baedeker).

The visceral fat may show the same changes as described for the subcutaneous fat (see p. 451).

Vascular changes usually are not conspicuous in SLE. In rare instances, however, there may be widespread vasculitis of the type seen in patients with periarteritis nodosa, causing rupture of some of the vessels and resulting in hemorrhage (Case Records, Massachusetts General Hospital). It is probable that SLE and periarteritis nodosa are present simultaneously in these cases.

A highly specific structure, the so-called hematoxylin bodies, can be found in SLE in various organs, but only on autopsy and not in biopsy specimens. They form through the action of the lupus erythematosus factor (LE factor), an antibody to whole nucleoprotein, on nuclei. However, the LE factor cannot penetrate nuclei during life but only after the cell has suffered damage through death. In penetrating the nucleus, the LE factor damages the chromatin pattern of the nucleus, so that the nucleus swells, becomes homogeneous in appearance, and stains reddish purple with hematoxylin-eosin (McDuffie). Hematoxylin bodies are found especially in the endocardium, the lumina of glomerular capillaries, the ovaries, the lymph nodes, and, occasionally, the skin (Worthington et al).

Histogenesis. The presence of multiple antibodies in the serum and tissues of patients with SLE has led to the concept of lupus erythematosus as an autoimmune disorder. Among the antibodies present in the serum may be anti-native DNA (anti-nDNA or anti-double stranded DNA) antibodies and antinucleoprotein antibodies, the latter being used in two diagnostic tests, the fluorescent antinuclear antibody (ANA) test (Carnabuci et al) and the LE cell test (McDuffie). Additional antinuclear antibodies that may be present are anti-single-stranded (ss) DNA antibodies and antinuclear ribonucleic acid protein (anti-nRNP) antibodies, the latter being found in about 33% of patients with SLE and in all patients with mixed connective tissue disease (Provost, 1979a). Occasionally, antinuclear antibodies are absent, and cytoplasmic antigens termed Ro and La are found, Ro being a cytoplasmic glycoprotein and La a cytoplasmic RNA protein (Provost, 1979a). Such cases are a special subset of SLE characterized by a severe photosensitivity eruption and multisystem disease but a low incidence

of nephritis and neuropsychiatric symptoms (Maddison et al). Many patients with anticytoplasmic antibodies present the clinical aspect of subacute cutaneous lupus erythematosus (Gilliam and Sontheimer). Among additional antibodies occasionally present in the serum of patients with SLE are antibodies against red cells causing hemolytic anemia, antibodies against platelets causing thrombocytopenia, and antibodies causing false-positive serologic tests for syphilis.

The fluorescent *ANA test* is a very sensitive test for SLE. With mouse liver sections used as tissue substrate and a serum dilution of 1:20, the test is positive in more than 90% of untreated SLE patients (Maddison et al). About half of those with a negative ANA test represent the above-mentioned special subset of SLE, which shows anticytoplasmic antibodies and is characterized by a photosensitivity eruption and a low frequency of renal disease. However, the test lacks specificity for SLE and thus can usually be used merely as a preliminary screening test. Only a titer of 1:160 or higher with a peripheral staining pattern can be regarded as virtually diagnostic of SLE (Nisengard et al). At a titer of 1:20, about 20% of patients with DLE, most patients with systemic scleroderma, and as many as 5% of normal persons have a positive reaction. Some differences exist in the pattern of nuclear fluorescence in SLE and systemic scleroderma: sera of patients with SLE are apt to produce either homogeneous or peripheral fluorescence of the substrate nuclei, whereas sera of patients with systemic scleroderma produce either speckled or nucleolar fluorescence (Burnham, 1978).

Two tests have a high specificity, being generally positive only in SLE: the LE cell test and the test for anti-nDNA antibodies. Since the latter test is as sensitive and specific as the LE cell test and has the advantages of being less time-consuming and easier to read, it has replaced the LE cell test. Nevertheless, because of its historic significance, a few words may be said about the LE cell test.

In the *LE cell test*, the patient's serum is incubated with normal white blood cells. If the LE factor, an antibody to whole nucleoprotein, is present in the patient's serum, it penetrates into the nuclei of some of the normal white blood cells and causes nuclear damage. The damaged nuclei, being leukotactic, are then phagocytized by some of the neutrophils that have escaped damage. If a smear of the incubated white blood cells is made and stained with the Wright stain, the phagocytized nuclear material may be observed within some of the neutrophils as a large, round, amorphous, smoky, basophilic body of such a large size that it presses the nucleus of the neutrophil against the cell membrane. This represents the LE cell (Fig. 25-7) (Hargraves et al; McDuffie; Zweiman and Hebert). In addition to LE cells, one also observes so-called rosettes (Fig. 25-7). They consist of disintegrated nuclear material surrounded by neutrophils that are phagocytizing this material.

Determination of the presence of *anti-nDNA antibodies*

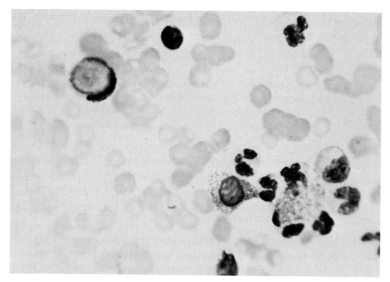

Fig. 25-7. Systemic lupus erythematosus, LE cell test
For the demonstration of the LE cell phenomenon, normal white blood cells are incubated with the patient's serum. In this positive test, an LE cell is seen in the upper left corner; it is a neutrophil containing a large smoky body. In the lower right corner, a rosette is seen consisting of amorphous material surrounded by phagocytizing neutrophils. ($\times 400$)

in the serum at various dilutions has replaced the LE cell test. Because it is associated with a high incidence of renal disease, the presence of anti-nDNA antibodies almost always indicates a severe prognosis. This frequent association is explained by the fact that anti-nDNA immune complexes are deposited in the renal glomeruli (see p. 452). Anti-nDNA antibodies are measured by one of three technics. These are counterimmunoelectrophoresis, radioimmunoassay, and an immunofluorescence technic employing *Crithidia luciliae* as a substrate (Provost, 1979a).

The presence of anti-nDNA antibodies in the serum is frequently associated not only with renal disease but also with hypocomplementemia, with the presence of antinuclear antibodies showing a peripheral staining pattern, and with a positive lupus band test in uninvolved skin (Prystowski and Gilliam; Provost, 1979a).

The *lupus band test* is of considerable value in lupus erythematosus. This test entails the direct immunofluorescence testing of involved and uninvolved, sun-exposed skin for the purpose of diagnosis, and of uninvolved, sun-protected skin for the purpose of prognosis (Harrist and Mihm). For these tests, 3- or 4-mm biopsy specimens of unfixed skin are submitted in one of three conditions: in a frozen state, wrapped in saline-impregnated gauze, or immersed in phosphate-buffered saline. They are snap-frozen in liquid nitrogen and stored at −70°C. The sections are cut in a cryostat and stained with fluorescein-conjugated antisera to IgA, IgM, IgG, and the third component of complement (C3) (Pohle and Tuffanelli; Provost et al). In a positive test, fluorescence is present as a continuous granular line or band along the dermal-epidermal junction.

When involved skin is tested for diagnosis, immunoglobulins, most commonly IgG and IgM, and complement are found in over 90% of the specimens of both DLE and SLE. Thus, direct immunofluorescence testing

of involved skin is more specific and sensitive than routine histologic studies of biopsy specimens (Tuffanelli, 1975). It should be noted, however, that lesions less than 2 months old may give negative results (Bean). This fact explains why, in some cases of subacute cutaneous lupus erythematosus with sudden exacerbation following sun exposure, no lupus band can be demonstrated in the lesions (Sontheimer et al; Wechsler and Stavrides).

When uninvolved, sun-exposed skin is tested for diagnostic purposes, the biopsy specimen is usually taken from the dorsal surface of the forearm. Whereas the lupus band test is almost always negative in DLE, it is positive in over 80% of untreated patients with SLE (Halevy et al; Provost et al).

When uninvolved, sun-protected skin is tested for prognostic purposes, the biopsy specimen is taken either from the buttock area or from the volar aspect of the forearm. A definite correlation is then found between the incidence of a lupus band and the severity of renal disease. Although the overall incidence of a lupus band in sun-protected skin of patients with SLE is about 50%, patients with diffuse renal disease in two series had a lupus band in 81% and 83% of the cases, respectively, whereas patients with mild, focal, or no renal disease showed a band in only 23% and 19% of the cases, respectively (Gilliam et al; Dantzig et al).

Whereas the normal-appearing skin of SLE shows only immune complex deposits, involved skin of both DLE and SLE also contains the terminal complement complex, or membrane attack complex, composed of C5b, C6, C7, C8, and C9. The latter mediates an inflammatory response and causes damage to the basement membrane (Biesecker et al).

The lupus band differs from the band seen in bullous and cicatricial pemphigoid and in herpes gestationis. Whereas the lupus band consists of coalescing granules and, even though it is located subepidermally, often shows irregular extensions into the uppermost dermis (Burnham and Fine; Nebe and Barthelmes), the "pemphigoid" band appears narrow, tubular, sharply demarcated, and immediately subepidermal in location (see p. 115) (Burnham and Fine).

Electron microscopic examination of the cutaneous lesions of both DLE and SLE shows marked changes in the basal cells and the basement membrane. The basal cells show vacuolization of their cytoplasm, which may progress to disintegration and necrosis of the cytoplasm. In addition, the basal cells show numerous greatly elongated, narrow cytoplasmic projections into the dermis, which, because of their irregular shape, often appear as cross sections (EM 36). The projections are surrounded by basement membrane, which therefore appears as an irregular and extensive network. This network persists even in areas in which the projections of the basal cells have disintegrated. The impression is thus gained that the basal cells are a primary site of damage in the cutaneous lesions of lupus erythematosus (Tuffanelli et al). The basement membrane may even invade the dermis deeply, without the participation of the basal cells, forming loops and labryinths; this, too, is regarded as a secondary phenomenon following repeated damage to the basal cells (Ogawa).

The colloid or Civatte bodies that may be seen in the epidermis as well as in the dermis are similar in appearance on electron microscopy to those observed in lichen planus (see p. 153 and EM 28). They are finely filamentous to amorphous granular in appearance and do not possess a delimiting membrane (Haustein).

The exact electron microscopic location of the subepidermal immune complexes in lupus erythematosus has been studied after staining of the complexes with peroxidase-labeled antihuman gamma-globulin. With this method, the antigen–antibody complexes are seen as irregular aggregates in the uppermost portion of the dermis, beneath the basement membrane located in the ground substance, and occasionally also on collagen fibrils, masking their cross banding (Ueki et al). In some instances, small amounts of reaction product are seen within the basement membrane and the lamina lucida (Pehamberger et al). Localization of the immune complexes in lupus erythematosus thus differs from their localization in bullous pemphigoid, in which they are situated in their entirety between the basement membrane and the basal cells (see p. 115).

The presence of intracytoplasmic *tubuloreticular structures* has been frequently observed in the cutaneous and renal lesions of SLE (Györkey et al) and in the cutaneous lesions of DLE, particularly in early, active lesions (Hashimoto and Thompson). At first, these structures were regarded as unenveloped nucleocapsids of a paramyxovirus. However, it soon became apparent that they are by no means specific for lupus erythematosus; they were found in several other diseases, including not only other connective tissue diseases, such as dermatomyositis and scleroderma (Hashimoto and Thompson;

Landry and Winkelmann), but also entirely unrelated disease entities, such as bullous pemphigoid (Macadam et al) and malignant atrophic papulosis (Stahl et al). In addition, tubuloreticular structures have been found within vascular endothelial cells of various epithelial tumors, such as seborrheic keratosis, basal cell epithelioma, and Bowen's disease (Maciejewski et al). In another study, tubuloreticular structures were observed quite frequently in the visibly normal skin of patients with SLE and, rarely in the normal skin of patients with DLE. Following a 10-day course of ultraviolet light irradiation to visibly normal skin, the incidence of tubuloreticular structures in the irradiated skin of patients with SLE or DLE increased significantly (Berk and Blank).

The fact that the tubuloreticular structures can be provoked by exposure to ultraviolet light suggests that they are a reaction product of metabolically active cells. The tubuloreticular structures consist either of a single highly convoluted unit or of a large number of individual short, intertwined units. The average diameter of the tubules is 16 nm (range, 12–21 nm), and the maximum dimension of an entire structure 1.9 μm (EM 37) (Macadam et al). The tubuloreticular structures are present in the cytoplasm of endothelial cells and fibroblasts. The fact that the structures usually lie within the rough endoplasmic reticulum of these cells suggests that they are a product of the cells, since the rough endoplasmic reticulum is the site of cellular synthesis of proteins destined for subsequent "export" and is never the location of materials that have been previously phagocytized by the cell (Macadam et al).

Lupus Erythematosus Profundus

In lupus erythematosus profundus, which is quite rare, one observes one or several firm, asymptomatic, often fairly large subcutaneous nodules as a manifestation of either SLE (Winkelmann; Tuffanelli, 1971) or DLE (Schirren and Eggert; Fountain). The nodules occur most commonly on the head and arms and may either precede or follow the development of cutaneous lesions by several years. The skin overlying the subcutaneous nodules often appears normal but, in some instances, shows cutaneous lesions of lupus erythematosus (Fountain; Tuffanelli, 1971). On healing, the subcutaneous lesions may leave behind a cup-shaped depression. In place of lupus erythematosus profundus, the term *lupus erythematosus panniculitis* is now often used for the subcutaneous nodules.

Histopathology.   The subcutaneous nodules may merely show a nonspecific panniculitis composed of lymphoid cells, plasma cells, and histiocytes. In some instances, lymphoid follicles are seen showing small lymphocytes surrounding a germinal center with larger, paler nuclei (Harris et al). As a rather characteristic feature, necrobiotic changes with fibrinoid deposits are occasionally observed in the subcutaneous tissue (Fountain; Tuffanelli, 1971). Subsequent hyalinization of fat lobules may lead to separation of the fat cells by homogeneous, glassy, eosinophilic collagen (Sánchez et al). The hyalinization of the connective tissue separating the fat lobules may result in broad septa subdividing the subcutaneous fat (Winkelmann). In some cases, mucinous changes and foci of calcification are seen (Winkelmann). There may be severe vasculitis, but this often represents merely secondary involvement of the vessels in the inflammatory process rather than a primary vasculitis (Fountain). Vessels thus affected show inflammatory infiltration and thickening of their walls with narrowing of their lumina (Schirren and Eggert).

Jessner's Lymphocytic Infiltration of the Skin

Jessner's lymphocytic infiltration of the skin, first described in 1953 (Jessner and Kanof), shows asymptomatic, well-demarcated, slightly infiltrated, reddish plaques. The lesions begin as papules and expand peripherally. There may be central clearing. The surface of the lesions appears normal and, in particular, shows no follicular plugging or atrophy. The most common location of the lesions is the face, but, in some instances, the neck or upper trunk is involved either alone or in addition to the face. There may be one, a few, or numerous lesions. After having persisted for several months or even several years, the lesions usually disappear without sequelae, but they may recur either at the previous sites or elsewhere. In some instances, the eruption is precipitated or aggravated by sunlight (Gottlieb and Winkelmann). Antimalarial drugs of the 4-aminoquinoline group, such as chloroquine, sometimes clear the eruption dramatically, but they do not do so consistently (Calnan).

In female carriers of chronic granulomatous disease, a cutaneous eruption referred to as arcuate dermal erythema may occur. This eruption is indistinguishable clinically as well as histologically from Jessner's lymphocytic infiltration of the skin (Nelson et al).

Histopathology. The epidermis may be normal but often appears slightly flattened. In the dermis, one observes large, fairly well circumscribed patches of a cellular infiltrate composed almost entirely of lymphoid cells (Fig. 25-8). In addition to the lymphoid cells, a few histiocytes and plasma cells are usually present. The infiltrate often shows a tendency to arrange itself around cutaneous appendages and blood vessels, and it may extend into the subcutaneous fat (Jessner and Kanof).

Histogenesis. No unanimity exists concerning the nosologic position of lymphocytic infiltration. The following four views have been expressed: (1) it represents an entity; (2) although some cases represent an entity,

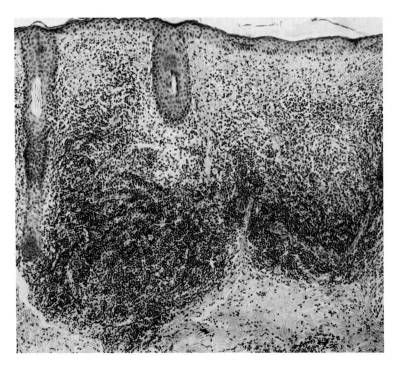

Fig. 25-8.   Jessner's lymphocytic infiltration of the skin
The epidermis is normal. The dermis contains large, fairly well demarcated patches of an inflammatory infiltrate composed almost entirely of lymphocytes. (×100)

others are DLE; (3) all cases are DLE; and (4) it represents an abortive or initial phase of any of the four other diseases with a patchy dermal infiltrate, that is, discoid lupus erythematosus, the plaque type of polymorphous light eruption, lymphocytoma cutis, and lymphocytic lymphoma (which together form the "five Ls," see p. 449).

First, several authors favor recognition of lymphocytic infiltration of the skin as an entity because of the extent to which its lesions differ from DLE: clinically by the absence of hyperkeratosis, healing without atrophy, an occasional lack of response to antimalarial drugs, and the fairly common occurrence of lesions on the back; and histologically by the absence of hydropic degeneration in the basal layer (Jessner and Kanof; Calnan; Bazex). To these criteria an additional characteristic has been added: a negative result on direct immunofluorescence testing for deposits of immunoglobulins and complement at the dermal-epidermal border (Barthelmes and Sönnichsen; Chorzelski et al). However, a positive test is obtained only in about 90% of the patients with DLE (see p. 454). This then leaves 10% of the cases of DLE with negative immunofluorescence findings, like Jessner's lymphocytic infiltration. Also, there has been a tendency to use the direct immunofluorescence test in cases of doubt as the criterion as to whether a case should be regarded as DLE or as lymphocytic infiltration of the skin (Chorzelski et al).

Second, the apparently close relationship of at least some cases of lymphocytic infiltration of the skin to DLE has persuaded some authors to regard a certain number of the cases reported as lymphocytic infiltration of the skin as instances of nonscarring DLE but other cases as a separate entity (Cabré and Steigleder; Gottlieb and Winkelmann).

A third group of authors holds the view that all cases of lymphocytic infiltration of the skin are instances of nonscarring DLE because of their clinical and histologic resemblance, the presence of photosensitivity common to the two, and their common response to antimalarial drugs (Bielicky and Trapl; Burnham, 1969).

Finally, a fourth view, which appears to be the most likely, regards the cases reported as lymphocytic infiltration of the skin as a heterogeneous group rather than as an entity. Accordingly, *lymphocytic infiltration of the skin* may be used as a preliminary diagnostic term until a more definitive diagnosis is possible. There seems to be little doubt that, unless the lesions subside spontaneously, most, if not all, cases of lymphocytic infiltration of the skin followed long enough can be reclassified, usually as DLE (Vivell) or the plaque type of polymorphous light eruption and occasionally as lymphocytoma cutis or, as described in one case, lymphocytic lymphoma (Calnan).

MIXED CONNECTIVE TISSUE DISEASE

In 1972, a syndrome was described that differs sufficiently from SLE in both clinical and laboratory features to have become recognized as a separate entity under the name *mixed connective tissue disease* (MCTD) (Sharp et al). The two decisive laboratory features are, first, the presence of very high titers of serum antibodies to an extractable nuclear antigen that characteristically is ribonuclease-sensitive and, second, epidermal nuclear staining of normal-appearing skin on direct immunofluorescence (Gilliam and Prystowsky).

The clinical manifestations, although somewhat variable, nevertheless are sufficiently distinctive in most cases to suggest the diagnosis of MCTD. The typical clinical pattern includes Raynaud's phenomenon, polyarthralgia, swelling of the hands leading to a sausage appearance and sclerodactyly of the fingers, esophageal hypomotility, inflammatory proximal myopathy, and pulmonary disease (Sharp and Anderson). About 85% of patients with MCTD have Raynaud's phenomenon, and this sign may precede all other manifestations.

Cutaneous lupus erythematosus lesions are found in approximately half of the patients, about as often as "sausage fingers" or sclerodactyly. They cover the entire spectrum of cutaneous lupus erythematosus. Most commonly, one observes diffuse, nonscarring, poorly demarcated subacute lesions, but some patients show acute malar eruptions as seen in SLE or persistent scarring lesions as seen in DLE (Prystowsky and Tuffanelli).

The prognosis is good in most patients, with a calculated mortality of only 7% (Sharp and Anderson). The reason for this good prognosis lies in the fact that only 10% of all patients with MCTD have renal disease, which, with few exceptions, is mild.

Histopathology. If cutaneous lesions of lupus erythematosus are present, the histologic findings correspond to the type of lesion, as described under DLE (see p. 446), subacute lupus erythematosus (see p. 448), and SLE (see p. 450).

Histogenesis. MCTD, in contrast with most cases of SLE, has no antibodies to DNA. The absence of such antibodies explains the rarity of renal disease.

High titers of antibodies to ribonucleoprotein in the serum occur not only in MCTD but occasionally also in SLE. It is characteristic of MCTD, however, that the saline-soluble (extractable) nuclear antigen is sensitive to ribonuclease. In contrast, the extractable nuclear antigen that may be found in SLE is resistant to ribonuclease and identical with the so-called Sm antigen (Prystowsky and Tuffanelli).

Direct immunofluorescence staining of normal skin shows deposition of IgG in a speckled (particulate) pattern in epidermal nuclei. Although this finding is typical of MCTD, it is found occasionally also in patients with SLE showing no extractable nuclear antigen or extractable ribonuclease-resistant nuclear antigen (Prystowski and Tuffanelli). In addition to showing epidermal nuclear immunofluorescence, patients with MCTD may show a subepidermal lupus band in normal skin. Such a band has been observed in sun-exposed, normal skin in about 40% and in sun-protected, normal skin in about 20% of the cases (Prystowski and Tuffanelli).

DERMATOMYOSITIS

In dermatomyositis, the skin and skeletal muscles are mainly affected, and only rarely are other organs involved. Polymyositis represents the same disease as dermatomyositis except for the absence of skin involvement (Bohan et al). Both dermatomyositis and polymyositis are fairly uncommon diseases, but their incidence is about the same (Bohan et al; Callen et al), and both occur most commonly either in childhood or in middle age (Winkelmann et al).

The cutaneous lesions consist of erythematous to purplish patches that show slight edema. Through gradual extension, fairly large areas of the skin may become involved. The face is most commonly affected, particularly the eyelids ("heliotrope erythema"); also, the upper chest, the extensor surfaces of the extremities, particularly the knees, elbows, and knuckles ("Gottron papules"), and the distal portions of the fingers may be affected (Callen). Often, the eruption greatly resembles the erythematous–edematous lesions seen in subacute or systemic lupus erythematosus; and, as in subacute and systemic lupus erythematosus, exposure to the sun may cause a flare-up. Not infrequently, the cutaneous lesions assume the appearance of poikiloderma atrophicans vasculare (see p. 460). In some instances, the cutaneous eruption precedes the development of muscular weakness by many months or even by several years (Krain).

Involvement of the skeletal muscles causes progressive weakness, vague muscular pain, and, later, atrophy of the muscles. The proximal muscles of the extremities and the anterior neck muscles often are the first to be involved. Involvement of the pharynx may result in dysphagia and aspiration of food, and involvement of the diaphragm and of the intercostal muscles may lead to respiratory failure. However, on the whole, the prognosis of dermatomyositis is favorable, especially when treatment with corticosteroids is used. Thus, the mortality was around 14% in some reported series (Rose and Walton; Bohan et al).

Areas of subcutaneous and periarticular calcification may occur and, if extensive, are referred to as dystrophic calcinosis universalis (see p. 420). Calcinosis is particularly common in children and is usually seen centered in the proximal muscles of the shoulders and pelvic girdle (Muller et al).

Proximal myopathy is occasionally found also in mixed connective tissue disease (MCTD). However, the additional clinical manifestations observed in MCTD, such as Raynaud's phenomenon and polyarthralgia, as well as laboratory findings, usually allow easy differentiation (see p. 457).

Histopathology. The erythematous–edematous lesions of the skin in dermatomyositis may show only nonspecific inflammation. However, quite frequently, the histologic changes are indistinguishable from those seen in SLE (see p. 450). In particular, one observes flattening of the epidermis, hydropic degeneration of the basal cell layer, edema of the upper dermis, a scattered inflammatory infiltrate, and often also PAS-positive fibrinoid deposits at the dermal-epidermal junction and around the capillaries of the upper dermis (Janis and Winkelmann).

Old cutaneous lesions with the clinical appearance of poikiloderma atrophicans vasculare usually show a bandlike infiltrate under a flattened epidermis (for details, see Poikiloderma Atrophicans Vasculare, p. 460).

In some instances, the dermis shows focal accumulations of mucin in the form of acid mucopolysaccharides demonstrable with alcian blue, either with or without an associated inflammatory infiltrate (Janis and Winkelmann).

The subcutaneous tissue may show focal areas of panniculitis associated with mucoid degeneration of fat cells in early lesions (Wainger and Lever). Extensive areas of calcification may be present in the subcutis at a later stage (see Calcinosis Cutis, p. 421) (Reich).

In selecting a site for muscle biopsy, it is advisable to choose a proximal muscle from an extremity, preferably one that is tender. Muscles merely showing weakness and atrophy are best avoided, since, in this end stage, the muscle fibers may have been replaced by fibrous connective tissue (Vignos et al). However, even if the site is carefully selected and a specimen of adequate size is taken for biopsy, it may happen that, owing to the fact that the muscle changes are often focal rather than diffuse, no abnormalities are found (Bohan et al). Muscles that are actively involved show degenerative changes and often also inflammation and signs of regeneration. It has been suggested that the degenerative changes represent infarctions resulting from a necrotizing vasculitis with subsequent occlusion of small perimysial and endomysial vessels by intimal hyperplasia and fibrin thrombi (Banker and Victor). However, some investigators have observed vascular changes in the muscles only very rarely (Bohan et al) or not at all (Janis and Winkelmann).

In areas of mild degeneration, the muscle fibers show loss of their transverse striation and hyalinization of the sarcoplasm. In areas of severe degeneration, they may additionally show fragmentation and granular and vacuolar degeneration as well as phagocytosis of degenerated muscle fragments by macrophages (Fig. 25-9). Regenerating muscle fibers characterized by basophilia and a reduction in diameter may also be present (Janis and Winkelmann). Interstitial inflammation in the muscles often is absent in areas of early degeneration, suggesting that inflammation occurs secondarily as a response to the parenchymal damage (O'Leary and Waisman). If present, the inflammatory reaction consists of patchy, perivascular, interstitial infiltrations of lymphoid cells and a few plasma cells. In addition, edema usually separates the muscle bundles in areas of active degenerative changes. Old lesions usually show a rather non-specific picture of atrophy of the muscle fibers and diffuse interstitial fibrosis with relatively little inflammation.

Systemic Lesions.   Changes in organs other than the skin and the striated muscles occur only rarely in dermatomyositis, in contrast to SLE and systemic scleroderma. The myocardium may show changes identical to those in the skeletal muscle but less severe (Kinney and Maher; O'Leary and Waisman; Wainger and Lever). Ulcerative lesions in the gastrointestinal tract, caused by vascular occlusions, have also been described (Horn; Wainger and Lever; Banker and Victor).

Association of Dermatomyositis with Malignant Tumors.   The association of dermatomyositis and malignant tumors has been much commented upon. Figures about the frequency of this occurrence vary. Nevertheless, it

seems that, on the average, the incidence of malignancy among adult patients with dermatomyositis lies around 15% (Williams; Barnes). A few series show significantly higher figures, such as 52%, 26%, and 23%, respectively (Arundel et al; Callen et al; Degos et al). In contrast, one series of 230 adult patients showed an incidence of only 7.8% (Christianson et al).

Two facts deserve emphasis: first, the incidence of malignancy apparently is significantly higher in dermatomyositis than in polymyositis, being 15% and 8.8%, respectively, in one series (Bohan et al) and 26% and 3.2%, respectively, in another series (Callen et al); second, in a review of the literature that included 167 cases of malignancy occurring in association with dermatomyositis, the malignancy preceded the onset of the dermatomyositis in 51, or nearly one third of the cases (Barnes).

Since the average incidence of malignancy in adult patients with dermatomyositis can be assumed to be about 15%, the incidence of malignancy preceding dermatomyositis would be one third of 15%, or about 5%, a figure not far off from the incidence actually seen in the average middle-aged population. However, the figure of 10% of malignancy developing after the onset of dermatomyositis, often within a short time after its onset, is higher than one would expect. It appears possible that the reduction in T lymphocytes that exists in some patients with dermatomyositis lowers the patient's immunologic defenses against malignancy (Weston and Thorne).

Histogenesis.   On *electron microscopic examination*, the degeneration of the muscle fibers in dermatomyositis

Fig. 25-9.   Dermatomyositis; muscle
The muscle bundles show various degrees of degeneration. In addition, one sees edema and focal collections of inflammatory cells. (×100)

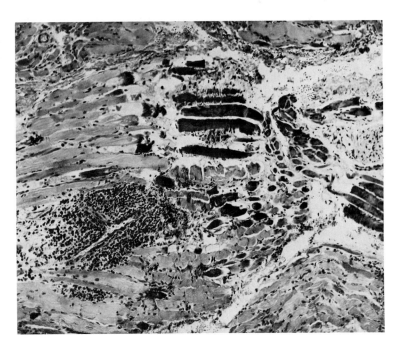

shows many similarities to the degenerative changes found in other diseases of muscle (Shafiq et al). The earliest change seen by electron microscopy seems to consist of focal disintegration of myofilaments and myofibrils resulting in areas of vacuolization and in the accumulation of lipid globules and lysosomes within muscle fibers (Gonzalez-Angulo et al; Hashimoto et al).

Intracytoplasmic tubuloreticular structures resembling paramyxovirus are frequently present in the skin and muscle lesions of dermatomyositis (Hashimoto et al; Landry and Winkelmann). As in lupus erythematosus, they probably represent a reaction product of metabolically active cells (see p. 455).

Differential Diagnosis.   Differentiation of the cutaneous lesions of dermatomyositis from those of subacute or systemic lupus erythematosus may be impossible on a histologic basis. It may also be impossible on clinical grounds in cases in which muscular weakness is mild or absent, as it may be in the early stage of dermatomyositis. In such cases, laboratory tests are of great value. The most important is the lupus band test, which is always negative in lesions of dermatomyositis (Harrist and Mihm), whereas, in lesions of lupus erythematosus, it is positive in 90% of the cases (see p. 454). Other tests that are usually negative in dermatomyositis and often positive in lupus erythematosus include urinalysis and renal function tests, as well as tests for antinuclear antibodies, anti-native DNA antibodies, and antibodies to ribonucleoprotein (see p. 453). The latter test, especially in conjunction with a negative result for antibodies to ribonuclease-sensitive extractable nuclear antigen, also excludes MCTD (see p. 457).

Poikiloderma Atrophicans Vasculare

Poikiloderma atrophicans vasculare may be seen in three different settings: (1) in association with three genodermatoses; (2) as an early stage of mycosis fungoides; and (3) in association with dermatomyositis and, less commonly, lupus erythematosus.

The three genodermatoses in which the cutaneous lesions have the appearance of poikiloderma atrophicans vasculare are (a) poikiloderma congenitale of Rothmund–Thomson (see p. 66), with the lesions of poikiloderma present largely on the face, hands, and feet and occasionally also on the arms, legs, and buttocks; (b) Bloom's syndrome (see p. 66), with poikilodermalike lesions on the face, hands, and forearms; and (c) dyskeratosis congenita (see p. 62), in which there may be extensive netlike pigmentation of the skin suggestive of poikiloderma atrophicans vasculare.

Poikilodermalike lesions as features of early mycosis fungoides may be seen in one of two clinical forms:

either as the large plaque type of parapsoriasis en plaques, also known as poikilodermatous parapsoriasis (see p. 142), or as parapsoriasis variegata, also called parakeratosis variegata, which, in its early state, shows papules arranged in a netlike pattern (see p. 149). Although these two types of parapsoriasis represent an early stage of mycosis fungoides, not all cases progress clinically into fully developed mycosis fungoides (Samman; Musger). Cases in which no progression toward mycosis fungoides is observed have been described also as idiopathic poikiloderma atrophicans vasculare (Dowling and Freudenthal; Downing et al; Steigleder).

The third group of diseases in which lesions of poikiloderma atrophicans vasculare occur is represented by dermatomyositis and SLE. Dermatomyositis is much more commonly seen as the primary disease than lupus erythematosus, and the association with dermatomyositis often is referred to as poikilodermatomyositis (Guy et al; Horn). In contrast to mycosis fungoides, in which poikilodermatous lesions are seen in the early stage, the lesions found in dermatomyositis and SLE generally represent a late stage.

Clinically, the term poikiloderma atrophicans vasculare is applied to lesions that, in the early stage, show erythema with slight, superficial scaling, a mottled pigmentation, and telangiectases. In the late stage, the skin appears atrophic, and the erythema is less pronounced than in the early stage, but the mottled pigmentation and the telangiectases are more pronounced. The clinical picture then resembles chronic radiodermatitis.

Histopathology.   Poikiloderma atrophicans vasculare, irrespective of whether it is associated with one of the genodermatoses, with early mycosis fungoides, or with dermatomyositis or SLE, in the early stage shows moderate thinning of the stratum malpighii, effacement of the rete ridges, and hydropic degeneration of the basal cells (Fig. 25-10). In the upper dermis, one finds a bandlike infiltrate, which in places invades the epidermis. The infiltrate consists mainly of lymphoid cells but also contains a few histiocytes. Melanophages filled with melanin as a result of pigmentary incontinence are found in varying numbers within the infiltrate. In addition, there is edema in the upper dermis, and the superficial capillaries are often dilated (Bonvalet et al; Vella Briffa et al; Janis and Winkelmann).

In the late stage, the epidermis is apt to be markedly thinned and flattened, but the basal cells still show hydropic degeneration. Melanophages and edema of the upper dermis are still present, and telangiectasia may be pronounced (Horn; Janis and Winkelmann).

The amount and type of dermal infiltrate vary with the underlying cause. In poikiloderma atro-

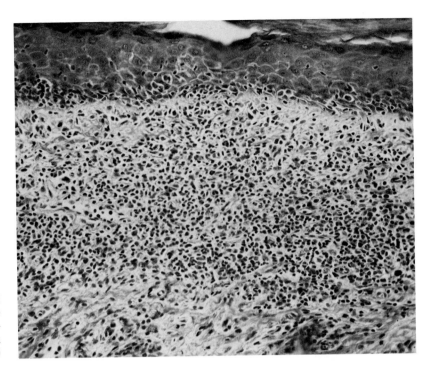

Fig. 25-10.
Poikilodermatomyositis, early stage
The epidermis appears flattened and shows hydropic degeneration of the basal cells. The upper dermis contains a bandlike infiltrate, which in places invades the epidermis. ($\times 200$)

phicans vasculare associated with one of the genodermatoses, the mononuclear infiltrate is mild and may be absent in the late stage (Braun-Falco and Marghescu). Similarly, in the late stage of poikiloderma seen in association with dermatomyositis or SLE, there is only slight dermal inflammation (Janis and Winkelmann). In contrast, the amount of inflammatory infiltrate seen in poikiloderma associated with early mycosis fungoides increases rather than decreases with time. In addition, cells with large, hyperchromatic nuclei, so-called mycosis cells, are apt to be present, and there is often marked epidermotropism of the infiltrate, which may result in Pautrier microabscesses (see p. 741) (Vella Briffa et al).

SCLERODERMA

Two types of scleroderma exist: circumscribed scleroderma (morphea), and systemic scleroderma (progressive systemic sclerosis). In addition, there are two variants of morphea: atrophoderma of Pasini and Pierini, and eosinophilic fasciitis of Shulman. The latter disease, however, differs sufficiently from scleroderma so that it will be discussed separately.

In morphea, the lesions usually are limited to the skin and to the subcutaneous tissue beneath the cutaneous lesions; however, occasionally, the underlying muscles are also affected. In systemic scleroderma, in addition

to extensive involvement of the skin and the subcutaneous tissue, visceral lesions are present, leading to death in about half of the patients.

On rare occasions, morphea and systemic scleroderma occur in the same patient. Usually in such instances, the manifestations of morphea arise first and are extensive, whereas those of systemic scleroderma are mild and nonprogressive (Tuffanelli et al; Weidner and Braun-Falco, cases 2 and 3; Korting and Brachtel; Ryckmanns and Konz; Diaz-Perez et al; Synkowski et al). Rarely, the manifestations of systemic scleroderma precede those of morphea (Weidner and Braun-Falco, case 1; Black et al; Ikai et al).

Morphea

Morphea, or circumscribed scleroderma, may be divided into five types: guttate, plaque, linear, segmental, and generalized.

Guttate lesions occur almost always in association with lesions of the plaque type. Guttate lesions are small and superficial; they resemble the lesions of lichen sclerosus et atrophicus but do not show hyperkeratosis or follicular plugging.

Lesions of the plaque type, the most common manifestation of morphea, are round or oval but through coalescence may assume an irregular configuration. They are indurated, have a smooth surface, and show an ivory color. As long as they are enlarging, they may show a violaceous border, the so-called lilac ring.

Lesions of the linear type occur predominantly on the extremities and on the anterior scalp. When one or several extremities are involved, there often is, in addition to induration of the skin, marked atrophy of the subcutaneous fat and of the muscles, resulting in contractures of muscles and tendons and ankyloses of joints (Christianson et al; Hickman and Sheils). On the anterior portion of the scalp and on the forehead, linear morphea often has the configuration of the stroke of a saber (coup de sabre) (Dilley and Perry).

Segmental morphea occurs on one side of the face, resulting in hemiatrophy. Occasionally, morphea en coup de sabre and facial hemiatrophy occur together (Dilley and Perry).

Generalized morphea comprises very extensive cases showing a combination of several of the four types just described. It is seen mainly in children, in whom it has been described as disabling pansclerotic morphea (Diaz-Perez et al) but it can also occur in adults (Stava, case 1; Synkowski et al). Rarely, bullous lesions are seen in patients with generalized morphea (Synkowski et al).

The occasional coexistence of lesions of morphea and lichen sclerosus et atrophicus is worthy of note (see p. 281).

Histopathology.   An early inflammatory and a late sclerotic stage exist in morphea. Most sections obtained routinely show a histologic picture intermediate between the two stages. It is of great importance that the specimen for biopsy include adequate amounts of subcutaneous tissue, since most of the diagnostic alterations are seen there.

In the early inflammatory stage, found particularly at the violaceous border of enlarging lesions, the reticular dermis shows thickened collagen bundles and a moderately severe inflammatory infiltrate, predominantly lymphocytic, between the collagen bundles and around the blood vessels (Fig. 25-11) (Reed et al). A much more pronounced inflammatory infiltrate than that seen in the dermis often involves the subcutaneous fat and its upward projections toward the eccrine glands. The trabeculae subdividing the subcutaneous fat are thickened because of the presence of an inflammatory infiltrate and the deposition of new collagen. Large areas of subcutaneous fat are replaced by newly formed collagen, which is composed of fine, wavy fibers rather than of bundles and which stains only faintly with hematoxylin-eosin (Fig. 25-12) (Fleischmajer and Nedwich). Vascular changes in the early inflammatory stage generally are mild both in the dermis and in the subcutaneous tissue. They may consist of endothelial swelling and edema of the walls of the vessels (O'Leary et al).

In the late sclerotic stage, as seen in the center of old lesions, the inflammatory infiltrate has disappeared almost completely, except in some areas of the subcutis. The epidermis is normal. The collagen bundles in the reticular dermis appear thickened and closely packed and stain more deeply eosinophilic than in normal skin. In the papillary dermis, where the collagen normally consists of loosely arranged fibers, the collagen may appear homogeneous (Reed et al). The eccrine glands

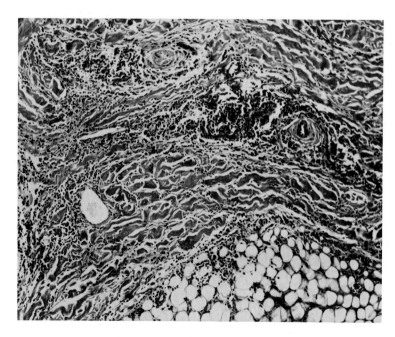

Fig. 25-11.   Scleroderma, early stage
A rather pronounced inflammatory infiltrate is present in the lower dermis and in the subcutaneous fat, where new collagen is being deposited; part of the collagen appears as closely packed, thick collagen bundles. (×100)

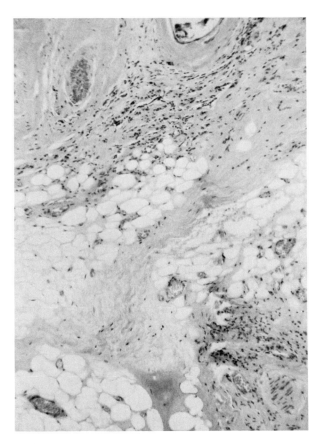

Fig. 25-12.   Scleroderma, early stage, subcutaneous fat
The trabeculae subdividing the subcutaneous fat are thickened. Large areas of subcutaneous fat are replaced by newly formed collagen fibers that show only faint staining. (×100)

appear markedly atrophic, and the fatty tissue normally surrounding them is greatly reduced in amount or absent. Instead, they are surrounded and appear tightly "bound down" by newly formed collagen (Fig. 25-13). Also, instead of lying, as they normally do, near the cutaneous–subcutaneous border, the sweat glands seem to lie well inside the dermis as a result of the replacement of most of the subcutaneous fat by newly formed collagen. The collagen that has largely replaced the fat cells in the subcutaneous tissue consists of thick, pale, sclerotic, homogeneous or hyalinized bundles with only few fibroblasts. Few blood vessels are seen within the sclerotic collagen; they often have a fibrotic wall and a narrowed lumen (Fleischmajer and Nedwich).

The fascia and striated muscles underlying lesions of morphea may be affected in the linear, segmental, and generalized types. The fascia shows fibrosis and sclerosis as seen in the subcutaneous tissue. The muscle fibers appear vacuolated and separated from one another by edema and focal collections of inflammatory cells (Hickman and Sheils).

Bullae, seen only on rare occasions in generalized morphea, arise subepidermally, probably as a result of lymphatic obstruction, causing subepidermal edema (Synkowski et al).

Differential Diagnosis. Histologic differentiation of the late stage of morphea from lichen sclerosus et atrophicus may cause difficulties, particularly in view of the fact that the two conditions may occur together (see p. 283). Both diseases can show homogenization of the papillary dermis and sclerosis of the reticular dermis. However, in lichen

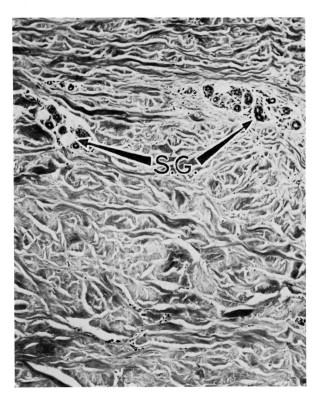

Fig. 25-13.   Scleroderma, late stage
Two groups of sweat glands (*S.G.*) appear markedly atrophic and are tightly "bound down" by newly formed collagen. Below the sweat glands, where subcutaneous fat was formerly located, the collagen consists of thick, closely packed, hyalinized bundles with only few fibroblasts. There is no longer any inflammatory infiltrate. (×100)

sclerosus et atrophicus, one observes, in addition, thinning of the rete malpighii, hydropic degeneration of the basal cells, and marked edema in the papillary dermis. Even though subepidermal bulla formation may be seen in morphea, it is more characteristic of lichen sclerosus et atrophicus (Anderson; Jablonska). Other points of differentiation are follicular plugging, which occurs exclusively in lichen sclerosus et atrophicus, and extension of the inflammatory reaction and fibrosis into the subcutaneous tissue, which is seen in morphea but does not occur in lichen sclerosus et atrophicus (Fleischmajer).

Systemic Scleroderma

In systemic scleroderma, the indurated lesions of the skin are not sharply demarcated or "circumscribed," as in morphea, although a few well-demarcated morphea-like patches may occasionally be seen (Black et al; Ikai et al).

Cutaneous involvement usually starts peripherally on the hands and face and gradually extends centripetally. This form is referred to as acrosclerosis. It is associated with Raynaud's phenomenon, which may precede other manifestations by months or even years. In about 5% of the cases, the cutaneous lesions first appear on the trunk as so-called *diffuse systemic scleroderma,* often sparing the peripheral portions of the extremities. Raynaud's phenomenon is absent in such patients (Tuffanelli and Winkelmann; Rowell). In both forms of systemic scleroderma, the skin in the involved areas is diffusely indurated and, as a result of diffuse fibrosis of the subcutaneous fat, becomes firmly bound to the underlying structures. The skeletal musculature is invariably affected, resulting in weakness and atrophy. Contractures of the muscles and tendons and ankyloses of the joints may develop.

Occasional manifestations pertaining to the skin include diffuse hyperpigmentation, which is seen mainly in diffuse systemic scleroderma, whereas macular telangiectasias on the face and hands, calcinosis cutis located on the extremities, and ulcerations, especially on the tips of the fingers and over the knuckles, occur predominantly in acrosclerosis.

Internal organs are usually affected, but their involvement varies greatly in extent and degree. Lesions in the esophagus may cause difficulties in deglutition. Involvement of the intestinal tract may lead to symptoms of malabsorption or, late in the disease, to ileus (Korting and Lachner). Lesions in the lungs may cause dyspnea and right-sided heart failure secondary to cor pulmonale (D'Angelo et al), and lesions in the kidneys may result in uremia (Fisher and Rodnan). A peculiar clinical feature of renal involvement in scleroderma is the rapidity with which either renal failure or "malignant" hypertension may develop. Renal failure and the cardiac complications

of "malignant" hypertension are the most common causes of death in scleroderma (Cannon et al). However, in quite a few patients, the disease ultimately comes to a standstill. Thus, in one series of 309 patients, the 7-year survival rate was 35% (Medsger et al). In another series of 267 patients, the 10-year survival rate was at least 47%, and, when only the traced patients were considered, it was 59% (Tuffanelli and Winkelmann).

A variant of acrosclerosis that frequently but not invariably has a favorable prognosis is the *Thibierge–Weissenbach syndrome,* also referred to as the *CRST syndrome,* consisting of **C**alcinosis cutis, **R**aynaud's phenomenon, **S**clerodactyly, and **T**elangiectases (Carr et al). Because of the frequent involvement of the **E**sophagus with dysphagia, it has also been called the *CREST syndrome* (Velayos et al). Death from visceral lesions of scleroderma is rather infrequent; it occurred in only 7 of 66 patients, or 11%, reported in five series (Carr et al; Medsger et al; Rowell; Velayos et al; Nielsen et al). It has also been pointed out that the frequency of polyarthritis is much lower in the CREST syndrome (15%) than in other forms of systemic scleroderma (65%) (Velayos et al).

Histopathology. The histologic appearance of the skin lesions in systemic scleroderma is similar to that of morphea, so that histologic differentiation of the two types is not possible. However, in early lesions of systemic scleroderma, the inflammatory reaction is less pronounced than in morphea, so that only a mild cellular infiltrate is present around the dermal vessels, around the eccrine coils, and in the subcutaneous tissue. The vascular changes in early lesions are slight, as in morphea. In contrast, in the late stage, systemic scleroderma shows more pronounced vascular changes than morphea, particularly in the subcutis. These changes consist of a paucity of blood vessels, thickening and hyalinization of their walls, and narrowing of the lumen (Fleischmajer et al, 1972). In the late stage of systemic sclerodema, in contrast with morphea, the epidermis may show disappearance of the rete ridges (O'Leary et al). Aggregates of calcium may also be seen in the late stage within areas of sclerotic, homogeneous collagen of the subcutaneous tissue (see also Calcinosis Cutis, p. 421) (Kanee).

Autopsy examination of the digital arteries in patients with Raynaud's phenomenon has revealed severe intimal fibrosis resulting in considerable narrowing of the lumina. Often, there is also adventitial fibrosis. These changes are similar to those present in the arcuate and interlobular renal arteries of patients with "scleroderma kidney" and in the small pulmonary arteries of patients with scleroderma who develop pulmonary arterial hypertension. However, accumulation of mucoid material in the intima is seen only in the arcuate and interlobular renal arteries (see below) (Rodnan et al).

Histologic examination of skeletal muscle in systemic scleroderma shows changes that are indistinguishable from those of dermatomyositis, although, as a rule, the degenerative changes are less pronounced, and atrophy and fibrosis predominate.

Systemic Lesions. Extensive areas of fibrosis and sclerosis may be found on autopsy, since these changes can occur wherever connective tissue normally exists (Piper and Helwig). Unless the involvement in a given organ is severe, it may be asymptomatic.

Obliterative vascular changes are of primary importance in producing the visceral lesions of systemic scleroderma, especially in the gastrointestinal tract, lungs, and kidneys (Alpert and Warner; Norton and Nardo; Toth and Alpert). The vessels primarily involved are the precapillary arterioles, which, in the earliest stage, show endothelial proliferation and perivascular inflammation. This is followed by marked intimal proliferation with narrowing of the lumen. Although widespread arteriolitis may be present in the early stage (Alpert and Warner), in rare instances only does the vascular disease in systemic scleroderma progress into a necrotizing arteriolitis, thus terminating as periarteritis nodosa (Toth and Alpert).

In the esophagus as well as in the stomach and intestinal tract, a variable amount of fibrosis is found, located chiefly in the submucosa but often involving and even replacing the muscularis. This is often associated with intimal thickening of the walls of vessels (Piper and Helwig).

In the lungs also, intimal thickening in the arterioles often seems to precede the development of interstitial fibrosis. In addition, it may lead to pulmonary hypertension, causing congestive heart failure. Cardiac insufficiency in systemic scleroderma usually is secondary to pulmonary fibrosis or hypertension rather than the result of myocardial fibrosis, which is rarely severe enough to produce clinical symptoms (D'Angelo et al). Severe interstitial fibrosis of the lungs may lead to degeneration of alveolar septa and formation of large and small cystic spaces, resulting in a so-called honeycomb lung (Getzowa). In several cases, secondary development of a pulmonary carcinoma has been reported. In most instances, the pulmonary carcinoma has been an alveolar cell or bronchiolar adenocarcinoma (Collins et al) but bronchogenic

squamous cell carcinoma (Tomkin) and oat cell carcinoma (Haqqani and Holti) have also been observed. Aside from the occasional development of malignancy in the lungs, no increased incidence of malignancy has been noted in systemic scleroderma, in contrast to dermatomyositis (see p. 459) (Talbott and Barrocas).

The histologic changes found in the kidneys in scleroderma are quite characteristic, differing from those of hypertensive disease. A primary distinguishing feature of renal scleroderma is the presence of adventitial fibrosis around the interlobar, arcuate, and interlobular arteries. Secondly, the interlobular arteries are the site of the most advanced vascular changes in scleroderma, whereas, in hypertensive disease, these vessels are normal, and the smaller arteries and arterioles are the site of pathologic changes (Cannon et al). Characteristically, in renal scleroderma, the arcuate and interlobular arteries show, regardless of whether the patients have a normotensive or hypertensive history, marked mucoid thickening of their intima, leading to narrowing or occlusion of their lumina (Fisher and Rodnan; Cannon et al). As a rule, the resulting cortical infarcts are larger in patients with scleroderma than in patients with hypertensive disease (Cannon et al).

Histogenesis. Two factors are recognized in the etiology of scleroderma: it is both a vascular disease and an autoimmune disorder (Rosenthal and Sack). In favor of an autoimmune etiology is the presence of antinuclear antibodies in the sera of about two thirds of the patients with systemic scleroderma. The titers of antibodies are frequently as high as in SLE (Rowell and Beck). The pattern usually evoked by the antinuclear antibodies in systemic scleroderma is either a speckled or a nucleolar fluorescence (Burnham). In addition, in some cases of systemic scleroderma, epidermal nucleolar IgG deposition is seen even in clinically normal skin as a result of high serum concentrations of antibody to nucleolar antigen (Prystowsky et al). Although subepidermal and vascular deposits are regularly absent in the skin (Tuffanelli), examination by direct immunofluorescence of kidney biopsies of patients with renal involvement shows diffuse vascular deposits of immunoglobulins, predominantly IgM, and/or of complement in the intima of the interlobular and arcuate arteries, which by light microscopy often exhibit fibromucinous alterations (see above) (Lapenas et al).

Electron microscopic examination in morphea and systemic scleroderma has shown significant changes in the small dermal blood vessels during the early stage of the disease, when light microscopy shows no vascular changes (Fleischmajer et al, 1976; Fleischmajer and Perlish). The main alterations are vacuolization and ultimate destruction of endothelial cells; reduplication of the basement membrane; a perivascular infiltrate of mononuclear cells; and the presence of fibroblasts and pericytes with enlarged rough endoplasmic reticulum, which is indicative of increased activity and is accompanied by perivascular fibrosis. Perivascular cellular infiltrates and endothelial cell damage appear to precede the stage of fibrosis (Fleischmajer and Perlish).

As a consequence of increased collagen synthesis in the skin in scleroderma, a considerable number of collagen fibrils have diameters smaller than those found in normal adult skin. Whereas the diameter of collagen fibrils normally varies between 70 nm and 140 nm, with an average width of 100 nm, 38% of the collagen fibrils in scleroderma in one study were found to have a diameter of less than 50 nm (Hayes and Rodnan).

Tissue culture and enzymatic studies have also indicated that there is an increase in the activity of fibroblasts and in the production of collagen during the active stage of scleroderma. Thus, cultures of fibroblasts show a higher rate than normal of DNA synthesis and an increase in collagen synthesis (Krieg et al). The activity of prolyl-hydroxylase is also increased in the skin, as is the incorporation of radioactive proline in the skin collagen (Bauer and Uitto). The relative proportions of type I and type III collagen are very similar to those found in normal adult dermis (Lovell et al).

Atrophoderma of Pasini and Pierini

In atrophoderma of Pasini and Pierini, one observes, usually on the trunk and particularly on the back, several areas in which the skin appears slightly depressed and has a slate-gray color but shows no other surface changes. The lesions are sharply but often irregularly demarcated and measure from 1 cm to 10 cm in diameter. They often show a "cliff-drop" border, which is largely an optical effect of the slate-gray discoloration. In old lesions, the center of the depressed area may feel slightly indurated.

Histopathology. The histologic changes in early lesions usually are slight and nonspecific, consisting of some thickening of the collagen bundles and a mild, scattered, chronic inflammatory infiltrate (Quiroga and Woscoff; Weiner and Gant). Older lesions show no inflammatory infiltrate, but, in the deeper layers of the dermis, they may show collagen bundles that not only are thickened but also appear tightly packed (Jablonska and Szczepanski). In addition, indurated areas may show homogeneous, hyalinized collagen bundles (Miller).

Since the collagen bundles in the skin of the back normally are rather thick, it may be difficult to determine whether the collagen shows any changes. It is therefore desirable to take a biopsy specimen not only from the lesion but also from normal skin, either from an area nearby or from the opposite side. Of course, subcutaneous fat should be included in the biopsy specimens.

Histogenesis. Some authors believe that atrophoderma of Pasini and Pierini is a disease entity, as suggested by the original describers. Those favoring this view regard the late induration occurring in some lesions as a pseudosclerosis (Canizares et al). It also has been pointed out that, in atrophoderma, the atrophy comes first and the sclerosis possibly later, whereas, in morphea, the sclerosis comes first and the atrophy later (Weiner).

In favor of the view that atrophoderma of Pasini and Pierini and morphea are identical speaks the fact that, in some instances, lesions of morphea appear either simultaneous with (Miller) or subsequent to atrophoderma (Kee et al). Even the transformation of lesions of morphea into those of atrophoderma has been observed (Rupec).

Some authors have suggested that there are two types of atrophoderma: an idiopathic type, and an atrophoscleroderma secondary to morphea (Kogoj; Pierini et al). Although this compromise may be acceptable to some, the impression remains that the two proposed types are one and the same disease. It may be pointed out that an atrophic form of morphea was first described in 1932 as forme lilacée non indurée (Gougerot). However, even though the atrophoderma of Pasini and Pierini probably represents morphea, the term should not be abandoned because of the typical clinical picture the disorder presents.

EOSINOPHILIC FASCIITIS (SHULMAN'S SYNDROME)

First described in 1974 (Shulman), eosinophilic fasciitis in most instances has an acute onset with tenderness affecting usually several extremities but occasionally only one (Krauser and Tuthill; Lupton and Goette). The involved limb or limbs appear diffusely swollen and on palpation are very firm, with the skin bound to the underlying tissue. Quite frequently, the skin in some of the affected areas shows surface irregularities characterized by depressions and ridges resulting in either a cobblestone appearance (Fleischmajer et al) or irregular dimpling of the skin (Weinstein and Schwartz). The induration may cause a decreased range of motion and, in severe cases, even joint contractures (Golitz). In only a few cases are there lesions on the trunk, and the face is almost invariably spared. On the trunk, the lesions may have the appearance of morphea (Weinstein and Schwartz; Chevrant-Breton et al; Michet et al). In most patients, moderate eosinophilia of the blood and hypergammaglobulinemia are present.

In many instances, there is gradual improvement and resolution of the lesions either under treatment with corticosteroids (Shulman) or spontaneously (Rodnan et al; Chevrant-Breton et al).

In nearly all reported cases, Raynaud's phenomenon and visceral lesions of scleroderma have been absent. Only very few instances of incontestable eosinophilic fasciitis have shown evidence of Raynaud's phenomenon (Barrière et al) or mild pulmonary fibrosis (Coyle and Chapman).

Histopathology. An elliptic biopsy deep enough to include the fascia overlying a muscle is required. In most cases, the adipose tissue shows no significant changes, except that the fibrous septa separating deeply located fat lobules are thicker, paler-staining, and more homogeneous and hyaline than normal dermal connective tissue (Torres and George). In other cases, however, the collagen in the lower reticular dermis appears pale and homogeneous, and the entire subcutaneous fat is replaced by horizontally oriented, thick, homogeneous collagen containing only few fibroblasts and merging with the fascia (Lupton and Goette). The fascia is markedly thickened, appears homogeneous, and is permeated by a chronic inflammatory infiltrate (Hintner et al). In some instances, the infiltrate in the fascia contains an admixture of eosinophils (Weinstein and Schwartz). The underlying skeletal muscle in some cases shows myofiber degeneration, severe inflammation with a component of eosinophils, and focal scarring (Lupton and Goette); in other cases, however, it is not involved (Shewmake et al).

Histogenesis. Whereas, at first, the impression prevailed that eosinophilic fasciitis was a new syndrome (Shulman; Rodnan et al), it soon became apparent that the disorder represents a variant of morphea (Golitz; Michet et al; Hintner et al). Eosinophilic fasciitis shares many features with generalized morphea; they may both show inflammation and fibrosis of the fascia, as well as blood eosinophilia and hypergammaglobulinemia (Fleischmajer et al; King et al). The term *morphea profunda* has been suggested, analogous to *lupus erythematosus profundus* (Su and Person). Nevertheless, because of its acute onset in most cases, its usual limitation to the structures underlying the skin, and its tendency to resolve, eosinophilic fasciitis deserves recognition as a distinct variant of morphea.

BIBLIOGRAPHY

Lupus Erythematosus

APPEL GB, SILVA FG, PIRANI CL et al: Renal involvement in systemic lupus erythematosus (SLE): A study of 56 patients emphasizing histologic classification. Medicine (Baltimore) 57:371–410, 1978

BALDWIN DS, GLUCK MC, LOWENSTEIN J et al: Lupus nephritis: Clinical course as related to morphologic forms and their transitions. Am J Med 62:12–30, 1977

BALDWIN DS, LOWENSTEIN J, ROTHFIELD NF et al: The clinical course of the proliferative and membranous forms of lupus nephritis. Ann Intern Med 73:929–942, 1970

BARTHELMES H, SÖNNICHSEN N: Differentialdiagnostische Untersuchungen zwischen Lupus erythematodes chronicus discoides und lymphocytärer Infiltration Jessner-Kanof mit Hilfe der Immunofluoreszenz-Histologie. Arch Klin Exp Dermatol 232:384–397, 1968

BAZEX A, SALVADOR R, DUPRÉ A et al: Ist es berechtigt, die lymphozytäre Infiltration der Haut von Jessner und Kanof als nosologische Einheit anzusehen? Hautarzt 16:250–254, 1965

BEAN SF: Proper biopsy technique for immunofluorescence test on skin. J Dermatol Surg 2:148–150, 1950

BELJAEWA HF, SMELOW NS, SJITSCH LI et al: Hautgefässe bei verschiedenen Formen des Lupus erythematosus im Laufe der Behandlung. Dermatol Wochenschr 154:631–636, 1968

BEN BASSAT M, ROSENFELD J, JOSHUA H et al: Lupus nephritis. Electron-dense and immunofluorescence deposits and their correlation with proteinuria and renal function. Am J Clin Pathol 72:186–193, 1979

BERK SH, BLANK H: Ultraviolet light and cytoplasmic tubules in lupus erythematosus. Arch Dermatol 109:364–366, 1974

BIELICKY T, TRAPL J: Nichtvernarbender chronischer Erythematodes. Arch Klin Exp Dermatol 217:438–456, 1963

BIESECKER G, LAVIN L, ZISKIND M et al: Cutaneous localization of the membrane attack complex in discoid and systemic lupus erythematosus. N Engl J Med 306:264–270, 1982

BLACK MM, HUDSON PM: Atrophie blanche lesions closely resembling malignant atrophic papulosis (Degos disease) in systemic lupus erythematosus. Br J Dermatol 95:649–652, 1976

BURNHAM TK: In discussion of Krieger BL: Lymphocytic infiltration of the skin (Jessner). Arch Dermatol 100:247–248, 1969

BURNHAM TK: Antinuclear antibodies. Arch Dermatol 114:1343–1344, 1978

BURNHAM TK, FINE G: The immunofluorescent "band" test for lupus erythematosus. Arch Dermatol 103:24–32, 1971

CABRÉ J, STEIGLEDER GK: Das Krankheitsbild der lymphozytären Infiltration (Lymphocytic Infiltration) im Sinne von Jessner und Kanof. Arch Klin Exp Dermatol 212:525–549, 1961

CALLEN JP: Chronic cutaneous lupus erythematosus. Arch Dermatol 118:412–416, 1982

CALNAN CD: Lymphocytic infiltration of the skin (Jessner). Br J Dermatol 69:169–173, 1957

CARNABUCI GI, LUSCOMBE HA, STOLOFF IL: ANA titers in lupus erythematosus and certain chronic dermatoses. Arch Dermatol 95:247–249, 1967

Case Records of the Massachusetts General Hospital, Case 18-1969. N Engl J Med 280:1009–1017, 1969

CAWLEY EP, MCMANUS JFA, LUPTON CH JR et al: An examination of skin from patients with collagen disease utilizing the combined alcian blue–periodic acid Schiff stain. J Invest Dermatol 27:389–394, 1956

CHORZELSKI T, JABLONSKA S, BLASZCZYK M: Diagnostischer und differentialdiagnostischer Wert der immunpathologischen Untersuchungen bei Erythematodes chronicus. Arch Klin Exp Dermatol 233:219–226, 1968

CLARK WH JR, REED RJ, MIHM MC: Lupus erythematosus. Histopathology of cutaneous lesions. Hum Pathol 4:157–163, 1973

COHEN AS, CANOSO JJ: Criteria for the classification of systemic lupus erythematosus—Status 1972. Arthritis Rheum 15:540–543, 1972

COPEMAN PWM, SCHROETER AL, KIERLAND RR: An unusual variant of lupus erythematosus or lichen planus. Br J Dermatol 83:269–272, 1970

DANTZIG PI, MAURO J, RAYHANZADEH S et al: The significance of a positive cutaneous immunofluorescence test in systemic lupus erythematosus. Br J Dermatol 93:531–537, 1975

DUBIN HV, STAWISKI MA: Systemic lupus erythematosus resembling malignant atrophic papulosis. Arch Intern Med 134:321–323, 1974

DUBOIS EL, CHANDOR S, FRIOU GS et al: Progressive systemic sclerosis (PSS) and localized scleroderma (morphea) with positive LE cell test and unusual systemic manifestations compatible with systemic lupus erythematosus (SLE). Medicine (Baltimore) 50:199–222, 1971

DUBOIS EL, TUFFANELLI DL: Clinical manifestations of systemic lupus erythematosus. JAMA 190:104–111, 1964

ERBSLÖH E, BAEDEKER WD: Lupus Myopathie. Dtsch Med Wochenschr 87:2464–2470, 1962

ESTES D, CHRISTIAN CL: The natural history of systemic lupus erythematosus by prospective analysis. Medicine (Baltimore) 50:85–95, 1971

FISHER DA, EPSTEIN JH, KAY DN et al: Polymorphous light eruption and lupus erythematosus. Arch Dermatol 101:458–461, 1970

FOUNTAIN RB: Lupus erythematosus profundus. Br J Dermatol 80:571–579, 1968

FRIES JF, PORTA J, LIANG MH: Marginal benefit of renal biopsy in systemic lupus erythematosus. Arch Intern Med 138:1386–1389, 1978

GILLIAM JN, CHEATUM DE, HURD ER et al: Immunoglobulins in clinically uninvolved skin in systemic lupus erythematosus. Association with renal disease. J Clin Invest 53:1434–1440, 1974

GILLIAM JN, SONTHEIMER RD: Distinctive cutaneous subsets in the spectrum of lupus erythematosus. J Am Acad Dermatol 4:471–475, 1981

GITLIN D, CRAIG JM, JANEWAY CA: Studies on the nature of fibrinoid in the collagen diseases. Am J Pathol 33:55–77, 1957

GOTTLIEB B, WINKELMANN RK: Lymphocytic infiltration of skin. Arch Dermatol 86:626–633, 1962

GYÖRKEY F, SINKOVICS JG, MIN KW et al: A morphologic study on the occurrence and distribution of structures resembling viral nucleocapsids in collagen diseases. Am J Med 53:148–158, 1972

HALEVY S, BEN-BASSAT M, JOSHUA H et al: Immunofluorescent and electron-microscopic findings in the uninvolved skin of patients with systemic lupus erythematosus. Acta Derm Venereol (Stockh) 59:427–433, 1979

HARGRAVES MM, RICHMOND H, MORTON RJ: Presentation of two bone marrow elements: The "tart" cell and the "LE" cell. Proc Mayo Clin 23:25–28, 1948

HARRIS RB, DUNCAN SC, ECKER RI et al: Lymphoid follicles in subcutaneous inflammatory disease. Arch Dermatol 115:442–443, 1979

HARRIST TJ, MIHM MC JR: Cutaneous immunopathology. The diagnostic use of direct and indirect immunofluorescence techniques in dermatologic diseases. (Review) Hum Pathol 10:625–653, 1979

HASHIMOTO K, THOMPSON DF: Discoid lupus erythematosus. Electron microscopic studies of paramyxovirus-like structures. Arch Dermatol 101:565–577, 1970

HAUSTEIN UF: Membranlose fibrilläre und amorph-granuläre Körper bei Lupus erythematodes. Dermatol Wochenschr 159:185–198, 1973

JESSNER M, KANOF NB: Lymphocytic infiltration of the skin. Arch Dermatol Syph 68:447–449, 1953

KANT KS, POLLACK VE, WEISS MA et al: Glomerular thrombosis in systemic lupus erythematosus: Prevalence and significance. Medicine (Baltimore) 60:71–86, 1981

KELLUM RE, HASERICK JR: Systemic lupus erythematosus: Statis-tical evaluation of mortality based on consecutive series of 299 patients. Arch Intern Med 113:200–207, 1964

KENNEDY C, GOLD SC: Subacute cutaneous lupus erythematosus. Clin Exp Dermatol 6:673–676, 1981

KLEMPERER P, POLLACK AD, BAEHR G: Pathology of disseminated lupus erythematosus. (Review of the pathology of visceral lesions) Arch Pathol 32:569–631, 1941

LANDRY M, WINKELMANN RK: Tubular cytoplasmic inclusions in dermatomyositis. Proc Mayo Clin 47:479–492, 1972

MACADAM RF, VETTERS JM, SAIKIA NK: A search for microtubular inclusions in endothelial cells in a variety of skin diseases. Br J Dermatol 92:175–182, 1975

MACIEJEWSKI W: Annular erythema as an unusual manifestation of chronic disseminated lupus erythematosus. Arch Dermatol 116:450–453, 1980

MACIEJEWSKI W, DABROWSKI J, JABLONSKA S et al: Virus-like tubular cytoplasmic inclusions in epithelial tumors. Dermatologica 146:141–148, 1973

MADDISON PJ, PROVOST TT, REICHLIN M: Serological findings in patients with "ANA-negative" systemic lupus erythematosus. Medicine (Baltimore) 60:87–94, 1981

MATTHAY RA, SCHWARZ MI, PETTY TL: Pulmonary manifestations of systemic lupus erythematosus: Review of 12 cases of acute lupus pneumonitis. Medicine (Baltimore) 54:397–409, 1975

MCCREIGHT WG, MONTGOMERY H: Cutaneous changes in lupus erythematosus. Arch Dermatol Syph 61:1–11, 1950

MCDUFFIE FC: Twenty years of the lupus erythematosus cell. Ann Intern Med 70:413–417, 1969

MILLARD LG, ROWELL NR: Abnormal laboratory test results and their relationship to prognosis in discoid lupus erythematosus. Arch Dermatol 115:1055–1058, 1979

MUEHRCKE RC, KARK RM, PIRANI CL et al: Lupus nephritis: A clinical and pathologic study based on renal biopsies. Medicine (Baltimore) 36:1–145, 1957

NEBE H, BARTHELMES H: Über den diagnostischen Wert der subepidermalen Immunoglobulin- und Komplementablagerungen beim Lupus erythematodes. Dermatol Monatsschr 159:594–603, 1973

NELSON CE, DAHL MV, GOLTZ RW: Arcuate dermal erythema in a carrier of granulomatous disease. Arch Dermatol 113:798–800, 1977

NISENGARD RJ, JABLONSKA S, CHORZELSKI T et al: Diagnosis of systemic lupus erythematosus. Importance of antinuclear antibody titers and peripheral staining patterns. Arch Dermatol 111:1298–1300, 1975

OGAWA K: Ultrastructure of cutaneous lesions in lupus erythematosus. J Dermatol (Tokyo) 8:175–186, 1981

O'LOUGHLIN S, SCHROETER AL, JORDON RE: A study of lupus erythematosus with particular reference to generalized discoid lupus. Br J Dermatol 99:1–11, 1978a

O'LOUGHLIN S, SCHROETER AL, JORDON RE: Chronic urticaria-like lesions in systemic lupus erythematosus. Arch Dermatol 114:879–883, 1978b

PANET-RAYMOND G, JOHNSON WC: Lupus erythematosus and polymorphous light eruption. Arch Dermatol 108:785–787, 1973

PEHAMBERGER H, KONRAD K, HOLUBAR K: Immunoelectron microscopy of skin in lupus erythematosus. J Cutan Pathol 5:319–328, 1978

PETERSON WC JR, FUSARO RM: Antinuclear factors in chronic discoid lupus erythematosus. Arch Dermatol 87:563–565, 1963

POHLE EL, TUFFANELLI DL: Study of cutaneous lupus erythematosus. Arch Dermatol 97:520–526, 1968

PROVOST TT: Subsets in systemic lupus erythematosus. J Invest Dermatol 72:110–113, 1979a

PROVOST TT: The relationship between discoid lupus erythematosus and systemic lupus erythematosus. Am J Dermatopathol 1:181–184, 1979b

PROVOST TT, ANDRES G, MADDISON PJ et al: Lupus band test in untreated SLE patients. J Invest Dermatol 74:407–412, 1980

PRUNIÉRAS M, MONTGOMERY H: Histopathology of cutaneous lesions in systemic lupus erythematosus. Arch Dermatol 74:177–190, 1956

PRYSTOWSKY SD, GILLIAM JN: Discoid lupus erythematosus as part of a larger disease spectrum. Arch Dermatol 111:1448–1452, 1975

ROPES M: Observations on the natural course of disseminated lupus erythematosus. Medicine (Baltimore) 43:387–391, 1964

SÁNCHEZ NP, PETERS MS, WINKELMANN RK: The histopathology of lupus erythematosus panniculitis. J Am Acad Dermatol 5:673–680, 1981

SCHIRREN CG, EGGERT D: Beitrag zum Erythematodes profundus (Kaposi-Irgang). Arch Klin Exp Dermatol 216:541–555, 1963

SCOTT A, REES EG: The relationship of systemic lupus erythematosus and discoid lupus erythematosus. Arch Dermatol 79:422–435, 1959

SHARP GC, ANDERSON PC: Current concepts in the classification of connective tissue diseases. Overlap syndromes and mixed connective tissue disease (MCTD). J Am Acad Dermatol 2:269–279, 1980

SONTHEIMER RD, THOMAS JR, GILLIAM JN: Subacute cutaneous lupus erythematosus. A cutaneous marker for a distinct lupus erythematosus subset. Arch Dermatol 115:1409–1415, 1979

STAHL D, THOMSEN K, HOU-JENSEN K: Malignant atrophic papulosis. Arch Dermatol 114:1687–1689, 1977

STOUGHTON R, WELLS G: A histochemical study on polysaccharides in normal and diseased skin. J Invest Dermatol 14:37–51, 1950

SÜMEGI I: Fibrinoid necrosis and downward motion of colloid bodies in lichen planus (apoptosis). Acta Derm Venereol (Stockh) 59:27–31, 1979

TUFFANELLI DL: Lupus erythematosus panniculitis (profundus). Arch Dermatol 103:231–242, 1971

TUFFANELLI DL: Cutaneous immunopathology: Recent observations. J Invest Dermatol 65:143–153, 1975

TUFFANELLI DL, KAY D, FUKUYAMA K: Dermal-epidermal junction in lupus erythematosus. Arch Dermatol 99:652–662, 1969

UEKI H: The application of the fluorescent antibody technique in dermatology. Jpn J Dermatol (Series B) 78:367–377, 1968

UEKI H, WOLFF HH, BRAUN-FALCO O: Cutaneous localization of human gamma globulins in lupus erythematosus. Arch Dermatol Forsch 248:297–314, 1974

UITTO J, SANTA-CRUZ DJ, EISEN AZ et al: Verrucous lesions in patients with discoid lupus erythematosus. Br J Dermatol 98:507–520, 1978

VIVELL K: Lymphozytäre Infiltration (Jessner-Kanof) mit Übergang in discoiden Lupus erythematodes. Z Hautkr 56:596–597, 1981

VON EICKSTEDT UM, HASSENPFLUG KH: Zur Kenntnis des Lupus erythematodes hypertrophicus (et profundus) Bechet. Arch Klin Exp Dermatol 214:471–481, 1962

WECHSLER HL, STAVRIDES A: Systemic lupus erythematosus with anti-Ro antibodies. J Am Acad Dermatol 6:73–83, 1982

WEIGAND DA, BURGDORF WHC, GREGG LJ: Dermal mucinosis in discoid lupus erythematosus. Arch Dermatol 117:735–738, 1981

WINKELMANN RK: Panniculitis and systemic lupus erythematosus. JAMA 211:472–475, 1970

WORTHINGTON JM, BAGGENSTOSS AH, HARGRAVES MM: Significance of hematoxylin bodies in the necropsy diagnosis of systemic lupus erythematosus. Am J Pathol 35:955–969, 1959

ZWEIMAN B, HEBERT J: The lupus erythematosus cell phenomenon: Mechanism and significance. Int J Dermatol 15:121–124, 1976

Mixed Connective Tissue Disease

GILLIAM JN, PRYSTOWSKY SD: Mixed connective tissue disease syndrome. Arch Dermatol 113:583–587, 1977

PRYSTOWSKY SD, TUFFANELLI DL: Speckled (particulate) epidermal nuclear IgG deposition in normal skin. Arch Dermatol 114:705–710, 1978

SHARP GC, ANDERSON PC: Current concepts in the classification of connective tissue diseases. J Am Acad Dermatol 2:269–279, 1980

SHARP GC, IRVIN WS, TAN EM et al: Mixed connective tissue disease: An apparently distinct rheumatic disease syndrome associated with a specific antibody to an extractable nuclear antigen (ENA). Am J Med 52:148–159, 1972

Dermatomyositis

ARUNDEL FD, WILKINSON RD, HASERICK JR: Dermatomyositis and malignant neoplasms in adults. Arch Dermatol 82:772–775, 1960

BANKER BQ, VICTOR M: Dermatomyositis (systemic angiopathy) of childhood. Medicine (Baltimore) 45:261–289, 1966

BARNES BE: Dermatomyositis and malignancy: A review of the literature. Ann Intern Med 84:68–76, 1976

BOHAN A, PETER JB, BOWMAN RL et al: A computer-assisted analysis of 153 patients with polymyositis and dermatomyositis. Medicine (Baltimore) 56:255–286, 1977

BONVALET D, COLAN-GOHM K, BELAICH S et al: Les différentes formes du parapsoriasis en plaques. Ann Dermatol Venereol 104:18–25, 1977

BRAUN-FALCO O, MARGHESCU S: Kongenitales teleangiektatisches Erythem (Bloom-Syndrom) mit Diabetes insipidus. Hautarzt 17:155–161, 1966

CALLEN JP: Dermatomyositis. (Review) Int J Dermatol 18:423–433, 1979

CALLEN JP, HYLA JF, BOLE GG et al: The relationship of dermatomyositis and polymyositis to internal malignancy. Arch Dermatol 116:295–298, 1980

CHRISTIANSON HB, BRUNSTING LA, PERRY HO: Dermatomyositis. Arch Dermatol 74:581–589, 1956

DEGOS R, CIVATTE J, BELAICH S et al: The prognosis of adult dermatomyositis. Trans St John's Hosp Dermatol Soc 57:98–104, 1971

DOWLING GB, FREUDENTHAL W: Dermatomyositis and poikiloderma atrophicans vasculare: A clinical and histological comparison. Br J Dermatol 50:519–539, 1938

DOWNING JB, EDELSTEIN JM, FITZPATRICK TB: Poikiloderma vasculare atrophicans. Arch Dermatol Syph 56:740–762, 1947

GONZALES-ANGULO A, FRAGA A, MINTZ G: Submicroscopic alterations in capillaries of skeletal muscles in polymyositis. Am J Med 45:873–879, 1968

GUY WH, GRAUER RC, JACOB FM: Poikilodermatomyositis. Arch Dermatol Syph 40:867–878, 1939

HARRIST TJ, MIHM MC JR: Cutaneous immunopathology. The diagnostic use of direct and indirect immunofluorescence techniques in dermatologic diseases. (Review) Hum Pathol 10:625–653, 1979

HASHIMOTO K, ROBINSON L, VELAYOS E et al: Dermatomyositis. Electron microscopic, immunologic, and tissue culture studies of paramyxovirus-like inclusions. Arch Dermatol 103:120–135, 1971

HORN RC JR: Poikilodermatomyositis. Arch Dermatol Syph 44:1086–1097, 1941

JANIS JF, WINKELMANN RK: Histopathology of the skin in dermatomyositis. Arch Dermatol 97:640–650, 1968

KINNEY TD, MAHER MM: Dermatomyositis. Am J Pathol 16:561–594, 1940

KRAIN LS: Dermatomyositis in six patients without initial muscle involvement. Arch Dermatol 111:241–245, 1975

LANDRY M, WINKELMANN RK: Tubular cytoplasmic inclusion in dermatomyositis. Mayo Clin Proc 47:479–492, 1972

MULLER SA, WINKELMANN RK, BRUNSTING LA: Calcinosis in dermatomyositis. Arch Dermatol 79:669–673, 1959

MUSGER A: Zur Frage nach der nosologischen Stellung der Parapsoriasis lichenoides Brocq. Hautarzt 17:280–284, 1966

O'LEARY PA, WAISMAN M: Dermatomyositis: A study of 40 cases. (Review) Arch Dermatol Syph 41:1001–1019, 1940

REICH H: Das Teutschlaender-Syndrom. Hautarzt 14:462–468, 1963

ROSE AL, WALTON JN: Polymyositis: A survey of 89 cases with particular reference to treatment and prognosis. Brain 89:747–768, 1966

SAMMAN PD: The natural history of parapsoriasis en plaques (chronic superficial dermatitis) and prereticulotic poikiloderma. Br J Dermatol 87:405–411, 1972

SHAFIQ SA, MILHORAT AT, GORYCKI MA: Electron microscope study of muscular degeneration and vascular changes in polymyositis. J Pathol Bacteriol 94:139–147, 1967

STEIGLEDER GK: Die Poikilodermien—Genodermien und Genodermatosen? Arch Dermatol Syph (Berlin) 194:461–475, 1952

VELLA BRIFFA D, WARIN AP, CALNAN CD: Parakeratosis variegata: A report of two cases and their treatment with PUVA. Clin Exp Dermatol 4:537–541, 1979

VIGNOS PJ, BOWLING GF, WATKINS MP: Polymyositis. Arch Intern Med 114:263–277, 1964

WAINGER CK, LEVER WF: Dermatomyositis: A report of three cases with postmortem observations. Arch Dermatol Syph 59:196–208, 1949

WESTON WL, THORNE EG: Profound T lymphopenia in dermatomyositis with cancer. N Engl J Med 291:208, 1974

WILLIAMS RC: Dermatomyositis and malignancy: A review of the literature. Ann Intern Med 50:1174–1181, 1959

WINKELMANN RK, MULDER DW, LAMBERT EH et al: Course of dermatomyositis-polymyositis. Mayo Clin Proc 43:545–556, 1968

Scleroderma

ALPERT LI, WARNER RR: Systemic sclerosis. Am J Med 45:468–473, 1968

ANDERSON CR: Bullous lichen sclerosus et atrophicus. Arch Dermatol Syph 49:423–426, 1944

BAUER EA, UITTO J: Collagen in cutaneous diseases. Int J Dermatol 18:251–270, 1979

BLACK MM, BOTTOMS E, SHUSTER S: Skin collagen content and thickness in systemic sclerosis. Br J Dermatol 83:552–555, 1970

BURNHAM TK: Antinuclear antibodies. Arch Dermatol 114:1343–1344, 1978

CANIZARES O, SACHS PM, JAIMOVICH L et al: Idiopathic atrophoderma of Pasini and Pierini. Arch Dermatol 77:42–60, 1958

CANNON PJ, HASSAR M, CASE DB et al: The relationship of hypertension and renal failure in scleroderma (progressive systemic sclerosis) to structural and functional abnormalities of the renal cortical circulation. Medicine (Baltimore) 53:1–46, 1974

CARR RD, HEISEL EB, STEVENSON TD: CRST syndrome. Arch Dermatol 92:519–525, 1965

CHRISTIANSON HB, DORSEY CS, O'LEARY P et al: Localized scleroderma. Arch Dermatol 74:629–639, 1956

COLLINS DH, DARKE CS, DODGE OG: Scleroderma with honeycomb lungs and bronchiolar carcinoma. J Pathol Bacteriol 76:531, 1958

D'ANGELO WA, FRIES JF, MASI AT et al: Pathologic observations in systemic sclerosis (scleroderma). Am J Med 46:428–440, 1969

DIAZ-PEREZ JL, CONNOLLY SM, WINKELMANN RK: Disabling pansclerotic morphea of children. Arch Dermatol 116:169–173, 1980

DILLEY JJ, PERRY HO: Bilateral linear scleroderma en coup de sabre. Arch Dermatol 97:688–689, 1968

FISHER ER, RODNAN GP: Pathologic observations concerning the kidney in progressive systemic sclerosis. Arch Pathol 65:29–39, 1958

FLEISCHMAJER R: Relationship between morphea and lichen sclerosus et atrophicus. Am J Dermatopathol 2:283–284, 1980

FLEISCHMAJER R, DAMIANO V, NEDWICH A: Alteration of subcutaneous tissue in systemic scleroderma. Arch Dermatol 105:59–66, 1972

FLEISCHMAJER R, NEDWICH A: Generalized morphea. I. Histology of the dermis and subcutaneous tissue. Arch Dermatol 106:509–514, 1972

FLEISCHMAJER R, PERLISH JS: Capillary alterations in scleroderma. J Am Acad Dermatol 2:161–170, 1980

FLEISCHMAJER R, PERLISH JS, SHAW KV et al: Skin capillary changes in early systemic scleroderma. Arch Dermatol 112:1553–1557, 1976

GETZOWA S: Cystic and compact pulmonary sclerosis in progressive scleroderma. Arch Pathol 40:99–106, 1945

GOUGEROT H: Sclérodermie atypique. La forme lilacée non indurée en plaques ou en bandes. Bull Soc Fr Dermatol Syph 39:1667–1669, 1932

HAQQANI MT, HOLTI G: Systemic sclerosis with pulmonary fibrosis and oat cell carcinoma. Acta Derm Venereol (Stockh) 53:369–374, 1973

HAYES RL, RODNAN GP: The ultrastructure of skin in progressive sclerosis (scleroderma). Am J Pathol 63:433–442, 1971

HICKMAN JW, SHEILS WS: Progressive facial hemiatrophy. Arch Intern Med 113:716–720, 1964

IKAI K, TAGAMI H, IMAMURA S et al: Morphea-like cutaneous changes in a patient with systemic scleroderma. Dermatologica 158:438–442, 1979

JABLONSKA S: Relationship between morphea and lichen sclerosus et atrophicus. Am J Dermatopathol 2:285, 1980

JABLONSKA S, SZCZEPANSKI A: Atrophoderma Pasini-Pierini: Is it an entity? Dermatologica 125:226–242, 1962

KANEE B: Scleropoikiloderma with calcinosis cutis, Raynaud-like syndrome and atrophoderma. Arch Dermatol Syph 50:254–260, 1944

KEE CE, BROTHERS WS, NEW W: Idiopathic atrophoderma of Pasini and Pierini with coexistent morphea. Arch Dermatol 82:100–103, 1960

KOGOJ F: Qu'est-ce que c'est que la maladie de Pasini-Pierini? Ann Dermatol Syph 88:247–256, 1961

KORTING GW, BRACHTEL R: Zur Raynaud Symptomatik bei circumscripter Sklerodermie. Hautarzt 23:273–275, 1972

KORTING GW, LACHNER H: Sclerodermia malabsorptiva. Hautarzt 23:12–16, 1972

KRIEG T, MÜLLER PK, GOERZ G: Fibroblasts from a patient with scleroderma reveal abnormal metabolism. Arch Dermatol Res 259:105–107, 1977

LAPENAS D, RODNAN GP, CAVALLO T: Immunopathology of the renal vascular lesion of progressive systemic sclerosis (scleroderma). Am J Pathol 91:243–256, 1978

LOVELL CR, NICHOLLS AC, DUANCE VC et al: Characterization of dermal collagen in systemic sclerosis. Br J Dermatol 100:359–369, 1979

MEDSGER TA, MASI AT, RODNAN GP et al: Survival with systemic sclerosis (Scleroderma). Ann Intern Med 75:369–376, 1971

MILLER RF: Idiopathic atrophoderma. (Review) Arch Dermatol 92:653–660, 1965

NIELSEN AO, BRUN B, SECHER L: Calcinosis in generalized scleroderma. Acta Derm Venereol (Stockh) 60:301–307, 1980

NORTON WL, NARDO JM: Vascular disease in progressive systemic sclerosis (scleroderma). Ann Intern Med 73:317–324, 1970

O'LEARY PA, MONTGOMERY H, RAGSDALE WE: Dermatohistopathology of various types of scleroderma. (Review) Arch Dermatol 75:78–87, 1957

PIERINI LE, ABULAFIA J, MOSTO SJ: Atrophodermie idiopathique progressive et états viosins. Ann Dermatol Syph 97:391–416, 1970

PIPER WN, HELWIG EB: Progressive systemic sclerosis. Arch Dermatol 72:535–546, 1955

PRYSTOWSKY SD, GILLIAM JN, TUFFANELLI D: Epidermal nucleolar IgG deposition in clinically normal skin. Arch Dermatol 114:536–538, 1971

QUIROGA ML, WOSCOFF A: L'atrophodermie idiopathique progressive (Pasini-Pierini) et la sclérodermie atypique lilacée non indurée (Gougerot). Ann Dermatol Syph 88:507–520, 1961

REED RJ, CLARK WH, MIHM MC: The cutaneous collagenoses. Hum Pathol 4:165–186, 1973

RODNAN GP, MYEROWITZ RL, JUSTH GO: Morphologic changes in the digital arteries of patients with progressive systemic sclerosis (scleroderma) and Reynaud phenomenon. Medicine (Baltimore) 59:393–408, 1980

ROSENTHAL DS, SACK B: Autoimmune hemolytic anemia in scleroderma. JAMA 216:2011–2012, 1971

ROWELL NR: The prognosis of systemic sclerosis. Br J Dermatol 95:57–60, 1976

ROWELL NR, BECK JS: The diagnostic value of an antinuclear antibody test in clinical dermatology. Arch Dermatol 96:290–295, 1967

RUPEC M: Über die Beziehungen der zirkumskripten Sklerodermie zum Morbus Pasini-Pierini. Z Hautkr 33:114–118, 1962

RYCKMANNS F, KONZ B: Disseminierte zirkumskripte Sklerodermie und diffuse Sklerodermie vom Typ der Akrosklerodermia. Hautarzt 31:86–90, 1980

STAVA Z: Zirkumskripte Sklerodermie. Dermatol Wochenschr 139:513–523, 1959

SYNKOWSKI DR, LOBITZ WC JR, PROVOST TT: Bullous scleroderma. Arch Dermatol 117:135–137, 1981

TALBOTT JH, BARROCAS M: Progressive systemic sclerosis (PSS) and malignancy, pulmonary and non-pulmonary. Medicine (Baltimore) 58:182–207, 1979

TOMKIN GH: Systemic sclerosis associated with carcinoma of the lung. Br J Dermatol 81:213–216, 1969

TOTH A, ALPERT LI: Progressive systemic sclerosis terminating as periarteritis nodosa. Arch Pathol 92:31–36, 1971

TUFFANELLI DL: Cutaneous immunopathology: Recent observations. J Invest Dermatol 65:143–153, 1975

TUFFANELLI DL, MARMELZAT WL, DORSEY CS: Linear scleroderma

with hemiatrophy: Report of three cases associated with collagen-vascular disease. Dermatologica 132:51–58, 1966

TUFFANELLI DL, WINKELMANN RK: Systemic scleroderma. Arch Dermatol 84:359–371, 1961

VELAYOS EE, MASI AT, STEVENS MB et al: The "CREST" syndrome. Comparison with SS (scleroderma). Arch Intern Med 139:1240–1244, 1979

WEIDNER F, BRAUN-FALCO O: Gleichzeitiges Vorkommen von Symptomen der circumscripten und progressiven Sklerodermie. Hautarzt 19:345–350, 1968

WEINER M: In discussion to Eshelman OM: Idiopathic atrophoderma of Pasini and Pierini. Arch Dermatol 92:737–738, 1965

WEINER MA, GANT JQ JR: Idiopathic atrophoderma of Pasini and Pierini in two brothers. Arch Dermatol 80:195–197, 1959

Eosinophilic Fasciitis (Shulman's Syndrome)

BARRIÈRE H, STALDER JF, BERGER M et al: Syndrome de Shulman. Ann Dermatol Venereol 107:643–646, 1980

CHEVRANT-BRETON J, MONDAUD M, SABOURAUD O et al: Le syndrome de Shulman: Fasciite avec éosinophilie; pseudo-sclérodermie à éosinophiles. A propos de deux cas. Ann Dermatol Venereol 104:616–621, 1977

COYLE HE, CHAPMAN RS: Eosinophilic fasciitis (Shulman syndrome) in association with systemic sclerosis. Acta Derm Venereol (Stockh) 60:181–182, 1980

FLEISCHMAJER R, JACOTOT AB, SHORE S et al: Scleroderma, eosinophilia, and diffuse fasciitis. Arch Dermatol 114:1320–1325, 1978

GOLITZ LE: Fasciitis with eosinophilia: The Shulman syndrome. Int J Dermatol 19:552–555, 1980

HINTNER H, TAPPEINER G, EGG D et al: Fasziitis mit Eosinophilie. Das Shulman Syndrom. Hautarzt 32:75–79, 1981

KING DF, DORE RK, GILBERT DJ et al: Generalized morphea with peripheral eosinophilia, fasciitis and myositis. Int J Dermatol 19:149–153, 1980

KRAUSER RE, TUTHILL RJ: Eosinophilic fasciitis. Arch Dermatol 113:1092–1093, 1977

LUPTON GP, GOETTE DK: Localized eosinophilic fasciitis. Arch Dermatol 115:85–87, 1979

MICHET CJ JR, DOYLE JA, GINSBURG WW: Eosinophilic fasciitis. Report of 15 cases. Mayo Clin Proc 56:27–34, 1981

RODNAN GP, DI BARTHOLOMEO AG, MEDSGER TA et al: Eosinophilic fasciitis: Report of seven cases of a newly recognized scleroderma-like syndrome. Arthritis Rheum 18:422–423, 1975

SHEWMAKE SW, LOPEZ PA, MCGLAMORY JC: The Shulman syndrome. Arch Dermatol 114:556–559, 1978

SHULMAN L: Diffuse fasciitis with hypergammaglobulinemia and eosinophilia: A new syndrome? (Abstr) J Rheumatol 1, Suppl 1:46, 1974

SU WPD, PERSON JR: Morphea profunda. Am J Dermatopathol 3:251–260, 1981

TORRES VM, GEORGE WM: Diffuse eosinophilic fasciitis. Arch Dermatol 113:1591–1593, 1977

WEINSTEIN D, SCHWARTZ RA: Eosinophilic fasciitis. Arch Dermatol 114:1047–1049, 1978

26

Tumors and Cysts of the Epidermis

CLASSIFICATION OF TUMORS OF THE EPIDERMIS

Epidermal tumors can be divided into tumors of the surface epidermis and tumors of the epidermal appendages. In each of the two classes, benign and malignant tumors occur.

Benign tumors in general are characterized by (1) uniformity in the appearance of the tumor cell nuclei; (2) architectural order in the arrangement of the tumor cell nuclei; (3) restraint in the ratio of growth; and (4) absence of metastases.

Malignant tumors, in contrast, are characterized by (1) atypicality in the appearance of the tumor cell nuclei, which show pleomorphism, that is, great variability in size and shape, and anaplasia, that is, hyperplasia and hyperchromasia; (2) architectural disorder in the arrangement of the tumor cell nuclei with loss of polarity; (3) rapid growth with the presence of mitoses, including atypical mitoses; and (4) potentiality to give rise to metastases.

Of the four criteria of malignancy just cited, only the potentiality to give rise to metastases is decisive evidence for the malignancy of a tumor. For metastases to form, the tumor cells must possess a degree of autonomy that nonmalignant cells do not have. This autonomy enables malignant tumor cells to induce foreign tissue to furnish the necessary stroma in which they can multiply.

In addition to malignant tumors, one finds in the surface epidermis so-called premalignant tumors, better regarded as tumors located largely in situ. Although cytologically malignant, they are biologically still benign.

The tumors of the surface epidermis may be classified as follows:

Benign tumors
  Linear epidermal nevus
  Nevus comedonicus
  Epidermolytic acanthoma
  Oral white sponge nevus
  Seborrheic keratosis
  Clear cell acanthoma
  Cysts
    Epidermal cyst
    Milia
    Trichilemmal cyst
    Steatocystoma multiplex
    Dermoid cyst
    Bronchogenic and thyroglossal duct cysts
    Cutaneous ciliated cyst
    Median raphe cyst of the penis
    Eruptive vellus hair cyst
  Warty dyskeratoma
  Keratoacanthoma
Precancerous tumors (located largely in situ)
  Solar keratosis
  Precancerous leukoplakia
  Oral florid papillomatosis
  Bowen's disease
  Erythroplasia of Queyrat
Carcinomas
  Squamous cell carcinoma
  Paget's disease

LINEAR EPIDERMAL NEVUS

Linear epidermal nevi, or verrucous nevi, may be either localized or systematized.

In the *localized type,* which is present usually but not invariably at birth, only one linear lesion is present. It consists of closely set, papillomatous, hyperkeratotic papules. It may be located anywhere—on the head, trunk, or extremities. Being located on only one side of the patient, it is often referred to as nevus unius lateris. In its configuration, the localized type of linear epidermal nevus resembles the inflammatory linear verrucous epidermal nevus (ILVEN), but the latter differs clinically by the presence of erythema and pruritus and histologically by the presence of inflammation and parakeratosis (see p. 158).

In the *systematized type,* papillomatous hyperkeratotic papules in a linear configuration are present not just as one linear lesion, as in the localized type, but as many linear lesions. These linear lesions often show a parallel arrangement, particularly on the trunk. They may be limited to one side of the patient or may have a bilateral, symmetric distribution. The term *ichthyosis hystrix* is occasionally used, perhaps unnecessarily, for instances of extensive bilateral lesions (Basler et al).

Localized and, more commonly, systematized linear epidermal nevi may be associated with skeletal deformities and central nervous system disease, such as mental retardation, epilepsy, and neural deafness (see also p. 536) (Solomon et al).

The presence of a basal cell epithelioma within a linear epidermal nevus has been observed occasionally, particularly on the head in cases in which the linear epidermal nevus has been associated with either a nevus sebaceus or a syringocystadenoma papilliferum (see pp. 537 and 545) (Winer and Levin). In areas other than the head, it is very rare (Horn et al). Similarly, development of a squamous cell carcinoma has been described only rarely (Dogliotti and Frenkel; Cramer et al).

Histopathology.   Nearly all cases of the localized type of linear epidermal nevus and some cases of the systematized type show the histologic picture of a benign papilloma (Basler et al). One observes considerable hyperkeratosis, papillomatosis, and acanthosis with elongation of the rete ridges (Fig. 26-1).

Occasionally in cases of the localized type, but quite frequently in cases of the systematized type, particularly those with a widespread distribution, one observes the rather striking histologic picture referred to either as epidermolytic hyperkeratosis (Ackerman) or as granular degeneration of the epidermis (Braun-Falco et al). It is the same process that was first recognized in all cases of bullous congenital ichthyosiform erythroderma and that is therefore often referred to as epidermolytic hyperkeratosis (see p. 58). It has since been found to

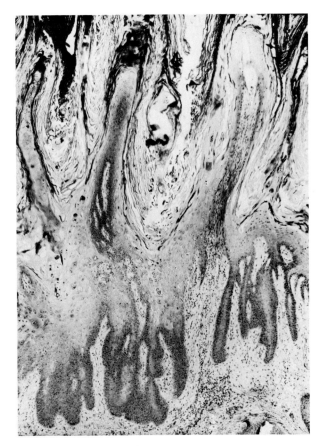

Fig. 26-1.   Linear epidermal nevus
There are considerable hyperkeratosis, papillomatosis, and acanthosis with elongation of the rete ridges. (×50)

occur in several other conditions as well (see Solitary and Disseminated Epidermolytic Acanthoma, p. 474).

The salient histologic features of epidermolytic hyperkeratosis are (1) perinuclear vacuolization of the cells in the stratum spinosum and in the stratum granulosum; (2) peripheral to the vacuolization, irregular cellular boundaries; (3) an increased number of irregularly shaped, large keratohyaline granules; and (4) compact hyperkeratosis in the stratum corneum (Zeligman and Pomeranz; Braun-Falco et al).

In some instances, histologic examination of unilateral linear lesions reveals features of acantholytic dyskeratosis as seen in Darier's disease (see p. 70). In some patients, these linear lesions have been present since birth or infancy (Demetree et al), but, in most instances, they have arisen in adult life (Starink and Woerdeman). Since acantholytic dyskeratosis is not specific for Darier's disease (see p. 72), the proposal has been made to designate such cases not as Darier's disease but as acantholytic dyskeratotic epidermal nevus (Star-ink and Woerdeman).

Differential Diagnosis.   The histologic picture of a benign papilloma, as found in most cases of linear epidermal nevus, can also be seen in seborrheic keratosis, verruca vulgaris, and acanthosis nigricans. Even though these four conditions have in common hyperkeratosis and papillomatosis, they can be differentiated easily in typical cases; however, one is occasionally unable to make a diagnosis any more specific than benign papilloma.

In the following three situations, clinical data are required for differentiation from linear epidermal nevus: (1) the hyperkeratotic type of seborrheic keratosis, which is characterized by the absence of basaloid cells and horn cysts and instead shows upward extension of epidermis-lined papillae (see p. 478); (2) old verrucae vulgares, which no longer show vacuolization of epidermal cells or columns of parakeratosis (see p. 371); and (3) acanthosis nigricans showing more pronounced acanthosis and greater elongation of the rete ridges than usual (see p. 430).

NEVUS COMEDONICUS

The lesions in nevus comedonicus consist of closely set, slightly elevated papules that have in their center a dark, firm, hyperkeratotic plug resembling a comedo. Nevus comedonicus, like linear epidermal nevus, usually has a linear configuration and occurs as a single lesion. In some instances, however, there are multiple bilateral linear lesions (Fritsch and Wittels) or lesions that are randomly distributed rather than linear (Paige and Mendelson). Lesions may be present on the palms and soles in addition to other areas (Wood and Thew). Occasionally, a unilateral linear lesion is limited either to a palm (Marsden et al) or to a sole (Abell and Read).

Histopathology.   Each comedo is represented by a wide, deep invagination of the epidermis filled with keratin. These invaginations resemble dilated hair follicles; in fact, as evidence that they actually represent rudimentary hair follicles, one occasionally finds in the lower portion of an invagination one or even several hair shafts (Fritsch and Wittels). One or two small sebaceous gland lobules may also be seen opening into the lower pole of invaginations (Paige and Mendelson).

In several instances, the keratinocytes composing the follicular epithelial wall have shown the typical changes of epidermolytic hyperkeratosis

(see below) (Barsky et al); in one case, these changes were seen also in the sebaceous ducts leading into the invagination (Plewig and Christophers).

In cases with lesions on the palms or soles, each invagination consists of a dilated eccrine duct containing a parakeratotic plug. The absence of the granular layer at the base of the plug together with the presence of epidermal cells showing vacuolization of their cytoplasm results in a histologic picture resembling that of porokeratosis (see p. 64) (Marsden et al; Abell and Read). The upper portion of the dermal eccrine duct beneath the plug is dilated and hyperplastic. The glandular portion, however, appears normal.

SOLITARY AND DISSEMINATED EPIDERMOLYTIC ACANTHOMA

Solitary epidermolytic acanthoma, histologically characterized by the presence of "epidermolytic hyperkeratosis," does not have a characteristic clinical appearance or location. It is a papillomatous lesion usually less than 1 cm in diameter (Shapiro and Baraf; Gebhart and Kidd; Niizuma).

Disseminated epidermolytic acanthoma occurs as numerous discrete, flat, brownish papules 2 mm to 6 mm in diameter resembling seborrheic keratoses. The upper trunk, especially the back, is the site of predilection (Hirone and Fukushiro; Miyamoto et al).

Histopathology.   In addition to hyperkeratosis and papillomatosis, one observes pronounced epidermolytic kyperkeratosis, also referred to as granular degeneration, throughout the stratum malpighii, sparing only the basal layer, just as seen in linear epidermal nevi with epidermolytic changes (see p. 473). One observes both intracellular and intercellular edema of the epidermal cells and keratohyaline granules that are coarser than normal and extend to a greater depth in the stratum malpighii (Shapiro and Baraf).

Differential Diagnosis.   Inclusion warts, caused by human papilloma virus type 1 (HPV-1) and referred to also as myrmecia warts, also show perinuclear vacuolization and an abundance of keratohyaline granules, representing a type of "granular degeneration" similar to that seen in epidermolytic hyperkeratosis. However, in inclusion warts, the keratohyaline granules are eosinophilic and coalesce in the upper layers of the epidermis to form large, homogeneous, eosinophilic "inclusion bodies" (see p. 373). In verrucae vulgares, caused by HPV-2, foci of vacuolated cells and clumped basophilic keratohyaline granules may be present, but these changes are limited to the upper layers of the epidermis (see p. 371). In addition, both inclusion warts and verrucae vulgares show focal parakeratosis, rather than orthokeratosis as seen in epidermolytic hyperkeratosis.

Incidental Epidermolytic Hyperkeratosis

Epidermolytic hyperkeratosis is seen not only in solitary and disseminated epidermolytic hyperkeratosis (see above) but also as a *regular* finding in epidermolytic hyperkeratosis, or bullous congenital ichthyosiform erythroderma (see p. 58), and epidermolytic keratosis palmaris et plantaris (see p. 61) and as an *occasional* finding in linear epidermal nevus (see p. 473) and nevus comedonicus (see p. 474). In addition, epidermolytic hyperkeratosis may represent an *incidental* histologic finding in many different types of lesions, largely but not exclusively tumors.

Histopathology. Epidermolytic hyperkeratosis may be seen throughout an entire lesion of solar keratosis (see p. 491) (Ackerman and Reed) and in the entire lining of a trichilemmal cyst (Ackerman, 1972). More commonly, however, the histologic features of epidermolytic hyperkeratosis are seen as a small focus, often limited to a single epidermal rete ridge, in such diverse lesions as sebaceous hyperplasia (Nagashima and Matsuoka), intradermal nevus, hypertrophic scar (Mehregan), seborrheic keratosis, the margin of a squamous cell carcinoma, lichenoid amyloidosis, and granuloma annulare (Ackerman, 1970). In some instances, the process is limited to one or two intraepidermal sweat duct units (Mehregan).

Incidental Focal Acantholytic Dyskeratosis

Analogous to epidermolytic hyperkeratosis, acantholytic dyskeratosis is seen as a *regular* histologic feature in Darier's disease (see p. 70), transient acantholytic dermatosis (see p. 127), and warty dyskeratoma (see p. 488). It also is an *occasional* finding in acantholytic dyskeratotic epidermal nevus, a variant of linear epidermal nevus (see p. 473). In addition, again like epidermolytic hyperkeratosis, focal acantholytic dyskeratosis is observed occasionally as an *incidental* histologic finding in a variety of lesions. It may also occur, though rarely, as focal acantholytic dyskeratoma, a solitary papular lesion showing as the only histologic change multiple foci of focal acantholytic dyskeratosis (Ackerman, 1972).

Histopathology. Focal suprabasal clefts with overlying acantholytic and dyskeratotic cells, some of which have the appearance of corps ronds, have been seen as a single focus in the epidermis overlying such diverse lesions as dermatofibroma, basal cell epithelioma, melanocytic nevus, and chondrodermatitis nodularis helicis (Ackerman, 1972), as well as in pityriasis rosea (Stern et al) and acral lentiginous malignant melanoma (Botet and Sánchez).

ORAL WHITE SPONGE NEVUS

First described in 1935 (Cannon), oral white sponge nevus has an autosomal dominant inheritance. It may be present at birth or have its onset in infancy, childhood, or adolescence (Jorgenson and Levin). Extensive areas of the oral mucosa and sometimes the entire oral mucosa have a thickened, folded, creamy white appearance. In some instances, the rectal mucosa (Cannon), vagina (Zegarelli et al), nasal mucosa (Witkop and Gorlin), or esophagus (Haye and Whitehead) is also involved. Malignant degeneration is not known to occur.

The oral lesions seen in pachyonychia congenita are both clinically and histologically indistinguishable from a white sponge nevus (see p. 62) (Witkop and Gorlin).

Histopathology. The oral epithelium shows hyperplasia with much more pronounced hydropic swelling of the epithelial cells than is normal for the oral mucosa. The swelling, though extensive, is focal (Cooke and Morgan). It extends into the rete ridges but spares the basal layer (Stüttgen et al). The nuclei appear smaller than normal (Jorgenson and Levin). The surface shows parakeratosis, as does the normal oral mucosa, and only rarely are there small accumulations of keratohyaline granules (Zegarelli et al).

Histogenesis. On *electron microscopic examination*, large cytoplasmic areas of the epithelial cells appear optically empty or contain only faint granular material. Tonofilaments are limited to the perinuclear and peripheral areas. The intercellular areas show irregular dilatation, and large, irregularly shaped vacuoles are present within the cytoplasm (Kuhlwein et al). A possibly fundamental disturbance is the presence of numerous intracellular Odland bodies or membrane-coating granules (see p. 14), which are not extruded into the intercellular spaces (Metz and Metz).

Differential Diagnosis. The histologic picture of oral white sponge nevus is identical not only to that seen in pachyonychia congenita (see above) but also to that of oral focal epithelial hyperplasia (see p. 378) (Kuhlwein et al) and of leukoedema of the oral mucosa (see below).

Leukoedema of the Oral Mucosa

Leukoedema of the oral mucosa is a common condition that, when pronounced, shows a clinical and histologic resemblance to oral white sponge nevus. However, leukoedema differs from white sponge nevus by being patchy rather than diffuse, by having exacerbations and remissions and adult onset, and by not being inherited (Duncan and Su).

Histopathology. In leukoedema of the oral mucosa, as in oral white sponge nevus, the suprabasal epithelial cells show marked intracellular edema. The nuclei appear smaller than normal.

Lingua Geographica

In geographic tongue, also referred to as superficial migratory glossitis, the dorsum of the tongue shows irregularly shaped red patches surrounded by a whitish, raised border a few millimeters wide. The patches change configuration from day to day.

Histopathology. Whereas the dorsum of the tongue normally shows a granular and a horny layer (see p. 11), these layers are absent in the red patches of lingua geographica. Along the whitish border, the epithelium shows irregular thickening and infiltration of neutrophils. In its upper portion, the epithelium shows collections of neutrophils within the interstices of a spongelike network formed by degenerated and thinned epithelial cells (Dawson; Marks and Radden). The histologic picture thus shows Kogoj's spongiform pustules, which are indistinguishable from those seen in pustular psoriasis.

Histogenesis. The presence of spongiform pustules generally is regarded as diagnostic of pustular psoriasis and as almost specific for it (see p. 145), even though it rarely occurs in other pustules, such as those caused by *Candida albicans* (Degos et al). It has therefore been suggested that geographic tongue represents a localized form of pustular psoriasis (O'Keefe et al). However, even though pustular psoriasis and lingua geographica may both show annular lesions on the tongue, pustular psoriasis of the mouth generally shows clinical evidence of pustules and is usually seen also in other areas of the mouth. It is therefore best to regard lingua geographica as a separate entity.

SEBORRHEIC KERATOSIS

Seborrheic keratoses are very common lesions. There may be only one lesion, but there are often many. They occur mainly on the trunk and face but also on the extremities, with the exception of the palms and soles. Seborrheic keratoses usually do not appear before middle age. They are sharply demarcated, brownish in color, and slightly raised, so that they often look as if they are stuck on the surface of the skin. Most of them have a verrucous surface, which has a soft, friable consistency. Some, however, have a smooth surface but characteristically show keratotic plugs. Although most lesions measure only a few millimeters in diameter, a lesion may occasionally reach a size of several centimeters. Crusting and an inflammatory base are found if the lesion has been subjected to trauma. Occasionally, seborrheic keratoses are pedunculated, especially on the neck and upper chest, and then clinically resemble soft fibromas (see p. 600).

Histopathology. Seborrheic keratoses show a considerable variety of histologic appearances. Six types are generally recognized: acanthotic, hyperkeratotic, reticulated, clonal, irritated, and melanoacanthoma. Often, more than one type is found in the same lesion. In addition, two clinical variants of seborrheic keratosis will be described. They are dermatosis papulosa nigra and stucco keratosis.

All types of seborrheic keratosis have in common hyperkeratosis, acanthosis, and papillomatosis. The acanthosis in most instances is due entirely to upward extension of the tumor. Thus, the lower border of the tumor is even and lies on a straight line that may be drawn from the normal epidermis at one end of the tumor to the normal epidermis at the other end (Fig. 26-2). Two types of cells are usually seen in the acanthotic epidermis: squamous cells and basaloid cells. The former have the appearance of squamous cells normally found in the epidermis, whereas the basaloid cells are small and uniform in appearance and have a relatively large nucleus. In areas of slight intercellular edema, intercellular bridges can be easily recognized (Andrade and Steigleder). Thus, they resemble the basal cells found normally in the basal layer of the epidermis.

Acanthotic Type. In the acanthotic type, the most common type of seborrheic keratosis, hyperkeratosis and papillomatosis often are slight, but the epidermis is greatly thickened. Although only narrow papillae are included in the thickened epidermis in some cases, one can see in other lesions a retiform pattern composed of thick, interwoven tracts of epithelial cells surrounding

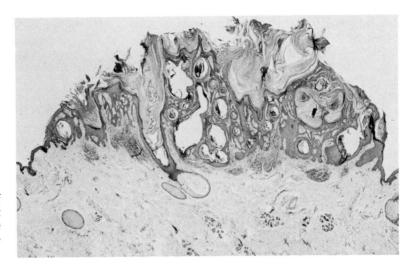

Fig. 26-2. Seborrheic keratosis, acanthotic type
Low magnification. The lower border of the tumor in general follows a straight line from the normal epidermis at one end of the tumor to the normal epidermis at the other end. (×25)

islands of connective tissue (Fig. 26-3). Horny invaginations that on cross sections appear as pseudo-horn cysts are numerous. In addition, there also are true horn cysts, which, like the pseudo-horn cysts, show sudden and complete keratinization. The true horn cysts begin as foci of orthokeratosis within the substance of the lesion (Sanderson). In time, they enlarge and are carried by the current of epidermal cells toward the surface of the lesion, where they unite with the invaginations of surface keratin. In the greatly thickened epidermis, basaloid cells usually outnumber squamous cells.

The amount of melanin in seborrheic keratoses of the acanthotic type is often greater than normal. Excess amounts of melanin are seen in about one third of the specimens stained with hematoxylin–eosin (Becker); staining with silver reveals excess amounts in about two thirds of the cases (Lennox). In dopa-stained sections, melanocytes are limited to the dermal-epidermal junctional layer present at the base of the tumor and at the interfaces between the tumor tracts and the islands of dermal stroma (Mevorah and Mishima). The melanin, largely present in keratinocytes, is in most instances also limited to keratinocytes located at the dermal-epidermal junction. Only deeply pigmented lesions show melanin widely distributed throughout the tumor within basaloid cells (Mishima and Pinkus).

A mononuclear inflammatory infiltrate is seen quite frequently in the dermis underlying a seborrheic keratosis. The inflammation may impinge on the tumor in a lichenoid or eczematous pattern. In the lichenoid pattern, a bandlike infiltrate is seen

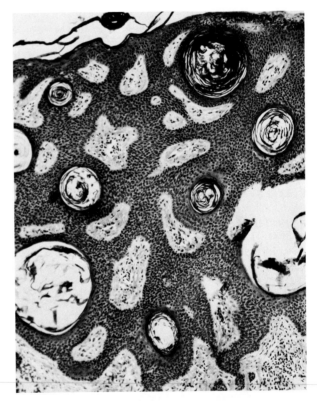

Fig. 26-3. Seborrheic keratosis, acanthotic type
High magnification. Thick, interwoven tracts of epidermal cells compose the tumor. Most of the epidermal cells have the appearance of epidermal basal cells and are referred to as basaloid cells. Interspersed are cystic inclusions of horny material representing either horn cysts, when they form within the tumor, or pseudo-horn cysts, when they consist of horny invaginations. (×100)

hugging the basal cell layer of the tumor. In the eczematous pattern, there is exocytosis leading to spongiosis. Squamous eddies, typical of irritated seborrheic keratoses, are only rarely seen in inflamed seborrheic keratoses (Berman and Winkelmann).

Formation of an in situ carcinoma within an acanthotic seborrheic keratosis, so-called bowenoid transformation, is seen occasionally (Rahbari; Baer et al). It seems to occur predominantly in lesions located in sun-exposed areas of the skin, so that sun damage may be a factor (Booth). In one reported case, a metastasis in a regional lymph node was found (Christeler and Delacrétaz). On rare occasions, a basal cell epithelioma may form within an acanthotic seborrheic keratosis and may extend from there into the underlying dermis (Balabanow and Angelow; Mikhail and Mehregan).

Histogenesis. *Electron microscopic examination* has confirmed the light microscopic impression that the small basaloid cells seen in the acanthotic type of seborrheic keratosis are related to cells of the epidermal basal cell layer rather than to the basalioma cells of basal cell epithelioma. They possess a fair number of desmosomes and a moderate number of tonofilaments that differ from those present in cells of the epidermal basal cell layer only by showing less orientation (Braun-Falco et al).

Hyperkeratotic Type. In the hyperkeratotic type, also referred to as the digitate or serrated type, hyperkeratosis and papillomatosis are pronounced, whereas acanthosis is not very conspicuous. The numerous digitate upward extensions of epidermis-lined papillae often resemble church spires. The histologic picture then resembles that seen in acrokeratosis verruciformis of Hopf (see p. 74). The epidermis consists largely of squamous

cells, although small aggregates of basaloid cells may be seen here and there. As a rule, no excess amounts of melanin are found.

Reticulated Type. In the reticulated or adenoid type of seborrheic keratosis, numerous thin tracts of epidermal cells extend from the epidermis and show branching and interweaving in the dermis. Many tracts are composed of only a double row of basaloid cells (Fig. 26-4). Horn cysts and pseudo-horn cysts are absent in purely reticulated lesions; however, the reticulated type often also shows areas of the acanthotic type, and horn cysts and pseudo-horn cysts are commonly seen in these areas. The basaloid cells of the reticulated type of seborrheic keratosis usually show marked hyperpigmentation.

There is both clinical and histologic evidence of a close relationship between lentigo senilis and the reticulated type of seborrheic keratosis. A lesion of lentigo senilis may even become a reticulated seborrheic keratosis through exaggeration of the process of downward budding of pigmented basaloid cells (see p. 697) (Mehregan, 1975).

Clonal Type. In the clonal, or nesting, type of seborrheic keratosis, well-defined nests of cells are located within the epidermis. In some instances, the nests resemble foci of basal cell epithelioma, since the nuclei appear small and dark-staining and intercellular bridges are seen in only a few areas (Fig. 26-5). The histologic picture in such cases has been erroneously interpreted by some authors as representing an intraepidermal epithelioma of Borst–Jadassohn (see p. 571) (Mehregan and Pinkus). In other instances of clonal seborrheic keratosis, the nests are composed of fairly large cells showing distinct intercellular bridges (Fig. 26-6).

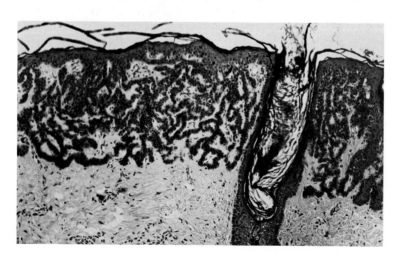

Fig. 26-4. Seborrheic keratosis, adenoid type

Thin, interwoven tracts composed of a double row of epidermal basal cells compose the tumor. No cystic inclusions of horny material are present. (× 100)

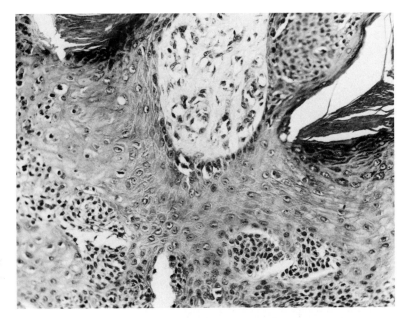

Fig. 26-5.   Seborrheic keratosis, clonal type
Well-defined nests of small basaloid cells are present. The nests resemble foci of basal cell epithelioma, but intercellular bridges can be recognized in some areas. (×200)

Fig. 26-6.   Seborrheic keratosis, clonal type
Well-defined nests of large cells with distinct intercellular bridges are present. (×200)

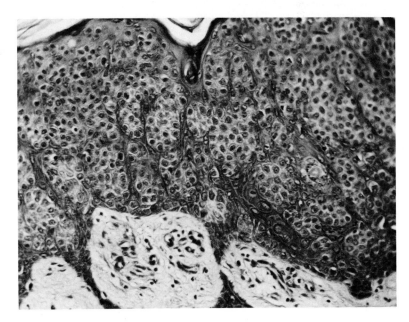

Irritated Type.   In the irritated, or activated, type of seborrheic keratosis, the characteristic feature is the presence of numerous whorls or eddies composed of eosinophilic flattened squamous cells arranged in an onion-peel fashion, thus resembling poorly differentiated horn pearls (Fig. 26-7). These "squamous eddies," however, are easily differentiated from the horn pearls of squamous cell carcinoma by their large number, small size, and circumscribed configuration. Irritated seborrheic keratoses, in addition, may show areas of downward proliferation breaking through the horizontal demarcation generally present in nonirritated seborrheic keratoses (Sim-Davis et al; Indianer). Frequently, some of these proliferations are seen to originate from the walls of keratin-filled invaginations. Inflammation beneath irritated seborrheic keratoses usually is mild or absent, indicating that irritated seborrheic keratoses are different from inflamed seborrheic keratoses (see p. 477).

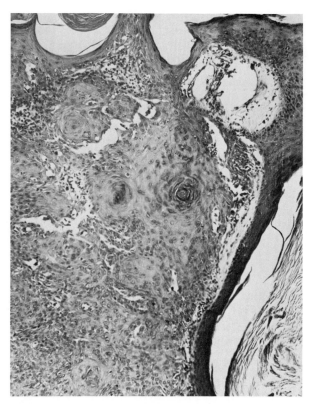

Fig. 26-7.   Irritated seborrheic keratosis
Numerous whorls of eosinophilic flattened squamous cells, so-called squamous eddies, are present. They differ from the horn pearls of squamous cell carcinoma by their large number, small size, and circumscribed configuration. (×200)

Histogenesis. Formation of numerous squamous eddies is the result of the "activation" of resting basaloid cells into squamous cells. This unique and highly diagnostic feature of irritated or activated seborrheic keratoses, as well as their downward proliferation, is the result of irritation. This has been proved experimentally by the excision of seborrheic keratoses either after a previous biopsy (Morales and Hu) or after irritation with croton oil (Mevorah and Mishima).

The identical histologic picture as seen in irritated seborrheic keratosis has been described under designations such as inverted follicular keratosis (Helwig; Mehregan, 1964) and follicular poroma (Duperrat and Mascaro; Grosshans and Hanau). As these terms indicate, the authors regard the keratin-filled invaginations as follicular infundibula and the proliferations arising from them as composed of cells of the follicular infundibulum. Aside from the fact that the follicular infundibulum consists of cells with the same type of keratinization as the surface epidermis, there is evidence that seborrheic keratoses may incorporate the cells of the infundibular portion of the hair follicle and even are partially derived

from these cells. Some seborrheic keratoses even contain aggregates of vellus hairs within the keratinous invaginations, an occurrence analogous to trichostasis spinulosa (see p. 202) (Kossard et al). Thus, whereas some authors merely concede that irritated seborrheic keratoses and inverted follicular keratoses may be histologically indistinguishable (Headington; Brownstein and Shapiro), others regard the two disorders as identical (Sim-Davis et al; Indianer; Kossard et al). Because of their histologic similarity and, particularly, because of the highly specific appearance of the squamous eddies that occur exclusively in these two conditions, they are best regarded as identical.

Melanoacanthoma.   In one rather rare histologic variant of seborrheic keratosis referred to as melanoacanthoma (Mishima and Pinkus), one finds numerous large, pigment-filled melanocytes distributed throughout the lesion. In some instances, they are apparent even in sections stained with hematoxylin-eosin (Mishima and Pinkus; Schlappner et al). In any case, staining with silver reveals numerous melanocytes possessing large dendrites and containing considerable amounts of melanin, whereas the keratinocytes contain hardly any melanin (Delacrétaz; Matsuoka et al). Thus, melanoacanthoma differs from the common pigmented seborrheic keratosis, in which there are only few melanocytes and the melanin is found almost entirely within the keratinocytes.

Histogenesis. It is obvious that at least a partial block in the transfer of melanin from melanocytes to keratinocytes exists in melanoacanthoma. Since some melanoacanthomas have the histologic appearance of an irritated seborrheic keratosis, it has been assumed that the transfer of melanin to keratinocytes is blocked as a result of the transformation of most basaloid cells into squamous cells. However, in a study in which seborrheic keratoses were changed into irritated seborrheic keratoses by croton oil or surgical trauma, no changes characteristic of melanoacanthoma were seen (Mevorah and Mishima). Thus, it appears likely that melanoacanthoma is a benign mixed tumor of melanocytes and keratinocytes, as first described (Mishima and Pinkus).

Leser–Trélat Sign

The Leser–Trélat sign is characterized by the sudden appearance of numerous seborrheic keratoses in association with a malignant tumor. Although several reports have appeared in recent years concerning this sign, the association may well be purely coincidental, and the validity of the sign is therefore not generally accepted (Gitlin and Pirozzi; Lambert et al). In the opinion of some, the Leser–Trélat sign applies only to cases in which the seborrheic keratoses are pruritic and the skin was previously free of them (Ronchese).

Although the malignant tumor in most of the reported cases consisted of an abdominal adenocarcinoma (Liddell et al), the associated malignant disease in some reports was leukemia (Kechijian et al) or mycosis fungoides (Lambert et al).

Histopathology. The histologic appearance of the seborrheic keratoses in the Leser–Trélat sign does not differ from that of other seborrheic keratoses (Schwartz and Burgess). Nevertheless, they have been interpreted as "an incomplete form of acanthosis nigricans" (Sneddon and Roberts) or as "potentially representing an early stage of acanthosis nigricans" (Ronchese). There are indeed cases in which the seborrheic keratoses seen in this sign were either accompanied (Schwartz and Burgess) or followed by acanthosis nigricans (Ronchese) (see p. 430).

Dermatosis Papulosa Nigra

Dermatosis papulosa nigra is found in about 35% of all adult blacks, and often has its onset during adolescence (Hairston et al). The lesions are located predominantly on the face, especially in the malar regions, but may also occur on the neck and upper trunk. They usually consist of small, smooth, pigmented papules, except on the neck and trunk, where some of them may be pedunculated.

Histopathology. The lesions have the histologic appearance of seborrheic keratoses but are smaller in size. Most lesions are of the acanthotic type and show thick interwoven tracts of epithelial cells. The cells are largely squamous in appearance, with only a few basaloid cells (Hairston et al). Horn cysts are quite common. An occasional lesion shows a reticulated pattern, in which the tracts are composed of a double row of basaloid cells. Melanin pigmentation is pronounced in all lesions.

Stucco Keratosis

Stucco keratoses are small, grayish white seborrheic keratoses 1 mm to 3 mm in diameter located in symmetric arrangement on the distal portions of the extremities, especially the ankles. They can easily be scraped off without any resultant bleeding.

Histopathology. Stucco keratoses have the appearance of the hyperkeratotic type of seborrheic keratosis, showing the church-spire pattern of upward-extending papillae (Willoughby and Soter; Braun-Falco and Weissmann). Horn cysts and basaloid cells are usually absent (Kocsard and Carter).

CLEAR CELL ACANTHOMA

Clear cell acanthoma, a tumor that is clinically and histologically quite distinct, was first described in 1962 (Degos et al). It is not rare, so that, by 1977, more than 200 cases had already been reported (Kerl).

In most instances, the lesion is solitary and is located on the legs. Usually, it consists of a slowly growing, sharply delineated, red nodule or plaque 1 cm to 2 cm in diameter. In most cases, it is covered with a thin crust and exudes some moisture. A collarette is often seen at the periphery. It has been said that the lesion appears stuck on, like a seborrheic keratosis, and is vascular, like a granuloma pyogenicum (Fine and Chernosky).

Histopathology. Within a sharply demarcated area of the epidermis, all epidermal cells, with the exception of cells of the basal cell layer, appear strikingly clear and slightly enlarged (Fig. 26-8). The nuclei of the clear epidermal cells appear normal. When staining is carried out with the periodic acid-Schiff (PAS) reaction, the presence of large amounts of glycogen is revealed within the cells (Degos et al; Wells and Wilson Jones).

Slight spongiosis is present between the clear cells. The rete ridges are elongated and may show intertwining (Kerl). The surface shows parakeratosis with few or no granular cells. The acrosyringia and acrotrichia within the tumor retain their normal stainability (Zak and Girerd). There is an absence of melanin within the tumor cells, but sparsely scattered, weakly dopa-positive melanocytes are present, and melanin can be seen within the melanocytes and their dendritic processes on silver staining (Wells and Wilson Jones).

A conspicuous feature in most lesions is the presence throughout the epidermis of numerous neutrophils, many of which show fragmentation of their nuclei (Fig. 26-9). The neutrophils often form microabscesses in the parakeratotic horny layer (Wilson Jones and Wells; Trau et al). Dilated capillaries are seen in the elongated papillae and often also in the dermis underlying the tumor (Wells and Wilson Jones). In addition, a mild to moderately severe cellular infiltrate composed largely of lymphoid cells is present in the dermis.

Beneath the tumor, some cases have shown hyperplasia of sweat ducts (Wilson Jones and Wells) or syringomalike proliferations (Cramer).

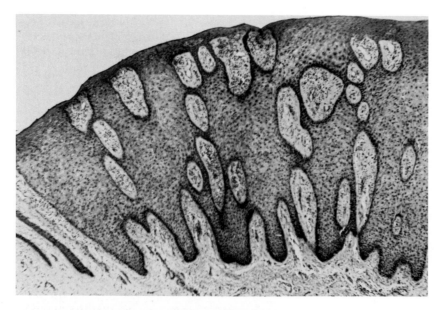

Fig. 26-8.   Clear cell acanthoma
Low magnification. The cells within the thickened epidermis appear strikingly clear because of the presence of large amounts of glycogen. (×100)

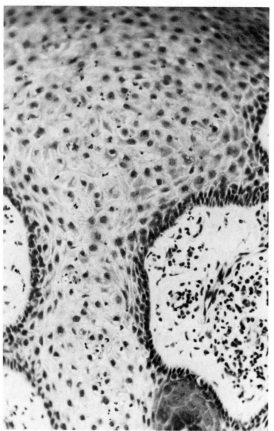

Fig. 26-9.   Clear cell acanthoma
High magnification. Neutrophils and nuclear dust are scattered through the tumor. At the lower border, part of an acrosyringium is visible with cells that have retained their normal stainability. (×400)

Histogenesis. On *histochemical examination,* phosphorylase is absent in clear cell acanthoma except for the basal cell layer. This enzyme normally is present in the epidermis and is necessary for the degradation of glycogen (Desmons et al).

Electron microscopy reveals glycogen granules in the tumor cells, except in the cells of the basal cell layer. In the lower portion of the tumor, the glycogen granules are seen largely around the nuclei. In the upper portion, however, the amount of glycogen is increased, and the granules are seen to infiltrate between the tonofilaments (Desmons et al).

Although the melanocytes, including their dendrites, contain melanosomes, hardly any melanosomes are present within the tumor cells, indicating a blockage in the transfer of melanosomes from the melanocytes to the tumor cells (Hu and Sisson).

EPIDERMAL CYST

Epidermal cysts are slowly growing, elevated, round, firm, intradermal or subcutaneous tumors that cease growing after having reached a size of 1 cm to 5 cm in diameter. They occur most commonly on the face, scalp, neck, and trunk. Although epidermal cysts in most instances arise spontaneously, they occasionally form as a result of the traumatic implantation of epidermis into the dermis or subcutis (Onuigbo; Leonforte). Usually, a patient has only one or a few epidermal cysts, rarely many. In Gardner's syndrome, however, numerous epidermal cysts occur, especially on the scalp and face (see p. 607).

Histopathology.   Epidermal cysts have a wall composed of true epidermis, as seen on the skin surface and in the infundibulum of hair follicles, the infundibulum being the uppermost part of the hair follicle that extends down to the entry of the sebaceous duct. In young epidermal cysts, several layers of squamous and granular cells can usually be recognized (Fig. 26-10). In older epidermal cysts, however, the wall often is markedly atrophic either in some areas or in the entire cyst and then may consist of only one or two rows of greatly flattened cells. The cyst is filled with horny material arranged in laminated layers. In sections stained with hematoxylin-eosin, melanocytes and melanin pigmentation of keratinocytes can be seen only rarely in epidermal cysts of Caucasoids but frequently in epidermal cysts of Negroids. Silver stains reveal that most of the melanin is located in the basal layer of the cyst lining, but some melanin is seen also in the contents of the cyst (Fieselman et al).

When an epidermal cyst ruptures and the contents of the cyst are released into the dermis, a considerable foreign body reaction with numerous

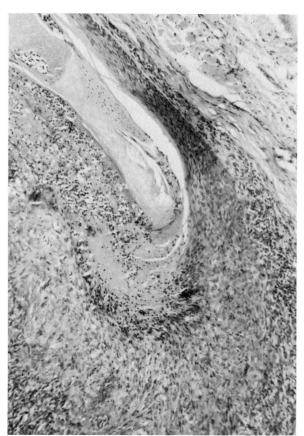

Fig. 26-11.   Epidermal cyst with squamous cell carcinoma
The squamous cell carcinoma present in the wall of the cyst is walled off by an inflammatory infiltrate. (×100)

multinucleated giant cells results. The foreign body reaction usually causes disintegration of the cyst wall. However, it may lead to a pseudocarcinomatous proliferation in remnants of the cyst wall, simulating a squamous cell carcinoma (Raab and Steigleder).

Development of a basal cell epithelioma (Delacrétaz), a lesion of Bowen's disease (Shelley and Wood), or a squamous cell carcinoma (McDonald) in epidermal cysts is a rare event. In cases of squamous cell carcinoma, the tumor is apt to be of low malignancy and does not metastasize (Fig. 26-11). It is likely that some cases that were regarded in the past as malignant degeneration of epidermal cysts now are interpreted either as pseudocarcinomatous hyperplasia in a ruptured epidermal cyst (Raab and Steigleder) or as proliferating trichilemmal tumor (see p. 532) (Wilson Jones).

Histogenesis. As seen by *electron microscopy*, the keratinization in epidermal cysts is identical to that in the

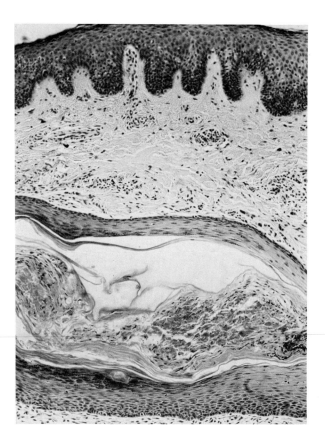

Fig. 26-10.   Epidermal cyst
The wall of the cyst is composed of true epidermis, that is, squamous, granular, and horn cells. The cyst is filled with horny material arranged in laminated layers. (×100)

surface epidermis and in the pilosebaceous infundibulum, since the keratin located within the keratinized cells consists of relatively electron-lucent tonofilaments embedded in an electron-dense interfilamentous substance derived from keratohyaline granules (see p. 13). The keratinized cells of the cyst content have a markedly flattened, elongated appearance and are surrounded by a thick marginal band rather than by a plasma membrane (see p. 14). The intercellular spaces between the fully keratinized cells is filled with moderately electron-dense material. Desmosomes are no longer present (McGavran and Binnington).

MILIA

Milia are multiple, superficially located, whitish, globoid, firm lesions generally only 1 mm to 2 mm in size. A distinction is made between primary milia, which arise spontaneously on the face in predisposed individuals, and secondary milia, which occur either in diseases associated with subepidermal bullae, such as bullous pemphigoid, dystrophic epidermolysis bullosa, porphyria cutanea tarda, and lichen sclerosus et atrophicus (Leppard and Sneddon), or after dermabrasion (Epstein and Kligman) and other trauma.

Histopathology. *Primary milia* of the face are derived from the lowest portion of the infundib-

ulum of vellus hairs at about the level of the sebaceous duct. The milia often are still connected with the vellus hair follicle by an epithelial pedicle. Primary milia are small cysts differing from epidermal cysts only in size. They are lined by a stratified epithelium a few cell layers thick and contain concentric lamellae of keratin (Epstein and Kligman).

Secondary milia have the same histologic appearance as primary milia (Epstein and Kligman). They may develop from any epithelial structure and on serial sections may still show a connection to the parent structure, whether a hair follicle, sweat duct, sebaceous duct, or epidermis (Leppard and Sneddon). Secondary milia that follow blistering arise in most instances from the eccrine sweat duct and very rarely from a hair follicle. In a certain percentage, however, no connection is found with any skin appendage, suggesting that the milia have developed from aberrant epidermis (Tsuji et al). In milia derived from eccrine sweat ducts, the sweat ducts are frequently seen to enter the cyst wall at the botton of the milium (Epstein and Kligman; Tsuji et al).

Histogenesis. Primary milia of the face represent a keratinizing type of benign tumor (Epstein and Kligman).

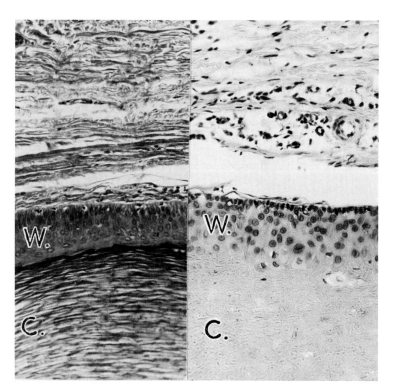

Fig. 26-12. Comparison of epidermal cyst with trichilemmal cyst
(*Left*) The wall (W.) of the epidermal cyst is composed of epidermis; the cystic cavity (C.) contains horny material arranged in laminated layers. (*Right*) The wall (W.) of the trichilemmal cyst shows distinct palisading of the peripheral cell layer and swelling of the cells close to the cystic cavity (C.). The content of the cysts consists of homogeneous horny material. (×200)

In contrast, secondary milia represent retention cysts caused by proliferative tendencies of the epithelium after injury (Pinkus).

TRICHILEMMAL CYST

Trichilemmal cysts are clinically indistinguishable from epidermal cysts. They differ from epidermal cysts, however, in frequency and distribution. In the first place, they are less common than epidermal cysts, constituting only about 25% of the combined material; in the second place, about 90% of trichilemmal cysts occur on the scalp. Additional differences are that trichilemmal cysts often show an autosomal dominant inheritance and are solitary in only 30% of the cases, with 10% of the patients having more than 10 cysts (Leppard and Sanderson). Furthermore, in contrast to epidermal cysts, trichilemmal cysts are easily enucleated and appear as firm, smooth, white-walled cysts (Leppard et al).

Histopathology. The wall of trichilemmal cysts is composed of epithelial cells possessing no clearly visible intercellular bridges. The peripheral layer of cells shows a distinct palisade arrangement not seen in epidermal cysts. The epithelial cells close to the cystic cavity appear swollen and are filled with pale cytoplasm (Fig. 26-12). These swollen cells do not produce a granular layer but generally undergo abrupt keratinization, although nuclear remnants are occasionally retained in a few cells. The content of the cysts consists of homogeneous eosinophilic material (McGavran and Binnington).

Whereas focal calcification of the cyst content does not occur in epidermal cysts, foci of calcification are seen in approximately one quarter of trichilemmal cysts (Fig. 26-13) (Leppard and Sanderson). In trichilemmal as in epidermal cysts, a considerable foreign body reaction results when the wall of the cyst ruptures, and the cyst may then undergo partial or complete disintegration.

Trichilemmal cysts frequently disclose small, acanthotic foci in their walls that are indistinguishable from trichilemmal tumors (Brownstein and Arluk). The association of a trichilemmal cyst with a trichilemmal tumor is also seen occasionally (see p. 532) (Leppard and Sanderson).

Histogenesis. Trichilemmal cysts, also referred to as pilar cysts, originally were called sebaceous cysts. The name was changed when it became apparent that the keratinization in them is analogous to the keratinization that takes place in the outer root sheath of the hair, or trichilemma (Pinkus). The outer root sheath of the hair does not keratinize wherever it covers the inner root sheath. It keratinizes normally in two areas: the follicular

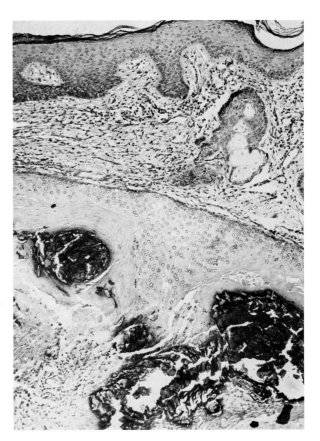

Fig. 26-13. Trichilemmal cyst with foci of calcification
The palisading of the basal layer makes it evident that this is a trichilemmal cyst. The cyst has ruptured, and fibrous tissue has proliferated into the lumen. (×100)

isthmus of anagen hairs and the sac surrounding catagen and telogen hairs, because, in these two regions, the inner root sheath has disappeared. The follicular isthmus of anagen hairs (see p. 27) is the short, middle portion of the hair follicle, extending upward from the attachment of the arrector pili muscle to the entrance of the sebaceous duct. At the lower end of the follicular isthmus, the inner root sheath sloughs off, exposing the outer root sheath, which, in its exposed portion, undergoes a specific type of homogeneous keratinization without the interposition of a granular layer. This type of trichilemmal keratinization also takes place in the sac surrounding catagen and telogen hairs, because hairs in these stages have lost their inner root sheath (see p. 28).

Electron microscopic examination of the epithelial lining of trichilemmal cysts shows that, on their way from the peripheral layer toward the center, the epithelial cells have an increasing number of filaments in their cytoplasm. The transition from nucleate to anucleate cells is abrupt and is associated with the loss of all cytoplasmic organelles. The junction between the keratinizing and keratinized cells shows interdigitations (Kimura). The keratinized cells are filled with tonofilaments and, unlike those in epidermal cysts, retain their desmosomal connections (McGavran and Binnington).

STEATOCYSTOMA MULTIPLEX

Steatocystoma multiplex is inherited in an autosomal dominant pattern. One observes numerous small, rounded, moderately firm, cystic nodules that are adherent to the overlying skin and usually measure 1 cm to 3 cm in diameter. When punctured, the cysts discharge an oily or creamy fluid and, in some instances, also small hairs (Contreras and Costello). They are found most commonly in the axillae, in the sternal region, and on the arms. Steatocystoma also occurs occasionally as a solitary, noninherited tumor in adults referred to as steatocystoma simplex (Brownstein).

Histopathology. Histologic examination reveals an intricately folded cyst wall consisting of several layers of epithelial cells. In areas of atrophy of the cyst wall, only two or three layers of flat cells may be present. Elsewhere is a basal layer in palisade arrangement, above which are two or three layers of swollen cells without recognizable intercellular bridges. Central to these cells, there is a thick, homogeneous, eosinophilic horny layer that protrudes irregularly into the lumen in a fashion simulating the decapitation secretion of apocrine glands (Fig. 26-14) (Hashimoto et al).

A characteristic feature seen in most lesions of steatocystoma is the presence of flattened sebaceous gland lobules either within or close to the cyst wall (Oyal and Nikolowski). Also, in some cysts, invaginations resembling hair follicles extend from the cyst wall into the surrounding stroma and, in rare instances, true hair shafts are seen within them, indicating that the invaginations represent the outer root sheath of hairs. In occasional cysts, the lumen contains clusters of hair, mainly of lanugo size but partially of intermediate character (Kligman and Kirschbaum). When stained with the PAS reaction, the cells of the cyst wall are found to be rich in glycogen.

Histogenesis. *Electron microscopic examination* has shown that the cyst wall consists of keratinizing cells. Nearest to the lumen, the cyst wall consists of several layers of flattened, very elongated horny cells interconnected by desmosomes.

It appears likely that differentiation in the cyst wall of steatocystoma multiplex is to a large extent in the direction of the outer root sheath of hair because (1) the cells of the cyst wall contain abundant glycogen and amylophosphorylase; (2) histologically, the homogeneous, eosinophilic horny layer seen adjacent to the lumen in steatocystoma multiplex greatly resembles the homogeneous, eosinophilic content of trichilemmal cysts; (3) keratinization in steatocystoma multiplex, as in trichilemmal cysts, takes place without the interposition of keratohyaline granules; and (4) on electron microscopy, the cells of the horny layer, like the keratinized cells in trichilemmal cysts (see above), are seen to retain their desmosomes (Hashimoto et al).

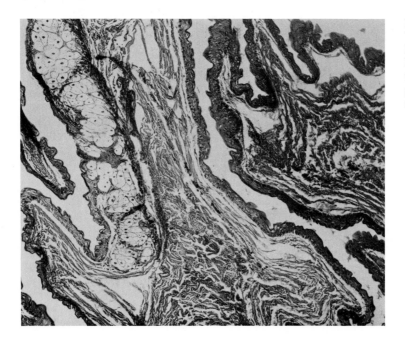

Fig. 26-14. Steatocystoma multiplex
The cyst wall shows intricate folding. The lining of the cyst consists of a homogeneous horny layer that protrudes irregularly into the lumen. On the left, flattened sebaceous gland lobules lie within, or close to, the cyst wall. (×100)

The presence of sebaceous gland lobules in many tumors indicates that differentiation toward sebaceous structures occurs frequently. It is apparent that this differentiation also includes the sebaceous duct, since an undulating surface is particularly evident in the horny layer of normal sebaceous ducts both by light microscopy and by electron microscopy (Kimura; Brownstein).

DERMOID CYST

Dermoid cysts are subcutaneous cysts that usually are present at birth. They occur most commonly on the head, mainly around the eyes, and occasionally on the neck. When located on the head, they often are adherent to the periosteum. Usually, they measure between 1 cm and 4 cm in size.

Histopathology. Dermoid cysts, in contrast to epidermal cysts, are lined by an epidermis that possesses various epidermal appendages. These appendages are as a rule fully matured. Hair follicles containing hairs that project into the lumen of the cyst are regularly present. In addition, the dermis of dermoid cysts contains nearly always sebaceous glands, often eccrine glands, and, in about one fifth of the cases, also apocrine glands (Brownstein and Helwig).

Histogenesis. Dermoid cysts are a result of the sequestration of skin along lines of embryonic closure.

BRONCHOGENIC AND THYROGLOSSAL DUCT CYSTS

Bronchogenic cysts are rare. They are small, solitary lesions seen most commonly in the skin or subcutaneous tissue just above the sternal notch. Rarely, they are located on the anterior aspect of the neck or on the chin. As a rule, they are discovered shortly after birth. They may show a draining sinus.

Thyroglossal duct cysts are clinically indistinguishable from bronchogenic cysts, except that they are usually located on the anterior aspect of the neck.

Histopathology. *Bronchogenic cysts* are lined by a mucosa consisting of a pseudostratified columnar epithelium (Fig. 26-15). Some of the epithelial cells show cilia extending into the lumen (Fig. 26-16). Varying numbers of goblet cells may be interspersed. The wall frequently contains smooth muscle and mucous glands but only rarely contains cartilage (Fraga et al).

Thyroglossal duct cysts differ from bronchogenic cysts in that they do not contain smooth muscle

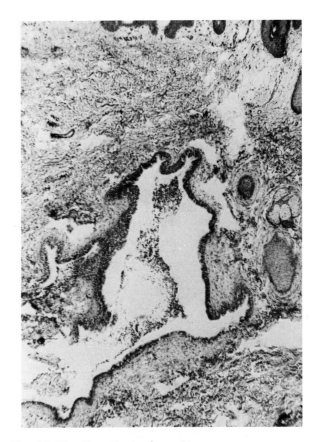

Fig. 26-15.   Bronchogenic cyst
Low magnification. The cyst located in the dermis is lined by a pseudostratified columnar epithelium. (×50)

Fig. 26-16.   Bronchogenic cyst
High magnification. Cilia are recognizable on several of the lining cells. (×400)

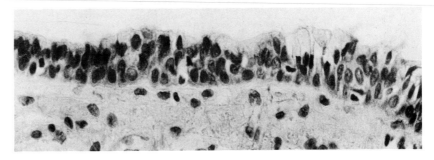

and in that they frequently show the presence of thyroid follicles (Ambiavagar and Rosen).

CUTANEOUS CILIATED CYST

Cutaneous ciliated cysts are found very rarely in females as a single lesion, largely on the lower extremities. They usually measure several centimeters in diameter. They are either unilocular or multilocular and are filled with clear or amber fluid.

Histopathology. Cutaneous ciliated cysts show numerous papillary projections lined by a simple cuboidal or columnar ciliated epithelium. Mucin-secreting cells are absent (Farmer and Helwig).

Histogenesis. The epithelial lining of the cysts resembles that seen in the fallopian tube. On electron microscopy, the cilia show two central filaments encircled by nine pairs of filaments (Clark).

MEDIAN RAPHE CYST OF THE PENIS

Median raphe cysts of the penis arise usually in young adults as the result of a developmental defect. They are located on the ventral aspect of the penis, most commonly on the glans. They are solitary and measure only a few millimeters in diameter (Cole and Helwig). It seems that, in some instances, median raphe cysts have been erroneously reported as apocrine cystadenoma of the penis (Ahmed and Jones; Powell et al).

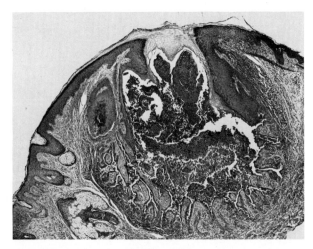

Fig. 26-17. Warty dyskeratoma
Low magnification. A large invagination is connected with the surface by a channel containing keratinous material. (×25) (Armed Forces Institute of Pathology, No. 57-6202)

Histopathology. The cysts are lined by pseudo-stratified columnar epithelium varying from one to four cells in thickness. Some of the epithelial cells have clear cytoplasm. Mucin-containing cells are found in only a few cases (Asarch et al).

ERUPTIVE VELLUS HAIR CYSTS

In eruptive vellus hair cysts, a condition first described in 1977 (Esterly et al), asymptomatic follicular papules 1 mm to 2 mm in diameter occur, most commonly on the chest but in some instances on the extremities or posterior trunk. Some of the papules have a crusted or umbilicated surface. The condition is usually seen in children and young adults, and spontaneous clearing may take place in a few years. Autosomal dominant inheritance has been described (Stiefler and Bergfeld; Piepkorn et al).

Histopathology. A cystic structure is usually seen in the middermis lined by squamous epithelium. It contains laminated keratinous material and varying numbers of transversely and obliquely cut vellus hairs (Esterly et al). In some cysts, vellus hairs are seen emerging from folliclelike invaginations of the cyst wall (Lee and Kim). In other cysts, a telogen hair follicle is seen extending from the lower surface towards the subcutis (Esterly et al). Crusted or umbilicated lesions show either a cyst communicating with the surface and extruding its contents (Burns and Calnan; Piepkorn et al) or partial destruction of a cyst by a granulomatous infiltrate and elimination of vellus hairs to the surface of the skin (Bovenmyer).

Histogenesis. Eruptive vellus hair cysts represent a developmental abnormality of vellus hair follicles, predisposing them to occlusion at their infundibular level. This results in retention of hairs, cystic dilatation of the proximal part of the follicle, and secondary atrophy of the hair bulbs (Esterly et al; Burns and Calnan).

WARTY DYSKERATOMA

Warty dyskeratoma, first described in 1957 (Szymanski), occurs nearly always as a solitary lesion, most commonly on the scalp, face, or neck. In several instances, it has been reported to occur in areas not customarily exposed to the sun, and it has been observed on several occasions on the oral mucosa, usually on the hard palate or an alveolar ridge (Gorlin and Peterson; Harrist et al). Although its clinical appearance is not always distinctive, it often occurs as a slightly elevated papule or nodule with a keratotic umbilicated center (Tanay and Mehregan). The lesion, after having reached a certain size, persists indefinitely.

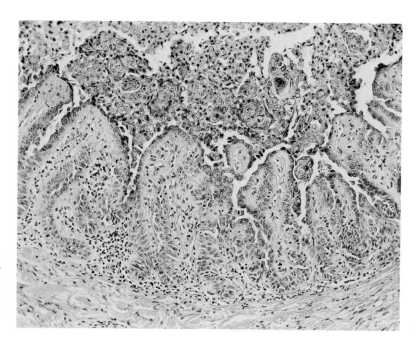

Fig. 26-18.   Warty dyskeratoma
The villi at the base of the invagination are covered with a single layer of epidermal cells. Acantholytic, dyskeratotic cells lie above the villi. (×100) (Armed Forces Institute of Pathology, No. 57-6203)

Histopathology.   The center of the lesion is occupied by a large, cup-shaped invagination connected with the surface by a channel. The channel is filled with keratinous material (Fig. 26-17). The large invagination contains numerous acantholytic, dyskeratotic cells in its upper portion. The lower portion of the invagination is occupied by numerous villi, that is, markedly elongated dermal papillae, that are often lined with only a single layer of basal cells and project upward from the base of the cupshaped invagination (Fig. 26-18). At the base of the upward-growing villi, one often observes an irregular downward growth of epidermal strands, often as a double layer of basal cells separated by a narrow slit containing a few dyskeratotic, acantholytic cells (Szymanski; Graham and Helwig; Delacrétaz; Metz and Schröpl). Typical corps ronds can usually be seen in the thickened granular layer lining the channel at the entrance to the invagination (Fig. 26-19) (Furtado and Szymanski; Tanay and Mehregan).

Histogenesis. The central cup-shaped invagination has been interpreted by several observers as a greatly dilated hair follicle, since, in early lesions, a hair follicle or sebaceous gland is often connected with the invagination (Graham and Helwig). Occasionally, two or three adjoining follicles seem to be involved (Tanay and Mehregan). Still, the fact that warty dyskeratoma can arise on the oral mucosa indicates that, as in Darier's disease, the dyskeratotic, acantholytic process is not always derived from a pilosebaceous structure.

Although attempts were made at first to correlate warty dyskeratoma either with Darier's disease or with solar keratosis, it is now generally agreed that warty dyskeratoma represents an entity, "a benign cutaneous tumor that resembles Darier's disease microscopically" (Szymanski).

In spite of the histologic resemblance, it is not likely that warty dyskeratoma is related to Darier's disease. First, there is no clinical resemblance, and the development of a warty dyskeratoma subsequent to Darier's disease has been reported in only one case (Kellum and Haserick), which was probably coincidental. Second, Darier's disease is not known to show such a deep invagination as warty dyskeratoma.

A relationship with solar keratosis, as was once suggested (Tritsch; Jablonska and Chorzelski), is unlikely despite the occasional presence of dyskeratosis and acantholysis in solar keratosis. The following observations speak against a relationship: warty dyskeratoma occasionally occurs in areas of the skin protected from the sun; warty dyskeratoma develops within a cup-shaped invagination into which solar rays are unlikely to penetrate; no corps ronds occur in solar keratosis; and an invasive squamous cell carcinoma has never been observed in warty dyskeratoma.

SOLAR KERATOSIS

Solar keratoses are also known as actinic keratoses. However, the adjective *solar* is more specific, since it refers to the sun as the cause, whereas the adjective *actinic* refers to a variety of rays (Brownstein and Rabinowitz).

Solar keratoses are usually seen as multiple lesions in

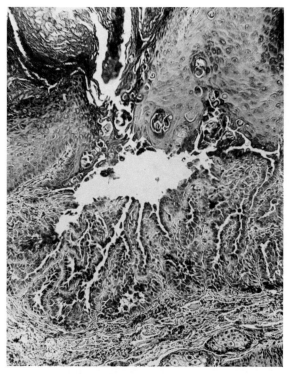

Fig. 26-19.   Warty dyskeratoma
Typical corps ronds are located in the thickened granular layer lining the channel that leads into the invagination. (×100)

sun-exposed areas of the skin in persons in or past middle life who have a fair complexion. Excessive exposure to sunlight over many years and inadequate protection against it are the essential predisposing factors. Solar keratoses are seen most commonly on the face and the dorsa of the hands and in the bald portions of the scalp in men.

Usually, the lesions measure less than 1 cm in diameter. They are erythematous, are often covered by adherent scales, and show little or no infiltration. Some solar keratoses are pigmented and show peripheral spreading, making clinical differentiation from lentigo maligna difficult (James et al). Occasionally, lesions show marked hyperkeratosis and then have the clinical aspect of cutaneous horns (see p. 493). A lesion analogous to solar keratosis occurs on the vermilion border of the lower lip as *solar cheilitis* and may show areas of erosion and hyperkeratosis (Koten et al; Mashkillejson; Cataldo and Doku).

Solar keratosis can develop into squamous cell carcinoma. However, the incidence of this transformation is difficult to determine, because the border line between solar keratosis and squamous cell carcinoma is not clearcut (see Histopathology). It has been estimated that in 20% of patients with solar keratoses squamous cell carcinoma develops in one or more of the lesions (Montgomery and Dörffel). Usually, squamous cell carcinomas arising either in solar keratoses or as such in sundamaged skin do not metastasize. The incidence of metastasis in different series varies from 0.5% (Lund) to 3% (Møller et al). In carcinoma of the vermilion border

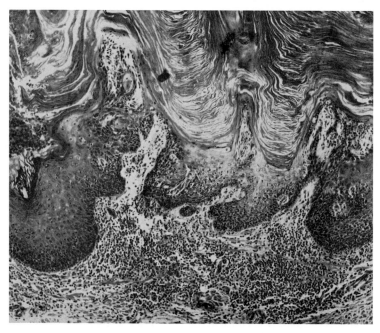

Fig. 26-20.   Solar keratosis, hypertrophic type
One observes hyperkeratosis and papillomatosis. The stratum malpighii demonstrates irregular hyperplasia in which the epidermal cells show a rather disorderly arrangement and some of the nuclei appear pleomorphic and atypical. The upper dermis shows a rather pronounced chronic inflammatory infiltrate.(×100)

of the lip, however, metastases have been found in 11% of the cases (see p. 499) (Møller et al).

Histopathology. Solar keratoses are squamous cell carcinomas in situ. This definition is preferable to their designation as precancerosis, because morphologically anaplastic cells are present. However, biologically, the lesions are still benign; invasion into the dermis, if present at all, is limited to the most superficial portion.

Five types of solar keratosis can be recognized histologically: hypertrophic, atrophic, bowenoid, acantholytic, and pigmented. Transitions and combinations among these five types occur. In addition, many cutaneous horns prove on histologic examination to be solar keratoses (see p. 493).

In the *hypertrophic type* of solar keratosis, hyperkeratosis is pronounced and is usually intermingled with areas of parakeratosis. Mild or moderate papillomatosis may be present. The epidermis is thickened in most areas and shows irregular downward proliferation, which, however, is limited to the uppermost dermis and thus does not represent frank invasion (Fig. 26-20). The cells of the entire stratum malpighii show a loss of polarity and thus a disorderly arrangement. Some of these cells show pleomorphism and atypicality ("anaplasia") of their nuclei, which appear large, irregular, and hyperchromatic. Often, the nuclei in the basal layer are closely crowded together. Some of the cells in the midportion of the epidermis show premature keratinization, resulting in dyskeratotic cells characterized by homogeneous, eosinophilic cytoplasm with or without a nucleus. It is worthy of note that, in contrast to the epidermal keratinocytes, the cells of the hair follicles and eccrine ducts that penetrate the epidermis within solar keratoses retain their normal appearance and keratinize normally (Halter; Pinkus, 1958). In some cases, abnormal keratinocytes extend downward on the outside of the follicular infundibulum to the level of the sebaceous duct and, less commonly, along the eccrine duct (Pinkus, 1958).

In rare instances of solar keratosis of the hypertrophic type, in addition to finding anaplastic nuclei in the lower epidermis, one finds areas of epidermolytic hyperkeratosis in the upper epidermis (Fig. 26-21). These changes are like those seen in bullous congenital ichthyosiform erythroderma, in linear epidermal nevus, and as incidental epidermolytic hyperkeratosis in a variety of lesions (see p. 475). In areas of epidermolytic hyperkeratosis, one observes in the upper epidermis clear spaces

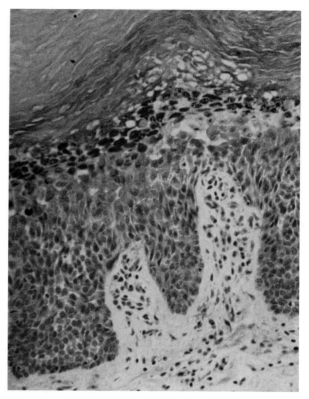

Fig. 26-21. Solar keratosis, hypertrophic type, showing epidermolytic hyperkeratosis
In addition to disorderly arrangement and anaplasia of the nuclei in the lower epidermis, epidermolytic hyperkeratosis, referred to also as *granular degeneration,* is present in the upper epidermis. One observes clear spaces around the nuclei and a thickened granular layer with large, irregularly shaped keratohyaline granules. (×200)

around the nuclei and a thickened granular layer with large, irregularly shaped keratohyaline granules (Ackerman and Reed).

In the *atrophic type* of solar keratosis, hyperkeratosis usually is slight. The epidermis is atrophic and devoid of rete ridges. Atypicality of the cells is found predominantly in the basal cell layer, which consists of cells with large hyperchromatic nuclei that lie close together (Fig. 26-22). The atypical basal layer may proliferate into the dermis as buds and ductlike structures. It may also surround as cell mantles the upper portion of pilosebaceous follicles and sweat ducts, the epithelium of which otherwise appears normal (Pinkus, 1958).

The *bowenoid type* of solar keratosis is histologically indistinguishable from Bowen's disease. As

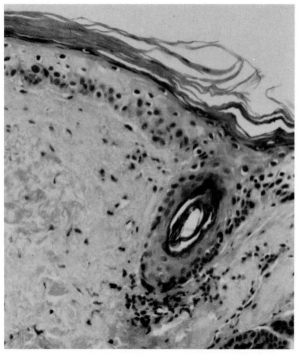

Fig. 26-22. Solar keratosis, atrophic type
Hyperkeratosis is mild. The epidermis is atrophic. The nuclei of the basal cells are anaplastic and appear closely crowded together. Anaplastic basal cells also line a hair follicle as a cell mantle. (×200)

in Bowen's disease, one observes within the epidermis considerable disorder in the arrangement of the nuclei, as well as clumping of nuclei and dyskeratosis (see p. 496).

In the *acantholytic type* of solar keratosis, one observes immediately above the atypical cells composing the basal cell layer clefts or lacunae similar to those seen in Darier's disease (see p. 70). These clefts form as a result of anaplastic changes in the lowermost epidermis, resulting in dyskeratosis and loss of the intercellular bridges (Fig. 26-23). A few acantholytic cells may be present within the clefts. Because the acantholysis is preceded by cellular changes, it is referred to as secondary acantholysis, in contrast to the primary acantholysis seen in the "acantholytic" diseases, such as pemphigus vulgaris and Darier's disease. Above the acantholytic clefts, the epidermis may show little or no atypicality. This can be explained by the fact that the normal adnexal epithelium proliferates in the manner of an umbrella over the anaplastic lower epidermis (Pinkus, 1958). The anaplastic cells of the basal cell layer frequently show extensions into the upper dermis as buds or short, ductlike structures.

In the *pigmented type* of solar keratosis, excessive amounts of melanin are present, especially in the basal cell layer. In some cases, the atypical keratinocytes appear well melanized, whereas, in others, almost all the melanin is retained within the

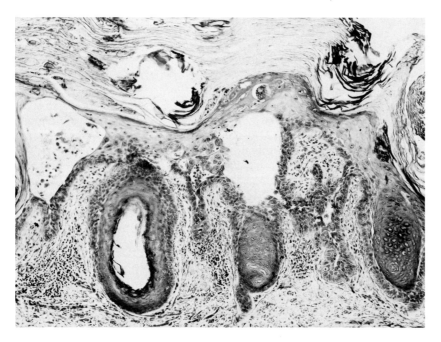

Fig. 26-23. Solar keratosis, acantholytic type
Nuclear atypicality is most pronounced in the basal layer, which proliferates into the dermis as short, ductlike structures. Suprabasal clefts and lacunae are present as a result of secondary acantholysis. (×150)

cell bodies and dendrites of the melanocytes, indicating some breakdown in melanin transfer. Numerous melanophages are seen in most cases in the superficial dermis (James et al).

In all five types of solar keratosis, the upper dermis usually shows a fairly dense, chronic inflammatory infiltrate composed predominantly of lymphoid cells but often also containing plasma cells. In some instances, the infiltrate lies close to the base of the lesion and thus shows a lichenoid pattern. Solar cheilitis, more frequently than solar keratosis of the skin, shows an inflammatory infiltrate in which plasma cells predominate (Koten et al). Although the upper dermis usually shows solar or basophilic degeneration, this may be absent in areas with a pronounced inflammatory reaction, probably because the inflammation has resulted in a regeneration of collagen.

In instances in which the histologic diagnosis is solar keratosis but the clinical diagnosis is squamous cell carcinoma, it is advisable to section more deeply into the block of tissue, because progression into squamous cell carcinoma may have taken place in another area. Because no sharp line of demarcation exists between the two conditions, it is not always possible to decide definitely whether a lesion can still be regarded as a solar keratosis or should be classified as an early squamous cell carcinoma. Such situations arise, for instance, when irregular branches of atypical cells descend from a hypertrophic solar keratosis fairly deeply into the dermis or when buds or ductlike structures extend quite deeply from an atrophic or acantholytic solar keratosis. However, as already pointed out, this decision is rarely a vital one, unlike the case of malignant melanoma in situ versus invasive malignant melanoma, because early squamous cell carcinoma arising in a solar keratosis rarely causes metastases although it may become deeply invasive and destructive through further growth. Since carcinomas arising in solar cheilitis have a significantly higher tendency to metastasize than carcinomas arising in solar keratosis (see p. 499), and since invasion of the dermis in solar cheilitis may be focal, lesions of solar cheilitis require thorough examination by means of step sections (Cataldo and Doku).

Differential Diagnosis.   In solar keratoses showing relatively slight atypicality, or anaplasia, of the tumor cells, diagnosis may be difficult. Thus, a hypertrophic solar keratosis with a lichenoid inflammatory infiltrate may show a close histologic resemblance to the lesion known as benign lichenoid keratosis (see p. 156). In fact, this lesion was at one time thought to be a variant of solar keratosis (Hirsch and Marmelzat; Pinkus, 1973). Benign lichenoid keratosis differs from solar keratosis by showing dissolution rather than atypicality of the basal cell layer, analogous to lichen planus (Shapiro and Ackerman; Scott and Johnson).

An atrophic solar keratosis may closely resemble lupus erythematosus, since both types of lesions show flattening of the epidermis. Although lupus erythematosus shows vacuolization, and solar keratosis shows atypicality of the cells in the basal layer, these two changes are not always easily distinguished from one another. Therefore, other findings, such as follicular plugging and a patchy, periappendageal infiltrate in lupus erythematosus, are necessary for differentiation (see p. 446).

A pigmented solar keratosis may resemble lentigo maligna, particularly if the melanin is seen largely within the melanocytes (James et al). Usually, however, lentigo maligna shows more flattening of the epidermis than pigmented solar keratosis and, most important, a great increase in the number of melanocytes, together with atypicality in the melanocytes but not in the basal keratinocytes (see p. 703).

Cutaneous Horn

Cutaneous horn, or *cornu cutaneum,* is the clinical term for a circumscribed, conical, markedly hyperkeratotic lesion in which the height of the keratotic mass amounts to at least half of its largest diameter (Bart et al). The term refers to a reaction pattern and not to a specific lesion (Brownstein and Shapiro).

Histopathology.   On histologic examination, different types of lesions can be seen at the base of the conical hyperkeratosis of a cornu cutaneum. Most commonly, a solar keratosis is encountered (Cramer and Kahlert). In some instances, a filiform verruca, a seborrheic keratosis, or a squamous cell carcinoma is found (Bart et al). On rare occasions, a trichilemmoma (Brownstein and Shapiro) or a basal cell epithelioma is seen (Sandbank).

LEUKOPLAKIA

The term *leukoplakia* was used in the past by dermatologists as well as gynecologists (McAdams and Kistner) to designate white patches of the oral mucosa or the vulva that showed early, that is, in situ, anaplastic changes, whereas the term *leukokeratosis* was used for patches with a histologically benign appearance. However, leukoplakia has been redefined on the basis of the concept proposed by oral pathologists (Shklar, 1967), and this concept has been accepted by the World Health Association (Pindborg).

According to this concept, the term *leukoplakia* carries no histologic connotation and is used only as a clinical description. It is defined as a white patch or plaque that will not rub off and that cannot be characterized clinically or histologically as any specific disease (*e.g.,* lichen planus, lupus erythematosus, candidiasis, white sponge nevus) (Waldron and Shafer). The reason for using the term *leukoplakia* as a purely clinical designation is that a distinction between benign leukoplakia and leukoplakia with anaplastic changes cannot be made on clinical grounds but only on histologic grounds. It is therefore essential that all white plaques that either are idiopathic in origin or persist for 3 to 4 weeks after any existing irritation has been eliminated be examined histologically (Hornstein). In many cases of oral leukoplakia, either chemical irritation through tobacco or mechanical irritation through dental stumps or ill-fitting dentures plays a role. Whereas the leukoplakia clears in some instances after the irritation has been removed, it persists in others. However, the transformation of a benign leukoplakia into a malignant leukoplakia is regarded as rare (Shklar, 1981). Vulvar leukoplakia usually develops as a result of involutional atrophy of the vulva.

Clinically, lesions of leukoplakia on the oral mucosa and vulva consist of one or several white patches that may not be raised and then appear ill defined. However, if they are slightly elevated, they appear sharply demarcated, with an irregular outline.

Erythroplakia of the oral mucosa consists of red, sharply delineated patches that vary greatly in size. Some of these lesions are sprinkled or intermingled with patches of leukoplakia and are then referred to as speckled erythroplakia (Shafer and Waldron).

On examination by histology, scraping, or culture, both leukoplakia and erythroplakia frequently show *Candida albicans* as a secondary invader, a finding that may give rise to an incorrect diagnosis of candidiasis (Grässel-Pietrusky and Hornstein). However, infection with *Candida albicans* may cause oral lesions that are clinically indistinguishable from leukoplakia (Cawson and Lehner).

Histopathology.   The whitish color of leukoplakia is the result of hydration of a thickened horny layer. On histologic examination, about 80% of the lesions of oral leukoplakia are found to be benign (Waldron and Shafer; Grässel-Pietrusky and Hornstein). Such lesions show hyperkeratotic or parakeratotic thickening of the horny layer, acanthosis, and a chronic inflammatory infiltrate. Of the remaining 20% of the cases, 17% show varying degrees of in situ anaplasia, and 3% show infiltrating squamous cell carcinoma (Waldron and Shafer). Ultimate development of carcinoma has been observed in 7% to 13% of all cases of leukoplakia (Pindborg).

In situ anaplasia, also referred to as precancerous leukoplakia, usually has the same histologic appearance as the hypertrophic type of solar keratosis (see p. 491). Thus, the most important features observed within a moderately acanthotic epithelium are, first, pleomorphism and atypicality of the nuclei, which appear large, irregular, and hyperchromatic, and, second, loss of polarity, resulting in a disorderly arrangement of the cells (Fig. 26-24). In some instances, one finds as additional features premature keratinization resulting in dyskeratotic cells in the midportion of the epithelium, crowding of nuclei in the basal cell layer, and irregular downward proliferations of the epithelium.

Erythroplakia of the oral mucosa, in contrast to leukoplakia, invariably shows nuclear atypicality. One observes in situ anaplasia in half of the cases and invasive carcinoma in the other half (Shafer and Waldron). The red appearance is explained by the absence of the normal surface covering of orthokeratin or parakeratin.

Differential Diagnosis.   A decision as to whether in situ anaplasia exists in a leukoplakia can be difficult, since some pleomorphism of nuclei and some loss of polarity of the cells can be seen occasionally also in various inflammatory conditions, including benign leukoplakia (Hornstein). In cases of doubt, step sections throughout the biopsy specimen are required, as well as, possibly, examination of additional biopsy specimens. The decision as to whether a leukoplakia is benign or shows in situ anaplasia and thus is "precancerous" is of considerable importance. In comparison with squamous cell carcinoma of the skin developing secondary to a solar keratosis, squamous cell carcinoma of the oral mucosa or the vulva developing secondary to a leukoplakia with in situ anaplasia has a much greater tendency to metastasize.

VERRUCOUS HYPERPLASIA, VERRUCOUS CARCINOMA OF THE ORAL MUCOSA

Verrucous hyperplasia of the oral mucosa consists of extensive verrucous, whitish patches that may arise as such or develop from lesions of leukoplakia. Verrucous hyperplasia and verrucous carcinoma are indistinguish-

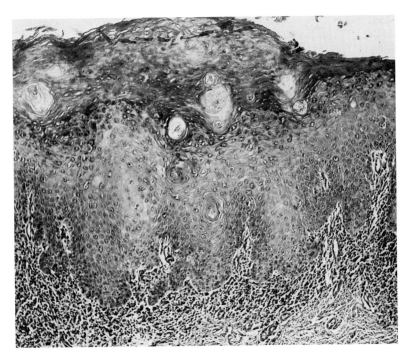

Fig. 26-24.   Leukoplakia of the oral leukoplakia with in situ anaplasia The lesion shows hyperkeratosis and acanthosis. In addition to disorder in the arrangement of the cells, there is nuclear atypicality. (×200)

able clinically. They may coexist, or verrucous carcinoma may develop from verrucous hyperplasia. In some instances, verrucous hyperplasia develops into frank squamous cell carcinoma rather than into verrucous carcinoma (Shear and Pindborg).

Verrucous carcinoma of the oral mucosa is also known as oral florid papillomatosis. Clinically, one observes whitish, cauliflowerlike lesions that may involve large areas of the oral mucosa and that gradually extend and coalesce. Extensive local tissue destruction may occur. However, metastases are rare and, if they occur, remain limited to the regional lymph nodes (Kraus and Perez-Mesa; Samitz et al; Grinspan and Abulafia).

Histopathology. *Verrucous hyperplasia* shows a hyperplastic epithelium with upward extension of verrucous projections located predominantly superficial to the adjacent epithelium (Shear and Pindborg).

Verrucous carcinoma (oral florid papillomatosis) differs in its early stage from verrucous hyperplasia by showing, in addition to the surface verrucous projections, extension of the lesion into the underlying connective tissue (Shear and Pindborg). The downward extensions of the epithelium are round and club-shaped and appear well demarcated from the surrounding stroma. Nuclear pleomorphism or hyperchromasia and formation of horn pearls are absent.

Some lesions of verrucous carcinoma persist in this stage for many years, although ultimately they show in the areas of deepest extension a moderate loss of polarity, increased cytoplasmic basophilia, nuclear hyperchromasia, and frequent mitotic figures. These features, however, do not suffice for a diagnosis of squamous cell carcinoma (Wechsler and Fisher). Other lesions show sufficient nuclear atypicality and loss of polarity in the downward proliferations to indicate the presence of a well-differentiated squamous cell carcinoma (Kanee). In about 10% of the cases of verrucous carcinoma, transformation into a classic squamous cell carcinoma takes place (Samitz et al; Grinspan and Abulafia). (For a more detailed discussion of verrucous carcinoma, see p. 505.)

NECROTIZING SIALOMETAPLASIA

One or occasionally two ulcers showing a rolled border and measuring 1 cm to 2 cm in diameter are found on the hard or soft palate. Spontaneous healing takes place within 6 to 12 weeks. The importance of necrotizing sialometaplasia, a rare condition first reported in 1973 (Abrams et al), lies in its clinical and histologic resemblance to carcinoma.

Histopathology. Histologic examination shows coagulative necrosis of salivary gland lobules and squamous metaplasia within adjacent viable lobules. The connective tissue framework of the necrotic glands remains intact, thereby preserving their lobular outline. Faintly basophilic material representing sialomucin is seen within the necrotic glands. This is both PAS-positive and alcian-blue-positive. Adjacent to the necrotic glands, one may see normal-appearing salivary gland acini. Other salivary gland structures show either partial squamous metaplasia, with a peripheral rim of squamous cells, or complete replacement by squamous epithelium. The squamous metaplasia also involves the salivary ducts (Raugi and Kessler; Piette et al).

Differential Diagnosis. To pathologists not familiar with this condition, the apparent irregular proliferation and deep extension of squamous epithelium may suggest a diagnosis of carcinoma. However, the confinement of cytologically benign squamous epithelium to the pre-existing lobular pattern of salivary glands should permit the correct diagnosis (Fechner).

EOSINOPHILIC ULCER OF THE TONGUE

An asymptomatic ulcer measuring 1 cm to 2 cm in diameter is found on the tongue. This ulcer heals spontaneously within a few weeks.

Histopathology. A dense cellular infiltrate is present at the base of the ulcer, extending through the submucosa into the striated muscle bundles of the tongue. Most of the cells are eosinophils, but there are also lymphocytes and histiocytes (Shapiro and Juhlin; Burgess et al).

Differential Diagnosis. This lesion differs from eosinophilic granuloma of histiocytosis X (see

p. 395) clinically by its tendency to heal rapidly and histologically by the smaller number and smaller size of the histiocytes (Shapiro and Juhlin).

BOWEN'S DISEASE

Bowen's disease usually but not always consists of a solitary lesion. It may occur on exposed or on unexposed skin. It may be caused on exposed skin by exposure to the sun and on unexposed skin by the ingestion of arsenic (see Histogenesis below and Arsenical Keratosis and Carcinoma, p. 267). Lesions of Bowen's disease also commonly form in lesions of epidermodysplasia verruciformis caused by HPV-5 (see p. 375).

Bowen's disease manifests itself as a slowly enlarging erythematous patch of sharp but irregular outline, showing little or no infiltration. Within the patch are generally areas of scaling and crusting. Although Bowen's disease may resemble a superficial basal cell epithelioma, it differs from it by the absence both of a fine pearly border and of a tendency to heal centrally. Lesions of Bowen's disease can occur on the glans penis, where they are referred to also as erythroplasia of Queyrat (see p. 498).

Bowenoid papulosis of the genitalia, because of its probable relationship to genital warts, is discussed on p. 377.

Histopathology. Bowen's disease is an intraepidermal squamous cell carcinoma referred to also as squamous cell carcinoma in situ. Thus, it represents biologically but not morphologically a *precancerous dermatosis,* under which designation it was described originally in 1912 (Bowen).

The epidermis shows acanthosis with elongation and thickening of the rete ridges, often to such a degree that the papillae located between the rete ridges are reduced to thin strands. Throughout the

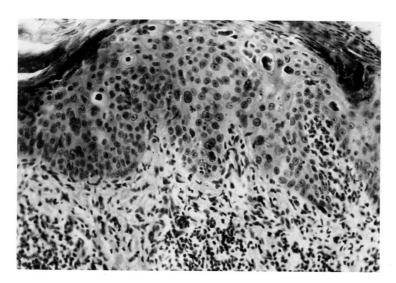

Fig. 26-25. Bowen's disease
The epidermis is thickened. The border between the epidermis and dermis appears sharp. The cells of the stratum malpighii lie in complete disorder, and many of them appear atypical, showing large, hyperchromatic nuclei. Several multinucleated epidermal cells are present. The stratum corneum shows parakeratosis. ($\times 200$)

epidermis, the cells lie in complete disorder. Many of them appear highly atypical, showing large, hyperchromatic nuclei. Multinucleated epidermal cells containing clusters of nuclei are often present (Fig. 26-25). The horny layer usually is thickened and consists largely of parakeratotic cells with atypical, hyperchromatic nuclei (Montgomery).

A common and rather characteristic feature is the presence of cells showing atypical individual cell keratinization (Fig. 26-26). Such dyskeratotic cells are large and round and have a homogeneous, strongly eosinophilic cytoplasm and a hyperchromatic nucleus. The infiltrate of Bowen's disease frequently extends into follicular infundibula and causes replacement of the follicular epithelium by atypical cells down to the entrance of the sebaceous duct (Brownstein and Rabinowitz).

Even though the marked atypicality of the epidermal cells includes the cells of the basal layer, the border between the epidermis and dermis everywhere appears sharp, and, on staining with the PAS reaction, the PAS-positive basement membrane zone is intact. The upper dermis usually shows a moderate amount of a chronic inflammatory infiltrate.

An occasional finding in Bowen's disease is vacuolization of the cells, especially in the upper portion of the epidermis (Montgomery and Waisman). Also, in exceptional cases, multiple nests of atypical cells are scattered through a normal epidermis, sometimes with sparing of the basal cell layer. This results in a histologic picture that used to be interpreted as intraepidermal epithelioma of Borst–Jadassohn (see p. 571) (Strayer and Santa Cruz; Brownstein and Rabinowitz).

In a small percentage of cases of Bowen's disease, an invasive squamous cell carcinoma develops. The figures given in the literature as to the frequency of this development vary. The highest incidence given is 11% (Graham and Helwig, 1959). On the opposite end is a statement that, in the vast majority of cases, Bowen's disease remains a carcinoma in situ for the lifetimes of those affected (Ackerman). If invasion happens, it usually takes place after many years's duration of the disease. The invasive tumor retains the cytologic characteristics of the intraepidermal tumor, and invasion may occur at first in only a limited area. In order not to miss such an area, it is advisable to examine representative sections throughout the entire tissue block. As soon as invasion has taken place, the prognosis changes. So long as Bowen's disease remains in its intraepidermal stage, metastases do not occur. However, once invasion of the dermis

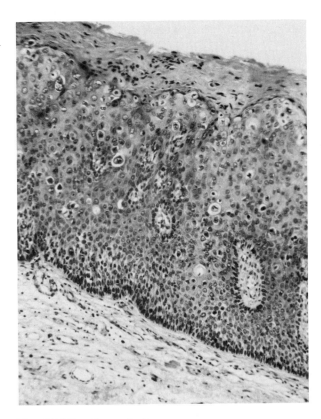

Fig. 26-26. Bowen's disease
In addition to the changes described for Figure 26-25, there are scattered cells within the stratum malpighii showing atypical individual cell keratinization or dyskeratosis. ($\times 200$)

has occurred, the likelihood of regional and even visceral metastases is great (Graham and Helwig, 1959).

Histogenesis. No agreement exists with regard to the frequency with which visceral carcinoma develops in patients with Bowen's disease. The first authors to point out an association between Bowen's disease and visceral cancer found that, of 35 patients with Bowen's disease who were known to have died, 20 (57%) had an associated internal cancer (Graham and Helwig, 1959). In a subsequent series, however, a significant increase in the incidence of associated internal cancer was observed only in patients in whom the lesions of Bowen's disease were located in areas not exposed to the sun (33%), whereas, in patients in whom the lesions were in exposed areas, the incidence of visceral cancer was low (5%) (Peterka et al). This suggested the possibility that at least some of the Bowen's lesions in unexposed areas, as well as the associated visceral cancer, were caused by the ingestion of arsenic. (See also Arsenical Keratosis and Carcinoma, p. 267.) Of two later series, one showed no significant increase in visceral carcinoma among patients with Bowen's disease, the incidence being 11% (Anderson et al), whereas the other showed a significantly increased incidence, 29%, without evidence of arsenic as a causative factor in most patients. No significant difference in the incidence of visceral cancer was found for Bowen's lesions in exposed or unexposed areas (Callen and Headington).

Electron microscopic examination of lesions of Bowen's disease has demonstrated the presence of many dyskeratotic cells. The perinuclear aggregation and condensation of tonofilaments in these dyskeratotic cells are similar to but more pronounced than in the dyskeratotic cells of Darier's disease (Seiji and Mizuno). Some of the markedly dyskeratotic cells in Bowen's disease disintegrate, and portions of such cells are phagocytized by other epidermal cells, which then contain, in addition to the phagocytized dyskeratotic material, phagocytized desmosomes in their cytoplasm (Seiji and Mizuno; Olson et al, 1969). In other instances, the intracellularly located desmosomes are not phagocytized but are drawn into the dyskeratotic cells of Bowen's disease together with aggregating tonofilaments (Sato and Seiji). The phenomenon of intracytoplasmic desmosomes, however, is not specific for Bowen's disease, although it is found most commonly in this condition. Thus, intracytoplasmic desmosomes have been observed within dyskeratotic keratinocytes in Darier's disease (Arai and Hori), squamous cell carcinoma (Klingmüller et al), and keratoacanthoma (Fisher et al); within nondyskeratotic keratinocytes in extramammary Paget's disease (Ishibashi et al) and malignant melanoma (Klug and Haustein); and even within normal keratinocytes in both the epidermis (Komura and Watanabe) and the oral mucosa (Schenk). It can be assumed that the occasional occurrence of invaginations of the plasma membrane is a normal event in keratinocytes and that the invaginated plasma membrane can contain desmosomal structures. These structures are more resistant to enzymatic destruction than the plasma membrane and thus may be found free in the cytoplasm (Schenk).

Two types of epidermal giant cells can be recognized in Bowen's disease. In one type, an entire dyskeratotic cell has been "cannibalized" by another keratinocyte and is located within the cytoplasm of the phagocytizing cell (Olson et al, 1968). In the second type, multiple nuclei lie in the center of the giant cell surrounded by dyskeratotic tonofilaments. It seems that, by becoming entangled with the spindles of the mitotic apparatus, the dyskeratotic tonofilaments interfere with the normal division of the cell so that nuclear division can take place but cellular division cannot (Seiji and Mizuno; Olson et al, 1969).

Differential Diagnosis.   No histologic difference exists between bowenoid solar keratosis and Bowen's disease. They differ merely in size, the bowenoid solar keratosis usually being smaller than Bowen's disease.

Paget's disease may share with Bowen's disease the presence of vacuolated cells but, in contrast with Bowen's disease, it shows no dyskeratosis. In addition, the material contained in Paget cells is often PAS-positive and diastase-resistant, whereas the PAS-positive material that is sometimes present in the vacuolated cells of Bowen's disease is glycogen and therefore diastase-labile (Raiten et al).

Erythroplasia of Queyrat (Bowen's Disease of the Glans Penis)

Erythroplasia of Queyrat is the term often used for carcinoma in situ located on the glans penis. Clinically and histologically, it is identical to Bowen's disease, and this designation would seem preferable for simplicity's sake. The only reason for keeping the term *erythroplasia of Queyrat* alive is that it was introduced in 1911 (Queyrat), 1 year before the description of Bowen's disease (Bowen). At one time, the term *erythroplasia of Queyrat* was used also for oral lesions, but this usage has been abandoned because of differences in histologic appearance and the frequent occurrence of invasion in oral lesions, which are now known as oral erythroplakia (see p. 494). The existence of a lesion of the female genitalia analogous to erythroplasia of the glans has also been questioned (Graham and Helwig, 1972), although Bowen's disease of the vulva exists.

Erythroplasia or Bowen's disease of the glans penis is seen almost exclusively in uncircumcised men. It manifests itself as an asymptomatic, sharply demarcated, bright red, shiny, very slightly infiltrated plaque on the glans penis or, less often, in the coronal sulcus or on the inner surface of the prepuce (Goette).

Histopathology.   Erythroplasia of Queyrat of the glans penis has the same histologic appearance as Bowen's disease. Progression into an invasive squamous cell carcinoma has been observed in up to 30% of the patients (Mikhail), with metastases in about 20% of the patients with invasive erythroplasia (Graham and Helwig, 1972). It thus has a greater tendency toward invasion and metastasis than Bowen's disease of the skin (Mikhail).

Differential Diagnosis.   A clinical diagnosis of erythroplasia of Queyrat requires histologic examination for confirmation, since differentiation from balanitis circumscripta plasmacellularis is not possible on a clinical basis.

Balanitis Circumscripta Plasmacellularis

A disorder first described in 1952 (Zoon), balanitis circumscripta plasmacellularis has the same clinical appearance as erythroplasia of Queyrat or Bowen's disease of the glans penis. In some instances, erosions with a tendency to bleed are present (Eberhartinger and Bergmann). Like erythroplasia, this disorder is seen almost exclusively in uncircumcised males (Souteyrand et al). On rare occasions, an analogous lesion referred to as vulvitis circumscripta plasmacellularis is observed on the vulva (Souteyrand et al; Mensing and Jänner).

Histopathology.   The epidermis appears thinned and often shows absence of its upper layers (Brodin). It may be partially detached as a result of subepidermal cleavage or even absent (Eberhartinger and Bergmann; Jonquières and de Lutzky). If present, the epidermis has a rather distinctive appearance; in addition to being thinned and flattened, it is composed of diamond- or lozenge-shaped, flattened keratinocytes that are separated from each other by uniform intercellular edema (Souteyrand et al). Erythrocytes may be seen permeating the epidermis. In some cases, the keratinocytes appear degenerated or necrotic (Brodin).

The upper dermis shows a banklike infiltrate in which numerous plasma cells are often seen (Zoon; Brodin). In some cases, however, their number is only moderate (Souteyrand et al) or even small (Jonquières and de Lutzky). In addition, the capillaries are dilated, and there may be extravasations of erythrocytes and deposits of hemosiderin (Nödl).

Histogenesis. It has been pointed out that plasma cells frequently predominate in the inflammatory response at mucocutaneous junctions in a variety of benign and malignant processes. Thus, the term *circumorificial plasmacytosis* was introduced for benign plasma cell infiltrates on the glans penis, vulva, and lips (Schuermann; Moldenhauer; Baughman et al). However, the combination of histologic and clinical features seen in balanitis circumscripta plasmacellularis, and probably also in vulvitis circumscripta plasmacellularis, is unique and deserves recognition as an entity (Brodin; Souteyrand et al; Mensing and Jänner).

SQUAMOUS CELL CARCINOMA

Squamous cell carcinoma may occur anywhere on the skin as well as on mucous membranes with squamous epithelium. It rarely arises from normal-appearing skin. Most commonly, it arises in sun-damaged skin, either as such or from a solar keratosis. Carcinomas arising in sun-damaged skin have a very low propensity to metastasize, the incidence amounting to only about 0.5% (Lund). This is in contrast to a metastatic rate of 2% to 3% for all patients with squamous cell carcinoma of the skin, with death resulting in about three quarters of the patients with metastases (Epstein et al; Møller et al).

Carcinomas of the lower lip, even though in most cases also induced by exposure to the sun, have a much higher incidence of metastasis, about 11% (Møller et al).

Cutaneous squamous cell carcinomas that arise secondary to inflammatory and degenerative processes have a much higher rate of metastasis than those developing in sun-damaged skin. Thus, the rate of metastasis was found to be 31% in squamous cell carcinomas arising in osteomyelitic sinuses (Sedlin and Fleming), 20% in radiation-induced skin cancer (Martin et al), and 18% in carcinomas developing in burn scars (Arons et al). Furthermore, carcinomas arising from modified skin, such as the glans penis and the vulva, and from the oral mucosa have a rather high rate of metastasis unless recognized and adequately treated at an early stage.

The incidence of squamous cell carcinomas, like that of other malignant neoplasms, is significantly increased in immunosuppressed patients (Hoxtell et al). Squamous cell carcinomas may also show greater aggressiveness in such patients (Turner and Callen).

Clinically, squamous cell carcinoma of the skin most commonly consists of a shallow ulcer surrounded by a wide, elevated, indurated border. Often, the ulcer is covered by a crust that conceals a red, granular base. Occasionally, raised, fungoid, verrucous lesions without ulceration occur.

Two variants of squamous cell carcinoma, *adenoid squamous cell carcinoma* and *verrucous carcinoma,* will be discussed later (see pp. 503 and 505).

Histopathology.   Squamous cell carcinoma is a true, invasive carcinoma of the surface epidermis. On histologic examination, one finds the tumor to consist of irregular masses of epidermal cells that proliferate downward into the dermis. The invading tumor masses are composed in varying proportions of normal squamous cells and of atypical (anaplastic) squamous cells (see p. 472). The more malignant the tumor, the greater is the number of atypical squamous cells. Atypicality of squamous cells expresses itself in such changes as great variation in the size and shape of the cells, hyperplasia and hyperchromasia of the nuclei, absence of intercellular bridges, keratinization of individual cells, and the presence of atypical mitotic figures.

Differentiation in squamous cell carcinoma is in the direction of keratinization. Keratinization often takes place in the form of horn pearls, which are very characteristic structures composed of concentric layers of squamous cells showing gradually increasing keratinization toward the center. The center shows usually incomplete and only rarely complete keratinization. Keratohyaline granules within the horn pearls are sparse or absent.

Grading and Grades.   A system of grading of cutaneous squamous cell carcinoma was introduced in 1921 (Broders). This system recognizes four grades of severity according to the proportion of mature, that is, differentiated, cells present in the tumor. In grade 1, more than 75% of the cells are differentiated; in grade 2, more than 50%; in grade 3, more than 25%; and in grade 4, less than 25%. Since differentiation is in the direction of keratinization, the degree of keratinization represents the essential feature in Broders' system of grading. However, it is now generally recognized that, in addition to the proportion of differentiated cells, the degree of atypicality of the tumor cells and the depth of penetration of the lesion are important factors in grading. It must also be kept in mind that different degrees of malignancy may be present in different fields of the same tumor. Therefore, it is advisable to examine several sections of every tumor that is to be graded and then grade according to the least differentiated portion (Edmundson).

In squamous cell carcinoma, grade 1 (Fig. 26-27), the tumor masses have not penetrated below the level of the sweat glands. They still show in some areas an intact basal layer at their periphery. In other areas, however, the basal layer has become disorganized and may no longer be present. In such areas, cell masses appear poorly demarcated from the surrounding stroma. Most cells of the invading cell masses show well-developed intercellular bridges, even though some of the cells show atypical nuclei. Horn pearls are present in fairly large number. Some are well developed and have nearly fully keratinized centers; others, however, show only slight keratinization of their centers, and the concentric arrangement of the cells is not distinct. Besides horn pearls, sheets of partially keratinized cells may be present. The dermis often shows a rather marked inflammatory reaction. It is noteworthy that the inflammatory reaction in the dermis is usually much more pronounced in solar keratosis and squamous cell carcinoma, grade 1, than in the more malignant forms of squamous cell carcinoma. This phenomenon, which probably represents an immune reaction, suggests that tissue invaded by malignant cells is able to react against the cells to some extent, provided that they are only moderately malignant (see Histogenesis). (The same observation can also be made in malignant melanoma; see p. 710.)

In squamous cell carcinoma, grade 2 (Fig. 26-28), the invading cell masses as a rule are poorly demarcated from the surrounding stroma. Keratinization is much less evident than in grade 1. There are only a few horn pearls, and those present show rather poorly keratinizing centers. A fairly large number of the squamous cells are atypical.

In squamous cell carcinoma, grade 3 (Fig. 26-29), keratinization is absent in many areas. Horn pearls are not found. Instead, keratinization occurs in small cell groups in which the cells possess a slightly eosinophilic cytoplasm and a few intercellular bridges. In addition, one may find individual cell keratinization in which the dyskeratotic cells are large and round and have a deeply eosinophilic cytoplasm and a hyperchromatic nucleus. The majority of the nuclei in the tumor cells are atypical. Mitotic figures are conspicuous, and many are atypical.

In squamous cell carcinoma, grade 4 (Fig. 26-30), keratinization is almost completely absent. Nearly all tumor cells are atypical and devoid of intercellular bridges. Thus, it is often difficult to arrive at the correct diagnosis as long as only individual fields are studied. The tumor may then suggest an amelanotic malignant melanoma in some instances and a fibrosarcoma in others. The latter diagnosis

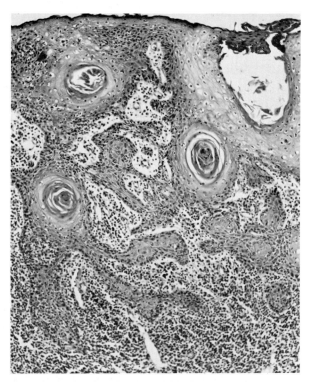

Fig. 26-27. Squamous cell carcinoma, grade 1
There is invasion of the dermis by epidermal masses, the cells of which are predominantly mature squamous cells showing relatively slight atypicality. Several horn pearls are present. The dermis shows a marked inflammatory reaction. (× 100)

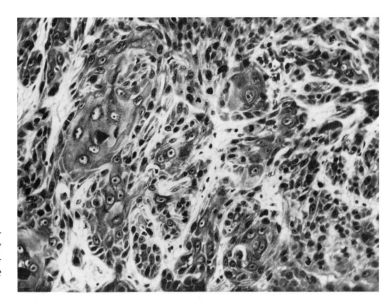

Fig. 26-28.   Squamous cell carcinoma, grade 2
The cell masses show much less keratinization than in grade 1. There are only a few horn pearls, and those present show incompletely keratinized centers. Atypical cells are conspicuous. (×200)

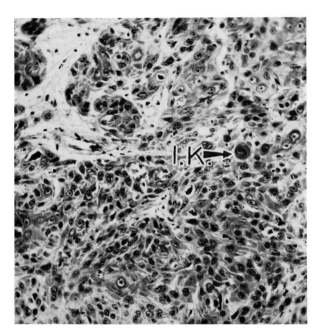

Fig. 26-29.   Squamous cell carcinoma, grade 3
No horn pearls are present. Keratinization occurs only in small cell groups. Many cells are atypical and devoid of prickles. To the right, a cell shows individual cell keratinization (*I.K.*). (×200)

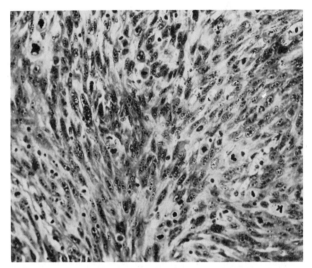

Fig. 26-30.   Squamous cell carcinoma, grade 4
Evidence of keratinization is absent. The tumor cells appear atypical and have no recognizable intercellular bridges. Because many tumor cells are elongated, the tumor suggests a fibrosarcoma more than a carcinoma. (×200)

may be particularly difficult to rule out when the cells are spindle-shaped, as in the so-called spindle cell squamous cell carcinoma.

Spindle cell squamous cell carcinomas arise mainly but not exclusively in areas of solar or radiation damage. In some instances, they contain areas in which the cells either show intercellular bridges and beginning keratinization or show evidence of origin from the epidermis. In other cases, however, such areas cannot be detected in spite of step sectioning, so that they have to be designated noncommittally as sarcomalike tumors (Evans and Smith). In both the spindle cell squamous cell carcinomas and the sarcomalike tumors of the skin, the spindle cells often appear highly anaplastic.

The spindle cells are intermingled with collagen and may be arranged in whorls (Manglani et al). Not infrequently, pleomorphic giant cells are seen (Fig. 26-31) (Evans and Smith). In such instances, distinction from atypical fibroxanthoma (see p. 611) may be impossible, and, indeed, some presumed atypical fibroxanthomas have been shown by electron microscopy or by demonstration of the presence of keratin to be spindle cell squamous cell carcinoma (see Histogenesis). The distinction between spindle cell squamous cell carcinomas and sarcomalike tumors is of little prognostic import per se, since the prognosis is primarily dependent on the depth of invasion (Evans and Smith).

Raised, verrucous lesions of squamous cell carcinoma may show a considerable histologic resemblance to keratoacanthoma (see p. 507) by having a central keratin-filled crater with peripheral buttresses. In most instances, however, one finds less cellular maturation and evidence of nuclear atypicality (Fig. 26-32).

Histogenesis. *Electron microscopy* of squamous cell carcinoma, in comparison with normal epidermal squamous cells, shows a reduction in the number of desmosomes on the cell surface. In their place, microvilli extend into the widened intercellular spaces. Desmosomes can be seen within the cytoplasm of some of the tumor cells, either by themselves or attached to bundles of tonofilaments (EM 38) (Klingmüller et al). Their intracytoplasmic location may be the result of either phagocytosis or invagination of the plasma membrane. However, it is not a specific finding for squamous cell carcinoma;

intracytoplasmic desmosomes can be found also in keratoacanthoma (see p. 508) and Bowen's disease, as well as in several unrelated epidermal proliferations and even in normal keratinocytes (see p. 498).

At the dermal-epidermal junction, the basement membrane shows sporadic discontinuities through which long cytoplasmic protrusions penetrate, indicating invasion of the dermis by epidermal keratinocytes (Kobayasi).

In early squamous cell carcinoma, lymphocytes are often seen in close contact with tumor cells, some of which show degenerative changes such as disruption of the plasma membrane, as well as fragmentation and subsequent release of organelles into the intercellular spaces. This can be interpreted as the cellular expression of an immune reaction against tumor cells (Boncinelli et al).

The epithelial nature of the sarcomalike cells in spindle cell squamous cell carcinoma is supported by electron microscopic findings, which have shown that these cells contain tonofilaments and occasional desmosomelike structures (Battifora; Manglani et al). Electron microscopy has also shown that structures diagnosed by light microscopy as atypical fibroxanthomas represent a heterogeneous group of neoplasms and that some are in actuality spindle cell squamous cell carcinomas (Barr et al; Evans and Smith). Also, prekeratin can be demonstrated in such tumors with the peroxidase–antiperoxidase method by use of an antibody raised against human prekeratin (Penneys et al).

Differential Diagnosis. The diagnosis of squamous cell carcinoma, although easily made in typical cases, may sometimes be difficult.

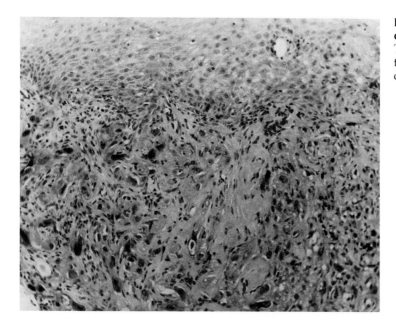

Fig. 26-31. Spindle cell squamous cell carcinoma with pleomorphic giant cells
The tumor resembles an atypical fibroxanthoma but in a few areas shows evidence of origin from the epidermis. (×200)

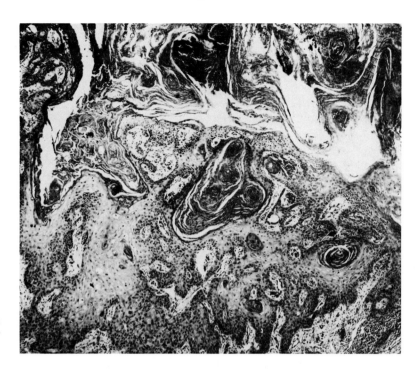

Fig. 26-32.   Squamous cell carcinoma
The tumor resembles a keratoacanthoma but shows less maturation and nuclear atypicality. (×100)

The differences between squamous cell carcinoma and solar keratosis lie in the degree rather than the type of changes. In both conditions, one finds atypicality of cells, with dyskeratosis of individual cells and downward proliferation of the epidermis. However, only in squamous cell carcinoma is there actual invasion of the dermis by tumor masses that may contain horn pearls. No sharp line of demarcation exists between the two conditions, and it is not infrequent on step sectioning for a lesion with the histologic appearance of solar keratosis to reveal one or several areas in which the changes have progressed to squamous cell carcinoma.

For discussions of differentiation of squamous cell carcinoma from pseudocarcinomatous hyperplasia, see p. 505; from keratoacanthoma, p. 507; and from basal cell epithelioma, p. 564.

Adenoid Squamous Cell Carcinoma

As a result of dyskeratosis and subsequent acantholysis, squamous cell carcinomas occasionally show tubular and alveolar formations on histologic examination. Clinically, such adenoid or pseudoglandular squamous cell carcinomas are found almost exclusively in sun-damaged skin of elderly patients, especially on the face and ears (Lever; Johnson and Helwig). They have also been seen on the vermilion border of the lower lip (Borelli). Two

instances of occurrence on the oral mucosa have been reported, but both were recurrences after radiation therapy (Takagi et al).

On sun-exposed skin, adenoid squamous cell carcinomas may arise as such or may develop from a solar keratosis (Chorzelski; Johnson and Helwig). In most instances, they do not differ in clinical appearance from the usual type of squamous cell carcinoma and thus commonly show a central ulceration surrounded by a raised, indurated border. Occasionally, they greatly resemble a keratoacanthoma in clinical appearance (Muller et al). Metastases are rare but were reported in 3 of 213 patients, resulting in the deaths of these patients (Johnson and Helwig).

Histopathology.   The adenoid changes may be seen in only a portion of a squamous cell carcinoma or throughout the lesion. Not infrequently, a solar keratosis of the acantholytic type is seen overlying the lesion. There are tubular and alveolar lumina lined with one or several layers of epithelium (Fig. 26-33). In areas in which the lumina are lined with a single layer of epithelium, the epithelial cells resemble glandular cells, but in areas with several layers of epithelium, squamous and partially keratinized cells usually form the inner layers. The lumina are filled with desquamated acantholytic cells, many of which are partially or fully keratinized (Delacrétaz et al; Muller et al; Johnson and Helwig). In some cases, the eccrine ducts at

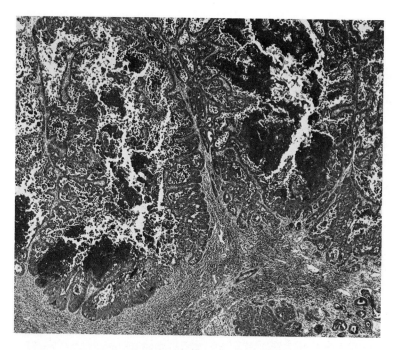

Fig. 26-33. Adenoid squamous cell carcinoma
Low magnification. The tumors shows large alveolar spaces into which papillary projections protrude. The alveolar spaces contain many desquamated, acantholytic cells, many of which appear dyskeratotic. (×50)

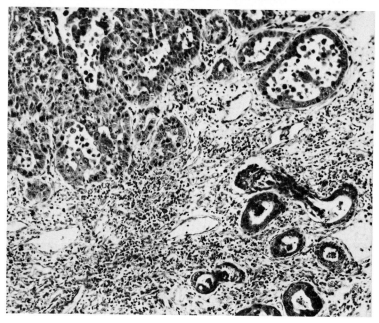

Fig. 26-34. Adenoid squamous cell carcinoma
High magnification of the base of the tumor shown in Figure 26-33. The tubular lumina of the tumor contain acantholytic, dyskeratotic cells. The sweat glands in the lower right corner show some epithelial proliferation, probably induced by the inflammatory infiltrate. (×200)

the periphery of these tumors show signs of dilatation and proliferation (Fig. 26-34) (Lever; Delacrétaz). These ductal changes probably are induced by the surrounding inflammatory infiltrate.

Histogenesis. These tumors represent squamous cell carcinomas of lobular growth in which there is considerable dyskeratosis with individual cell keratinization

resulting in acantholysis in the center of the lobular formations. This process is analogous to the suprabasal clefts seen in some solar keratoses (Muller et al). Adenoid squamous cell carcinomas differ from adenosquamous carcinomas as described for the vulva, in which the single row of cuboidal cells lining the lumina consists of true glandular cells (Lasser et al; Underwood et al). The latter type of tumor is highly malignant and has a low survival rate.

Verrucous Carcinoma

Verrucous carcinoma is a low-grade squamous cell carcinoma first described in 1948 (Ackerman) as occurring in the oral cavity. The diagnosis of verrucous carcinoma requires evaluation of the clinical and microscopic appearance and biologic behavior of the neoplasm. It is a slowly growing, at first exophytic, verrucous, and fungating tumor that may ultimately penetrate deep into the tissue. However, it causes regional metastases only very late, if at all. Because of its high degree of histologic differentiation, it is often not recognized as a carcinoma for a long time. Three major forms of verrucous carcinoma are recognized, all of them occurring in areas of maceration.

Verrucous carcinoma of the oral cavity, also called oral florid papillomatosis, shows whitish, cauliflowerlike lesions that may involve large areas of the oral mucosa (see p. 495).

Verrucous carcinoma of the genitoanal region, also called giant condylomata acuminata of Buschke and Loewenstein, most commonly occurs on the glans penis and foreskin of uncircumcised males, where it consists of papillomatous proliferations. Ultimately, it may penetrate into the urethra. It may also occur on the vulva in females and in the anal region (see p. 376).

Plantar verrucous carcinoma, also called epithelioma cuniculatum (Aird et al), at first shows a striking resemblance to an intractable plantar wart. As the exophytic mass grows, it shows a great tendency toward deep, penetrating growth, resulting in numerous deep crypts filled with horny material and pus. The crypts resemble the burrows of rabbits, hence the name *cuniculatum*. The tumor ultimately penetrates the plantar fascia (Brown and Freeman) and may even destroy metatarsal bones and invade the skin of the dorsum of the foot (Reingold et al).

The occurrence of verrucous carcinoma has also been described in pre-existing lesions, such as chronic ulcers and draining sinuses of hidradenitis suppurativa (Klima et al).

Histopathology. For the diagnosis of verrucous carcinoma, a large, deep biopsy is essential. The superficial portions generally resemble a verruca by showing hyperkeratosis, parakeratosis, and acanthosis. The keratinocytes appear well differentiated, stain lightly with eosin, and possess a small nucleus. The tumor invades with broad strands that often contain keratin-filled cysts in their center. There are large, bulbous, downward proliferations that compress the collagen bundles and push them aside. Thus, the tumor has been said to invade by "bulldozing rather than stabbing" (Mohs and Sahl). Even in the deep portions of the tumor, nuclear atypia, individual cell keratinization, and horn pearls are absent (Brodin and Mehregan).

However, in some instances, particularly in the oral cavity (Kanee; Samitz et al) but occasionally also in the genitoanal region (Dawson et al) and on the plantar surface (Seehafer et al; McKee et al, 1981b), verrucous carcinoma may ultimately show sufficient nuclear atypicality and loss of polarity to indicate the development of a true squamous cell carcinoma. In rare instances, the development of regional lymph node metastases has been observed in verrucous carcinoma of the mouth (Grinspan and Abulafia), the genitals (Dawson et al), and the soles of the feet (McKee et al, 1981b). Radiation therapy has led in some instances of oral verrucous carcinoma to anaplastic transformation and extensive metastases (Perez et al).

Histogenesis. In some cases of verrucous carcinoma, development from viral warts has been suspected. Whereas a viral etiology for oral verrucous carcinoma or giant condylomata acuminata has not been proved, coexistence of plantar verrucous carcinoma with a plantar wart has been described in one case (Wilkinson et al), and, in 5 of 13 reported cases, viruslike particles were found on electron microscopy in the superficial epithelium of the plantar verrucous tumors (McKee et al, 1981a).

Pseudocarcinomatous Hyperplasia

Pseudocarcinomatous hyperplasia or *pseudoepitheliomatous hyperplasia,* as it is often called, represents a considerable downward proliferation of the epidermis into the dermis. Clinically as well as histologically, this downward proliferation may suggest a squamous cell carcinoma. It occurs occasionally (1) in chronic proliferative inflammatory processes, such as bromoderma, blastomycosis, blastomycosislike pyoderma (pyoderma vegetans) (Su et al), or hidradenitis suppurativa (Sommerville), and (2) at the edges of chronic ulcers, as seen in the following conditions: after burns or in stasis dermatitis (Winer), pyoderma gangrenosum, basal cell epithelioma (Freeman), lupus vulgaris, scrofuloderma, gumma, and granuloma inguinale. In addition, granular cell tumor is known to evoke quite frequently a pseudocarcinomatous hyperplasia.

Histopathology. Histologically, pseudocarcinomatous hyperplasia shows an epithelial hyperplasia that often closely resembles squamous cell carcinoma, grade 1 or 2. Although squamous cell carcinoma may develop at the edges of chronic ulcers, it is likely that some cases that are regarded as such actually represent pseudocarcinomatous hyperplasia. Nevertheless, a lesion starting out as pseudocarcinomatous hyperplasia at the edge of an ulcer may eventually develop into a squamous cell carcinoma and even metastasize (Ju).

The histologic picture of pseudocarcinomatous hyperplasia shows irregular invasion of the dermis by uneven, jagged, often sharply pointed epidermal cell masses and strands with horn-pearl formation and often numerous mitotic figures (Fig. 26-35). These irregular proliferations of the epidermis may extend below the level of the sweat glands, where they appear in sections as isolated islands of epidermal tissue (Sommerville). However, the squamous cells usually are well differentiated, and atypicalities, such as individual cell keratinization and nuclear hyperplasia and hyperchromasia, are minimal or absent. Furthermore, one often sees invasion of the epithelial proliferations by leukocytes and disintegration of some of the epidermal cells in pseudocarcinomatous hyperplasia, findings that usually are absent in squamous cell carcinoma (Winer). Nevertheless, even when all of these criteria are taken into account, it may still be difficult to differentiate squamous cell carcinoma from pseudocarcinomatous hyperplasia by the study of just one histologic section (Sommerville). Multiple biopsies and detailed clinical data may be necessary for differentiation.

In every section in which a diagnosis of squamous cell carcinoma, grade 1 or 2, is contemplated, it is worthwhile to study the inflammatory infiltrate for the possible presence of granulomas, as seen in tuberculosis and the deep mycoses, or intraepidermal abscesses, as seen in bromoderma. If such evidence is found, one may be dealing with pseudocarcinomatous hyperplasia instead of squamous cell carcinoma.

Differential Diagnosis. Differentiation of pseudocarcinomatous hyperplasia from verrucous carcinoma rarely causes difficulties, because, in verrucous carcinoma, one observes verrucous upward proliferation as well as downward proliferation. Also, verrucous carcinoma shows more pronounced keratinization in the downward extensions, which, in addition, appear bulbous rather than sharply pointed.

KERATOACANTHOMA

Two types of keratoacanthoma exist: solitary and multiple.

Solitary Keratoacanthoma

Only since 1950 (Rook and Whimster, 1950; Musso and Gordon) has solitary keratoacanthoma, a common lesion, been recognized as an entity and differentiated from squamous cell carcinoma, which it often resembles clinically and histologically. Solitary keratoacanthoma occurs in elderly persons usually as a single lesion; however, occasionally, there are several lesions, or new lesions develop. The lesion consists of a firm, dome-shaped nodule 1 cm to 2.5 cm in diameter with a horn-filled crater in its center. The sites of predilection are exposed areas, where about 95% of solitary keratoacanthomas occur (Ghadially, 1979), but they may occur on any hairy cutaneous site. They have not been reported on the palms, soles, or mucous surfaces, although, in rare instances, they occur subungually (see below). Keratoacanthomas located on the vermilion border of the lip probably arise from hair follicles in the adjacent skin (Silberberg et al). Keratoacanthomas usually reach their

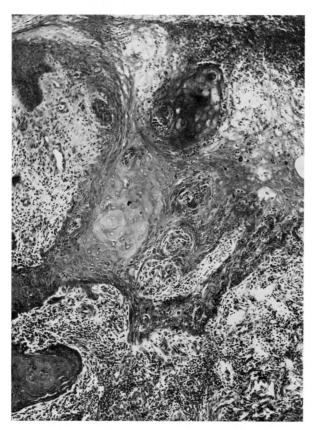

Fig. 26-35. Pseudocarcinomatous hyperplasia in bromoderma
There is downward proliferation of the epidermis analogous to squamous cell carcinoma, grade 1. In the field shown, it is impossible to rule out carcinoma. Note, however, the permeation of the epidermis in many areas by inflammatory cells. (× 100)

full size within 6 to 8 weeks and involute spontaneously, generally in less than 6 months. Healing takes place with a slightly depressed scar. In some instances, a keratoacanthoma increases in size for more than 2 months and takes up to 1 year to involute (Ghadially, 1979).

An increased incidence of keratoacanthoma is observed in immunosuppressed patients (Sullivan and Colditz). Also, keratoacanthomas commonly occur in Torre's syndrome of sebaceous neoplasms associated with visceral carcinomas, and there are often several lesions (see p. 539) (Housholder and Zeligman).

There are three rare clinical variants of solitary keratoacanthoma. In two forms, giant keratoacanthoma and keratoacanthoma centrifugum marginatum, the keratoacanthoma attains a large size. In *giant keratoacanthoma*, the growth rapidly reaches a size of 5 cm or more and may cause destruction of underlying tissues. Nevertheless, spontaneous involution takes place after several months, often accompanied by detachment of a large keratotic plaque. The most common sites are the nose (Rapaport; Bart et al) and the eyelids (Kallos; Obermayer; Sullivan and Colditz). In *keratoacanthoma centrifugum marginatum*, the lesion may even reach a size of 20 cm in diameter. There is no tendency toward spontaneous involution; instead, there is peripheral extension with a raised, rolled border and atrophy in the center of the lesion. The most common locations are the dorsa of the hands (Belisario; Miedzinski and Kozakiewicz) and the legs (Weedon and Barnett; Heid et al). The third rare variant is *subungual keratoacanthoma*, which shows a destructive crateriform lesion with keratotic excrescences under the distal portion of a fingernail. It fails to regress spontaneously, is tender, and by roentgenogram shows damage to the terminal phalanx by pressure erosion (Macaulay; Stoll and Ackerman).

Claims have been made that keratoacanthoma can undergo transformation into a squamous cell carcinoma either spontaneously (Belisario; Rook and Whimster, 1979) or as a result of immunosuppression (Sullivan and Colditz; Poleksic and Yeung). It appears more likely, however, that the squamous cell carcinoma existed from the beginning in such instances (see Differential Diagnosis) (Ghadially, 1979; Kern and McCray).

Histopathology. The architecture of the lesion in a keratoacanthoma is as important to the diagnosis as the cellular characteristics. Therefore, if the lesion cannot be excised in its entirety, it is advisable that a fusiform specimen be excised for biopsy from the center of the lesion and that this specimen include the edge at least of one side and preferably of both sides of the lesion (Popkin et al). A shave biopsy is inadvisable, since the histologic changes at the base of the lesion are often of great importance in differentiation from squamous cell carcinoma.

In the early proliferative stage, one observes a horn-filled invagination of the epidermis from which strands of epidermis protrude into the dermis. These strands are poorly demarcated from the surrounding stroma in many areas and may contain cells showing nuclear atypia (Wade and Ackerman) as well as many mitotic figures (de Moragas et al). Even atypical mitoses may be seen occasionally (Giltman). Dyskeratotic cells, that is, cells showing individual cell keratinization, may also be seen in areas that otherwise do not show advanced keratinization. However, even at this early stage, some of the tumor areas show a fairly pronounced degree of keratinization, giving them an eosinophilic, glassy appearance. In the dermis, a rather pronounced inflammatory infiltrate is present (de Moragas et al). Perineural invasion is occasionally seen in the proliferative phase of keratoacanthoma and should not be misinterpreted as evidence of malignancy (Janecka et al; Lapins and Helwig).

A fully developed lesion shows in its center a large, irregularly shaped crater filled with keratin (Fig. 26-36). The epidermis extends like a lip or a buttress over the sides of the crater. At the base of the crater, irregular epidermal proliferations extend both upward into the crater and downward from the base of the crater. These proliferations may still appear somewhat atypical, but less so than in the initial stage; the keratinization is extensive and fairly advanced, with only a thin shell of one or two layers of basophilic, nonkeratinized cells at the periphery of the proliferations, whereas the cells within this shell appear eosinophilic and glassy as a result of keratinization (Fig. 26-37). There are many horn pearls, most of which show complete keratinization in their center. The base of a fully developed keratoacanthoma appears regular and well demarcated and usually does not extend below the level of the sweat glands. A rather dense inflammatory infiltrate is present at the base of the lesion (Levy et al; Ghadially, 1979).

In the involuting stage, proliferation has ceased, and most cells at the base of the crater have undergone keratinization. There may be shrunken, eosinophilic cells analogous to colloid or Civatte bodies among the tumor cells located nearest to the stroma as well as in the stroma, suggesting that cell degeneration followed by apoptosis contributes to the involution of the keratoacanthoma (Weedon and Barnett). Gradually, the crater flattens and finally disappears during healing.

Histogenesis. It is generally agreed that the lesion starts with hyperplasia of the infundibulum of one or several adjoining hair follicles and with squamous metaplasia

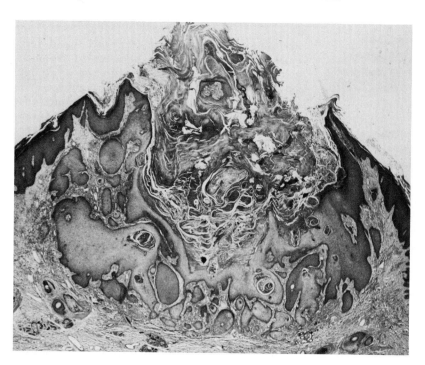

Fig. 26-36. Keratoacanthoma
Low magnification. There is a large, central keratin-filled crater. On the right, the epidermis extends like a buttress over the side of the crater. Irregular epidermal proliferations extend downward from the base of the crater into the dermis. (×25)

of the attached sebaceous glands (Calnan and Haber). The application of cutaneous carcinogens to the skin of animals frequently produces, among other tumors, lesions with the histologic appearance of keratoacanthomas, and these tumors also have their origin in the infundibulum of one or several hair follicles (Ghadially, 1961).

The cause of keratoacanthoma is not known. The theory of a viral genesis has not been confirmed. The electron microscopic findings are largely nonspecific. It is of interest, however, that keratoacanthomas, like squamous cell carcinomas and lesions of Bowen's disease, often show the presence of fairly numerous intracytoplasmic desmosomes (Takaki et al; von Bülow and Klingmüller).

Differential Diagnosis. Differentiation of typical, mature lesions of keratoacanthoma from squamous cell carcinoma generally is not difficult. In favor of a diagnosis of keratoacanthoma are the architecture of a crater surrounded by buttresses and the high degree of keratinization, which is manifested by the eosinophilic, glassy appearance of many of the cells. Clinical data are also of great value: rapid development of an exophytic lesion showing a central, horn-filled crater speaks for keratoacanthoma rather than for squamous cell carcinoma.

The greatest difficulties in the differentiation of a keratoacanthoma from a squamous cell carcinoma are encountered in very early lesions, since a horn-filled invagination may be seen in squamous cell carcinoma (see Fig. 26-32) and cells with an atypical appearance may occur in a keratoacanthoma. Occasionally, an early keratoacanthoma shows a greater degree of nuclear atypia than do some squamous cell carcinomas (Chalet et al). Also, individual cell keratinization can occur in keratoacanthoma. On rare occasions, even adenoid formations caused by dyskeratosis and acantholysis can occur in keratoacanthoma (Stevanovic). Thus, it was found on reclassification in one study that in only 81% of the cases of keratoacanthoma could a diagnosis of squamous cell carcinoma be fully excluded and that in only 86% of the cases of squamous cell carcinoma could keratoacanthoma be ruled out with certainty. These findings explain why, on rare occasions, lesions classified as keratoacanthoma cause metastases (Kern and McCray).

Since it is widely agreed that squamous cell carcinomas can masquerade as keratoacanthomas not only clinically but also histologically (Nikolowski; Ghadially, 1979), it is best to err on the safe side in a case of doubt and to proceed on the assumption that the lesion is a squamous cell carcinoma.

Multiple Keratoacanthoma

There are two variants of multiple keratoacanthoma: the multiple self-healing epitheliomas of the skin, or Fer-

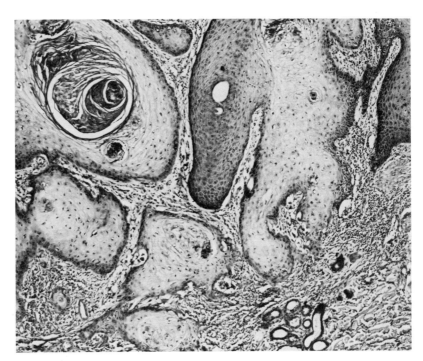

Fig. 26-37. Keratoacanthoma
Higher magnification of the epidermal proliferations at the base of the crater shows their resemblance to squamous cell carcinoma. However, there is more keratinization than is usually seen in squamous cell carcinoma, giving the tumor islands a glassy appearance. (× 100)

guson Smith type, and the eruptive keratoacanthomas, or Grzybowski type. Both variants are rare in comparison with solitary keratoacanthoma.

In *multiple self-healing epitheliomas* of the skin, lesions begin to appear in childhood or adolescence on any part of the skin, including the palms and soles, but especially on the face and the extremities. Subungual lesions have also been described (Stoll and Ackerman). Generally, there are no more than a dozen lesions at any one time (Sullivan et al). The lesions may reach the same size as solitary keratoacanthomas and after a few months heal with a depressed scar (Ferguson Smith; Tarnowski). In some patients, the condition is inherited (Sommerville and Milne).

In *eruptive keratoacanthoma,* lesions do not appear until adult life. Many hundreds of follicular papules are present, measuring from 2 mm to 3 mm in diameter (Grzybowski). The oral mucosa and larynx may be involved (Rossman et al; Winkelmann and Brown).

Histopathology. The histologic appearance of the lesions of multiple self-healing epitheliomas of the skin is similar to that of solitary keratoacanthoma (Tarnowski; Sullivan et al). The cutaneous lesions in eruptive keratoacanthoma show less crater formation than those in solitary keratoacanthoma. The mucosal lesions lack a crater and can easily be misinterpreted as squamous cell carcinoma (Rossman et al; Winkelmann and Brown).

Histogenesis. It appears likely that multiple keratoacanthoma basically represents the same condition as

solitary keratoacanthoma and that predisposition or genetic factors are responsible for the greater number of lesions (Rook and Moffat). In multiple as in solitary keratoacanthoma, lesions arising in hair-bearing parts of the skin have their onset in the upper portion of a hair follicle, whereas the site of origin of lesions arising on the palms, the soles, and the mucous membranes is not apparent (Rossman et al).

PAGET'S DISEASE

Paget's disease of the breast occurs almost exclusively in women. Only a few instances of its occurrence in the male breast have been described (Chrichlow and Czernobilsky). Of interest is its occurrence in the male breast after treatment of a carcinoma of the prostate with estrogen (Hadlich et al). The cutaneous lesion in Paget's disease of the breast begins either on the nipple or the areola of the breast and extends slowly to the surrounding skin. It is always unilateral and consists of a sharply defined, slightly infiltrated area of erythema showing scaling, oozing, and crusting. There may or may not be ulceration or retraction of the nipple.

The cutaneous lesion is regularly associated with carcinoma of the breast, and, in more than half of the patients, a mass can be felt on palpation of the breast. Metastases in the axillary lymph nodes were found by one group of investigators in about two thirds of their patients with a palpable mass and in one third of those without a palpable mass (Ashikari et al). This contrasts with the experience of others, who encountered no

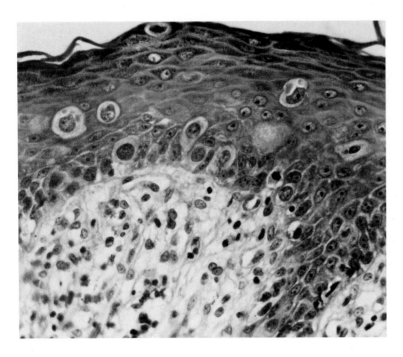

Fig. 26-38. Paget's disease of the breast
Only a few Paget cells are scattered through the epidermis. They are large, rounded cells devoid of intercellular bridges, with ample, pale-staining cytoplasm. ($\times 400$)

axillary metastases in the absence of a palpable mass (Paone and Baker).

A clinical picture indistinguishable from that of early Paget's disease of the nipple is seen in erosive adenomatosis of the nipple, a benign neoplasm of the major nipple ducts (see p. 547) (Lewis et al).

Histopathology.   In early lesions of Paget's disease of the breast, the epidermis usually shows only a few scattered Paget cells (Fig. 26-38). They are large, rounded cells that are devoid of intercellular bridges and contain a large nucleus and ample cytoplasm. The cytoplasm of these cells stains much lighter than that of the adjacent squamous cells. As the number of Paget cells increases, they compress the squamous cells to such an extent that the latter may merely form a network, the meshes of which are filled with Paget cells lying singly and in groups. In particular, one often observes flattened basal cells lying between Paget cells and the underlying dermis (Fig. 26-39).

Histochemical staining of the Paget cells within the epidermis in Paget's disease of the breast has given inconsistent results. In some cases, one observes Paget cells that stain with the PAS reaction (Fig. 26-40). This reaction is diastase-resistant, indicating the presence of neutral mucopolysaccharides rather than of glycogen (Fisher and Beyer; Dupré et al). Often, however, neutral mucopolysaccharides can be shown to be present in only a few Paget cells (Wood and Culling), and, occa-

sionally, they are completely absent (Hopsu-Havu and Sonck). In some cases in which the Paget cells contain neutral mucopolysaccharides, they also contain acid mucopolysaccharides, as demonstrated by a positive stain with alcian blue (Fisher and Beyer; Dupré et al). Metachromasia on staining with methylene blue or thionin is found to be absent (Fisher and Beyer). Occasionally, Paget cells contain some melanin (Culberson and Horn); however, they are dopa-negative (Helwig and Graham).

The dermis in Paget's disease shows a moderately severe chronic inflammatory reaction. Although Paget cells do not invade the dermis from the epidermis, they may be seen extending from the epidermis into the epithelium of hair follicles (Orr and Parish).

Histologic examination of the mammary ducts and glands nearly always shows malignant changes in some of them. At first, the carcinoma is confined within the walls of the ducts and glands (Fig. 26-41), but the tumor cells ultimately invade the connective tissue. From then on, lymphatic spread and metastases occur, just as in other types of mammary carcinoma.

Histogenesis. On the basis of light microscopic findings, a few authors have maintained that the intraepidermal Paget cell in mammary Paget's disease represents a modified keratinocyte (Montgomery). Most authors, however, regard the intraepidermal Paget cell as a mammary gland cell. In favor of the view that the Paget cell is a mammary gland cell and that the epidermal involvement in Paget's disease of the breast is due to the presence of an "epidermotropic mammary carcinoma" (Pinkus and Mehregan) are the following observations: (1) Paget cells act like foreign cells in the epidermis and therefore do not invade from the epidermis into the underlying dermis, whereas they do invade from the mammary glands into the surrounding tissue; (2) Paget cells, like apocrine and mammary gland cells, frequently contain neutral mucopolysaccharides (Fisher and Beyer); and (3) in rare instances, a primary breast carcinoma and its metastases may directly invade the epidermis and produce a lesion with the histopathologic appearance of Paget's disease (Greenwood and Minkowitz). It is likely that the initial lesion in Paget's disease of the breast is an intraductal carcinoma arising in one or several mammary ducts. The primary ductal carcinoma extends from its site of origin downward within the epithelium of the mammary ducts and glands and upward into the epidermis, where it causes the cutaneous lesion (Muir).

Electron microscopic study of Paget's disease of the breast has led to various interpretations. Often, the Paget cells show relatively little differentiation, so that their identification with any mature cell type is difficult. According to one view, the intraepidermal Paget cells must be derived from keratinocytes, since desmosomes are present between neighboring Paget cells as well as between Paget cells and keratinocytes (Sagebiel). However, this view does not give consideration to the fact that scattered desmosomes are normally found connecting the cells of the mammary ducts (Ebner). Some authors favor the origin of the mammary Paget cells from the luminal cells of mammary ducts because of the presence of secretory granules and their frequent arrangement around lumina in areas in which several Paget cells lie together in the epidermis (Ebner; Caputo and Califano).

The glandular derivation of the Paget cells in the epidermis of both mammary and extramammary Paget's disease has found strong support by the recent demonstration with a peroxidase–antiperoxidase technic that these cells contain carcinoembryonic antigen, a substance that is present in the cells of both eccrine and apocrine glands (Penneys et al).

Enzyme histochemistry in Paget's disease of the breast has shown the presence of an apocrine enzymatic pattern in the intraepidermal Paget cells, that is, a strong reactivity for acid phosphatase and esterase and only a weakly positive reaction for aminopeptidase and succinic dehydrogenase (Belcher). This finding suggests that the intraepidermal Paget cells in Paget's disease of the breast are derived from mammary gland cells, since the mammary gland represents a modified apocrine gland.

Differential Diagnosis. Paget's disease of the breast must be differentiated from Bowen's disease and the superficial spreading or "pagetoid" type of malignant melanoma in situ. Although vacuo-

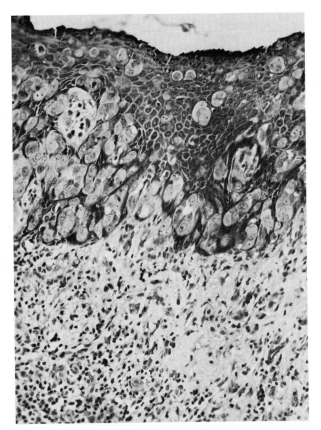

Fig. 26-39. Paget's disease of the breast
Low magnification. The epidermis is permeated with numerous Paget cells lying singly and in groups. There is no invasion of the dermis by Paget cells. Flattened basal cells lie between the tumor cells and the dermis in many places, a finding that aids in the differentiation of Paget's disease from malignant melanoma in situ. (× 200)

lated cells may occur in both Paget's disease and Bowen's disease, one observes clear-cut transitions between the vacuolated cells and epidermal cells only in Bowen's disease. Furthermore, one may observe in Bowen's disease but not in Paget's disease clumping of nuclei within multinucleated epidermal cells and individual cell keratinization. In addition, even though the PAS reaction is often positive both in Paget cells and in Bowen's disease, it is abolished by diastase digestion only in Bowen's disease (Fisher and Beyer).

In the superficial spreading or pagetoid type of malignant melanoma in situ, as in the epidermis of Paget's disease of the breast, one observes large, vacuolated cells scattered through the epidermis (Hopsu-Havu and Sonck). The difficulty in distinguishing between the two types of cells may be

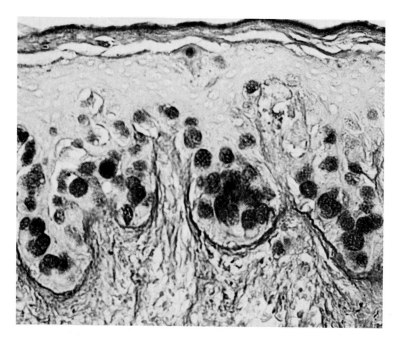

Fig. 26-40. Paget's disease of the breast
PAS stain. The cytoplasm of the Paget cells gives a positive PAS reaction that is diastase-resistant. (×200)

Fig. 26-41. Paget's disease of the breast
Intraductal carcinoma is present in the mammary ducts. (×200)

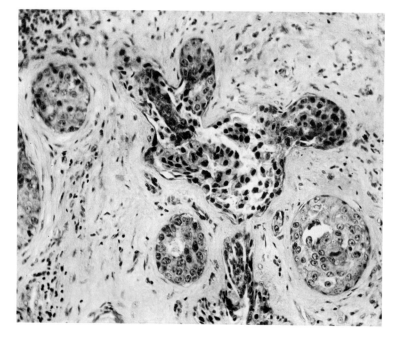

increased by the fact that Paget cells occasionally also contain melanin (Culberson and Horn). The most important points to remember in differentiating the two types of cells are as follows: (1) Paget cells are separated in many areas from the dermis by flattened basal cells, whereas melanoma cells border directly on the dermis; (2) Paget cells do not invade the dermis, whereas melanoma cells often do; (3) in many Paget cells, the PAS reaction is positive and diastase-resistant, and the alcian blue stain is often also positive, whereas, in malignant melanoma, these staining reactions are almost invariably negative (Fisher and Beyer; Helwig and Graham); and (4) Paget cells are dopa-negative, unlike melanoma cells.

Extramammary Paget's Disease

Extramammary Paget's disease most commonly affects the vulva, less commonly the male genital area (Murrell and McMullan) or the perianal area (Helwig and Graham), and, in exceptional cases only, the axillae, the region of the ceruminal glands (Fligiel and Kaneko), or that of Moll's glands (Whorton and Patterson). In cases with involvement of the axillae, the genital area may also be affected (Duperrat and Mascaro; Kawatsu and Miki). Thus, extramammary Paget's disease involves areas in which apocrine glands are normally encountered. Only very few cases of an association between mammary and vulvar Paget's disease have been described (Fetissoff et al). In rare instances, extramammary Paget's disease is a secondary event caused by extension of an adenocarcinoma either of the rectum to the perianal region or of the cervix to the vulvar region (Helwig and Graham; McKee and Hertogs).

In extramammary as in mammary Paget's disease, the clinical picture shows a slowly enlarging reddish patch with oozing and crusting. The patch resembles an eczematous lesion but has a sharp border. In extramammary Paget's disease, in contrast to the mammary type, itching is common.

Histopathology. Extramammary Paget's disease shares with Paget's disease the presence of varying numbers of Paget cells within the epidermis. Frequently, Paget cells can also be identified in the epithelium of the epidermal adnexa, particularly within the epithelium of some hair follicles or eccrine sweat ducts (Jones et al). In addition, an adnexal adenocarcinoma can be found in the dermis in some cases. Although the origin of this adenocarcinoma cannot always be clearly established and may be the result of a breakthrough of an in situ adnexal carcinoma, as in mammary Paget's disease, the dermal adenocarcinoma in most instances is the result of dermal invasion by epidermal Paget cells (Hart and Millman; Jones et al; Gunn and Gallager). In this respect, extramammary Paget's disease differs from mammary Paget's disease, in which invasion of the dermis from the overlying epidermis does not occur (Orr and Parish). Also, glandular clusters with a central lumen, generally absent in mammary Paget's disease, may be seen in the lower epidermis in extramammary Paget's disease (Lee et al; Jones et al).

On histochemical staining, the Paget cells seen in the epidermis and in the adnexa show a positive reaction for neutral mucopolysaccharides and for acid mucopolysaccharides more frequently and more extensively in extramammary Paget's disease than in mammary Paget's disease (Lee et al; Jones et al). Nevertheless, these stains can be negative in cases of extramammary as well as of mammary Paget's disease (Hopsu-Havu and Sonck).

In cases of "secondary" extramammary Paget's disease, the process extends either from a mucus-secreting adenocarcinoma of the rectum to the perianal skin (Yoell and Price; Helwig and Graham; Wood and Culling) or from a mucus-secreting endocervical carcinoma to the vulva (McKee and Hertogs). In such cases, the Paget cells in the perianal or vulvar skin are derived from the pre-existing carcinoma and contain mucus that always is PAS-positive and diastase-resistant and always shows a positive staining reaction with alcian blue that is hyaluronidase-resistant. The mucus thus represents sialomucin, a nonsulfated acid mucopolysaccharide (Helwig and Graham). The prognosis in cases of secondary extramammary Paget's disease is poor.

The prognosis of "primary" extramammary Paget's disease generally is better than that of mammary Paget's disease. In two large combined series of 123 patients with vulvar Paget's disease, only 26 patients (21%) showed an underlying invasive carcinoma in the dermis at the time of operation (Hart and Millman; Jones et al). In the other 79%, the Paget cells were present only within the epidermis and the epithelium of the cutaneous appendages, so that the process was still in situ. However, the rate of local recurrence is high even after seemingly adequate excision. The reasons for this are not only that the extent of histologically demonstrable disease is often far greater than that of the visible lesion but also that extramammary Paget's disease, in contrast to mammary Paget's disease, can arise multifocally even in clinically normal-appearing areas of the skin (Gunn and Gallager).

Histogenesis. Two opposing views exist with regard to the histogenesis of primary extramammary Paget's disease. According to one view, the Paget cells in the epidermis are there as a result of an in situ upward extension of an in situ adenocarcinoma of sweat glands along eccrine or apocrine ducts (Koss and Brockunier; Lee et al). This view is analogous to the generally accepted theory that secondary extramammary Paget's disease represents an extension of a rectal or cervical mucus-secreting adenocarcinoma and to the widely accepted view that the development of mammary Paget's disease is an extension of an "epidermotropic mammary carcinoma" (see p. 511) (Pinkus and Mehregan). The fact that an underlying in situ adenocarcinoma often cannot be demonstrated is explained by the anatomic differences between the breast, which has only 20 large, conspicuous lactiferous ducts, and the genital skin, which has thousands of small apocrine and eccrine glands, making location of the particular small gland involved by carcinoma technically difficult (Lee et al).

According to the other view, extramammary Paget's disease has a multifocal primary origin within the epidermis and its related appendages and thus does not represent an epidermotropic spread or metastasis from an underlying sweat gland carcinoma (Hart and Millman). Careful subserial total sectioning of excised lesions of vulvar Paget's disease has shown that the lesions within the epidermis and its appendages have a multifocal origin (Gunn and Gallager). Another pertinent argument in favor of the independence of the epidermal foci from any appendageal foci is the observation that in cases with extensive epidermal lesions, involvement of eccrine ducts and glands is often sparse and involvement of apocrine ducts and glands almost invariably absent, even though some Paget cells form apocrine glandular structures in the epidermis (Jones et al). Also, even if there is continuity between the epidermal and the ductal foci, there is no certain way of determining whether the extension is in an upward or downward direction. However, the clinching argument in favor of the autonomy of the epidermal foci in primary extramammary Paget's disease is the fact that, in contrast to mammary Paget's disease, dermal invasion generally originates from the epidermis rather than from ductal or glandular structures (Hart and Millman; Jones et al).

If extramammary Paget's disease is believed to arise within the epidermis and to extend from there at a later date into the adnexa and still later from the epidermis into the dermis, the question is, which cell gives rise to the Paget cell? Two possibilities have been suggested, although proof for either is lacking. The first is that the Paget cell arises within the poral portion of an apocrine duct (Pinkus and Mehregan). The second is that, since the disease tends to occur in areas rich in apocrine glands and since there is in some cases unequivocal evidence of apocrine differentiation in the epidermis, intraepidermal Paget cells may be formed by pluripotential germinative cells within the epidermis that go awry in their attempt to form apocrine structures (Murrell and McMullan; Jones et al).

Electron microscopic studies of Paget cells in extramammary Paget's disease have given conflicting results. Several authors have observed cells that they regarded as intermediate to keratinocytes and Paget cells and have therefore postulated that the derivation of the intraepidermal Paget cells is epidermal (Piérard and Kint; Medenica and Sahihi). Other authors have interpreted the genital Paget cells as apocrine secretory cells because of the presence of a prominent Golgi zone and an abundant and dilated rough-surfaced endoplasmic retic-

ulum, as seen in glandular cells and not in keratinocytes, and because of the presence of secretory cells (Caputo and Califano; Demopoulos). Still other authors having observed two types of cells, one of them with secretory granules and intercellular canaliculi, have assumed that the Paget cells in genital Paget's disease are eccrine secretory cells (Koss and Brockunier; Belcher). In any case, the presence of carcinoembryonic antigen favors an origin from glandular, rather than from epidermal, cells (see p. 511).

Enzyme histochemistry in one case of vulvar Paget's disease has revealed in the Paget cells strongly positive reactions for eccrine enzymes, especially amylophosphorylase and leucine aminopeptidase, and minimal to absent reactions to apocrine enzymes, such as acid phosphatase, beta-glucuronidase, and esterase (Belcher). This observation contrasts with findings by the same author of a prevalence of apocrine enzymes in mammary Paget cells (see p. 511).

Differential Diagnosis. Extramammary Paget's disease, like Paget's disease of the breast, must be differentiated from Bowen's disease and especially from superficial spreading or pagetoid malignant melanoma in situ (see Paget's Disease, Differential Diagnosis).

BIBLIOGRAPHY

Linear Epidermal Nevus
ACKERMAN AB: Histopathologic concept of epidermolytic hyperkeratosis. Arch Dermatol 102:253–259, 1970

BASLER RSW, JACOBS SI, TAYLOR WB: Ichthyosis hystrix. Arch Dermatol 114:1059–1060, 1978

BRAUN-FALCO O, PETZOLDT D, CHRISTOPHERS E et al: Die granulöse Degeneration bei Naevus verrucosus bilateralis. Arch Klin Exp Dermatol 235:115–137, 1969

CRAMER SF, MANDEL MA, HAULER R et al: Squamous cell carcinoma arising in linear epidermal nevus. Arch Dermatol 117:222–224, 1981

DEMETREE JW, LANG PG, ST CLAIR JT: Unilateral linear zosteriform epidermal nevus with acantholytic dyskeratosis. Arch Dermatol 115:875–877, 1979

DOGLIOTTI, M, FRENKEL A: Malignant change in a verrucous nevus. Int J Dermatol 17:225–227, 1978

HORN MS, SAUSKER WF, PIERSON DL: Basal cell epithelioma arising in a linear epidermal nevus. Arch Dermatol 117:247, 1981

SOLOMON LM, FRETZIN DF, DEWALD RL: The epidermal nevus syndrome. Arch Dermatol 97:273–285, 1968

STARINK TM, WOERDEMAN MJ: Unilateral systematized keratosis follicularis. A variant of Darier's disease or an epidermal nevus (acantholytic dyskeratotic epidermal naevus)? Br J Dermatol 105:207–214, 1981

WINER LH, LEVIN GH: Pigmented basal-cell carcinoma in verrucous nevi. Arch Dermatol 83:960–964, 1961

ZELIGMAN I, POMERANZ J: Variations of congenital ichthyosiform erythroderma. Arch Dermatol 91:120–125, 1965

Nevus Comedonicus
ABELL E, READ SI: Porokeratotic eccrine ostial and dermal duct nevus. Br J Dermatol 103:435–441, 1980

BARSKY S, DOYLE JA, WINKELMANN RK: Nevus comedonicus with epidermolytic hyperkeratosis. Arch Dermatol 117:86–88, 1981

FRITSCH P, WITTELS W: Ein Fall von bilateralem Naevus comedonicus. Hautarzt 22:409–412, 1971

MARSDEN RA, FLEMING K, DAWBER RPR: Comedo naevus of the palm. A sweat duct naevus? Br J Dermatol 101:717–722, 1979

PAIGE TN, MENDELSON CG: Bilateral nevus comedonicus. Arch Dermatol 96:172–175, 1967

PLEWIG G, CHRISTOPHERS E: Nevoid follicular epidermolytic hyperkeratosis. Arch Dermatol 111:223–226, 1975

WOOD MG, THEW MA: Nevus comedonicus. Arch Dermatol 98:111–116, 1968

Solitary and Disseminated Epidermolytic Acanthoma, Incidental Epidermolytic Hyperkeratosis, Incidental Focal Acantholytic Dyskeratosis

ACKERMAN AB: Histopathologic concept of epidermolytic hyperkeratosis. Arch Dermatol 102:253–259, 1970

ACKERMAN AB: Focal acantholytic dyskeratosis. Arch Dermatol 106:702–706, 1972

ACKERMAN AB, REED RJ: Epidermolytic variant of solar keratosis. Arch Dermatol 107:104–106, 1973

BOTET MV, SÁNCHEZ JL: Vesiculation of focal acantholytic dyskeratosis in acral lentiginous malignant melanoma. J Dermatol Surg Oncol 5:798–800, 1979

GEBHART W, KIDD RL: Das solitäre epidermolytische Akanthom. Z Hautkr 47:1–4, 1972

HIRONE T, FUKUSHIRO R: Disseminated epidermolytic acanthoma. Acta DermVenereol (Stockh) 53:393–402, 1973

MEHREGAN A: Epidermolytic hyperkeratosis. J Cutan Pathol 5:76–80, 1978

MIYAMOTO Y, UEDA K, SATO M et al: Disseminated epidermolytic acanthoma. J Cutan Pathol 6:272–279, 1979

NAGASHIMA M, MATSUOKA S: So-called granular degeneration as incidental histopathological finding. Jpn J Dermatol (Series B) 81:494–497, 1971

NIIZUMA K: Isolated epidermolytic acanthoma. Dermatologica 159:30–36, 1979

SHAPIRO L, BARAF CS: Isolated epidermolytic acanthoma. Arch Dermatol 101:220–223, 1970

STERN JK, WOLF JE JR, ROSEN T: Focal acantholytic dyskeratosis in pityriasis rosea. Arch Dermatol 115:497, 1979

Oral White Sponge Nevus, Leukoedema of the Oral Mucosa, Geographic Tongue

CANNON AB: White sponge nevus of the mucosa (naevus spongiosus albus mucosae). Arch Dermatol Syph 31:365–370, 1935

COOKE BED, MORGAN J: Oral epithelial nevi. Br J Dermatol 71:134–138, 1959

DAWSON TAJ: Microscopic appearance of geographic tongue. Br J Dermatol 81:827–828, 1969

DEGOS R, GARNIER G, CIVATTE J: Pustulose par Candida albicans avec lésions psoriasiformes rappelant le psoriasis pustuleux. Bull Soc Fr Dermatol Syph 69:231–233, 1962

DUNCAN SC, SU WPD: Leukoedema of the oral mucosa. Arch Dermatol 116:906–908, 1980

HAYE KR, WHITEHEAD FIH: Hereditary leukokeratosis of the mucous membranes. Br J Dermatol 80:529–533, 1968

JORGENSON RJ, LEVIN S: White sponge nevus. Arch Dermatol 117:73–76, 1981

KUHLWEIN A, NASEMANN T, JÄNNER M: Nachweis von Papillomviren bei fokaler epithelialer Hyperplasic Heck und die Differentialdiagnose zum weissen Schleimhautnävus. Hautarzt 32:617–621, 1981

MARKS R, RADDEN BG: Geographic tongue. Aust J Dermatol 22:75–79, 1981

METZ J, METZ G: Der Naevus spongiosus albus mucosae. Z Hautkr 54:604–612, 1979

O'KEEFE E, BRAVERMAN IM, COHEN I: Annulus migrans: Identical lesions in pustular psoriasis, Reiter's syndrome, and geographic tongue. Arch Dermatol 107:240–244, 1973

STÜTTGEN G, BERRES HH, WILL W: Leukoplakische epitheliale Naevi der Mundschleimhaut. Arch Klin Exp Dermatol 221:433–446, 1965

WITKOP CJ JR, GORLIN RJ: Four hereditary mucosal syndromes. Arch Dermatol 84:762–771, 1961

ZEGARELLI EV, EVERETT FG, KUTSCHER AH et al: Familial white folded dysplasia of the mucous membranes. Arch Dermatol 80:59–65, 1959

Seborrheic Keratosis, Dermatosis Papulosa Nigra, Stucco Keratosis

ANDRADE R, STEIGLEDER GK: Contribution à l'étude histologique et histochimique de la verrue seborrhéique (papillome basocellulaire). Ann Dermatol Syph 86:495–505, 1959

BAER RL, GARCIA RL, PARTSALIDOU V et al: Papillated squamous cell carcinoma in situ arising in a seborrheic keratosis. J Am Acad Dermatol 5:561–565, 1981

BALABANOW K, ANGELOW N: Ein Fall von Verruca seborrhoica mit Übergang in Epitheliom. Dermatol Wochenschr 150:683–687, 1964

BECKER SW: Seborrheic keratosis and verruca with special reference to the melanotic variety. Arch Dermatol Syph 63:358–372, 1951

BERMAN A, WINKELMANN RK: Inflammatory seborrheic keratoses with mononuclear cell infiltration. J Cutan Pathol 5:353–360, 1978

BOOTH JC: Atypical seborrheic keratosis. Aust J Dermatol 18:10–14, 1977

BRAUN-FALCO O, KINT A, VOGELL W: Zur Histogenese der Verruca seborrhoica. II. Mitteilung. Elektronenmikroskopische Befunde. Arch Klin Exp Dermatol 217:627–651, 1963

BRAUN-FALCO O, WEISSMANN I: Stukkokeratosen. Hautarzt 29:573–577, 1978

BROWNSTEIN MH, SHAPIRO L: The pilosebaceous tumors. Int J Dermatol 16:340–352, 1977

CHRISTELER A, DELACRÉTAZ J: Verrues séborrhéiques et transformation maligne. Dermatologica 133:33–39, 1966

DELACRÉTAZ J: Mélano-acanthome. Dermatologica 151:236–240, 1975

DUPERRAT B, MASCARO JM: Une tumeur développée aux dépens de l'acrotrichium ou partie intraépidermique du follicule pilaire: Porome folliculaire. Dermatologica 126:291–310, 1963

GITLIN MC, PIROZZI DJ: The sign of Leser-Trélat. Arch Dermatol 111:792–793, 1975

GROSSHANS E, HANAU D: L'adénome infundibulaire: Un porome folliculaire à différenciation sebacée et apocrine. Ann Dermatol Venereol 108:59–66, 1981

HAIRSTON MA JR, REED RJ, DERBES VJ: Dermatosis papulosa nigra. Arch Dermatol 89:655–658, 1964

HEADINGTON JT: Tumors of the hair follicle. A review. Am J Pathol 85:480–514, 1976

HELWIG EB: Inverted follicular keratosis. In Seminar on the Skin: Neoplasms and Dermatoses. Proceedings of the 20th Seminar of the American Society of Clinical Pathologists, Washington, DC, 1954, pp 38–42. Washington, DC, American Society of Clinical Pathologists, 1955

INDIANER L: Controversies in dematopathology. J Dermatol Surg Oncol 5:321–328, 1979

KECHIJIAN P, SADICK NS, MARIGLIO J et al: Cytarabine-induced inflammation in the seborrheic keratoses of Leser-Trélat. Ann Intern Med 91:868–869, 1979

KOCSARD E, CARTER JJ: The papillomatous keratoses. The nature and differential diagnosis of stucco keratosis. Aust J Dermatol 12:80–88, 1971

KOSSARD S, BERMAN A, WINKELMANN RK: Seborrheic keratoses and trichostasis spinulosa. J Cutan Pathol 6:492–495, 1979

LAMBERT D, FORT M, LEGOUX A et al: Le signe de Leser-Trélat. Ann Dermatol Venereol 107:1035–1041, 1980

LENNOX B: Pigment patterns in epithelial tumors of the skin. J Pathol Bacteriol 61:587–598, 1949

LIDDELL K, WHITE JE, CALDWELL JW: Seborrheic keratoses and carcinoma of the large bowel. Br J Dermatol 92:449–452, 1975

MATSUOKA LY, GLASSER S, BARSKY S: Melanoacanthoma of the lip. Arch Dermatol 115:1116–1117, 1979

MEHREGAN AH: Inverted follicular keratosis. Arch Dermatol 89:229–235, 1964

MEHREGAN AH: Lentigo senilis and its evolutions. J Invest Dermatol 65:429–433, 1975

MEHREGAN AH, PINKUS H: Intraepidermal carcinoma: A critical study. Cancer 17:609–636, 1964

MEVORAH B, MISHIMA Y: Cellular response of seborrheic keratosis following croton oil irritation and surgical trauma. Dermatologica 131:452–462, 1965

MIKHAIL GR, MEHREGAN AH: Basal cell carcinoma in seborrheic keratosis. J Am Acad Dermatol 6:500–506, 1982

MISHIMA Y, PINKUS H: Benign mixed tumor of melanocytes and malpighian cells. Arch Dermatol 81:539–550, 1960

MORALES A, HU F: Seborrheic verruca and intraepidermal basal cell epithelioma of Jadassohn. Arch Dermatol 91:342–344, 1965

RAHBARI H: Bowenoid transformation of seborrheic verrucae (keratoses). Br J Dermatol 101:459–463, 1979

RONCHESE F: Keratoses, cancer and the sign of Leser-Trélat. Cancer 18:1003–1006, 1965

SANDERSON KF: The structure of seborrheic keratoses. Br J Dermatol 80:588–593, 1968

SCHLAPPNER OLA, ROWDEN G, PHILLIPS TM et al: Melanoacanthoma. Ultrastructural and immunological studies. J Cutan Pathol 5:127–141, 1978

SCHWARTZ RA, BURGESS GH: Florid cutaneous papillomatosis. Arch Dermatol 114:1803–1806, 1978

SIM-DAVIS D, MARKS R, WILSON JONES E: The inverted follicular keratosis. Acta Derm Venereol (Stockh) 56:337–344, 1976

SNEDDON IB, ROBERTS JBM: An incomplete form of acanthosis nigricans. Gut 3:269–272, 1962

WILLOUGHBY C, SOTER NA: Stucco keratosis. Arch Dermatol 105:859–861, 1972

Clear Cell Acanthoma

CRAMER HJ: Klarzellenakanthom (Degos) mit syringomatösen und Naevus-sebaceus-artigen Anteilen. Dermatologica 143:265–270, 1971

DEGOS R, CIVATTE J: Clear-cell acanthoma: Experience of 8 years. Br J Dermatol 83:248–254, 1970

DESMONS F, BREUILLARD F, THOMAS P et al: Multiple clear-cell acanthoma (Degos). Int J Dermatol 16:203–213, 1977

FINE RM, CHERNOSKY ME: Clinical recognition of clear-cell acanthoma (Degos). Arch Dermatol 100:559–563, 1969

HU F, SISSON JK: The ultrastructure of pale cell acanthoma. J Invest Dermatol 52:185–188, 1969

KERL H: Das Klarzellenakanthom. Hautarzt 28:456–462, 1977

TRAU H, FISHER BK, SCHEWACH-MILLET M: Multiple clear cell acanthomas. Arch Dermatol 116:433–434, 1980

WELLS GC, WILSON JONES E: Degos' acanthoma (acanthome à cellules claires). Br J Dermatol 79:249–258, 1967

WILSON JONES E, WELLS GC: Degos' acanthoma (acanthome à cellules claires). Arch Dermatol 94:286–294, 1966

ZAK FG, GIRERD RJ: Das blasszellige Akanthom (Degos). Hautarzt 19:559–561, 1968

Epidermal Cyst

DELACRÉTAZ J: Keratotic basal-cell carcinoma arising from an epidermoid cyst. J Dermatol Surg Oncol 3:310–311, 1977

FIESELMAN DW, REED RJ, ICHINOSE H: Pigmented epidermal cyst. J Cutan Pathol 1:256–259, 1974

LEONFORTE JF: Palmoplantare Epidermiszyste. Hautarzt 29:657–658, 1978

MCDONALD LW: Carcinomatous change in cysts of skin. Arch Dermatol 87:208–211, 1963

MCGAVRAN MH, BINNINGTON B: Keratinous cysts of the skin. Arch Dermatol 94:499–508, 1966

ONUIGBO WIB: Vulval epidermoid cysts in the Igbos of Nigeria. Arch Dermatol 112:1405–1406, 1976

RAAB W, STEIGLEDER GK: Fehldiagnosen bei Horncysten. Arch Klin Exp Dermatol 212:606–615, 1961

SHELLEY WB, WOOD MG: Occult Bowen's disease in keratinous cysts. Br J Dermatol 105:105–108, 1981

WILSON JONES E: Proliferating epidermoid cysts. Arch Dermatol 94:11–19, 1966

Milia

EPSTEIN W, KLIGMAN AM: The pathogenesis of milia and benign tumors of the skin. J Invest Dermatol 26:1–11, 1956

LEEPARD B, SNEDDON IB: Milia occurring in lichen sclerosus et atrophicus. Br J Dermatol 92:711–714, 1975

PINKUS H: In discussion of Epstein W, Kligman AM: J Invest Dermatol 26:10–11, 1956

TSUJI T, SUGAI T, SUZUKI S: The mode of growth of eccrine duct milia. J Invest Dermatol 65:388–393, 1975

Trichilemmal Cyst

BROWNSTEIN MH, ARLUK DJ: Proliferating trichilemmal cysts: Analysis of 50 new cases. (Abstr) Arch Dermatol 115:1347, 1979

KIMURA S: Trichilemmal cysts. Dermatologica 157:164–170, 1978

LEPPARD BJ, SANDERSON KV: The natural history of trichilemmal cysts. Br J Dermatol 94:379–390, 1976

LEPPARD BJ, SANDERSON KV, WELLS RS: Hereditary trichilemmal cysts. Clin Exp Dermatol 2:23–32, 1977

MCGAVRAN MH, BINNINGTON B: Keratinous cysts of the skin. Arch Dermatol 94:499–508, 1966

PINKUS H: "Sebaceous cysts" are trichilemmal cysts. Arch Dermatol 99:544–555, 1969

Steatocystoma Multiplex

BROWNSTEIN MH: Steatocystoma simplex. A solitary steatocystoma. Arch Dermatol 118:409–411, 1982

CONTRERAS MA, COSTELLO MJ: Steatocystoma multiplex with embryonal hair formation. Arch Dermatol 76:720–725, 1957

HASHIMOTO K, FISHER BK, LEVER WF: Steatocystoma multiplex. Hautarzt 15:299–305, 1964

KIMURA S: An ultrastructural study of steatocystoma multiplex and the normal pilosebaceous apparatus. J Dermatol (Tokyo) 8:459–465, 1981

KLIGMAN AM, KIRSCHBAUM JD: Steatocystoma multiplex: A dermoid tumor. J Invest Dermatol 42:383–387, 1964

OYAL H, NIKOLOWSKI W: Sebocystomatosen. Arch Klin Exp Dermatol 204:361–373, 1957

Dermoid Cyst

BROWNSTEIN MH, HELWIG EB: Subcutaneous dermoid cysts. Arch Dermatol 107:237–239, 1973

Bronchogenic and Thyroglossal Duct Cysts

AMBIAVAGAR PC, ROSEN Y: Cutaneous ciliated cyst on the chin. Probable bronchogenic cyst. Arch Dermatol 115:895–896, 1979

FRAGA S, HELWIG EB, ROSEN SH: Bronchogenic cysts in the skin and subcutaneous tissue. Am J Clin Pathol 56:230–238, 1971

Cutaneous Ciliated Cyst

CLARK JV: Ciliated epithelium in a cyst of the lower limb. J Pathol 98:289–291, 1969

FARMER ER, HELWIG EB: Cutaneous ciliated cysts. Arch Dermatol 114:70–73, 1978

Median Raphe Cyst of the Penis

AHMED A, JONES AW: Apocrine cystadenoma. Br J Dermatol 81:899–901, 1969

ASARCH RG, GOLITZ LE, SAUSKER WF et al: Median raphe cysts of the penis. Arch Dermatol 115:1084–1086, 1979

COLE LA, HELWIG EB: Mucoid cysts of the penile skin. J Urol 115:397–400, 1976

POWELL RF, PALMER CH, SMITH EB: Apocrine cystadenoma of the penile shaft. Arch Dermatol 113:1250–1251, 1977

Eruptive Vellus Hair Cysts

BOVENMYER DA: Eruptive vellus hair cysts. Arch Dermatol 115:338–339, 1979

BURNS DA, CALNAN CD: Eruptive vellus hair cysts. Clin Exp Dermatol 6: 209–213, 1981

ESTERLY NB, FRETZIN DF, PINKUS H: Eruptive vellus hair cysts. Arch Dermatol 113:500–503, 1977

LEE S, KIM JG: Eruptive vellus hair cyst. Arch Dermatol 115:744–746, 1979

PIEPKORN MW, CLARK L, LOMBARDI DL: A kindred with congenital vellus hair cysts. J Am Acad Dermatol 5:661–665, 1981

STIEFLER RE, BERGFELD WF: Eruptive vellus hair cysts, an inherited disorder. J Am Acad Dermatol 3:425–429, 1980

Warty Dyskeratoma

DELACRÉTAZ J: Dyskératomes verruqueux et kératoses séniles dyskératosiques. Dermatologica 127:23–32, 1963

FURTADO TA, SZYMANSKI FJ: Étude histologique du dyskératose verruqueux. Ann Dermatol Syph 88:633–640, 1961

GORLIN RJ, PETERSON WC JR: Warty dyskeratoma. A note concerning its occurrence in the oral mucosa. Arch Dermatol 95:292–293, 1967

GRAHAM JH, HELWIG EB: Isolated dyskeratosis follicularis. Arch Dermatol 77:377–389, 1958

HARRIST TJ, MURPHY GF, MIHM MC JR: Oral warty dyskeratoma. Arch Dermatol 116:929–931, 1980

JABLONSKA S, CHORZELSKI T: Dyskeratoma and epithelioma (carcinoma) dyskeratoticum segregans. Dermatologica 123:24–37, 1961

KELLUM RE, HASERICK JR: Localized linear keratosis follicularis. Arch Dermatol 86:450–454, 1962

METZ J, SCHRÖPL F: Zur Nosologie des Dyskeratoma segregans ("Warty dyskeratoma"). Arch Klin Exp Dermatol 238:21–37, 1970

SZYMANSKI FJ: Warty dyskeratoma. Arch Dermatol 75:567–572, 1957

TANAY A, MEHREGAN AH: Warty dyskeratoma. (Review) Dermatologica 138:155–164, 1969

TRITSCH H: Beitrag zur Darier-ähnlichen Atypie des Keratoma senile (sogenanntes warziges Dyskeratom). Arch Klin Exp Dermatol 210:280–290, 1960

Solar Keratosis (Actinic Keratosis)

ACKERMAN AB, REED RJ: Epidermolytic variant of solar keratosis. Arch Dermatol 107:104–106, 1973

BART RS, ANDRADE R, KOPF AW: Cutaneous horn. Acta Derm Venereol (Stockh) 48:507–515, 1968

BROWNSTEIN MH, RABINOWITZ AD: The precursors of cutaneous squamous cell carcinoma. Int J Dermatol 18:1–16, 1979

BROWNSTEIN MH, SHAPIRO EE: Trichilemmal horn: Cutaneous horn overlying trichilemmoma. Clin Exp Dermatol 4:59–63, 1979

CATALDO E, DOKU HC: Solar cheilitis. J Dermatol Surg Oncol 7:989–993, 1981

CRAMER HJ, KAHLERT G: Das Cornu cutaneum. Selbständiges Krankheitsbild oder klinisches Symptom? Dermatol Wochenschr 150:521–531, 1964

HALTER K: Über ein wenig beachtetes histologisches Kennzeichen des Keratoma senile. Hautarzt 3:215–216, 1952

HIRSCH P, MARMELZAT WL: Lichenoid actinic keratosis. Dermatol Int 6:101–103, 1967

JAMES MP, WELLS GC, WHIMSTER IW: Spreading pigmented actinic keratosis. Br J Dermatol 98:373–379, 1978

KOTEN JW, VERHAGEN ARHB, FRANK GL: Histopathology of actinic cheilitis. Dermatologica 135:465–471, 1967

LUND HZ: How often does squamous cell carcinoma of the skin metastasize? Arch Dermatol 92:635–637, 1965

MASHKILLEJSON AL: Über die Vorkrebserkrankung der Lippen. Dermatol Monatsschr 155:103–111, 1969

MØLLER R, REYMANN F, HOU-JENSEN K: Metastases in dermatological patients with squamous cell carcinoma. Arch Dermatol 115:703–705, 1979

MONTGOMERY H, DÖRFFEL J: Verruca senilis und Keratoma senile. Arch Dermatol Syph (Berlin) 166:286–296, 1932

PINKUS H: Keratosis senilis. Am J Clin Pathol 29:193–207, 1958

PINKUS H; Lichenoid tissue reactions. Arch Dermatol 107:840–846, 1973

SANDBANK M: Basal cell carcinoma at the base of cutaneous horn (cornu cutaneum). Arch Dermatol 104:97–98, 1971

SCOTT MA, JOHNSON WC: Lichenoid benign keratosis. J Cutan Pathol 3:217–221, 1976

SHAPIRO L, ACKERMAN AB: Solitary lichen planus-like keratosis. Dermatologica 132:386–392, 1966

Leukoplakia

CAWSON RA, LEHNER T: Chronic hyperplastic candidiasis: Candidal leukoplakia. Br J Dermatol 80:9–16, 1968

GRÄSSEL-PIETRUSKY R, HORNSTEIN OP: Histologische Untersuchungen zur Häufigkeit des Candidabefalls präkanzeröser oraler Leukoplakien. Hautarzt 31:21–25, 1980

HORNSTEIN OP: Klinik, Ätiologie und Therapie der oralen Leukoplakien. Hautarzt 30:40–50, 1979

MCADAMS AJ JR, KISTNER RW: The relationship of chronic vulvar disease, leukoplakia, and carcinoma in situ to carcinoma of the vulva. Cancer 11:740–757, 1958

PINDBORG JJ: Pathology of oral leukoplakia. Am J Dermatopathol 2:277–278, 1980

SHAFER WG, WALDRON CA: Erythroplakia of the oral cavity. Cancer 36:1021–1028, 1975

SHKLAR G: Oral leukoplakia—Studies in enzyme histochemistry. J Invest Dermatol 48:153–158, 1967

SHKLAR G: Modern studies and concepts of leukoplakia in the mouth. J Dermatol Surg Oncol 7:996–1003, 1981

WALDRON CA, SHAFER WG: Leukoplakia revisited. A clinicopathologic study of 3256 leukoplakias. Cancer 36:1386–1392, 1975

Verrucous Hyperplasia, Verrucous Carcinoma of the Oral Mucosa

GRINSPAN D, ABULAFIA J: Oral florid papillomatosis (verrucous carcinoma). Int J Dermatol 18:608–622, 1979

KANEE B: Oral florid papillomatosis complicated by verrucous squamous carcinoma. Arch Dermatol 99:196–202, 1969

KRAUS FT, PEREZ-MESA C: Verrucous carcinoma. Cancer 19:26–38, 1966

SAMITZ MH, ACKERMAN AB, LANTIS LR: Squamous cell carcinoma arising at the site of oral florid papillomatosis. Arch Dermatol 96:286–289, 1967

SHEAR M, PINDBORG JJ: Verrucous hyperplasia of the oral mucosa. Cancer 46:1855–1862, 1980

WECHSLER HL, FISHER ER: Oral florid papillomatosis. Arch Dermatol 86:480–492, 1962

Necrotizing Sialometaplasia

ABRAMS AM, MELROSE RJ, HOWELL FV: Necrotizing sialometaplasia. A disease simulating malignancy. Cancer 32:130–135, 1973

FECHNER RE: Necrotizing sialometaplasia. A source of confusion with carcinoma of the palate. Am J Clin Pathol 67:315–317, 1977

PIETTE F, SAUQUE E, PELLERIN P et al: Sialométaplasie nécrosante. Ann Dermatol Venereol 107:821–824, 1980

RAUGI GJ, KESSLER S: Necrotizing sialometaplasia: A condition simulating malignancy. Arch Dermatol 115:329–331, 1979

Eosinophilic Ulcer of the Tongue

BURGESS GH, MEHREGAN AH, DRINNAN AJ: Eosinophilic ulcer of the tongue. Arch Dermatol 113:644–645, 1977

SHAPIRO L, JUHLIN EA: Eosinophilic ulcer of the tongue. Dermatologica 140:242–250, 1970

Bowen's Disease, Erythroplasia of Queyrat, Balanitis Circumscripta

ACKERMAN AB: Reply to Mascaro JM: Bowenoid papulosis. J Am Acad Dermatol 4:608, 1981

ANDERSEN SL, NIELSEN H, RAYMANN F: Relationship between Bowen's disease and internal malignant tumors. Arch Dermatol 108:367–370, 1973

ARAI Y, HORI Y: An ultrastructural observation of intracytoplasmic desmosomes in Darier's disease. J Dermatol (Tokyo) 4:223–234, 1977

BAUGHMAN RD, BERGER P, PRINGLE WM: Plasma cell cheilitis. Arch Dermatol 110:725–726, 1974

BOWEN JT: Precancerous dermatosis. J Cutan Dis 30:241–255, 1912

BRODIN M: Balanitis circumscripta plasmacellularis. J Am Acad Dermatol 2:33–35, 1980

BROWNSTEIN MH, RABINOWITZ AD: The precursors of cutaneous squamous cell carcinoma. (Review) Int J Dermatol 18:1–16, 1979

CALLEN JP, HEADINGTON J: Bowen's and non-Bowen's squamous intraepidermal neoplasia of the skin. Arch Dermatol 116:422–426, 1980

EBERHARTINGER C, BERGMANN M: Balanoposthitis chronica circumscripta plasmacellularis Zoon und Phimose. Z Hautkr 46:251–254, 1971

FISHER ER, MCCOY MM II, WECHSLER HL: Analysis of histopathologic and electron microscopic determinants of keratoacanthoma and squamous cell carcinoma. Cancer 29:1387–1397, 1972

GOETTE DK: Erythroplasia of Queyrat. Arch Dermatol 110:271–273, 1974

GRAHAM JH, HELWIG EB: Bowen's disease and its relationship to systemic cancer. Arch Dermatol 80:133–159, 1959

GRAHAM JH, HELWIG EB: Erythroplasia of Queyrat. In Graham JH, Johnson WC, Helwig EB (eds): Dermal Pathology, pp 597–606. Hagerstown, MD, Harper & Row, 1972

ISHIBASHI Y, NIIMURA M, KLINGMÜLLER G: Elektronenmikroskopischer Beitrag zur Morphologie von Paget-Zellen. Arch Dermatol Forsch 245:402–416, 1972

JONQUIÈRES EDL, DE LUTZKY FK: Balanites et vulvites pseudo-érythroplasiques chroniques. Ann Dermatol Venereol 107:173–180, 1980

KLINGMÜLLER G, KLEHR HU, ISHIBASHI Y: Desmosomen im Cytoplasma entdifferenzierter Keratinocyten des Plattenepithelcarcinoms. Arch Klin Exp Dermatol 238:356–365, 1970

KLUG H, HAUSTEIN UF: Vorkommen von intrazytoplasmatischen Desmosomen in Keratinozyten. Dermatologica 148:143–153, 1974

KOMURA J, WATANABE S: Desmosome-like structures in the cytoplasm of normal human keratinocyte. Arch Dermatol Res 253:145–149, 1975

MENSING H, JÄNNER M: Vulvitis plasmacellularis Zoon. Z Hautkr 56:728–732, 1981

MIKHAIL GR: Cancers, precancers, and pseudocancers on the male genitalia. J Dermatol Surg Oncol 6:1027–1035, 1980

MOLDENHAUER E: Die Cheilitis plasmacellularis. Ein Beitrag zur Plasmocytosis circumorificialis. Dermatol Wochenschr 152:636–640, 1966

MONTGOMERY H: Precancerous dermatosis and epithelioma in situ. Arch Dermatol Syph 39:387–408, 1939

MONTGOMERY H, WAISMAN M: Epithelioma attributable to arsenic. J Invest Dermatol 4:365, 1941

NÖDL F: Zur Klinik und Histologie der Balanoposthitis chronica circumscripta benigna plasmacellularis. Arch Dermatol Syph (Berlin) 198:557–566, 1954

OLSON RL, NORDQUIST R, EVERETT MA: An electron microscopic study of Bowen's disease. Cancer Res 28:2078–2085, 1968

OLSON RL, NORDQUIST R, EVERETT MA: Dyskeratosis in Bowen's disease. Br J Dermatol 81:676–680, 1969

PETERKA ES, LYNCH FW, GOLTZ RW: An association between Bowen's disease and internal cancer. Arch Dermatol 84:623–629, 1961

QUEYRAT L: Erythroplasie du gland. Bull Soc Fr Dermatol Syph 22:378–382, 1911

RAITEN K, PANIAGO-PEREIRA C, ACKERMAN AB: Pagetoid Bowen's disease vs. extramammary Paget's disease. J Dermatol Surg Oncol 2:24–25, 1976

SATO A, SEIJI M: Electron microscopic observations of malignant dyskeratosis in leukoplakia and Bowen's disease. Acta Derm Venereol (Stockh) 53 (Suppl 73):101–110, 1973

SCHENK P: Desmosomale Strukturen im Cytoplasma normaler und pathologischer Keratinocyten. Arch Dermatol Res 253:23–42, 1975

SCHUERMANN H: Plasmocytosis circumorificialis. Dtsch Zahnaerztl Z 15:601–611, 1960

SEIJI M, MIZUNO F: Electron microscopic study of Bowen's disease. Arch Dermatol 99:3–16, 1969

SOUTEYRAND P, WONG E, MACDONALD DM: Zoon's balanitis (balanitis circumscripta plasmacellularis). Br J Dermatol 105:195–199, 1981

STRAYER DS, SANTA CRUZ DJ: Carcinoma in situ of the skin: A review of histopathology. J Cutan Pathol 7:244–259, 1980

ZOON JJ: Balanoposthite chronique circonscrite bénigne à plasmocytes. Dermatologica 105:1–7, 1952

Squamous Cell Carcinoma, Pseudocarcinomatous Hyperplasia

ACKERMAN LV: Verrucous carcinoma of the oral cavity. Surgery 23:670–678, 1948

AIRD I, JOHNSON HD, LENNOX B et al: Epithelioma cuniculatum. A variety of squamous carcinoma peculiar to the foot. Br J Surg 42:245–250, 1954

ARONS MS, LYNCH JB, LEWIS SR et al: Scar tissue carcinoma. I. A clinical study with special reference to burn scar carcinoma. Ann Surg 161:170–188, 1965

BARR RJ, WUERKER RB, GRAHAM JH: Ultrastructure of atypical fibroxanthoma. Cancer 40:736–743, 1977

BATTIFORA H: Spindle cell carcinoma. Ultrastructural evidence of squamous origin and collagen production by the tumor cells. Cancer 37:2275–2282, 1976

BONCINELLI U, FORNIERI C, MUSCATELLO U: Relationship between leukocytes and tumor cells in precancerous and cancerous lesions of the lip. A possible expression of immune reaction. J Invest Dermatol 71:407–411, 1978

BORELLI D: Aspetti pseudoglandolari nell'epitelioma discheratosico: "Adenoacanthoma of sweat glands" di Lever. Dermatologica 97:193–207, 1948

BRODERS AC: Squamous-cell epithelioma of the skin. Ann Surg 73:141–160, 1921

BRODIN MB, MEHREGAN AH: Verrucous carcinoma. Arch Dermatol 116:987, 1980

BROWN SM, FREEMAN RG: Epithelioma cuniculatum. Arch Dermatol 112:1295–1296, 1976

CHORZELSKI T: Ein Fall von Übergang einer Keratosis senilis mit Dyskeratose vom Typ des Morbus Darier in ein dyskeratotisches Spinaliom. Hautarzt 14:37–38, 1963

DAWSON DF, DUCKWORTH JK, BERNHARDT H et al: Giant condyloma and verrucous carcinoma of the genital area. Arch Pathol 79:225–231, 1965

DELACRÉTAZ J, MADJEDI AS, LORETAN R: Epithelioma spinocellulare segregans. Über die sogenannten "Adenoacanthome der Schweissdrüsen" (Lever). Hautarzt 8:512–518, 1957

EDMUNDSON WF: Microscopic grading of cancer and its practical implication. Arch Dermatol Syph 57:141–150, 1948

EPSTEIN E, EPSTEIN NN, BRAGG K et al: Metastases from squamous cell carcinomas of the skin. Arch Dermatol 97:245–251, 1968

EVANS HL, SMITH JL: Spindle cell squamous carcinoma and sarcoma-like tumors of the skin. Cancer 45:2687–2697, 1980

FREEMAN RG: On the pathogenesis of pseudoepitheliomatous hyperplasia. J Cutan Pathol 1:231–237, 1974

GRINSPAN D, ABULAFIA J: Oral florid papillomatosis (verrucous carcinoma). Int J Dermatol 18:608–622, 1979

HOXTELL EO, MANDEL JS, MURRAY SS et al: Incidence of skin carcinoma after renal transplantation. Arch Dermatol 113:436–438, 1977

JOHNSON WC, HELWIG EB: Adenoid squamous cell carcinoma (adenoacanthoma). Cancer 19:1639–1650, 1966

JU DMC: Pseudoepitheliomatous hyperplasia of the skin. Dermatol Int 6:82–92, 1967

KANEE B: Oral florid papillomatosis complicated by verrucous squamous carcinoma. Arch Dermatol 99:196–202, 1969

KLIMA M, KURTIS B, JORDAN PH JR: Verrucous carcinoma of the skin. J Cutan Pathol 7:88–98, 1980

KLINGMÜLLER G, KLEHR HU, ISHIBASHI Y: Desmosomen im Cytoplasma entdifferenzierter Keratinocyten des Plattenepithelcarcinoms. Arch Klin Exp Dermatol 238:356–365, 1970

KOBAYASI T: Dermo-epidermal junction in invasive squamous cell carcinoma. Acta Derm Venereol (Stockh) 49:445–448, 1969

LASSER A, CORNOG JL, MORRIS J MCL: Adenoid squamous cell carcinoma of the vulva. Cancer 33:224–227, 1974

LEVER WF: Adenoacanthoma of sweat glands. Arch Dermatol Syph 56:157–171, 1947

LUND HZ: How often does squamous cell carcinoma of the skin metastasize? Arch Dermatol 92:635–637, 1965

MANGLANI KS, MANALIGOD JR, RAY B: Spindle cell carcinoma of the glans penis. Cancer 46:2266–2272, 1980

MARTIN H, STRONG E, SPIRO RH: Radiation-induced skin cancer of the head and neck. Cancer 25:61–71, 1970

MCKEE PH, WILKINSON JD, BLACK MM et al: Carcinoma (epithelioma) cuniculatum. Histopathology 5:425–436, 1981a

MCKEE PH, WILKINSON JD, CORBETT MF et al: Carcinoma cuniculatum: A case metastasizing to skin and lymph nodes. Clin Exp Dermatol 6:613–618, 1981b

MOHS FE, SAHL WJ: Chemosurgery for verrucous carcinoma. J Dermatol Surg Oncol 5:302–306, 1979

MØLLER R, REYMANN F, HOU-JENSEN K: Metastases in dermatological patients with squamous cell carcinoma. Arch Dermatol 115:703–705, 1979

MULLER SA, WILHELMJ CM JR, HARRISON EG JR et al: Adenoid squamous cell carcinoma (adenoacanthoma of Lever). Arch Dermatol 89:589–597, 1964

PENNEYS NS, NADJI M, ZIEGELS-WEISSMAN et al: Prekeratin in spindle cell tumors of the skin. Arch Dermatol, in press

PEREZ CA, KRAUS FT, EVANS JC et al: Anaplastic transformation in verrucous carcinoma of the oral cavity after radiation therapy. Radiology 86:108–115, 1966

REINGOLD IM, SMITH BP, GRAHAM JH: Epithelioma cuniculatum pedis, a variant of squamous cell carcinoma. Am J Clin Pathol 69:561–565, 1978

SAMITZ MH, ACKERMAN AB, LANTIS LR: Squamous cell carcinoma arising at the site of oral florid papillomatosis. Arch Dermatol 96:286–289, 1967

SEDLIN ED, FLEMING JL: Epidermal carcinoma arising in chronic osteomyelitic foci. J Bone Joint Surg 45:827–837, 1963

SEEHAFER JR, MULLER SA, DICKEN CH et al: Bilateral verrucous carcinoma of the feet. Arch Dermatol 115:1222–1223, 1979

SOMMERVILLE J: Pseudo-epitheliomatous hyperplasia. Acta Derm Venereol (Stockh) 33:236–251, 1953

SU WPD, DUNCAN SC, PERRY HO: Blastomycosis-like pyoderma. Arch Dermatol 115:170–173, 1979

TAKAGI M, SAKOTA Y, TAKAYAMA S et al: Adenoid squamous cell carcinoma of the oral mucosa. Report of two autopsy cases. Cancer 40:2250–2255, 1977

TURNER JE, CALLEN JP: Aggressive behavior of squamous cell carcinoma in a patient with preceding lymphocytic lymphoma. J Am Acad Dermatol 4:446–450, 1981

UNDERWOOD JW, ADCOCK LL, OKAGARI T: Adenosquamous carcinoma of skin appendages (adenoid squamous cell carcinoma, pseudoglandular squamous cell carcinoma, adenoacanthoma of sweat glands of Lever) of the vulva. Cancer 42:1851–1858, 1978

WILKINSON JD, MCKEE PH, BLACK MM et al: A case of carcinoma cuniculatum with coexistent viral plantar wart. Clin Exp Dermatol 6:619–623, 1981

WINER LH: Pseudoepitheliomatous hyperplasia. Arch Dermatol Syph 42:856–867, 1940

Keratoacanthoma

BART RS, POPKIN GL, KOPF AW et al: Giant keratoacanthoma. J Dermatol Surg 1(2):49–55, 1975

BELISARIO JC: Brief review of keratoacanthoma and description of keratoacanthoma centrifugum marginatum. Aust J Dermatol 8:65–72, 1965

CALNAN CD, HABER H: Molluscum sebaceum. J Pathol Bacteriol 69:61–66, 1955

CHALET MD, CONNORS RC, ACKERMAN AB: Squamous cell carcinoma vs. keratoacanthoma: Criteria for histologic differentiation. J Dermatol Surg 1(1):16–17, 1975

DE MORAGAS JM, MONTGOMERY H, MCDONALD JR: Keratoacanthoma versus squamous-cell carcinoma. Arch Dermatol 77:390–395, 1957

FERGUSON SMITH J: A case of multiple primary squamous-celled carcinomata of the skin in a young man with spontaneous healing. Br J Dermatol 46:267–272, 1934

GHADIALLY FN: The role of the hair follicle in the origin and evolution of some cutaneous neoplasms of man and experimental animals. Cancer 14:801–816, 1961

GHADIALLY FN: Keratoacanthoma. In Fitzpatrick TB, Eisen AZ, Wolff K et al (eds): Dermatology in General Medicine, 2nd ed, pp 383–389. New York, McGraw-Hill, 1979

GILTMAN LI: Tripolar mitosis in a keratoacanthoma. Acta Derm Venereol (Stockh) 61:362–363, 1981

GRZYBOWSKI M: A case of peculiar generalized epithelial tumours of the skin. Br J Dermatol 62:310–313, 1950

HEID E, GROSSHANS E, LAZRAK B et al: Keratoacanthoma centrifugum marginatum. Ann Dermatol Venereol 106:367–370, 1979

HOUSHOLDER MS, ZELIGMAN I: Sebaceous neoplasms associated with visceral carcinomas. Arch Dermatol 116:61–64, 1980

JANECKA IP, WOLFF M, CRIKELAIR GF et al: Aggressive histological features of keratoacanthoma. J Cutan Pathol 4:342–348, 1978

KALLOS A: Giant keratoacanthoma. Arch Dermatol 78:207–209, 1958

KERN WH, MCGRAY MK: The histopathologic differentiation of keratoacanthoma and squamous cell carcinoma of the skin. J Cutan Pathol 7:318–325, 1980

LAPINS NA, HELWIG EB: Perineural invasion by keratoacanthoma. Arch Dermatol 116:791–793, 1980

LEVY EJ, CAHN MM, SHAFFER B et al: Keratoacanthoma. JAMA 155:562–564, 1954

MACAULAY WL: Subungual keratoacanthoma. Arch Dermatol 112:1004–1005, 1976

MIEDZINSKI F, KOZAKIEWICZ J: Das Keratoakanthoma centrifugum, eine besondere Varietät des Keratoakanthoms. Hautarzt 13:348–352, 1962

MUSSO L, GORDON H: Spontaneous resolution of molluscum sebaceum. Proc Roy Soc Med 43:838–839, 1950

NIKOLOWSKI W: Zur Problematik des Keratoakanthoms. Dermatol Monatsschr 156:148–153, 1970

OBERMAYER ME: Das Keratoakanthom: Seine zur Gewebsdestruktion führende Wachstumskapazität. Hautarzt 15:628–630, 1964

POLEKSIC S, YEUNG KY: Rapid development of keratoacanthoma and accelerated transformation into squamous cell carcinoma of the skin. Cancer 41:12–16, 1978

POPKIN GL, BRODIE SJ, HYMAN AB et al: A technique of biopsy recommended for keratoacanthoma. Arch Dermatol 94:191–193, 1966

RAPAPORT J: Giant keratoacanthoma of the nose. Arch Dermatol 111:73–75, 1975

ROOK A, MOFFAT JL: Multiple self-healing epithelioma of Ferguson Smith type. Arch Dermatol 74:525–532, 1956

ROOK A, WHIMSTER IW: Le kératoacanthome. Arch Belg Dermatol Syph 6:137–146, 1950

ROOK A, WHIMSTER I: Keratoacanthoma, a 30-year retrospect. Br J Dermatol 100:41–47, 1979

ROSSMAN RE, FREEMAN RG, KNOX JM: Multiple keratoacanthomas. Arch Dermatol 89:374–381, 1964

SILBERBERG I, KOPF A, BAER RL: Recurrent keratoacanthoma of the lip. Arch Dermatol 86:44–53, 1962

SOMMERVILLE J, MILNE JA: Familial primary self-healing squamous epithelioma of the skin (Ferguson Smith type). Br J Dermatol 62:485–490, 1950

STEVANOVIC DV: Keratoacanthoma dyskeratoticum and segregans. Arch Dermatol 92:666–669, 1965

STOLL DM, ACKERMAN AB: Subungual keratoacanthoma. Am J Dermatopathol 2:265–271, 1980

SULLIVAN JJ, COLDITZ GA: Keratoacanthoma in a subtropical climate. Aust J Dermatol 20:34–42, 1979

SULLIVAN JJ, DONOGHUE MF, KYNASTON B et al: Multiple keratoacanthomas. Aust J Dermatol 21:16–24, 1980

TAKAKI Y, MASUTANI M, KAWADA A: Electron microscopic study of keratoacanthoma. Acta Derm Venereol (Stockh) 51:21–26, 1971

TARNOWSKI WM: Multiple keratoacanthomata. Arch Dermatol 94:74–80, 1966

VON BÜLOW M, KLINGMÜLLER G: Elektronenmikroskopische Untersuchungen des Keratoakanthoms. Arch Dermatol Forsch 241:292–304, 1971

WADE TR, ACKERMAN AB: The many faces of keratoacanthoma. J Dermatol Surg Oncol 4:498–501, 1978

WEEDON D, BARNETT L: Keratoacanthoma centrifugum marginatum. Arch Dermatol 111:1024–1026, 1975

WINKELMANN RK, BROWN J: Generalized eruptive keratoacanthoma. Arch Dermatol 97:615–623, 1968

Paget's Disease

ASHIKARI R, PARK K, HUVOS AG et al: Paget's disease of the breast. Cancer 26:680–685, 1970

BELCHER RW: Extramammary Paget's disease. Enzyme histochemical and electron microscopic study. Arch Pathol 94:59–64, 1972

CAPUTO R, CALIFANO A: Ultrastructural features of extramammary Paget's disease. Arch Klin Exp Dermatol 236:121–132, 1970

CHRICHLOW RW, CZERNOBILSKY B: Paget's disease of the male breast. Cancer 24:1031–1040, 1969

CULBERSON JD, HORN RC JR: Paget's disease of the nipple. Arch Surg 72:224–231, 1956

DEMOPOULOS RI: Fine structure of the extramammary Paget's cell. Cancer 27:1202–1210, 1971

DUPERRAT B, MASCARO JM: Maladie de Paget abdomino-scrotale (3ᵉ présentation). Apparition d'un épithéliome apocrine de l'aisselle et de lésions de maladie de Paget sur la peau axillaire sus-jacente. Bull Soc Fr Dermatol Syph 71:176–177, 1964

DUPRÉ A, BONAFÉ JL, VANCINA S et al: Maladie de Paget du mamelon. Ann Dermatol Venereol 107:367–374, 1980

EBNER H: Zur Ultrastruktur des Morbus Paget mamillae. Z Hautkr 44:297–304, 1969

FETISSOFF, F, ARBEILLE-BRASSART B, LANSAC J et al: Association d'une maladie de Paget mammaire et vulvaire. Ann Dermatol Venerol 109:43–50, 1981

FISHER ER, BEYER F JR: Differentiation of neoplastic lesions characterized by large vacuolated intraepidermal (pagetoid) cells. Arch Pathol 67:140–145, 1959

FLIGIEL Z, KANEKO M: Extramammary Paget's disease of the external ear canal in association with ceruminous gland carcinoma. Cancer 36:1072–1076, 1975

GREENWOOD SM, MINKOWITZ S: Paget's disease in metastatic breast carcinoma. Arch Dermatol 14:312–315, 1971

GUNN RA, GALLAGER HS: Vulvar Paget's disease. Cancer 46:590–594, 1980

HADLICH J, GÖRING HD, LINSE R: Morbus Paget beim Mann nach Östrogenbehandlung. Dermatol Monatsschr 167:305–308, 1981

HART WR, MILLMAN JB: Progression of intraepithelial Paget's disease of the vulva to invasive carcinoma. Cancer 40:2333–2337, 1977

HELWIG EB, GRAHAM JH: Anogenital (extramammary) Paget's disease: A clinicopathologic study. Cancer 16:387–403, 1963

HOPSU-HAVU VK, SONCK CE: The problem of extramammary Paget's disease. Report of four cases with "pagetoid" cells. Z Hautkr 46:41–50, 1971

JONES RE JR, AUSTIN C, ACKERMAN AB: Extramammary Paget's disease. Am J Dermatopathol 1:101–132, 1979

KAWATSU T, MIKI V: Triple extramammary Paget's disease. Arch Dermatol 104:316–319, 1971

KOSS LG, BROCKUNIER A JR: Ultrastructural aspects of Paget's disease of the vulva. Arch Pathol 87:592–600, 1969

LEE SC, ROTH LM, EHRLICH C et al: Extramammary Paget's disease of the vulva. Cancer 39:2540–2549, 1977

LEWIS HM, OVITZ ML, GOLITZ LE: Erosive adenomatosis of the nipple. Arch Dermatol 112:1427–1428, 1976

MCKEE PH, HERTOGS KT: Endocervical adenocarcinoma and vulval Paget's disease: A significant association. Br J Dermatol 103:443–448, 1980

MEDENICA M, SAHIHI T: Ultrastructural aspects of Paget's disease of the vulva. Arch Dermatol 105:236–243, 1972

MONTGOMERY H: Dermatopathology, Vol. 2, pp. 1007–1016. New York, Paul B Hoeber, 1967

MUIR R: Further observations on Paget's disease of the nipple. J Pathol Bacteriol 49:299–312, 1939

MURRELL TW JR, MCMULLAN FH: Extramammary Paget's disease. Arch Dermatol 85:600–613, 1962

ORR JW, PARISH DJ: The nature of the nipple changes in Paget's disease. J Pathol Bacteriol 84:201–208, 1962

PAONE JF, BAKER RR: Pathogenesis and treatment of Paget's disease of the breast. Cancer 48:825–829, 1981

PENNEYS NS, NADJI M, MORALES A: Carcinoembryonic antigen in benign sweat gland tumors. Arch Dermatol 118:225–227, 1982

PIÉRARD J, KINT A: Maladie de Paget extramammaire. Étude d'un cas en microscopie électronique. Arch Belg Dermatol 24:335–347, 1968

PINKUS H, MEHREGAN AH: A Guide to Dermatopathology, 3rd ed, pp 471–475. New York, Appleton-Century-Crofts, 1981

SAGEBIEL RW: Ultrastructural observations on epidermal cells in Paget's disease of the breast. Am J Pathol 57:49–64, 1969

WHORTON CM, PATTERSON JB: Carcinoma of Moll's glands with extramammary Paget's disease of the eyelid. Cancer 8:1009–1015, 1955

WOOD WS, CULLING CFA: Perianal Paget disease. Arch Pathol 99:442–445, 1975

YOELL JH, PRICE WG: Paget's disease of the perianal skin with associated adenocarcinoma. Arch Dermatol 82:986–991, 1960

27

Tumors of the Epidermal Appendages

CLASSIFICATION OF THE APPENDAGE TUMORS

The benign tumors differentiating in the direction of epidermal appendages can be divided into four groups: those differentiating toward hair, toward sebaceous glands, toward apocrine glands, and toward eccrine glands.

Besides the benign tumors differentiating toward epidermal appendages, there are carcinomas of epidermal appendages. Three types of carcinoma are recognized: carcinoma of sebaceous glands, eccrine sweat glands, and apocrine glands.

Classification of the Benign Appendage Tumors. The four groups of benign appendage tumors with differentiation toward hair, sebaceous glands, apocrine glands, and eccrine glands can be divided, according to the decreasing degree of differentiation observed in them, into four subgroups: hyperplasias, adenomas, benign epitheliomas, and primordial epitheliomas or basal cell epitheliomas. Arrangement of the appendage tumors according to their degree and direction of differentiation then results in a "kind of periodic table" (Kligman and Pinkus). This table was first published in 1948 (Lever) and has been modified over the years (Table 27-1).

Of the four subgroups into which the benign appendage tumors can be divided, the hyperplasias are composed of mature or nearly mature structures. The adenomas show less differentiation than the hyperplasias; nonetheless, well-developed, glandlike structures are present. The benign epitheliomas are a further step down with regard to degree of differentiation, and it is usually difficult to recognize the type of structure that the tumor is attempting to form. The primordial epitheliomas, or basal cell epitheliomas, are the least differentiated of the benign appendage tumors. According to the concept set forth here, basal cell epitheliomas are not carcinomas, being composed of immature rather than of anaplastic cells (see p. 572).

Although most of the benign appendage tumors fit well into one of the entities listed in Table 27-1, tumors in an intermediate stage of differentiation are occasionally encountered. Also, because of differentiation in more than one direction, combinations of several tumor types occur, so that one may find within the same tumor, for instance, differentiation toward sebaceous as well as apocrine structures (Wechsler and Fisher).

Histogenesis of the Benign Appendage Tumors. In 1948, the thesis was advanced that cutaneous tumors differentiating toward hair, sebaceous glands, or apocrine glands developed from primary epithelial germ cells and, as such, were primary epithelial germ tumors; and, further, that the hyperplasias, adenomas, and benign epitheliomas arose from primary epithelial germ cells that had attained a certain degree of differentiation before the onset of neoplasia, whereas the basal cell epitheliomas arose from primary epithelial germ cells that had attained little or no differentiation (Lever).

522

TABLE 27-1.   Classification of the Benign Appendage Tumors

	Hair Differentiation	Sebaceous Differentiation	Apocrine Differentiation	Eccrine Differentiation
Hyperplasias (Hamartomas)		Nevus sebaceus Sebaceous hyper-plasia Fordyce's condition	Apocrine nevus	Eccrine nevus
Adenomas	Trichofolliculoma Dilated pore Pilar sheath acan-thoma Multiple fibrofol-liculomas Multiple trichodis-comas	Sebaceous adenoma	Apocrine hidrocys-toma Hidradenoma papil-liferum Apocrine syringo-cystadenoma papilliferum Tubular apocrine adenoma Erosive adenomato-sis of the nipple	Eccrine hidrocys-toma Syringoma (Eccrine syringo-cystadenoma papilliferum)
Benign Epithe-liomas	Trichoepithelioma Desmoplastic tricho-epithelioma Trichoadenoma Generalized hair follicle hamar-toma Pilomatricoma Proliferating trichi-lemmal tumor Trichilemmoma Tumor of the follic-ular infundibu-lum	Sebaceous epithe-lioma	Apocrine cylin-droma (Apocrine chon-droid syringoma)	(Eccrine cylin-droma) Eccrine poroma Mucinous syringo-metaplasia Eccrine spirade-noma Clear cell hidrade-noma Eccrine chondroid syringoma
Primordial Epithe-liomas	Keratotic basal cell epithelioma	Cystic basal cell epi-thelioma	Adenoid basal cell epithelioma	Basal cell epithe-lioma with ec-crine differentia-tion

In the case of benign appendage tumors that are present at birth, such as the nevus sebaceus, one can assume that such tumors are actually derived from embryonic primary epithelial germ cells. In all other instances, it is likely that the benign appendage tumors arise from pluripotential cells that have formed during life and possess the potentiality, as do primary epithelial germ cells, of differentiating into tumors with hair, sebaceous gland, or apocrine structures (Pinkus). It is of interest in this respect that basal cell epitheliomas ultrastructurally have more features in common with fetal hair follicles than with fetal or adult epidermis and thus seem to mimic fetal primary epithelial germs (Kumakiri and Hashimoto). Similarly, eccrine sweat gland tumors arise from pluripotential cells that form during adult life and possess the potentiality of differentiating into tumors with eccrine gland structures. In genetically determined appendage tumors, such as multiple cylindromas, multiple trichoepitheliomas, and the nevoid basal cell epithelioma syndrome, one may assume that the genes regulating the development of pluripotential cells into cutaneous appendages are abnormal and sooner or later modify the growth of pluripotential cells into appendage tumors rather than into mature appendages. It appears unlikely, however, that any benign appendage tumors arise from mature structures. For this reason, it is useless to search for any connection between, for instance, a benign eccrine gland tumor and a pre-existing eccrine gland.

In the original classification of the appendage tumors presented in 1948, several tumors that are now regarded as eccrine, such as syringoma, were classified as apocrine. The reason for this lies in the fact that enzyme histochemical and electron microscopic methods that were not yet available in 1948 have since proved of great value in distinguishing eccrine from apocrine differentiation (Hashimoto and Lever).

Terminology. The terms *nevus* and *epithelioma* used in the classification of the benign appendage tumors require definition.

Nevus. The term *nevus* is used in the literature in two different ways, referring (1) to a tumor composed of nevus cells (nevocellular nevus, melanocytic nevus, pigmented nevus), or (2) to a lesion that is usually present at birth and is composed of mature or nearly mature structures (connatal hyperplasias, such as nevus sebaceus, eccrine nevus, nevus verrucosus, and nevus flammeus). In order to avoid confusion, it is advisable when referring to a connatal hyperplasia always to use the term *nevus* with a qualifying adjective, so that *nevus* without a qualifying adjecting designates a tumor composed of nevus cells.

The term *hamartoma* would seem appropriate for those nevi that have no nevus cells and, like congenital hyperplasias, are composed of mature or nearly mature structures. *Hamartoma*, derived from the Greek word *hamartanein* (to fail, to err), was chosen as the designation for "tumorlike malformations showing a faulty mixture of the normal components of the organ in which they occur" (Albrecht).

Epithelioma. The term *epithelioma* is used by many authors as a synonym for *carcinoma*. However, since the literal meaning of the word is "tumor of the epithelium," the term may be employed as a designation of benign as well as of malignant tumors of the epithelium, provided that a qualifying adjective is added (Jadassohn). It seems best, however, to reserve the term *epithelioma* for benign epithelial tumors and the term *carcinoma* for malignant epithelial tumors (Becker).

TUMORS WITH DIFFERENTIATION TOWARD HAIR STRUCTURES

TRICHOFOLLICULOMA

Trichofolliculoma occurs in adults as a solitary lesion, usually on the face but occasionally on the scalp or neck. It consists of a small, skin-colored, dome-shaped nodule. Frequently, there is a central pore. If such a central pore is present, a woollike tuft of immature, usually white hairs may be seen emerging from it, a highly diagnostic clinical feature (Pinkus and Sutton).

Histopathology. On histologic examination, the dermis contains a large cystic space that is lined by squamous epithelium and contains horny material and frequently also fragments of birefringent hair shafts (Gray and Helwig). In cases with a central pore, the large cystic space is continuous with the surface epidermis, an indication that it represents an enlarged, distorted hair follicle. In some cases, one or two additional cystic spaces are present in the dermis. Radiating from the wall of these "primary" hair follicles, one sees many small but usually fairly well differentiated "secondary"' hair follicles. Well-developed secondary hair follicles often show a hair papilla. Furthermore, they usually show an outer and an inner root sheath, the latter of which may contain eosinophilic trichohyaline granules and, located in the center, a fine hair (Fig. 27-1). These fine hairs are visualized best where the secondary hair follicles appear in cross sections. Small groups of sebaceous gland cells may be embedded in the walls of the secondary hair follicles (Hyman and Clayman). In some of the more rudimentary secondary follicles, one observes in place of a hair a central horn cyst, as seen also in trichoepithelioma (Sanderson). The stroma is rich in fibroblasts and is oriented in parallel bundles of fibers that encapsulate the epithelial proliferations in a manner resembling that of the normal fibrous root sheath (Kligman and Pinkus). Large amounts of glycogen can be demonstrated in the outer root sheath of the secondary hair follicles, just as it is seen in the outer root sheath of mature hair structures (Gray and Helwig).

In all trichofolliculomas, epithelial strands interconnect the secondary hair follicles. Since these epithelial strands differentiate in the direction of the outer root sheath, the peripheral cell row shows palisading, and because of their glycogen content, the cells within the strands appear large and vacuolated (Kligman and Pinkus).

Sebaceous Trichofolliculoma

A variant of trichofolliculoma, sebaceous trichofolliculoma occurs in areas rich in sebaceous follicles, such as

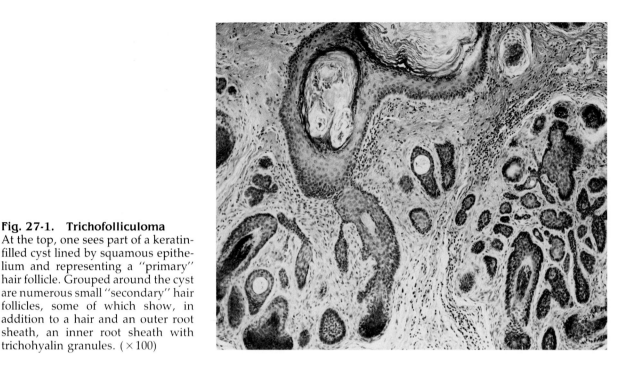

Fig. 27-1. Trichofolliculoma
At the top, one sees part of a keratin-filled cyst lined by squamous epithelium and representing a "primary" hair follicle. Grouped around the cyst are numerous small "secondary" hair follicles, some of which show, in addition to a hair and an outer root sheath, an inner root sheath with trichohyalin granules. (×100)

the nose. It is a centrally depressed lesion with a fistula-like opening from which terminal hairs and vellus hairs protrude (Plewig).

Histopathology.   There is a rather large, irregularly shaped, centrally located cavity lined by squamous epithelium. Many radially arranged pilosebaceous follicles connect to the cavity. These contain sebaceous ducts and numerous well-differentiated, large sebaceous lobules, as well as hair follicles containing partially terminal and partially vellus hairs (Plewig).

DILATED PORE, PILAR SHEATH ACANTHOMA

Dilated pore and pilar sheath acanthoma share with trichofolliculoma clinically the presence of a central pore and histologically the presence of a large cystic space that is continuous with the surface epidermis, lined by squamous epithelium, and filled with keratinous material.

The *dilated pore*, described in 1954 (Winer), occurs on the face, usually as a solitary lesion and predominantly in adult males. It has the appearance of a giant comedo and does not possess any palpable induration.

The *pilar sheath acanthoma*, described in 1978 (Mehregan and Brownstein), is usually found on the skin of the upper lip of adults. It is seen elsewhere on the face only rarely. It occurs as a solitary skin-colored nodule with a central porelike opening.

Histopathology.   The *dilated pore* shows a markedly dilated pilar infundibulum lined by an epidermis that is atrophic near the ostium but hypertrophic deeper in the cystic cavity, where it shows many rete ridges and irregular thin proliferations into the surrounding stroma. The keratin-filled cystic cavity may extend into the subcutaneous fat. In the lower portion, small sebaceous gland lobules and vellus hair follicles may be attached to the lining epidermis (Winer).

The *pilar sheath acanthoma* differs from the dilated pore by showing a larger, irregularly branching cystic cavity. In place of thin proliferations, as seen in the dilated pore, numerous lobulated masses of tumor cells radiate from the wall of the cystic cavity into the dermis and the subcutaneous tissue (Mehregan and Brownstein). The tumor cells in some areas show peripheral palisading and contain varying amounts of glycogen. They thus resemble outer root sheath epithelium (Bhawan).

MULTIPLE FIBROFOLLICULOMAS, MULTIPLE TRICHODISCOMAS

Multiple fibrofolliculomas have been described not only in association with trichodiscomas and acrochordons (Birt et al; Fujita et al) but also in association with a large connective tissue nevus (Weintraub and Pinkus).

Fibrofolliculomas consist of multiple 2- to 4-mm large, yellowish white, smooth, dome-shaped lesions. In patients who also have trichodiscomas and acrochordons, the lesions are present in considerable number mainly on the face and neck. In such cases, the trichodiscomas are clinically indistinguishable from the fibrofolliculomas (Birt et al). In a reported patient with a large connective tissue nevus, fibrofolliculomas were present in large numbers within as well as around the connective tissue nevus.

Multiple trichodiscomas, besides occurring in association with multiple fibrofolliculomas, also occur without them, as small papules either widely disseminated (Pinkus et al) or localized to one area (Grosshans et al).

Histopathology. *Fibrofolliculomas* show in their center a hair follicle that often appears distorted. It is surrounded by a thick mantle of basophilic, mucoid stroma. Numerous thin, anastomosing bands of follicular epithelium extend into this stroma (Birt et al; Weintraub and Pinkus).

Trichodiscomas show in a subepidermal location within a circumscribed area fine fibrillary connective tissue containing thick-walled blood vessels with a small lumen. A hair follicle is usually found at the margin of the lesion (Birt et al). Trichodis-

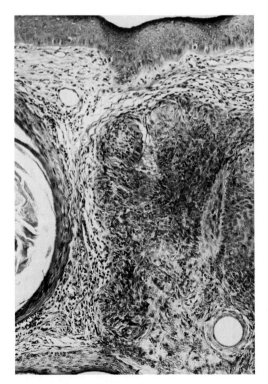

Fig. 27-2.   Trichoepithelioma
The two major components are horn cysts of varying sizes and formations resembling basal cell epithelioma. (×200)

comas are regarded as hamartomas of the mesodermal component of hair disks (Pinkus et al).

The pedunculated acrochordons seen in association with multiple fibrofolliculomas may contain only dermal connective tissue. However, in some instances, they contain thin, anastomosing strands of epithelium; they are then fibrofolliculomas displaying the configuration of an acrochordon (Fujita et al).

TRICHOEPITHELIOMA

The name *trichoepithelioma* is preferable to other designations, such as *epithelioma adenoides cysticum* and *multiple benign cystic epithelioma,* since it indicates that the differentiation in this tumor is directed toward hair structures. Trichoepithelioma occurs either in multiple lesions or as a solitary lesion.

Multiple trichoepithelioma is transmitted as an autosomal dominant trait (Gaul). In most instances, the first lesions appear in childhood and gradually increase in number (Gray and Helwig). One observes numerous rounded, skin-colored, firm papules and nodules usually between 2 mm and 8 mm in size and located mainly in the nasolabial folds but also on the nose, forehead, and upper lip. Occasionally, lesions are seen also on the scalp, neck, and upper trunk. Ulceration of the lesions occurs very rarely, in contrast with basal cell epithelioma and the nevoid basal cell epithelioma syndrome. Transformation into multiple basal cell epitheliomas does not occur (Howell and Anderson), although, in exceptional cases, there may be a solitary, large, ulcerating basal cell epithelioma (Ziprkowski and Schewach-Millet). The simultaneous presence of lesions of trichoepithelioma and cylindroma, the latter of which is also dominantly inherited, has been observed repeatedly (see Cylindroma, p. 548).

Solitary trichoepithelioma occurs more commonly than multiple trichoepitheliomas (Gray and Helwig). It is not inherited and consists of a firm, elevated, flesh-colored nodule usually less than 2 cm in size. Its onset usually is in childhood or early adult life (Zeligman). Most commonly, the lesion is seen on the face, but it may occur elsewhere. The presence within the same tumor of a solitary trichoepithelioma and an apocrine adenoma has been described (Müller-Hess and Delacrétaz).

Histopathology.   As a rule, the lesions of multiple trichoepithelioma appear well circumscribed on histologic examination. Horn cysts represent the most characteristic histologic feature, although they may be absent in some lesions. They consist of a fully keratinized center surrounded by basophilic cells that have the same appearance as the cells in basal cell epithelioma ("basalioma cells") (Fig. 27-2). The keratinization is abrupt and complete, not gradual and incomplete as in the horn pearls of squamous cell carcinoma. Quite frequently, one observes one or a few layers of cells with eosinophilic cytoplasm and large, oval, pale, vesicular nuclei situated between the basophilic cells and the horn cysts (Gray and Helwig).

As the second major component of multiple trichoepitheliomas besides the horn cysts, one finds tumor islands composed of basophilic cells of the same appearance as basalioma cells, arranged usually in a lacelike or adenoid network but occasionally also as solid aggregates. These tumor islands show peripheral palisading of their cells and are surrounded by a stroma with a moderate number of fibroblasts. Both the adenoid and the solid aggregates show invaginations, which contain numerous fibroblasts and thus resemble hair papillae (Fig. 27-3).

Additional findings, observed in some but not all multiple trichoepitheliomas, are the presence of a foreign body giant cell reaction in the vicinity of ruptured horn cysts and of calcium deposits either within the foci of the foreign body reaction or within intact horn cysts (Gray and Helwig).

Occasionally, some lesions in patients with multiple trichoepithelioma show relatively little differentiation toward hair structures. Then they contain only a few horn cysts but many areas with the appearance of basal cell epithelioma (Gray and Helwig). Such lesions are indistinguishable from those of a keratotic basal cell epithelioma, which may also show horn cysts (Fig. 27-4) (see p. 565). Thus, on a histologic basis, no sharp line of demarcation can be drawn between multiple trichoepithelioma and basal cell epithelioma, and, to arrive at a diagnosis in a given case, it may be necessary to have knowledge of clinical data, such as the number and distribution of the lesions and the presence of hereditary transmission.

Solitary trichoepithelioma is used as a histologic designation only for lesions showing a high degree of differentiation toward hair structures. Solitary lesions with relatively little differentiation toward hair structures are best classified as keratotic basal cell epithelioma. Thus, if a lesion is to qualify for the diagnosis of solitary trichoepithelioma, it should contain numerous horn cysts as well as abortive hair papillae and show only few areas with the appearance of basal cell epithelioma (Zeligman).

Histogenesis. It can be assumed that the basophilic cells surrounding horn cysts are analogous to hair matrix cells and that the horn cysts represent attempts at hair shaft formation. The eosinophilic cells seen occasionally around

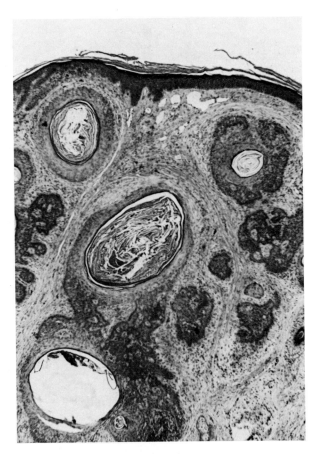

Fig. 27-3. Trichoepithelioma
The walls of the horn cysts in this case are formed by a few layers of cells with eosinophilic cytoplasm and large vesicular nuclei. Some of the basophilic cells are arranged in an adenoid network. (× 100)

horn cysts probably represent cells with initial keratinization and are similar to the nucleated cells seen in normal hair shafts at the keratogenous zone.

Electron microscopic study has confirmed that the horn cysts of trichoepithelioma represent immature hair structures, with abrupt development of the horn cells from hair matrix cells (Kyllönen et al).

Histochemical staining with the Gomori stain for alkaline phosphatase has shown positive staining in many invaginations at the periphery of tumor islands and strands, indicative of a differentiation toward hair papillae (see p. 26) (Kopf).

The close relationship between trichoepithelioma and basal cell epithelioma can be explained on the basis of the assumption that they have a common genesis from pluripotential cells, which, like primary epithelial germ cells, may develop toward hair structures (Lever). Thus, the two types of tumor differ merely in the degree of maturity of their cells. Since cells of various degrees of maturity may occur in the same lesion, one may find in

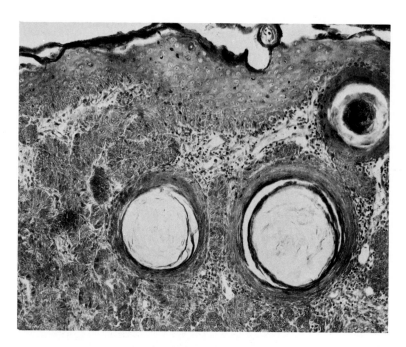

Fig. 27-4. Basal cell epithelioma with horn cysts
Histologically, this tumor is in an intermediate stage of differentiation between basal cell epithelioma and trichoepithelioma. Clinically, the lesion was a basal cell epithelioma. (×200)

trichoepithelioma areas consistent with the histologic picture of basal cell epithelioma and vice versa.

The occasional association of multiple trichoepithelioma with cylindroma, an appendage tumor with differentiation probably toward apocrine structures (see p. 548), and of a solitary trichoepithelioma with an apocrine adenoma (see p. 526) also speaks in favor of the development of trichoepithelioma from immature cells with the potential to differentiate toward primary epithelial germ structures.

Differential Diagnosis. The difficulty of differentiating multiple trichoepithelioma from keratotic basal cell epithelioma on histologic grounds has been pointed out, and the need for clinical data has been stressed.

The differentiation of multiple trichoepithelioma from the nevoid basal cell epithelioma syndrome on histologic grounds can be just as difficult. This, too, often requires clinical data. Although both diseases are dominantly inherited and have multiple lesions, the lesions in trichoepithelioma are present mainly in the nasolabial fold, remain small, and hardly ever ulcerate, whereas the lesions in the nevoid basal cell epithelioma syndrome are haphazardly distributed and, especially in the late, "neoplastic" phase, can grow to considerable size, ulcerate deeply, and show severely destructive growth. In addition, patients with the nevoid basal cell epithelioma syndrome almost invariably show multiple skeletal and central nervous system anomalies and frequently show multiple palmar and plantar pits. (See Nevoid Basal Cell Epithelioma Syndrome, p. 563.)

Desmoplastic Trichoepithelioma

A solitary lesion, desmoplastic trichoepithelioma was formerly considered a solitary trichoepithelioma (Zeligman; Gray and Helwig). However, it has sufficient clinical and histologic characteristics to be regarded as a distinct variant of trichoepithelioma. The term *desmoplastic trichoepithelioma* (Brownstein and Shapiro) appears preferable to the designation *sclerosing epithelial hamartoma* (MacDonald et al), since it stresses the relationship of the lesion to solitary trichoepithelioma.

Clinically, the tumor almost always is located on the face, measures from 3 mm to 8 mm in diameter, and is markedly indurated. In many instances, there is a raised, annular border and a depressed nonulcerated center, causing the lesion to resemble granuloma annulare (Brownstein and Shapiro). Most commonly, the lesion appears in early adulthood, but it quite frequently appears already in the second decade of life (MacDonald et al). It is much more common in females than in males (Brownstein and Shapiro).

Histopathology. The three characteristic histologic features are narrow strands of tumor cells, horn cysts, and a desmoplastic stroma (Fig. 27-5) (Brownstein and Shapiro). The tumor strands usually are from one to three cells thick and are composed of small basaloid cells with prominent oval nuclei and scant cytoplasm. Usually, there are numerous horn cysts, which in some cases are large (Dupré et al). Considerable amounts of densely collagenous and hypocellular stroma are present. Large aggregates of tumor cells are not seen. Foreign body granulomas at the site of ruptured horn cysts and areas of calcification within some of the horn cysts are seen in many tumors.

Differential Diagnosis.   The resemblance of desmoplastic trichoepithelioma to fibrosing basal cell epithelioma is great; however, in fibrosing basal cell epithelioma, horn cysts are absent.

Trichoadenoma

A rare, solitary tumor first described in 1958 (Nikolowski), trichoadenoma usually occurs on the face and varies from 3 mm to 15 mm in diameter. It may arise any time during adult life.

Histopathology.   Numerous horn cysts are present. They are surrounded by eosinophilic cells, which greatly resemble the eosinophilic cells that are often seen in trichoepithelioma located between the basophilic cells and the central horn cysts (Fig. 27-6). In some instances, a single layer of flattened granular cells is interpolated between the horn cysts and the surrounding eosinophilic cells (Rahbari et al; Nikolowski, 1978). Some islands consist only of eosinophilic epithelial cells without central keratinization. Sparse intercellular bridges have been observed between the eosinophilic cells (Nikolowski, 1958). Foci of foreign body granuloma are present at the sites of ruptured horn cysts (Nikolowski, 1958).

Histogenesis.   The general architecture of trichoadenoma greatly resembles that of trichoepithelioma and thus suggests the development of immature hair structures. However, because the cyst wall consists of epidermoid cells and the keratinization may take place with formation of keratohyalin, it has been suggested that the tumor differentiates largely toward the infundibular portion of the pilosebaceous canal (Rahbari et al).

GENERALIZED HAIR FOLLICLE HAMARTOMA

Only two cases have been described of generalized hair follicle hamartoma, a distinctive condition characterized by progressive generalized alopecia starting in adulthood and by diffuse papules and plaques of the face. In

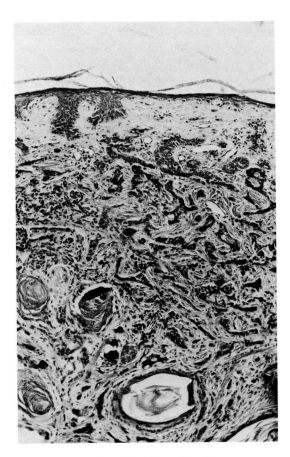

Fig. 27-5.   Desmoplastic trichoepithelioma
The three characteristic features are narrow strands of basaloid tumor cells, horn cysts, and desmoplastic stroma. (×100)

addition, myasthenia gravis was present in both patients (Brown et al; Ridley and Smith).

Histopathology.   The gradually extending hair loss is the result of damage inflicted on each hair follicle by gradually growing "hair follicle hamartomas."

Areas of alopecia without papules or plaques reveal more or less advanced replacement of the hair follicles by solid islands and branching cords of basaloid cells resembling trichoepithelioma (Brown et al).

The papules and plaques of the face show a complete lack of hair structures and extensive proliferations of basaloid cells embedded in a cellular stroma with formation of horn cysts in some areas. Thus, the histologic appearance is indistinguishable from that of trichoepithelioma (Ridley and Smith).

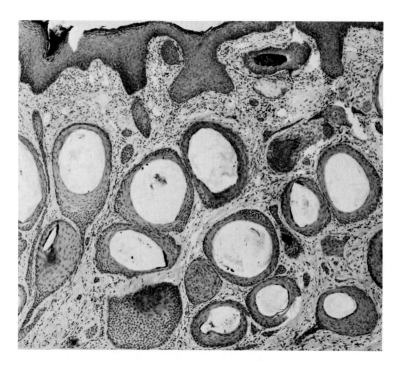

Fig. 27-6. Trichoadenoma
Numerous horn cysts are present surrounded by eosinophilic cells. Some islands consist entirely of eosinophilic epithelial cells. (×100)

PILOMATRICOMA (CALCIFYING EPITHELIOMA)

Pilomatricoma, or calcifying epithelioma of Malherbe, is a tumor with differentiation toward hair cells, particularly hair cortex cells. Most commonly, it manifests itself as a firm, deep-seated nodule that is covered by normal skin. Occasionally, however, the tumor is more superficially located, causing a bluish red discoloration of the overlying skin, and, rarely, it protrudes as a sharply demarcated, dark red nodule (Hadlich and Linse). Pilomatricoma occurs usually as a solitary lesion. The face and the upper extremities are the most common sites. Generally, the tumor varies in size from 0.5 cm to 3 cm, but it may be as large as 5 cm. The tumors may arise in persons of any age, but about 40% of them arise in children under the age of 10, and about 60% in persons in the first two decades of life (Moehlenbeck). Although, as a rule, pilomatricoma is not hereditary, there are a few instances of familial occurrence, and, in some of these cases, the tumor is associated with myotonic dystrophy (Chiaramonti and Gilgor).

Histopathology. The tumor is sharply demarcated and often surrounded by a connective tissue capsule. It is usually located in the lower dermis and extends into the subcutaneous fat. Embedded in a rather cellular stroma, irregularly shaped islands of epithelial cells are present. As a rule, two types of cells, *basophilic cells* and *shadow cells*, compose the islands (Fig. 27-7). In some tumors,

however, basophilic cells are absent. The basophilic cells possess round or elongated, deeply basophilic nuclei and scanty cytoplasm, so that the nuclei lie close together. The cellular borders of the basophilic cells often are indistinct, so that it appears as if the nuclei were embedded in a symplasmic mass. The basophilic cells are arranged either on one side or along the periphery of the tumor islands. In some areas, the transition of basophilic cells into shadow cells is abrupt, whereas in others, the transition is gradual. In areas of gradual transition, one observes cells showing a gradual loss of nuclei and ultimately appearing as faintly eosinophilic, keratinized shadow cells. The shadow cells have a distinct border and possess a central unstained area as a shadow of the lost nucleus. In tumors of recent origin, numerous areas of basophilic cells usually are present. As the lesion ages, the number of basophilic cells decreases, owing to development into shadow cells, and, in tumors of long standing, few or no basophilic cells remain.

In many tumors, small, round, eosinophilic centers of keratinization are seen within areas of basophilic cells or within aggregates of shadow cells. The keratinization within these centers is abrupt and complete (Lever and Griesemer). In some tumors, melanin is present. It is found most commonly in shadow cells or within melanophages of the stroma, but in some instances is seen also

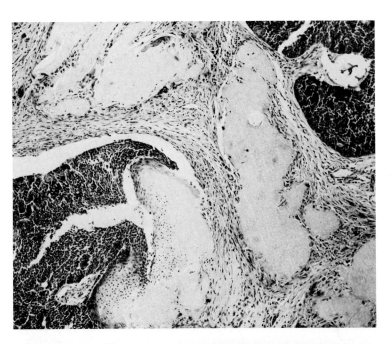

Fig. 27-7. Pilomatricoma (calcifying epithelioma)
The tumor consists of irregularly shaped islands embedded in a rather cellular stroma. Two types of cells compose the islands: basophilic cells and shadow cells. The basophilic cells resemble hair matrix cells. The shadow cells show a central, unstained shadow at the site of the lost nucleus. In the center of the field, one can see transformation of the basophilic cells into shadow cells. The stroma contains numerous multinucleated giant cells. (×100)

Fig. 27-8. Pilomatricoma (calcifying epithelioma)
Small and large areas of calcification are present within the lobules of shadow cells. (×100)

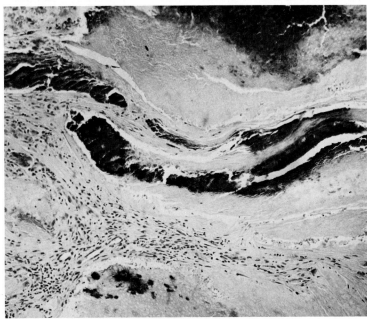

in dendritic melanocytes located in islands of basophilic cells (Cazers et al). The stroma of the tumor usually shows a considerable foreign body giant cell reaction adjacent to the shadow cells.

With the von Kossa stain, calcium deposits are found in approximately three fourths of the tumors (Peterson and Hult). Usually, the calcium is already apparent as deeply basophilic deposits in sections stained with hematoxylin-eosin. Most of the tumors containing calcium are composed largely of shadow cells. The calcium is seen either as fine basophilic granules within the cytoplasm of the shadow cells or as large sheets of amorphous, basophilic material replacing the shadow cells (Fig. 27-8). Occasionally, foci of calcification are seen also in the stroma of the tumors (Forbis and

Helwig). Areas of ossification are seen in 15% to 20% of the cases (Forbis and Helwig; Peterson and Hult). Ossification takes place in the stroma next to areas of shadow cells, probably through metaplasia of fibroblasts into osteoblasts (Fig. 27-9) (Geiser). Calcium-rich shadow cells thereby act as inducing factor (Wiedersberg).

Histogenesis. Calcifying epithelioma was originally described in 1880 as calcified epithelioma of sebaceous glands (Malherbe and Chenantais); however, it was recognized in 1942 that the cells of the tumor differentiate in the direction of hair cortex cells (Turhan and Krainer), a finding that was subsequently confirmed by electron microscopic studies. On this basis, the designation *pilomatricoma* was suggested (Forbis and Helwig).

Histochemical studies have revealed in most tumor cells a strongly positive reaction with the performic acid-Schiff stain for sulfhydryl or disulfide groups. This reaction is indicative of keratinization (Peterson and Hult; Hashimoto et al). As further evidence of keratinization, the shadow cells show strong birefringence in polarized light (Lever and Hashimoto). A very similar birefringence is seen in the keratogenous zone of hair

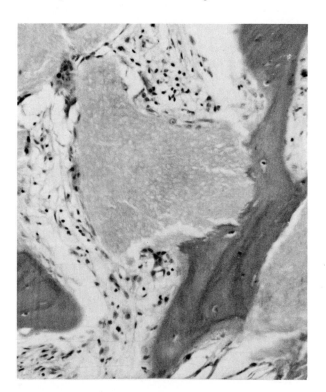

Fig. 27-9. Pilomatricoma (calcifying epithelioma) with ossification
Elongated, irregularly shaped areas of ossification are present in the stroma. In the center, an island of shadow cells is seen. (× 200)

(Forbis and Helwig). Also, the regular presence of citrulline in the cells of pilomatricoma is indicative of the formation of hair keratin rather than of keratin of the type formed in the epidermis (see p. 573) (Holmes).

Electron microscopic examination has revealed a few desmosomes and a moderate number of tonofilaments in the areas of basophilic cells (McGavran). In cells that are in transition to shadow cells, numerous tonofilaments are seen aggregated into thick keratin fibrils. They thus form keratin without the appearance of keratohyaline granules. A striking resemblance exists between cells that are in transition to shadow cells and cells in the keratogenous zone of normal hair, because both types of cells show thick keratin fibrils concentrically arranged around a faintly visible nucleus. Fully developed shadow cells show numerous fused, electron-dense keratin fibrils surrounding the empty nuclear area (Hashimoto et al; Hashimoto and Lever).

Differential Diagnosis.   The wall of trichilemmal cysts also contains basophilic cells, which, as they keratinize, gradually lose their nuclei and often undergo calcification. The peripheral layer of basophilic cells in trichilemmal cysts, however, shows a palisading pattern, whereas the basophilic cells of pilomatricoma do not. Furthermore, shadow cells characterized by a central unstained area at the site of the disintegrated nucleus are seen in no tumor other than pilomatricoma.

Pilomatrix Carcinoma

On rare occasions, pilomatricomas show invasive growth (Lopansri and Mihm; Weedon et al). Such tumors are not necessarily larger than those of benign pilomatricoma but tend to recur after excision. No metastases have been reported.

Histopathology.   Many areas, especially at the periphery of the tumor, show proliferations of large, anaplastic, hyperchromatic basophilic cells with numerous mitoses (Lopansri and Mihm). Toward the center of the tumor, there is transformation of basophilic cells into eosinophilic shadow cells of the type seen in pilomatricomas (Weedon et al).

PROLIFERATING TRICHILEMMAL TUMOR

Proliferating trichilemmal tumor is a solitary tumor referred to also as pilar tumor of the scalp. About 90% of the cases occur on the scalp, with the residual 10% occurring mainly on the back. More than 80% of the patients are women, most of them elderly (Bloch and

Müller). Starting as a subcutaneous nodule suggestive of a wen, the tumor may grow into a large, elevated, lobulated mass that may undergo ulceration. The tumor may occur in association with one or even several trichilemmal cysts of the scalp (Holmes; Korting and Hoede). There is evidence that a proliferating trichilemmal tumor may develop from a trichilemmal cyst (Leppard and Sanderson; Brownstein and Arluk). However, the tumor may also give rise to one or several trichilemmal cysts, which ultimately may separate from it (Hanau and Grosshans). There have been two reported instances of a regional lymph node metastasis (Peden; Holmes). In both instances, the patients were alive and well after 11 years and 5 years, respectively (Leppard and Sanderson).

Histopathology. The tumor usually is well demarcated from the surrounding tissue (Wilson Jones). It is composed of variably sized lobules composed of squamous epithelium. Some of the lobules are surrounded by a vitreous layer and show palisading of their peripheral cell layer (Hanau and Grosshans). Characteristically, the epithelium in the center of the lobules abruptly changes into eosinophilic amorphous keratin (Fig. 27-10). This amorphous keratin is of the same type as that seen in the cavity of trichilemmal cysts (Reed and Lamar). In addition to showing trichilemmal keratinization, some proliferating trichilemmal tumors exhibit changes resembling the keratinization of the follicular infundibulum. These changes consist of epidermoid keratinization resulting in horn pearls, some of which resemble "squamous eddies" (Brownstein and Arluk).

The tumor cells in many areas show a slight degree of nuclear anaplasia, as well as individual cell keratinization, which at first glance suggests a squamous cell carcinoma (Fig. 27-11) (Holmes; Dabska). The tumor differs from a squamous cell carcinoma, however, by its rather sharp demarcation from the surrounding stroma as well as by its abrupt mode of keratinization (Wilson Jones). Foci of calcification, although generally small, are often present in the areas of amorphous keratin (Fig. 27-11) (Wilson Jones; Korting and Hoede). Some tumors show vacuolization or clear cell formation of some of the tumor cells as a result of glycogen storage (Reed and Lamar; Holmes).

Histogenesis. Because all proliferating trichilemmal tumors show the presence of nuclear anaplasia, it has been suggested that they are low-grade carcinomas (Holmes). However, the propensity for regional metastases is so low that, for practical purposes, the tumor can be regarded as biologically benign.

Keratinization in proliferating trichilemmal tumors is of the same type as in trichilemmal cysts (see p. 485). The keratinization in both of these trichilemmal tumors is analogous to that of the outer root sheath as seen normally at the follicular isthmus above the zone of sloughing of the inner root sheath (Pinkus) and in the sac surrounding the lower end of the telogen hair (Holmes; Pinkus). Analogous to the keratinization of the outer root sheath, proliferating trichilemmal tumors show (1) an abrupt change of squamous epithelium into amorphous keratin; (2) vacuolated cells containing glycogen, like the cells of the outer root sheath; and (3) a prominent glassy layer of collagen surrounding some

Fig. 27-10. Proliferating trichilemmal tumor
The tumor is composed of irregularly shaped lobules of squamous epithelium undergoing abrupt change into amorphous keratin. A large area of amorphous keratin is present in the center. (×200)

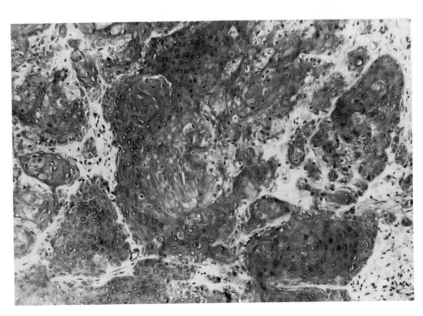

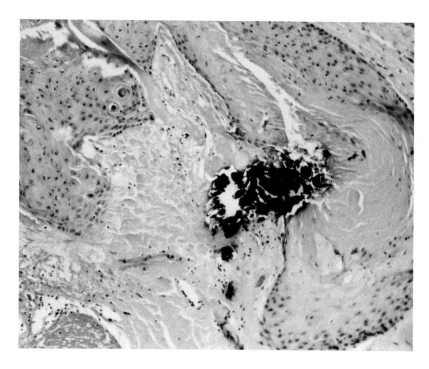

Fig. 27-11.   Proliferating trichilemmal tumor
An area of calcification is present in the center. On the right side, an area of amorphous keratin is seen. On the left, two dyskeratotic cells are located in a lobule of squamous epithelium. (×200)

tumor formations (Reed and Lamar). Focal calcification within the amorphous keratin is a feature that proliferating trichilemmal tumors and trichilemmal cysts have in common.

Differential Diagnosis.   The presence of numerous sharply demarcated areas of amorphous eosinophilic keratin in the center of the tumor strands and lobules usually permits easy differentiation from squamous cell carcinoma.

TRICHILEMMOMA

Trichilemmoma is a fairly common solitary tumor. In addition, multiple facial trichilemmomas are specifically associated with Cowden's disease.

Solitary Trichilemmoma

Solitary trichilemmoma, first recognized as an entity in 1962 (Headington and French), is a small tumor, generally 3 mm to 8 mm in diameter, occurring usually on the face and occasionally on the neck (Brownstein and Shapiro, 1973). It has no characteristic clinical appearance. In some instances, it is found at the base of a cutaneous horn (Brownstein and Shapiro, 1979).

Histopathology.   One or several lobules are seen descending from the surface epidermis into the dermis. In some instances, the lobules are oriented about a central hair-containing follicle (Headington and French). A variable number of tumor cells have the appearance of clear cells owing to their content of glycogen (Fig. 27-12). The periphery of the tumor lobules usually shows palisading of columnar cells and a distinct, often thickened basement membrane zone resembling the vitreous layer surrounding the lower portion of normal hair follicles (Brownstein and Shapiro, 1973). Trichilemmomas do not show the trichilemmal type of keratinization seen in trichilemmal cysts and proliferating trichilemmal tumors. Rather, at the surface, trichilemmomas display epidermoid keratinization, which is frequently pronounced and may even lead to the formation of an overlying cutaneous horn (Brownstein and Shapiro, 1979).

Differential Diagnosis.   In instances with relatively few clear cells and marked hypergranulosis and hyperkeratosis, differentiation from a verruca vulgaris may be difficult. A periodic acid-Schiff (PAS) stain for the demonstration of glycogen may aid in the differentiation. Nevertheless, the view has been expressed that trichilemmomas, both the solitary and the multiple types, represent verrucae vulgares with secondary trichilemmal proliferation of the hair follicle (Ackerman and Wade).

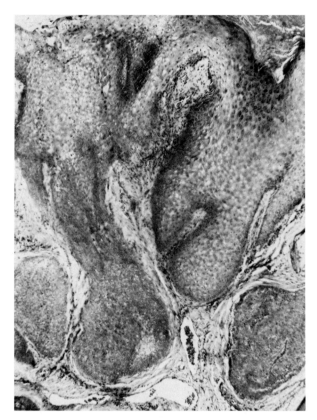

Fig. 27-12. Trichilemmoma
The tumor shows lobular formations extending into the dermis. As a result of their differentiation toward outer root sheath cells, many cells appear clear. (×50)

Fig. 27-13. Tumor of the follicular infundibulum
A platelike growth of pale-staining epithelial cells extends parallel to the epidermis in the upper dermis and shows multiple connections with the epidermis. The peripheral cell layer of the tumor plate shows palisading. (×100)

Multiple Trichilemmomas in Cowden's Disease

Cowden's disease, or multiple hamartoma syndrome, is an autosomal dominant genodermatosis with distinctive cutaneous findings. Recognition of Cowden's disease is important because of the high incidence of breast cancer in women. The multiple trichilemmomas precede the development of breast cancer and thus can identify women with a high risk of developing this cancer (Brownstein et al, 1978). Other visceral malignancies also occasionally occur in Cowden's disease, but most of the internal lesions are fibrous hamartomas, especially of the breasts, thyroid, and gastrointestinal tract (Allen et al).

Multiple trichilemmomas are found in all patients with Cowden's disease (Brownstein et al, 1979). They are limited to the face, where they are found mainly about the mouth, nose, and ears. They consist of flesh-colored, pink, or brown papules that may resemble verrucae vulgares (Thyresson and Doyle). In addition, there may be closely set oral papules, giving the lips, gingiva, and tongue a characteristic "cobblestone" appearance, as well as multiple small acral keratoses.

Histopathology. It may require multiple biopsy specimens to find the diagnostic histologic picture of trichilemmoma in the facial lesions. Thus, in one series, only 29 of 53 facial lesions showed findings consistent with trichilemmoma (Brownstein et al, 1979).

The oral lesions may show a fibromatous nodule composed of relatively acellular fibers patterned in whorls (Weary et al) or fibrovascular tissue with acanthosis (Brownstein et al, 1979).

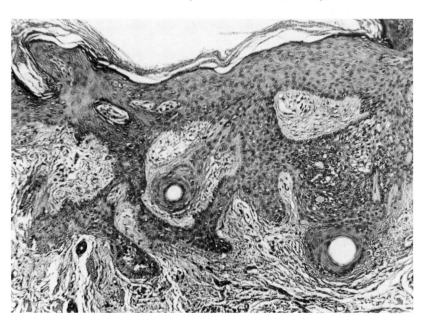

Differential Diagnosis. See Differential Diagnosis under Solitary Trichilemmoma.

TUMOR OF THE FOLLICULAR INFUNDIBULUM

Besides the lobular type of trichilemmoma just described, there is a second type of trichilemmoma. This type, which shows platelike growth, was first described in 1961 as tumor of the follicular infundibulum (Mehregan and Butler). It usually occurs as a solitary flat, keratotic papule on the face (Mehregan). Rarely, multiple papules are present (Johnson and Hookerman).

Histopathology. One finds a platelike growth of epithelial cells in the upper dermis extending parallel to the epidermis and showing multiple connections with the lower margin of the epidermis (Fig. 27-13). The peripheral cell layer of the tumor plate shows palisading, and the centrally located cells show a pale-staining cytoplasm as a result of their content of glycogen. Small hair follicles enter the tumor plate from below and lose their identity and then are no longer recognizable (Mehregan). Along the lower margin of the plate, there may be invaginations that resemble hair papillae (Johnson and Hookerman).

Differential Diagnosis. The platelike growth with multiple connections to the epidermis resembles superficial basal cell epithelioma, which may also show peripheral palisading. However, the cells of the tumor of the follicular infundibulum possess a greater amount of cytoplasm, in which, furthermore, PAS-positive material is present (Chan et al).

Trichilemmocarcinoma

A malignant variant of the tumor of the follicular infundibulum has been described occurring as an extensive ulcerated lesion on the ear (Ten Seldam).

Histopathology. The tumor replaces the surface epidermis with a wide band of tumor cells and shows numerous buds and downward extensions suggesting pilar structures. The tumor cells possess atypical nuclei and clear cytoplasm that, like glycogen, is PAS-positive and diastase-sensitive (Ten Seldam).

TUMORS WITH SEBACEOUS DIFFERENTIATION

NEVUS SEBACEUS

Nevus sebaceus of Jadassohn is as a rule located on the scalp or the face as a single lesion and is present already at birth. In childhood, it consists of a circumscribed, only slightly raised, hairless plaque that is often linear in configuration but may be round or irregularly shaped. In puberty, the lesion becomes verrucous and nodular (Mehregan and Pinkus).

In rare instances, nevus sebaceus consists of multiple extensive plaques not limited to the head. Usually, at least some of the lesions have a linear configuration (Lentz et al). In addition, some patients with extensive nevus sebaceus show as evidence of a "neurocutaneous syndrome" epilepsy and mental retardation (Schimmelpenning; Feuerstein and Mims; Marden and Venters), neurologic defects (Wauschkuhn and Rohde), or skeletal deformities (Hornstein and Knickenberg). In some patients, the linear nevus is partially a linear nevus sebaceus and partially a linear epidermal nevus (Wauschkuhn and Rohde; Hornstein and Knickenberg). Thus, the "neurocutaneous syndrome" that is associated with nevus sebaceus overlaps with the abnormalities associated with the epidermal nevus syndrome, in which skeletal deformities and central nervous system abnormalities may also occur (see p. 473) (Solomon et al). The involvement of the central nervous system that may be seen in extensive cases of both linear nevus sebaceus and linear epidermal nevus closely resembles that of tuberous sclerosis by computed tomography and x-ray studies (see p. 603) (Kuokkanen et al).

Histopathology. The sebaceous glands in nevus sebaceus follow the pattern of normal sebaceous glands during infancy, childhood, and adolescence. In the first few months of life, they are well developed (Steigleder and Cortes; Lantis et al). Thereafter, through childhood, the sebaceous glands in nevus sebaceus are underdeveloped and, therefore, greatly reduced in size and number (Fig. 27-14). Thus, the diagnosis of nevus sebaceus may be missed. However, the presence of incompletely differentiated hair structures is typical of nevus sebaceus. There often are cords of undifferentiated cells resembling the embryonic stage of hair follicles (Mehregan and Pinkus). Some hair

about two thirds of the patients at puberty and sometimes at a younger age (Mehregan and Pinkus; Bourlond et al; Wilson Jones and Heyl). These glands are located deep in the dermis beneath the masses of sebaceous gland lobules (Fig. 27-15).

Quite commonly, in addition to the infantile and adolescent phases, there is a third stage in adulthood during which various types of appendage tumors develop secondarily within lesions of nevus sebaceus. A syringocystadenoma papilliferum has been found in 8% to 19% of the lesions of nevus sebaceus (Wilson Jones and Heyl; Mehregan and Pinkus). Less commonly found appendage tumors include nodular hidradenoma, syringoma, and sebaceous epithelioma (Mehregan and Pinkus). A basal cell epithelioma that is clinically evident has been observed in 5% to 7% of the cases of nevus sebaceus (Fig. 27-16) (Brownstein and Shapiro; Wilson Jones and Heyl). In many

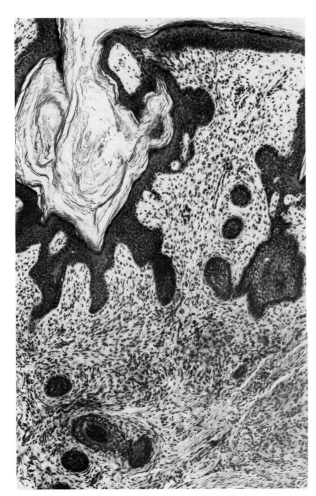

Fig. 27-14. Nevus sebaceus from the scalp of a child
There are two dilated, keratin-filled infundibula showing multiple buds of undifferentiated cells representing malformed hair germs. The dermis contains many fibroblasts and one immature hair structure; sebaceous glands are absent in childhood. (×100) (Courtesy of Benjamin K. Fisher, M.D.)

structures consist of dilated, keratin-filled infundibula showing multiple buds of undifferentiated cells.

At puberty, the lesion assumes its diagnostic histologic appearance. This is brought on by the presence of large numbers of mature or nearly mature sebaceous glands and by papillomatous hyperplasia of the epidermis. The hair structures remain small except for occasional dilated infundibula. There are often buds of undifferentiated cells that resemble foci of basal cell epithelioma and represent malformed hair germs (Wilson Jones and Heyl). Ectopic apocrine glands develop in

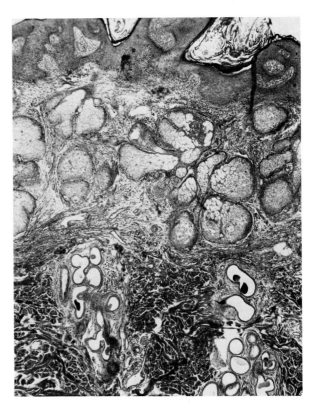

Fig. 27-15. Nevus sebaceus from the scalp of an adult
Hyperkeratosis and papillomatosis are present. Numerous mature sebaceous glands lie in the upper dermis. Mature apocrine glands are located in the lower dermis. (×50)

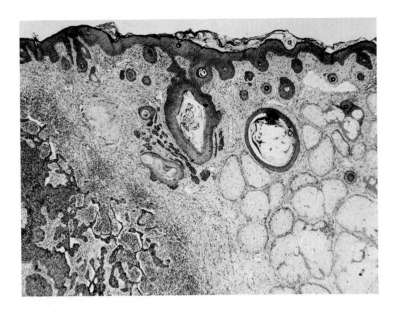

Fig. 27-16. Nevus sebaceus
A basal cell epithelioma has arisen within the lesion. The nevus sebaceus shows numerous tiny hair structures and two large, keratin-filled infundibula. (×25)

instances, however, basal cell epitheliomas are found that are small and clinically not apparent and that show no aggressive growth pattern (Wilson Jones and Heyl). It is not always possible to differentiate histologically between a basal cell epithelioma and "basaloid proliferations" that arise in malformed hair germs and are seen in as many as half of all cases of nevus sebaceus (Brownstein and Shapiro).

In only rare instances does a squamous cell carcinoma develop within a nevus sebaceus. This may be associated either with a regional lymph node metastasis (Schirren and Pfirstinger) or with generalized metastases (Domingo and Helwig). Also, apocrine carcinomas have been seen to develop in nevi sebacei, and they, too, may lead to regional or even generalized metastases (Domingo and Helwig).

Histogenesis. The frequent association of nevus sebaceus with other appendage tumors as well as with apocrine glands suggests that nevus sebaceus is derived from the primary epithelial germ (Haber; Wilson Jones and Heyl). Thus, the development of a basal cell epithelioma in a nevus sebaceus should not be interpreted as malignant degeneration (Michalowski). Rather, it represents a decrease in the degree of differentiation of the primary epithelial germ cells present in the lesion and, as a consequence, an increase in the rate of proliferation (Lever; Schirren and Pfirstinger).

SEBACEOUS HYPERPLASIA

The lesions of sebaceous hyperplasia occur on the face, chiefly on the forehead and cheeks, in persons past middle age. Either one or, more commonly, several elevated, small, soft, yellowish, slightly umbilicated papules are present. Their usual size is 2 mm to 3 mm in diameter.

Histopathology. Most lesions consist of a single greatly enlarged sebaceous gland composed of numerous lobules grouped around a centrally located, wide sebaceous duct (Fig. 27-17). Its opening to the surface corresponds to the central umbilication of the lesion. Serial sections show that all sebaceous lobules grouped around the central duct are connected with that duct (Gilman). Large lesions may consist of several enlarged sebaceous glands and contain several ducts, with sebaceous lobules grouped around each of them (Braun-Falco and Thianprasit). Whereas some sebaceous gland lobules appear fully mature, others show more than one peripheral row of undifferentiated, generative cells in which there are few or no lipid droplets (Luderschmidt and Plewig).

Histogenesis. Labeling with tritiated thymidine has shown that the migration of sebocytes from the basal cell area to the center of the sebaceous lobules and into the sebaceous duct is distinctly slower in cases of sebaceous hyperplasia than in normal sebaceous glands (Luderschmidt and Plewig).

In sebaceous hyperplasia, in contrast to rhinophyma, only one sebaceous gland or, at the most, a few sebaceous glands are enlarged. This makes it appear likely that the lesions of sebaceous hyperplasia represent a hamartoma rather than a hypertrophy, as in rhinophyma.

Differential Diagnosis. In rhinophyma, which also shows large sebaceous glands and ducts, there

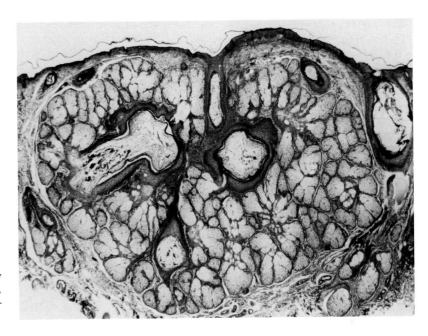

Fig. 27-17.   Sebaceous hyperplasia
The lesion consists of a single, greatly enlarged sebaceous gland with a wide, branching sebaceous duct in the center. (×25)

is no grapelike grouping of the sebaceous lobules around the ducts, and the lesion is not sharply demarcated. In nevus sebaceus, ductal structures are less apparent than in sebaceous hyperplasia, and apocrine glands are often found beneath the sebaceous glands.

FORDYCE'S CONDITION

In Fordyce's condition, groups of minute yellowish globoid lesions are observed on the vermilion border of the lips or on the oral mucosa. The incidence of the disorder increases with age, so that 70% to 80% of elderly persons show such lesions, which represent ectopic sebaceous glands (Miles).

Histopathology.   Each globoid lesion consists of a group of small but mature sebaceous lobules situated around a small sebaceous duct leading to the surface epithelium (Chambers; Miles). Because of the small size of the sebaceous duct, serial sections may be required to demonstrate the presence of the duct.

SEBACEOUS ADENOMA

Sebaceous adenoma represents an organoid tumor of variable size and location possessing no diagnostic clinical features. Up to 1968, sebaceous adenoma was regarded as a rare solitary tumor, and there were few publications about it (Woolhandler and Becker; Lever; Groterjahn; Essenhigh et al).

Torre's Syndrome.   Since 1968, when the first publication appeared concerning the coexistence of *multiple sebaceous tumors* and usually *multiple visceral carcinomas* (Torre), at least 15 reports have been published (12 of them reviewed by Housholder and Zeligman) in which this coexistence, now known as *Torre's syndrome* (Housholder and Zeligman; Schwartz et al) or the *Muir–Torre syndrome* (Worret et al; Fahmy et al), is described. However, only 21 of the 23 patients described in the 15 publications had multiple sebaceous tumors; two had only solitary sebaceous adenomas on the scalp and an ear, respectively (Sciallis and Winkelmann; Housholder and Zeligman). All patients with multiple sebaceous tumors had multiple sebaceous adenomas, but most of them also had other types of sebaceous tumors, such as sebaceous epithelioma, sebaceous hyperplasia, and, in four instances, sebaceous carcinoma (Housholder and Zeligman). However, all four tumors classified as sebaceous carcinoma remained localized and did not metastasize (Torre; Leonard and Deaton; Housholder and Zeligman; Worret et al). In addition, keratoacanthomas, often multiple, were frequently present (Housholder and Zeligman). All patients had lesions on the head, but most patients also had lesions on the trunk (Leonard and Deaton).

Some authors have included in Torre's syndrome cases of patients who had no sebaceous tumors but only multiple keratoacanthomas in association with multiple visceral malignancies (Poleksic; Stewart et al). The frequent coexistence of sebaceous tumors and keratoacanthomas in Torre's syndrome is explained by the fact that both types of tumors are derived from pilosebaceous follicles (Woret et al).

The multiple visceral carcinomas generally are of low-grade malignancy and, with rare exceptions, do not metastasize (Rulon and Helwig). Although a malignant visceral tumor precedes the development of the cutaneous lesions in most instances, the cutaneous lesions appear first in some patients and then suggest the existence of Torre's syndrome. Torre's syndrome is also occasionally associated with a family history of carcinoma (Lynch et al).

Histopathology. On histologic examination, sebaceous adenoma is sharply demarcated from the surrounding tissue (Woolhandler and Becker). It is composed of incompletely differentiated sebaceous lobules that are irregular in size and shape (Fig. 27-18) (Groterjahn; Housholder and Zeligman). Two types of cells are present in the lobules. The cells of the first type are identical to the cells present at the periphery of normal sebaceous glands and represent undifferentiated germinative cells. The cells of the second type are mature sebaceous cells (Schwartz et al). In addition, there often are some cells in a transitional stage between these two types. Distribution of the germinative and sebaceous cells within the lobules varies. Some lobules contain predominantly germinative cells. Other lobules contain mainly sebaceous cells and thereby resemble mature sebaceous lobules. In most lobules, however, the two types of cells occur in approximately equal proportions, often arranged in such a way that groups of sebaceous cells are surrounded by germinative cells (Lever). Fat stains reveal the presence of lipid material in the seba-

ceous and transitional cells. Some large lobules contain cystic spaces in their center formed by the disintegration of mature sebaceous cells. Also, there may be foci of squamous epithelium with keratinization (Essenhigh et al). These foci probably represent areas with differentiation toward sebaceous duct structures.

Differential Diagnosis. In degree of differentiation, sebaceous adenoma stands between sebaceous hyperplasia (see p. 538), in which the sebaceous lobules appear fully or nearly fully matured, and sebaceous epithelioma (see below), in which the tumor is composed not of lobules but of irregularly shaped cell masses and the percentage of tumor cells with differentiation to sebaceous cells is far less than 50%.

SEBACEOUS EPITHELIOMA

Clinically, sebaceous epitheliomas have the appearance of basal cell epitheliomas and may show ulceration (Zackheim). Some of the lesions possess a yellowish color. Usually, they occur on the face or the scalp as solitary lesions. In one reported instance, however, a lesion was located on the sole of the foot (Raab). In addition to occurring as a primary lesion, a sebaceous epithelioma occasionally arises within a nevus sebaceus

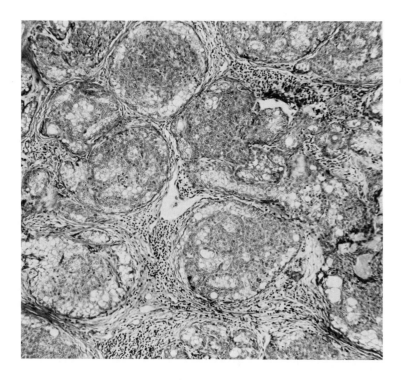

Fig. 27-18. Sebaceous adenoma
The tumor is composed of lobules of irregular size and shape. In the lobules, two types of cells can be recognized: generative and sebaceous. (×100)

(Zackheim; Mehregan and Pinkus; Wilson Jones and Heyl). Sebaceous epitheliomas may also be found among the multiple sebaceous neoplasms that occur in association with multiple visceral carcinomas and are referred to as Torre's syndrome (see p. 539).

Histopathology.   Sebaceous epithelioma, in contrast to sebaceous adenoma, is not a well-circumscribed tumor but rather grows in irregularly shaped cell masses (Fig. 27-19). Thus, it grows like a basal cell epithelioma, but its cells have undergone considerable differentiation toward sebaceous cells (McMullan). As a rule, the majority of cells are undifferentiated cells that, when arranged in a palisade fashion at the periphery of a cell mass, resemble the germinative cells of sebaceous glands but, when lying in aggregates, are indistinguishable from the cells of a basal cell epithelioma (McMullan; Urban and Winkelmann). In addition, there is a fairly large number of transitional cells showing beginning fatty vacuolization of the cytoplasm. Groups of mature sebaceous cells lie in the center of most cell masses. Cysts formed by the disintegration of cells and filled with amorphous material may be present in some of the tumor masses (Urban and Winkelmann).

Histogenesis.   In degree of differentiation, sebaceous epithelioma stands between sebaceous adenoma, in which there are typical sebaceous lobules, and a certain type of cystic basal cell epithelioma that represents a basal cell epithelioma with only slight differentiation toward sebaceous cells (see p. 566).

It is generally agreed that, in sebaceous adenoma, three types of cells are present: germinative cells of sebaceous glands, sebaceous cells, and cells transitional between these two types (see p. 540). It appears likely that, in sebaceous epithelioma, in addition to these three types of cells, also cells of lower differentiation are present, approximating the cells seen in basal cell epithelioma (Lever; McMullan; Raab; Urban and Winkelmann; Rulon and Helwig). In the view of some authors, however, sebaceous epitheliomas originate from germinative cells of sebaceous glands, which are thus the

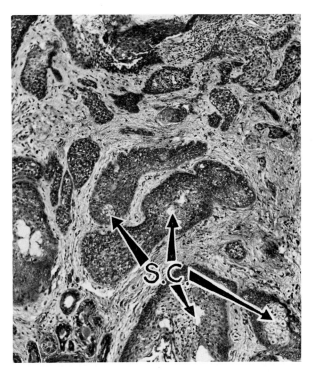

Fig. 27-19.   Sebaceous epithelioma
The tumor is composed of irregularly shaped cell masses. The majority of cells are of the same type as in basal cell epithelioma, but many cells show differentiation toward sebaceous cells (*S.C.*). (×100)

least differentiated cells found in sebaceous epithelioma (Zackheim; Niizuma; Hori et al). In two electron microscopic studies, no cells with lower differentiation than germinative cells were seen (Niizuma; Hori et al); it is possible, however, that the two tumors studied were sebaceous adenomas.

Differential Diagnosis.   For a discussion of differentiation of sebaceous epithelioma from sebaceous carcinoma, which may cause metastases, see p. 575.

TUMORS WITH APOCRINE DIFFERENTIATION

APOCRINE NEVUS

Large numbers of mature apocrine secretory lumina are frequently present in scalp lesions of nevus sebaceus (see p. 537) and syringocystadenoma papilliferum (see p. 544). Pure apocrine nevi, however, are very rare. The

few reported cases have had no uniform clinical appearance. In two cases, a small nodule was present on the scalp (Civatte et al); in one case, a soft mass was found in each axilla (Rabens et al); and, in still another case, multiple firm papules were seen in the sternal region (Vakilzadeh et al).

Histopathology. In all cases, numerous mature apocrine glands were seen, situated largely in the reticular layer of the dermis but extending into the subcutis (Rabens et al; Vakilzadeh et al). In one case, basaloid proliferations of the epidermis were also seen (Civatte et al).

APOCRINE HIDROCYSTOMA

Apocrine hidrocystoma occurs usually as a solitary translucent nodule of cystic consistency. The size varies between 3 mm and 15 mm (Mehregan). Quite frequently, instead of being skin-colored, the lesion has a bluish hue and then resembles a blue nevus. The usual location of apocrine hidrocystoma is on the face, but it is occasionally seen on the ears, scalp, chest, or shoulders (Smith and Chernosky; Benisch and Peison). Multiple apocrine hidrocystomas are only rarely encountered (Smith and Chernosky; Kruse et al). Lesions described as occurring on the penis have been reclassified as median raphe cysts (see p. 488) (Asarch et al).

Histopathology. The dermis contains one or several large cystic spaces into which papillary projections often extend. The inner surface of the wall and the papillary projections are lined by a row of secretory cells of variable height showing "decapitation" secretion indicative of apocrine secretion (Fig. 27-20). Peripheral to the layer of secretory cells are elongated myoepithelial cells, their long axes running parallel to the cyst wall (Smith and Chernosky). In some cases, one finds superficially located lumina lined by a double layer of ductal epithelium in addition to the cysts lined by secretory cells (Mehregan).

Histogenesis. The apocrine nature of the secretion of the luminal cells has been proved not only by the presence of numerous large PAS-positive, diastase-resistant granules in the secretory cells (Mehregan) but also by electron microscopy.

Electron microscopic examination shows abundant secretory granules of moderate density and uniform internal structure in the secretory cells of apocrine hidrocystoma, particularly in their luminal portion (Gross; Hassan et al). Although some secretory granules are discharged by merocrine secretion, there is also apocrine decapitation secretion (Hassan et al) just as seen in normal apocrine secretory cells (see p. 24) (Schaumburg-Lever and Lever). During decapitation secretion, a large, apical cap forms, followed first by the formation of a dividing membrane at the base of the cap and then by the separation of the apical cap from the rest of the cell. During the process of separation, two new cell membranes form above the dividing membrane: one at the base of the apical cap, and one along the upper border of the remaining portion of the cell. Numerous secretory granules are seen within the detaching apical cap (Hassan et al).

The bluish color seen in some of the cysts is not fully explained. According to some authors, it is a Tyndall effect caused by the scattering of light in a colloidal

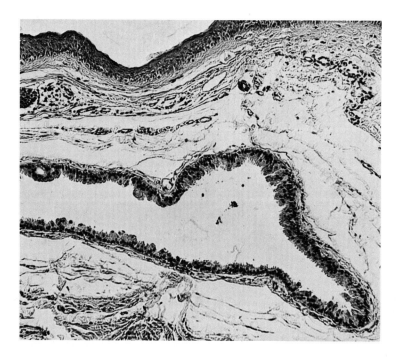

Fig. 27-20. Apocrine hidrocystoma
The dermis contains a cyst lined by a row of secretory cells showing secretion of the apocrine type, so-called decapitation secretion. Peripheral to the row of secretory cells are elongated myoepithelial cells. (×100)

system and the resultant reflection of blue light (Smith and Chernosky; Kruse et al). There are only occasional cases in which the fluid contained in the cysts is brownish. It has been postulated that this fluid may be lipofuscin (Cramer). Although the presence of hemosiderin and melanin has been excluded by several authors (Mehregan), melanocytes have been identified in the cyst wall in one case (Bhawan et al). The bluish color has also been attributed to the presence of extravasated erythrocytes in the surrounding stroma (Hashimoto and Lever).

The apocrine hidrocystoma can be regarded as an adenoma rather than as a retention cyst because the secretory cells do not appear flattened, as they would be in a retention cyst, and because papillary projections extend into the lumen of the cystic spaces (Mehregan).

Differential Diagnosis.   Eccrine hidrocystomas, which are lined by ductal cells, differ from apocrine hidrocystomas by the absence of decapitation secretion, of PAS-positive granules, and of myoepithelial cells (see p. 550). However, those portions of an apocrine hidrocystoma in which the cystic spaces are lined by ductal epithelium have the same appearance as the cystic spaces in eccrine hidrocystomas, except that the latter usually are unilocular, whereas apocrine hidrocystomas are often multilocular. Median raphe cysts of the penis, which have been mistakenly reported as apocrine hidrocystomas, show a pseudostratified columnar cyst wall without evidence of decapitation secretion and without a row of myoepithelial cells (Asarch et al).

HIDRADENOMA PAPILLIFERUM

Hidradenoma papilliferum occurs only in women, usually on the labia majora or in the perineal or perianal region. In rare instances, it has occurred on the nipple (Tappeiner and Wolff) and on the upper eyelid (Santa Cruz et al). The tumor usually is covered by normal skin and measures only a few millimeters in diameter. Malignant changes have been reported in only one patient, in whom a metastasizing, fatal squamous cell carcinoma developed within a perianally located hidradenoma papilliferum (Shenoy).

Histopathology.   The tumor represents an adenoma with apocrine differentiation (Meeker et al). It is located in the dermis, is well circumscribed, is surrounded by a fibrous capsule, and, in most instances, shows no connection with the overlying epidermis. Some tumors have a peripheral epithelial wall showing areas of keratinization (Hashimoto). Within the tumor, one observes tubular and cystic structures (Fig. 27-21). Papillary folds

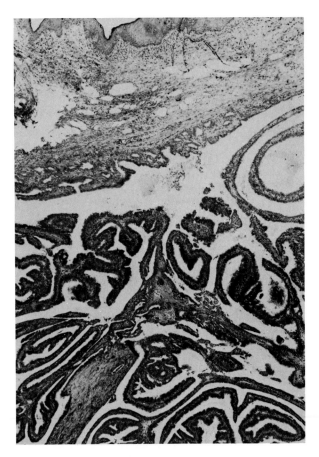

Fig. 27-21.   Hidradenoma papilliferum
Low magnification. The tumor consists of a large cystic space. Numerous papillary folds project into the cystic lumen. (×50)

project into the cystic spaces. The lumina are lined occasionally with only a single row of columnar cells, which show an oval, pale-staining nucleus located near the base, a faintly eosinophilic cytoplasm, and active decapitation secretion as seen in the secretory cells of apocrine glands (Fig. 27-22). Usually, however, the lumina are surrounded by a double layer of cells consisting not only of a luminal layer of secretory cells but also of an outer layer of small cuboidal cells with deeply basophilic nuclei. These represent myoepithelial cells (Tappeiner and Wolff; Hashimoto).

Histogenesis.   The apocrine nature of the secretion in hidradenoma papilliferum has been established by histochemical, enzyme histochemical, and electron microscopic examinations.

Histochemically, the luminal cells contain many large, PAS-positive, diastase-resistant granules as encountered

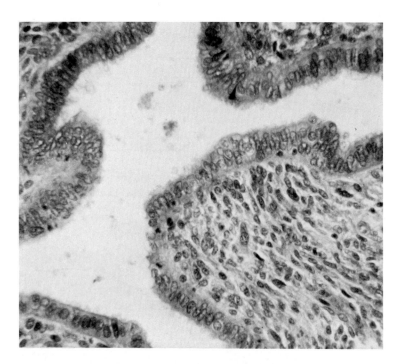

Fig. 27-22.   Hidradenoma papilliferum
High magnification of Figure 27-21. The papillary folds are lined by one layer of high cylindric cells, which show evidence of active "decapitation" secretion like that seen in apocrine glands. (×400)

in the secretory cells of apocrine glands. In addition, the luminal cells are positive for nonspecific esterase and acid phosphatase, the so-called apocrine enzymes, and negative for phosphorylase, a typical eccrine enzyme. Furthermore, the outer row of cells stains positive for alkaline phosphatase, as myoepithelial cells normally do (Tappeiner and Wolff).

Electron microscopic examination shows in the luminal cells two features that are regarded as characteristic of the secretory cells of apocrine glands. First, numerous membrane-limited, secretory granules that are of varying size and density and that contain lipid droplets are present in the apical portion of these cells (Tappeiner and Wolff). Second, as evidence of decapitation secretion, portions of apical cytoplasm containing large secretory granules are released into the lumen (Hashimoto). The peripheral layer of cells contains numerous myofilaments.

SYRINGOCYSTADENOMA PAPILLIFERUM

Syringocystadenoma papilliferum occurs most commonly on the scalp or the face. However, in about one fourth of the cases, it is seen elsewhere (Helwig and Hackney). It is usually first noted at birth or in early childhood and consists of either one papule or several papules in a linear arrangement (Rostan and Waller), or of a solitary plaque. The lesion increases in size at puberty, becoming papillomatous and often crusted (Pinkus). On the scalp, syringocystadenoma papilliferum frequently arises around puberty within a nevus sebaceus that has been present since birth (see p. 537).

Histopathology.   The epidermis shows varying degrees of papillomatosis. One or several cystic invaginations extend downward from the epidermis (Fig. 27-23). The upper portion of the invaginations and, in some instances, large segments of the cystic invaginations are lined by squamous, keratinizing cells similar to those of the surface epidermis (Hashimoto). In the lower portion of the cystic invaginations, numerous papillary projections extend into the lumina of the invaginations. The papillary projections and the lower portion of the invaginations are lined by glandular epithelium often consisting of two rows of cells (Fig. 27-24). The luminal row of cells consists of high columnar cells with oval nuclei and faintly eosinophilic cytoplasm. Occasionally, some of these cells show active decapitation secretion, and cellular debris is found in the lumina (Lever; Fusaro and Goltz; Krinitz). The outer row of cells consists of small cuboidal cells with round nuclei and scanty cytoplasm. In some areas, the cells of the luminal layer are arranged in multiple layers and form a lacelike pattern resulting in multiple small, tubular lumina (Fig. 27-24) (Helwig and Hackney).

Beneath the cystic invaginations, deep in the dermis, one can find in many cases groups of tubular glands with large lumina (Fig. 27-25). The cells lining the large lumina often show evidence of active decapitation secretion (Fig. 27-26), suggesting that they are apocrine glands (Lever; Appel;

Grund; Pinkus; Krinitz). Connections of the apocrine glands deep in the dermis with the cystic invaginations in the upper dermis can be traced when step sections are carried out (Lever; Krinitz).

A highly diagnostic feature is the almost invariable presence of a fairly dense cellular infiltrate composed almost entirely of plasma cells in the stroma of this tumor, especially in the papillary projections.

Frequently, one finds malformed sebaceous glands and hair structures in the lesions of syringocystadenoma papilliferum (Pinkus). In about one third of the cases, syringocystadenoma papilliferum is associated with a nevus sebaceus. In about one tenth of the cases, a basal cell epithelioma develops, but this is noted only in lesions that also exhibit a nevus sebaceus (Helwig and Hackney).

Histogenesis. There is no unanimity about the direction of differentiation in syringocystadenoma papilliferum. On the basis of light microscopic examinations alone, many authors have concluded that this lesion is an apocrine tumor because of the occasional presence of decapitation secretion in some of the luminal cells of the tumor (Lever; Fusaro and Goltz; Krinitz) and the frequent presence of tubular glands with large lumina and decapitation secretion beneath the tumor (Lever; Appel; Grund; Pinkus; Krinitz). The possibility has been conceded, however, that, in some lesions of syringocystadenoma papilliferum in which there are no apocrine glands in the deep dermis, the papilliferous structures represent eccrine proliferations (Pinkus). It has also been suggested that, under pathologic conditions, apparent decapitation secretion in the glands deep in the dermis cannot be taken as unequivocal evidence that the lesion is basically of apocrine origin, and the fact that 90% of all lesions occur on body surfaces, where apocrine glands normally do not occur, would also favor the theory of an eccrine derivation (Helwig and Hackney). However, the latter argument is not valid if it is assumed that, rather than arising from mature structures, syringocystadenoma papilliferum arises from pluripotential cells with the potential to develop into primary epithelial germ structures. It may also be pointed out that apocrine hidrocystoma generally arises on the face, an area in which apocrine glands normally do not occur.

So far, only two *electron microscopic studies* have been published on syringocystadenoma papilliferum, with contradictory results. One tumor proved to be eccrine in its differentiation (Hashimoto). Although composed largely of ductal structures, it showed two types of secretory cells, light and dark, like the secretory cells of eccrine glands. The secretory granules in the dark secretory cells, in contrast to apocrine secretory granules, were small and did not coalesce. None of the cuboidal cells showed myofilaments. The other tumor, however, showed differentiation toward both intrafollicular and

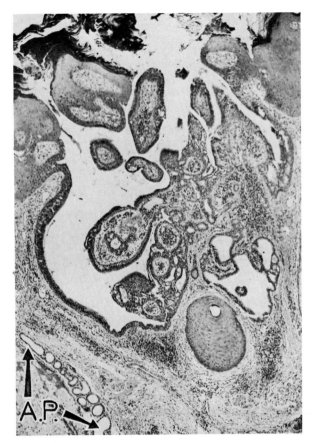

Fig. 27-23. Syringocystadenoma papilliferum
Low magnification. A cystic invagination extends downward from the epidermis. Numerous papillary projections extend into the lumen of the cystic invagination. A group of aprocrine glands (*A.P.*) is present in the left lower corner. (×50)

intradermal ducts of embryonic apocrine sweat glands (Niizuma).

Histochemical studies have been similarly inconclusive. In several instances, the luminal cells lining the villi have given a positive Turnbull blue reaction for iron, which is suggestive of apocrine glands (Pinkus). The presence of large amounts of PAS-positive, diastase-resistant material throughout the luminal cells, and of alcian-blue-positive material in their apical portion, also favors apocrine differentiation (Fusaro and Goltz). So far, only two "preliminary" enzyme histochemical studies have been published (Hashimoto and Lever; Landry and Winkelmann). In the first study, the presence of phosphorylase and succinic dehydrogenase activity suggested eccrine differentiation. In the second study, phosphorylase activity was absent except for a few foci, a factor in favor of apocrine differentiation.

In conclusion, the view expressed by Pinkus probably is correct that, although most lesions of syringocystad-

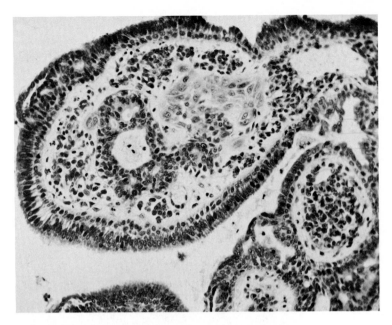

Fig. 27-24. Syringocystadenoma papilliferum
High magnification of Figure 27-23. The papillary projections are lined by two rows of cells. The luminal row of cells consists of columnar cells with evidence of active "decapitation" secretion like that seen in apocrine glands. The outer row of cells consists of small, cuboidal cells. (×200)

enoma papilliferum are apocrine in differentiation, some are eccrine. The differentiation in either case may be predominantly ductal or secretory.

TUBULAR APOCRINE ADENOMA

First described in 1972 (Landry and Winkelmann), six additional cases of tubular apocrine adenoma have been reported since (Umbert and Winkelmann; Civatte et al; Okun et al, case 2). The 14 cases described in 1977 by Rulon and Helwig under the designation *papillary eccrine adenoma* have the same histologic appearance as that described for tubular apocrine adenoma and thus can be regarded as identical with it (Civatte et al).

This tumor consists of a well-defined nodule without any typical location. Most tumors have a smooth surface and are under 2 cm in size, although one reported lesion located on the scalp measured 7 cm by 4 cm (Landry and Winkelmann), and another on the back 4 cm by 3 cm (Civatte).

Histopathology. The characteristic feature of this tumor is the presence of numerous irregularly shaped tubular structures that are usually lined by two layers of epithelial cells. The peripheral layer consists of cuboidal or flattened cells, whereas the luminal layer is composed of columnar cells (Landry and Winkelmann). Some of the tubules have a dilated lumen with papillary projections extending into it (Umbert and Winkelmann; Rulon and Helwig). Decapitation secretion of the luminal cells is seen in many areas (Landry and Winkelmann; Okun et al). In addition, cellular fragments are seen in some lumina (Umbert and Winkelmann; Rulon and Helwig; Civatte et al).

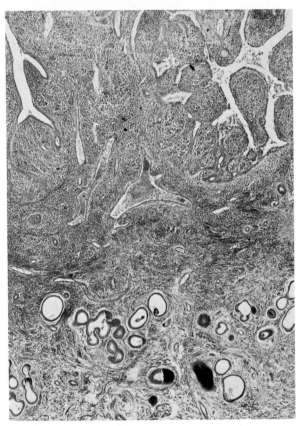

Fig. 27-25. Syringocystadenoma papilliferum
Low magnification. In the upper dermis, numerous papillary projections extend into cystic spaces. A marked inflammatory infiltrate containing many plasma cells is present around the cystic invaginations. The lower dermis contains numerous apocrine glands. (×50)

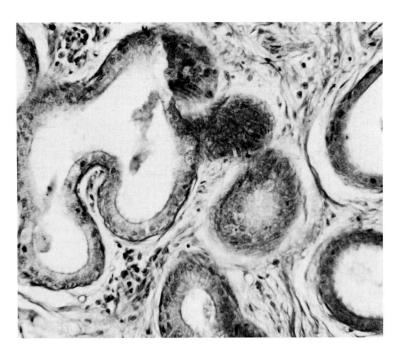

Fig. 27-26. Syringocystadenoma papilliferum
High magnification of Figure 27-25. The secretory cells of the apocrine cells show evidence of active "decapitation" secretion. (×400)

Histogenesis. *Electron microscopy* has revealed secretory granules in the luminal cells. Some of the granules are of considerable size and contain lipid droplets (Landry and Winkelmann). Some of the luminal cells show decapitation secretion with formation of an apical cap and an underlying dividing membrane (Umbert and Winkelmann), as seen in apocrine secretory cells (see p. 24). In contrast to hidradenoma papilliferum, the peripheral cell layer contains no myofilaments.

Enzyme histochemistry has indicated the absence of phosphorylase, an eccrine enzyme, and the presence of indoxyl esterase and acid phosphatase, two apocrine enzymes (Landry and Winkelmann).

Differential Diagnosis. In tubular apocrine adenomas with marked papillary proliferations, there may be some nuclear pleomorphism, which is suggestive either of a "sweat gland carcinoma" (Rulon and Helwig) or of a metastatic adenocarcinoma (Umbert and Winkelmann; Okun et al). However, the presence of a peripheral layer of cuboidal or flattened cells is a feature favoring benignity (Okun et al).

EROSIVE ADENOMATOSIS OF THE NIPPLE

Erosive adenomatosis of the nipple represents an adenoma of the major nipple ducts. In the early stage, the nipple appears eroded and inflamed and often shows a serous discharge. During this early erosive phase, clinical differentiation from Paget's disease of the breast may be impossible (Lewis et al; Smith and Wilson Jones; Undeutsch and Nikolowski). At a later stage, when the nipple shows nodular thickening, differentiation from Paget's disease is easy (Lewis et al).

Histopathology. Extending downward from the epidermis are irregular, dilated tubular structures greatly resembling those seen in tubular apocrine adenoma (see p. 546). The tubules are lined by a peripheral layer of cuboidal cells and a luminal layer of columnar cells that in some areas show secretory projections at their luminal border (Smith and Wilson Jones; Marsch and Nürnberger). Within some of the tubules are papillary projections of the luminal cells into the lumen (Lewis et al; Undeutsch and Nikolowski). This proliferation of cells may be so pronounced as to nearly fill the entire lumen (Smith et al; Albrecht-Nebe et al). In other areas, detached, partially necrotic cells may be seen in the tubular lumina (Undeutsch and Nikolowski). In some lesions, considerable acanthosis of the epidermis is seen, with extension of squamous epithelium into some of the superficial ductal structures (Smith and Wilson Jones; Undeutsch and Nikolowski).

Differential Diagnosis. Erosive adenomatosis of the nipple must be differentiated from intraductal carcinoma, which shows larger cuboidal cells and atypicality of the nuclei (Undeutsch and Nikolowski).

CYLINDROMA

Cylindroma represents a tumor in which differentiation is probably in most cases in the direction of apocrine structures but is in some instances toward eccrine structures (see Histogenesis). It occurs at least as commonly as a solitary lesion as it does as multiple lesions (Crain and Helwig). Cases with multiple lesions are dominantly inherited and show numerous dome-shaped, smooth nodules of various sizes on the scalp. Occasionally, scattered nodules are also present on the face and, in rare instances, on the trunk and the extremities (Kleine-Natrop; Baden). The lesions begin to appear in early adulthood and increase in number and size throughout life. They vary in size from a few millimeters to several centimeters. Nodules on the scalp may be present in such large numbers as to cover the entire scalp like a turban. For this reason, they are referred to occasionally as *turban tumors*.

Cylindromas occasionally undergo malignant degeneration. Eight cases are on record. Autopsy revealed visceral metastases in three patients with multiple cylindromas (Luger; Gertler; Korting et al) and in one patient with solitary cylindroma (Bourlond et al). In one patient, death was assumed to be due to visceral metastases (Greither and Rehrmann). One patient had multiple metastases to superficial lymph nodes (Lausecker). In one patient, the malignant degeneration led to invasion

of the skull and a fatal hemorrhage (Zontschew), and in another to invasion of the brain and a fatal meningitis (Lyon and Rouillard).

The association of multiple lesions of cylindroma with multiple lesions of trichoepithelioma is quite common (Lausecker; Guggenheim and Schnyder; Crain and Helwig; Bandmann et al; Welch et al; Gottschalk et al; Headington et al; Knoth). In cases with such association, the lesions of the scalp are cylindromas, and those elsewhere are partially cylindromas and partially trichoepitheliomas. The association of these two types of tumors, both of which are dominantly inherited, is also of interest in regard to their histogenesis (see below).

Solitary cylindromas are not inherited; they appear in adulthood and occur either on the scalp or the face. Their histologic appearance is the same as that of multiple cylindromas (Crain and Helwig).

Histopathology. The tumors of cylindroma are composed of numerous islands of epithelial cells. Varying considerably in size and shape and lying close together, separated often only by their hyaline sheath and a narrow band of collagen, the islands of epithelial cells seem to fit together like pieces of a jigsaw puzzle (Fig. 27-27). The hyaline sheath surrounding the tumor islands, like a cylinder, is quite variable in thickness. In addition, droplets

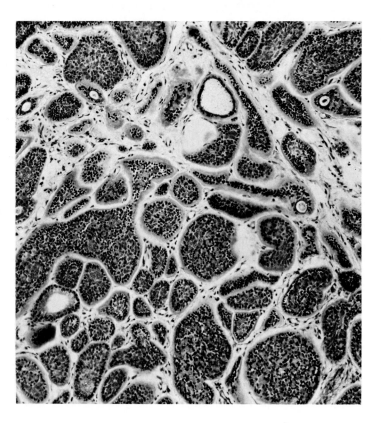

Fig. 27-27. Cylindroma
Low magnification. The tumor is composed of irregularly shaped islands that fit together like pieces of a jigsaw puzzle. The islands are surrounded by a hyaline sheath. Several islands in the lower right quadrant contain droplets of hyalin. (×75)

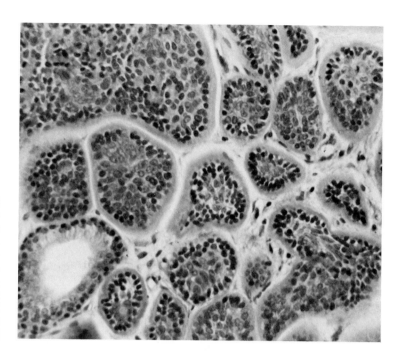

Fig. 27-28. Cylindroma
High magnification of Figure 27-27. Two types of epithelial cells compose the islands. There are cells with small, dark nuclei, representing undifferentiated cells, and cells with large, pale nuclei, representing cells with a certain degree of differentiation toward ductal or secretory cells. In the lower left corner, a glandular lumen is lined by two rows of cells. The cells of the inner row show active secretion, like the secretory cells of apocrine glands. (×200)

of hyalin are present in many islands, and some islands consist largely of hyalin and contain only a few cells. The hyalin is PAS-positive and diastase-resistance and does not stain with alcian blue, indicating that it contains only neutral and no acid mucopolysaccharides (Fusaro and Goltz).

Two types of cells constitute the islands: cells with small, dark-staining nuclei are present predominantly at the periphery of the islands, often in a palisade arrangement, and cells with large, light-staining nuclei lie in the center of the islands (Fig. 27-28). In addition, tubular lumina are often present. In some cases, they are quite numerous, whereas, in others, only a few are found after a thorough search. The lumina are lined by cells that usually have the appearance of ductal cells (Urbach et al). Occasionally, however, the luminal cells show active secretion, like the secretory cells of apocrine glands (Fig. 27-28) (Lever). Often, amorphous material is found within the lumina; it contains both neutral and acid mucopolysaccharides, as shown by the fact that it stains positively both with the PAS reaction and with alcian blue (Fusaro and Goltz).

In the eight reported cases of malignant degeneration occurring in lesions of cylindroma, the areas of malignant degeneration were characterized by islands of cells showing marked anaplasia and pleomorphism of the nuclei, many atypical mitotic figures, loss of the hyaline sheath, loss of palisading

at the periphery, and invasion into the surrounding tissue (Lyon and Rouillard; Bourland; Greither and Rehrmann).

Histogenesis. No agreement exists about whether the direction of differentiation in cylindroma is eccrine or apocrine. Histochemical and enzyme histochemical examinations have not led to clear-cut conclusions, although electron microscopic findings are somewhat in favor of apocrine differentiation.

The fact that the amorphous material within the tubular lumina contains neutral as well as acid mucopolysaccharides allows no conclusion, since both the mucoid secretory cells of eccrine glands and the apocrine secretory cells excrete granules containing neutral and acid mucopolysaccharides.

Enzyme histochemical staining in cylindroma has revealed little or no activity for phosphorylase, an "eccrine" type of enzyme. There are weak reactions for acid phosphatase and beta-glucuronidase and a negative reaction for indoxyl esterase, all "apocrine" enzymes (Holubar and Wolff; Hashimoto and Lever). The absence of significant enzyme reactions may be due to the immaturity of the tumor cells.

Electron microscopic examination, similar to examination by light microscopy, has revealed two major types of cells: undifferentiated basal cells with small, dark nuclei, and differentiating cells with large, pale nuclei. Most of the differentiating cells still appear immature as "indeterminate cells," but some show a certain degree of differentiation toward secretory or ductal cells and are in part arranged around lumina. In the view of some authors, the differentiation of the secretory cells is eccrine, since they contain secretory vacuoles resembling those seen in the dark mucoid cells of the eccrine gland (Munger et al; Urbach et al). Other authors have observed within the secretory cells two types of secretory granules similar to the secretory cells of apocrine glands; one type is large and contains lipid globules, and the other type contains central cristae, suggesting a mitochondrial origin (Hashimoto and Lever). Decapitation secretion indicative of apocrine secretory activity has also been observed (Tsambaos et al).

In addition to the electron microscopic findings, the common association of trichoepithelioma and cylindroma speaks in favor of apocrine differentiation in cylindroma, since an origin from pluripotential cells with the potentiality of primary epithelial germ cells would explain the formation of both hair structures and apocrine structures. Also, a study of two large pedigrees has led to the conclusion that cylindromas and trichoepitheliomas are different expressions of the same disorder and not merely examples of genetic linkage (Welch et al). In contrast, the coexistence of cylindroma and eccrine spiradenoma in a few instances has been interpreted as evidence for the theory that cylindroma is of an eccrine nature (Crain and Helwig; Goette et al).

The thick hyalin band surrounding the tumor islands of cylindroma shows two intermingled components. First, there is an amorphous to finely filamentous material representing a greatly thickened basement membrane that is connected with the tumor cells by half-desmosomes. Second is a fibrous component consisting of anchoring fibrils as well as of collagen fibrils. These fibrils vary in maturity and thus also in width. They show a range of periodicity from 15 nm to 69 nm (Hashimoto and Lever; Gebhart et al). It is likely, in view of the findings in hyalinosis cutis et mucosae (see p. 415), that the amorphous and thin, filamentous material represents type IV collagen, as found in basement membranes. The hyaline material within the tumor islands represents inclusions of the surrounding hyalin band into the tumor islands. The amorphous material and the fine filaments representing type IV collagen are secreted by the tumor cells, whereas the thicker collagen fibrils, representing types I and III collagen, and the anchoring fibrils are synthesized by fibroblasts (see p. 31).

TUMORS WITH ECCRINE DIFFERENTIATION

ECCRINE NEVUS

Eccrine nevi are very rare. They may show a circumscribed area of hyperhidrosis (Arnold; Goldstein; Martius), a solitary sweat-discharging pore (Herzberg), or a small, circumscribed plaque (Pippione et al).

In the so-called eccrine angiomatous hamartoma, there may be one or several nodules (Hyman et al; Challa and Jona) or a solitary large plaque (Zeller and Goldman). Hyperhidrosis may not be apparent (Challa and Jona).

Histopathology.   Eccrine nevi show an increase in the size of the eccrine coil in cases with only one eccrine duct (Herzberg), whereas, in cases with multiple ducts, they show an increase in both the size and the number of coils (Arnold; Goldstein; Martius). In addition, the epidermis may show basaloid proliferations (Pippione et al).

Eccrine angiomatous hamartomas show not only increased numbers of eccrine structures but also numerous capillary channels either surrounding the eccrine structures (Hyman et al; Zeller and Goldman) or intermingled with them (Challa and Jona).

ECCRINE HIDROCYSTOMA

In this condition, usually one lesion, but occasionally several, and rarely numerous lesions are present on the face (Smith and Chernosky). As in apocrine hidrocystoma, the lesion consists of a small, translucent, cystic nodule 1 mm to 3 mm in diameter that often has a bluish hue. In some patients with numerous lesions, the number of cysts increases in warm weather and decreases during winter (Dostrovsky and Sagher; Ebner and Erlach; Cordero and Montes).

Histopathology.   Eccrine hidrocystoma shows a single cystic cavity located in the dermis. The cyst wall usually shows two layers of small, cuboidal epithelial cells (Smith and Chernosky). In some areas, however, only a single layer of flattened epithelial cells can be seen, their nuclei extending parallel to the cyst wall (Ebner and Erlach). Papillary projections extending into the cavity of the cyst are observed only rarely, and, if present, are small (Hassan and Khan). Eccrine secretory tubules and ducts are often located below the cyst and in close approximation to it (Cordero and Montes), and, on serial sections, one may find an eccrine duct leading into the cyst from below (Herzberg; Hashimoto and Lever; Ebner and Erlach). However, no connection can be found between the cyst and the epidermis.

Histogenesis. *Electron microscopy* of eccrine hidrocystoma has established that the cyst wall is composed of ductal cells, since the luminal cell membrane shows numerous microvilli and no secretory activity. In addition, no secretory granules are present. Tonofilaments are seen in the luminal portion of the cells, and desmosomes interconnect the cells (Ebner and Erlach; Hassan and Khan).

Enzyme histochemistry in a case with numerous cysts revealed the presence of phosphorylase and of succinic dehydrogenase, that is, of eccrine enzymes (Ebner and Erlach).

It is likely that malformations of the eccrine ducts lead to either temporary or permanent retention of sweat (Herzberg; Ebner and Erlach).

Differential Diagnosis. For a discussion of differentiation of eccrine from apocrine hidrocystoma, see p. 543.

SYRINGOMA

According to histochemical and electron microscopic findings, syringoma represents an adenoma of intraepidermal eccrine ducts. It occurs predominantly in women at puberty or later in life. Although occasionally solitary, the lesions usually are multiple and may be present in great numbers. They are small, skin-colored or slightly yellowish, soft papules usually only 1 mm or 2 mm in size. In many patients, the lesions are limited to the lower eyelids. Other sites of predilection are the cheeks, axillae, abdomen, and vulva (Thomas et al). In so-called eruptive hidradenoma or syringoma, the lesions arise in large numbers in successive crops on the anterior trunk of young persons (Hashimoto et al, 1967). Rarely, the lesions of syringoma show a unilateral, linear arrangement (Yung et al).

Histopathology. Embedded in a fibrous stroma are numerous small ducts (Fig. 27-29), the walls of which are lined usually by two rows of epithelial cells. In most instances, these cells are flat. Occasionally, however, the cells of the inner row appear vacuolated. The lumina of the ducts contain amorphous debris. Some of the ducts possess small, commalike tails of epithelial cells, giving them the appearance of tadpoles. In addition, there are solid strands of basophilic epithelial cells independent of the ducts.

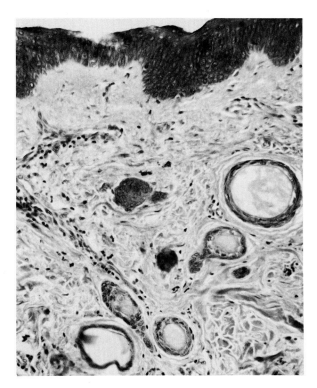

Fig. 27-29. Syringoma
The dermis contains several small ducts. The walls of the ducts are lined predominantly by two rows of epithelial cells. Two of the ducts have commalike tails, giving them the appearance of tadpoles. (×200)

Near the epidermis, there may be cystic ductal lumina filled with keratin and lined by cells containing keratohyaline granules (Fig. 27-30). These keratin cysts may rupture, whereupon they produce a marked foreign body giant cell reaction that is occasionally followed by calcification (Hashimoto et al, 1967).

In rare instances, many of the tumor cells appear as clear cells as a result of glycogen accumulation (Headington et al). In such cases, one observes only few ductal structures and epithelial cords but predominantly cell islands that are irregular in shape and of varying size. With the occasional exception of the peripheral cell layer, these islands are composed entirely of clear cells (Fig. 27-31).

Histogenesis. The frequent onset of syringoma at puberty, its rather common location in apocrine areas, and the interpretation of the amorphous material in the ducts as products of secretion had in the past suggested differentiation toward apocrine structures (Lever). However, enzyme histochemical and electron microscopic studies have established syringoma as a tumor with differentiation toward intraepidermal eccrine sweat ducts.

The *enzyme pattern* in the cells of syringoma shows a prevalence of eccrine enzymes such as succinic dehydrogenase (Mustakallio), as well as phosphorylase and

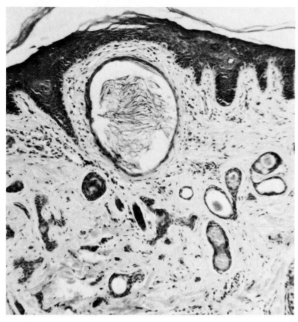

Fig. 27-30.   Syringoma
Near the epidermis, the lumen of a cystic duct is filled with keratin. (×100)

leucine aminopeptidase (Winkelmann and Muller). In contrast to apocrine structures, syringomas react only weakly to lysosomal, apocrine enzymes such as acid phosphatase and beta-glucuronidase, except in a narrow, lysosome-rich periluminal zone (Hashimoto et al, 1967).

Electron microscopic examination reveals that the lumina of the ducts are lined not by secretory but by ductal cells showing numerous short microvilli, interconnecting desmosomes, a periluminal band of tonofilaments, and many lysosomes (EM 39). In some tumor cells, intracytoplasmic cavities are formed by lysosomal action. Coalescence of several such intracytoplasmic cavities to form an intercellular lumen is the mode by which the ductal lumina are formed in syringoma; this is identical with the mode of formation of the embryonic as well as the regenerating intraepidermal eccrine ducts (see p. 6) (Hashimoto et al, 1966, 1967; Hashimoto and Lever).

The finding of cystic ductal lumina filled with keratin near the epidermis is compatible with the natural keratinizing propensity of the luminal cells of the intraepidermal eccrine sweat duct toward the upper strata of the epidermis (Hashimoto et al, 1967).

The occasional presence of large amounts of glycogen in the cells of syringoma is analogous to that in nodular hidradenoma, a tumor that usually shows eccrine differentiation and often contains clear cells and then is referred to as clear cell hidradenoma (see p. 557) (Headington et al).

Differential Diagnosis. The solid strands of basophilic epithelial cells embedded in a fibrous stroma seen in some cases of syringoma have an appearance similar to that of the strands seen in

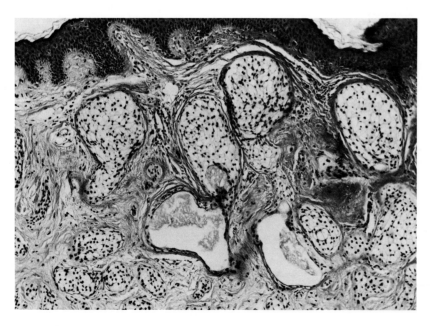

Fig. 27-31.   Syringoma
In this rare variant, the tumor islands consist largely of clear cells as a result of glycogen accumulation. (×100)

D. D BCC
Trichoep (Desmoplastic)
Microcytic Adnexal Ca

fibrosing basal cell epithelioma (see p. 569). The latter tumor, however, lacks ductal structures containing amorphous material. The horn cysts near the epidermis in syringoma resemble those occurring in trichoepithelioma, and their presence in syringoma was formerly misinterpreted as the occurrence of both types of tumors within the same lesion (Lever). Although trichoepithelioma shows solid strands of basophilic epithelial cells and horn cysts, it lacks ductal structures.

ECCRINE POROMA

Eccrine poroma, first described in 1956 (Pinkus et al), is a fairly common solitary tumor. In about two thirds of the cases, it is found on the sole or the sides of the foot (Hyman and Brownstein), occurring next in frequency on the hands and fingers. Eccrine poroma has also been observed in many other areas of the skin, such as the neck, chest, and nose (Okun and Ansell; Penneys et al). Eccrine poroma generally arises in middle-aged persons. The tumor has a rather firm consistency, is raised and often slightly pedunculated, is asymptomatic, and usually measures less than 2 cm in diameter.

Two unusual clinical variants have been described: eccrine poromatosis, and acrosyringial nevus. In *eccrine poromatosis*, more than 100 papules may be observed on the palms and soles (Goldner); in one reported case, the papular poromas, in addition to involving the palms and soles, showed a widespread, diffuse distribution (Wilkinson et al). In *acrosyringeal nevus*, there may be either a linear lesion extending along a lower extremity (Ogino) or a solitary verrucous plaque (Weedon and Lewis).

Histopathology. In its typical form, eccrine poroma arises within the lower portion of the epidermis, from where it extends downward into the dermis as tumor masses that often consist of broad, anastomosing bands. The border between epidermis and tumor is readily apparent because of the distinctive appearance of the tumor cells: they are smaller than squamous cells, have a uniform cuboidal appearance and a round, deeply basophilic nucleus, and are connected by intercellular bridges (Fig. 27-32). These cells show no tendency to keratinize within the tumor, but they are able to keratinize on the surface of the tumor in instances in which the tumor has replaced the overlying epidermis. Although the border between tumor formations and the stroma is sharp, tumor cells located at the periphery show no palisading.

As a characteristic feature, the tumor cells contain significant amounts of glycogen, usually in an uneven distribution (Freeman et al). Melanocytes and melanin often are absent (Pinkus et al), al-

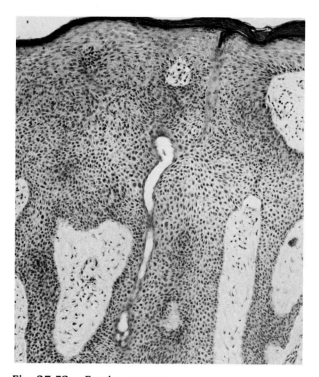

Fig. 27-32. Eccrine poroma
The tumor consists of broad, anastomosing bands. The cells composing the tumor have a uniformly small, cuboidal appearance and are connected by intercellular bridges. A ductal lumen extends through the tumor in a vertical direction. It is lined by an eosinophilic cuticle and a single row of luminal cells. ($\times 150$)

though they may be present in tumors encountered in blacks (Knox and Spiller), Mongols (Yasuda et al), and occasionally even whites (Krinitz, 1967).

In most but not in all eccrine poromas, narrow ductal lumina and occasionally cystic spaces are found within the tumor bands (Freeman et al). They are lined by an eosinophilic, PAS-positive, diastase-resistant cuticle similar to that lining the lumina of eccrine sweat ducts and by a single row of luminal cells.

Poromas are occasionally located entirely within the epidermis, where they appear as discrete aggregates. Such intraepidermal poromas were first described under the designation *hidroacanthoma simplex* in 1956 (Smith and Coburn), the same year in which poroma was first described (Pinkus et al). A few ductal lumina lined by an eosinophilic cuticle can often be seen within the intraepidermal islands (Mehregan and Levson). However, eccrine poromas may also be located largely or entirely within the dermis, where they consist of variously shaped tumor islands containing ductal lumina. They are then referred to as dermal duct tumor (Winkelmann and McLeod).

Acrosyringeal nevus differs slightly in its histologic appearance from eccrine poroma in showing areas in which the tumor cells are arranged in thin, long, anastomosing cords of cells in a pattern similar to that seen in fibroepithelioma (Ogino). Eccrine duct lumina are seen within the thin cords of tumor cells, and some of the cords connect with underlying eccrine ducts (Weeden and Lewis).

Histogenesis. Enzyme histochemical staining has shown the prevalence in eccrine poroma of eccrine enzymes, particularly phosphorylase but also succinic dehydrogenase (Sanderson and Ryan; Hashimoto and Lever, 1964; Winkelmann and McLeod).

Electron microscopic examination reveals that the tumor cells, except for the luminal cells, contain a moderate number of tonofilaments, are connected with each other by desmosomes, and appear identical to the cells that compose the outer layer of the intraepidermal eccrine duct (poral epithelial cells) (Hashimoto and Lever, 1964). The luminal cells show a periluminal filamentous zone and, extending into the lumen, numerous tortuous microvilli coated with amorphous material that forms the eosinophilic cuticle seen by light microscopy. Small intracytoplasmic ductal lumina surrounded by numerous lysosomes are occasionally seen within tumor cells (Hashimoto and Lever, 1964; Mishima). Since it is characteristic of embryonic as well as of regenerating intraepidermal eccrine ducts to be located initially within the cytoplasm of cells (Hashimoto et al), eccrine poroma can be regarded as a tumor differentiating in the direction of intraepidermal eccrine ducts. In some areas, however, electron microscopic examination shows slitlike separations between tumor cells resembling intradermal duct formation (Hashimoto and Lever, 1969). Thus, some of the tumor cells in eccrine poroma and most, if not all, of the tumor cells in the dermal duct tumor, are differentiating toward dermal duct cells (Hu et al). (For a description of embryonic intraepidermal and dermal eccrine duct formation, see p. 6.)

Differential Diagnosis. Eccrine poroma must be differentiated from basal cell epithelioma and seborrheic keratosis. In basal cell epithelioma, the cells have no visible intercellular bridges, are more variable in size, often show peripheral palisading, and contain little or no glycogen. The cells of eccrine poroma greatly resemble the small basaloid cells of seborrheic keratosis, especially since they, too, possess clearly visible intercellular bridges. However, seborrheic keratoses have an even demarcation at their lower border; moreover, their cells have the potential to keratinize, and, when they keratinize, they form horn cysts. Also, both basal cell epithelioma and seborrheic keratosis lack lumina lined with an eosinophilic cuticle. Furthermore, these two types of tumors hardly ever occur on the sole of the foot.

Malignant Eccrine Poroma

Malignant eccrine poroma, or porocarcinoma, may arise as such (Pinkus and Mehregan; Mishima and Morioka), but usually it develops in an eccrine poroma of long standing (Krinitz, 1972; Bardach; Gschnait et al; Mohri et al). In some instances, the malignant eccrine poroma is still localized, manifesting itself as a nodule (Bardach), plaque (Mishima and Morioka), or ulcerated tumor (Ishikawa; Mohri et al); in other cases, there are multiple cutaneous metastases, which are usually associated with visceral metastases, resulting in death (Pinkus and Mehregan; Krinitz, 1972; Miura; Gschnait et al). The propensity to form multiple cutaneous metastases is a unique feature of malignant eccrine poroma.

Histopathology. Malignant eccrine poroma may be seen adjoining a typical eccrine poroma (Mohri et al) or a purely intraepidermal eccrine poroma (Bardach). In such cases, one observes areas composed of eccrine poroma cells with a benign appearance adjoining areas of anaplastic cells (Fig. 27-33). The malignant cells have large, hyperchromatic, irregularly shaped nuclei and may be multinucleated (Mohri et al). They are rich in glycogen (Pinkus and Mehregan).

In the primary tumor, the malignant cells may be limited to the epidermis (Mishima and Morioka; Bardach) or may extend into the dermis (Krinitz, 1972; Mohri et al). Some islands of tumor cells may lie free in the dermis (Ishikawa). The epidermis often shows considerable acanthosis as a result of the proliferation of numerous well-defined tumor cell nests within it (Krinitz, 1972). Cystic lumina may be seen within the epidermal and dermal tumor nests (Krinitz, 1972; Ishikawa).

In the cutaneous metastases, numerous nests of tumor cells are present in both the epidermis and the dermis. In the epidermis, sharply defined small and large nests of tumor cells are seen surrounded by the squamous cells of the hyperplastic epidermis, resulting in a "pagetoid" pattern (Pinkus and Mehregan; Krinitz, 1972). Some of the tumor nests in the dermis are located within dilated lymphatic vessels, suggesting spread of the tumor in the lymphatics of the skin (Pinkus and Mehregan; Miura). From the lymphatics, the tumor cells invade the overlying epidermis because of the "epidermotropic" nature of the acrosyringeal tumor cells.

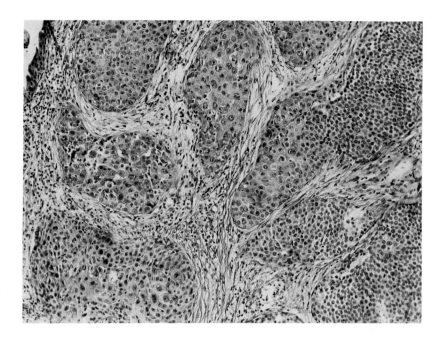

Fig. 27-33. Malignant eccrine poroma
On the right side, the tumor has an appearance similar to that of an eccrine poroma; on the left side, the tumor lobules are composed of cells showing anaplastic nuclei and dyskeratosis. (×100)

MUCINOUS SYRINGOMETAPLASIA

A rare condition first described in 1974 (Kwittken), mucinous syringometaplasia usually occurs on the sole of the foot as a solitary lesion resembling a plantar wart. With pressure, serous fluid can be expressed (King and Barr).

Histopathology.   An invagination lined by squamous epithelium extends deeply into the dermis. One or several eccrine ducts lead into the invagination. They are lined in part by mucin-laden goblet cells (King and Barr). In addition, there may be mucinous metaplasia in the underlying eccrine coils (Mehregan). The epithelial mucin is PAS-positive and alcian-blue-reactive, suggesting that it is sialomucin.

Histogenesis. It is not clear whether mucinous syringometaplasia represents a reactive process or a neoplasia (Mehregan).

ECCRINE SPIRADENOMA

As a rule, eccrine spiradenoma occurs, as a solitary intradermal nodule measuring 1 cm to 2 cm in diameter. Occasionally, there are several nodules (Munger et al; Hashimoto et al), and, rarely, there are numerous small nodules in a zosteriform pattern (Nödl; Shelley and Wood) or large nodules, up to 5 cm in size, in a linear arrangement (Tsur et al). In most instances, eccrine spiradenoma arises in early adulthood. It has no char-

acteristic location. The nodules are often tender and occasionally painful.

Histopathology.   The tumor may consist of one large, sharply demarcated lobule, but, more commonly, there are several such lobules located in the dermis without connections to the epidermis. The lobules are evenly and sharply demarcated and may be encapsulated. On low magnification, the tumor lobules often appear deeply basophilic because of the close aggregation of the nuclei (Fig. 27-34).

On higher magnification, the epithelial cells within the tumor lobules are found to be arranged in intertwining cords (Lever; Kersting and Helwig). These cords may enclose small, irregularly shaped islands of edematous connective tissue (Castro and Winkelmann). Two types of epithelial cells are present in the cords, both of which possess only scant amounts of cytoplasm. The cells of the first type possess small, dark nuclei; they are generally located at the periphery of the cellular aggregates. The cells of the second type have large, pale nuclei; they are located in the center of the aggregates and may be arranged partially around small lumina (Fig. 27-35). The lumina frequently contain small amounts of a granular, eosinophilic material that is PAS-positive and diastase-resistant (Kersting and Helwig). In the absence of lumina, the cells with pale nuclei may show a rosettelike arrangement. Glycogen is absent in the tumor cells or is present in insignificant amounts.

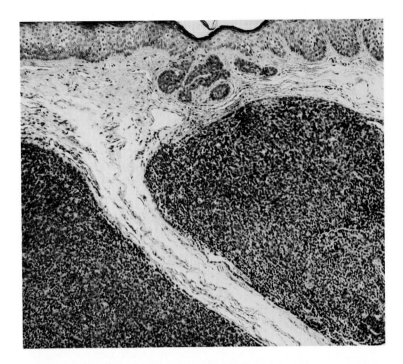

Fig. 27-34. Eccrine spiradenoma
Low magnification. Two large masses of tumor cells composed of two types of cells are shown. (×100)

Fig. 27-35. Eccrine spiradenoma
High magnification. The epithelial cells are arranged in intertwining bands. Two types of cells can be seen. Cells with small, dark nuclei lie at the periphery of the bands; they represent undifferentiated cells. Cells with large, pale nuclei lie in the center of the bands and around small lumina. (×400)

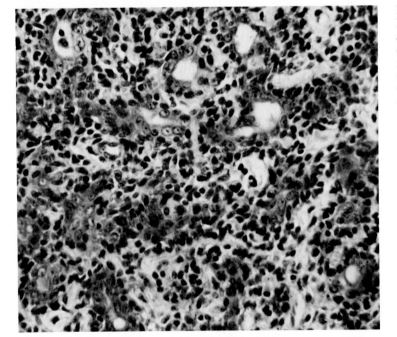

In some cases of eccrine spiradenoma, hyaline material is present in the stroma that surrounds the cords of tumor cells. In addition, hyalin may be seen within some of the cords among the tumor cells as hyalin droplets (Kersting and Helwig). The stroma surrounding the tumor lobules occasionally shows lymphedema with greatly dilated blood or lymph capillaries (Kersting and Helwig).

Histogenesis. Enzyme histochemical staining has revealed a prevalence of eccrine enzymes in eccrine spiradenoma, but the reactions are not as strong by far as in syringoma or eccrine poroma. The most characteristic eccrine enzyme, phosphorylase, was seen in one case only in the peripheral cells of the tumor islands (Hashimoto et al) and in three other cases was absent (Winkelmann and Wolff; Castro and Winkelmann). However, respiratory enzymes such as succinic dehydrogenase and diphosphopyridine nucleotide (DPNH) diaphorase, found also largely in eccrine structures, are present. Stains for alkaline phosphatase are negative, indicating the absence of a significant number of mature, functioning myoepithelial cells (Hashimoto et al).

Electron microscopic examination, similar to light microscopic examination, has shown two types of cells: undifferentiated basal cells with small, dark nuclei, and differentiating cells with large, pale nuclei. Most of the differentiating cells are immature ("indeterminate cells") and, in some tumors, may show no further differentiation (Castro and Winkelmann). In most instances, however, there is some degree of differentiation toward intradermal eccrine ductal cells or toward eccrine secretory cells. As evidence of the immaturity of the tumor, one may observe lumina lined by cells with different degrees and directions of differentiation. Thus, around the same lumen, some cells may show numerous microvilli and a well-developed periluminal zone of tonofilaments and thus resemble ductal cells, whereas other cells have only a few thin microvilli and thus resemble secretory cells (Hashimoto et al; Hashimoto and Lever). Some of the secretory cells show abundant ergastoplasmic sacs with endoplasmic reticulum, as seen in the mucoid cells of the eccrine secretory segment, but secretory granules are absent (Munger et al). A few myoepithelial cells with typical myofilaments are present occasionally at the periphery of tubular structures (Hashimoto et al).

It can be concluded that differentiation in eccrine spiradenoma is in the direction of both the dermal duct and the secretory segment of the eccrine sweat gland. However, the weakness and inconsistency of the enzyme histochemical reactions, the presence largely of undifferentiated and indeterminate cells, and the absence of secretory granules in the secretory cells indicate a rather low degree of differentiation.

Malignant Eccrine Spiradenoma

Only few cases are on record describing the formation of a carcinoma in long-standing lesions of eccrine spiradenoma (Evans et al). In one instance, a regional lymph node metastasis was present.

Histopathology. Two distinct components are seen: typical benign eccrine spiradenoma, and carcinoma, with areas of transitions. The carcinoma may be undifferentiated or may show gland formation in some areas (Evans et al).

CLEAR CELL HIDRADENOMA

Clear cell hidradenoma, referred to in the past as clear cell myoepithelioma (see Histogenesis), is presently also called nodular hidradenoma (Lund), eccrine sweat gland adenoma of the clear cell type (O'Hara et al; O'Hara and Bensch), solid cystic hidradenoma (Winkelmann and Wolff, 1967, 1968), and eccrine acrospiroma (Johnson and Helwig).

Clear cell hidradenoma, now generally regarded as an eccrine sweat gland tumor on the basis of its enzyme histochemical and electron microscopic features, occurs as a solitary tumor in most instances; however, rarely, several lesions are present (Efskind and Eker). The tumors present themselves as intradermal nodules and in most instances measure between 0.5 cm and 2 cm in diameter, although they may be larger. They are usually covered by intact skin, but some tumors show superficial ulceration (Winkelmann and Wolff, 1968) and discharge serous material (Johnson and Helwig). Whereas, clinically, the tumor only rarely gives the impression of being cystic, gross examination of the specimen often reveals the presence of cysts (Lever and Castleman; Johnson and Helwig).

Histopathology. The tumor seems well circumscribed and may appear encapsulated. It is composed of lobulated masses located in the dermis and extending into the subcutaneous fat. Within the lobulated masses, tubular lumina of various sizes are often present (Fig. 27-36). However, such lumina may be absent or may be few in number, so that they are found only on step sectioning. The tubular lumina in some instances show branching. There are often cystic spaces, which may be of considerable size and contain a faintly eosinophilic, homogeneous material (Fig. 27-37) (Winkelmann and Wolff, 1968). The tubular lumina are lined by cuboidal ductal cells or by columnar secretory cells. Occasionally, the secretory cells show active secretion suggestive of decapitation secretion (Fig. 27-36) (Lever and Castleman; Efskind and Eker; Okun and Edelstein; Gartmann and Pullmann). The wide cystic spaces are only rarely lined by a single row of luminal cells; more frequently, they are bordered by tumor cells that show no particular orientation and occasionally show degenerative changes (Lever and Castleman). This suggests that the cystic spaces form as a result of degeneration of tumor cells.

In solid portions of the tumor, two types of cells can be recognized (Lever and Castleman; Kersting; Hashimoto et al; Winkelmann and Wolff, 1968). The proportion of these two types of cells varies considerably in different tumors. One type of cell is usually polyhedral with a rounded nucleus and

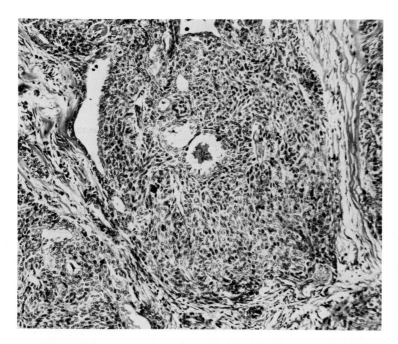

Fig. 27-36.   Clear cell hidradenoma
The tumor consists of lobular masses composed of cells with clear cytoplasm. Small and large lumina are present lined either by cuboidal ductal cells or by columnar secretory cells. (×200)

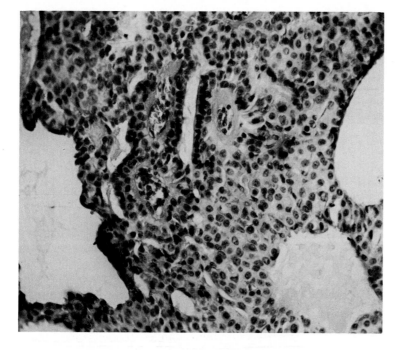

Fig. 27-37.   Clear cell hidradenoma
Tubular lumina and cystic spaces are present within the tumor. The cystic spaces seem to form as a result of degeneration of tumor cells. (×200)

slightly basophilic cytoplasm. Some of these cells may appear fusiform and show an elongated nucleus (Fig. 27-38). The second type of cell is usually round and contains very clear cytoplasm, so that the cell membrane is distinctly visible. Its nucleus appears small and dark (Fig. 27-39). There also are cells transitional between these two varieties; these cells usually show a rather light, eosinophilic cytoplasm. The clear cells contain considerable amounts of glycogen, but they may show, in addition, significant amounts of PAS-positive, diastase-resistant material along their periphery (Kersting). In some tumors, keratinizing cells with formation of horn pearls are present (Lever and Castleman;

O'Hara et al). In other tumors, groups of squamous cells are arranged around small lumina that are lined with a well-defined eosinophilic cuticle and thus resemble the intraepidermal portion of the eccrine duct (Kersting; Johnson and Helwig).

In most cases, no connections of the tumor lobules with the surface epidermis are noted; however, in some instances, the tumor replaces the epidermis centrally and merges with the acanthotic epidermis at the periphery of the tumor (Lever and Castleman; O'Hara et al; Johnson and Helwig).

Histogenesis. The polyhedral and fusiform cells, because of their location peripheral to the luminal cells and because of their shape, were originally regarded as cells differentiating in the direction of myoepithelial cells (Lever and Castleman; Efskind and Eker). However, the absence of alkaline phosphatase and, ultrastructurally, of myofilaments has disproved their relationship to myoepithelial cells.

Enzyme histochemical staining has established the presence in clear cell hidradenoma of high concentrations of eccrine enzymes, particularly phosphorylase and respiratory enzymes, including succinic dehydrogenase and

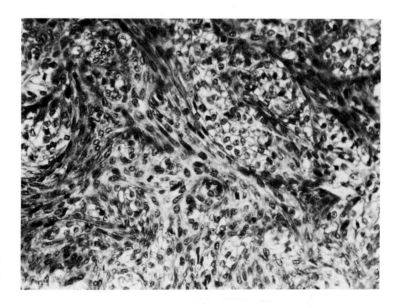

Fig. 27-38.   Clear cell hidradenoma
The tumor contains polyhedral cells, some of which appear fusiform. Others show a clear cytoplasm. (×200)

Fig. 27-39.   Clear cell hidradenoma
There are numerous clear cells and, in addition, tubular lumina lined by a single layer of cuboidal ductal cells. (×200)

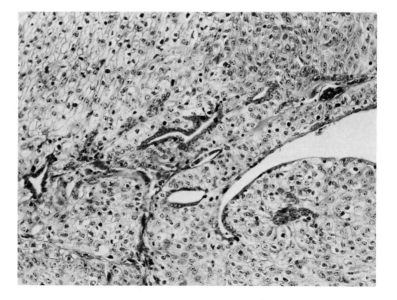

diphosphopyridine nucleotide (DPNH) diaphorase (Hashimoto et al; Winkelmann and Wolff, 1967).

Electron microscopic examination has shown a fair number of tonofilaments in the polyhedral and fusiform cells and an abundance of glycogen in the clear cells. These two types of tumor cells resemble the tumor cells of eccrine poroma and consequently also resemble the cells that compose the outer layers of the intraepidermal eccrine duct (Hashimoto et al). In addition, four types of luminal cells can be recognized (Hashimoto et al). One type shows, as evidence of active secretion, pinched-off microvilli disintegrating in the lumen. These secretory cells, as in normal eccrine glands, either are glycogen-rich or are glycogen-free with a moderate number of secretory granules. The second type of luminal cell contains a periluminal filamentous zone and thus appears dermal–ductal in differentiation. The third type of cell shows not only a periluminal filamentous zone but also lysosomes and, occasionally, keratohyaline granules, indicative of epidermal–ductal differentiation. The fourth type appears to be immature and intermediary in differentiation between a ductal and a secretory cell. It can be concluded that clear cell hidradenoma shows differentiation toward intraepidermal as well as intradermal eccrine structures ranging from the poral epithelium to the secretory segment (Hashimoto et al). Thus, ultrastructurally clear cell hidradenoma seems to be intermediate between eccrine poroma, with its largely intraepidermal ductal differentiation, and eccrine spiradenoma, with its dermal–ductal and secretory differentiation. From this point of view, the clear cells represent immature poral epithelial cells, and the horn-pearl formation can be regarded as the keratinization of poral epithelial cells.

According to another ultrastructural study, the clear cells in clear cell hidradenoma closely resemble the clear type of eccrine secretory cells not only in that they have a high glycogen content but also in that they possess a similar system of intracellular organelles and a similar complex intercellular canalicular system (O'Hara and Bensch).

Even though an occasional clear cell hidradenoma shows luminal cells with decapitation secretion on light microscopic examination, none of the clear cell hidradenomas that have been studied by enzyme histochemistry or electron microscopy have shown evidence of apocrine differentiation.

Differential Diagnosis. Clear cell hidradenoma shares with trichilemmoma the presence of clear cells rich in glycogen. Foci of keratinization may also be found in both. However, only clear cell hidradenoma usually shows the presence of large cystic spaces and of tubular lumina, and only trichilemmoma shows peripheral palisading of its tumor cells.

Malignant Clear Cell Hidradenoma

Malignant clear cell hidradenomas are rare. Usually, they are malignant from the beginning. They tend to metastasize, and they may cause death (Keasbey and Hadley; Santler and Eberhartinger; Hernández-Pérez and Cruz).

Histopathology. In contrast to benign clear cell hidradenomas, which are well demarcated, malignant clear cell hidradenomas show invasion into the surrounding tissue (Kersting; Santler and Eberhartinger). There may be angiolymphatic invasion (Headington et al). However, nuclear anaplasia may be only slight to moderate (Headington et al) or even absent (Hernández-Pérez and Cruz) in both the primary tumor and the metastases. Nuclear anaplasia, if present, may be limited to the clear cells (Santler and Eberhartinger) or affect both the polyhedral and the clear cells (Headington et al).

CHONDROID SYRINGOMA

The term *chondroid syringoma,* introduced in 1961 (Hirsch and Helwig), has widely replaced the old designation *mixed tumor of the skin* because of the recognition that the tumor is epithelial with merely secondary changes in the stroma. Chondroid syringomas are firm intradermal or subcutaneous nodules. Although the overlying skin may be attached to the tumor, it otherwise appears normal. Mixed tumors occur most commonly on the head and neck (Hirsch and Helwig). Their usual size is between 0.5 cm and 3 cm.

Histopathology. Histologically, two types of chondroid syringomas can be recognized: one with tubular and cystic, partially branching lumina, and the other with small, tubular lumina (Headington). The former type is much more common than the latter.

Chondroid syringoma with tubular, branching lumina shows marked variation in the size and shape of the tubular lumina; it also shows cystic dilatation and branching (Fig. 27-40). Embedded in an abundant stroma, the tubular lumina are lined by two layers of epithelial cells: a luminal layer of cuboidal cells, and a peripheral layer of flattened cells (Kresbach). Furthermore, there are large and small aggregates of epithelial cells without lumina as well as single epithelial cells widely scattered through the stroma. One gains the impression that cells from the peripheral cell layer of the tubular struc-

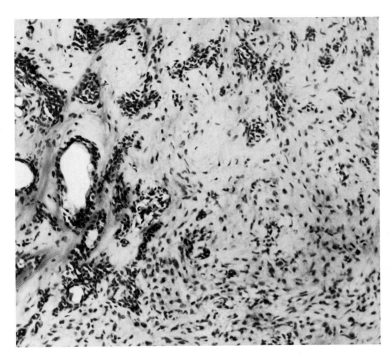

Fig. 27-40.   Chondroid syringoma with tubular, cystic lumina
Embedded in an abundant stroma, the tubular lumina are lined by two layers of cells: a luminal layer of cuboidal cells and a peripheral layer of flattened cells. Cells from the peripheral layer proliferate into the stroma, which has a mucoid, faintly basophilic appearance. (×200)

tures and from the solid aggregates proliferate into the stroma (Hirsch and Helwig). In most instances, the tubular lumina contain small amounts of amorphous, eosinophilic material that is PAS-positive and resistant to digestion with diastase. In general, the tubular structures are suggestive of eccrine differentiation (Hirsch and Helwig). Occasionally, however, the impression is gained that the luminal cells show an apocrine type of decapitation secretion, at least in some areas (Headington; Tsoitis et al; Gartmann and Pullmann, 1979b; Welke and Goos).

The abundant stroma in many areas has a mucoid, faintly basophilic appearance. As a result of shrinkage of the mucoid substance, the fibroblasts and epithelial cells that are scattered through it are surrounded by a halo, so that they resemble the cells of cartilage. The mucoid stroma stains with alcian blue, mucicarmine, and aldehyde–fuchsin. The alcian blue material is not appreciably decreased by predigestion with hyaluronidase (Hirsch and Helwig). Furthermore, on staining with toluidine blue or the Giemsa stain, there is distinct metachromasia (Gartmann and Pullmann, 1979a). Therefore, it can be concluded that the mucin consists largely of sulfated acid mucopolysaccharides, that is, chondroitin sulfate. The stroma thus is histochemically similar to normal cartilage

(Hirsch and Helwig). In a few areas, the stroma may appear homogeneous and eosinophilic, like hyalin, and is PAS-positive and diastase-resistant (Hirsch and Helwig; Kresbach; Varela-Duran et al).

Chondroid syringoma with small, tubular lumina shows numerous small ducts as well as small groups of epithelial cells and solitary epithelial cells scattered through a mucoid stroma (Fig. 27-41). The tubular lumina are lined by only a single layer of flat epithelial cells, from which small, commalike proliferations often extend into the stroma (Headington). The mucoid stroma contains acid mucopolysaccharides that stain metachromatically with toluidine blue.

Histogenesis. *Electron microscopy* has shown eccrine differentiation in the three cases examined so far (Hernandez; Varela-Duran et al). Both ductal and secretory lumina are present, with the secretory lumina lined by clear and dark cells as in eccrine secretory lumina (Hernandez). The cells of the outer layer of the tubuloalveolar and ductal structures, like myoepithelial cells, contain numerous filaments and extend into the chondroid matrix, which they apparently produce (Varela-Duran et al). No chondrocytes were seen in the chondroid matrix in one study (Varela-Duran et al). In another study, however, the stroma showed not only epithelial cells and fibroblasts embedded in a fibrocollagenous matrix but also islands of cartilaginous tissue containing

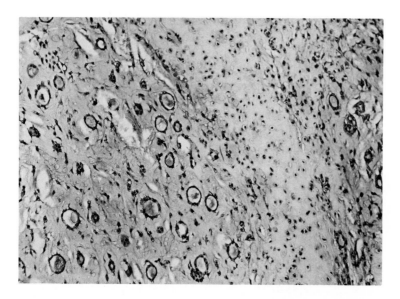

Fig. 27-41. Chondroid syringoma with small, tubular lumina
There are numerous small, tubular lumina lined with a single layer of epithelial cells. There also are small groups of epithelial cells and solitary epithelial cells. The epithelial structures are embedded in a mucoid stroma. (×100)

chondrocytes with ultrastructural features similar to mature cartilage (Hernandez). In this particular case, foci of ossification were also observed, indicating that metaplasia into cartilage and bone had taken place.

Malignant Chondroid Syringoma

In the rare cases of malignant chondroid syringoma that occur, anaplastic changes apparently are present from the beginning (Harrist et al). The degree of malignancy varies. There may be only a local recurrence (Botha and Kahn), but some cases have shown regional lymph node metastases (Hilton and Blackwell), an osseous metastasis (Harrist et al), and even fatal visceral metastases (Matz et al).

Histopathology. The malignant tumor and its metastases are recognizable as chondroid syringoma through their chondroid stroma and tubular structures. However, tubular differentiation is much less evident than in benign lesions (Matz et al). Most of the epithelial cells in the malignant tumor are arranged in irregular cords (Botha and Kahn). The tumor cells appear atypical and hyperchromatic (Hilton and Blackwell). In addition, an increased mitotic rate, invasion of surrounding tissue, and necrosis are noted (Harrist et al).

BASAL CELL EPITHELIOMA

Basal cell epitheliomas are seen almost exclusively on hair-bearing skin, especially on the face. Except in the nevoid basal cell epithelioma syndrome (see p. 563),

they rarely occur on the palms (Johnson; Hyman and Barsky) or on the soles (Hyman and Michaelides; Lewis et al). Their occurrence on the mucous membrane is doubted; instances of basal cell epithelioma of the oral mucosa reported in the literature (Williamson et al) probably are in reality ameloblastomas (Small and Waldron).

Basal cell epitheliomas usually occur as single lesions, although the occurrence of several lesions either simultaneously or subsequently is not infrequent. About 40% of patients who have had a basal cell epithelioma will have one or more basal cell epitheliomas within 10 years (Schubert et al). Basal cell epitheliomas generally occur in adults, though, in rare instances, they may be seen in children (Murray and Cannon; Maron; Milstone and Helwig). However, there are two rare forms of basal cell epithelioma, the linear unilateral basal cell nevus, and the nevoid basal cell epithelioma syndrome (see below), in which numerous lesions are present at birth and in childhood, respectively.

PREDISPOSING FACTORS. Although basal cell epitheliomas may arise without apparent reason, there are several predisposing factors. The most common of them is a light skin color in association with prolonged exposure to strong sunlight (Gellin et al). The predisposing effect of sun exposure is particularly evident in patients with xeroderma pigmentosum, in whom both basal cell epithelioma and squamous cell carcinoma are common (see p. 64). Additional factors that predispose a person to develop both basal cell epithelioma and squamous cell carcinoma are large doses of roentgen rays (Anderson and Anderson; Schwartz et al) and, less commonly, burn scars (Gaughan et al; Margolis) and other scars (Wechsler et al). In contrast, most carcinomas of the skin caused by the prolonged intake of inorganic arsenic are squamous cell carcinomas, which often, as Bowen's disease, are located in situ (Montgomery and Waisman; Hundeiker and Petres). Occasionally, however, basal cell epitheliomas, particularly superficial basal cell epitheliomas, can result (Fierz; Yeh) (see Arsenical Keratosis and Carcinoma, p. 267).

OCCURRENCE OF METASTASES. As a rule, basal cell epitheliomas do not metastasize. However, there are exceptions. The incidence of metastasis has been calculated to be 0.0028% (Paver et al). A review published in 1977 revealed only 78 proved cases (Mikhail et al). The typical case history of a metastatic basal cell epithelioma is that of a large, ulcerated, locally invasive and destructive primary lesion that has recurred despite repeated surgical procedures or radiotherapy (Amonette et al). Most observers have found no specific histologic type of basal cell epithelioma that is more capable of metastasizing than others (Assor; Wermuth and Fajardo). However, some authors assert that the metatypical or basosquamous type of basal cell epithelioma (see p. 571) is the most likely to metastasize (Farmer and Helwig).

In nearly half of the reported cases, metastasis was limited to the regional lymph nodes, and, in 10%, the metastases were limited to the lungs or bones. Metastases to the liver as well as other viscera and to the skin also occurred. However, these areas were usually involved only when at least one of the three major sites of metastasis was also affected. Metastasis to a single site occurred in 70.5% of the cases, and to multiple sites in 29.5% (Mikhail et al). The average survival time after metastasis to the lungs, bones, or internal organs is reported to be about 10 months (Safai and Good). Although cell-mediated immunity was found to be deficient in some patients with metastases (Safai and Good), it was normal in others (Mikhail et al).

Clinical Appearance. Five clinical types of basal cell epithelioma occur: (1) nodulo-ulcerative basal cell epithelioma, including rodent ulcer, by far the most common type; (2) pigmented basal cell epithelioma; (3) morphealike or fibrosing basal cell epithelioma; (4) superficial basal cell epithelioma; and (5) fibroepithelioma. In addition, there are three clinical syndromes in which basal cell epitheliomas play an important part. They are (1) the nevoid basal cell epithelioma syndrome; (2) the linear unilateral basal cell nevus; and (3) the Bazex syndrome, showing follicular atrophoderma with multiple basal cell epitheliomas.

Nodulo-ulcerative basal cell epithelioma begins as a small, waxy nodule that often shows a few small telangiectatic vessels on its surface. The nodule usually increases slowly in size and often undergoes central ulceration. A typical lesion then consists of a slowly enlarging ulcer surrounded by a pearly, rolled border. This represents the so-called rodent ulcer.

Most rodent ulcers possess a limited potential for growth; however, in rare instances, they can be aggressive and then can reach considerable size and invade deeply. On the face, they may destroy the eyes and nose (Dvoretzky and Fisher), or they may penetrate the skull and invade the dura mater (Gormley and Hirsch). Death may then ensue. (Such destructive basal cell epitheliomas are seen occasionally also in the nevoid basal cell epithelioma syndrome; see below.)

Pigmented basal cell epithelioma differs from the nodulo-ulcerative type only by the brown pigmentation of the lesion.

Morphealike or fibrosing basal cell epithelioma manifests itself as a solitary, flat or slightly depressed, indurated, yellowish plaque. The surface is smooth and shiny. The border is often ill defined. The overlying skin remains intact for a long time before ulceration finally occurs.

Superficial basal cell epithelioma consists of one or several erythematous, scaling, only slightly infiltrated patches that slowly increase in size by peripheral extension. The patches are often surrounded, at least in part, by a fine, threadlike, pearly border. The patches usually show small areas of superficial ulceration and crusting. In addition, their center may show smooth, atrophic scarring. Whereas the three types of basal cell epithelioma previously described are commonly situated on the face, superficial basal cell epithelioma occurs predominantly on the trunk.

Fibroepithelioma consists of one or several raised, moderately firm, often slightly pedunculated nodules, covered by smooth, slightly reddened skin. Clinically, they resemble fibromas. The most common location is the back.

The *nevoid basal cell epithelioma syndrome* is an autosomal dominant disorder with low penetration. During childhood and, at the latest, in puberty, small nodules appear, of which there may be hundreds or thousands. During the "nevoid" stage, the nodules slowly increase in number and size. They are haphazardly distributed over the face and body. Often during adulthood, many of the basal cell epitheliomas undergo ulceration, and later in life, the disease sometimes enters a "neoplastic" stage, in which some of the basal cell epitheliomas, especially of the face, become invasive, destructive, and mutilating. Occasionally, even death occurs as the result of invasion, first, of an orbit and, later on, of the brain (Taylor et al; Southwick and Schwartz; Berendes). There also may be metastases to the lung (Taylor et al).

Half of the adult patients with the nevoid basal cell epithelioma syndrome show numerous palmar and plantar pits 1 mm to 3 mm in diameter. These pits usually develop during the second decade of life and represent *formes frustes* of basal cell epithelioma (see Histopathology) (Howell and Mehregan).

Aside from showing cutaneous lesions, nearly all patients show multiple skeletal and central nervous system anomalies (Southwick and Schwartz), among which are odontogenic keratocysts of the jaws, anomalies of the ribs, scoliosis, mental retardation, and calcification of the falx cerebri (Totten). In several reported cases, there has also been a cerebellar medulloblastoma (Hermans et al) or a fibrosarcoma of a mandible or maxilla (Reed). In the jaw cysts, an ameloblastoma may arise (Happle).

The *linear unilateral basal cell nevus* is very rare. There is an extensive unilateral linear or zosteriform eruption, usually present since birth, consisting of closely set nodules of basal cell epithelioma (Anderson and Best). They may be interspersed with comedones (Carney; Horio and Komura) and striaelike areas of atrophy (Bleiberg and Brodkin). The lesions do not increase in size with aging of the patient.

The *Bazex syndrome*, first described in 1966 (Bazex et al), is dominantly inherited and shows as its main features, first, follicular atrophoderma characterized by widened follicular openings like "ice-pick marks" mainly on the extremities and, second, multiple small basal cell epitheliomas on the face first arising in childhood, adolescence, or early adulthood (Viksnins and Berlin). In addition, there may be localized anhidrosis and/or generalized hypohidrosis, and congenital hypotrichosis on the scalp as well as elsewhere (Plosila et al).

Histopathology.   The characteristic cells of basal cell epithelioma, referred to by some as basalioma cells, have a large, oval or elongated nucleus and relatively little cytoplasm. Often, the cytoplasm of individual cells is poorly defined, so that it may appear as if their nuclei are embedded in a symplasmic mass. The nuclei resemble those of basal cells of the epidermis, but basalioma cells differ from basal cells by having a larger ratio of nucleus to cytoplasm (Rupec et al, 1975) and by not showing intercellular bridges. The nuclei in basal cell epitheliomas as a rule have a rather uniform and not an anaplastic appearance. Thus, they show no pronounced variation in size or intensity of staining and no abnormal mitoses, even in the rare instances of basal cell epithelioma with metastases. In the exceptional cases of basal cell epithelioma in which one finds, interspersed among the usual cells of basal cell epithelioma, cells with large hyperchromatic nuclei, multiple nuclei, and bizarre "starburst" mitoses, the clinical course is not different from that of the usual basal cell epithelioma (Okun and Blumental; Rupec et al, 1969). Nevertheless, there are histologic indications of aggressive behavior in some basal cell epitheliomas. Aside from the depth invasion, these are the presence of small groups of cells displaying an irregular, spiky appearance, and infiltration of cells in thin cords only one or two layers thick (Jacobs et al).

The connective tissue stroma proliferates with the tumor and is arranged in parallel bundles around the tumor masses, so that a mutual relationship seems to exist between the parenchyma of the tumor and its stroma (Pinkus, 1953, 1965). The stroma adjacent to the tumor masses often shows numerous young fibroblasts; in addition, it may appear mucinous (Fanger and Barker; Moore

et al). Since mucin shrinks during the process of fixation and dehydration of the specimen, the stroma frequently shows retraction from the tumor islands, so that tumor islands in processed sections may be partially or completely detached from the surrounding stroma (see Fig. 27-52). Although this retraction represents an artifact caused by shrinkage during processing, it is quite typical of basal cell epithelioma and may aid in its differentiation from other tumors, such as squamous cell carcinoma. Also, stromal or intratumor deposits of amyloid are found quite frequently (see Histogenesis, p. 574) (Weedon and Shand). A mild inflammatory infiltrate is often seen in the stroma of nonulcerated basal cell epitheliomas but may be entirely lacking. If ulceration occurs, there usually is a rather pronounced inflammatory reaction.

From a histologic point of view, basal cell epitheliomas can be divided into two groups: undifferentiated and differentiated. Those of the latter group show a slight degree of differentiation toward the cutaneous appendages, that is, hair, sebaceous glands, apocrine glands, or eccrine glands. A sharp dividing line between the two groups cannot be drawn, because many undifferentiated basal cell epitheliomas show differentiation in some areas, and most differentiated basal cell epitheliomas show areas lacking differentiation. By correlating the clinical classification with the histologic classification, it can be stated that the nodulo-ulcerative type of basal cell epithelioma, as well as the lesions of the nevoid basal cell epithelioma syndrome, the linear unilateral basal cell nevus, and the Bazex syndrome, may either show differentiation or show no differentiation, whereas the other four types of basal cell epithelioma—pigmented basal cell epithelioma, fibrosing basal cell epithelioma, superficial basal cell epithelioma, and fibroepithelioma—usually show little or no differentiation.

Basal cell epitheliomas showing no differentiation are called *solid* basal cell epitheliomas. Those with differentiation toward hair structures are called *keratotic;* toward sebaceous glands, *cystic;* and toward apocrine or eccrine glands, *adenoid* basal cell epitheliomas. In many differentiated basal cell epitheliomas, differentiation is directed toward more than one of these cutaneous appendages. For example, areas of keratinization may be found in a tumor that also shows adenoid structures. No difference exists in the rate of growth between undifferentiated and differentiated basal cell epitheliomas.

Solid basal cell epithelioma, which has also been

called the *primordial* type of basal cell epithelioma (Foot), shows tumor masses of various sizes and shapes embedded in the dermis (Fig. 27-42). In more than 90% of basal cell epitheliomas, a connection between tumor cell formations and the surface epidermis can be shown to exist (Hundeiker and Berger). Occasionally, a tumor mass is found in contact with an outer root sheath. The peripheral cell layer of the tumor masses often shows a palisade arrangement, whereas the nuclei of the cells inside lie in a haphazard fashion.

Some basal cell epitheliomas, though they show little or no structural differentiation toward any of the epidermal appendages, nevertheless show two types of cells: a large cell with an oval, pale nucleus, and a small cell with an elongated, dark nucleus (Fig. 27-43) (Reidbord et al).

Keratotic basal cell epithelioma, also called the *pilar* type (Foot), shows parakeratotic cells and horn cysts in addition to undifferentiated cells (Fig. 27-44). The parakeratotic cells possess elongated nuclei and a slightly eosinophilic cytoplasm, in contrast to the deeply basophilic cytoplasm of undifferentiated cells. The parakeratotic cells may lie in strands, in concentric whorls, or around the horn cysts. It is likely that they are cells with initial keratinization somewhat similar to the nucleated cells in the keratogenic zone of normal hair shafts. The horn cysts, which are composed of fully keratinized cells, represent attempts at hair shaft formation (Foot). Just as in the keratinization of the hair shaft, the horn cysts form without the interposition of granular cells. Some keratotic basal

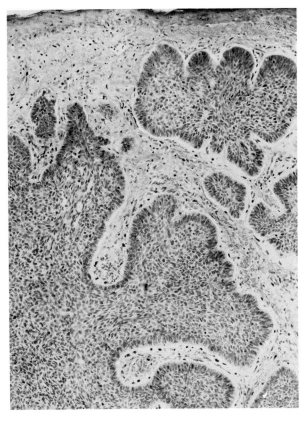

Fig. 27-42. Solid basal cell epithelioma
There are masses of various shapes and sizes composed of basal cell epithelioma cells or basalioma cells. The peripheral cell layer of the tumor masses shows a palisade arrangement of the nuclei. (×100)

Fig. 27-43. Basal cell epithelioma with differentiation into two types of cells
One type of cell is large and has an oval, pale nucleus; the other type of cell is small and has an elongated, dark nucleus. (×400)

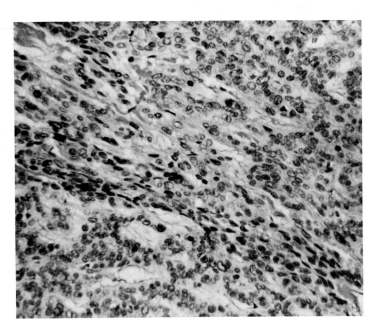

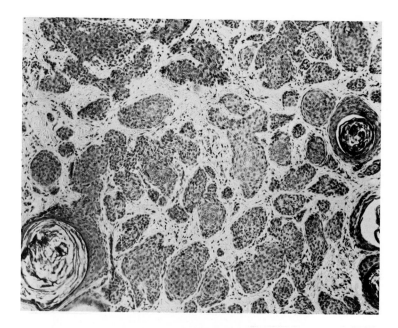

Fig. 27-44. Keratotic basal cell epithelioma
In addition to undifferentiated tumor cells, there are parakeratotic cells and horn cysts. The parakeratotic cells possess an elongated nucleus and a slightly eosinophilic cytoplasm; they lie in strands, in concentric whorls, or around the horn cyst. (×100)

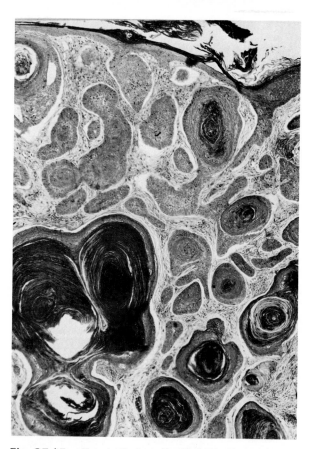

Fig. 27-45. Keratotic basal cell epithelioma
This tumor contains unusually large horn cysts. (×50)

cell epitheliomas possess horn cysts of considerable size (Fig. 27-45).

Keratotic basal cell epithelioma shares with trichoepithelioma the presence of horn cysts, and it is sometimes difficult to decide whether a lesion represents a keratotic basal cell epithelioma or a trichoepithelioma (see p. 527). Clinical data may be necessary for a decision to be reached. Also, the horn cysts must not be confused with the horn pearls that occur in squamous cell carcinoma (see Differential Diagnosis).

Cystic basal cell epithelioma shows one or several cystic spaces within tumor lobules. In most instances, the cysts form as a result of necrobiotic changes in the centrally located tumor cells (Reidbord et al). In rare instances, the cells in the center of tumor islands assume a vesicular appearance before disintegrating, suggesting differentiation into sebaceous cells (Fig. 27-46) (Foot). The disintegration is then analogous to that of sebaceous cells in the process of forming their secretion. In some instances, fat stains have demonstrated the presence of lipid material in the vacuolated cells (Urban and Winkelmann).

The diagnosis of basal cell epithelioma with sebaceous cell differentiation has been applied to basal cell epitheliomas that show, either with or without cysts, groups of mature or nearly mature sebaceous cells enclosed in the lobules of a basal cell epithelioma (Urban and Winkelmann; Rulon and Helwig). Such tumors blend into sebaceous epithelioma (see (p. 541) without a sharp dividing line.

Adenoid basal cell epithelioma shows formations suggesting tubular, glandlike structures. The cells are arranged in intertwining strands and radially around islands of connective tissue, resulting in a lacelike patterning of the tumor (Fig. 27-47). In rare instances, one may find lumina surrounded by cells that have the appearance of secretory cells (Fig. 27-48). The lumina may be filled with a colloidlike substance or with an amorphous granular material, but definite evidence of secretory activity of the cells lining the lumina cannot be obtained, even with histochemical methods. Sim-

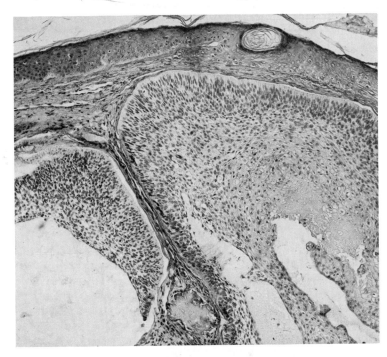

Fig. 27-46.   Cystic basal cell epithelioma
The cyst on the right side has formed by disintegration of cells with sebaceous differentiation. (×100)

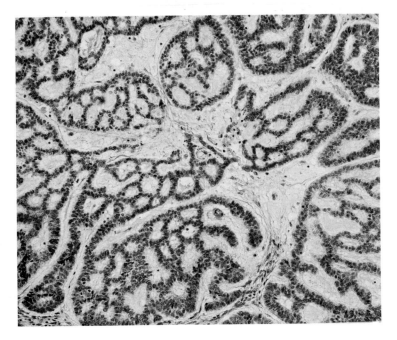

Fig. 27-47.   Adenoid basal cell epithelioma
The strands of epithelial cells present a lacelike pattern. The stroma has a mucoid appearance. (×200)

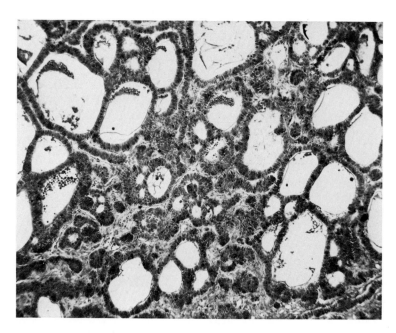

Fig. 27-48.   Adenoid basal cell epithelioma
The tumor contains lumina surrounded by cells that have the appearance of glandular cells. (×200)

ilarly, because of the low degree of differentiation of the cells, histochemical reactions that would indicate either apocrine or eccrine differentiation are negative (Wood et al).

However, there is one rather rare type of adenoid basal cell epithelioma, referred to as eccrine epithelioma, in which differentiation toward eccrine ductal structures is quite evident. In most instances, the tumor is located on the scalp, is quite large, may ulcerate (Baer et al), and may infiltrate so deeply that it invades underlying bone (Sanchez and Winkelmann). Eccrine epithelioma resembles syringoma by showing ductal as well as cystic and commalike epithelial components and by containing eccrine enzymes, such as phosphorylase and succinic dehyrogenase (Freeman and Winkelmann). The difference between eccrine epithelioma and syringoma lies in the large size of eccrine epithelioma and the depth of its invasion.

Two uncommon histologic variants of basal cell epithelioma have been described, the adamantoid and the granular types. Neither has a characteristic clinical appearance. *Adamantoid basal cell epithelioma* shows a great histologic resemblance to dental ameloblastoma or adamantinoma (Lerchin and Rahbari). One observes solid masses of basalioma cells with palisading at the periphery. Inside this layer, the cells show elongated nuclei and stellate cytoplasm stretched as thin, connecting bridges across empty spaces, as seen in adamantinoma. In *granular basal cell epithelioma,* some of the tumor

cells have the usual appearance of basalioma cells, whereas others show a gradual transition to granular cells. The granular cells show in their cytoplasm numerous eosinophilic granules with a tendency to coalesce (Barr and Graham). The eosinophilic granules greatly resemble those seen in granular cell tumor (see p. 674).

Nodulo-ulcerative Basal Cell Epithelioma. Nodulo-ulcerative basal cell epithelioma, clinically the most common type of basal cell epithelioma, may on histologic examination appear solid, keratotic, cystic, or adenoid. The histologic descriptions given above for solid, keratotic, cystic, and adenoid basal cell epithelioma apply in general to the nodulo-ulcerative type of basal cell epithelioma.

Pigmented Basal Cell Epithelioma. Although three fourths of all basal cell epitheliomas are found on staining with dopa to contain melanocytes, and although melanin is present in one fourth of them (Deppe et al), large amounts of melanin are encountered only rarely. The presence of melanin in basal cell epitheliomas can be explained by the fact that melanocytes are present not only in the surface epidermis but also in the hair matrix and therefore may also be found in tumors with pilar differentiation (see p. 26).

Basal cell epitheliomas with large amounts of melanin are shown on staining with silver to contain melanocytes interspersed between the tumor cells. These melanocytes have numerous melanin granules in their cytoplasm, as well as in their dendrites (Streitmann). This contrasts with normal epidermal melanocytes of Caucasoids, in which, as a rule, one finds only a few rather small melanin granules (Zelickson et al). The tumor cells usually contain very little melanin, but there are many melanophages in the connective tissue stroma surrounding the tumor masses (Streitmann; Sanderson). The reason for the presence of pigment-laden melanocytes and melanophages lies in the inability of the tumor cells to accept more than a small amount of melanin. (For details, see Electron Microscopy, p. 574.)

Morphealike or Fibrosing Basal Cell Epithelioma. Connective tissue participation is much greater in the morphealike variant than in the other types of basal cell epithelioma. Embedded in a dense fibrous stroma are innumerable groups of tumor cells arranged in elongated strands (Fig. 27-49) (Caro and Howell). Most of the strands are narrow, often only one layer of cells thick, so that they resemble the narrow strands of tumor cells seen in the skin in metastatic scirrhous carcinoma of the breast. However, on searching, one usually finds at least a few larger aggregates of tumor cells as well as some strands of tumor cells showing branching. The strands of tumor cells often extend deep into the dermis.

Superficial Basal Cell Epithelioma. Superficial basal cell epithelioma shows buds and irregular proliferations of tumor tissue attached to the undersurface of the epidermis (Fig. 27-50). The peripheral cell layer of the tumor formations often shows palisading. In most cases, there is little penetration into the dermis. The overlying epidermis usually shows atrophy. Fibroblasts, often in a fairly large number, are arranged around the tumor cell proliferations. In addition, a mild to moderate amount of a nonspecific chronic inflammatory infiltrate is present in the upper dermis.

Some superficial basal cell epitheliomas, after having persisted as such for various lengths of time, become invasive basal cell epitheliomas. Since this change may be limited at first to a few areas,

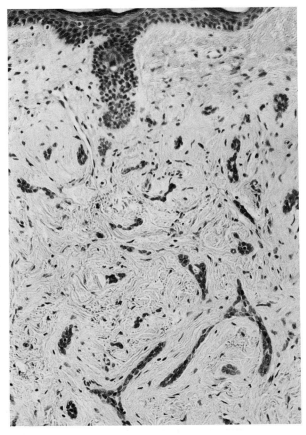

Fig. 27-49. Morphealike or fibrosing basal cell epithelioma
Innumerable small groups of closely packed tumor cells, many of them arranged in elongated strands, are embedded in a dense fibrous stroma. (×100)

Fig. 27-50. Superficial basal cell epithelioma
The tumor shows buds and irregular proliferations of tumor tissue attached to the undersurface of the epidermis. Note the similarity between the tumor buds in this illustration and the primary epithelial germ buds in the embryonal skin shown in Figure 2-1. (×100)

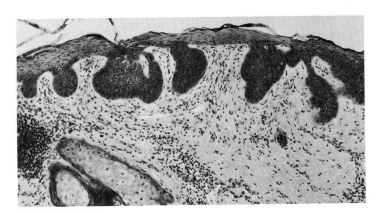

representative sections throughout the entire block should be examined. For a discussion of the question of whether superficial basal cell epithelioma is unicentric or multicentric in origin, see Histogenesis.

Fibroepithelioma. In fibroepithelioma, first described in 1953 (Pinkus), long, thin, branching, anastomosing strands of basal cell epithelioma are embedded in a fibrous stroma (Fig. 27-51) (Pinkus, 1953; Hornstein). Many of the strands show connections with the surface epidermis. Here and there, small groups of dark-staining cells showing a palisade arrangement of the peripheral cell layer may be seen along the epithelial strands, like buds on a branch. Usually, the tumor is quite superficial in location and is well demarcated at its lower border. Fibroepithelioma combines features of the intracanalicular fibroadenoma of the breast, the

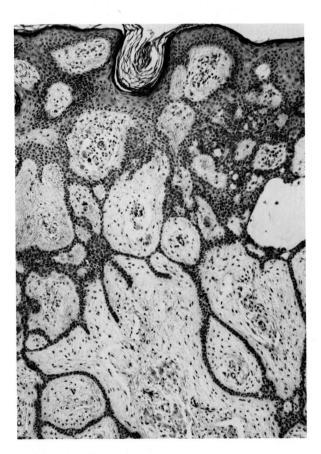

Fig. 27-51.   Fibroepithelioma
Long, thin, branching, anastomosing strands of basal cell epithelioma are embedded in a fibrous stroma. Here and there, small buds of basophilic cells are seen along the epithelial strands. (×100)

reticulated type of seborrheic keratosis, and superficial basal cell epithelioma (Pinkus, 1953). Fibroepithelioma can change into an invasive and ulcerating basal cell epithelioma (Degos and Hewitt).

Nevoid Basal Cell Epithelioma Syndrome. The multiple basal cell epitheliomas seen in the nevoid basal cell epithelioma syndrome present no features that distinguish them from ordinary basal cell epithelioma, even while they are still in the early nevoid stage and have not yet become invasive and destructive, as they may be later in the neoplastic stage (Howell and Caro). All the diverse features of basal cell epithelioma, such as solid, adenoid, cystic, keratotic, superficial, and fibrosing formations, can be seen in the lesions of the nevoid basal cell epithelioma syndrome (Mason et al). Usually, a histologic distinction between the nevoid basal cell epithelioma syndrome and typical trichoepithelioma is easy, since keratotic cysts are more prominent in the latter. However, some lesions of trichoepithelioma show relatively few horn cysts (see p. 526), and a histologic distinction in such cases may be impossible (Jablonska). Clinical data will then be necessary (see p. 528).

The palmar and plantar pits are a result of the premature desquamation of most of the horny layer (Howell and Freeman). On histologic examination, the epidermal rete ridges beneath the pits are found to be crowded with cells resembling those of basal cell epithelioma. Overlying these rete ridges, one finds a markedly thinned granular layer topped by a very thin layer of loose keratin (Howell and Mehregan). In some patients, the pits actually show at their base the presence of small basal cell epitheliomas (Holubar et al). In rare instances, one or several clinically visible basal cell epitheliomas arise on the palms or soles in patients with palmar and plantar pits (Ward; Taylor and Wilkins; Howell and Freeman).

The jaw cysts represent odontogenic keratocysts. They are lined by keratinizing squamous epithelium and contain laminated keratin (Totten). Each jaw cyst may consist of either one large cyst or multiple microcysts (Mason et al).

Linear Unilateral Basal Cell Nevus. The basal cell epitheliomas in linear unilateral basal cell nevus have a variable histologic appearance. The tumor formations may be solid, adenoid, keratotic, or cystic (Carney; Horio and Komura). In addition, there may be areas resembling trichoepithelioma (Anderson and Best) or eccrine spiradenoma (Blanchard et al). The walls of the comedones show numerous buds of basal cell epithelioma extending into the surrounding dermis (Carney; Bleiberg and Brodkin).

Bazex Syndrome. The basal cell epitheliomas encountered in the Bazex syndrome have a variable histologic appearance. Some of them are indistinguishable from trichoepithelioma (Viksnins and Berlin; Plosila et al). The areas of follicular atrophoderma show a dilated follicular ostium leading into a distorted and underdeveloped pilosebaceous unit (Plosila et al).

Intraepidermal Epithelioma of Borst–Jadassohn. Originally, the Borst–Jadassohn tumor was thought to be an intraepidermal basal cell epithelioma, because the cells composing the intraepidermal islands usually are small and have a deeply basophilic cytoplasm (Sims and Parker). However, on careful examination, it subsequently became evident that the cells composing the intraepidermal islands in the presumed intraepidermal basal cell epitheliomas possess intercellular bridges and in reality are seborrheic keratoses of the clonal type (see p. 478) (Morales and Hu). The existence of an intraepidermal basal cell epithelioma is also unlikely because the close relationship that exists between tumor and stroma in basal cell epithelioma excludes the formation of intraepidermal nests, which would lack any contact with the stroma (Holubar and Wolff).

However, there are several types of tumors, some benign and some malignant, that on occasion show well-defined islands of cells within the epidermis that differ in their appearance from the surrounding epidermal cells (Mehregan and Pinkus). This is referred to as the Jadassohn phenomenon. Among the tumors that occasionally have an intraepidermal location are the following:

Clonal seborrheic keratosis. Some of these tumors show intraepidermal aggregates of basaloid cells suggestive of a basal cell epithelioma in situ (see Fig. 26-5) (Morales and Hu), whereas others show intraepidermal islands of an irritated seborrheic keratosis simulating a squamous cell carcinoma in situ.

Bowen's disease. Occasionally, one observes clonal aggregates of Bowen's disease within the epidermis (Okun and Edelstein). At a later stage, there may be dermal invasion (Berger and Baughman).

Intraepidermal poroma, also referred to as hidroacanthoma simplex (Smith and Coburn; Mehregan and Levson).

Intraepidermal malignant eccrine poroma (Bardach). In cases of intraepidermal metastases of malignant eccrine poroma, the tumor masses extend through the superficial lymphatics from the dermis into the epidermis (see p. 554) (Pinkus and Mehregan).

The concept of intraepidermal tumors has been extended also to include Paget's disease of the breast (see p. 510), extramammary Paget's disease (see p. 513), intraepidermal junction nevus (see p. 682), and superficial spreading malignant melanoma in situ, which is also referred to as pagetoid malignant melanoma in situ (see p. 705) (Mehregan and Pinkus).

It should be mentioned that some authors regard the intraepidermal epithelioma of Jadassohn as a distinct entity that may invade the dermis and on rare occasions cause metastases (Graham and Helwig; Cook and Ridgway). It has been postulated that this tumor arises from acrosyringium keratinocytes or pluripotential adnexal cells (Graham and Helwig). It seems possible, however, that it represents Bowen's disease with intraepidermal clonal aggregates.

Basal Squamous Cell Epithelioma. The existence of basal cell epitheliomas with features of squamous cell carcinoma was first postulated in 1922 (Darier and Ferrand). Two types of basal squamous cell epitheliomas, referred to as metatypical epitheliomas, were recognized: a mixed and an intermediary type. The mixed type was described as showing focal keratinization consisting of pearls with a colloidal or parakeratotic center, and the intermediary type as showing within a network of narrow strands two kinds of cells, an outer row of dark-staining basal cells, and an inner layer of cells appearing larger, lighter, and better defined than the basal cells and regarded as intermediate in character between basal and squamous cells.

Several authors have accepted the existence of basal squamous cell epitheliomas or metatypical epitheliomas (Montgomery, 1928; Gertler; Borel; Farmer and Helwig). They are considered to represent a transition from basal cell epithelioma to squamous cell carcinoma. It has been stated that a continuum extends from basal cell carcinoma at one extreme to squamous cell carcinoma at the other (Borel). The incidence of basal squamous cell carcinomas among basal cell epitheliomas has been judged to be 3% (Borel), 8% (Gertler), and even 12% (Montgomery, 1928). It has also been stated that basal squamous cell epitheliomas show a greater tendency to metastasize than basal cell epitheliomas (Montgomery, 1928; Borel; Farmer and Helwig).

However, the existence of basal squamous cell epitheliomas is questioned by many (Welton et al;

Lennox and Wells; Smith and Swerdlow; Pinkus, 1965; Holmes et al; Freeman). It would seem that the entirely different genesis of squamous cell carcinoma, a true anaplastic carcinoma of the epidermis, and basal cell epithelioma, an appendage tumor composed of immature rather than anaplastic cells, makes the occurrence of transitional forms quite unlikely (see Histogenesis). It can be assumed that the so-called mixed type of basal squamous cell epithelioma represents a keratotic basal cell epithelioma (see Fig. 27-44) and that the intermediate type represents a basal cell epithelioma with differentiation into two types of cells (see Fig. 27-43 and p. 565).

Mixed Carcinoma. Mixed carcinoma shows a squamous cell carcinoma contiguous to a basal cell epithelioma as a so-called collision tumor (Fig. 27-52). It is likely that, in most instances, the squamous cell carcinoma develops secondary to the basal cell epithelioma. Like other chronic ulcerative lesions, such as burns and stasis ulcers, basal cell epithelioma may stimulate the development of a squamous cell carcinoma. Before making a diagnosis of mixed carcinoma, however, one must rule out the possibility of pseudocarcinomatous hyperplasia occurring in a basal cell epithelioma (see p. 505).

Histogenesis. Krompecher, the original describer of basal cell epithelioma, stated in 1903 that he regarded this tumor as a carcinoma of the basal cells of the epidermis and that those tumors that show a tendency

toward gland formation are imitating the potential of the basal cells to form cutaneous glands. Krompecher's view is still supported by some (Montgomery, 1967; Teloh and Wheelock; Ten Seldam and Helwig). According to Geschickter and Koehler, only those basal cells with a potential to develop into glandular cells give rise to basal cell epithelioma. They suggested the designation *appendage cell carcinoma.* Mallory held the opinion that basal cell epitheliomas are carcinomas of hair matrix cells. In 1947, Foot expressed the view that basal cell epitheliomas are carcinomas that have developed from distorted primordia of dermal adnexa rather than from ordinary epidermal basal cells. He stated that the tumors imitate the embryonal development of any one type or of all three types of adnexal primordia, that is, hair, sebaceous gland, and sweat gland.

The first author to express doubts that basal cell epitheliomas are carcinomas was Adamson; in 1914, he stated that, in his opinion, basal cell epitheliomas are nevoid tumors originating "from latent embryonic foci aroused from their dormant state at a later period in life." He believed that the latent embryonic foci usually are embryonic pilosebaceous follicles but occasionally are embryonic sweat ducts. Several other authors have since reached similar conclusions, among them Wallace and Halpert, who stated in 1950 that they regarded basal cell epitheliomas as benign tumors arising from cells of the matrix differentiated to form the hair follicle. They proposed the term *trichoma* for them.

In 1948, Lever expressed his belief that basal cell epitheliomas are not carcinomas and are not derived from basal cells, but rather are nevoid tumors, or hamartomas, derived from primary epithelial germ cells. In other words, basal cell epitheliomas originate from incompletely differentiated, immature cells and not from

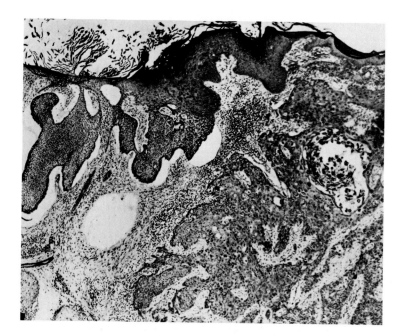

Fig. 27-52.   Mixed carcinoma
A basal cell epithelioma (*left*) and a squamous cell carcinoma (*right*) lie side by side. (×50)

anaplastic cells. They thus represent the least differentiated of the appendage tumors. (See Classification and Histogenesis of the Benign Appendage Tumors, p. 522; see also Table 27-1, p. 523.)

It was originally assumed, analogous to Adamson's view, that the primary epithelial germ cells giving rise to basal cell epithelioma are in all instances embryonic cells that lay dormant until the onset of neoplasia. Even though this view applies to the linear unilateral basal cell nevus, which is usually present from birth (see p. 570), it is likely that, as suggested by Pinkus (1953), basal cell epitheliomas occurring later in life arise not from dormant embryonic primary epithelial germ cells but from pluripotential cells that form continuously during life and, like embryonic primary epithelial germ cells, have the potentiality of forming hair, sebaceous glands, and apocrine glands. The fact that basal cell epitheliomas may arise in sun-exposed areas and in areas of radiodermatitis supports this view.

PILAR DIFFERENTIATION. Differentiation in basal cell epithelioma is predominantly toward pilar keratin. The presence of citrulline in keratinized structures indicates that the origin of such keratin is the hair matrix, since epidermal keratin contains no citrulline (Holmes et al). However, not all keratin of hair matrix origin contains citrulline. The hair cortex and hair cuticle do not contain it, whereas the medulla of the hair and the inner root sheath do. The outer root sheath, being of epidermal origin, is also free of citrulline. Thus, citrulline is regularly present in pilomatricoma (see p. 532) but absent in trichilemmal cysts and proliferating trichilemmal tumors, which are composed of outer root sheath cells (see p. 533). Keratotic basal cell epitheliomas contain both citrulline-positive and citrulline-negative keratin, reflecting the different lines of differentiation inherent in the hair matrix (Holmes et al).

ECCRINE DIFFERENTIATION. Basal cell epitheliomas can arise not only from immature pluripotential cells differentiating toward primary epithelial germ structures but also from immature pluripotential cells differentiating toward eccrine glands. The occurrence of eccrine epitheliomas bears out this theory (see p. 568). The rarity of basal cell epitheliomas on the palms and soles implies that cells with the potential to differentiate toward eccrine glands rarely participate in the formation of basal cell epitheliomas. The fact that the palmar and plantar pits of the nevoid basal cell epithelioma very rarely show a full-fledged basal cell epithelioma suggests that the palms and soles do not possess the stromal factor necessary for the formation of appendage tumors of the pilosebaceous type (Covo).

STROMAL FACTOR. In addition to the rarity of basal cell epithelioma on the palms and soles, there is experimental evidence indicating the importance of the stromal factor in the development of basal cell epithelioma: autotransplants of basal cell epitheliomas survive only when they include connective tissue stroma (Van Scott and Reinertson).

LACK OF AUTONOMY. Basal cell epitheliomas, when transplanted to the anterior chamber of the rabbit's eye together with their connective tissue stroma, fail to grow, in contrast to squamous cell carcinoma (Gerstein). This observation suggests a lack of autonomy of the cells of basal cell epithelioma. Since autonomy of the tumor cell is a prerequisite for the formation of metastases and represents a characteristic feature of malignant tumors (Greene), the absence of autonomy in basal cell epithelioma indicates that this tumor is not a true carcinoma.

SITE OF ORIGIN. The usual site of origin of basal cell epithelioma is the surface epidermis (Hundeiker and Berger). Occasionally, however, the tumor may originate from the outer root sheath of a hair follicle (Zackheim; Brown et al).

Of particular interest is the manner of growth of superficial basal cell epithelioma. Routine sectioning carried out perpendicular to the skin surface shows seemingly independent nests of basal cell epithelioma suggestive at times of the growth of primary epithelial germs in the embryonic skin (see Fig. 2-1). Thus, it was at one time widely assumed that the peripheral extension seen in superficial basal cell epithelioma was based on a "multicentric" growth characterized by the formation of new buds of tumor tissue at the periphery. However, on the basis of findings in serial sections and in wax reconstructions of superficial basal cell epitheliomas, Madsen has favored the theory of a "unicentric" origin. Madsen (1941, 1955, 1965) was able to show that the tumor strands are continuous but are attached to the undersurface of the epidermis only at intervals, like garlands. Madsen found not only in his wax reconstructions but also in sections cut parallel to the surface of the skin that individual tumor islands are interconnected. Oberste-Lehn, using a technic of separating the epidermis from the dermis by maceration, could not find such interconnections, but the possibility could not be excluded, as Madsen pointed out, that the interconnections had ruptured as a result of the maceration. It was subsequently shown when trypsin was used for the separation of the epidermis from the dermis that interconnections exist between tumor cell nests in superficial basal cell epithelioma (Kimura).

ELECTRON MICROSCOPY. The predominant cell in undifferentiated basal cell epithelioma is characterized by a large nucleus, poorly developed desmosomes, and rather sparse tonofilaments. Thus, the tumor cells differ from normal epidermal basal cells. They resemble the cells of the undifferentiated hair matrix (Zelickson, 1962) or the immature basal cells of the embryonic epidermis, particularly those of the primary epithelial germ (Lever and Hashimoto; Kumakiri and Hashimoto). In addition to the prevalent large, light cells, a few cells that are smaller, darker, and more irregularly shaped can be found (Lever and Hashimoto; Reidbord et al). The darkness of the latter cells is due to the abundance of ribonucleoprotein particles in their cytoplasm. A well-developed basement membrane separates the tumor from the dermis (Zelickson, 1962). Processes from the tumor cells do not usually penetrate the basement membrane in basal cell epithelioma, in contrast to squamous cell carcinoma, in which processes extend through a fragmented basement membrane into the stroma (Cutler et al).

Keratinization is commonly observed by electron microscopy in basal cell epithelioma, especially in the keratotic type. In addition to well-developed desmosomes and many thick bundles of tonofilaments, dense clumps of homogeneous, dyskeratotic material are present in many keratinizing cells (EM 40). A small number of keratohyaline granules are often seen. They probably represent trichohyaline granules, which occur in the process of keratinization of the inner root sheath and its cuticle (Lever and Hashimoto).

Some basal cell epitheliomas show areas of adenoid differentiation in which cells are grouped around glandlike lumina. Such cells may show pronounced infolding of the plasma membrane at their lateral borders as seen normally in eccrine ductal cells (see p. 22) (Reidbord et al).

In pigmented basal cell epitheliomas, most of the melanin is found not within the tumor cells but within melanocytes of the tumor and in melanophages located in the connective tissue stroma. The reason for this distribution of melanin is the following: although numerous melanosomes are present in the dendrites of the melanocytes, the tumor cells generally do not phagocytize the melanin-containing dendrites, resulting in a blockage of the transfer of melanin from melanocytes to the tumor cells (Zelickson, 1967; Bleehen). This is analogous to the blocked transfer from melanocytes to tumor cells in some pigmented seborrheic keratoses referred to as melanoacanthoma (see p. 480). Nevertheless, in occasional instances of pigmented basal cell epithelioma, some transfer of melanosomes to the tumor cells takes place. The tumor cells then contain melanosomes, which are located largely as melanosome complexes within lysosomes (EM 41) (Lever and Hashimoto).

PRESENCE OF AMYLOID. Cell proliferation in basal cell epithelioma is considerable. The experimentally determined cell-doubling time of 9 days, however, does not conform with the clinical observation that basal cell epithelioma, as a rule, is a very slowly growing tumor (Weinstein and Frost). This suggests that there must be cell death. In addition to phagocytosis by neighboring tumor cells and macrophages (Kerr and Searle), apoptosis of tumor cells also often takes place, with transformation of the cells into colloid bodies and subsequently into amyloid (Weedon and Shand; Hashimoto and Kobayashi). This conversion of epithelial cells into amyloid is analogous to that occurring in lichenoid and macular amyloidosis (see p. 411). Colloid bodies, demonstrable by direct immunofluorescence for immuno-

globulin M (IgM), have been found in 89% of basal cell epitheliomas (Weedon and Shand). Amyloid has been observed in the stroma and inside the tumor islands both by histochemistry and by electron microscopy in as many as 65% of basal cell epitheliomas (Hashimoto and Brownstein; Weedon and Shand). This amyloid shows positive staining with antikeratin antiserum, indicating that it is derived from tonofilaments (Masu et al).

Differential Diagnosis. Differentiation of basal cell epithelioma from squamous cell carcinoma can sometimes be difficult, so difficult that some authors believe that intermediate forms (basal squamous cell epitheliomas) occur. However, as a rule, differentiation is fairly easy. One of the best points of differentiation is that most cells of basal cell epithelioma stain deeply basophilic, whereas most cells of squamous cell carcinoma, at least in grades 1 and 2, have an eosinophilic tint owing to partial keratinization. The cells in squamous cell carcinoma, grades 3 and 4, may appear basophilic because of the absence of keratinization. However, they then differ from basal cell epithelioma by showing much greater atypicality of their nuclei and their mitotic figures. It is important to remember that keratinization is not a prerogative of squamous cell carcinoma; it occurs also in basal cell epithelioma with differentiation toward hair structures (see Keratotic Basal Cell Epithelioma, p. 565). Keratinization in basal cell epitheliomas may be partial and then result in parakeratotic bands and whorls, or it may be complete and result in horn cysts. The keratinization seen in the horn cysts differs from that seen in the horn pearls of squamous cell carcinomas by being abrupt and complete rather than gradual and incomplete. The fairly common presence in basal cell epithelioma of areas of retraction of the tumor cell masses from the surrounding connective tissue (see p. 564) also aids in the differentiation of this tumor from squamous cell carcinoma, in which such areas of retraction are rarely found.

The differential diagnosis of basal cell epithelioma from trichoepithelioma has already been discussed (see p. 527). Of particular importance is the differentiation of fibrosing basal cell epithelioma from the only recently described desmoplastic trichoepithelioma (see p. 528). Both tumors have in common thin strands of small basaloid cells embedded in a dense, fibrous stroma, but desmoplastic trichoepithelioma shows, in addition, a considerable number of horn cysts. A fairly high percentage of tumors originally diagnosed as basal cell epitheliomas in children and teenagers could be reclassified as desmoplastic trichoepithelioma (Rahbari and Mehregan).

CARCINOMA OF SEBACEOUS GLANDS

Carcinomas of the sebaceous glands occur most frequently on the eyelids, where they originate usually from the meibomian glands and less commonly from the glands of Zeis. However, they may occur elsewhere on the skin. On the eyelids, sebaceous carcinoma may be easily mistaken for chronic blepharoconjunctivitis or a chalazion (Dixon et al). On the skin, sebaceous carcinoma usually manifests itself as a nodule that may or may not be ulcerated (Urban and Winkelmann; King et al). Sebaceous carcinomas of the eyelids quite frequently cause regional metastases. Also, there may be orbital invasion, and, in 14% of the cases reported in one study, death resulted from visceral metastases (Boniuk and Zimmerman). Sebaceous carcinomas of the skin also may cause regional metastases (Rulon and Helwig; Hernández-Pérez and Baños; Mellette et al). However, visceral metastasis resulting in death is very rare, although it has been described (King et al). The sebaceous carcinomas that may be found among the multiple sebaceous neoplasms occurring in association with multiple visceral carcinomas in Torre's syndrome do not metastasize (see p. 539) (Leonard and Deaton).

Histopathology. One observes irregular lobular formations with great variation in the size of the lobules (Fig. 27-53). Although many cells are undifferentiated, distinct sebaceous cells showing a foamy cytoplasm are present in the center of most lobules (King et al). Many undifferentiated cells and sebaceous cells appear atypical, showing considerable variation in the shape and size of their nuclei (Rulon and Helwig). Also, many of the undifferentiated cells have an eosinophilic cytoplasm, and, when fat stains are used on frozen sections, are found to contain fine lipid globules (Dixon et al). Some of the large lobules show areas composed of atypical keratinizing cells, as seen in squamous cell carcinoma (Urban and Winkelmann).

Sebaceous carcinoma of the eyelids may show a pagetoid spread of malignant cells in the overlying epithelium. Recognition of the pagetoid growth pattern in biopsy material can be essential to recognition of the existence of an underlying sebaceous carcinoma (Russell et al).

Differential Diagnosis. Sebaceous carcinomas must be differentiated from sebaceous epithelioma, which represents a basal cell epithelioma with considerable differentiation of the cells toward

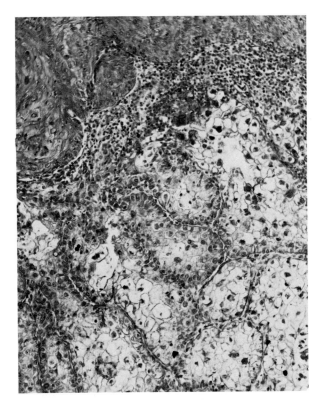

Fig. 27-53. Carcinoma of sebaceous glands
Irregular, lobular formations are composed of sebaceous and undifferentiated cells showing considerable variation in the shape and size of their nuclei. The undifferentiated cells differ from the undifferentiated cells of sebaceous epithelioma by showing greater atypicality of their nuclei and an eosinophilic rather than a basophilic cytoplasm. (×200)

sebaceous gland cells (see p. 541). Sebaceous carcinoma, in contrast with sebaceous epithelioma, shows no areas of basal cell epithelioma. The undifferentiated cells of sebaceous carcinoma differ from those of basal cell epithelioma by showing greater atypicality and a more eosinophilic cytoplasm (Beach and Severance).

CARCINOMA OF ECCRINE SWEAT GLANDS

Carcinomas of the eccrine sweat glands do not possess a characteristic clinical appearance or location. Although they may arise on the palms (Grant; Fresen; Hashimoto and Lever) or on the soles (Teloh et al), they more commonly arise elsewhere, particularly in the head and neck region (El-Domeiri et al).

Histopathology. Several histologic types of eccrine sweat gland carcinoma are recognized. In addition to a *classic* type, there is a *mucinous* carcinoma of eccrine glands and an *adenoid cystic* carcinoma of eccrine glands. It should also be pointed out that the malignant eccrine poroma (see p. 554) as well as the malignant eccrine spiradenoma (see p. 557), the malignant clear cell hidradenoma (see p. 560), and the malignant chondroid syringoma (see p. 562) are variants of eccrine sweat gland carcinoma.

Classic Type.   The classic type of eccrine gland carcinoma has a high incidence of metastases. Of 68 patients followed for 5 years or more, 29 had regional lymph node metastases, and visceral metastases were present in 26 (El-Domeiri et al).

The histologic configuration in the classic type of eccrine gland carcinoma varies from fairly well differentiated tubular structures in some areas to anaplastic cells in other areas, not recognizable by themselves as eccrine sweat gland structure (Teloh et al). The tubular structures usually show only small lumina that are lined by either a single layer (Fresen) or a double layer of cells (Teloh et al). In some areas, the lumina are lined by secretory cells, which appear large and vacuolated owing to the presence of glycogen and, in addition, often contain PAS-positive, diastase-resistant granules (Hashimoto and Lever; Dave). In other areas, an eosinophilic, PAS-positive, diastase-resistant cuticle may be seen lining some of the lumina. It is analogous to the cuticle seen in eccrine ducts (Fig. 27-54) (Orbaneja et al).

It is often difficult to differentiate the classic type of eccrine sweat gland carcinoma from a metastatic adenocarcinoma. Therefore, the diagnosis of metastatic adenocarcinoma should always be given serious consideration before a diagnosis of eccrine sweat gland carcinoma is decided upon. So-called eccrine enzymes, such as amylophosphorylase and succinic dehydrogenase, may be present in moderate amounts and aid in the recognition of the tumors as eccrine rather than as metastatic (Hashimoto and Lever; Orbaneja et al).

Mucinous Carcinoma.   In the rather uncommon mucinous carcinoma of eccrine glands, first described in 1971 (Mendoza and Helwig), regional lymph node metastases occur occasionally (Santa Cruz et al). However, widespread metastases have been described very rarely (Yeung and Stinson).

The histologic appearance is highly characteristic. The tumor is divided into numerous compartments by strands of fibrous tissue. In each compartment, abundant amounts of pale-staining mucin surround nests or cords of moderately anaplastic epithelial cells, some of which show a tubular lumen (Fig. 27-55) (Mendoza and Helwig; Headington). The mucin shows strongly positive reactions with both PAS and colloidal iron. The mucinous material is resistant to diastase and hyaluronidase but is sensitive to digestion with sialidase. The reaction with alcian blue is position at pH 2.5 but negative at pH 0.4, which indicates that the mucin is nonsulfated. It can thus be concluded that the mucin represents sialomucin,

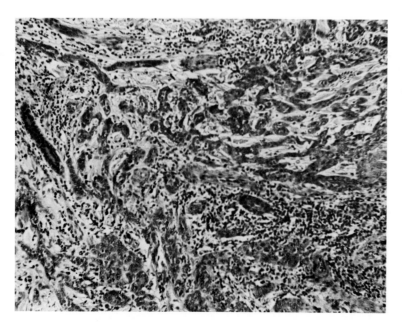

Fig. 27-54.   Carcinoma of eccrine glands
The tumor consists largely of tubular structures. Some of the tubules show a narrow lumen lined with an eosinophilic cuticle analogous to eccrine ducts. ($\times$100)

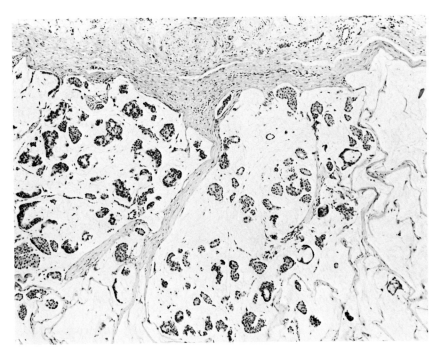

Fig. 27-55. Mucinous carcinoma of eccrine glands
The tumor is divided into numerous compartments. In each compartment, abundant amounts of mucin surround small islets of tumor cells, some of which show a lumen. (×25) (Headington JT: Cancer 39:1055–1063, 1977)

an epithelial mucin (Mendoza and Helwig; Headington).

Enzyme histochemical examination has revealed a prevalence of enzymes of the eccrine type (Headington). Electron microscopy has revealed two types of secretory cells in the tumor, dark and light, analogous to the two types normally encountered in eccrine coils. The sialomucin is secreted by the dark cells (Wright and Font).

Adenoid Cystic Carcinoma. The rarest type of eccrine sweat gland carcinomas is the adenoid cystic carcinoma, first described in 1975 (Boggio). Thus far, lymph node metastases have not been observed (Headington et al).

Histologic examination reveals large cell masses with an adenoid or cribiform pattern and, in addition, many small, solid epithelial islands (Fig. 27-56). Through the accumulation of mucin, the adenoid spaces may be transformed into multiple cystic spaces lined by a flattened cuboidal epithelium. The adenoid and cystic spaces contain pale-staining mucin that is readily removed by hyaluronidase digestion (Headington et al). Additional features that are occasionally present are ductal structures resembling eccrine ducts and invasion of perineural spaces (Boggio).

Adenoid cystic carcinoma of eccrine glands must be distinguished from the adenoid type of basal cell epithelioma, from which it differs by lack of continuity with the epidermis or hair sheath and by the absence of palisading (Headington et al).

TRABECULAR CARCINOMA (MERKEL CELL CARCINOMA)

Trabecular carcinoma, originally described as a sweat gland carcinoma in 1972 (Toker), was identified as a Merkel cell tumor by means of electron microscopy in 1978 (Tang and Toker). In most instances, a solitary nodule is present, but multiple lesions have been observed, either localized in one area (Taxy et al) or widely distributed (Abaci and Zak; Wong et al). There generally is no tendency to ulceration. Although half of the neoplasms reported have arisen in the skin of the head and neck, they may occur in many other areas (Sidhu et al). Metastatic spread to regional lymph nodes occurs in more than half of the patients, and widespread metastases resulting in death have been observed in 17% of the cases (Sidhu et al).

Histopathology. The histologic picture is quite distinct. Anastomosing cords and bands as well as clusters of tumor cells are seen in the dermis extending into the subcutis but usually showing no contact with the epidermis (Fig. 27-57). The tumor cells have a uniform appearance showing closely spaced, round, vesicular nuclei and scanty, ill-defined cytoplasm, so that the cell boundaries

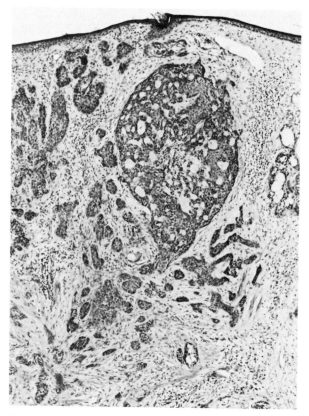

Fig. 27-56. Adenoid cystic carcinoma of eccrine glands
A large cell mass shows an adenoid or cribiform pattern. In addition, many small, solid epithelial islands are present. (×25) (Headington JT: Arch Dermatol 114:421–424, 1978)

are not discernible. Usually, numerous mitotic figures are present (Fig. 27-58) (Toker).

The granules in the tumor cells are argyrophilic (see p. 16); therefore, impregnation with a silver nitrate solution will stain them black, provided that large numbers of granules are present (de Wolf-Peeters et al; Iwasaki et al). However, in most instances, the number of granules is too small for them to be apparent with silver impregnation.

Histogenesis. On *electron microscopic examination,* one observes in the cytoplasm scattered, membrane-bound, round, dense-core granules 120 nm to 210 nm in diameter. They show a distinct halo underneath their limiting membrane (Tang and Toker; Sidhu et al; Iwasaki et al) and are indistinguishable from those seen in Merkel cells (see p. 20) and in other cells differentiating from the neurocrest as cells of the APUD system (*a*mine *p*recursor *u*ptake and *d*ecarboxylation). The concentration of the granules is variable. Whereas some tumors contain only a few granules, others contain numerous aggregates of granules (Tang and Toker; Sidhu et al). As with Merkel cells, occasional desmosomes are usually seen between the tumor cells (Tang and Toker; Wong et al).

Differential Diagnosis. The uniformity of the tumor cells and their immature aspect may suggest a "blastic" type of lymphoma (de Wolf-Peeters et al) or a metastatic carcinoma, especially one originating from an oat cell carcinoma of the lung. In the latter case, the tumor cells also contain dense-core granules (Taxy et al). Although the "trabecular" arrangement of some of the tumor cells in anastomosing cords and bands is typical for a

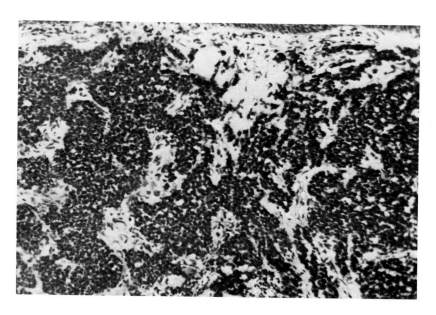

Fig. 27-57. Trabecular carcinoma (Merkel cell carcinoma)
Anastomosing cords and bands as well as clusters of tumor cells having a rather uniform appearance are present in the dermis. They show no contact with the epidermis. (×100)

trabecular carcinoma, electron microscopic examination may be desirable for confirmation of the diagnosis (Pollack and Goslen).

CARCINOMA OF APOCRINE GLANDS

Carcinomas of apocrine glands have been described only rarely. By 1970, a total of 18 cases had been described (Baes and Suurmond). Since then, ten additional cases have been reported (Warkel and Helwig). Their occurrence has been reported mainly in the axillae (Kipkie and Haust; Futrell et al; Warkel and Helwig). Occasionally, however, they arise in other areas endowed with apocrine glands, such as the vulva. They may also occur on the eyelids and in the external auditory meatus (Neldner), where Moll's glands and the ceruminal glands, respectively, are found as modified apocrine glands.

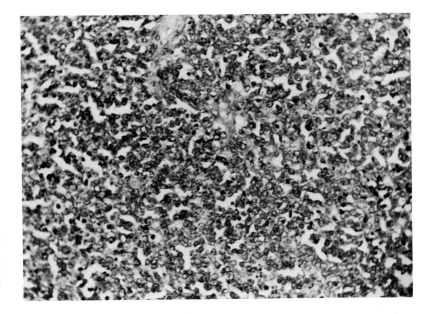

Fig. 27-58.   Trabecular carcinoma (Merkel cell carcinoma)
The tumor cells have closely spaced, round, vesicular nuclei and scanty, ill-defined cytoplasm. Numerous mitotic figures are present, showing a small, dark center surrounded by a clear space. ($\times 200$)

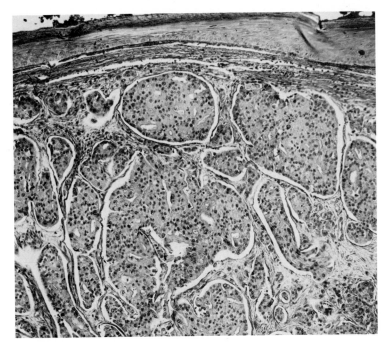

Fig. 27-59.   Apocrine carcinoma of the vulva
The tumor consists of atypical glandular cells with eosinophilic cytoplasm and active "decapitation" secretion. ($\times 100$)

Rarely, apocrine gland carcinomas arise in areas in which apocrine glands are normally absent, such as the forehead (Smith) and chest (Baes and Suurmond). Whereas some cases of carcinoma of apocrine glands show only local invasiveness (Neldner; Warkel and Helwig), others metastasize to regional lymph nodes (Futrell et al), and some patients have died from widespread metastases (Baes and Suurmond; Warkel and Helwig).

Histopathology.   The histologic picture is that of an adenocarcinoma that is fairly well, moderately, or poorly differentiated (Warkel and Helwig).

In fairly well differentiated apocrine gland carcinomas, nuclear atypicality and invasiveness are limited in degree. Well-developed glandular lumina are present (Fig. 27-59). The lumina may be cystic and show branching (Warkel and Helwig). The cytoplasm of the tumor cells is strongly eosinophilic. Evidence of decapitation secretion, typical of apocrine glands, is present at least in some areas (Futrell et al). In addition, the cytoplasm of the tumor cells contains PAS-positive, diastase-resistant granules (Elliot and Ramsey) and, often, iron-positive granules (Kipkie and Haust; Warkel and Helwig). Myoepithelial cells are absent.

In moderately or poorly differentiated apocrine gland carcinomas, recognition of an apocrine genesis may be difficult, although even poorly differentiated tumors often show fairly good differentiation in some areas (Warkel and Helwig).

Histogenesis. Enzyme histochemical determinations are of value in establishing an apocrine genesis, since apocrine gland carcinomas show strong activity of apocrine enzymes, such as acid phosphatase and indoxyl acetate esterase, and low activity or absence of eccrine enzymes, such as phosphorylase and succinic dehydrogenase (Neldner; Baes and Suurmond).

Differential Diagnosis.   Apocrine gland carcinoma of the axilla must be differentiated from a carcinoma arising in ectopic breast tissue. Features that favor the diagnosis of a carcinoma of apocrine glands are the presence of neoplastic glands high in the dermis, apocrine glands near the tumor, and intracytoplasmic granules of iron (Warkel and Helwig).

BIBLIOGRAPHY

Classification of the Appendage Tumors
ALBRECHT E: Uber Hamartome. Verh Dtsch Ges Pathol 7:153–157, 1904

BECKER SW: Seborrheic keratosis and verruca, with special reference to the melanotic variety. Arch Dermatol Syph 63:358–372, 1951

HASHIMOTO K, LEVER WF: Appendage Tumors of the Skin. Springfield, IL, Charles C Thomas, 1968

JADASSOHN J: Die benignen Epitheliome. Arch Dermatol Syph (Berlin) 117:705–716, 833–846, 1914

KLIGMAN AM, PINKUS H: The histogenesis of nevoid tumors of the skin. Arch Dermatol 81:922–930, 1960

KUMAKIRI M, HASHIMOTO K: Ultrastructural resemblance of basal cell epithelioma to primary epithelial germ. J Cutan Pathol 5:53–67, 1978

LEVER WF: Pathogenesis of benign tumors of cutaneous appendages and of basal cell epithelioma. Arch Dermatol Syph 57:679–724, 1948

PINKUS H: Premalignant fibroepithelial tumors of the skin. Arch Dermatol Syph 67:598–615, 1953

WECHSLER HL, FISHER ER: A combined polymorphic and adnexal tumor in nevus unius lateris. Dermatologica 130:158–164, 1964

Trichofolliculoma
GRAY HR, HELWIG EB: Trichofolliculoma. Arch Dermatol 86:619–625, 1962

HYMAN AB, CLAYMAN SJ: Hair follicle nevus. Arch Dermatol 75:678–684, 1957

KLIGMAN AM, PINKUS H: The histogenesis of nevoid tumors of the skin. Arch Dermatol 81:922–930, 1960

PINKUS H, SUTTON RL JR: Trichofolliculoma. Arch Dermatol 91:46–49, 1965

PLEWIG G: Sebaceous trichofolliculoma. J Cutan Pathol 7:394–403, 1980

SANDERSON KV: Hair follicle naevus. Trans St John's Hosp Dermatol Soc 47:154–156, 1961

Dilated Pore, Pilar Sheath Acanthoma
BHAWAN J: Pilar sheath acanthoma. J Cutan Pathol 6:438–440, 1979

MEHREGAN AH, BROWNSTEIN MH: Pilar sheath acanthoma. Arch Dermatol 114:1495–1497, 1978

WINER L: The dilated pore, a trichoepithelioma. J Invest Dermatol 23:181–188, 1954

Multiple Fibrofolliculomas, Multiple Trichodiscomas
BIRT AR, HOGG GR, DUBÉ J: Hereditary multiple fibrofolliculomas with trichodiscomas and acrochordons. Arch Dermatol 113:1674–1677, 1977

FUJITA WH, BARR RJ, HEADLEY JL: Multiple fibrofolliculomas with trichodiscomas and acrochordons. Arch Dermatol 117:32–35, 1981

GROSSHANS E, DUNGLER T, HANAU D: Le trichodiscome de Pinkus. Ann Dermatol Venereol 108:837–846, 1981

PINKUS H, COSKEY R, BURGESS GH: Trichodiscoma. A benign tumor related to the *Haarscheibe* (hair disk). J Invest Dermatol 63:212–218, 1974

WEINTRAUB R, PINKUS H: Multiple fibrofolliculomas (Birt-Hogg-Dubé) associated with a large connective tissue nevus. J Cutan Pathol 4:289–299, 1977

Trichoepithelioma, Trichoadenoma
BROWNSTEIN MH, SHAPIRO L: Desmoplastic trichoepithelioma. Cancer 40:2979–2986, 1977

DUPRÉ A, BONAFÉ, JL, LASSÈRE J: Hamartome épithélial sclérosant: Forme clinique du tricho-épithéliome. Ann Dermatol Venereol 107:649–654, 1980

GAUL LE: Heredity of multiple benign cystic epithelioma. Arch Dermatol Syph 68:517–524, 1953

GRAY HR, HELWIG EB: Epithelioma adenoides cysticum and solitary trichoepithelioma. Arch Dermatol 87:102–114, 1963

HOWELL JB, ANDERSON DE: Transformation of epithelioma adenoides cysticum into multiple rodent ulcers: Fact or fallacy? Br J Dermatol 95:233–242, 1976

KOPF AW: The distribution of alkaline phosphatase in normal and pathologic human skin. Arch Dermatol 75:1–37, 1957

KYLLÖNEN AP, STENBÄCK F, VÄÄNÄNEN R: Trichoepitheliomatous tumors: Morphology and ultrastructure. (Abstr) J Cutan Pathol 8:167–168, 1981

LEVER WF: Pathogenesis of benign tumors of cutaneous appendages and of basal cell epithelioma. Arch Dermatol Syph 57:679–724, 1948

MACDONALD DM, WILSON JONES E, MARKS R: Sclerosing epithelial hamartoma. Clin Exp Dermatol 2:153–160, 1977

MÜLLER-HESS S, DELACRÉTAZ J: Trichoepitheliom mit Strukturen eines apokrinen Adenoms. Dermatologica 146:170–176, 1973

NIKOLOWSKI W: Tricho-adenom. Arch Klin Exp Dermatol 207:34–45, 1958

NIKOLOWSKI W: Trichoadenom. Z Hautkr 53:87–90, 1977

RAHBARI H, MEHREGAN A, PINKUS H: Trichoadenoma of Nikolowski. J Cutan Pathol 4:90–98, 1977

ZELIGMAN I: Solitary trichoepithelioma. Arch Dermatol 82:35–40, 1960

ZIPRKOWSKI L, SCHEWACH-MILLET M: Multiple trichoepithelioma in a mother and two children. Dermatologica 132:248–256, 1966

Generalized Hair Follicle Hamartoma

BROWN AC, CROUNSE RG, WINKELMANN RK: Generalized hair-follicle hamartoma. Arch Dermatol 99:478–493, 1969

RIDLEY CM, SMITH N: Generalized hair follicle hamartoma associated with alopecia and myasthenia gravis: Report of a second case. Clin Exp Dermatol 6:283–289, 1981

Pilomatricoma (Calcifying Epithelioma)

CAZERS JS, OKUN MR, PEARSON SH: Pigmented calcifying epithelioma. Arch Dermatol 110:773–774, 1974

CHIARAMONTI A, GILGOR RS: Pilomatricomas associated with myotonic dystrophy. Arch Dermatol 114:1363–1365, 1978

FORBIS R JR, HELWIG EB: Pilomatrixoma (calcifying epithelioma). Arch Dermatol 83:606–618, 1961

GEISER JD: L'épithélioma calcifié de Malherbe. Ann Dermatol Syph 86:383–403, 1959

HADLICH J, LINSE R: Zur klinischen Diagnostik des Epithelioma calcificans Malherbe. Dermatol Monatsschr 165:432–439, 1979

HASHIMOTO K, LEVER WF: Histogenesis of skin appendage tumors. Arch Dermatol 100:356–369, 1969

HASHIMOTO K, NELSON RG, LEVER WF: Calcifying epithelioma of Malherbe. Histochemical and electron microscopic studies. J Invest Dermatol 46:391–408, 1966

HOLMES EJ: A histochemical test for citrulline. Adaptation of the carbamidodiacetyl reaction to histologic sections with positive results in pilomatrixomas (calcifying epitheliomas). J Histochem Cytochem 16:136–146, 1968

LEVER WF, GRIESEMER RD: Calcifying epithelioma of Malherbe. Arch Dermatol Syph 59:506–518, 1949

LEVER WF, HASHIMOTO K: Die Histogenese einiger Hautanhangstumoren im Lichte histochemischer und elektronenmikroskopischer Befunde. Hautarzt 17:161–173, 1966

LOPANSRI S, MIHM MC JR: Pilomatrix carcinoma or calcifying epitheliocarcinoma of Malherbe. Cancer 45:2368–2373, 1980

MALHERBE A, CHENANTAIS J: Note sur l'épithéliome calcifié des glandes sébacées. Prog Med 8:826–828, 1880

MCGAVRAN MH: Ultrastructure of pilomatrixoma (calcifying epithelioma). Cancer 18:1445–1456, 1965

MOEHLENBECK F: Pilomatrixoma (calcifying epithelioma). Arch Dermatol 108:532–534, 1973

PETERSON WC JR, HULT AM: Calcifying epithelioma of Malherbe. Arch Dermatol 90:404–410, 1964

TURHAN B, KRAINER L: Bemerkungen über die sogenannten verkalkenden Epitheliome der Haut und ihre Genese. Dermatologica 85:73–90, 1942

WEEDON D, BELL J, MAYZE J: Matrical carcinoma of the skin. J Cutan Pathol 7:39–42, 1980

WIEDERSBERG H: Das Epithelioma calcificans Malherbe. Dermatol Monatsschr 157:867–883, 1971

Proliferating Trichilemmal Tumor

BLOCH PH, MÜLLER HD: Pilartumor der Kopfhaut. Hautarzt 30:84–88, 1979

BROWNSTEIN MH, ARLUK DJ: Proliferating trichilemmal cyst. Cancer 48:1207–1214, 1981

DABSKA M: Giant hair matrix tumor. Cancer 28:701–706, 1971

HANAU D, GROSSHANS E: Trichilemmal tumor undergoing specific keratinization. J Cutan Pathol 6:463–475, 1979

HOLMES EJ: Tumors of lower hair sheath. The common histogenesis of certain so-called "sebaceous cysts," adenomas, and "sebaceous carcinomas." Cancer 21:234–248, 1968

KORTING GW, HOEDE N: Zum sogenannten "Pilar Tumor of the Scalp." Arch Klin Exp Dermatol 234:409–419, 1969

LEPPARD BJ, SANDERSON KV: The natural history of trichilemmal cysts. Br J Dermatol 94:379–390, 1976

PEDEN JC: Carcinoma developing in sebaceous cysts. Ann Surg 128:1136–1147, 1948

PINKUS H: "Sebaceous cysts" are trichilemmal cysts. Arch Dermatol 99:544–555, 1969

REED RJ, LAMAR LM: Invasive hair matrix tumors of the scalp. Arch Dermatol 94:310–316, 1966

WILSON JONES E: Proliferating epidermoid cysts. Arch Dermatol 94:11–19, 1966

Trichilemmoma

ACKERMAN AB, WADE TR: Tricholemmoma. Am J Dermatopathol 2:207–224, 1980

ALLEN BS, FITCH MH, SMITH JG JR: Multiple hamartoma syndrome. J Am Acad Dermatol 2:303–308, 1980

BROWNSTEIN MH, MEHREGAN AH, BIKOWSKI B et al: The dermatopathology of Cowden's syndrome. Br J Dermatol 100:667–673, 1979

BROWNSTEIN MH, SHAPIRO L: Trichilemmoma. Arch Dermatol 107:866–869, 1973

BROWNSTEIN MH, SHAPIRO EE: Trichilemmal horn: Cutaneous horn overlying trichilemmoma. Clin Exp Dermatol 4:59–63, 1979

BROWNSTEIN MH, WOLF, M, BIKOWSKI JB: Cowden's disease. A cutaneous marker of breast cancer. Cancer 41:2393–2398, 1978

HEADINGTON JT, FRENCH AJ: Primary neoplasms of the hair follicle. Arch Dermatol 86:430–441, 1962

THYRESSON HN, DOYLE JA: Cowden's disease (multiple hamartoma syndrome). (Review) Mayo Clin Proc 56:179–184, 1981

WEARY PE, GORLIN RJ, GENTRY WC JR et al: Multiple hamartoma syndrome (Cowden's disease). Arch Dermatol 106:682–690, 1972

Tumor of the Follicular Infundibulum, Trichilemmocarcinoma

CHAN P, WHITE SW, PIERSON DL et al: Trichilemmoma. J Dermatol Surg Oncol 5:58–59, 1979

JOHNSON WC, HOOKERMAN BJ: Basal call hamartoma with follicular differentiation. Arch Dermatol 105:105–106, 1972

MEHREGAN AH: Tumor of follicular infundibulum. Dermatologica 142:177–183, 1971

MEHREGAN AH, BUTTLER JD: A tumor of follicular infundibulum. Arch Dermatol 83:924–927, 1961

TEN SELDAM REJ: Tricholemmocarcinoma. Aust J Dermatol 18:62–72, 1977

Nevus Sebaceus

BOURLOND A, DEMEERSMAN E, FIERENS F: Polymorphisme clinique et histologique du naevus sébacé. Arch Belg Dermatol Syph 25:337–344, 1969

BROWNSTEIN MH, SHAPIRO L: The pilosebaceous tumors. Int J Dermatol 16:340–352, 1977

DOMINGO J, HELWIG EB: Malignant neoplasms associated with nevus sebaceus of Jadassohn. J Am Acad Dermatol 1:545–556, 1979

FEUERSTEIN R, MIMS L: Linear nevus sebaceus with convulsions and mental retardation. Am J Dis Child 104:675–679, 1962

HABER H: Verrucous naevi. Trans St John's Hosp Dermatol Soc 34:20–28, 1955

HORNSTEIN OP, KNICKENBERG M: Zur Kenntnis des Schimmelpenning-Feuerstein-Mims-Syndroms. Arch Dermatol Forsch 250:33–50, 1974

KUOKKANEN K, KOIVIKKO M, ALAVAIKKO M: Organoid nevus phakomatosis. Acta Derm Venereol (Stockh) 60:534–537, 1980

LANTIS S, LEYDEN J, THEW M et al: Nevus sebaceus of Jadassohn, Part of a new neurocutaneous syndrome. Arch Dermatol 98:117–123, 1968

LENTZ CL, ALTMAN J, MOPPER C: Nevus sebaceus of Jadassohn. Arch Dermatol 97:294–296, 1968

LEVER WF: Pathogenesis of benign tumors of cutaneous appendages and of basal cell epithelioma. Arch Dermatol Syph 57:679–724, 1948

MARDEN PM, VENTERS HD: A new neurocutaneous syndrome. Am J Dis Child 112:79–81, 1966

MEHREGAN AH, PINKUS H: Life history of organoid nevi. Arch Dermatol 91:574–588, 1965

MICHALOWSKI R: Naevus sébacé de Jadassohn—Un état précancéreux. Dermatologica 124:326–340, 1962

SCHIMMELPENNING GW: Klinischer Beitrag zur Symptomatologie der Phakomatosen. Fortschr Roentgenstr 87:716–720, 1957

SCHIRREN CG, PFIRSTINGER H: Zur Entwicklung von Plattenepithelcarcinomen auf dem Boden des Naevus sebaceus (Jadassohn). Hautarzt 14:397–401, 1963

SOLOMON LW, FRETZIN DF, DEWALD RL: The epidermal nevus syndrome. Arch Dermatol 97:273–285, 1968

STEIGLEDER G, CORTES AC: Verhalten der Talgdrüsen im Talgdrüsennaevus während des Kindesalters. Arch Klin Exp Dermatol 239:323–328, 1971

WAUSCHKUHN J, ROHDE B: Systematisierte Talgdrüsen-, Pigment-, und epitheliale Naevi mit neurologischer Symptomatik; Feuerstein-Mimssches neuroektodermales Syndrom. Hautarzt 22:10–33, 1971

WILSON JONES E, HEYL T: Naevus sebaceus. Br J Dermatol 82:99–117, 1970

Sebaceous Hyperplasia

BRAUN-FALCO O, THIANPRASIT M: Über die circumscripte senile Talgdrüsenhyperplasie. Arch Klin Exp Dermatol 221:207–231, 1965

GILMAN RL: Adenomatoid sebaceous tumors with particular reference to adenomatoid hyperplasia. Arch Dermatol Syph 35:633–642, 1937

LUDERSCHMIDT C, PLEWIG G: Circumscribed sebaceous gland hyperplasia: Autoradiographic and histoplanometric studies. J Invest Dermatol 70:207–209, 1978

Fordyce's Condition

CHAMBERS SO: The structure of Fordyce's disease as demonstrated by wax reconstruction. Arch Dermatol Syph 18:666–672, 1928

MILES AEW: Sebaceous glands in the lip and cheek mucosa of man. Br Dent J 105:235–248, 1958

Sebaceous Adenoma

ESSENHIGH DM, JONES D, RACK JH: A sebaceous adenoma. Br J Dermatol 76:330–340, 1964

FAHMY A, BURGDORF WHC, SCHLOSSER RH et al: Muir-Torre syndrome. Cancer 49:1898–1903, 1982

GROTERJAHN A: Die Talgdrüsengeschwülste mit besonderer Berücksichtigung des Talgdrüsenadenoms. Hautarzt 1:319–321, 1950

HOUSHOLDER MS, ZELIGMAN I: Sebaceous neoplasms associated with visceral carcinoma. Arch Dermatol 116:61–64, 1980

LEONARD DD, DEATON WR JR: Multiple sebaceous gland tumors and visceral carcinomas. Arch Dermatol 110:917–920, 1974

LEVER WF: Sebaceous adenoma, review of the literature and report of a case. Arch Dermatol Syph 57:102–111, 1948

LYNCH HT, LYNCH PM, PESTER J et al: The cancer family syndrome. Rare cutaneous phenotypic linkage of Torre's syndrome. Arch Intern Med 141:607–611, 1981

POLEKSIC S: Keratoacanthoma and multiple carcinomas. Br J Dermatol 91:461–463, 1974

RULON DB, HELWIG EB: Multiple sebaceous neoplasms of the skin. An association with multiple visceral carcinomas, especially of the colon. Am J Clin Pathol 60:745–752, 1973

SCHWARTZ RA, FLEIGER DN, SAIED NK: The Torre syndrome with gastrointestinal polyposis. Arch Dermatol 116:312–314, 1980

SCIALLIS GF, WINKELMANN RK: Multiple sebaceous adenomas and gastrointestinal carcinoma. Arch Dermatol 110:913–916, 1974

STEWART WM, LAURET P, HEMET J et al: Keratoacanthomes multiples et carcinomes visceraux. Syndrome de Torre. Ann Dermatol Venereol 104:622–626, 1977

TORRE D: Multiple sebaceous tumors. Arch Dermatol 98:549–551, 1968

WOOLHANDLER HW, BECKER WS: Adenoma of sebaceous glands (adenoma sebaceum). Arch Dermatol Syph 45:734–756, 1942

WORRET WI, BURGDORF WHC, FAHMY A et al: Torre-Muir Syndrom. Hautarzt 32:519–524, 1981

Sebaceous Epithelioma

HORI M, EGAMI K, MAEJIMA K et al: Electron microscopic study of sebaceous epithelioma. J Dermatol 5:139–147, 1978

LEVER WF: Sebaceous adenoma. Arch Dermatol Syph 57:102–111, 1948

MCMULLAN FH: Sebaceous epithelioma. Arch Dermatol Syph 71:725–727, 1955

MEHREGAN AH, PINKUS H: Life history of organoid nevi. Arch Dermatol 91:574–588, 1965

NIIZUMA K: An electron microscopic study of sebaceous epithelioma. Dermatologica 154:98–106, 1977

RAAB W: Talgdrüsenepitheliom. Arch Klin Exp Dermatol 216:325–333, 1964

RULON DB, HELWIG EB: Cutaneous sebaceous neoplasms. Cancer 33:82–102, 1974

URBAN FH, WINKELMANN RK: Sebaceous malignancy. Arch Dermatol 84:63–72, 1961

WILSON JONES E, HEYL T: Naevus sebaceus. Br J Dermatol 82:99–117, 1970

ZACKHEIM HS: The sebaceous epithelioma. Arch Dermatol 89:711–724, 1964

Apocrine Nevus

CIVATTE J, TSOITIS G, PRÉAUX J: Le naevus apocrine. Ann Dermatol Syph 101:251–261, 1974

RABENS SF, NANESS JI, GOTTLIEB BF: Apocrine gland organic hamartoma (apocrine nevus). Arch Dermatol 112:520–522, 1976

VAKILZADEH F, HAPPLE R, PETERS P et al: Fokale dermale Hypoplasie mit apokrinen Naevi und streifenförmiger Anomalie der Knochen. Arch Dermatol Res 256:189–195, 1976

Apocrine Hidrocystoma

ASARCH RG, GOLITZ LE, SAUSKER WF et al: Median raphe cysts of the penis. Arch Dermatol 115:1084–1086, 1979

BENISCH B, PEISON B: Apocrine hidrocystoma of the shoulder. Arch Dermatol 113:71–72, 1977

BHAWAN J, MALHOTRA R, FRANKS SB: Pigmented apocrine hidrocystoma. (Abstr) Arch Dermatol 116:1392, 1980

CRAMER HJ: Das schwarze Hidrocystom (Monfort). Dermatol Monatsschr 166:114–118, 1980

GROSS BG: The fine structure of apocrine hidrocystoma. Arch Dermatol 92:706–712, 1965

HASHIMOTO K, LEVER WF: Appendage Tumors of the Skin, pp. 52–54. Springfield, IL, Charles C Thomas, 1968

HASSAN MO, KHAN JA, KRUSE TV: Apocrine cystadenoma. Arch Dermatol 115:194–200, 1979

KRUSE TV, KHAN MA, HASSAN MO: Multiple apocrine cystadenomas. Br J Dermatol 100:675–681, 1979

MEHREGAN AH: Apocrine cystadenoma. Arch Dermatol 90:274–279, 1964

SCHAUMBURG-LEVER G, LEVER WF: Secretion from human apocrine glands. J Invest Dermatol 64:38–41, 1975

SMITH JD, CHERNOSKY ME: Apocrine hidrocystoma (cystadenoma). Arch Dermatol 109:700–702, 1974

Hidradenoma Papilliferum

HASHIMOTO K: Hidradenoma papilliferum. An electron microscopic study. Acta Derm Venereol (Stockh) 53:22–30, 1973

MEEKER JH, NEUBECKER RD, HELWIG EG: Hidradenoma papilliferum. Am J Clin Pathol 37:182–195, 1962

SANTA CRUZ DJ, PRIOLEAU PG, SMITH ME: Hidradenoma papilliferum of the eyelid. Arch Dermatol 117:55–56, 1981

SHENOY YMV: Malignant perianal papillary hidradenoma. Arch Dermatol 83:965–967, 1961

TAPPEINER J, WOLFF K: Hidradenoma papilliferum. Eine enzymhistochemische und elektronenmikroskopische Studie. Hautarzt 19:101–109, 1969

Syringocystadenoma Papilliferum

APPEL B: Nevus syringadenomatosus papilliferus. Arch Dermatol Syph 61:311–318, 1950

FUSARO RM, GOLTZ RW: Histochemically demonstrable carbohydrates of appendageal tumors of the skin. II. Benign apocrine gland tumors. J Invest Dermatol 38:137–142, 1962

GRUND JL: Syringocystadenoma papilliferum and nevus sebaceus (Jadassohn) occurring as a single tumor. Arch Dermatol Syph 65:340–347, 1952

HASHIMOTO K: Syringocystadenoma papilliferum. An electron microscopic study. Arch Dermatol Forsch 245:353–369, 1972

HASHIMOTO K, LEVER WF: Appendage Tumors of the Skin, p 47. Springfield IL, Charles C Thomas, 1968

HELWIG EB, HACKNEY VC: Syringadenoma papilliferum. Arch Dermatol 71:361–372, 1955

KRINITZ K: Naevus syringocystadenomatosus papilliferus in linearer Anordnung. Hautarzt 17:260–265, 1966

LANDRY M, WINKELMANN RK: An unusual tubular apocrine adenoma. Arch Dermatol 105:869–879, 1972

LEVER WF: Pathogenesis of benign tumors of cutaneous appendages and of basal cell epithelioma. Arch Dermatol Syph 57:679–724, 1948

NIIZUMA K: Syringocystadenoma papilliferum: Light and electron microscopic studies. Acta Derm Venereol (Stockh) 56:327–336, 1976

PINKUS H: Life history of naevus syringadenomatosus papilliferus. Arch Dermatol Syph 69:305–322, 1954

ROSTAN SE, WALLER JD: Syringocystadenoma papilliferum in an unusual location. Arch Dermatol 112:835–836, 1976

Tubular Apocrine Adenoma

CIVATTE J, BELAICH S, LAURET P: Adénome tubulaire apocrine. Ann Dermatol Venereol 106:665–669, 1979

LANDRY M, WINKELMANN RK: An unusual tubular adenoma. Arch Dermatol 105:869–879, 1972

OKUN MR, FINN R, BLUMENTAL G: Apocrine adenoma versus apocrine carcinoma. J Am Acad Dermatol 2:322–326, 1980

RULON DB, HELWIG EB: Papillary eccrine adenoma. Arch Dermatol 113:596–598, 1977

UMBERT P, WINKELMANN RK: Tubular apocrine adenoma. J Cutan Pathol 3:75–87, 1976

Erosive Adenomatosis of the Nipple

ALBRECHT-NEBE H, THORMANN T, WINTER H et al: Das Mamillenadenom (Pseudo-Paget). Dermatol Monatsschr 167:169–174, 1981

LEWIS HM, OVITZ ML, GOLITZ LE: Erosive adenomatosis of the nipple. Arch Dermatol 112:1427–1428, 1976

MARSCH WC, NÜRNBERGER F: Das Mamillenadenom. Z Hautkr 54:1067–1072, 1979

SMITH EJ, KRON SD, GROSS PR: Erosive adenomatosis of the nipple. Arch Dermatol 102:330–332, 1970

SMITH NP, WILSON JONES E: Erosive adenomatosis of the nipple. Clin Exp Dermatol 2:79–84, 1977

UNDEUTSCH W, NIKOLOWSKI J: Papillomatöses Milchgangsadenom (Pseudo-Paget der Mamille). Hautarzt 30:371–375, 1979

Cylindroma

BADEN H: Cylindromatosis simulating neurofibromatosis. N Engl J Med 267:296–297, 1962

BANDMANN HJ, HAMBURGER D, ROMITI N: Bericht zur Brooke-Spieglerschen Phakomatose. Hautarzt 16:450–453, 1965

BOURLOND A, CLERENS A, SIGART H: Cylindrome malin. Dermatologica 158:203–207, 1979

CRAIN RC, HELWIG EB: Dermal cylindroma (dermal eccrine cylindroma). Am J Clin Pathol 35:504–515, 1961

FUSARO RM, GOLTZ RW: Histochemically demonstrable carbohydrates of appendageal tumors of the skin. J Invest Dermatol 38:137–142, 1962

GEBHART W, KOKOSCHKA WM, WICK J: The cylindroma: A model for human epithelial basement membrane. (Abstr) J Invest Dermatol 64:286, 1975

GERTLER W: Spieglersche Tumoren mit Übergang in metastasierendes Spinaliom. Dermatol Wochenschr 128:673–674, 1953

GOETTE DK, MCCONNELL MA, FOWLER VR: Cylindroma and eccrine spiradenoma coexistent in the same lesion. Arch Dermatol 118:273–274, 1982

GOTTSCHALK HR, GRAHAM JH, ASTON EE IV: Dermal eccrine cylindroma, epithelioma adenoides cysticum, and eccrine spiradenoma. Arch Dermatol 110:473–474, 1974

GREITHER A, REHRMANN A: Spiegler-Karzinome mit assoziierten Symptomen. Dermatologica 160:361–370, 1980

GUGGENHEIM W, SCHNYDER UW: Zur Nosologie der Spiegler-Brooke'schen Tumoren. Dermatologica 122:274–278, 1961

HASHIMOTO K, LEVER WF: Histogenesis of skin appendage tumors. Arch Dermatol 100:356–369, 1969

HEADINGTON JT, BATSAKIS JG, BEALS TF et al: Membranous basal cell adenoma of parotid gland, dermal cylindromas, and trichoepitheliomas. Cancer 39:2460–2469, 1977

HOLUBAR K, WOLFF K: Zur Histogenese des Cylindroms. Eine enzym-histochemische Studie. Arch Klin Exp Dermatol 229:205–216, 1967

KLEINE-NATROP HE: Gleichzeitige Generalisation gutartiger Basaliome der beiden Typen Spiegler und Brooke. Arch Klin Exp Dermatol 209:45–55, 1959

KNOTH W: Epitheliomatöse Phakomatose Brooke-Spiegler (Epithelioma adenoides cysticum und Zylindrome). Dermatol Monatsschr 164:63–64, 1978

KORTING GW, HOEDE N, GEBHARDT R: Kurzer Bericht über einen maligne entarteten Spiegler-Tumor. Dermatol Monatschr 156:141–147, 1970

LAUSECKER H: Beitrag zu den Naevo-epitheliomen. Arch Dermatol Syph (Berlin) 194:639–662, 1952

LEVER WF: Pathogenesis of benign tumors of cutaneous appendages and of basal cell epithelioma. Arch Dermatol Syph 57:679–724, 1948

LUGER A: Das Cylindrom der Haut und seine maligne Degeneration. Arch Dermatol Syph (Berlin) 188:155–180, 1949

LYON JB, ROUILLARD LM: Malignant degeneration of turban tumour of scalp. Trans St John's Hosp Derm Soc 46:74–77, 1961

MUNGER BL, GRAHAM JH, HELWIG EB: Ultrastructure and histochemical characteristics of dermal eccrine cylindroma (turban tumor). J Invest Dermatol 39:577–594, 1962

TSAMBAOS D, GREITHER A, ORFANOS CE: Multiple malignant Spiegler tumors with brachydactyly and racket-nails. J Cutan Pathol 6:31–41, 1979

URBACH F, GRAHAM JH, GOLDSTEIN J, MUNGER BL: Dermal eccrine cylindroma. Arch Dermatol 88:880–894, 1963

WELCH JP, WELLS RS, KERR CB: Ancell-Spiegler cylindromas (turban tumors) and Brooke-Fordyce trichoepitheliomas: Evidence for a single genetic entity. J Med Genet 5:29–35, 1968

ZONTSCHEW P: Cylindroma capitis mit maligner Entartung. Zentralbl Chir 86:1875–1879, 1961

Eccrine Nevus

ARNOLD HL: Nevus seborrheicus et sudoriferus. Arch Dermatol 51:370–372, 1945

CHALLA VR, JONA J: Eccrine angiomatous hamartoma: A rare skin lesion with diverse histological features. Dermatologica 155:206–209, 1977

GOLDSTEIN N: Ephidrosis (local hyperhidrosis), nevus sudoriferus. Arch Dermatol 96:67–68, 1967

HERZBERG JJ: Ekkrines Syringocystadenom. Arch Klin Exp Dermatol 214:600–621, 1962

HYMAN AB, HARRIS H, BROWNSTEIN MH: Eccrine angiomatous hamartoma. NY State J Med 68:2803–2806, 1968

MARTIUS I: Lokalisierte ekkrine Schweissdrüsenhyperplasie. Dermatol Monatsschr 165:327–330, 1979

PIPPIONE M, DEPAOLI MA, SARTORIS S: Naevus eccrine. Dermatologica 152:40–46, 1976

ZELLER DJ, GOLDMAN RL: Eccrine-pilar angiomatous hamartoma. Dermatologica 143:100–104, 1971

Eccrine Hidrocystoma

CORDERO AA, MONTES LF: Eccrine hidrocystoma. J Cutan Pathol 3:292–293, 1976

DOSTROVSKY A, SAGHER F: Experimentally induced disappearance and reappearance of lesions of hidrocystoma. J Invest Dermatol 5:167–172, 1942

EBNER H, ERLACH E: Ekkrine Hidrozystome. Dermatol Monatsschr 161:739–744, 1975

HASHIMOTO K, LEVER WF: Appendage Tumors of the Skin, pp 19–25. Springfield, IL, Charles C Thomas, 1968

HASSAN MO, KHAN MA: Ultrastructure of eccrine cystadenoma. Arch Dermatol 115:1217–1221, 1979

HERZBERG JJ: Ekkrines Syringocystadenom. Arch Klin Exp Dermatol 214:600–621, 1962

SMITH JD, CHERNOSKY ME: Hidrocystomas. Arch Dermatol 108:676–679, 1973

Syringoma

HASHIMOTO K, DIBELLA, BORSUK GM et al: Eruptive hidradenoma and syringoma. Arch Dermatol 96:500–519, 1967

HASHIMOTO K, GROSS BG, LEVER WF: Syringoma: Histochemical and electron microscopic studies. J Invest Dermatol 46:150–166, 1966

HASHIMOTO K, LEVER WF: Histogenesis of skin appendage tumors. Arch Dermatol 100:356–369, 1969

HEADINGTON JT, KOSKI J, MURPHY PJ: Clear cell glycogenosis in multiple syringomas. Arch Dermatol 106:353–356, 1972

LEVER WF: Pathogenesis of benign tumors of cutaneous appendages and of basal cell epithelioma. Arch Dermatol Syph 57:679–724, 1948

MUSTAKALLIO KK: Succinic dehyrogenase activity of syringomas. Acta Dermatol 89:827–831, 1964

THOMAS J, MAJMUDAR B, GORELKIN L: Syringoma localized to the vulva. Arch Dermatol 115:95–96, 1979

WINKELMANN RK, MULLER SA: Sweat gland tumors. Arch Dermatol 89:827–831, 1964

YUNG CW, SOLTANI K, BERNSTEIN JE et al: Unilateral linear nevoidal syringoma. J Am Acad Dermatol 4:412–416, 1981

Eccrine Poroma, Malignant Eccrine Poroma

BARDACH H: Hidroacanthoma simplex with in situ porocarcinoma. J Cutan Pathol 5:236–248, 1978

FREEMAN RG, KNOX JM, SPILLER WF: Eccrine poroma. Am J Clin Pathol 36:444–450, 1961

GOLDNER R: Eccrine poromatosis. Arch Dermatol 101:606–608, 1970

GSCHNAIT F, HORN F, LINDLBAUER R et al: Eccrine porocarcinoma. J Cutan Pathol 7:349–353, 1980

HASHIMOTO K, GROSS BG, LEVER WF: The ultrastructure of the skin of human embryos. I. The intraepidermal eccrine sweat duct. J Invest Dermatol 45:139–151, 1965

HASHIMOTO K, LEVER WF: Eccrine poroma. Histochemical and electron microscopic studies. J Invest Dermatol 43:237–247, 1964

HASHIMOTO K, LEVER WF: Histogenesis of skin appendage tumors. Arch Dermatol 100:356–369, 1969

HU CH, MARQUES AS, WINKELMANN RK: Dermal duct tumor. Arch Dermatol 114:1659–1664, 1978

HYMAN AB, BROWNSTEIN MH: Eccrine poroma. An analysis of 45 new cases. Dermatologica 138:29–38, 1969

ISHIKAWA K: Malignant hidroacanthoma simplex. Arch Dermatol 104:529–532, 1971

KNOX JM, SPILLER WF: Eccrine poroma. Arch Dermatol 77:726–729, 1958

KRINITZ K: Ein Beitrag zur Klinik und Histologie des ekkrinen Poroms. Hautarzt 18:504–508, 1967

KRINITZ K: Malignes intraepidermales ekkrines Porom. Z Hautkr 47:9–17, 1972

MEHREGAN AH, LEVSON DN: Hidroacanthoma simplex. Arch Dermatol 100:303–305, 1969

MISHIMA Y: Epitheliomatous differentiation of the intraepidermal eccrine sweat duct. J Invest Dermatol 52:233–246, 1969

MISHIMA Y, MORIOKA S: Oncogenic differentiation of the intraepidermal eccrine sweat duct: Eccrine poroma, poroepithelioma and porocarcinoma. Dermatologica 138:238–250, 1969

MIURA Y: Epidermotropic eccrine carcinoma. Jpn J Dermatol (Series B) 78:226–230, 1968

MOHRI S, CHIKA K, SAITO I et al: A case of porocarcinoma. J Dermatol (Tokyo) 7:431–434, 1980

OGINO A: Linear eccrine poroma. Arch Dermatol 112:841–844, 1976

OKUN MR, ANSELL HB: Eccrine poroma. Arch Dermatol 88:561–566, 1963

PENNEYS NS, ACKERMAN AB, INDGIN SN et al: Eccrine poroma. Br J Dermatol 82:613–615, 1970

PINKUS H, MEHREGAN AH: Epidermotropic eccrine carcinoma. Arch Dermatol 88:597–606, 1963

PINKUS H, ROGIN JR, GOLDMAN P: Eccrine poroma. Arch Dermatol 74:511–521, 1956

SANDERSON KV, RYAN EA: The histochemistry of eccrine poroma. Br J Dermatol 75:86–88, 1963

SMITH JLS, COBURN JG: Hidroacanthoma simplex. Br J Dermatol 68:400–418, 1956

WEEDON D, LEWIS J: Acrosyringeal nevus. J Cutan Pathol 4:166–168, 1977

WILKINSON RD, SCHOPFLOCHER P, ROZENFELD M: Hidrotic ectodermal dysplasia with diffuse eccrine poromatosis. Arch Dermatol 113:472–476, 1977

WINKELMANN RK, MCLEOD WA: The dermal duct tumor. Arch Dermatol 94:50–55, 1966

YASUDA T, KAWADA A, YOSHIDA K: Eccrine poroma. Arch Dermatol 90:428–431, 1964

Mucinous Syringometaplasia

KING DT, BARR RJ: Syringometaplasia: Mucinous and squamous variants. J Cutan Pathol 6:284–291, 1979

KWITTKEN J: Muciparous epidermal tumors. Arch Dermatol 109:554–555, 1974

MEHREGAN AH: Mucinous syringometaplasia. Arch Dermatol 116:988–989, 1980

Eccrine Spiradenoma, Malignant Eccrine Spiradenoma

CASTRO C, WINKELMANN RK: Spiradenoma. Histochemical and electron microscopic study. Arch Dermatol 109:40–48, 1974

EVANS HL, SU WPD, SMITH JL et al: Carcinoma arising in eccrine spiradenoma. Cancer 43:1881–1884, 1979

HASHIMOTO K, GROSS BG, NELSON RG et al: Eccrine spiradenoma. Histochemical and electron microscopic studies. J Invest Dermatol 46:347–365, 1966

HASHIMOTO K, LEVER WF: Histogenesis of skin appendage tumors. Arch Dermatol 100:356–369, 1969

KERSTING DW, HELWIG EB: Eccrine spiradenoma. Arch Dermatol 73:199–227, 1956

LEVER WF: Myoepithelial sweat gland tumor: Myoepithelioma. Arch Dermatol Syph 57:332–347, 1948

MUNGER BL, BERGHORN BM, HELWIG EB: A light- and electron-microscopic study of a case of multiple eccrine spiradenoma. J Invest Dermatol 38:289–297, 1962

NÖDL F: Zur Histogenese der ekkrinen Spiradenome. Arch Klin Exp Dermatol 221:323–335, 1965

SHELLEY WB, WOOD MG: A zosteriform network of spiradenoma. J Am Acad Dermatol 2:59–61, 1980

TSUR H, LIPSKIER E, FISHER BK: Multiple linear spiradenomas. Plast Reconstr Surg 68:100–102, 1981

WINKELMANN RK, WOLFF K: Histochemistry of hidradenoma and eccrine spiradenoma. J Invest Dermatol 49:173–180, 1967

Clear Cell Hidradenoma, Malignant Clear Cell Hidradenoma

EFSKIND J, EKER R: Myo-epitheliomas of the skin. Acta Derm Venereol (Stockh) 34:279–283, 1954

GARTMANN H, PULLMANN H: Apokriner und ekkriner Mischtumor der Kopfhaut. Z Hautkr 54:952–958, 1979

HASHIMOTO K, DI BELLA RJ, LEVER WF: Clear cell hidradenoma. Histologic, histochemical, and electron microscopic study. Arch Dermatol 96:18–38, 1967

HEADINGTON JT, NIEDERHUBER JE, BEALS TF: Malignant clear cell acrospiroma. Cancer 41:641–647, 1978

HERNÁNDEZ-PÉREZ E, CRUZ FA: Clear cell hidradenocarcinoma. Dermatologica 153:249–252, 1976

JOHNSON BL JR, HELWIG EB: Eccrine acrospiroma. Cancer 23:641–657, 1969

KEASBEY LE, HADLEY GC: Clear-cell hidradenoma. Report of three cases with widespread metastases. Cancer 7:934–952, 1954

KERSTING DW: Clear cell hidradenoma and hidradenocarcinoma. Arch Dermatol 87:323–333, 1963

LEVER WF, CASTLEMAN B: Clear cell myoepithelioma of the skin. Am J Pathol 28:691–699, 1952

LUND HZ: Tumors of the Skin. In Atlas of Tumor Pathology, Section I, Fascicle 2. Washington, DC, Armed Forces Institute of Pathology, 1957

O'HARA JM, BENSCH KG: Fine structure of eccrine sweat gland adenoma, clear cell type. J Invest Dermatol 49:261–272, 1967

O'HARA JM, BENSCH K, IOANNIDES G et al: Eccrine sweat gland adenoma, clear cell type. Cancer 19:1438–1450, 1966

OKUN MR, EDELSTEIN LM: Gross and Microscopic Pathology of the Skin, Vol 2, pp 726–729. Boston, Dermatopathology Foundation Press, 1976

SANTLER R, EBERHARTINGER C: Malignes Klarzellen-Myoepitheliom. Dermatologica 130:340–347, 1965

WINKELMANN RK, WOLFF K: Histochemistry of hidradenoma and eccrine spiradenoma. J Invest Dermatol 49:173–180, 1967

WINKELMANN RK, WOLFF K: Solid-cystic hidradenoma of the skin. Arch Dermatol 97:651–661, 1968

Chondroid Syringoma, Malignant Chondroid Syringoma

BOTHA JBC, KAHN LB: Aggressive chondroid syringoma. Arch Dermatol 114:954–955, 1978

GARTMANN H, PULLMANN H: Chondroides Syringom. Z Hautkr 54:908–913, 1979a

GARTMANN H, PULLMANN H: Apokriner und ekkriner Mischtumor der Kopfhaut. Z Hautkr 54:952–958, 1979b

HARRIST TJ, ARETZ TH, MIHM MC JR et al: Malignant chondroid syringoma. Arch Dermatol 117:719–724, 1981

HEADINGTON JT: Mixed tumors of the skin: Eccrine and apocrine types. Arch Dermatol 84:989–996, 1961

HERNANDEZ FJ: Mixed tumors of the skin of the salivary gland type: A light and electron microscopic study. J Invest Dermatol 66:49–52, 1976

HILTON JMN, BLACKWELL JB: Metastasizing chondroid syringoma. J Pathol 109:167–170, 1973

HIRSCH P, HELWIG EB: Chondroid syringoma. Arch Dermatol 84:835–847, 1961

KRESBACH H: Ein Beitrag zum sogenannten Mischtumor der Haut. Arch Klin Exp Dermatol 221:59–74, 1964

MATZ LR, MCCULLY DJ, STOKES BAR: Metastasizing chondroid syringoma: Case report. Pathology 1: 77–81, 1969

TSOITIS G, BRISOU B, DESTOMBES: Mummified cutaneous mixed tumor. Arch Dermatol 111:194–196, 1975

VARELA-DURAN J, DIAZ-FLORES L, VARELA-NUNEZ R: Ultrastructure of chondroid syringoma. Cancer 44:148–156, 1979

WELKE S, GOOS M: Das chondroide Syringom. Hautarzt 33:15–17, 1982

Basal Cell Epithelioma

ADAMSON HG: On the nature of rodent ulcer: Its relationship to epithelioma adenoides cysticum of Brooke and to other trichoepitheliomata of benign nevoid character; its distinction from malignant carcinoma. Lancet 1:810–814, 1914

AMONETTE RA, SALASCHE SJ, CHESNEY T MCC et al: Metastatic basal cell carcinoma. J Dermatol Surg 7:397–400, 1981

ANDERSON NP, ANDERSON HE: Development of basal cell epithelioma as a consequence of radiodermatitis. Arch Dermatol Syph 63:586–596, 1951

ANDERSON TE, BEST PV: Linear basal cell nevus. Br J Dermatol 74:20–23, 1962

ASSOR D: Basal cell carcinoma with metastasis to bone. Cancer 20:2125–2137, 1967

BAER RL, ROBBINS P, MENN HW et al: Ekkrines Epitheliom. Behandlung mittels Chemochirurgie nach Mohs. Hautarzt 22:241–244, 1971

BARDACH H: Hidroacanthoma simplex with in situ porocarcinoma. J Cutan Pathol 5:236–248, 1978

BARR RJ, GRAHAM JH: Granular cell basal cell carcinoma. Arch Dermatol 115:1064–1067, 1979

BAZEX A, DUPRÉ A, CHRISTOL B: Atrophodermie folliculaire, proliférations basocellulaires et hypotrichose. Ann Dermatol Syph 93:241–254, 1966

BERENDES U: Die klinische Bedeutung der onkotischen Phase des Basalzellnaevus-Syndroms. Hautarzt 22:261–263, 1971

BERGER P, BAUGHMAN R: Intra-epidermal epithelioma. Report of a case with invasion after many years. Br J Dermatol 90:343–349, 1974

BLANCHARD L, HODGE SJ, OWEN LG: Linear eccrine nevus with comedones. Arch Dermatol 117:357–359, 1981

BLEEHEN SS: Pigmented basal cell epithelioma. Br J Dermatol 93:361–370, 1975

BLEIBERG J, BRODKIN RH: Linear unilateral basal cell nevus with comedones. Arch Dermatol 100:187–190, 1969

BOREL DM: Cutaneous basosquamous carcinoma. Review of the literature and report of 35 cases. Arch Pathol 95:293–297, 1973

BROWN AC, CROUNSE RG, WINKELMANN RK: Generalized hair-follicle hamartoma. Arch Dermatol 99:478–493, 1969

CARNEY RG: Linear unilateral basal cell nevus with comedones. Arch Dermatol Syph 65:471–476, 1952

CARO MR, HOWELL JB: Morphea-like epithelioma. Arch Dermatol Syph 63:471–476, 1952

COOK MG, RIDGWAY HA: The intra-epidermal epithelioma of Jadassohn: A distinct entity. Br J Dermatol 101:659–667, 1979

COVO JA: The pits in the nevoid basal cell carcinoma syndrome. Arch Dermatol 103:568–569, 1971

CUTLER B, POSALAKY Z, KATZ I: Cell processes in basal cell carcinoma. J Cutan Pathol 7:310–314, 1980

DARIER J, FERRAND M: L'épithéliome pavimenteux mixte et intermédiaire. Ann Dermatol Syph 82:124–139, 1955

DEGOS R, HEWITT J: Tumeurs fibro-épithéliales prémalignes de Pinkus et épithélioma baso-cellulaire. Ann Dermatol Syph 82:124–139, 1955

DEPPE R, PULLMANN H, STEIGLEDER GK: Dopa-positive cells and melanin in basal cell epithelioma. Arch Dermatol Res 256:79–83, 1976

DVORETZKY I, FISHER BK, HAKER O: Mutilating basal cell epithelioma. Arch Dermatol 114:239–240, 1978

FANGER H, BARKER BE: Histochemical studies of some keratotic and proliferating skin lesions. Arch Pathol 64:143–147, 1957

FARMER ER, HELWIG EB: Metastatic basal cell carcinoma: A clinicopathologic study of 17 cases. Cancer 46:748–757, 1980

FIERZ U: Katamnestische Untersuchunger über die Nebenwirkungen der Therapie mit anorganischem Arsen bei Hautkrankheiten. Dermatologica 131:41–58, 1965

FOOT NC: Adnexal carcinoma of the skin. Am J Pathol 23:1–27, 1947

FREEMAN RG: Histopathologic considerations in the management of skin cancer. J Dermatol Surg 2:215–219, 1976

FREEMAN RG, WINKELMANN RK: Basal cell tumor with eccrine differentiation. Arch Dermatol 100:234–242, 1969

GAUGHAN LJ, BERGERON JR, MULLINS JF: Giant basal cell epithelioma developing in acute burn site. Arch Dermatol 99:594–595, 1969

GELLIN GA, KOPF AW, GARFINKEL L: Basal cell epithelioma. Arch Dermatol 91:38–45, 1965

GERSTEIN W: Transplantation of basal cell epithelioma to the rabbit. Arch Dermatol 88:834–836, 1963

GERTLER W: Zur Epithelverbundenheit der Basaliome. Dermatol Wochenschr 151:673–677, 1965

GESCHICKTER CF, KOEHLER HP: Ectodermal tumors of the skin. Am J Cancer 23:804–836, 1935

GORMLEY DE, HIRSCH P: Aggressive basal cell carcinoma of the scalp. Arch Dermatol 114:782–783, 1978

GRAHAM JH, HELWIG EB: Intraepidermal epithelioma of Jadassohn. In Graham JH, Johnson WC, Helwig EB (eds): Dermal Pathology, pp 613–623. Hagerstown, MD, Harper & Row, 1972

GREENE HSN: The heterologous transplantation of embryonic mammalian tissue. Cancer Res 3:809–822, 1943

HAPPLE R: Naevobasaliom und Ameloblastom. Hautarzt 24:290–294, 1973

HASHIMOTO K, BROWNSTEIN MH: Localized amyloidosis in basal cell epithelioma. Acta Derm Venereol (Stockh) 53:331–339, 1973

HASHIMOTO K, KOBAYASHI H: Histogenesis of amyloid in the skin. Am J Dermatopathol 2:165–171, 1980

HERMANS EH, GROSFELD JCM, SPAAS JAJ: The fifth phakomatosis. Dermatologica 130:446–476, 1965

HOLMES EJ, BENNINGTON JL, HABER SL: Citrulline-containing basal cell carcinomas. Cancer 22:663–670, 1968

HOLUBAR K, MATRAS H, SMALIK AV: Multiple palmar basal cell epitheliomas in basal cell nevus syndrome. Arch Dermatol 101:679–682, 1970

HOLUBAR K, WOLFF K: Intraepidermal eccrine poroma. Cancer 23:626–635, 1969

HORIO T, KOMURA J: Linear unilateral basal cell nevus with comedo-like lesions. Arch Dermatol 114:95–97, 1978

HORNSTEIN O: Über die Pinkussche Varietät der Basaliome. Hautarzt 8:406–411, 1957

HOWELL JB, CARO MR: The basal-cell nevus. Arch Dermatol 79:67–80, 1959

HOWELL JB, FREEMAN RG: Structure and significance of the pits with their tumors in the nevoid basal cell carcinoma syndrome. J Am Acad Dermatol 2:224–238, 1980

HOWELL JB, MEHREGAN AH: Pursuit of the pits in the nevoid basal cell carcinoma syndrome. Arch Dermatol 102:586–597, 1970

HUNDEIKER M, BERGER H: Zur Morphogenese der Basaliome. Arch Klin Exp Dermatol 231:161–169, 1968

HUNDEIKER M, PETRES J: Morphogenese und Formenreichtum der arseninduzierten Präkanzerosen. Arch Klin Exp Dermatol 231:355–365, 1968

HYMAN AB, BARSKY AJ: Basal cell epithelioma of the palm. Arch Dermatol 92:571–573, 1965

HYMAN AB, MICHAELIDES P: Basal-cell epithelioma of the sole. Arch Dermatol 87:481–485, 1963

JABLONSKA S: Basaliome naevoider Abkunft. Hautarzt 12:147–157, 1961

JACOBS GH, RIPPEY JJ, ALTINI M: Prediction of aggressive behavior in basal cell carcinoma. Cancer 49:533–537, 1982

JOHNSON DE: Basal-cell epithelioma of the palm. Arch Dermatol 82:253–255, 1960

KERR JFR, SEARLE J: A suggested explanation for the paradoxically slow growth rate of basal-cell carcinoma that contain numerous mitotic figures. J Pathol 107:41–44, 1972

KIMURA S: Three-dimensional architecture of epithelial skin tumors: An application of epidermal separation. J Dermatol (Tokyo) 8:13–19, 1981

KROMPECHER E: Der Basalzellenkrebs. Jena, Gustav Fischer, 1903

KUMAKIRI M, HASHIMOTO K: Ultrastructural resemblance of basal cell epithelioma to primary epithelial germ. J Cutan Pathol 5:53–67, 1978

LENNOX B, WELLS AL: Differentiation in the rodent ulcer group of tumours. Br J Cancer 5:195–212, 1951

LERCHIN E, RAHBARI H: Adamantinoid basal cell epithelioma. Arch Dermatol 111:586–588, 1975

LEVER WF: Pathogenesis of benign tumors of cutaneous appendages and of basal cell epithelioma. Arch Dermatol Syph 57:679–724, 1948

LEVER WF, HASHIMOTO K: Electron microscopic and histochemical findings in basal cell epithelioma, squamous cell carcinoma and some appendage tumors. XIII Congressus Internat Dermatol, Vol 1, pp 3–8. Berlin, Springer-Verlag, 1968

LEWIS HM, STENSAAS CO, OKUN MR: Basal cell epithelioma of the sole. Arch Dermatol 91:623–624, 1965

MADSEN A: De l'épithélioma baso-cellulaire superficiel. Acta Derm Venereol (Stockh) 22, Suppl 7:1–161, 1941

MADSEN A: The histogenesis of superficial basal-cell epithelioma. Arch Dermatol 72:29–30, 1955

MADSEN A: Studies on basal-cell epithelioma of the skin. Acta Pathol Microbiol Suppl 177, 1965

MALLORY FB: Recent progress in the microscopic anatomy and differentiation of cancer. JAMA 55:1513–1518, 1910

MARGOLIS MH: Superficial multicentric basal cell epithelioma arising in thermal burn scar. Arch Dermatol 102:474–476, 1970

MARON H: Basaliom bei Kindern. Dermatol Wochenschr 147:545–550, 1963

MASON JK, HELWIG EB, GRAHAM JH: Pathology of the nevoid basal cell carcinoma syndrome. Arch Pathol 79:401–409, 1965

MASU S, HOSOKAWA M, SEIJI M: Amyloid in localized cutaneous amyloidosis: Immunofluorescence studies with anti-keratin antiserum especially concerning the difference between systemic and localized cutaneous amyloidosis. Acta Derm Venereol (Stockh) 61:381–384, 1981

MEHREGAN AH, LEVSON DN: Hidroacanthoma simplex. Arch Dermatol 100:303–305, 1969

MEHREGAN AH, PINKUS H: Intraepidermal epithelioma: A critical study. Cancer 17:609–636, 1964

MIKHAIL GR, NIMS LP, KELLY AP JR et al: Metastatic basal cell carcinoma. (Review) Arch Dermatol 113:1261–1269, 1977

MILSTONE EB, HELWIG EB: Basal cell carcinoma in children. Arch Dermatol 108:523–527, 1973

MONTGOMERY H: Basal squamous cell epithelioma. Arch Dermatol Syph 18:50–73, 1928

MONTGOMERY H: Dermatopathology, pp 923–934. New York, Harper & Row, 1967

MONTGOMERY H, WAISMAN M: Epithelioma attributable to arsenic. J Invest Dermatol 4:365–383, 1941

MOORE RD, STEVENSON J, SCHOENBERG MD: The response of connective tissue associated with tumors of the skin. Am J Clin Pathol 34:125–130, 1960

MORALES A, HU F: Seborrheic verruca and intraepidermal basal cell epithelioma of Jadassohn. Arch Dermatol 91:342–344, 1965

MURRAY JE, CANNON B: Basal-cell cancer in children and young adults. N Engl J Med 262:440–443, 1960

OBERSTE-LEHN H: Zur Histogenese des Basalioms. Z Hautkr 16:334–339, 1954

OKUN MR, BLUMENTAL G: Basal cell epithelioma with giant cells and nuclear atypicality. Arch Dermatol 89:598–600, 1964

OKUN MR, EDELSTEIN LM: Gross and Microscopic Pathology of the Skin, Vol 2, pp 618–619. Boston, Dermatopathology Foundation Press, 1976

PAVER K, POYZEN K, BURRY N et al: The incidence of basal cell carcinoma and their metastases in Australia and New Zealand. Aust J Dermatol 14:53, 1973

PINKUS H: Premalignant fibroepithelial tumors of the skin. Arch Dermatol Syph 67:598–615, 1953

PINKUS H: Epithelial and fibroepithelial tumors. Arch Dermatol 91:24–37, 1965

PINKUS H, MEHREGAN AH: Epidermotropic eccrine carcinoma. Arch Dermatol 88:597–606, 1963

PLOSILA M, KIISTALA R, NIEMI KM: The Bazex syndrome: Follicular atrophoderma with multiple basal cell carcinoma, hypotrichosis and hypohidrosis. Clin Exp Dermatol 6:31–41, 1981

RAHBARI H, MEHREGAN AH: Basal cell epithelioma (carcinoma) in children and teenagers. Cancer 49:350–353, 1982

REED JC: Nevoid basal cell carcinoma syndrome with associated fibrosarcoma of the maxilla. Arch Dermatol 97:304–306, 1968

REIDBORD HE, WECHSLER HL, FISHER ER: Ultrastructural study of basal cell carcinoma and its variants with comments on histogenesis. Arch Dermatol 104:132–140, 1971

RULON DB, HELWIG EB: Cutaneous sebaceous neoplasms. Cancer 33:82–102, 1974

RUPEC M, KINT A, HIMMELMANN GW et al: Zur Ultrastruktur des soliden Basalioms. Dermatologica 151:288–295, 1975

RUPEC M, VAKILZADEH F, KORB G: Über das Vorkommen von mehrkernigen Riesenzellen in Basaliomen. Arch Klin Exp Dermatol 235:198–202, 1969

SAFAI B, GOOD RA: Basal cell carcinoma with metastasis. Arch Pathol 101:327–331, 1977

SANCHEZ NP, WINKELMANN RK: Basal cell tumor with eccrine differentiation (eccrine epithelioma). J Am Acad Dermatol 6:514–518, 1982

SANDERSON KV: The architecture of basal-cell carcinoma. Br J Dermatol 73:455–474, 1961

SCHUBERT H, WOLFRAM G, GÜLDNER G: Basaliomrezidive nach Behandlung. Dermatol Monatsschr 165:89–96, 1979

SCHWARTZ RA, BURGESS GH, MILGROM H: Breast carcinoma and basal cell epitheliomas after x-ray therapy for hirsutism. Cancer 44:1601–1605, 1979

SIMS CF, PARKER RL: Intraepidermal basal cell epithelioma. Arch Dermatol Syph 59:45–49, 1949

SMALL IA, WALDRON C: Ameloblastomas of the jaws. Oral Surg 8:281–297, 1955

SMITH JLS, COBURN JG: Hidroacanthoma simplex. Br J Dermatol 68:400–418, 1956

SMITH OD, SWERDLOW MA: Histogenesis of basal-cell epithelioma. Arch Dermatol 74:286–292, 1956

SOUTHWICK GJ, SCHWARTZ RA: The basal cell nevus syndrome. Disasters occurring among a series of 36 patients. Cancer 44:2294–2305, 1979

STREITMANN B: Zur Klinik der pigmentierten Epitheliome. Z Hautkr 26:279–287, 1959

TAYLOR WB, ANDERSON DE, HOWELL JB et al: The nevoid basal cell carcinoma syndrome. Arch Dermatol 98:612–614, 1968

TAYLOR WB, WILKINS JW JR: Nevoid basal cell carcinoma of the palm. Arch Dermatol 102:654–655, 1970

TELOH HA, WHEELOCK MC: Histogenesis of basal cell carcinoma. Arch Pathol 48:447–461, 1949

TEN SELDAM REJ, HELWIG EB: Histological Typing of Skin Tumours, pp 48–49. Geneva, World Health Organization, 1974

TOTTEN JR: The multiple nevoid basal cell carcinoma syndrome. Cancer 46:1456–1462, 1980

URBAN FH, WINKELMANN RK: Sebaceous malignancy. Arch Dermatol 84:63–72, 1961

VAN SCOTT EJ, REINERTSON RP: The modulating influence of stromal environment on epithelial cells studied in human autotransplants. J Invest Dermatol 36:109–117, 1961

VIKSNINS P, BERLIN A: Follicular atrophoderma and basal cell carcinomas. Arch Dermatol 113:948–951, 1977

WALLACE SA, HALPERT B: Trichoma: Tumor of hair anlage. Arch Pathol 50:199–208, 1950

WARD WH: Nevoid basal cell carcinoma associated with a dyskeratosis of the palms and soles. Aust J Dermatol 5:204–208, 1960

WECHSLER HL, KRUGH FJ, DOMONKOS AN et al: Polydysplastic epidermolysis bullosa and development of epidermal neoplasms. Arch Dermatol 102:374–380, 1970

WEEDON D, SHAND E: Amyloid in basal cell carcinomas. Br J Dermatol 101:141–146, 1979

WEINSTEIN GO, FROST P: Cell proliferation in human basal cell carcinoma. Cancer Res 30:724–728, 1970

WELTON DG, ELLIOTT JA, KIMMELSTIEL P: Epithelioma. Arch Dermatol Syph 60:277–293, 1949

WERMUTH BM, FAJARDO LF: Metastatic basal cell carcinoma. Arch Pathol 90:458–462, 1970

WILLIAMSON JJ, COHNEY BC, HENDERSON BM: Basal cell carcinoma of the mandibular gingiva. Arch Dermatol 95:76–80, 1967

WOOD MG, PRANICH K, BEERMAN H: Investigation of possible apocrine gland component in basal-cell epithelioma. J Invest Dermatol 30:273–281, 1958

YEH S: Skin cancer in chronic arsenicism. Human Pathol 4:469–485, 1973

ZACKHEIM HS: Origin of the human basal cell epithelioma. J Invest Dermatol 40:283–297, 1963

ZELICKSON AS: An electron microscope study of the basal cell epithelioma. J Invest Dermatol 39:183–187, 1962

ZELICKSON AS: The pigmented basal cell epithelioma. Arch Dermatol 96:524–527, 1967

ZELICKSON AS, GOLTZ RW, HARTMANN JF: A histologic and electron microscopic study of a pigmenting basal cell epithelioma. J Invest Dermatol 36:299–302, 1961

Carcinoma of Sebaceous Glands

BEACH A, SEVERANCE AO: Sebaceous gland carcinoma. Ann Surg 115:258–266, 1942

BONIUK M, ZIMMERMAN LE: Sebaceous carcinoma of the eyelid, eyebrow, caruncle and orbit. Trans Am Acad Opthalmol Otolaryngol 72:619–642, 1968

DIXON RS, MIKHAIL GR, SLATER HC: Sebaceous carcinoma of the eyelid. J Am Acad Dermatol 3:241–243, 1980

HERNÁNDEZ-PÉREZ E, BAÑOS E: Sebaceous carcinoma: Report of two cases with metastasis. Dermatologica 156:184–188, 1978

KING DT, HIROSE FM, GUREVITCH AW: Sebaceous carcinoma of the skin with visceral metastases. Arch Dermatol 115:862–863, 1979

LEONARD DD, DEATON WR JR: Multiple sebaceous gland tumors and visceral carcinomas. Arch Dermatol 110:917–920, 1974

MELLETTE JR, AMONETTE RA, GARDNER JH et al: Carcinoma of sebaceous glands on the head and neck. J Dermatol Surg Oncol 7:404–407, 1981

RULON DB, HELWIG EB: Cutaneous sebaceous neoplasms. Cancer 33:83–102, 1974

RUSSELL WG, HOUGH AG, ROGERS LW: Sebaceous carcinoma of meibomian gland origin. Am J Clin Pathol 73:504–511, 1980

URBAN FH, WINKELMANN RK: Sebaceous malignancy. Arch Dermatol 84:63–72, 1961

Carcinoma of Eccrine Sweat Glands

BOGGIO R: Adenoid cystic carcinoma of the scalp. Arch Dermatol 111:793–794, 1975

DAVE VK: Eccrine sweat gland carcinoma with metastases. Br J Dermatol 86:95–97, 1972

EL-DOMEIRI AA, BRASFIELD RD, HUVOS AG et al: Sweat gland carcinoma. Ann Surg 173:270–274, 1971

FRESEN O: Über das Carcinom der Hautdrüsen am Beispiel eines Schweissdrüsenkrebses der Hohlhand. Hautarzt 11:15–23, 1960

GRANT RA: Sweat gland carcinoma with metastases. JAMA 173:490–492, 1960

HASHIMOTO K, LEVER WF: Appendage Tumors of the Skin, pp 150–151. Springfield, IL, Charles C Thomas, 1968

HEADINGTON JT: Primary mucinous carcinoma of the skin. Cancer 39:1055–1063, 1977

HEADINGTON JT, TESARS R, NIEDERHUBER JE et al: Primary adenoid cystic carcinoma of the skin. Arch Dermatol 114:421–424, 1978

MENDOZA S, HELWIG EB: Mucinous (adenocystic) carcinoma of the skin. Arch Dermatol 103:68–78, 1971

ORBANEJA JG, YUS ES, DIAZ-FLORES L et al: Adenocarcinom der ekkrinen Schweissdrüsen. Hautarzt 24:197–202, 1973

SANTA CRUZ DJ, MEYERS JH, GNEPP DR et al: Primary mucinous carcinoma of the skin. Br J Dermatol 98:645–653, 1978

TELOH HA, BALKIN RB, GRIER JP: Metastasizing sweat gland carcinoma. Arch Dermatol 76:80–86, 1957

WRIGHT JD, FONT RL: Mucinous sweat gland adenocarcinoma of eyelid. Cancer 44:1757–1768, 1979

YEUNG KY, STINSON JC: Mucinous (adenocystic) carcinoma of sweat glands with widespread metastases. Cancer 39:2556–2562, 1977

Trabecular Carcinoma (Merkel Cell Carcinoma)

ABACI IF, ZAK FG: Multicentric amyloid containing cutaneous trabecular carcinoma. J Cutan Pathol 6:292–303, 1979

DE WOLF-PEETERS C, MARIEN K, MEBIS J et al: A cutaneous APUDoma or Merkel cell tumor. Cancer 46:1810–1816, 1980

IWASAKI H, MITSUI T, KIKUCHI M et al: Neuroendocrine carcinoma (trabecular carcinoma) of the skin with ectopic ACTH production. Cancer 48:753–756, 1981

POLLACK SV, GOSLEN JB: Small-cell neuroepithelial tumor of the skin: A Merkel-cell neoplasm. J Dermatol Surg Oncol 8:116–122, 1982

SIDHU GS, MULLINS JD, FEINER H et al: Merkel cell neoplasms. Am J Dermatopathol 2:101–119, 1980

TANG CK, TOKER C: Trabecular carcinoma of the skin. Cancer 42:2311–2321, 1978

TAXY JB, ETTINGER DS, WHARAM MD: Primary small cell carcinoma of the skin. Cancer 46:2308–2311, 1980

TOKER C: Trabecular carcinoma of the skin. Arch Dermatol 105:107–110, 1972

WONG SW, DAO AH, GLICK AD: Trabecular carcinoma of the skin: A case report. Hum Pathol 12:838–840, 1981

Carcinoma of Apocrine Glands

BAES H, SUURMOND D: Apocrine sweat gland carcinoma. Br J Dermatol 83:483–486, 1970

ELLIOT GB, RAMSEY DW: Sweat gland carcinoma. Ann Surg 144:99–106, 1956

FUTRELL JW, KRUEGER GR, CHRETIEN PB et al: Multiple primary sweat gland carcinoma. Cancer 28:686–691, 1971

KIPKIE GG, HAUST MD: Carcinoma of apocrine glands. Arch Dermatol 78:440–445, 1958

NELDNER KH: Ceruminoma. Arch Dermatol 98:344–348, 1968

SMITH CCK: Metastasizing carcinoma of the sweat glands. Br J Surg 43:80–84, 1955

WARKEL RL, HELWIG EB: Apocrine gland adenoma and adenocarcinoma of the axilla. Arch Dermatol 114:198–203, 1978

28

Metastatic Carcinoma and Carcinoid

INCIDENCE AND DISSEMINATION OF METASTATIC CARCINOMA

Cutaneous metastases are quite uncommon; of 2298 patients reported who had died of internal carcinoma, only 2.7% had cutaneous metastases (Gates). The incidence of the various tumors metastatic to the skin in men and women correlates well with the frequency of occurrence of the primary malignant tumor in each sex.

Review of 724 patients with cutaneous metastases gave the following results (Brownstein and Helwig). In women, commensurate with the great frequency of carcinoma of the breast, 69% of all cutaneous metastases had their origin in the breast. Carcinoma of the large intestine accounted for 9% of cutaneous metastases, and carcinoma of the lungs, carcinoma of the ovary, and malignant melanoma each accounted for 4% to 5%. In contrast, among men with cutaneous metastases, carcinoma of the lung was the primary tumor in 24% of the cases, carcinoma of the large intestine in 19%, malignant melanoma in 13%, carcinoma of the oral cavity in 12%, and carcinoma of the kidney and of the stomach each in 6%.

Owing to the relative rarity of these types of carcinoma, cutaneous metastases are infrequently encountered in carcinomas of the thyroid gland (Barr and Dann), pancreas (Chakraborty et al), liver (Reingold and Smith), bladder (Hollander and Grots), endometrium (Rasbach et al), prostate (Peison), or testis (Price and Kopf).

Dissemination may take place through the lymphatics or through the blood stream. In carcinomas of the breast and of the oral cavity, metastases reach the skin largely through lymphatic channels and are often located in the overlying skin. In contrast, cutaneous metastatic lesions in other carcinomas usually are the result of hematogenous dissemination and may appear in any area of the skin (Brownstein and Helwig).

CUTANEOUS METASTASIS FROM CARCINOMA OF THE BREAST

Four types of cutaneous metastases occur in carcinoma of the breast by way of the lymphatics. A fifth, rather rare, type of metastasis takes place through the blood stream.

The four types of cutaneous metastases that occur through lymphatic dissemination are: inflammatory carcinoma, telangiectatic carcinoma, nodular carcinoma, and carcinoma en cuirasse. Several of these four types may be present in the same patient. If dissemination of the tumor cells takes place through the lymphatics of the entire dermis and even of the subcutaneous tissue, inflammatory carcinoma results. If dissemination occurs only through the superficial lymphatics and blood vessels of the dermis, telangiectatic carcinoma occurs. In nodular carcinoma and in cancer en cuirasse, the tumor cells disseminate largely along tissue spaces and only to a minor degree through lymphatic vessels.

In *inflammatory carcinoma*, the skin of the affected breast and the adjoining skin is red, warm, and slightly indurated, with well-demarcated borders similar to those seen in erysipelas (Leavell and Tillotson).

In *telangiectatic carcinoma*, the skin contains numerous purplish papules and hemorrhagic pseudovesicles resembling a hemolymphangioma (Leavell and Tillotson).

In *nodular carcinoma*, asymptomatic, firm nodules are located in the skin and subcutaneous tissue. Those located in the skin may cause ulceration of the skin.

In *cancer en cuirasse*, the skin of the breast affected by the carcinoma and, often, also the surrounding skin show diffuse induration.

In *hematogenous dissemination* of carcinoma of the breast, only a single distant metastasis is usually found (Brownstein and Helwig); however, in some instances, there are multiple metastases (Peled et al). A fairly common site for one or several hematogenous metastases is the scalp. In the beginning, before the metastases in the scalp become elevated above the level of the skin, they may resemble patches of alopecia areata except for a reduction in the number of hair follicles. They are then referred to as alopecia neoplastica (Cohen et al).

Histopathology.   In *inflammatory carcinoma*, histologic examination of the skin reveals extensive invasion of the dermal and often also of the subcutaneous lymphatics by groups and cords of tumor cells (Fig. 28-1) (Leavell and Tillotson). The tumor cells are similar to those of the primary growth and atypical in character, with large, pleomorphic, hyperchromatic nuclei. There is marked capillary congestion (the reason for the clinical appearance of inflammation). In addition, one observes edema and a slight perivascular lymphoid infiltrate in the dermis, but no fibrosis (Siegel). The extensive lymphatic dissemination is caused by retrograde lymphatic spreading into the skin

secondary to blockage of the deep lymphatics and of the lymph nodes (Zala and Jenni).

In *telangiectatic carcinoma*, one observes carcinomatous permeation of dilated small blood vessels and lymphatics in the upper dermis. The blood vessels contain, in addition to the neoplastic aggregates, numerous red blood cells (Ingram). The location of many of the dilated blood vessels immediately beneath the epidermis causes the clinical resemblance of the lesion to hemorrhagic vesicles.

In *nodular carcinoma*, the nodules show large and small groups of tumor cells in the dermis surrounded by fibrosis (Fig. 28-2) (Leavell and Tillotson). Some of the groups of tumor cells may show a glandular arrangement.

In *cancer en cuirasse*, also referred to as scirrhous carcinoma, the indurated areas show fibrosis and usually contain only a few tumor cells, which may easily be overlooked because of their resemblance to fibroblasts. Like fibroblasts, the tumor cells have elongated nuclei, but their nuclei are often larger, more angular, and more deeply basophilic than the nuclei of fibroblasts. Also, even though the tumor cells often lie singly, in some areas they lie in small groups or in single-row lines between thickened collagen bundles. This arrangement in single-row lines, referred to as Indian filing, is of particular diagnostic importance (Fig. 28-3).

In *hematogenous metastases*, the histologic picture varies with the clinical presentation. Nodular lesions show infiltration of the dermis with large

Fig. 28-1.   Cutaneous metastasis from carcinoma of the breast
Inflammatory carcinoma. The dermal lymphatics are filled with clusters of tumor cells. ($\times 100$)

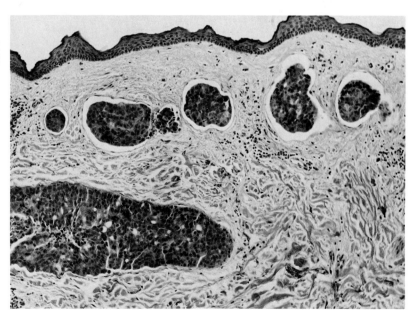

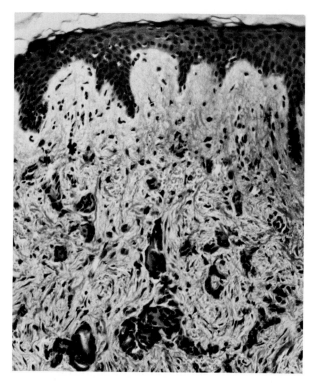

Fig. 28-2. Cutaneous metastasis from carcinoma of the breast
Nodular carcinoma. There are scattered islands of tumor cells and fibrosis of the dermis. Some of the tumor islands show a suggestive glandular arrangement of tumor cells. (×200)

and small groups of tumor cells, similar to what is seen in metastatic nodular carcinoma (Peled et al). The tumor cells may show a glandular arrangement (Baran). Flat lesions, as seen in alopecia neoplastica, may show a histologic picture resembling that described for cancer en cuirasse; in both, one encounters single files of tumor cells between thickened collagen bundles (Cohen et al; Baum et al). Atrophy of the hair follicles is a result of the fibrosis (Cohen et al).

Carcinoma of the Inframammary Crease

In rare instances, the first manifestation of carcinoma of the breast is a raised, indurated, nodular lesion in the inframammary crease that may undergo central ulceration (Waisman).

Histopathology. Islands of epithelial cells with hyperchromatic nuclei are seen contiguous with the epidermis and in the dermis. If only a small biospy is taken, the findings are easily misinterpreted as representing a basal cell epithelioma (Dowlati and Nedwich; Waisman). An adequate biopsy, however, shows a carcinoma of the breast extending into the dermis.

CUTANEOUS METASTASIS FROM CARCINOMAS OTHER THAN BREAST CARCINOMA

In carcinomas other than those of the breast or mouth, cutaneous metastases are almost always caused by hem-

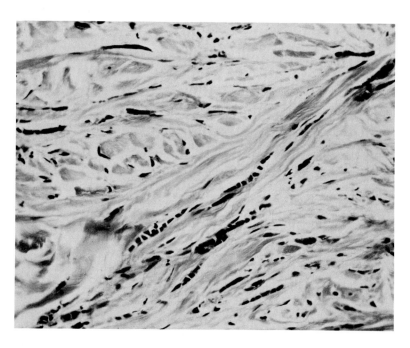

Fig. 28-3. Cutaneous metastasis from carcinoma of the breast
Cancer en cuirasse. Only a few tumor cells are present. They lie embedded between collagen bundles in single-row lines, a pattern referred to as Indian filing. Because of their small number and size, the tumor cells can easily be overlooked. (×400)

atogenous spread. In rare instances, inflammatory carcinoma of the chest wall caused by lymphatic spread occurs in patients with carcinoma of the bronchus (Ingram) or pulmonary adenocarcinoma (Hazelrigg and Rudolph). This is then analogous to the inflammatory carcinoma seen in carcinoma of the breast.

Cutaneous metastases caused by hematogenous dissemination from a visceral carcinoma often are apparent before recognition of the primary tumor. This is true particularly of carcinomas of the lung and of the kidney, in which, in over half of the cases with cutaneous metastases, the existence of the primary carcinoma was not known prior to the appearance of the cutaneous metastases (Ehlers and Krause; Brownstein and Helwig). Not infrequently, in instances of early metastasis, only one or, at the most, a few cutaneous nodules are encountered (Winer and Wright; Kahn et al; Samitz; Batres et al). In patients in whom the cutaneous metastases appear late, they are often multiple, and duration of life then averages only 3 months after the appearance of the skin tumors (Reingold).

Histopathology. In cutaneous metastases caused by hematogenous dissemination, large and small groups of anaplastic tumor cells are present in the dermis and often extend into the subcutaneous tissue. In most instances, it is not possible to recognize from a histologic examination of the metastasis the organ in which the primary tumor is situated, and it is possible to classify the metastatic carcinoma only as an adenocarcinoma, a squamous cell carcinoma, or an undifferentiated carcinoma. However, in four types of carcinoma, it is often possible to recognize the site of the primary neoplasm from the histologic characteristics of the metastatic lesion in the skin. These four types are carcinoma of the gastrointestinal tract, of the kidney, and of the liver, and choriocarcinoma (see below).

As pointed out by several authors, the development of a solitary cutaneous metastasis or of a few metastases in a patient, especially a male, without known existence of a carcinoma should immediately raise the suspicion of carcinoma of the lung (Ehlers and Krause; Brownstein and Helwig). The cutaneous metastases of a pulmonary carcinoma show a wide variety of histologic patterns, including squamous cell carcinoma and adenocarcinoma of varying degrees of differentiation, but, most commonly, they show an undifferentiated carcinoma composed of small, closely packed "oat cells." Even if the initial examination reveals no evidence of pulmonary carcinoma because of the small size of the tumor, further examinations, including bronchoscopy, are advisable.

In *carcinoma of the gastrointestinal tract*, the tumor cells of the cutaneous metastases, like the primary tumor, often contain mucin (Winer and Wright; Samitz). The mucin-containing cells present in the metastases may lie in glandular formations (Fig. 28-4), or they may be grouped irregularly as so-called signet-ring cells, that is, as large, round cells filled with mucin, which presses the nucleus against the cellular wall (Fig. 28-5). The mucin, being epithelial mucin of the sialomucin type, contains both neutral and acid mucopolysaccha-

Fig. 28-4. Cutaneous metastasis from an adenocarcinoma
Numerous glandular lumina are present. (×100)

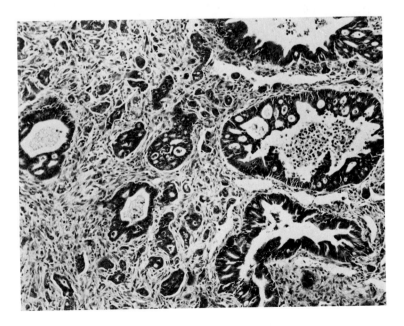

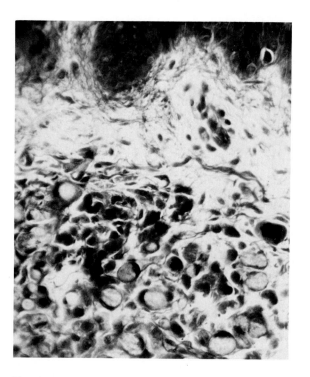

Fig. 28-5. Cutaneous metastasis from carcinoma of the gastrointestinal tract
Many of the tumor cells are so-called signet-ring cells, in which, because of the presence of mucin in the cytoplasm, the nucleus is pressed against the wall. (×400)

rides. The mucin thus (1) is PAS-positive and diastase-resistant, (2) stains with alcian blue at pH 2.5 but not at pH 0.4, indicating that the acid mucopolysaccharides in the sialomucin are non-sulfated, and (3) is hyaluronidase-resistant (Winer and Wright; Cawley et al; Mendoza and Helwig).

In *carcinoma of the kidney,* the cutaneous metastases contain large polyhedral cells arranged in tubular, glandlike structures. The tumor cells have light-staining, centrally located nuclei and abundant, pale cytoplasm (Fig. 28-6). The pale appearance of the cytoplasm is due, at least in part, to the presence of glycogen (Rosenthal and Lever). The stroma of the metastases often is richly vascular, leading to the extravasation of erythrocytes into the lumina of the glandlike structures (Connor et al).

In *carcinoma of the liver,* the tumor may be either a hepatocellular carcinoma or an adenocarcinoma (cholangiocarcinoma), or a mixture of the two. Metastases of hepatocellular carcinoma may be recognized as such because of the arrangement of the malignant hepatocytes in irregular columns (Reingold and Smith). Identification of the tumor as a liver metastasis is fully assured if there are acinar structures containing bile in some of the lumina (Kahn et al).

In *choriocarcinoma,* the cutaneous metastases show the two types of cells that arise from the fetal trophoblast: cytotrophoblasts and syncytiotroph-

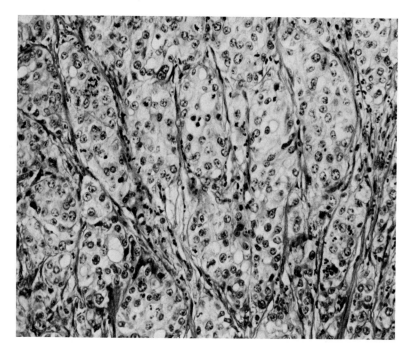

Fig. 28-6. Cutaneous metastasis from carcinoma of the kidney
The tumor cells possess abundant pale cytoplasm and are arranged in tubular, glandlike structures. (×400)

oblasts. The cytotrophoblasts usually grow in clusters, and the cells appear cuboidal with large, vesicular nuclei and a pale cytoplasm. The syncytiotrophoblasts, which have large and irregular nuclei and a basophilic cytoplasm, grow around the clusters of cytotrophoblasts in a plexiform pattern resembling chorionic villi (Cosnow and Fretzin). Patients with choriocarcinoma excrete large amounts of chorionic gonadotropin in their urine.

METASTATIC CUTANEOUS CARCINOID

The carcinoid syndrome occurs in 20% to 40% of patients with a malignant carcinoid tumor (Kurtz et al). Generally, extensive metastases, especially to the liver, are present in such patients. In rare instances, however, a large carcinoid of the ovary may produce the manifestations of the carcinoid syndrome without the presence of metastases (Kierland et al). Clinically, the carcinoid syndrome is characterized by periodic attacks of flushing and of abdominal cramps associated with diarrhea.

Malignant carcinoid tumors and their metastases produce excessive amounts of 5-hydroxytryptamine (serotonin). An excessive excretion of 5-hydroxyindolacetic acid in the urine is diagnostic of the carcinoid syndrome. Since the carcinoid tumor and its metastases divert much tryptophan toward serotonin and thus away from niacin, the endogenous niacin production is depressed. If, in addition, diarrhea reduces the availability of exogenous niacin, pellagra, caused by niacin deficiency, may result (Castiello and Lynch). (For a discussion of pellagra, see p. 433.)

The metastases caused by malignant carcinoid tumors are found most commonly in the regional lymph nodes and the liver but may occur in many other organs. Cutaneous metastases occur occasionally. They may consist of a solitary cutaneous nodule (Norman et al; Keane et al), which may be the first manifestation of the disease (Brody et al). In other cases, there are one or several subcutaneous nodules (Steele; Rudner et al) or numerous cutaneous and subcutaneous nodules (Reingold and Escovitz; Hyman and Wells). In a review of the English language literature published in 1980 (Keane et al), 17 cases of cutaneous or subcutaneous metastases from carcinoid tumors are discussed. In nine cases, the primary site was the bronchus, and in six cases the small intestines, including the appendix. In two patients, the primary site could not be determined. In addition, one patient had a solitary cutaneous carcinoid tumor that appeared to be primary rather than metastatic (van Dijk and Ten Seldam). The relatively high incidence of cutaneous metastases originating from a bronchial carcinoid is interesting, since only about 12% of all carcinoids are bronchial (Godwin). Only one of the nine patients with bronchial carcinoid and two of the six patients with intestinal carcinoid who had metastases to the skin had symptoms of the carcinoid syndrome.

Histopathology. Carcinoid metastases in the skin and subcutaneous tissue consist of solid islands, nests, and cords of tumor cells. As a rule, the cells appear quite uniform in size and shape, with small, round nuclei and abundant clear to eosinophilic cytoplasm occasionally containing numerous eosinophilic granules (Reingold and Escovitz; van Dijk and ten Seldam; Brody et al). In some instances, however, the nuclei are hyperchromatic (Keane et al), and there may even be areas in which the nuclei show anaplasia by being irregularly shaped, large, and hyperchromatic (Reingold and Escovitz).

Carcinoids of the bronchus are of foregut origin (type 1) and usually contain *argyrophil* granules, which can be impregnated with silver, whereas carcinoids of the small intestine are of midgut origin (type 2) and almost invariably contain *argentaffin* granules, which stain with the Fontana–Masson stain (see p. 16) (Brody et al). Although the cutaneous metastases of intestinal carcinoids often contain cells with argentaffin granules (Norman et al), the cutaneous metastases of bronchial carcinoids may have neither argyrophil nor argentaffin granules (Keane et al).

Histogenesis. On *electron microscopy*, the cells of the cutaneous metastases of carcinoid tumors are seen to contain numerous dense core granules in their cytoplasm, even when they are found to be devoid of argyrophil or argentaffin granules on light microscopy (Keane et al). The granules range from 100 nm to 250 nm in diameter and, like the granules in Merkel cells (see p. 20) and trabecular carcinoma (see p. 578), show peripheral to their dense core an electron-lucid halo and a limiting membrane (Serratoni and Robboy). These neurosecretory granules are capable of synthesizing and storing various polypeptide hormones. The cells of carcinoids thus belong to the APUD (*a*mine *p*recursor *u*ptake and *d*ecarboxylation) cell series and as such are derived from the neural crest (Brody et al).

The chemical mediation of the carcinoid syndrome is not fully clarified. Although the release of serotonin may produce the diarrhea (Kurtz et al), the flushing phenomenon is probably due to elevated blood levels of bradykinin (Norman et al).

Differential Diagnosis. Even though the cells of carcinoid tumors have a fairly characteristic appearance, with small, uniform nuclei and abundant cytoplasm, they may be mistaken for a sweat gland carcinoma or a glomus tumor because of their arrangement in well-defined islands (Reingold and Escovitz). The absence of lumina and of spaces lined by endothelial cells aids in the distinction.

BIBLIOGRAPHY

Incidence and Dissemination of Metastatic Carcinoma

BARR R, DANN F: Anaplastic thyroid carcinoma metastatic to skin. J Cutan Pathol 1:201–206, 1974

BROWNSTEIN MH, HELWIG EB: Patterns of cutaneous metastasis. Arch Dermatol 105:862–868, 1972

CHAKRABORTY AK, REDDY AN, GROSBERG SJ et al: Pancreatic carcinoma with dissemination to umbilicus and skin. Arch Dermatol 113:838–839, 1977

GATES O: Cutaneous metastasis of malignant diseases. Am J Cancer 30:718–730, 1937

HOLLANDER A, GROTS IA: Oculocutaneous metastases from carcinoma of the urinary bladder. Arch Dermatol 97:678–684, 1968

PEISON B: Metastasis of carcinoma of the prostate to the scalp. Arch Dermatol 104:301–303, 1971

PRICE NM, KOPF AW: Metastases to skin from occult malignant neoplasms. Cutaneous metastases from a teratocarcinoma. Arch Dermatol 109:547–550, 1974

RASBACH D, HENDRICKS A, STOLTZNER G: Endometrial adenocarcinoma metastatic to the scalp. Arch Dermatol 114:1708–1709, 1978

REINGOLD IM, SMITH BR: Cutaneous metastases from hepatomas. Arch Dermatol 114:1045–1046, 1978

Cutaneous Metastases from Carcinoma of the Breast

BARAN R: Les métastases alopéciantes scléro-atrophiques des cancers mammaires. Dermatologica 138:169–181, 1969

BAUM EM, OMURA EF, PAYNE RR et al: Alopecia neoplastica, a rare form of cutaneous metastasis. J Am Acad Dermatol 4:688–694, 1981

BROWNSTEIN MH, HELWIG EB: Metastatic tumors of the skin. Cancer 29:1298–1307, 1972

COHEN I, LEVY E, SCHREIBER H: Alopecia neoplastica due to breast carcinoma. Arch Dermatol 84:490–492, 1961

DOWLATI Y, NEDWICH A: Carcinoma of mammary crease simulating basal cell epithelioma. Arch Dermatol 107:628–629, 1973

INGRAM JT: Carcinoma erysipelatodes and carcinoma telangiectaticum. Arch Dermatol 77:227–231, 1958

LEAVELL UW JR, TILLOTSON FW: Metastatic cutaneous carcinoma from the breast. Arch Dermatol Syph 64:774–782, 1951

PELED IJ, OKON E, WESCHLER Z et al: Distant, late metastases to skin of carcinoma of the breast. J Dermatol Surg Oncol 8:192–195, 1982

SIEGEL JM: Inflammatory carcinoma of the breast. Arch Dermatol Syph 66:710–716, 1952

WAISMAN M: Carcinoma of the inframammary crease. Arch Dermatol 114:1520–1521, 1978

ZALA L, JENNI C: Das Carcinoma erysipelatodes. Dermatologica 160:80–89, 1980

Cutaneous Metastasis from Carcinomas Other Than Breast Carcinoma

BATRES E, KNOX JM, WOLF JE JR: Metastatic renal cell carcinoma resembling a pyogenic granuloma. Arch Dermatol 114:1082–1083, 1978

BROWNSTEIN MH, HELWIG EB: Patterns of cutaneous metastasis. Arch Dermatol 105:862–868, 1972

CAWLEY EP, HSU YT, WEARY PE: The evaluation of neoplastic metastoses of the skin. Arch Dermatol 90:262–265, 1964

CONNOR DH, TAYLOR HB, HELWIG EB: Cutaneous metastasis of renal cell carcinoma. Arch Pathol 76:339–346, 1963

COSNOW I, FRETZIN DF: Choriocarcinoma metastatic to skin. Arch Dermatol 109:551–553, 1974

EHLERS G, KRAUSE W: Über cutane Metastasen maligner Tumoren innerer Organe. Hautarzt 21:66–75, 1970

HAZELRIGG DE, RUDOLPH AH: Inflammatory metastatic carcinoma. Carcinoma erysipeloides. Arch Dermatol 113:69–70, 1977

INGRAM JT: Carcinoma erysipelatodes and carcinoma telangiectaticum. Arch Dermatol 77:227–231, 1958

KAHN JA, SINHAMOHAPATRA SB, SCHNEIDER AF: Hepatoma presenting as a skin metastasis. Arch Dermatol 104:299–300, 1971

MENDOZA S, HELWIG EB: Mucinous (adenocystic) carcinoma of the skin. Arch Dermatol 103:68–78, 1971

REINGOLD IM: Cutaneous metastases from internal carcinoma. Cancer 19:162–168, 1966

REINGOLD IM, SMITH BR: Cutaneous metastases from hepatomas. Arch Dermatol 114:1045–1046, 1978

ROSENTHAL AL, LEVER WF: Involvement of the skin in renal carcinoma. Arch Dermatol 76:96–102, 1957

SAMITZ MH: Umbilical metastasis from carcinoma of the stomach. Arch Dermatol 111:1478–1479, 1975

WINER LM, WRIGHT ET: Über den sekundären (metastatischen) Hautkrebs. Hautarzt 11:23–27, 1960

Metastatic Cutaneous Carcinoid

BRODY HJ, STALLINGS WP, FINE RM et al: Carcinoid in an umbilical nodule. Arch Dermatol 114:570–572, 1978

CASTIELLO RJ, LYNCH PJ: Pellagra and the carcinoid syndrome. Arch Dermatol 105:574–577, 1972

GODWIN JD II: Carcinoid tumors: An analysis of 2837 cases. Cancer 36:560–569, 1975

HYMAN GA, WELLS J: Bronchial carcinoid with osteoblastic metastases. Arch Intern Med 114:541–546, 1964

KEANE J, FRETZIN DF, JAO W et al: Bronchial carcinoid metastatic to skin. J Cutan Pathol 7:43–49, 1980

KIERLAND RK, SAUER WG, DEARING WH: The cutaneous manifestations of the functioning carcinoid. Arch Dermatol 77:86–90, 1958

KURTZ RC, SHERLOCK P, WINAWER SJ: Dermatologic abnormalities associated with gastrointestinal malignant and premalignant diseases. Int J Dermatol 17:14–19, 1978

NORMAN JL, CUNNINGHAM PJ, CLEVELAND BR: Skin and subcutaneous metastases from gastrointestinal carcinoid tumors. Arch Surg 103:767–769, 1971

REINGOLD IM, ESCOVITZ WE: Metastatic cutaneous carcinoid. Arch Dermatol 82:971–975, 1960

RUDNER EJ, LENTZ C, BROWN J: Bronchial carcinoid tumor with skin metastases. Arch Dermatol 92:73–75, 1965

SERRATONI FT, ROBBOY SJ: Ultrastructure of primary and metastatic ovarian carcinoids. Cancer 36:157–160, 1975

STEELE CW: Malignant carcinoid. Arch Intern Med 110:763–768, 1962

VAN DIJK, TEN SELDAM REJ: A possible primary cutaneous carcinoid. Cancer 36:1016–1020, 1975

Tumors of Fibrous Tissue 29

DERMATOFIBROMA

Dermatofibromas are known also as fibrous histiocytomas, histiocytomas, and sclerosing hemangiomas (see Histogenesis). They occur in the skin as firm, indolent, single or multiple nodules. Usually, the nodules arise in adults. They are situated most commonly on the extremities but may occur elsewhere. They are seen only rarely on the palms and soles (Bedi et al). Although they are as a rule only a few millimeters in diameter, they occasionally measure 2 cm to 3 cm in size. Rarely, as a result of hemorrhage into the tumor, they may attain a larger size (Hairston and Reed). Most lesions have a reddish color, but they may be reddish brown because of hyperpigmentation of the overlying skin or, rarely, bluish black because of the presence of large amounts of hemosiderin within the tumor. In the latter case, the clinical appearance resembles that of a malignant melanoma. The lesions of dermatofibroma usually persist indefinitely, although, in a few instances, spontaneous involution has been observed (Niemi).

Histopathology. Dermatofibromas are composed to varying degrees of fibroblasts, young collagen, mature collagen, capillaries, and histiocytes. On this basis, dermatofibromas have been divided into "fibrous" lesions composed entirely or almost entirely of fibroblasts and collagen and "cellular" lesions composed to a significant degree of phagocytic cells with the appearance of histiocytes (Rentiers and Montgomery). Lesions intermediate in character also occur (Niemi). Some authors recognize as a third variety lesions with a vascular component (Vilanova and Flint). In all large series, the percentage of fibrous tumors has been significantly higher than that of cellular tumors.

In fibrous dermatofibromas, the cells have the appearance of fibroblasts showing elongated nuclei and hardly any cytoplasm. Much of the collagen is young and thus, instead of staining bright red with hematoxylin-eosin, stains a pale blue; and further, instead of being assembled in firm bundles, the collagen in many areas consists of individual fibers (Plate 3, facing p. 612). As a rule, the collagen is irregularly arranged in intertwining and anastomosing bands, a so-called storiform (matlike) pattern (Fig. 29-1). Occasionally, the fibroblasts and the collagen they produce radiate from a central point, or "hub," of condensed collagen in a whorl-like fashion, giving the appearance of a cartwheel (Niemi). The nodule shows poor demarcation on both sides, so that the fibroblasts and the young basophilic collagen of the tumor extend between the mature, eosinophilic collagen bundles of the dermis and surround them, thus trapping normal collagen bundles at the periphery of the nodule. At the lower border, the demarcation is usually fairly sharp, but irregular penetration into the subcutaneous fat can be observed in some cases (Bandmann). At the upper border, the tumor is usually, but not always, separated from the overlying epidermis by a narrow band of collagen (Fig. 29-2). If present, this band consists of young collagen composed of individual fibers rather than of bundles.

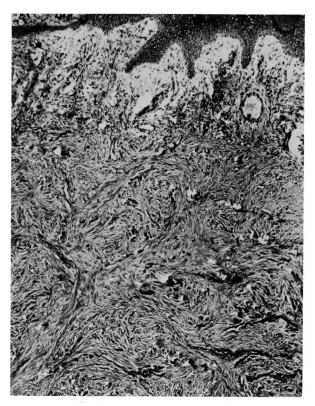

Fig. 29-1.   Dermatofibroma, fibrous type
The collagen is irregularly arranged in intertwining, anastomosing bands. Some of the collagen, instead of being assembled in firm bundles, lies in individual fibers. There is a moderate increase in the number of fibroblasts. (×50)

In cellular dermatofibromas, often referred to as histiocytomas, many cells, in contrast to those of the fibrous type, possess round to oval nuclei and ample, well-defined cytoplasm, thus resembling histiocytes rather than fibroblasts (Niemi). The cells produce only small amounts of collagen, which is present almost exclusively as individual fibers rather than as bundles (Fig. 29-3).

In both the fibrous type and the cellular type of dermatofibroma, scattered small capillaries with prominent endothelial cells are usually present. In some instances, capillaries are quite numerous, giving the lesion an angiomatous component (Vilanova and Flint). Such lesions have been referred to as sclerosing hemangiomas (Gross and Wolbach). Small areas of hemorrhage may be seen in such vascular tumors (Niemi). Rarely, large, blood-filled tissue spaces are present (Hairston and Reed; Santa Cruz and Kyriakos).

In about one third of all dermatofibromas, special staining reveals deposits of lipid or hemosiderin within tumor cells (Cramer). Significant deposits are more apt to be found in cellular than in fibrous dermatofibromas. In routinely stained sections, the lipid-containing tumor cells, depending on the amount of lipid present, either have a pale, irregularly vacuolated cytoplasm or appear as true foam cells. The lipid is often doubly refractile on polariscopic examination (Arnold and Tilden). In some instances, one also finds multinucleated giant cells. These cells may or may not contain lipid material. If they do, they may have the appearance of Touton giant cells (Frenk; Niemi). Intracellular deposits of hemosiderin are often present in tumors that also contain lipid (Rentiers and Montgomery). Usually, the areas of hemosiderin deposits are small (Niemi). Large amounts of hemosiderin both intracellularly and extracellularly may be seen in the vicinity of areas of hemorrhage (Santa Cruz and Kyriakos).

A significant hyperplasia of the overlying epidermis in the center of the lesion occurs in more than 80% of the lesions of dermatofibroma, irrespective of whether they are of the fibrous or the cellular type (Steigleder et al; Schoenfeld). The presence of such hyperplasia often has considerable value in the diagnosis of dermatofibroma. Most commonly, the hyperplasia consists of a regular elongation of the rete ridges, which may be associated with hyperpigmentation of the basal cell layer. In some cases, the epidermal hyperplasia is reminiscent of a seborrheic keratosis through the interlacing of thickened rete ridges. Occasionally, downward proliferations are present that imitate the hair matrix to the point of having a connective tissue papilla (Steigleder et al). In 2% to 5% of the lesions, the downward proliferations are indistinguishable from those of a superficial basal epithelioma (Fig. 29-2) (Cramer and Cramer; Bryant). Even though the proliferations in most of these instances are to be regarded as basal-cell-epithelioma-like, in rare instances, a truly invasive nodular basal cell epithelioma associated with ulceration develops (Thies and Hennies; Goette and Helwig; Buselmeier and Uecker).

Histogenesis. Dermatofibroma was originally described as fibroma simplex by Unna in 1894; In 1932, Woringer and Kviatkowski showed that some dermatofibromas contain phagocytizing cells, which they regarded as histiocytes. They proposed the term *histiocytoma* for such tumors. In 1936, Senear and Caro injected colloidal iron under six dermatofibromas prior to excision and found that all of them phagocytized iron. They therefore

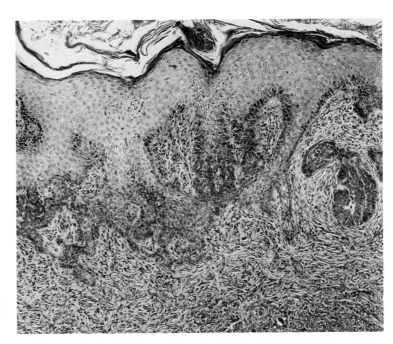

Fig. 29-2.   Dermatofibroma, fibrous type
The overlying epidermis shows budding proliferations resembling a superficial basal cell epithelioma. (×100)

Fig. 29-3.   Dermatofibroma, cellular type (histiocytoma)
Many cells possess round to oval nuclei and ample cytoplasm and thus resemble histiocytes. Only small amounts of collagen are present, largely as individual fibers rather than as bundles. Many capillaries with prominent endothelial cells are seen. Several cells have a foamy cytoplasm; two particularly large foam cells (*F.C.*) are located in the upper left corner. (×400)

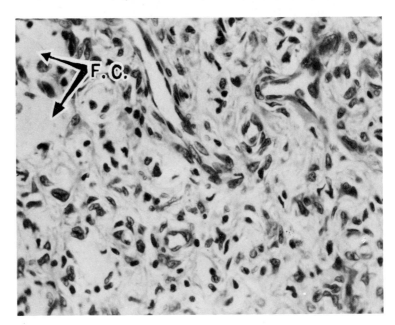

concluded that all dermatofibromas are histiocytomas. In contrast, Rentiers and Montgomery regarded the presence of phagocytizing histiocytes within dermatofibromas as a secondary event "originating in response to hemorrhage, inflammatory changes and local tissue destruction in the nodules."

Although no full agreement existed about the relationship between histiocytes and fibroblasts, it became a widely accepted practice to refer to tumors composed predominantly of collagen fibers as dermatofibromas, and to tumors with significant deposits of lipids or hemosiderin in the tumor cells as histiocytomas (Niemi).

In recent years, several authors have stressed the essential unity of dermatofibroma and histiocytoma. Frenk came to the conclusion that even the tumors showing phagocytosis of iron or lipid are dermatofibromas, since phagocytosis lies within the functional potential of the fibroblast. Klaus and Winkelmann found acid phosphatase activity as evidence of a phagocytic potential within the cells of all nine dermatofibromas examined by them, irrespective of whether they showed a predominance of stromal proliferation ("dermatofibromas") or were predominantly cellular ("histiocytomas").

ELECTRON MICROSCOPY. Electron microscopic examination of dermatofibromas has shown that even some lesions showing phagocytosis are composed of fibroblasts. Carrington and Winkelmann, having examined by electron microscopy two dermatofibromas with numerous lipid and hemosiderin inclusions, stated that the "histiocytes of this lesion resembled fibroblasts, having more of an oval nucleus, a prominent rough endoplasmic reticulum, and, in some, perinuclear fibrillar structures." Mihatsch-Konz et al examined eight dermatofibromas of the fibrous type by electron microscopy and found that fibroblasts were the essential cell and were engaged in both collagen production and lipid storage (EM 42). When blood was injected into one lesion 24 hr prior to excision, fragments of polymorphonuclear cells were visible within large phagolysosomes, demonstrating the ability of the fibroblasts to carry out phagocytosis.

Additional electron microscopic studies have shown the presence of many histiocytes in cellular dermatofibromas (Auböck). In one study, aside from some fibroblastlike and histiocytelike cells, the majority of cells had the appearance of myofibroblasts (see p. 601) (Katenkamp and Stiller).

In conclusion, it seems very likely, as proposed by Rentiers and Montgomery (see above), that the fibroblast is the primary cell type in dermatofibroma and that the presence of phagocytizing histiocytes is a secondary event. It is of interest that the phagocytic histiocytes in dermatofibroma do not contain lysozyme, in contrast to histiocytes of the bone-marrow-derived monocyte–macrophage system. This makes it likely that both the fibroblastic and histiocytic cells in dermatofibroma arise from primitive mesenchymal elements (Burgdorf et al). (For a more detailed discussion, see Histogenesis under Malignant Fibrous Histiocytoma, p. 613.)

NEOPLASM VERSUS FIBROSIS. The view has been expressed that dermatofibromas are not tumors at all, but rather represent a reactive proliferation of fibroblasts subsequent to a trauma. Thus, Rentiers and Montgomery as well as Klaus and Winkelmann refer to them as nodular subepidermal fibrosis. However, the fact that the lesions, with very few exceptions, show no tendency to regress but persist indefinitely speaks in favor of a neoplastic rather than a reactive, inflammatory genesis (Bandmann).

DERMATOFIBROMA VERSUS SCLEROSING HEMANGIOMA. The view expressed by Gross and Wolbach in 1943 that dermatofibromas are actually sclerosing hemangiomas still has adherents among general pathologists. According to Gross and Wolbach, early dermatofibromas show proliferating capillaries surrounded by fibroblasts and proliferating endothelial cells with phagocytic ability that attempt to form new capillaries but do not always succeed and instead become engulfed by regressive fibrosis. In an electron microscopic study, an attempt has been made to support this theory (Carstens and Schrodt). The investigators found cell clusters composed of endothelial cells, identifiable as such by the presence of Weibel–Palade bodies. The finding that some spaces, regarded as obliterated vascular spaces, were lined by cells with ultrastructural characteristics of fibroblasts was explained by the assumption that endothelial cells "may obtain an ultrastructural similarity to fibroblasts." In conclusion, it seems unlikely that the fibrosis in dermatofibromas represents a "regressive process," since dermatofibromas do not regress but persist indefinitely.

HYPERPLASIA OF THE EPIDERMIS. The hyperplasia of the epidermis overlying dermatofibromas can be explained by the presence of young collagen and of abundant amounts of metachromatic ground substance in the subepidermal region. This material, which resembles embryonic mesenchyme, stimulates the epidermis in a fashion similar to that of embryonic mesenchyme, thus causing the formation of immature hair structures and even of primary epithelial germs. Because the dermatofibroma prevents their downward growth, the immature hair structures, including the primary epithelial germ formations, proliferate in the narrow space between the epidermis and the tumor (Pinkus). The primary epithelial germ proliferations resemble the proliferations of a basal cell epithelioma and in rare instances even give rise to a true basal cell epithelioma.

Differential Diagnosis. Rarely, dermatofibromas show a considerable number of nuclei, some of them arranged in a whorled or cartwheel pattern. In such cases, differentiation from dermatofibrosarcoma protuberans (see p. 609) may cause difficulties. However, the lack of atypicality in the appearance of the nuclei, the absence of mitotic figures, the absence of ulceration, and the presence of significant epidermal hyperplasia rule out fibrosarcoma.

A dermatofibroma with many foam cells but without hemosiderin or significant fibroblastic proliferation may be indistinguishable from a xanthoma tuberosum in a regressive, fibrosing stage (Arnold and Tilden). In such cases, clinical data, such as the number and location of the lesions and the presence or absence of elevated serum lipid values, are necessary for the correct diagnosis to be reached.

SOFT FIBROMA

Soft fibromas, also called acrochordons or cutaneous tags, occur in three types: (1) as multiple small, furrowed papules, especially on the neck and in the axillae, generally only 1 mm to 2 mm in width and length; (2) as single or multiple filiform, smooth growths in varying locations, about 2 mm in width and 5 mm in length; and (3) as usually solitary baglike, pedunculated growths, usually about 1 cm in size but occasionally much larger, seen most commonly on the lower trunk (Flegel and Tessmann; Field). (For a discussion of acrochordon in association with fibrofolliculomas and trichodiscomas, see p. 526.)

Histopathology. The multiple small, furrowed papules usually show papillomatosis, hyperkeratosis, and regular acanthosis and occasionally also horn cysts within their acanthotic epidermis. Thus, there is often considerable resemblance to a pedunculated seborrheic keratosis.

The filiform, smooth growths show slight to moderate acanthosis and, occasionally, mild papillomatosis. The connective tissue stalk is composed of loose collagen fibers and often contains numerous dilated capillaries filled with erythrocytes (Fig. 29-4) (Flegel and Tessmann). Nevus cells are found in as many as 30% of the filiform growths, indicating that some of them represent involuting melanocytic nevi (Stegmaier).

The baglike, soft fibromas generally show a flattened epidermis. The dermis, like that of the filiform soft fibromas, is composed of loosely arranged collagen fibers. Mature fat cells form the center (Field). In some instances, the dermis is quite thin, so that the fat cells compose a significant portion of the tumor. The tumor may then be regarded as a lipofibroma (Cramer).

RECURRENT INFANTILE DIGITAL FIBROMA

In recurrent infantile digital fibroma, single or multiple fibrous nodules are present on the fingers or toes. They may be present at birth but they usually appear during the first year of life or, less commonly, later in childhood. The nodules involute spontaneously. In about 75% of the cases, recurrences are observed during early childhood (Santa Cruz and Reiner).

Histopathology. The dermis shows numerous spindle-shaped fibroblasts and collagen bundles arranged in interlacing fascicles. There may be extension deep into the subcutaneous tissue (Mehregan et al). A valuable diagnostic feature is the presence of characteristic eosinophilic cytoplasmic inclusion bodies within many of the fibroblasts, often in the paranuclear region. These inclusion bodies measure from 3 μm to 10 μm in diameter (Shapiro). They are best visualized either with phosphotungstic acid-hematoxylin, which stains them a deep red, or with Masson's trichrome, which stains them purple (Santa Cruz and Reiner).

Histogenesis. *Electron microscopic study* shows that most of the fibroblasts contain one or two narrow bundles of filaments running longitudinally within the cell. Distributed along each bundle are dense bodies such as seen in the contractile apparatus of smooth muscle cells. Some of these bundles are attached to the cell membrane. It can thus be concluded that the tumor cells are myofibroblasts and that the bundles are composed of myofilaments (Bhawan et al). Myofibroblasts are modified

Fig. 29-4. Soft fibroma, filiform type
This type of soft fibroma shows a hyperplastic epidermis. The connective tissue stalk contains loosely arranged collagen fibers and many capillaries. (×50)

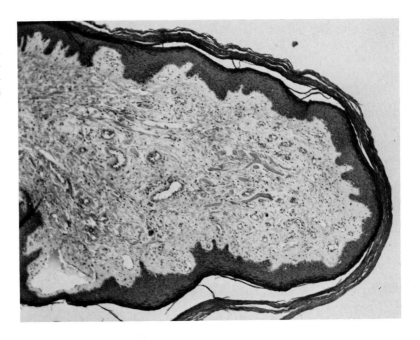

fibroblasts originally observed in granulation tissue (Majno et al; Ryan et al) but subsequently seen in various fibroblastic tumors, including dermatofibromas (see p. 600) and desmoid tumors (see p. 607). However, in recurrent infantile digital fibroma, all or nearly all fibroblasts are myofibroblasts, so that the designation *infantile digital myofibroblastoma* has been suggested (Bhawan et al).

The cytoplasmic inclusion bodies consist in the center of a dense aggregate of electron-dense filaments; at the periphery, the filaments are more loosely arranged (Gebhart et al). The inclusion bodies seem to form by accretion of myofilaments, since they are often continuous with bundles of myofilaments. Also, the filaments in the inclusion bodies and in the bundles of myofilaments have the same range of diameter, varying from 5 nm to 12 nm (Bhawan et al). In addition, dense bodies are frequently seen in the bundles of filaments extending from the inclusion bodies (Iwasaki et al).

ACQUIRED DIGITAL FIBROKERATOMA

A solitary rounded, firm, more or less hyperkeratotic projection is seen most commonly on a finger or toe but occasionally on the palms or soles (Verallo). The outgrowth is either elongated or dome-shaped and, if dome-shaped, often slightly pedunculated. It arises out of a collarette of slightly raised skin. In contrast to recurrent infantile digital fibroma, acquired digital fibrokeratoma occurs in adults.

Histopathology.   The epidermis shows marked hyperkeratosis and acanthosis with thickened, often branching rete ridges. The core of the lesion is formed by thick, interwoven bundles of collagen predominantly oriented in the direction of the vertical axis of the lesion (Bart et al). Elastic fibers are usually present but are apt to be thin and scanty (Hare and Smith). Many tumors are highly vascular (Verallo).

Differential Diagnosis.   Although acquired digital fibrokeratoma may resemble a rudimentary supernumerary digit in its clinical and histologic appearance, rudimentary polydactyly almost always occurs at the base of the fifth finger, is present from birth, and is often bilateral. Histologically, rudimentary polydactyly differs from digital fibrokeratoma by the presence of numerous nerve bundles, especially at the base of the lesion (Bart et al).

MULTIPLE PERIFOLLICULAR FIBROMAS

Multiple perifollicular fibromas, a rare condition, shows numerous skin-colored perifollicular papules, some of which have a central comedo (Belaich et al). The eruption is usually limited to the face and neck (Zackheim and Pinkus), but it may extend to the upper trunk (Vakilzadeh and Manegold) or may even be generalized (Hornstein and Knickenberg). In the latter case, the condition may be familial and associated with polyps of the colon.

Histopathology.   The hair follicles are either normal (Zackheim and Pinkus) or dilated and filled with keratinous material (Belaich et al). The follicles are surrounded by concentrically arranged young collagen showing numerous spindle-shaped nuclei (Zackheim and Pinkus).

Differential Diagnosis.   The angiofibromas of tuberous sclerosis usually show vascular dilatation and perivascular fibrosis, in addition to perifollicular fibrosis. Fibrous papule of the face usually shows no perifollicular arrangement of the fibroblasts, but, if it does, distinction is possible only on a clinical basis (Zackheim and Pinkus). Fibrofolliculomas, which are often associated with trichodiscomas and acrochordons, show epithelial strands extending from the infundibulum of the hair follicle into the mantle of connective tissue (Birt et al) (see p. 525). Trichodiscomas do not show a concentric, perifollicular arrangement of the collagen (Pinkus et al).

FIBROUS PAPULE OF THE FACE (NOSE)

Fibrous papule of the face, a common lesion, occurs nearly always as a solitary lesion on the face, especially on the nose, in mature persons. It is usually dome-shaped, firm, and small, not exceeding 5 mm in diameter. In most cases, it is skin-colored, but it may be reddish or pigmented. Described at first as solitary perifollicular fibroma (Zackheim and Pinkus; Pinkus), the lesion has been regarded by subsequent authors either as an involuting melanocytic nevus (Graham et al; Saylan et al; Altmeyer; McGibbon and Wilson Jones) or as a solitary angiofibroma analogous to the multiple angiofibromas of tuberous sclerosis (Reed et al; Reed; Meigel and Ackerman; Santa Cruz and Prioleau; Ragaz and Berezowsky). It seems most likely that the so-called fibrous papule of the nose or face is not an entity. Whereas most cases represent solitary angiofibromas, others are involuting melanocytic nevi or, in rare instances, solitary perifollicular fibromas. A histologic distinction between an angiofibroma and an involuting nevus may in some cases be impossible.

Histopathology.   In cases representing *solitary angiofibromas*, variable numbers of spindle-shaped, plump, stellate, and occasionally also multinucleated cells are present in the dermis and are regarded as fibroblasts. In addition, melanophages are often present in the upper dermis. Numerous vellus hair follicles are commonly seen surrounded by coarse collagen fibers in a concentric array. The blood vessels are usually increased in number and dilated and are occasionally surrounded by fibrosis (Meigel and Ackerman). There may be an increase in the number and size of the basal melanocytes in the epidermis (Reed).

Histogenesis. In two *electron microscopic studies* involving a total of seven cases, the dermal cells had the appearance of fibroblasts rather than of melanocytes, possessing a well-developed rough endoplasmic reticulum, microfilaments, and some primary lysosomes but no melanosomes or basement membrane (Santa Cruz and Prioleau; Ragaz and Berezowsky).

In cases representing *fibrosing melanocytic nevi,* melanocytic hyperplasia is often pronounced in the overlying epidermis. Stellate and multinucleated cells resembling nevus cells rather than fibroblasts are present, and, in some instances, typical nesting of cells is seen, as in melanocytic nevi. Also, there is often telangiectasia. However, there is neither capillary proliferation, as often seen in angiofibroma, nor perifollicular fibrosis, as seen in perifollicular fibroma (Graham et al; Saylan et al; Altmeyer; McGibbon and Wilson Jones).

A small percentage of fibrous papules of the face fulfill the criteria of *solitary perifollicular fibromas* (see p. 602) (Zackheim and Pinkus; Pinkus).

TUBEROUS SCLEROSIS

Tuberous sclerosis, a dominantly inherited disorder, is characterized by the triad of mental deficiency, epilepsy, and angiofibromas of the face. The triad is not necessarily complete. The angiofibromas consist of numerous small, reddish, smooth papules in symmetric distribution in the nasolabial folds, on the cheeks, and on the chin.

Additional cutaneous manifestations that may be present include asymmetrically arranged, large, raised, soft, brownish fibromas on the face and the scalp; subungual and periungual fibromas; and so-called shagreen patches, usually found in the lumbosacral region and consisting of slightly raised and slightly thickened areas of the skin. Scattered hypopigmented, leaf-shaped areas are present in more than half of the patients with tuberous sclerosis. They are best visualized with the aid of Wood's light. Their diagnostic significance lies in the fact that they either are present at birth or appear very early in life and thus are the earliest cutaneous sign of tuberous sclerosis (Fitzpatrick et al).

Histopathology. In the past, the symmetrically distributed, small, reddish angiofibromas of the face were mistakenly called adenoma sebaceum of Pringle. However, the sebaceous glands are generally atrophic, and the main findings are dermal fibrosis and dilatation of some of the capillaries. In some lesions, the fibrosis has a "glial" appearance because of the large size and stellate shape of the fibroblasts. Occasionally, multinucleated giant cells are also present. In some cases, one observes vascular proliferation and perivascular proliferation of fibroblasts in addition to vascular dilatation (Nickel and Reed). In old lesions, there may be perifollicular proliferation of collagen leading to the compression of atrophic hair follicles by concentric layers of collagen. Elastic tissue is absent in the angiofibromas.

The larger, asymmetric fibromas on the face and scalp show markedly sclerotic collagen arranged in thick, concentric layers around atrophic pilosebaceous follicles (Fig. 29-5). In contrast to the smaller lesions, dilated capillaries usually are absent.

The ungual fibromas show fibrosis, usually without but occasionally with capillary dilatation. The areas of fibrosis may have a glial appearance due to the presence of large stellate fibroblasts (Nickel and Reed).

The shagreen patches show two somewhat different types of changes in the collagen. In the more common variety, a dense, sclerotic mass of very broad collagenous bundles are seen in the lower dermis, mimicking the appearance of morphea. In the other type, normal-appearing collagen bundles throughout the dermis are seen in an interwoven pattern, so that some bundles are cut across and others lengthwise. The elastic tissue in some instances shows fragmentation and clumping (Nickel and Reed) but generally is reduced in amount (Kobayasi et al).

The hypopigmented, leaf-shaped areas show a normal number of melanocytes with the dopa reaction. However, the reaction is less intense than normal. On electron microscopy, the melanosomes within the melanocytes and keratinocytes show a decrease from normal in the degree of melanization and a diminution in size (Fitzpatrick et al; Tilgen).

Systemic Lesions. Multiple tumors are commonly found in the brain, retina, heart, and kidneys. The "tuberous" tumors of the brain, which are up to 3 cm in size, are gliomas; they are often calcified and are then visible on x-ray examination (Reed et al). Prior to calcification, they may be visualized by computed tomography, often already in infancy (Burkhart and El-Shaar). The retinal tumors are also gliomas. Because of their peripheral location, they cause no visual disturbances. They are either flat or extend as mulber-

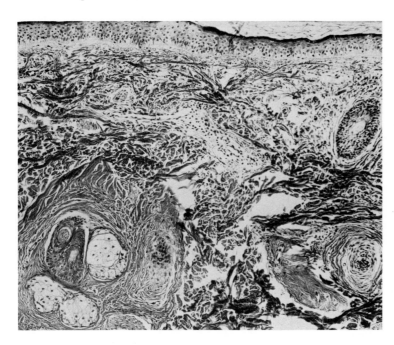

Fig. 29-5.   Tuberous sclerosis
A fibromatous lesion shows markedly sclerotic collagen arranged in thick concentric layers around atrophic pilosebaceous structures. (×100)

rylike growths into the vitreous (Scheig and Bornstein). The cardiac tumors are rhabdomyomas in which the striated muscle cells appear markedly vacuolated as a result of the intracellular accumulation of glycogen (Morales). The renal tumors are angiomyolipomas, which occur exclusively in tuberous sclerosis. They may be large or small and solitary or multiple, and they are bilateral. Rarely, they lead to renal failure by gradually replacing renal tissue (Chonco et al). Histologically, there is a mixture of adipose tissue, blood vessels, and smooth muscle. Although there may be a slight degree of pleomorphism of some of the smooth muscle cells, the tumors always remain benign (Price and Mostofi).

Differential Diagnosis.   The angiofibromas of tuberous sclerosis are histologically indistinguishable from the solitary angiofibroma manifesting itself as fibrous papule of the face or nose (see p. 602). The shagreen patches of tuberous sclerosis differ from other connective tissue nevi by the regular absence of any increase in elastic tissue (see p. 77).

HYPERTROPHIC SCAR AND KELOID

Hypertrophic scars and keloids initially have the same clinical appearance: they are red, raised, and firm and possess a smooth, shiny surface. Whereas hypertrophic scars flatten spontaneously in the course of one or several

years, keloids persist and may even extend beyond the site of the original injury.

Keloids usually follow an injury, but patients sometimes have no recollection of prior injury. This is particularly true in the case of presternal keloids. Occasionally, there is a familial predilection for keloid formation (Murray et al). Also, keloids are much more common in blacks than in whites (Onwukwe). In the rare Rubinstein–Taybi syndrome, keloids are apt to develop spontaneously in adolescence or early adulthood. This syndrome is characterized by microcephaly, mental retardation, beaking of the nose, and characteristic broadening of the terminal phalanges of the thumbs and first toes (Kurwa).

Histopathology.   Hypertrophic scars and keloids are indistinguishable from one another on histologic examination, since both show formation of whorls and nodules. Whereas the whorls and nodules persist in keloid, they ultimately flatten out in hypertrophic scars (Linares et al).

The difference between normal wound healing and healing with a hypertrophic scar or keloid lies not only in the length of time over which new collagen is formed but also in the arrangement of the newly formed collagen. Normal wound healing proceeds through an early inflammatory stage to a "fibroblastic" stage in which one finds granulation tissue composed of numerous capillaries, fibroblasts, and collagen fibers. The collagen fibers in the reticular dermis show a parallel, wavy orientation (Linares and Larson). Usually after

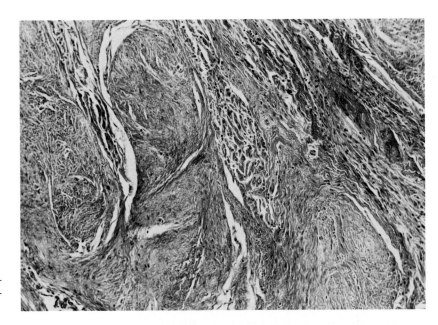

Fig. 29-6.   Keloid
Highly compacted hyalinized collagen is present in nodular formations. (×50)

5 weeks, the number of capillaries and fibroblasts has decreased, and the collagen lies as thick hyalinlike bundles in parallel arrangement (Mancini and Quaife).

In hypertrophic scars and keloids, the formation of new collagen following the inflammatory stage extends over a much longer period of time than in normally healing wounds. Even in the early period of the fibroblastic stage, one can already see that the collagen fibers in the granulation tissue are arranged in a whorllike or nodular pattern (Linares and Larson). The nodules gradually increase in size and ultimately show thick, highly compacted, hyalinized bands of collagen lying in a concentric arrangement (Fig. 29-6) (Linares et al).

Depending upon whether the nodular condensation of the collagen encroaches upon the papillary dermis, the epidermis appears either flattened or normal (Nikolowski).

In keloids, the nodular condensation of the collagen persists indefinitely; in contrast, in hypertrophic scars, the thick and hyalinized collagen bundles in the nodules gradually become thinner and straighten out, so that the orientation of the collagen bundles begins to parallel the free surface of the skin (Fig. 29-7).

Histogenesis. Myofibroblasts (see p. 601) were first observed in granulation tissue (Majno et al; Ryan et al), and it has been assumed that they aid in the gradual contraction of granulation tissue. Since early keloids contain granulation tissue, it is not surprising that many fibroblasts in them have the appearance of myofibro-

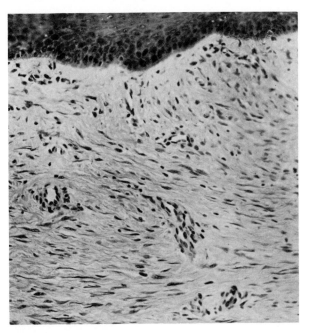

Fig. 29-7.   Hypertrophic scar
In contrast to keloid and young hypertrophic scars, in which the collagen is in a nodular arrangement, resolving hypertrophic scars show thick, hyalinized collagen bundles lying parallel to the free surface of the skin. (×200)

blasts, containing myofilaments with dense bodies (James et al). In mature keloids, only some of the fibroblasts show structural alterations toward myofibroblasts (Katenkamp and Stiller).

GIANT CELL TUMOR OF TENDON SHEATH

The giant cell tumor of tendon sheath occurs most commonly on the fingers, hands, and wrists, where it is attached to a tendon sheath. It is firm in consistency and measures from 1 cm to 3 cm in diameter. There is no tendency toward spontaneous involution. The tumor may extend to the synovium of an adjacent joint space and, on rare occasions, may even extend into the overlying skin (King et al).

Histopathology. The tumor is often lobulated, with the lobules surrounded by dense, hyalinized collagen. The cellularity within the tumor varies. In cellular areas, most cells have the appearance of histiocytes showing vesicular nuclei. Often, they contain hemosiderin or lipid. Some of the lipid-laden cells have the appearance of foam cells. Less cellular areas show fibroblasts within a fibrous or hyalinized stroma (Fort and Rodman; King et al). The characteristic giant cells, often of considerable size, are found scattered through both the cellular and fibrous areas. Their cytoplasm is deeply eosinophilic and irregularly demarcated and contains a variable number of haphazardly distributed nuclei (Carstens).

A variant of the giant cell tumor of tendon sheath is called fibroma of tendon sheath (Chung and Enzinger). The two are clinically indistinguishable from one another. Fibroma of the tendon sheath lacks lipophages and siderophages and only rarely shows a few multinucleated giant cells. It contains relatively few cellular areas that resemble those seen in a fibrous dermatofibroma as well as cell-poor areas containing only few fibroblasts embedded in a homogeneous collagenized stroma.

Histogenesis. The prevalence of fibroblasts and histiocytes is analogous to that seen in dermatofibroma (see p. 597) (Foster; King et al). However, the nature of the giant cells is not clear.

GIANT CELL EPULIS

Giant cell epulis occurs as a solitary gingival tumor in children and young adults. It grows outward and thus does not invade the bone. It is found only in the vicinity of deciduous teeth, such as the bicuspids and the anterior teeth. The lesion is benign. It usually measures from 1 cm to 2 cm in diameter, is moderately firm and dark red in color, and has a smooth surface.

Histopathology. The lesion is well circumscribed but not encapsulated. It consists of dense accumulations of fibroblasts, scattered among which are numerous large, multinucleated giant cells (Fig. 29-8). The giant cells possess ample amounts of homogeneous, eosinophilic cytoplasm and numerous irregularly arranged nuclei. Mitotic figures are absent (Sachs and Garbe).

Histogenesis. Because of the association of the giant cell epulis with deciduous teeth, it has been assumed that the giant cells within the tumor are derived from odontoclasts, which are multinucleated cells causing loosening of the deciduous teeth prior to their replacement by permanent teeth (Geschickter and Copeland).

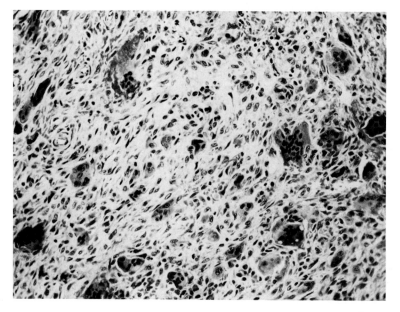

Fig. 29-8. Giant cell epulis
Numerous large, irregularly shaped, multinucleated giant cells are present. ($\times 200$)

DESMOID TUMOR

Desmoid tumors are benign fibrous neoplasms that arise from a muscular aponeurosis and tend to invade the muscle. They are firm, nontender masses. Although their rate of growth is slow, they may attain considerable size, as large as 25 cm in diameter (Gonatas). They are usually solitary but may be multiple (Goellner and Soule).

Desmoid tumors may occur in children, but they are seen mainly in young adults, particularly women. The most common type of desmoid tumor arises in women from the rectus abdominis muscle following a pregnancy. In some instances, desmoid tumors develop in scars resulting from abdominal operations. However, they may arise as extra-abdominal desmoid tumors within any skeletal muscle (Gonatas).

In addition, desmoid tumors occur in the rare, dominantly transmitted *Gardner's syndrome*. This syndrome consists of (1) intestinal polyposis, which is usually limited to the large intestine and which, in about half of the cases, results in a malignant transformation of one or several adenomatous polyps into adenocarcinoma; (2) epidermal cysts, especially on the face and scalp; (3) osteomatosis with a predilection for the membranous bones of the head; and (4) fibrous tissue tumors consisting either of well-demarcated fibromas located in the skin, the subcutaneous tissue, or the abdominal cavity or of desmoid tumors that invade adjacent muscles. The latter arise either in an abdominal scar following colectomy or spontaneously at other sites (Weary et al).

Histopathology. Desmoid tumors are composed of fibroblasts that produce abundant collagen. Although most desmoid tumors are quite cellular, at least in some areas, and show arrangement of their fibroblasts in interlacing bundles, the nuclei are regular and not particularly hyperchromatic, mitoses are infrequent, and giant cells are absent (Goellner and Soule).

Desmoid tumors show a great tendency to infiltrate adjacent striated muscle bundles. Isolated degenerating and sometimes multinucleated muscle fibers are frequently found entrapped in the tumors (Gonatas).

Histogenesis. Desmoid tumors are regarded as tumors by most authors, although some investigators believe that they represent a hyperplasia of connective tissue analogous to keloids (Gonatas). They differ from keloids, however, by their location, their invasive tendency, their potential to occur without trauma, and their histopathologic appearance.

On *electron microscopic examination*, desmoid tumors, like keloids (see p. 604), are found to contain myofibroblasts (see p. 601). Not infrequently, the majority of the fibroblasts are myofibroblasts (Stiller and Katenkamp; Goellner and Soule). This might reflect an abnormal persistence and proliferation of myofibroblasts, which

normally disappear gradually in the late stages of wound healing (Goellner and Soule).

CONGENITAL GENERALIZED FIBROMATOSIS

Congenital generalized fibromatosis is a rare entity in which nodules or masses are present at birth. There are two types: multiple fibromatosis, with involvement limited to the subcutaneous tissue, and generalized fibromatosis, with widespread involvement of the viscera as well as the musculoskeletal system and subcutaneous tissue (Roggli et al).

In infants with visceral involvement, particularly of the lungs, death may occur in the first few months of life (Roggli et al). In infants who survive, spontaneous involution of the lesions takes place, often within the first year of life (Benjamin et al, 1977).

Histopathology. In cellular areas, the subcutaneous nodules show fibroblasts with oval to spindle-shaped nuclei arranged in interlacing bundles or in a whorled pattern (Roggli et al). In less cellular areas, the stroma may appear mucoid and show capillary proliferation (Benjamin et al, 1977).

Histogenesis. Electron microscopy shows that virtually all fibroblasts are myofibroblasts (see p. 601). It may be concluded that myofibroblasts as fibrocontractile cells play a role in the shrinkage and eventual disappearance of the nodules (Benjamin et al, 1978).

FIBROUS HAMARTOMA OF INFANCY

In fibrous hamartoma of infancy, usually one and rarely two subcutaneous nodules are present at birth or develop before the end of the first year of life (Enzinger). After an initial period of growth, there is no further increase in the size of the nodule.

Histopathology. The nodule consists of rather cell-poor fibrous trabeculae, whorls of immature-appearing spindle cells in a mucoid matrix, and mature adipose tissue (Enzinger; King et al).

JUVENILE HYALIN FIBROMATOSIS

A rare, recessively inherited disorder, juvenile hyalin fibromatosis starts in early infancy with flexural contractures, innumerable skin nodules that gradually increase in size, and a hypertrophic gangiva. The largest nodes are usually seen on the scalp (Puretić et al).

Histopathology. The nodules are composed to varying degrees of cells and ground substance. Small, newly developed tumors are more cellular, whereas larger tumors contain much more ground substance (Kitano et al). The cells have elliptic nuclei and abundant, light cytoplasm containing fine, eosinophilic granules. The ground substance appears homogeneous and eosinophilic with some wavy filaments and is strongly PAS-positive and diastase-resistant, analogous to hyalin (Kitano).

Histogenesis. On *electron microscopy,* the tumor cells, analogous to fibroblasts, show a dilated rough endoplasmic reticulum in which the ground substance is apparently produced (Kitano et al).

NODULAR PSEUDOSARCOMATOUS FASCIITIS

Although nodular pseudosarcomatous fasciitis is quite common, this subcutaneous nodular lesion was not recognized as an entity until 1955 (Konwaler et al). A considerable number of publications about the lesion have appeared since then, among which are four dealing with more than 50 cases each (Price et al; Soule; Stout; Hutter et al).

The lesion is nearly always solitary. It consists of a rapidly developing subcutaneous nodule that reaches its ultimate size of 1 cm to 5 cm within a few weeks. The lesion is self-limited in duration and thus, even if it is incompletely excised, regresses, usually within a few months (Soule; Hutter et al). The longest known duration of a nodule is 26 months (Soule). Often, the lesion is slightly tender. Although the arm is the most common site, the lesion may occur in any subcutaneous area. The overlying skin is freely movable over the nodule. Although most patients are middle-aged, about 5% are infants or children (Stout).

The cause is unknown. Trauma does not seem to play a role. The general view is that nodular fasciitis represents a reactive fibroblastic and vascular proliferation.

Histopathology. The lesion is usually attached to the fascia from which it arises and extends into the subcutaneous fat in an irregular fashion. In rare instances, it infiltrates into the underlying muscle (Price et al). Also rarely, the lesion arises not from a fascia but from fibrous septa of the subcutaneous fat (Chung and Enzinger).

An outstanding feature of the lesion is the infiltrative manner of growth along several of the thin fibrous septa of the subcutaneous fat, resulting in a serrated appearance (Soule). The nodule consists of numerous large, pleomorphic fibroblasts growing haphazardly in a stroma that is often highly vascularized and contains varying amounts of mucoid ground substance, argyrophilic reticulum fibers, and collagen fibers (Fig. 29-9) (Price et al; Röckl and Schubert). The vascular component consists partially of well-formed capillaries and partially of slitlike spaces. Erythrocytes are present not only in the capillaries and slitlike spaces but also free in the tissue (Price et al). The fibroblasts show a fair number of mitoses, which, however,

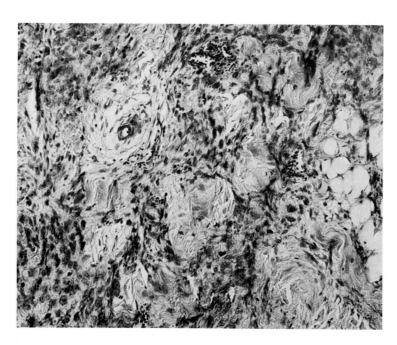

Fig. 29-9. Nodular pseudosarcomatous fasciitis
Numerous large pleomorphic fibroblasts are present. They are embedded in a mucoid ground substance on the right and are forming collagen on the left. A few fat cells of the invaded subcutaneous layer are still seen on the right. (× 200)

do not appear atypical. In about half of the cases, small, spindle-shaped giant cells are found containing two to six centrally placed nuclei (Soule). In some cases, another type of giant cell is seen that resembles ganglion cells, showing an abundant, irregularly outlined, basophilic cytoplasm with one or two large vesicular nuclei (Chung and Enzinger). Both types of giant cells represent modified fibroblasts. In some instances, degenerated muscle fibers have the appearance of multinucleated giant cells (Bernstein and Lattes). A scattered chronic inflammatory infiltrate is often present, particularly at the periphery of the nodule (Mehregan). In older lesions, the fibroblasts appear more mature, showing a more compact arrangement of spindle cells with increased production of collagen (Soule).

Histogenesis. The fibroblasts in lesions of nodular pseudosarcomatous fasciitis are found on *electron microscopy* to be myofibroblasts (see p. 601) (Wirman). It may be concluded that myofibroblasts play a role in the eventual disappearance of the lesion, as they do in recurrent infantile digital fibroma (see p. 601) and in congenital generalized fibromatosis (see p. 607).

Differential Diagnosis. Unfamiliarity with this lesion would result in a diagnosis of fibrosarcoma because of the presence of numerous large, pleomorphic fibroblasts and the infiltrative type of growth. Aside from clinical data, such as rapid growth and tenderness, the combination of fibroblastic and vascular proliferation is the most helpful diagnostic feature. Other findings suggesting the diagnosis of nodular fasciitis are the presence of a mucoid ground substance and of an inflammatory infiltrate, especially near the margin of the lesion. Since nodular fasciitis as a reactive lesion does not recur, the recurrence of a lesion originally diagnosed as such should spur a careful reappraisal of the histologic findings (Bernstein and Lattes).

Cranial Fasciitis of Childhood

Cranial fasciitis of childhood is an unusual variant of nodular pseudosarcomatous fasciitis that occurs in infants and children. One observes a rapidly growing mass in the subcutaneous tissue of the scalp that extends into the underlying cranium. No recurrence has been reported after excision of the mass with resection or curettage of the underlying bone (Lauer and Enzinger).

Histopathology. The histologic features closely resemble those of nodular pseudosarcomatous fas-

ciitis. An origin in one of the deep fascial layers of the scalp appears likely (Lauer and Enzinger).

DERMATOFIBROSARCOMA PROTUBERANS

Dermatofibrosarcoma protuberans represents a slowly growing tumor originating in the dermis. It usually begins as an indurated plaque on which multiple nodules subsequently arise. The nodules are reddish or bluish in color and firm in consistency, and, as they slowly increase in size, they may ulcerate. The trunk is the most frequent location, followed by the extremities, particularly their proximal regions; the scalp, neck, and face are only rarely involved (McPeak et al; Sauter and De Feo; Korom). Occurrence on the palms or soles has not been reported (Brenner et al). In about 10% of the cases, the tumor arises in childhood; it is rarely evident already at birth (Metz).

Although the tumor is locally invasive, it gives rise to metastases only rarely and then generally only after many years' duration. Of more than 400 cases of dermatofibrosarcoma protuberans documented in the literature up to 1978, only 27 showed metastases. There were 7 instances of metastases to regional lymph nodes and 17 instances of hematogenous metastases, largely to the lungs but occasionally to abdominal organs, the brain, or the bones. In addition, in three cases, both regional lymph node metastases and pulmonary metastases were present (Kahn et al).

Histopathology. The histologic appearance of the tumor is that of a fairly well differentiated fibrosarcoma (Mopper and Pinkus). Even though the degree of differentiation varies in different tumors and may even vary in different areas of the same tumor, the tumor is composed predominantly of cells with large, spindle-shaped nuclei embedded in varying amounts of collagen. The cells generally are arranged in irregular, intertwining bands, resulting in a storiform (matlike) pattern. In some areas, the cells radiate from a central hub of fibrous tissue in a whorllike fashion, resulting in a cartwheel pattern (Fig. 29-10) (Taylor and Helwig). Although storiform and cartwheel patterns may also be seen in the fibrous type of dermatofibroma, dermatofibrosarcoma protuberans differs from dermatofibroma by having a greater degree of cellularity, larger nuclei that show a moderate degree of atypicality, and, generally, scattered mitotic figures. In addition, the size of the tumor is significantly larger, so that it commonly penetrates deep into the subcutaneous fat. Infiltration into the underlying fascia and muscle is a late event (Taylor and Helwig). However, lateral extension of irregular strands of tumor tissue is often pronounced and frequently results in

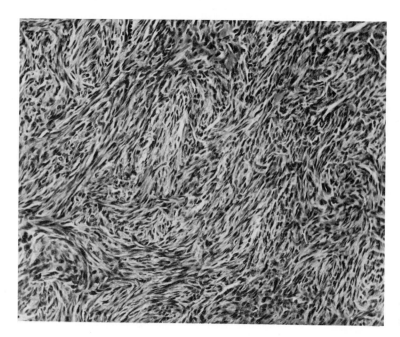

Fig. 29-10.   Dermatofibrosarcoma protuberans
The nuclei of the fibroblasts lie in irregular strands and whorls. In some areas, they form cartwheels, with the fibroblasts arranged radially about a small central hub of fibrous tissue. Some of the nuclei show a slight degree of atypicality. In contrast with the more malignant subcutaneous fibrosarcoma, formation of collagen is well in evidence. (×200)

recurrences after presumably adequate resection (Kahn et al). The epidermis may show atrophy of ulceration (Fig. 29-11). Occasionally, the epidermis is mildly hyperplastic, showing changes that resemble those often observed in dermatofibromas (Hashimoto et al).

Giant cells are either absent or present in small numbers. If present, they do not appear atypical (Vargas-Cortes, et al; Hausner et al). In some instances, lipid-laden foam cells, hemosiderin-laden macrophages, and even Touton-type giant cells are present focally in the lesion (Kahn et al).

Histogenesis. On the basis of *electron microscopic* findings, most observers regard the tumor cells as fibroblasts, since they show active synthesis of collagen in a well-developed endoplasmic reticulum (Auböck; Alguacil-Garcia et al; Zina and Bundino). A distinctive feature of the tumor cells is the cerebriform, deeply lobulated appearance of their nuclei. This is regarded as a morphologic correlate of the semimalignant nature of the tumor by some (Auböck) but not by others (Zina and Bundino). In some tumors, many cells show interrupted basement-membrane-like material along the cell membrane, suggesting that the tumor cells are modified fibroblasts possessing features of perineural and endoneural cells (Hashimoto et al). However, the presence of such interrupted basement-membrane-like material is not a constant feature (Alguacil-Garcia et al; Hausner et al; Zina and Bundino). The occasional presence of phagocytic cells (see above) can be regarded as a secondary event, as in dermatofibroma (see p. 600).

Some authors regard dermatofibrosarcoma protuberans as a histiocytic tumor, but their reasons are not very

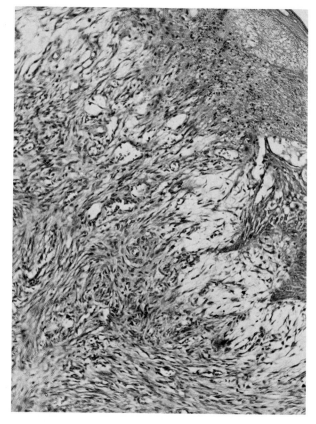

Fig. 29-11.   Dermatofibrosarcoma protuberans
The tumor nuclei show only a mild degree of atypicality. However, the tumor cells are invading and destroying the epidermis, causing ulceration. (×100)

convincing. Thus, one author concluded that dermatofibrosarcoma protuberans is a fibrous histiocytic tumor because he observed some evidence of histiocytic differentiation in the fibroblastic cells (Hausner et al). Another author observed ameboid outgrowth in explants of tumor cells obtained from dermatofibrosarcoma protuberans and regarded these outgrowths as indicative of histiocytes (Ozzello and Hamels).

ATYPICAL FIBROXANTHOMA OF THE SKIN

A fairly common lesion, atypical fibroxanthoma of the skin was first described in 1963 (Helwig). At first, it was interpreted as a benign, reactive lesion (Fretzin and Helwig; Kroe and Pitcock). However, because of the occasional occurrence of metastases in regional lymph nodes, it is now widely regarded as a neoplasm of low-grade malignancy related to malignant fibrous histiocytoma (see p. 612), which it resembles histologically (Barr et al; Enzinger). Its more favorable prognosis is the result of its small size and superficial location (Enzinger).

Originally, atypical fibroxanthoma was described as a raised, nodular lesion in a sun-exposed area of the head or neck of an elderly person. Subsequently, however, it became apparent that atypical fibroxanthoma occurs also on the trunk and extremities, usually in younger persons (Vargas-Cortes et al; Dahl). In some instances, the site at which the lesion subsequently arose had been irradiated with roentgen rays (Samitz; Jacobs et al).

In most reported cases, the nodule was of recent origin, but, in some reports, it had been present for several years (Levan et al; Vargas-Cortes et al). Some lesions are covered by normal skin, whereas others are eroded (Goette and Odom) or ulcerated (Kempson and McGavran). The size of the lesion rarely exceeds 2 cm in diameter.

Histopathology. A highly cellular dermal infiltrate extends to the epidermis or to the ulcerated surface of the lesion. It may also extend into the subcutaneous fat. The infiltrate is composed of cells with pleomorphic, often hyperchromatic nuclei in an irregular arrangement. Some cells are spindle-shaped and lie in small bundles, thus resembling fibroblasts. Other cells appear polygonal and have ample, sometimes foamy and vacuolated cytoplasm; these cells resemble histiocytes. There also are cells that are intermediate between these two types (Kemp et al; Barr et al). A striking feature in most tumors is the presence of large, bizarre, multinucleated giant cells showing marked nuclear atypicality (Fig. 29-12) (Kroe and Pitcock; Vargas-Cortes et al). Many mitoses are present, some of them atypical in appearance (Enzinger). Only small amounts of collagen are seen.

Four cases of atypical fibroxanthoma with metastasis to regional lymph nodes are on record. In the first case, vascular invasion by the tumor was noted (Fretzin and Helwig). In the second case, the tumor arose in an area of x-irradiation, recurred three times, and invaded the nasal cartilage (Jacobs et al). The third patient had chronic lymphocytic leukemia, which may have altered the immunologic status of the patient (Kemp et al). In the

Fig. 29-12. Atypical fibroxanthoma
The lesion shows a dense infiltrate of highly pleomorphic, often hyperchromatic nuclei, many of them elongated. As a characteristic feature, large, bizarre, multinucleated giant cells are present. In addition, there are mitotic figures, some of them atypical. The lesion is located in the dermis, in contrast to malignant fibrous histiocytoma, which arises in the subcutaneous layer or even deeper structures. (×200)

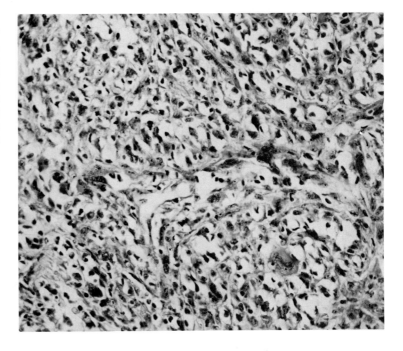

fourth patient, however, the tumor did not differ clinically or histologically from other atypical fibroxanthomas of the skin (Dahl).

Histogenesis. On *electron microscopy*, the tumor cells appear quite undifferentiated, often with only few organelles. In some cells, cisternae of the rough endoplasmic reticulum are distended and contain amorphous material as seen in fibroblasts (Alguacil-Garcia et al). Other cells show pinocytotic activity and contain membrane-bound vacuoles as seen in histiocytes (Barr et al). Lipid inclusions are seen in many cells.

For discussion of the histogenesis of atypical fibroxanthoma, see Malignant Fibrous Histiocytoma, to which atypical fibroxanthoma is related (see p. 614).

Differential Diagnosis.   In general, the diagnosis of atypical fibroxanthoma is easily made in lesions that contain the characteristic bizarre giant cells. Malignant fibrous histiocytoma differs from atypical fibroxanthoma only by its deeper location and larger size (see below).

In lesions with relatively few and not so bizarre giant cells, it may be difficult and even impossible to exclude malignant melanoma, metastatic carcinoma, and particularly spindle cell squamous cell carcinoma (Barr et al). In spindle cell squamous cell carcinoma, there are usually areas of continuity between the tumor and the overlying epidermis and occasionally also areas of keratinization (see Fig. 26-31). Also, the presence of tonofilaments and desmosomes may be demonstrated by electron microscopy (Feldman and Barr) and the presence of prekeratin by an immunoperoxidase technic (Penneys et al).

MALIGNANT FIBROUS HISTIOCYTOMA

Malignant fibrous histiocytoma, also referred to as fibroxanthosarcoma (Kempson and Kyriakos), is a pleomorphic sarcoma that probably represents the most common soft tissue sarcoma of middle and late adulthood (Weiss and Enzinger, 1978). Many tumors previously diagnosed as pleomorphic variants of liposarcoma, fibrosarcoma, or rhabdomyosarcoma are now interpreted as examples of malignant fibrous histiocytoma.

Since, aside from its volume, the tumor's depth of location affects survival, malignant fibrous histiocytoma has been subdivided into superficial and deep tumors (Kearney et al). Superficial tumors are confined to the subcutaneous tissue, although they may be attached to the fascia. Only rarely do such tumors invade the skin secondarily, resulting in ulceration (Kempson and Kyriakos). Deep tumors either lie entirely within the muscle or have extended from the subcutaneous tissue through the fascia into the muscle. Deep tumors, which are twice

as common as superficial tumors, show a poorer 4-year survival rate than superficial tumors: 40% survival versus 65%, respectively (Kearney et al). Aside from regional lymph node metastases, pulmonary metastases are frequent and are the usual cause of death.

The most common site of involvement is the thigh, including the buttock, where more than one third of all malignant fibrous histiocytomas occur (Weiss and Enzinger, 1978; Kearney et al). The other soft tissues show no significant difference in predilection, except that the hands, feet, and head are only rarely involved. The tumors are often of considerable size. Because of poor demarcation, local recurrences occur in nearly half of the cases after presumably adequate excision (Weiss and Enzinger, 1978).

Histopathology.   Malignant fibrous histiocytoma is a highly cellular tumor with a pleomorphic appearance. Some of the cells have elongated to spindle-shaped nuclei arranged in an intertwining, storiform pattern with only little cytoplasm. These cells thus appear fibroblastlike, and small amounts of collagen may be seen among them (Fig. 29-13). Other cells have a polygonal outline with irregularly shaped nuclei and ample cytoplasm that is either eosinophilic or vacuolated. Such cells appear histiocytelike, and some of them have such pronounced vacuolization as a result of lipid storage that they appear as foam cells. In addition, there are multinucleated giant cells showing bizarrely shaped, large, hyperchromatic nuclei. Mitotic figures are common, and some of them are atypical (Fu et al; Hardy et al). Some tumors show numerous foam cells and, in addition, bizarre giant cells with a foamy cytoplasm (Fig. 29-14). Such tumors have been referred to as fibroxanthosarcoma (Kempson and Kyriakos).

Several variants of malignant fibrous histiocytoma have been described: a myxoid, an inflammatory, an angiomatoid, and a giant cell variant (Kearney et al).

In the *myxoid variant*, large areas are relatively hypocellular and show widely spaced, bizarre, spindle-shaped and stellate cells in a myxoid matrix that is rich in acid mucopolysaccharides (Weiss and Enzinger, 1977; Weimar and Ceilley).

In the *inflammatory variant*, a diffuse, intense infiltrate of neutrophils is seen unassociated with tissue necrosis. In some of the inflammatory malignant fibrous histiocytomas, numerous foam cells and lipid-containing bizarre giant cells are present, as seen in fibroxanthosarcoma (Fig. 29-14) (Kyriakos and Kempson).

In the *angiomatoid variant*, large areas of hemorrhage are seen within cystlike spaces, and thin-

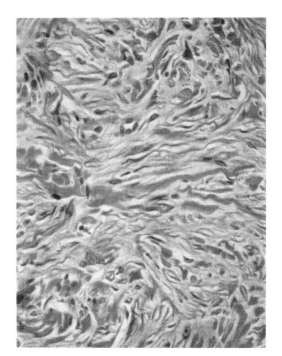

Dermatofibroma. Most of the collagen is young and stains faintly basophilic, instead of deeply eosinophilic as mature collagen does. There are numerous spindle-shaped fibroblasts. Several capillaries lined by prominent endothelial cells are present. (See p. 597.) (×175)

Kaposi's sarcoma. An area of spindle cell formation is shown. In addition to proliferations of spindle-shaped cells, there are narrow vascular slits filled with erythrocytes and areas of extravasation of erythrocytes. (See p. 639.) (×100)

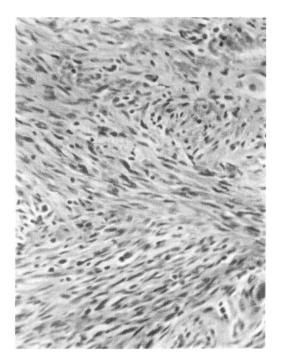

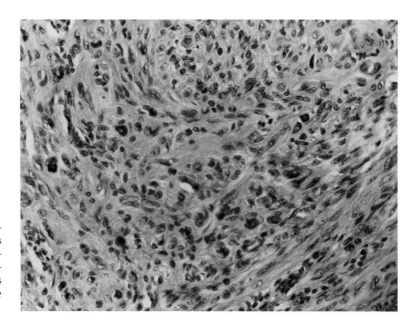

Fig. 29-13.   Malignant fibrous histiocytoma
There are some fibroblastlike cells, although the majority of cells possess irregularly shaped nuclei and ample cytoplasm and therefore appear histiocytelike. A few multinucleated giant cells showing hyperchromatic nuclei are present. (×200)

Fig. 29-14.   Malignant fibrous histiocytoma (fibroxanthosarcoma)
The tumor contains numerous foam cells and lipid-containing bizarre giant cells indicative of fibroxanthosarcoma. In addition, there is a neutrophilic infiltrate as seen in the inflammatory variant of malignant fibrous histiocytoma. (×200)

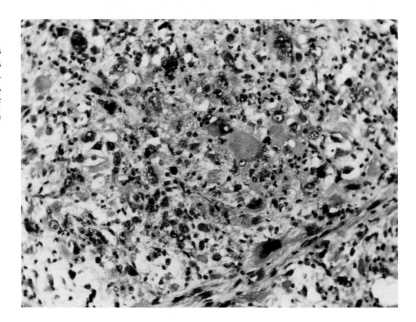

walled vascular spaces are evident nearby (Enzinger, 1979a).

In the *giant cell variant,* one observes, in addition to giant cells of the pleomorphic malignant type, osteoclastlike giant cells with abundant cytoplasm and numerous vesicular nuclei of uniform size (Angervall et al).

Histogenesis. It was originally assumed that malignant fibrous histiocytoma was composed of malignant histio-

cytes capable of acting as "facultative fibroblasts" (Soule and Enriquez; McCarthy et al). This view was based on tissue culture studies on malignant fibrous histiocytomas in which the explanted cells at first had the appearance of stellate histiocytelike cells. These cells gradually transformed into bipolar, spindle-shaped, fibroblastlike cells (Ozzello et al). However, the existence of a tissue histiocyte, the "resting wandering cell" of Maximow, has become questionable since it was established that histiocytes or macrophages are derived from circulating monocytes originating in the bone marrow (see p. 51)

(Fu et al). In contrast to the histiocytes of the bone-marrow-derived monocyte–macrophage system, the tumor cells of malignant fibrous histiocytoma do not contain lysozyme (Burgdorf et al).

Electron microscopic studies have indicated that the progenitor cell in malignant fibrous histiocytoma is not a histiocyte but an undifferentiated mesenchymal cell that is capable of differentiating in both a "histiocytic" and a fibroblastic direction (Fu et al; Taxy and Battifora). This undifferentiated cell is small and has a round nucleus and only a thin rim of cytoplasm with few organelles. The presence of small lysosomes distinguishes it from a lymphocyte, which it otherwise resembles (Fu et al). In favor of a derivation of the tumor cells from a common progenitor cell is also the presence of cells sharing some of the morphologic features of both the fibroblastlike and the histiocytelike cells (Hardy et al; Alguacil-Garcia et al).

The fibroblastlike cells in malignant fibrous histiocytoma generally are spindle-shaped and have a large, elongated nucleus. They possess a well-developed rough endoplastic reticulum with dilated cisternae. Occasional lipid droplets are seen within the cytoplasm (Fu et al; Hardy et al). The organelles of the histiocytelike cells show a more variable structure than those of the fibroblastlike cells. Generally, they have an oval to stellate shape and an irregular cell membrane forming a few pseudopodia. The nucleus often appears kidney-shaped. The ample cytoplasm usually contains extensive smooth endoplasmic reticulum and lysosomes as well as phagolysosomes and myelin figures. Varying amounts of droplets and vacuoles at the site of extracted lipid are present. Those with many lipid droplets and vacuoles correspond to foam cells (Fu et al; Hardy et al).

It is entirely possible that some of the histiocytelike cells are not tumor cells but actually are macrophages derived from circulating monocytes that have their origin in the bone marrow and have migrated into the tumor for the purpose of phagocytosis (Alguacil-Garcia et al).

It appears likely that atypical fibroxanthoma (see p. 611) has the same histogenesis as malignant fibrous histiocytoma and is also derived from an undifferentiated mesenchymal cell. Both tumors have similar histologic features. The more favorable prognosis of atypical fibroxanthoma is the result of its small size and superficial location (Enzinger, 1979b).

Differential Diagnosis. Although atypical fibroxanthoma and malignant fibrous histiocytoma are related tumors, their prognosis differs greatly, and differentiation between them is therefore very important. This usually is not difficult. Atypical fibroxanthoma is a relatively small growth originating in the dermis without a tendency toward uninhibited growth. In addition, a storiform pattern is commonly seen in malignant fibrous histiocytoma and is absent in atypical fibroxanthoma.

For differentiation of malignant fibrous histiocytoma from epithelioid sarcoma, see below; for differentiation from fibrosarcoma, see p. 616.

EPITHELIOID SARCOMA

Epithelioid sarcoma most commonly arises as a slowly growing intradermal or subcutaneous nodule on the volar surface of the fingers or on the palms, forearms, or feet (Sugarbaker et al). Less commonly, it arises as a deep-seated intramuscular tumor in the proximal regions of the extremities (Prat et al). Only rarely do cutaneous tumors occur in areas other than the extremities, such as the gluteal area (Frable et al) or the glans penis (Moore et al).

In tumors located on the distal portions of the extremities, the local recurrence rate after supposedly adequate excision is about 85% because of the insidious spreading of the tumor longitudinally along tendons, fascial planes, nerves, or blood vessels (Enzinger). The spreading often results in the appearance of multiple ulcerated nodules or annular plaques along the forearm (Saxe and Botha; Ratnam and Naik; Reymond et al). Metastases to lymph nodes may occur early, but metastases to the lungs usually are a late event (Prat et al).

Histopathology. One observes irregular nodular aggregates of tumor cells embedded in fibrous tissue (Fig. 29-15). Often, the center of the cellular aggregates shows evidence of necrosis, with palisading of tumor cells around the area of necrosis (Prat et al). Two types of tumor cells are present, both showing atypical nuclei. Cells of the first type predominate; they have a polygonal shape and abundant eosinophilic cytoplasm, thus resembling epithelioid cells. Cells of the second type appear spindle-shaped and may show an arrangement in a storiform pattern within larger nodular aggregates (Prat et al). Transitions between the two types of cells are frequently seen. Binucleate cells are very rarely seen and, if present, are neither large nor bizarre in appearance (Prat et al). An admixture of lymphocytes is frequently observed, mainly at the periphery of cellular aggregates but in some places also among tumor cells (Medenica et al).

In surgical specimens, the invasive character of the tumor is clearly evident and one frequently observes vascular and perineural invasion (Prat et al; Moore et al).

Histogenesis. It appears likely that the tumor cells are of synovial origin, since, like synovial cells, they possess an outer coat of finely granular material (Patchefsky et al; Reymond et al) and show interdigitations of cell membranes and occasional desmosomes between neighboring cells (Medenica et al).

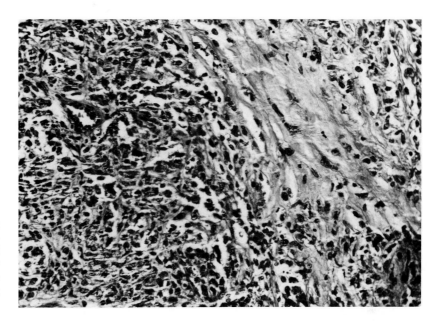

Fig. 29-15. Epithelioid sarcoma
The tumor cells lie in nodular aggregates. They have polygonal nuclei and abundant cytoplasm, thereby resembling epithelioid cells. However, the nuclei are hyperchromatic and appear atypical. (×200)

Differential Diagnosis.   At first glance, the tumor may suggest a granulomatous process because of the resemblance of most of the tumor cells to epithelioid cells and because of the presence of necrosis, fibrosis, and inflammatory cells. However, the atypical appearance of the nuclei indicates that the tumor is malignant (Enzinger).

Although epithelioid sarcoma shares with malignant fibrous histiocytoma the presence of two types of cells, one polygonal in shape and the other spindle-shaped, the absence in epithelioid sarcoma of large, bizarre multinucleated cells as well as of foam cells makes differentiation between the two possible.

FIBROSARCOMA

Fibrosarcoma used to be considered the most commonly occurring soft tissue sarcoma. However, many lesions formerly regarded as fibrosarcomas are now classified into other categories, such as malignant fibrous histiocytoma, synovial sarcoma, leiomyosarcoma, rhabdomyosarcoma, and liposarcoma (Pritchard et al).

Fibrosarcoma is a poorly circumscribed soft tissue tumor that infiltrates to varying degrees subcutaneous fat, muscle, fascia, and tendons. The skin may become tense, shiny, and red but ulcerates only very rarely (Soule and Pritchard). There is no obvious site of predilection. The tendency toward local recurrences and subsequent metastases is considerable in adults. However, aggressive local surgical technics can lead to a 5-year survival of 50% (Pritchard et al).

Fibrosarcoma may occur in infants and children and may even be present at birth (Chung and Enzinger). In children who are less than 5 years old when the tumor arises, the prognosis is fairly good, with metastases in only 8% of the cases (Chung and Enzinger); in contrast, in children 10 years old or older, the metastatic rate is 50% at a 5-year follow-up, a figure closely approximating that for adults (Soule and Pritchard).

Histopathology.   Fibrosarcoma is a spindle cell lesion in which the cells are arranged in fascicles and often in a herring-bone pattern (Fig. 29-16). Varying degrees of cellular anaplasia are present, but obvious pleomorphism is not seen, since polygonal and, in particular, giant cells are usually absent (Pritchard et al).

The degree of spindling decreases with the degree of cellular anaplasia. The anaplastic cells tend to have plump nuclei, whereas the better differentiated cells are more slender. Mitotic activity is usually more pronounced in the less differentiated lesions (Soule and Pritchard). Depending on the degree of fibroblastic differentiation, the amount of collagen production varies (Chung and Enzinger). A fine pattern of reticulum fibers around individual tumor cells is present even in the least differentiated tumors (Soule and Pritchard).

In some tumors, an indistinct storiform pattern is seen. A considerable amount of myxoid ground substance is also occasionally seen between the immature fibroblasts (Chung and Enzinger).

Differential Diagnosis.   A fairly well differentiated fibrosarcoma may resemble a dermatofibro-

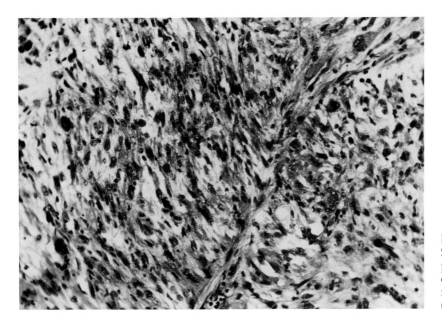

Fig. 29-16. Fibrosarcoma
Spindle-shaped tumor cells lie in parallel rows and, as seen in the center of the figure, are often arranged in a herring-bone pattern. (×200)

sarcoma protuberans (see p. 609). However, aside from having its primary location in the dermis, dermatofibrosarcoma protuberans shows a much more pronounced storiform pattern and often also cartwheel formations. Malignant fibrous histiocytoma (see p. 612), in contrast with fibrosarcoma, is a pleomorphic sarcoma showing bizarre giant cells. For a discussion of differentiation of fibrosarcoma from nodular pseudosarcomatous fasciitis, see p. 608.

FOCAL MUCINOSIS

In focal mucinosis, a solitary, asymptomatic, flesh-colored nodule is usually found on the face, trunk, or extremities. The nodule usually measures about 1 cm in diameter. Occasionally, there is some fluctuation.

Histopathology. Within a localized but not sharply circumscribed area of the dermis, the collagen is replaced to varying degrees by homogeneous mucinous material in which scattered fibroblasts are seen. The number of fibroblasts is increased in early lesions mainly in the center, whereas, in older lesions, after mucin has accumulated, the increase in fibroblasts is evident largely at the base and on the sides of the lesion (Decroix et al). Some of the fibroblasts have a stellate shape with fibrillar processes, thus having the appearance of mucoblasts. In some instances, cleftlike spaces or small cavities are present within the mucinous material

(Johnson and Helwig). The mucinous material stains pale blue with hematoxylin-eosin. It also stains with alcian blue and with colloidal iron before but not after exposure to hyaluronidase, indicating that the mucin consists largely of hyaluronic acid (Johnson and Helwig).

Differential Diagnosis. Lichen myxedematosus (papular mucinosis) differs from focal mucinosis by showing a larger number of fibroblasts, more collagen, less mucin, and no cleftlike spaces. Digital mucous cysts do not differ from focal mucinosis in their initial stage, but, at a later stage, they show a single large cavity, which does not occur in focal mucinosis.

DIGITAL MUCOUS CYST

Usually solitary lesions, digital mucous cysts occur most commonly on the dorsal aspect of the distal phalanx of a finger. Rarely, they are found on the dorsum of a toe. They consist of a small, semiglobular, translucent, slightly fluctuating nodule usually less than 1 cm in size and slightly tender. When it is punctured, a clear mucinous fluid exudes. The lesion has no tendency toward spontaneous disappearance.

Histopathology. Very early lesions have the same histologic appearance as seen in focal mucinosis, namely, an ill-defined area of mucinous material. Subsequently, multiple cleftlike spaces form and then coalesce into one large cystic space containing mucin (Fig. 29-17). The mucin stains pale blue with hematoxylin-eosin. Like the mucin in focal mucinosis, it is composed largely of hyaluronic acid and thus stains with alcian blue and colloidal iron (Johnson et al). The cystic space in early lesions is separated from the epidermis by mucinous stroma but in older lesions is found in a subepidermal location with thinning of the overlying epidermis. The collagen at the periphery of the cyst appears compressed. No lining of the cyst wall is apparent (Götz and Koch; Johnson et al; Goldman et al).

Histogenesis. Two views exist on the cause of digital mucous cysts. According to one view, the cysts result from an overproduction of hyaluronic acid by fibroblasts associated with a decrease in or absence of collagen formation (Götz and Koch; Johnson et al). Their formation would thus be analogous to that of focal mucinosis. According to the other view, the hyaluronic acid is derived from the joint fluid of the distal interphalangeal joint. The joint fluid is extruded into the tissue of the finger, where it forms a cystlike mass. This view is supported by two observations: (1) after the injection of methylene blue into the volar aspect of the distal interphalanageal joint space, the digital mucous cyst regularly contains the dye (Newmeyer et al; Goldman); and (2) on surgical exploration, a pedicle or stalk is found connecting the cyst with the distal interphalangeal joint (Kleinert et al; Goldman et al). This pedicle, in contrast to the cyst itself, shows a mesotheliumlike lining (Goldman et al).

Fig. 29-17.   Digital mucous cyst
Early stage, prior to actual cyst formation. The dermis contains much mucin. Through coalescence, the cleftlike spaces will later form a large cystic space. (×200)

MUCOUS CYST OF THE ORAL MUCOSA

Mucous cysts of the oral mucosa, also known as mucoceles, occur as solitary asymptomatic lesions, usually on the mucous surface of the lower lip and only rarely elsewhere on the oral mucosa, such as the buccal mucosa (Lattanand et al) or the tongue (Braun-Falco). The cysts usually measure less than 1 cm in diameter, appear dome-shaped, are translucent, and contain a clear, viscous fluid. The cysts may disappear spontaneously, with or without evacuating their mucous content (Nikolowski).

Mucous cysts of the oral mucosa usually are the result of a minor trauma causing rupture of a mucous duct and an outpouring of sialomucin into the tissue. Although most patients with an oral mucous cyst have no pre-existing abnormality, mucous cysts of the lower lip may occur in patients with *cheilitis glandularis*, a condition in which the labial mucous glands and ducts are hyperplastic (see p. 233) (Weir and Johnson).

Histopathology.   In early lesions, one finds multiple small spaces filled with sialomucin and surrounded by or intermixed with granulation tissue. Older lesions show either a solitary large cystic space or several large spaces lined by a thick layer of granulation tissue composed of neutrophils, lymphocytes, fibroblasts, macrophages, and capillaries (Fig. 29-18) (Braun-Falco; Ehlers; Lattanand et al). The macrophages contain prominent vacuoles representing phagocytized sialomucin (Braun-Falco). The wall of some cysts shows a ruptured

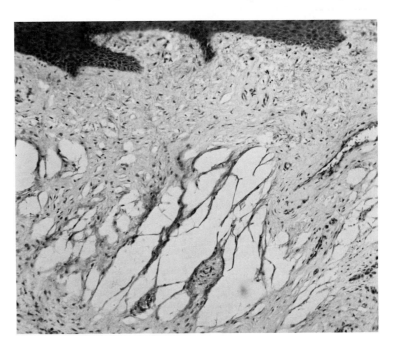

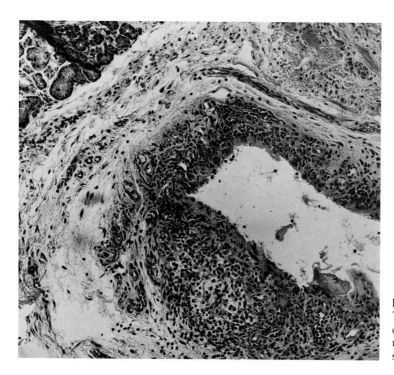

Fig. 29-18.   Mucous cyst of oral mucosa
The cyst is a result of the rupture of a salivary duct. It possesses a wall composed of granulation tissue. Parts of a salivary gland are seen in the upper left corner. (×100)

salivary duct opening into the cavity (Lattanand et al).

The sialomucin within the cysts appears as amorphous, slightly eosinophilic material in routinely stained sections. It is PAS-positive and diastase-resistant. It also stains with alcian blue and colloidal iron, both of which are hyaluronidase-resistant (Lattanand et al). Thus, sialomucin as an epithelial mucin contains both nonsulfated acid mucopolysaccharides and neutral mucopolysaccharides, the latter a glycoprotein (Nikolowski; Lattanand et al). (For a discussion of the presence of sialomucin in the skin, see also the sections on extramammary Paget's disease, p. 513, and cutaneous metastasis of carcinoma of the gastrointestinal tract, p. 593.)

MYXOSARCOMA

Tumors with the histologic appearance of a myxosarcoma arise only very rarely in the skin (Kopf and Bart) or in the subcutaneous tissue or fascia (Stout; Korting and Nürnberger). Although metastases are rare (Stout), they may occur (Kopf and Bart).

Histopathology.   Myxosarcomas show fairly numerous nuclei, some of them stellate in shape, embedded in a mucinous stroma. Many of these nuclei appear atypical (Sponsel et al), and even atypical multinucleated giant cells may be present (Korting and Nürnberger).

Before making a diagnosis of myxosarcoma, it is important to rule out sarcomas of various types in which a mucinous transformation of the stroma has taken place. This may occur in fibrosarcomas, malignant fibrous histiocytomas, extraskeletal chondrosarcomas, and, especially, liposarcomas (Weiss and Enzinger; Enterline et al). Since mucinous transformation occurs, as a rule, in only parts of the tumor, histologic examination of other parts of the tumor usually establishes the dominant tissue. In mucin-containing tumors in which a diagnosis of liposarcoma is being considered, fat stains are indicated; if significant amounts of fat are present, the tumor should be referred to as myxoid liposarcoma (Enterline et al). However, in some instances, myxosarcomas also contain some intracellular lipid as a result of necrobiotic changes (Korting and Nürnberger).

Histogenesis.   Since it is the function of the fibroblast to produce mucinous ground substance in addition to collagenous and elastic fibers, it appears likely that most myxosarcomas are basically fibrosarcomas (see p. 615).

BIBLIOGRAPHY

Dermatofibroma

ARNOLD HL JR, TILDEN IL: Histiocytoma cutis: A variant of xanthoma. Arch Dermatol Syph 47:498–516, 1943

AUBÖCK L: Zur Ultrastruktur fibröser und histiocytärer Haut-tumoren. Virchows Arch A (Pathol Anat) 368:253–274, 1975

BANDMANN HJ: Ein Beitrag zur morphologischen Pathologie des Dermatofibroma lenticulare bzw. des Histiocytoms. Arch Klin Exp Dermatol 204:584–603, 1957

BEDI TR, PANDHI RK, BHUTANI LK: Multiple palmoplantar histiocytomas. Arch Dermatol 112:1001–1003, 1976

BRYANT J: Basal cell carcinoma overlying longstanding dermatofibromas. Arch Dermatol 113:1445–1446, 1977

BURGDORF W, MORELAND A, WASIK R: Negative immunoperoxidase staining for lysozyme in nodular subepidermal fibrosis. Arch Dermatol 118:241–243, 1982

BUSELMEIER TJ, UECKER JH: Invasive basal cell carcinoma with metaplastic bone formation associated with a long-standing dermatofibroma. J Cutan Pathol 6:496–500, 1979

CARRINGTON SG, WINKELMANN RK: Electron microscopy of histiocytic diseases of the skin. Acta Derm Venereol (Stockh) 52:161–178, 1972

CARSTENS PHB, SCHRODT GR: Ultrastructure of sclerosing hemangioma. Am J Pathol 77:377–386, 1974

CRAMER HJ: Zur Histologie und Histochemie des xanthomatösen Histiocytoms. Arch Klin Exp Dermatol 232:138–147, 1968

CRAMER R, CRAMER HJ: Über die pseudobasaliomatöse Epithelhyperplasie der Haut. Arch Klin Exp Dermatol 216:231–245, 1963

FRENK E: Zur Histologie der Fibrome und Histiocytome der Haut. Hautarzt 12:15–19, 1961

GOETTE DK, HELWIG EB: Basal cell carcinomas and basal cell carcinoma-like changes overlying dermatofibroma. Arch Dermatol 111:589–591, 1975

GROSS RE, WOLBACH SB: Sclerosing hemangiomas: Their relationship to dermatofibroma, histiocytoma, xanthoma and to certain pigmented lesions of the skin, Am J Pathol 19:533–551, 1943

HAIRSTON MA JR, REED RJ: Aneurysmal sclerosing hemangioma of skin. Arch Dermatol 93:439–442, 1966

KATENKAMP D, STILLER D: Cellular composition of the so-called dermatofibroma (histiocytoma cutis). Virchows Archiv (Pathol Anat) 367:325–336, 1975

KLAUS SN, WINKELMANN RK: The enzyme histochemistry of nodular subepidermal fibrosis. Br J Dermatol 78:398–402, 1966

MIHATSCH-KONZ B, SCHAUMBURG-LEVER G, LEVER WF: Ultrastructure of dermatofibroma. Arch Dermatol Forsch 246:181–192, 1973

NIEMI KM: The benign fibrohistiocytic tumours of the skin. (Review) Acta Derm Venereol (Stockh) 50, Suppl 63:1–66, 1970

PINKUS H: Pathobiology of the pilary complex. Jpn J Dermatol (Series B) 77:304–330, 1967

RENTIERS PL, MONTGOMERY H: Nodular subepidermal fibrosis (dermatofibroma versus histiocytoma). Arch Dermatol Syph 59:568–583, 1949

SANTA CRUZ DJ, KYRIAKOS M: Aneurysmal ("angiomatoid") fibrous histiocytoma of the skin. Cancer 47:2053–2061, 1981

SCHOENFELD RJ: Epidermal proliferations overlying histiocytomas. Arch Dermatol 90:266–270, 1964

SENEAR FE, CARO MR: Histiocytoma cutis. Arch Dermatol Syph 33:209–226, 1936

STEIGLEDER GK, NICKLAS H, KAMEI Y: Die Epithelveränderungen beim Histiocytom, ihre Genese und ihr Erscheinungsbild. Dermatol Wochenschr 146:457–468, 1962

THIES W, HENNIES T: Über die Assoziation eines Histiocytoms mit einem Basaliom. Hautarzt 19:163–167, 1968

UNNA PG: Histopathologie der Hautkrankheiten, pp 839–842. Berlin, August Hirschwald, 1894

VILANOVA JR, FLINT A: The morphological variations of fibrous histiocytoma. J Cutan Pathol 1:155–164, 1974

WORINGER F, KVIATKOWSKI S: L'histiocytome de la peau. Ann Dermatol Syph 3:998–1010, 1932

Soft Fibroma

CRAMER HJ: Histochemische Untersuchungen mit dem sauren Hämateintest nach Baker an pathologisch veränderter Haut. Arch Klin Exp Dermatol 228:438–444, 1967

FIELD LM: A giant pendulous fibrolipoma. J Dermatol Surg Oncol 8:54–55, 1982

FLEGEL H, TESSMANN K: Gibt es ein weiches Fibrom der Haut? Hautarzt 18:251–256, 1967

STEGMAIER OC: Natural regression of the melanocytic nevus. J Invest Dermatol 32:413–419, 1959

Recurrent Infantile Digital Fibroma

BHAWAN J, BACCHETTA C, JORIS I et al: A myofibroblastic tumor. Infantile digital fibroma. Am J Pathol 94:19–36, 1979

GEBHART W, JASCHKE E, REICHEL K: Rezidivierende Digitalfibrome im Kindesalter. II. Mitteilung: Ultrastruktur. Z Hautkr 51:109–116, 1976

IWASAKI H, KIKUCHI M, MORI R et al: Infantile digital fibromatosis. Cancer 46:2238–2247, 1980

MAJNO G, GABBIANI G, HIRSCHEL BJ et al: Contraction of granulation tissue in vitro: Similarity to smooth muscle. Science 173:548–550, 1971

MEHREGAN AH, NABAI H, MATTHEWS JE: Recurring digital fibrous tumor of childhood. Arch Dermatol 106:375–378, 1972

RYAN GB, CLIFF WJ, GABBIANI G et al: Myofibroblasts in human granulation tissue. Hum Pathol 5:55–67, 1974

SANTA CRUZ DJ, REINER CB: Recurrent digital fibroma of childhood. J Cutan Pathol 5:339–346, 1978

SHAPIRO L: Infantile digital fibromatosis and aponeurotic fibroma. Arch Dermatol 99:37–42, 1969

Acquired Digital Fibrokeratoma

BART RS, ANDRADE R, KOPF AW et al: Acquired digital fibrokeratomas. Arch Dermatol 97:120–129, 1968

HARE PJ, SMITH PAJ: Acquired (digital) fibrokeratoma. Br J Dermatol 81:667–670, 1969

VERALLO VVM: Acquired digital fibrokeratomas. Br J Dermatol 80:730–736, 1968

Multiple Perifollicular Fibromas

BELAICH S, CIVATTE J, BONVALET D et al: Fibromes perifolliculaires multiples du visage et du cou posant le problème des adénomas sébacés symétriques blancs et fibreux. Ann Dermatol Venereol 105:959–960, 1978

BIRT AR, HOGG GR, DUBÉ J: Hereditary multiple fibrofolliculomas with trichodiscomas and acrochordons. Arch Dermatol 113:1674–1677, 1977

HORNSTEIN OP, KNICKENBERG M: Perifollicular fibromatosis cutis with polyps of the colon. Arch Dermatol Res 253:161–175, 1975

PINKUS H, COSKEY R, BURGESS GH: Trichodiscoma. A benign tumor related to the *Haarscheibe* (hair disk). J Invest Dermatol 63:212–218, 1974

VAKILZADEH, F, MANEGOLD HG: Perifolliküläre Fibrome. Z Hautkr 51:1039–1041, 1976

ZACKHEIM HS, PINKUS H: Perifollicular fibromas. Arch Dermatol 82:913–917, 1960

Fibrous Papule of the Face (Nose)

ALTMEYER P: Die fibrösen Nasenpapeln, eine klinische und histologische Entität? Hautarzt 28:416–420, 1977

GRAHAM JH, SANDERS JB, JOHNSON WC et al: Fibrous papule of the nose. J Invest Dermatol 45:194–203, 1965

MCGIBBON DH, WILSON JONES E: Fibrous papule of the face (nose). Fibrosing nevocytic nevus. Am J Dermatopathol 1:345–348, 1979

MEIGEL WN, ACKERMAN AB: Fibrous papule of face. Am J Dermatopathol 1:329–340, 1979

PINKUS H: Perifollicular fibromas. Pure periadnexal adventitial tumors. Am J Dermatopathol 1:341–342, 1979

RAGAZ A, BEREZOWSKY V: Fibrous papule of the face. A study of five cases by electron microscopy. Am J Dermatopathol 1:353–355, 1979

REED RJ: Fibrous papule of the face. Melanocytic angiofibroma. Am J Dermatopathol 1:343–344, 1979

REED RJ, HAIRSTON MA, PALOMEQUE FE: The histologic identity of adenoma sebaceum and solitary melanocytic angiofibroma. Dermatol Int 5:3–11, 1966

SANTA CRUZ DJ, PRIOLEAU PG: Fibrous papule of the face. An electron-microscopic study of two cases. Am J Dermatopathol 1:349–352, 1979

SAYLAN T, MARKS R, WILSON JONES E: Fibrous papule of the nose. Br J Dermatol 85:111–118, 1971

ZACKHEIM HS, PINKUS H: Perifollicular fibromas. Arch Dermatol 82:913–917, 1960

Tuberous Sclerosis

BURKHART CG, EL-SHAAR A: Computerized axial tomography in the early diagnosis of tuberous sclerosis. J Am Acad Dermatol 4:59–63, 1981

CHONCO AM, WEISS SM, STEIN JH et al: Renal involvement in tuberous sclerosis. Am J Med 56:124–132, 1974

FITZPATRICK TB, SZABO G, HORI Y et al: White leaf-shaped macules. Arch Dermatol 98:1–6, 1968

KOBAYASI T, WOLF-JÜRGENSEN P, DANIELSEN L: Ultrastructure of shagreen patch. Acta Derm Venereol (Stockh) 53:275–278, 1973

MORALES JB: Congenital rhabdomyoma, tuberous sclerosis, and splenic histiocytosis. Arch Pathol 71:485–493, 1961

NICKEL WR, REED WB: Tuberous sclerosis. (Review of cutaneous lesions) Arch Dermatol 85:209–226, 1962

PRICE EB JR, MOSTOFI FK: Symptomatic angiomyolipoma of the kidney. Cancer 18:761–767, 1965

REED WB, NICKEL WR, CAMPION G: Internal manifestations of tuberous sclerosis. (Review) Arch Dermatol 87:715–728, 1963

SCHEIG RL, BORNSTEIN P: Tuberous sclerosis in the adult. Arch Intern Med 108:789–795, 1961

TILGEN W: Zur Ultrastruktur der sogenannten White leaf-shaped macules bei der tuberösen Hirnsklerose Bourneville-Pringle. Arch Dermatol Forsch 248:13–27, 1973

Hypertrophic Scar and Keloid

JAMES WD, BESANCENEY CD, ODOM RB: The ultrastructure of a keloid. J Am Acad Dermatol 3:50–57, 1980

KATENKAMP D, STILLER D: Untersuchungen zur Ultrastruktur des Keloids. Zentralbl Allg Pathol 122:312–324, 1978

KURWA AR: Rubinstein-Taybi syndrome and spontaneous keloid. Clin Exp Dermatol 4:251–254, 1978

LINARES HA, KISCHER CW, DOBRKOVSKY M et al: The histiotypic organization of the hypertrophic scar in humans. J Invest Dermatol 59:323–331, 1972

LINARES HA, LARSON DL: Early differential diagnosis between hypertrophic and nonhypertrophic healing. J Invest Dermatol 62:514–516, 1974

MAJNO G, GABBIANI G, HIRSCHEL BJ et al: Contraction of granulation tissue in vitro: Similarity to smooth muscle. Science 1973:548–550, 1971

MANCINI RE, QUAIFE JV: Histogenesis of experimentally produced keloids. J Invest Dermatol 38:143–181, 1962

MURRAY JC, POLLACK SV, PINNEL SR: Keloids: A review. J Am Acad Dermatol 4:461–470, 1981

NIKOLOWSKI W: Pathogenese, Klink und Therapie des Keloids. Arch Klin Exp Dermatol 212:550–569, 1961

ONWUKWE MF: Classification of keloids. J Dermatol Surg Oncol 4:534–536, 1978

RYAN GB, CLIFF WJ, GABBIANI G et al: Myofibroblasts in human granulation tissue. Hum Pathol 5:55–67, 1974

Giant Cell Tumor of Tendon Sheath

CARSTENS PHB: Giant cell tumors of tendon sheath. Arch Pathol 102:99–103, 1978

CHUNG EB, ENZINGER FM: Fibroma of tendon sheath. Cancer 44:1945–1954, 1979

FORT SL, RODMAN OG: Erythema elevatum diutinum. Arch Dermatol 113:819–825, 1977

FOSTER LN: The benign giant cell tumor of tendon sheaths. An example of sclerosing hemangioma. Am J Pathol 23:567–584, 1947

KING DT, MILLMAN AJ, GUREVITCH AW et al: Giant cell tumor of the tendon sheath involving the skin. Arch Dermatol 114:944–946, 1978

Giant Cell Epulis

GESCHICKTER CF, COPELAND MM: Tumors of bone, 2nd ed. New York, Am J Cancer, 1936

SACHS W, GARBE W: Multinucleated (giant) cell tumor of the gum (epulis). Arch Dermatol Syph 38:603–614, 1938

Desmoid Tumor

GOELLNER JR, SOULE EH: Desmoid tumors. An ultrastructural study of eight cases. Hum Pathol 11:43–50, 1980

GONATAS NK: Extra-abdominal desmoid tumors. Arch Pathol 71:214–221, 1961

STILLER D, KATENKAMP D: Cellular features in desmoid fibromatosis and well differentiated fibrosarcomas: An electron microscopic study. Virchows Arch (Pathol Anat) 369:155–164, 1975

WEARY PE, LINTHICUM A, CAWLEY EP et al: Gardner's syndrome. Arch Dermatol 90:20–30, 1964

Congenital Generalized Fibromatosis

BENJAMIN SP, MERCER RD, HAWK WA: Myofibroblastic contraction in spontaneous regression of multiple congenital mesenchymal hamartomas. Cancer 40:2343–2352, 1977

BENJAMIN SP, MERCER RD, HAWK WA et al: Multiple congenital myofibroblastic hamartomas (congenital generalized fibromatosis) of infancy. (Abstr) Arch Dermatol 114:1833, 1978

ROGGLI VL, KIM HS, HAWKINS E: Congenital generalized fibromatosis with visceral involvement. Cancer 45:954–960, 1980

Fibrous Hamartoma of Infancy

ENZINGER F: Fibrous hamartoma of infancy. Cancer 18:241–248, 1965

KING DF, BARR RJ, HIROSE FM: Fibrous hamartoma of infancy. J Dermatol Surg Oncol 5:482–483, 1979

Juvenile Hyalin Fibromatosis

KITANO Y: Juvenile hyalin fibromatosis. Arch Dermatol 112:86–88, 1976

KITANO Y, HORIKI M, AOKI T et al: Two cases of juvenile hyalin fibromatosis. Arch Dermatol 106:877–883, 1972

PURETIĆ S, PURETIĆ B, FISER-HERMAN M et al: A unique form of mesenchymal dysplasia. Br J Dermatol 74:8–19, 1962

Nodular Pseudosarcomatous Fasciitis

BERNSTEIN KE, LATTES R: Nodular (pseudosarcomatous) fasciitis, a nonrecurrent lesion. Cancer 49:1668–1678, 1982

CHUNG EB, ENZINGER FM: Proliferative fasciitis. Cancer 36:1450–1458, 1975

HUTTER RVP, STEWART FW, FOOTE FW JR: Fasciitis. Cancer 15:992–1003, 1962

LAUER DH, ENZINGER FM: Cranial fasciitis of childhood. Cancer 45:401–406, 1980

KONWALER BE, KEASBEY L, KAPLAN L: Subcutaneous pseudosarcomatous fibromatosis (fasciitis). Am J Clin Pathol 25:241–252, 1955

MEHREGAN AH: Nodular fasciitis. Arch Dermatol 93:204–210, 1966

PRICE EB JR, SILIPHANT WM, SHUMAN R: Nodular fasciitis, a clinico-pathologic analysis of 65 cases. Am J Clin Pathol 35:122–136, 1961

RÖCKL H, SCHUBERT E: Fasciitis nodularis pseudosarcomatosa. Hautarzt 22:150–153, 1971

SOULE EH: Proliferative (nodular) fasciitis. Arch Pathol 73:437–444, 1962

STOUT AP: Pseudosarcomatous fasciitis in children. Cancer 14:1216–1222, 1961

WIRMAN JA: Nodular fasciitis, a lesion of myofibroblasts. Cancer 38:2378–2389, 1976

Dermatofibrosarcoma Protuberans

ALGUACIL-GARCIA A, UNNI KH, GOELLNER JR: Histogenesis of dermatofibrosarcoma protuberans. An ultrastructural study. Am J Clin Pathol 69:427–434, 1978

AUBÖCK L: Zur Ultrastruktur fibröser und histiocytärer Hauttumoren (Dermatofibrom, Dermatofibrosarcoma protuberans, Fibroxanthom und Histiocytom). Virchows Archiv (Pathol Ant) 368:253–274, 1975

BRENNER V, SCHAEFLER K, CHABRA H et al: Dermatofibrosarcoma protuberans metastatic to regional lymph nodes. Cancer 36:1897–1902, 1975

HASHIMOTO K, BROWNSTEIN MH, JACOBIEC FA: Dermatofibrosarcoma protuberans. Arch Dermatol 110:874–885, 1974

HAUSNER RJ, VARGAS-CORTES F, ALEXANDER RW: Dermatofibrosarcoma protuberans with lymph node involvement. Arch Dermatol 114:88–91, 1978

KAHN LB, SAXE N, GORDON W: Dermatofibrosarcoma protuberans with lymph node and pulmonary metastases. Arch Dermatol 114:599–601, 1978

KOROM I: Seit 20 Jahren bestehendes Dermatofibrosarcoma protuberans. Z Hautkr 51:583–586, 1976

MCPEAK CJ, CRUZ T, NICASTRI AD: Dermatofibrosarcoma protuberans: An analysis of 86 cases—5 with metastasis. Ann Surg 166 (Suppl 2):803, 1967

METZ G: Dermatofibrosarcoma protuberans im Kindesalter. Hautarzt 29:435–438, 1978

MOPPER C, PINKUS H: Dermatofibrosarcoma protuberans. Am J Clin Pathol 20:171–176, 1950

OZZELLO L, HAMELS J: The histiocytic nature of dermatofibrosarcoma protuberans. Am J Clin Pathol 65:136–148, 1976

SAUTER LS, DE FEO CP: Dermatofibrosarcoma protuberans of the face. Arch Dermatol 104:671–673, 1971

TAYLOR HB, HELWIG EB: Dermatofibrosarcoma protuberans. Cancer 15:717–725, 1961

VARGAS-CORTES F, WINKELMANN RK, SOULE EH: Atypical fibroxanthomas of the skin. Mayo Clin Proc 48:211–218, 1973

ZINA AM, BUNDINO S: Dermatofibrosarcoma protuberans. An ultrastructural study of five cases. J Cutan Pathol 6:265–271, 1979

Atypical Fibroxanthoma of the Skin

ALGUACIL-GARCIA A, UNNI KK, GOELLNER JR et al: Atypical fibroxanthoma of the skin. An ultrastructural study of two cases. Cancer 40:1471–1480, 1977

BARR RJ, WUERKER RB, GRAHAM JH: Ultrastructure of atypical fibroxanthoma. Cancer 40:736–743, 1977

DAHL I: Atypical fibroxanthoma of the skin. Acta Pathol Microbiol Scand (A), 84:183–197, 1976

ENZINGER FM: Atypical fibroxanthoma and malignant fibrous histiocytoma. Am J Dermatopathol 1:185, 1979

FELDMAN PS, BARR RJ: Ultrastructure of spindle cell squamous cell carcinoma. J Cutan Pathol 3:17–24, 1976

FRETZIN DFJ, HELWIG EB: Atypical fibroxanthoma of the skin. Cancer 31:1541–1552, 1973

GOETTE DK, ODOM RB: Atypical fibroxanthoma masquerading as pyogenic granuloma. Arch Dermatol 112:1155–1157, 1976

HELWIG EB: Atypical fibroxanthoma. Tex State J Med 59:664–667, 1963

JACOBS DS, EDWARDS WD, YE RC: Metastatic atypical fibroxanthoma of skin. Cancer 35:457–463, 1975

KEMP JD, STENN KS, ARONS M et al: Metastasizing atypical fibroxanthoma. Arch Dermatol 114:1533–1535, 1978

KEMPSON RL, MCGAVRAN MH: Atypical fibroxanthomas of the skin. Cancer 17:1463–1471, 1964

KROE OJ, PITCOCK JA: Atypical fibroxanthoma of the skin. Am J Clin Pathol 51:487–492, 1969

LEVAN NE, HIRSCH P, KWONG MQ: Pseudosarcomatous dermatofibroma. Arch Dermatol 88:908–912, 1963

PENNEYS NS, NADJI M, ZIEGELS-WEISSMAN J et al: Prekeratin in spindle cell tumors of the skin. Arch Dermatol, in press

SAMITZ MH: Pseudosarcoma. Arch Dermatol 96:283–285, 1967

VARGAS-CORTES F, WINKELMANN RK, SOULE EH: Atypical fibroxanthoma of the skin. Mayo Clin Proc 48:211–218, 1973

Malignant Fibrous Histiocytoma

ALGUACIL-GARCIA A, UNNI KK, GOELLNER JR: Malignant fibrous histiocytoma. Am J Clin Pathol 69:121–129, 1978

ANGERVALL L, HAGMAR B, KINDBLOM LG et al: Malignant giant cell tumor of soft tissue. Cancer 47:736–747, 1981

BURGDORF WHC, DURAY P, ROSAI J: Immunohistochemical identification of lysozyme in cutaneous lesions of alleged histiocytic nature. Am J Clin Pathol 75:162–167, 1981

ENZINGER FM: Angiomatoid malignant fibrous histiocytoma. Cancer 44:2147–2157, 1979a

ENZINGER FM: Atypical fibroxanthoma and malignant fibrous histiocytoma. Am J Dermatopathol 1:185, 1979b

FU YS, GABBIANI G, KAYE GI et al: Malignant soft tissue tumors of probable histiocytic origin (malignant fibrous histiocytoma). Cancer 35:176–198, 1975

HARDY TJ, AN T, BROWN PW et al: Postirradiation sarcoma (malignant fibrous histiocytoma) of axilla. Cancer 42:118–124, 1978

KEARNEY MM, SOULE EH, IVINS JC: Malignant fibrous histiocytoma. Cancer 45:167–178, 1980

KEMPSON RL, KYRIAKOS M: Fibroxanthosarcoma of the soft tissues. A type of malignant fibrous histiocytoma. Cancer 29:961–976, 1972

KYRIAKOS M, KEMPSON RL: Inflammatory fibrous histiocytoma. Cancer 37:1584–1606, 1976

MCCARTHY EF, MATSUNO T, DORFMAN HD: Malignant fibrous histiocytoma of bone. Hum Pathol 10:57–70, 1979

OZZELLO, L, STOUT AP, MURRAY MR: Cultural characteristics of malignant histiocytomas and fibrous xanthomas. Cancer 16:331–344, 1963

SOULE EH, ENRIQUEZ P: Atypical fibrous histiocytoma, malignant fibrous histiocytoma, malignant histiocytoma, and epithelioid sarcoma. A comparative study of 65 tumors. Cancer 30:128–143, 1972

TAXY JB, BATTIFORA H: Malignant fibrous histiocytoma. Cancer 40:254–267, 1977

WEIMAR VM, CEILLEY RI: A myxoid variant of malignant fibrous histiocytoma. J Dermatol Surg Oncol 5:16–18, 1979

WEISS SW, ENZINGER FM: Myxoid variant of malignant fibrous histiocytoma. Cancer 39:1672–1685, 1977

WEISS SW, ENZINGER RM: Malignant fibrous histiocytoma. Cancer 41:2250–2266, 1978

Epithelioid Sarcoma

ENZINGER FM: Epithelioid sarcoma. A sarcoma simulating a granuloma or a carcinoma. Cancer 26:1029–1041, 1970

FRABLE WJ, KAY S, LAWRENCE W et al: Epithelioid sarcoma. Arch Pathol 95:8–12, 1973

MEDENICA M, CASAS C, LORINCZ AL et al: Epithelioid sarcoma. Acta Derm Venereol (Stockh) 59:333–339, 1979

MOORE SW, WHEELER JE, HEFTER LG: Epithelioid sarcoma masquerading as Peyronie's disease. Cancer 35:1706–1710, 1975

PATCHEFSKY AS, SORIANO R, KOSTIANOVSKY M: Epithelioid sarcoma. Cancer 39:143–152, 1977

PRAT J, WOODRUFF JM, MARCOVE RC: Epithelioid sarcoma. Cancer 41:1472–1487, 1978

RATNAM AV, NAIK KG: Epithelioid sarcoma, a case report. Br J Dermatol 99:451–453, 1978

REYMOND JL, STOEBNER P, AMBLARD P et al: Sarcome épithélioide. Ann Dermatol Venereol 106:1013–1018, 1979

SAXE N, BOTHA JBC: Epithelioid sarcoma. Arch Dermatol 113:1106–1108, 1977

SUGARBAKER PH, AUDA S, WEBBER BL et al: Early distant metastases from epithelioid sarcoma of the hand. Cancer 48:852–855, 1981

Fibrosarcoma

CHUNG EB, ENZINGER FM: Infantile fibrosarcoma. Cancer 38:729–739, 1976

PRITCHARD DJ, SOULE EH, TAYLOR WF et al: Fibrosarcoma, a clinicopathologic and statistical study of 199 tumors of the soft tissues of the extremities and trunk. Cancer 33:888–897, 1974

SOULE EH, PRITCHARD DJ: Fibrosarcoma in infants and children. A review of 110 cases. Cancer 40:1711–1721, 1977

Focal Mucinosis

DECROIX J, GUILMOT-BRUNEAU MM, DEFRESNE C: Myxome cutané ou mucinose focale cutanée. Dermatologica 162:368–371, 1981

JOHNSON WC, HELWIG EB: Cutaneous focal mucinosis. Arch Dermatol 93:13–20, 1966

Digital Mucous Cyst

GOLDMAN JA, GOLDMAN L, JAFFE MS et al: Digital mucinous pseudocysts. Arthr Rheum 20:997–1002, 1977

GÖTZ H, KOCH R: Zur Klinik, Pathogenese und Therapie der sogenannten "Dorsalcysten." Hautarzt 7:533–537, 1956

JOHNSON WC, GRAHAM JH, HELWIG EB: Cutaneous myxoid cyst. JAMA 191:15–20, 1965

KLEINERT HE, KUTZ JE, FISHMAN JH et al: Etiology and treatment of the so-called mucous cyst of the finger. J Bone Joint Surg (Am) 54:1455–1458, 1972

NEWMEYER WL, KILGORE ES JR, GRAHAM WP III: Mucous cysts: The dorsal distal interphalangeal joint ganglion. Plast Reconstr Surg 53:313–315, 1974

Mucous Cyst of the Oral Mucosa

BRAUN-FALCO O: Über ein Schleimgranulom der Zunge. Hautarzt 11:131–133, 1960

EHLERS G: Zur Histogenese der Lippenschleimcysten. Z Hautkr 34:77–92, 1963

LATTANAND A, JOHNSON WC, GRAHAM JH: Mucous cyst (mucocele). Arch Dermatol 101:673–678, 1970

NIKOLOWSKI W: Schleimcysten und sogenanntes Schleimgranulom der Unterlippe. Arch Klin Exp Dermatol 203:246–255, 1956

WEIR TW, JOHNSON WC: Cheilitis glandularis. Arch Dermatol 103:433–437, 1971

Myxosarcoma

ENTERLINE HT, CULBERSON JD, ROCHLIN DB et al: Liposarcoma. Cancer 13:932–950, 1960

KOPF AW, BART RS: Tumor on shoulder arising after excision of a cyst: J Dermatol Surg 2:196–198, 1976

KORTING GW, NÜRNBERGER F: Zur Frage des Lipidgehaltes von Myxosarkomen. Arch Klin Exp Dermatol 230:172–182, 1967

SPONSEL KH, MCDONALD JR, GHORMLEY RK: Myxoma and myxosarcoma of the soft tissues of the extremities. J Bone Joint Surg (Am) 34:820–826, 1952

STOUT AP: Myxoma, the tumor of primitive mesenchyme. Ann Surg 127:706–719, 1948

WEISS SW, ENZINGER FM: Myxoid variant of malignant fibrous histiocytoma. Cancer 39:1672–1685, 1977

Tumors of Vascular Tissue

30

CONGENITAL HEMANGIOMAS

Three types of congenital hemangioma are recognized, aside from angiokeratoma circumscriptum, which will be discussed with the other types of angiokeratoma (see p. 626). The three types of congenital hemangioma are nevus flammeus, capillary hemangioma, and cavernous hemangioma.

Nevus Flammeus

Nevus flammeus, or nevus telangiectaticus, the so-called port-wine nevus, is present at birth. It is characterized by one or several dull red or bluish red patches of irregular outline not elevated above the level of the skin. Two types occur. The *medially located nevus flammeus* is seen most commonly in the occipital region and in the center of the face. It may fade with age, never becomes raised, and is not associated with other abnormalities (Schnyder, 1954). The *laterally located nevus flammeus* is usually unilateral in location but in rare instances is bilateral and is most commonly found on one or both sides of the face or on one or several extremities. On the face, it generally darkens with age and may become raised and nodular. The laterally located nevus flammeus is frequently associated with malformations of other blood vessels (Schnyder, 1954). Depending on which blood vessels are involved, the term *Sturge–Weber* or *Klippel–Trenaunay syndrome* is used.

In the *Sturge–Weber syndrome* (leptomeningeal nevus flammeus), the presence of leptomeningeal angiomatosis leads to progressive calcification in the underlying cortex. Epilepsy occurs in 80% of the patients, manifesting itself in 50% before the end of the first year of life. Contralateral hemiparesis may occur. Half of the patients with the Sturge–Weber syndrome have ocular involvement, which may be in the form of angiomatosis of the conjunctiva, iris, or choroid. The latter may result in congenital or late-onset glaucoma or in retinal detachment (Bluefarb; Person and Perry).

In the *Klippel–Trenaunay syndrome* (osteohypertrophic nevus flammeus), one observes hypertrophy of the soft tissues and bones on one or several extremities affected with a nevus flammeus. Associated with this are varicosities or arteriovenous fistulas or both (Mullins et al; Lindenauer). It is assumed that the osteohypertrophy is a result of venous hypertension caused by the fistulas (Defauw).

In some instances of the Klippel–Trenaunay syndrome associated with arteriovenous fistulas, one finds, in addition to the reddish areas of the nevus flammeus, painful violaceous nodules or plaques on the toes, feet, or legs that may undergo ulceration (Bluefarb and Adams; Earhart et al; Rosen et al). The cutaneous lesions simulate Kaposi's sarcoma both clinically and histologically, so that these lesions are referred to as pseudo-Kaposi sarcoma.

Histopathology. In the *medially located nevus flammeus*, no abnormalities are observed in early life. In adults, dilatation of blood vessels limited to the subpapillary area is seen (Schnyder, 1954).

In the *laterally located nevus flammeus*, no telangiectases are apparent histologically until the patient has reached an age of about 10 years (Miescher; Schnyder, 1954). The capillary ectasias thereafter gradually increase with age. Ultimately, when the lesion is raised or nodular, not only the superficial

623

capillaries but also some of the blood vessels in the deeper layers of the dermis and in the subcutaneous layer are dilated (Fig. 30-1). No proliferation of endothelial cells is seen, but loosely arranged collagenous fibers surround the ectatic vessels (Schnyder, 1954). Many ectatic vessels are filled with red blood cells (Finley et al).

In the lesions of so-called *pseudo-Kaposi sarcoma*, which is associated with the arteriovenous fistulas of the Klippel–Trenaunay syndrome, one observes a proliferation of capillaries and fibroblasts, extravasation of red cells, and deposition of hemosiderin in the dermis. In contrast with Kaposi's sarcoma, so-called vascular slits and atypicality of the nuclei of endothelial cells and spindle cells are absent (Bluefarb and Adams; Earhart et al).

Histogenesis. Since no histologic abnormalities are present early in life in nevus flammeus and no endothelial proliferation is ever seen, it appears likely that the nevus flammeus is the result of a congenital weakness of the capillary walls (Schnyder, 1954; Barsky et al). Thus, the nevus flammeus represents a telangiectasia and not a true angioma.

Capillary Hemangioma

Capillary hemangioma, or strawberry mark, consists of one or several bright red, soft, lobulated tumors. They vary greatly in size, may extend into the subcutaneous tissue, and are occasionally located largely in the subcutaneous tissue (Schnyder, 1957). In rare instances, large areas are involved and show numerous, closely aggregated lesions (Wilson and Haggard). Capillary hemangiomas usually first appear between the third week and the fifth week of life, increase in size for several months up to 1 year, and then, unlike the other two forms of congenital hemangioma, start to regress. Complete spontaneous resolution is common, occurring in about 70% of capillary hemangiomas by the time the patient has reached the age of 7 years. Continued improvement after this age is common, so that, ultimately, only about 6% of capillary hemangiomas constitute a cosmetic handicap (Bowers et al).

Kasabach–Merritt Syndrome. The association of extensive capillary hemangiomas in infants with thrombocytopenia and purpura was first described in 1940 (Kasabach and Merritt). However, this syndrome is also seen occasionally in adults with numerous or very large cavernous hemangiomas (Straub et al; Lang and Dubin) or with extensive glomangiomas (see p. 633). The purpura is not just a result of thrombocytopenia, as had been assumed at first, but represents a consumption coagulopathy in which blood coagulation and the associated fibrin formation within the hemangioma cause a consumption of platelets, fibrinogen, prothrombin, and plasminogen. This then results in disseminated intravascular coagulation with extensive bleeding (see p. 166) (Inceman and Yucel; Lang and Dubin).

Histopathology. During their period of growth in early infancy, capillary hemangiomas show considerable proliferation of their endothelial cells. The endothelial cells are large and are aggregated predominantly in solid strands and masses in which one observes only a few small capillary

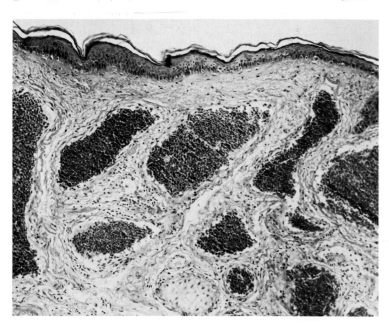

Fig. 30-1.   Congenital hemangioma: nevus flammeus, late stage
The capillaries are greatly dilated, engorged with blood, and lined by a single layer of endothelial cells. Loosely arranged collagenous fibers surround the ectatic vessels. (×100)

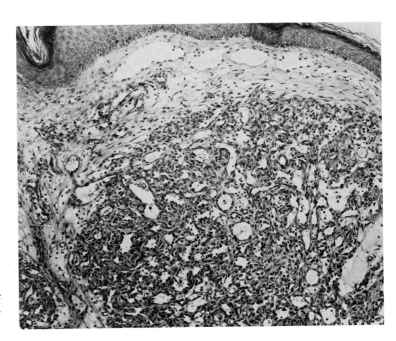

Fig. 30-2. Congenital hemangioma: capillary hemangioma, mature lesion
One observes considerable proliferation of endothelial cells and numerous capillary lumina. (×100)

lumina. In maturing lesions, the capillary lumina are wider, and the endothelial cells lining them appear flatter (Fig. 30-2). In mature lesions, some of the lumina may be greatly dilated (Walsh and Tompkins; Schnyder, 1957). In the involuting phase, deposits of hyalin are observed in the walls of the capillaries, leading to narrowing and occlusion of the capillary lumina. This is followed by involution of the capillaries and their replacement by edematous collagen (Nakayama).

Cavernous Hemangioma

Cavernous hemangioma consists of one or, more commonly, multiple deep dermal and subcutaneous nodules that are often compressible. They may appear in infancy, childhood, or adulthood. Cavernous hemangioma may be associated with an overlying capillary hemangioma. In a few instances, a unilateral dermatomal distribution has been noted (Steinway and Fretzin; Wilkin). There are two rare conditions in which numerous cavernous hemangiomas occur: Maffucci's syndrome, and the blue rubber-bleb nevus.

Maffucci's Syndrome. The outstanding features in Maffucci's syndrome are dyschondroplasia resulting in defects in ossification; fragility of the bones, causing severe deformities; and osteochondromas, which may develop into chondrosarcomas. In addition, large, compressible subcutaneous cavernous hemangiomas may be present at birth (Mullins and Livingood) or appear in childhood (Bean, 1955) or early adulthood (Sakurane et al).

Blue Rubber-Bleb Nevus. In the blue rubber-bleb nevus, cavernous hemangiomas are present at birth but may subsequently increase in size and number. They have a distinct appearance (Bean, 1958). Most of the hemangiomas are protuberant, dark blue, soft, and compressible, and some are pedunculated. They vary from a rather small size to 3 cm in diameter. In addition, subcutaneous hemangiomas are felt on palpation. There also are oral hemangiomas (Fretzin and Potter). The regular presence of hemangiomas in the intestinal tract causes chronic bleeding and anemia. Autopsy may reveal many visceral hemangiomas in addition to those of the intestinal tract (Rice and Fischer).

Histopathology. Cavernous hemangiomas show in the lower dermis and the subcutaneous tissue large, irregular spaces containing red blood cells and fibrinous material. The spaces are lined by a single layer of thin endothelial cells. The fibrous walls of the large vascular spaces are of variable thickness (Steinway and Fretzin; Wilkin). If they are thick, it is generally as a result of an increase in the number of adventitial cells. In some instances, smooth muscle cells are also present, giving the vascular spaces the appearance of large veins (Steinway and Fretzin). Some cases show, within some of the large lumina, aggregates of endothelial cells containing a few capillary lumina (Wilkin).

In *Maffucci's syndrome,* most cavernous hemangiomas show large, irregular spaces lined by a thin endothelial layer (Mullins and Livingood). In some lesions, however, one observes proliferations of endothelial cells around sparse, small, poorly defined vascular spaces (Kuzma and King).

In the *blue rubber-bleb nevus*, the cavernous hemangiomas also show, as a rule, a thin layer of endothelial cells and a thin rim of fibrous tissue (Rice and Fischer). However, some of the subcutaneous hemangiomas have lumina lined by a thick fibrous wall. In addition, some of the superficially located vessels show some endothelial proliferation tending to form small lumina (Fretzin and Potter). Also, in some cases, the thin walls of superficial vascular spaces directly adjoin the surface epidermis (Rice and Fischer).

Differential Diagnosis. Cavernous hemangioma, including the blue rubber-bleb nevus, may resemble the lesions of glomangioma. However, careful examination reveals a small number of glomus cells peripheral to the endothelial cells in at least some of the dilated vascular spaces of glomangioma (see p. 633).

ANGIOKERATOMA

Five types of angiokeratoma occur (Lynch and Kosanovich; Johnson): (1) the generalized systemic type—angiokeratoma corporis diffusum of Fabry (already discussed on p. 389); (2) the bilateral form occurring on the dorsa of the fingers and toes—angiokeratoma of Mibelli; (3) the localized scrotal form—angiokeratoma of Fordyce; (4) the usually solitary papular angiokeratoma; and (5) the plaque-like angiokeratoma circumscriptum, the only form of angiokeratoma that is apt to be present at birth.

Angiokeratoma Mibelli, Angiokeratoma Scroti, Papular Angiokeratoma

In *angiokeratoma Mibelli*, several dark red papules with a slightly verrucous surface are seen on the dorsa of the fingers and toes. Usually, the lesions appear in childhood or adolescence and measure from 3 mm to 5 mm in diameter (Haye and Rebello).

In *angiokeratoma of the scrotum,* multiple vascular papules 2 mm to 4 mm in diameter are seen on the scrotum. They arise in middle or later life. Early lesions are red, soft, and compressible, whereas, later, they become bluish, keratotic, and noncompressible (Agger and Osmundsen).

In *papular angiokeratoma,* usually one and occasionally several papular lesions arise in young adults, most commonly on the lower extremities. Their size ranges

from 2 mm to 10 mm in diameter, the average being 3 mm. Early lesions appear bright red and soft, but they later become bluish to black, firm, and hyperkeratotic (Imperial and Helwig, 1967a). Bluish to black lesions are occasionally misdiagnosed as malignant melanoma (Goldman et al).

Histopathology. The histologic findings are essentially the same in all three above-mentioned types of angiokeratoma (Imperial and Helwig, 1967a). They represent telangiectasias and are not true hemangiomas.

Early lesions show dilated capillaries in the uppermost dermis partially enclosed by elongated rete ridges. Older lesions are hyperkeratotic, and some of the dilated capillaries may be completely encircled by rete ridges. In papular angiokeratoma, organized or organizing thrombi are occasionally observed within the dilated capillaries. In some instances, the dilatation of vessels is not limited to the uppermost dermis and is present also in the middermis, but not below this level (Imperial and Helwig, 1967a).

Angiokeratoma Circumscriptum

Angiokeratoma circumscriptum in its early stage consists of one or occasionally several aggregates of purplish papules and blood-filled, cystic nodules that gradually become verrucous and coalesce into one or several plaques. If several plaques are present, they may show a linear arrangement. Usually, the lesions are present at birth (Imperial and Helwig, 1967b), but, in some cases, they do not appear until childhood (Dammert) or adulthood (Knoth et al). Commonly, the plaques enlarge in size as the patient grows older, and new lesions may appear (Maekawa and Arao). In most instances, the lesions measure only a few centimeters, but, in rare cases, they may be of considerable size and extent (Knoth et al; Maekawa and Arao). The clinical resemblance between angiokeratoma circumscriptum and lymphangioma circumscriptum is often great (see p. 631), and intermediate forms occur in which some of the superficial cystic nodules contain blood and others lymph fluid (Dammert).

Angiokeratoma circumscriptum may be associated with a nevus flammeus (Dammert) or with a cavernous hemangioma (Knoth et al; Lynch and Kosanovich). In addition, angiokeratoma circumscriptum has been observed in association with the Klippel–Trenaunay syndrome consisting of osteohypertrophy of one leg (see p. 623) (Fischer and Friederich). The so-called *Cobb syndrome* consists of a combination of an angiokeratoma circumscriptum or nevus flammeus and an angioma in the spinal cord within a segment or two of the dermatome involved (Jessen et al; Zala and Mumenthaler).

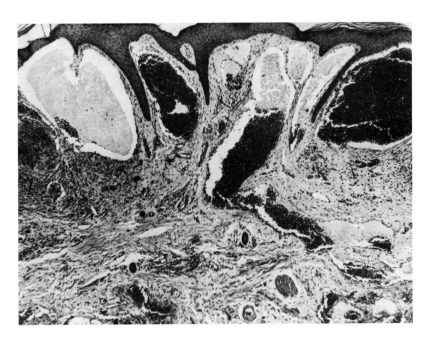

Fig. 30-3. Angiokeratoma circumscriptum
Greatly dilated capillary spaces are seen in both the papillary and the reticular dermis. Although most lumina contain erythrocytes, some are filled with lymph fluid. (×50)

Histopathology. In angiokeratoma circumscriptum, varying degrees of hyperkeratosis, papillomatosis, and irregular acanthosis are present. Greatly dilated capillary spaces are seen just beneath, or enclosed within, the papillomatous epidermis. Although, in most instances, all lumina contain only erythrocytes, thin-walled, lymph-filled spaces are occasionally intermingled with the blood-filled spaces (Fig. 30-3) (Dammert). Thrombi may be present in some of the dilated capillaries (Bruce). In contrast to papular angiokeratoma, which is purely a superficial telangiectasia, angiokeratoma circumscriptum shows vascular changes extending into the subcutaneous tissue. These changes vary from ectatic, blood-filled vessels in the reticular dermis and the subcutaneous fat (Fischer and Friederich; Dammert) to endothelial proliferations in the dermis and subcutis (Bruce; Imperial and Helwig, 1967b; Maekawa and Arao) and to large, clinically evident subcutaneous cavernous hemangiomas (Knoth et al; Lynch and Kosanovich).

VENOUS (ARTERIOVENOUS) HEMANGIOMA

Venous hemangioma occurs as a usually solitary dark red papule or nodule on the face or, less commonly, on the extremities. Although first described in 1956 (Biberstein and Jessner), it has become generally known only recently (Girard et al; Carapeto et al). Most of the lesions measure less than 1 cm in diameter.

Histopathology. Within a circumscribed area, usually limited to the dermis, one observes densely aggregated, thick-walled and thin-walled vessels lined by a single layer of endothelial cells (Fig. 30-4). The walls of the thick-walled vessels consist mainly of fibrous tissue but in most instances contain also some smooth muscle (Girard et al; Carapeto et al, Wade et al). Many vessels contain red blood cells, and thrombi are occasionally seen (Girard et al).

Histogenesis. It seems likely that both the thick-walled and the thin-walled vessels represent veins, since apparent transitions between them can be seen (Wade et al). Some authors, however, regard the thick-walled vessels as arteries (Biberstein and Jessner; Girard et al), even though the lesions show no pulsation. Still others regard them as transitional vascular channels analogous to those seen in the Suquet–Hoyer canal of the glomus (Carapeto et al); however, glomus cells are absent.

GENERALIZED ESSENTIAL TELANGIECTASIA

Widespread linear telangiectases, mainly on the extremities, may develop gradually in adults, predominantly in women (McGrae and Winkelmann). In some instances, the conjunctivae and oral mucosa may also be involved (Gentele and Lodin).

Histopathology. Dilated vessels, often filled with blood, are seen in the upper part of the dermis.

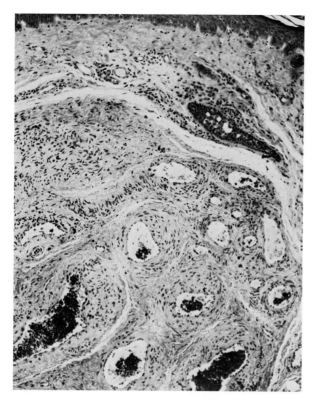

Fig. 30-4. Venous (arteriovenous) hemangioma
Within a circumscribed area of the dermis, one observes densely aggregated, thick-walled and thin-walled vessels lined by a single layer of endothelial cells. These vessels most likely represent veins. (×100)

The walls of the vessels are composed only of endothelium. The absence of alkaline phosphatase activity suggests that it is the venous portion of the capillary loop that participates in the disease process (McGrae and Winkelmann).

UNILATERAL NEVOID TELANGIECTASIA

Although unilateral nevoid telangiectasia may be congenital, it is in most instances related to high estrogen levels, with or without liver disease as a contributing factor (Wilkin). The telangiectases, which are largely punctate and stellate rather than linear, may involve the oral and gastric mucosa in addition to the skin (Anderton and Smith).

Histopathology. Numerous dilated vessels without endothelial proliferation are seen in the upper and middle dermis and, to a lesser extent, in the deeper part of the dermis (Anderton and Smith).

ANGIOMA SERPIGINOSUM

Angioma serpiginosum shows as primary lesions deeply red, nonpalpable puncta that are grouped closely together in a macular or netlike pattern. The disorder is asymptomatic. It usually begins in adolescence and extends slowly for several years (Frain-Bell). Irregular extension at the periphery of the macules may cause them to have a serpiginous border. Women are more commonly affected than men. The lower extremities are most frequently involved. The deeply red puncta represent dilated capillaries. Even though they usually do not blanch completely, they do not represent purpura and bleed freely when pricked (Barker and Sachs).

Histopathology. Dilated capillaries are seen in some of the dermal papillae. Each affected papilla contains either a single greatly dilated capillary (Marriott et al; Chavaz and Laugier) or a cluster of moderately dilated capillaries (Kumakiri et al). In addition, some subpapillary capillaries are dilated. All dilated capillaries show thickening of their walls (Kumakiri et al; Chavaz and Laugier).

Histogenesis. On *electron microscopic examination*, it is apparent that the thickening of the capillary walls is caused by a heavy precipitate of basement-membrane-like material admixed with thin collagen fibers and an increased number of concentrically arranged pericytes (Chavaz and Laugier). In addition, some of the dilated capillaries show slitlike protrusions of their lumina and endothelial lining into the surrounding thickened vessel walls (Kumakiri et al). Thus, angioma serpiginosum is not just a simple telangiectasia but rather represents a vascular malformation with a delayed onset, analogous to hereditary hemorrhagic telangiectasia (see below) (Chavez and Laugier).

HEREDITARY HEMORRHAGIC TELANGIECTASIA (OSLER'S DISEASE)

Osler's disease is inherited as an autosomal dominant trait. Although epistaxis may already begin in childhood, the characteristic telangiectases on the skin and the mucous membranes of the nose and mouth do not begin to appear until adolescence. The telangiectases may be punctate, stellate, or linear, and they blanch on pressure.

More or less widely disseminated telangiectases may exist in many viscera, especially in the gastrointestinal tract. Asymptomatic gastrointestinal bleeding occurs in about 15% of the patients, especially in later life. Severe melena may ultimately be the cause of death (Smith et al). Hepatomegaly is a frequent finding, and, on autopsy, the liver may show a pattern of patchy fibrosis with telangiectatic vessels but without significant parenchymal damage or an inflammatory reaction (Daly and Schiller). Patients with Osler's disease may show malformations of large blood vessels, such as arteriovenous fistulae in the lungs (Chandler) or the brain (Waller et al).

Histopathology. Irregularly dilated capillaries and venules are seen in the papillary and subpapillary dermis. They are lined only by flattened endothelial cells and show no pericytes. The perivascular connective tissue appears degenerated (Laugier). Dilated capillaries in the oral mucosa may form irregular convolutions and extend through a degenerating epithelium at sites of hemorrhage (Muggia).

Histogenesis. On *electron microscopy*, the dilated vessels in the skin and oral mucosa are seen to be small venules that normally do not possess pericytes. They show a defect in the perivascular supportive tissue consisting of an increased amount of amorphous and fine filamentous material and of abnormally large collagen fibrils with an irregular banding pattern (Hashimoto and Pritzker). This defective perivascular tissue is held responsible for the breakdown of the junctions between adjoining endothelial cells and thus for the hemorrhage. In the oral mucosa, the dilated vessels show many endothelial gaps that are filled with thrombi composed of fibrin and platelets (Hashimoto and Pritzker).

NEVUS ARANEUS

Nevus araneus, or spider nevus, shows a central, slightly elevated, red punctum from which blood vessels radiate. Occasionally, pulsation can be observed. The face is the most common site. Although spider nevi often arise spontaneously, pregnancy and cirrhosis of the liver are factors predisposing to their appearance. At the end of the pregnancy, they may disappear spontaneously.

Histopathology. In the center of the lesion is an ascending artery the wall of which shows either smooth muscle cells or, rarely, several layers of glomus cells (see p. 35) (Bean; Schuhmachers-Brendler). The artery widens into a subepidermal, thin-walled ampulla. Delicate arterial branches radiate from the ampulla and divide into capillaries (Whiting et al).

GRANULOMA PYOGENICUM

Granuloma pyogenicum occurs as a single lesion with but few exceptions (Juhlin et al). It consists of a dull red, soft or moderately firm, raised, slightly pedunculated nodule. It grows rapidly to a size of usually 0.5 cm but occasionally up to 2 cm and then remains unchanged. The surface may be smooth, but it often shows superficial ulceration and crusting. The lesion bleeds easily when traumatized. Although a granuloma

pyogenicum may occur anywhere on the skin, it is found most commonly on the fingers and the face. The oral cavity, particularly the gingiva, is a rather common site for granuloma pyogenicum, with pregnancy often as a precipitating factor (Leyden and Master).

In a few instances, the development of multiple small, angiomatous satellite lesions has been observed following the removal of a granuloma pyogenicum (Coskey and Mehregan; Warner and Wilson Jones). This may occur either with or without recurrence of the primary lesion. When left untreated, the satellite lesions either involute or remain unchanged. In a few instances, satellite lesions have appeared following mechanical irritation of a granuloma pyogenicum (Zaynoun et al). It is of interest that nearly all reported instances of multiple satellites around a lesion of granuloma pyogenicum have occurred on the trunk, particularly in the scapular region, although this is a rather rare location for granuloma pyogenicum. Also, most instances have occurred in children, even though granuloma pyogenicum in general shows no special predilection for children (Warner and Wilson Jones).

Histopathology. On histologic examination, one finds a circumscribed lesion covered by a flattened epidermis and showing, often in a lobulated arrangement, endothelial proliferations with formation of capillary lumina (Fig. 30-5). Whereas solid aggregates of endothelial cells are seen in the least matured areas, capillary lumina are evident in most areas, varying from small and cleftlike to markedly ectatic (Davies et al). Many lumina are lined by prominent endothelial cells projecting into the lumina of the vessels. The stroma in which the capillary proliferations are embedded appears edematous and does not contain mature collagen bundles. The epidermis as a rule shows inward growth at the base of the lesion and thus produces a so-called epidermal collarette, causing slight pedunculation of the lesion. Capillary proliferations are often also seen beneath the level of the collarette (Nödl).

In early lesions, one finds no inflammatory reaction (Nödl; Oehlschlaegel and Müller). In older lesions, because of erosion of the thinned epidermis, secondary inflammatory changes are often present in the stroma.

The satellite lesions seen following the removal or irritation of a granuloma pyogenicum usually have the same histologic appearance as the primary lesion of granuloma pyogenicum,, although early satellite nodules may lack a collarette and then simulate a simple capillary hemangioma (Warner and Wilson Jones; Zaynoun et al).

Histogenesis. It was formerly widely assumed that granuloma pyogenicum was caused by pyogenic infec-

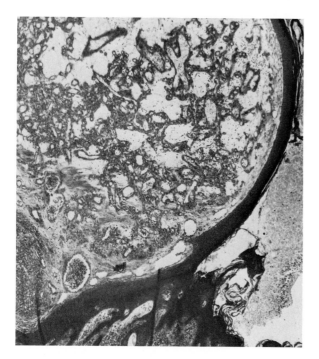

Fig. 30-5.   Granuloma pyogenicum
The lesion is pedunculated and covered by a flattened epidermis. One observes considerable proliferation of endothelial cells and numerous capillary lumina. The stroma is edematous and free of inflammatory infiltration. (×50)

tion of a small wound. However, the histologic picture of an early lesion with its endothelial proliferation is that of a capillary hemangioma (Nödl; Oehlschlaegel and Müller) and even an older, eroded lesion showing a pronounced inflammatory infiltrate in its superficial portion retains the appearance of a capillary hemangioma in its deeper portions. Therefore, the term *eruptive hemangioma* (Marsch) is more suitable for this lesion than granuloma pyogenicum.

Electron microscopic examination shows endothelial cells with numerous organelles, thereby also favoring the theory that the lesion is a capillary hemangioma (Marsch). Of interest is the nearly complete absence of Weibel–Palade bodies in the endothelial cells (Davies et al; Marsch).

Differential Diagnosis.   Differentiation of granuloma pyogenicum from the type of capillary hemangioma that occurs in infancy is usually easy because of the collarette formation at the base of the tumor and the edema of the stroma.

Lesions of granuloma pyogenicum with a fairly pronounced inflammatory infiltrate may greatly resemble granulation tissue; however, granuloma pyogenicum possesses a flattened epidermis with collarette formation and in its deeper layers shows

no inflammatory reaction but only vascular proliferation (Oehlschlaegel and Müller).

Early lesions of Kaposi's sarcoma, like granuloma pyogenicum, may show vascular proliferation and an inflammatory infiltrate. However, Kaposi's sarcoma shows no collarette formation. Furthermore, on careful searching or deeper sectioning, areas of spindle cell proliferation and of extravasations of red cells can be found. Differentiation of granuloma pyogenicum from angiosarcoma may cause difficulties in early lesions with pronounced endothelial proliferation; however, in angiosarcoma, the endothelial cells show pronounced atypicality and invasion into surrounding tissue as solid cords. For a discussion of differentiation from papular angioplasia, see p. 631.

CHERRY HEMANGIOMA

Cherry hemangiomas are bright red lesions varying in size from a hardly visible punctum to a soft, raised, dome-shaped lesion measuring several millimeters in diameter. This very common lesion, often present in large numbers, may already start appearing in early adulthood, and the number of lesions increases with age. Cherry hemangiomas may occur anywhere on the skin, but the trunk is the most common site.

Histopathology.   In their early stage of development, cherry hemangiomas have the appearance of true capillary hemangiomas, being composed of numerous newly formed capillaries with narrow lumina and prominent endothelial cells arranged in a lobular fashion in the subpapillary region (Schnyder and Keller). As the lesion ages, the capillaries become dilated. In a fully matured cherry hemangioma, one observes numerous moderately dilated capillaries lined by flattened endothelial cells. The intercapillary stroma shows edema and homogenization of the collagen. The epidermis is thinned and often surrounds most of the angioma as a collarette (Sălamon et al).

Differential Diagnosis.   In its early stage, cherry angioma, like granuloma pyogenicum, shows capillary proliferation; however, endothelial proliferation is much less pronounced than in granuloma pyogenicum, so that solid aggregates of endothelial cells are not seen.

PAPULAR ANGIOPLASIA

Multiple soft, purplish, vascular papules measuring only a few millimeters in diameter are seen on the face. Their number varies from 2 to 30. They may involute spontaneously (Wilson Jones and Marks).

The term *papular angioplasia* was suggested in 1970 (Wilson Jones and Marks). Two such cases were previously published, one with the diagnosis of Kaposi's sarcoma (Winer and Levin) and the other as atypical pyogenic granuloma (Peterson et al).

Histopathology. Atypical vascular proliferations are seen in the dermis. Small capillary lumina are lined by large, protruding, columnar endothelial cells (Winer and Levin), which occasionally form a double layer (Peterson et al). The stroma between the vessels contains numerous cells. Some of them resemble endothelial cells, and others fibroblastic cells; many appear atypical, being hyperchromatic and occasionally multinucleated (Wilson Jones and Marks). Extravasated erythrocytes may be found in the stroma (Peterson et al).

Differential Diagnosis. Without adequate clinical data, it is difficult to exclude a diagnosis of Kaposi's sarcoma or angiosarcoma. The lesion differs from granuloma pyogenicum by showing fewer lumina and endothelial cells and more intervascular stroma with cellular proliferation.

VENOUS LAKES

Venous lakes are small, dark blue, slightly raised, soft lesions occurring on the exposed skin of elderly persons. They can usually be emptied of most of their blood by sustained pressure. Usually, several lesions are present. The face, ears, and lips are the most common sites.

Histopathology. Venous lakes are not true hemangiomas but rather represent dilated veins or venules. In the upper dermis, close to the epidermis, they show either one greatly dilated space or several interconnected dilated spaces filled with erythrocytes and lined by a single layer of flattened endothelial cells and a thin wall of fibrous tissue (Bean and Walsh).

THROMBOSED CAPILLARY OR VEIN

In thrombosed capillary or vein, also referred to as *capillary aneurysm,* a dome-shaped or slightly lobulated, moderately firm, blue black nodule arises either abruptly or gradually. There may be a rim of erythema or brownish pigmentation around it. In most instances, the patient has not been aware of a pre-existing lesion (Epstein et al). The size of the nodule varies usually between 2 mm and 10 mm. The face is the most common site, but other areas may be involved, including the oral mucosa

(Weathers and Fine). The lesion is of significance largely because of its clinical resemblance to a malignant melanoma.

Histopathology. The upper dermis shows one or several greatly dilated vascular lumina filled with thrombi (Epstein et al; Weiner). The thrombi may show invasion by fibroblasts in one or several areas, indicating beginning organization (Epstein et al). Extravasated red cells and hemosiderin may be present in the upper dermis around the thrombosed lumina.

When several adjoining vascular lumina are thrombosed and such thrombosed lumina are present not only in the dermis but also in the epidermis, it is obvious that the pre-existing lesion was a papular angiokeratoma (see p. 626) (Hayen; Weiner). In other instances, when a solitary thrombosed lumen is surrounded by a venous wall, the pre-existing lesion may have been a venous lake of the face (Epstein et al). It is not possible in all cases, however, to identify the nature of the pre-existing lesion.

LYMPHANGIOMA

Three types of lymphangioma exist: (1) localized lymphangioma circumscriptum, corresponding to papular angiokeratoma; (2) the "classic" type of lymphangioma circumscriptum, corresponding to angiokeratoma circumscriptum; and (3) cavernous lymphangioma, including the cystic hygroma, corresponding to cavernous hemangioma (Peachey et al). Occasionally, the classic type of lymphangioma circumscriptum is seen in conjunction with cavernous lymphangioma (Whimster; Flanagan and Helwig). In addition, lymphangiectasia, which is indistinguishable from classic lymphangioma circumscriptum, may occur, though rarely, in association with congenital or acquired lymphedema (Fisher and Orkin; Prioleau and Santa Cruz).

Localized Lymphangioma Circumscriptum

The lesion of localized lymphangioma circumscriptum consists clinically of a single small patch of thick-walled vesicles that resemble frogs' spawn if they are filled solely with lymph fluid. In many cases, however, some of the vesicles have a purplish color because of an admixture of blood. The lesion often appears later in life and usually measures less than 1 cm in diameter (Peachey et al).

Histopathology. Cystically dilated lymph vessels lined by a single layer of endothelium are

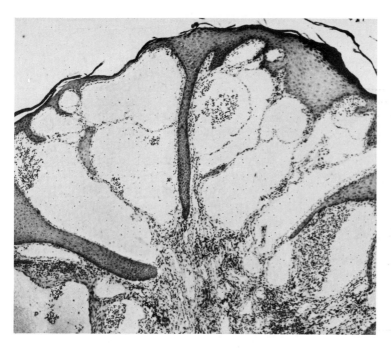

Fig. 30-6. Lymphangioma circumscriptum
Greatly dilated lymph vessels lined by a single layer of endothelial cells are present in the upper dermis. The epidermis shows downward growth and more or less surrounds some of the lymph vessels. There is moderate hyperkeratosis. (×50)

present in the uppermost portion of the dermis (Fig. 30-6). Occasionally, these lymph vessels contain some erythrocytes in addition to lymph. The epidermis varies in thickness. Over some of the lymph cysts, it is thinned; elsewhere, it may show acanthosis, papillomatosis, hyperkeratosis, and irregular downward growth. Some of the dilated lymph vessels may appear to be enclosed in the epidermis. The dilatation of lymph vessels may extend as far down as the middermis, but only one or two dilated lymphatics are seen deep in the dermis (Peachey et al).

Lymphangioma Circumscriptum

In the classic type of lymphangioma circumscriptum, one or several large patches with translucent vesicles are present, and the condition may be quite extensive. The lesions are present at birth or appear early in life. In many instances, there is a mild degree of diffuse swelling of the subcutaneous tissue beneath the vesicular lesions, and, in rare instances, there is associated enlargement of a whole limb (Peachey et al; Palmer et al). Some of the vesicles contain an admixture of blood. The skin surface between and even on top of some of the vesicles may be verrucous in appearance.

Histopathology. The histologic appearance of the epidermis and upper dermis in lymphangioma circumscriptum is similar to that described for localized lymphangioma circumscriptum, although the degree of hyperkeratosis and papillomatosis is usually greater. However, dilatation of the lymph vessels extends to the deeper zones of the dermis and into the subcutaneous fat. The lymph vessels in the subcutaneous fat are often of large caliber and form one or several large "cisterns" with a well-developed muscular coat. Lymphangiography shows that the cisterns and the overlying lymphangioma are not filled by the contrast medium (Whimster). In the rare cases with associated diffuse edema of a limb, lymphangiography shows widespread lymphectasia without connection to the lymphangioma (Palmer et al).

Cavernous Lymphangioma

Cavernous lymphangioma, also referred to as *cystic hygroma* when located on the neck, manifests itself as soft, circumscribed or diffuse swelling of the subcutaneous tissue with the consistency of a lipoma or cyst. Just as a subcutaneous hemangioma cavernosum may be associated with an overlying capillary hemangioma, lymphangioma cavernosum may be seen in conjunction with lymphangioma circumscriptum (Flanagan and Helwig).

Histopathology. Large, irregularly shaped cystic spaces are seen in the subcutaneous tissue lined by a single layer of endothelium. The periendothelial connective tissue varies in amount and composition. There may be loose stroma, compact stroma, or marked fibrosis. In some instances, especially in the case of large cystic spaces, bundles of smooth muscle cells are seen in the wall (Flanagan and Helwig). Large cavernous lymphangiomas, particularly in areas such as the lip or tongue, may extend between the muscle bundles, separating them from one another (Peachey et al).

Lymphangiectasia

In rare instances, lesions that are clinically similar to lymphangioma circumscriptum develop in an arm showing postmastectomy lymphedema (Plotnick and Richfield; Prioleau and Santa Cruz) or in a lower extremity affected with congenital lymphedema (Burstein). This is an even rarer event than the development of a lymphangiosarcoma in lymphedema (see p. 642).

Histopathology. The histologic appearance of lymphangiectasia secondary to lymphedema is identical to that of lymphangioma circumscriptum (Prioleau and Santa Cruz).

GLOMUS TUMOR

Two types of glomus tumors exist: solitary and multiple. The more common *solitary type* shows a purplish nodule measuring only a few millimeters in diameter. The nodule is tender and often gives rise to severe paroxysmal pains. Most commonly, the nodule is situated on the extremities, especially in the nail bed.

Multiple glomus tumors, or glomangiomas, are much less common than solitary tumors. In contrast to the solitary type, which is not inherited, the multiple type is in some instances dominantly transmitted (Schnyder; Rycroft et al). The lesions are either localized to one area (Laymon and Peterson) or generalized (McEvoy et al). As a rule, they are asymptomatic, but, occasionally, tenderness (Ishibashi et al) and even paroxysmal attacks of pain (Gupta et al) have been described in some or even in all of them. The lesions may be intracutaneous or subcutaneous in location. Although most of the nodules in the multiple type are small, some may reach a size of several centimeters in diameter (McEvoy et al). Cases of multiple glomus tumors in which the lesions have been large enough to be raised, soft, and compressible have been mistakenly diagnosed as blue rubber-bleb nevus even though intestinal bleeding has been absent (Fine et al; Mukhtar and Pfleger). Patients with generalized glomus tumors may show evidence of the Kasabach–Merritt syndrome, seen most commonly in extensive capillary hemangiomas (see p. 624) (McEvoy et al).

Histopathology. *Solitary glomus tumors* are surrounded by a fibrous capsule. They contain numerous small vascular lumina that are lined by a single layer of flattened, often elongated endothelial cells. Peripheral to the endothelial cells are a few to many layers of glomus cells (Fig. 30-7). The glomus cells have a faintly eosinophilic cytoplasm and large, pale, round to oval nuclei of a rather uniform appearance. The glomus cells thus resemble epithelioid cells. In many areas, the glomus cells are seen to extend irregularly from the vascular walls into the connective tissue stroma of the tumor. This stroma appears edematous and contains scattered fibroblasts and fairly numerous mast cells (Murad et al). Staining with the Bodian stain shows a considerable number of nerve fibers in the perivascular stroma of solitary tumors (Shugart et al).

Multiple glomus tumors possess no capsule and show much larger vascular spaces than the solitary glomus tumor. Because of their conspicuous vascular component, multiple glomus tumors are referred to also as *glomangiomas* (Laymon and Peterson). The large vascular spaces usually have an irregular shape. Just as in the solitary glomus tumor, the vascular spaces are lined by a single layer of flat endothelial cells, but the number of glomus cells located peripheral to the endothelial cells is much smaller than in the solitary glomus tumor (Fig. 30-8). Usually, the glomus cells form only a narrow rim of one to three layers. They may even be absent around part of the vessel walls, and some of the vascular spaces may show no glomus cells (Laymon and Peterson). Rarely, a patient may show glomus cells in only some of his tumors and none in others (Schnyder). With the Bodian stain, only few nerve fibers are seen in the connective tissue surrounding the vascular formations of multiple glomus tumors (Gordon and Hyman; Chandon et al).

Histogenesis. Both solitary and multiple glomus tumors are related to the arterial segment of the cutaneous glomus, the so-called Suquet–Hoyer canal (see p. 35). By light microscopy, the normal Suquet–Hoyer canal is seen to have a narrow lumen surrounded by a single layer of endothelial cells and four to six layers of glomus cells (see p. 35). On *electron microscopy*, normal glomus cells are found to be vascular smooth muscle cells (Goodman). Similarly, the glomus cells of glomus tumors are shown by electron microscopy to be smooth muscle cells, both in the solitary glomus tumor (Murad et al) and in multiple glomus tumors (Tarnowski and Hashimoto; Lüders et al; Goodman and Abele). However, the smooth muscle cells seen in glomus tumors are polyhedral in shape instead of their usual elongated form

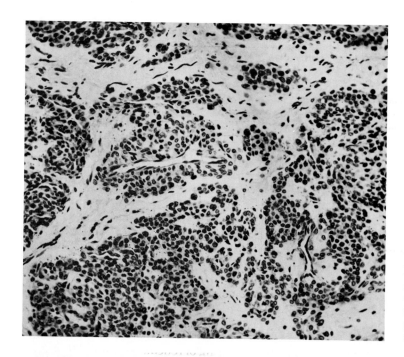

Fig. 30-7. Solitary glomus tumor
There are several narrow vascular lumina lined by a single layer of flattened, elongated endothelial cells. Peripheral to the endothelial cells are multiple rows of glomus cells. In addition, there are masses of glomus cells in which no vascular lumen can be seen. (×200)

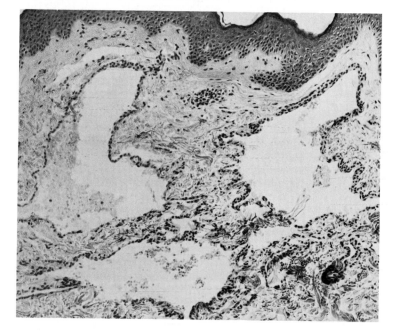

Fig. 30-8. Multiple glomus tumor (glomangioma)
Greatly dilated vascular spaces are lined by a single layer of flat endothelial cells. Glomus cells are seen in most, but not all, areas peripheral to the endothelial cells as a narrow rim of one to three layers. (×100)

(Murad et al). Being smooth muscle cells, glomus cells are surrounded by a filamentous basement membrane. A well-developed basement membrane also separates the glomus cells from the endothelial cell layer. Glomus cells contain numerous myofilaments, which measure about 5 nm in diameter and are arranged in bundles (EM 43) (Goodman and Abele). So-called dense bodies representing condensations that hold bundles of myofil-

aments together are distributed at random in the cytoplasm and are also present on the inner surface of the plasma membrane. Many of the longitudinally sectioned glomus cells show the typically compressed and scalloped nuclei that are associated with contraction (Tarnowski and Hashimoto). Whereas nerve fibers are easily demonstrated in solitary glomus tumors (Murad et al; Ishibashi et al), in multiple glomus tumors, sparse nonmyelinated axons have been found embedded in the cytoplasm of Schwann cells and in close contact with glomus cells by some authors (Lüders et al; Ishibashi et al) but not by others (Tarnowski and Hashimoto).

It has been noted in several instances of multiple glomus tumors that some of the glomus cells contain relatively few myofilaments limited to the periphery of the glomus cells (Lüders et al); in other instances, the myofilaments are not held together in bundles by dense bodies and therefore extend in different directions. It seems doubtful that the latter type of cell can effectively contract (Ishibashi et al).

Differential Diagnosis. Hemangiopericytoma differs from the solitary type of glomus tumor by its larger size, the irregular proliferation of its cells, and the presence of spindle-shaped rather than epithelioid-shaped cells.

Multiple glomus tumors differ from the lesions of the blue rubber-bleb nevus by the presence of glomus cells in nearly all tumors. Also in contrast to the lesions of the blue rubber-bleb nevus, multiple glomus tumors do not occur in the gastrointestinal tract and thus are not associated with gastrointestinal bleeding (Chandon et al).

HEMANGIOPERICYTOMA

Hemangiopericytoma, a tumor first described in 1942 (Stout and Murray), may arise wherever there are capillaries. It is found most commonly in the somatic soft tissue, especially of the extremities, such as muscle, fascia, subcutaneous tissue, and, rarely, skin. Subcutaneous lesions may be small and clinically resemble a lipoma (Cole et al) but, in most instances, they attain considerable size (Sims et al) and may invade underlying structures (Bianchi et al). Cutaneous lesions appear as red, indurated, large plaques (Reich, 1956) or nodules (Schneider and Undeutsch) that are often invasive. Aside from the subcutaneous and muscular tissue, the extradural, paraspinal, and retroperitoneal tissue may be involved (McMaster et al).

The tendency of hemangiopericytomas to metastasize is widely regarded as unpredictable. It was at one time thought that the location of the tumor was a more important factor to its prognosis than its histologic appearance and that tumors in the deep tissues of the thigh and retroperitoneum were most apt to metastasize (Stout, 1955; Reich, 1973). Recent histologic studies, however, have established that a fairly good correlation exists between degree of maturity of the cells and prognosis (Enzinger and Smith; McMaster et al). Small, superficially located tumors limited to the skin and subcutaneous tissue have a fairly good prognosis, because they usually have a less malignant histologic appearance than large, deep-seated tumors.

The mortality rate of hemangiopericytoma on adequate follow-up is about 50% (O'Brien and Brasfield; McMaster et al). Death is usually caused by pulmonary metastases. The rate of survival for children is not better than that for adults (Hollmann et al). However, hemangiopericytomas that are present at birth or arise in the first 7 months of life do not metastasize and therefore have an excellent prognosis, even though their histologic appearance usually is rather ominous (Altmeyer and Nödl; Enzinger and Smith). It may be added that such infantile hemangiopericytomas occur exclusively as cutaneous-subcutaneous plaques (Altmeyer and Nödl) or as subcutaneous, multinodular lesions (Cole et al; Eimoto).

Histopathology. The tumor is characterized by the presence of endothelium-lined tubes and sprouts surrounded by irregularly proliferating, closely packed pericytes with spindle-shaped nuclei (Fig. 30-9) (Stout, 1949; O'Brien and Brasfield). In some cases, one may observe dividing vessels with an antlerlike configuration (Enzinger and Smith). Reticulum fibers encircle the capillary endothelium, so that, in sections stained for reticulum fibers, the tumor cells are seen to be located peripheral to the periendothelial ring of reticulum. Thus, a reticulum stain is often of considerable value in the diagnosis of this tumor. In some instances, a reticulum stain also reveals that some of the individual tumor cells are surrounded by a delicate network of reticulum fibers (Forrester and Houston; Reich, 1956; Nunnery et al).

Hemangiopericytomas can be divided on a histologic basis into benign, borderline malignant, and malignant (McMaster et al). The benign tumors do not metastasize. They show a prominent vascular pattern, mostly spindle-shaped pericytes, and either no mitoses or only an occasional mitosis. The borderline tumors are more cellular than the benign tumors, and the cells are more plump, but anaplasia is not a prominent feature. Occasional mitoses are present, and the vascular spaces often appear compressed and poorly outlined. The tumor cells of the malignant tumors show a varying degree of anaplasia and varying numbers of mitoses. One third of the borderline tumors and three quarters of the tumors regarded as malignant have been found to metastasize.

Histogenesis. Hemangiopericytomas are tumors of the pericyte, a cell that is found in the walls of capillaries and venules as a discontinuous layer lying between the endothelium and the adventitial connective tissue. Pericytes are completely surrounded by the capillary basement membrane, which stains positive with reticulum stains (see p. 30). Pericytes thus share with glomus cells the location peripheral to endothelial cells and envelopment by the basement membrane; however, they

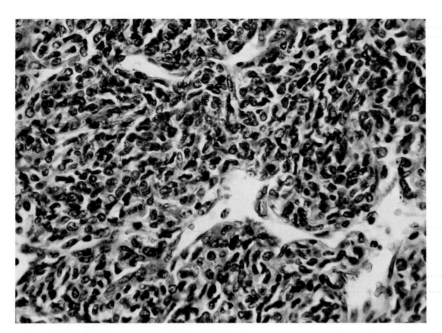

well circumscribed
No pallisading
"Staghorn" Vessels

Fig. 30-9.
Hemangiopericytoma —*spindle cell Tumor*
The capillary lumina are lined with a single layer of endothelial cells and are surrounded by irregularly proliferating, closely packed pericytes. Most of the pericytes are spindle-shaped. (× 400)

differ from glomus cells (1) by their presence in the walls of capillaries and venules, rather than in the wall of the arterial Suquet–Hoyer canal; (2) by their ubiquitous distribution throughout the body; and (3) as seen on electron microscopy, by their lack of bundles of myofilaments with so-called dense bodies (Meade et al). Some pericytes, however, show small bundles of filaments adjacent to the cell membrane and dense material resembling dense bodies clumped against the cell membrane (Kuhn and Rosai). In addition, transitional forms between pericytes and smooth muscle cells have been observed in the walls of small arterioles (Hahn et al; Weber and Braun-Falco).

Electron microscopic examination of hemangiopericytomas has revealed that some of them are composed of rather poorly differentiated cells showing no distinct basement membrane but only basement-membrane-like material around the cells (Ramsey; Murad et al). Other tumors, however, have shown well-defined basement membranes around the tumor cells (Hahn et al; Battifora). In addition, cytoplasmic filaments have been observed in several instances, and even occasional dense body formation in association with these filaments has been seen in some cases (Hahn et al; Nunnery et al). In one instance, in addition to containing pericytes, the tumor contained typical smooth muscle cells as well as cells transitional between pericytes and smooth muscle cells (Kuhn and Rosai). It thus presented "some kind of hybrid between classical glomus tumor and hemangiopericytoma" (Lattes).

Differential Diagnosis. For a discussion of differentiation of hemangiopericytoma from the solitary type of glomus tumor, see p. 633. Kaposi's sarcoma shows more conspicuous vascular proliferation with more prominent endothelial cells and, almost always, extravasations of erythrocytes. In angiosarcoma, vascular lumina are more prominent and often more irregularly demarcated than in hemangiopericytoma. Also, in staining the periendothelial basement membrane, a reticulum stain shows that the tumor cells in hemangiopericytoma are located peripheral to the periendothelial ring of reticulum; in contrast, in angiosarcoma, whenever such a ring of reticulum can be recognized at all, the tumor cells, being endothelial cells, lie inside this ring.

KAPOSI'S SARCOMA

Kaposi's sarcoma, or multiple idiopathic hemorrhagic sarcoma, is characterized by the presence of bluish red or dark brown plaques and nodules, particularly on the distal portion of the lower extremities. In some patients, the initial manifestation consists of annular, serpiginous, bluish red patches (Schwartz et al). In the late stage, some of the nodules and plaques may undergo ulceration. Lymphedema of the lower extremities is then common. Occasionally, spontaneous involution of some of the lesions occurs. In some instances, Kaposi's sarcoma is localized to one area (Cox et al), or it consists of a single lesion without a tendency to progress (Cox and Helwig). Excision of a solitary lesion appears to result in a cure (O'Brien and Brasfield). As a rule, however, the disease is slowly progressive.

Next to the skin, the most common sites of involvement are the subcutaneous lymph nodes, which become enlarged (Amazon and Rywlin). The lymph nodes are involved in about 10% of all cases (Duperrat and Pacot). In rare instances, they are the only site of involvement (Ecklund and Valaitis).

Visceral lesions are encountered in only about 10% of the patients (Tedeschi; Feuerman and Potruch-Eisenkraft). The most common sites of visceral involvement, in order of frequency, are the gastrointestinal tract, liver, lungs, abdominal lymph nodes, and heart (Temime et al). In rare instances, the disease is found exclusively in visceral organs (Tedeschi et al; Anthony and Koneman; Cox and Helwig).

Except in African blacks and in young homosexual men (see below), Kaposi's sarcoma causes death in only 10% to 20% of those affected (Cox and Helwig; Reynolds et al; Feuerman and Potruch-Eisenkraft). Death may result from hemorrhages caused by lesions in the gastrointestinal tract or the lungs, from extensive cutaneous dissemination, from severe infiltration and ulceration of the lower extremities, or from lymphoma. The mean duration of the disease in those dying from it is 9 years (O'Brien and Brasfield).

Three aspects pertaining to Kaposi's sarcoma have received considerable attention: its association with lymphoma and immunosuppression, its prevalence in Africa south of the Sahara, and its common occurrence in young homosexual men.

The relatively common association of Kaposi's sarcoma with lymphoma and leukemia has been recognized for many years, with an incidence varying between 6% (Cox and Helwig; Reynolds et al) and 12% (O'Brien and Brasfield). More recently, the development of Kaposi's sarcoma has been noted in some patients on long-term immunosuppressive treatment, particularly after a renal transplant (Straehley et al; Harwood et al). In some of these patients, remission of Kaposi's sarcoma was noted upon discontinuance of the immunosuppressive therapy (Stribling et al). It can thus be concluded that the association of lymphoma and leukemia with Kaposi's sarcoma occurs on the basis of a deficiency in cellular immunity, which is common in patients with lymphoma or leukemia (Ulbright and Santa Cruz).

Kaposi's sarcoma is a common neoplasm among blacks in sub-Sahara Africa, whereas, elsewhere in the world, it is quite rare. Also in Africa, men are predominantly affected, but often at middle age rather than advanced age, and visceral involvement, in addition to cutaneous lesions, is much more common than elsewhere (Templeton). In young children, the disease may show extensive involvement of subcutaneous lymph nodes without skin lesions. It is then rapidly fatal as the result of extensive visceral involvement. In contrast, in children who present mainly with cutaneous lesions, there is no rapid progression of the disease (Slavin et al).

A high incidence of a rapidly progressive, extensively disseminated, and quickly fatal form of Kaposi's sarcoma in young homosexual men has been noted in recent years in the United States (Gottlieb et al; Friedman-Kien). The disease in these men closely resembles the African variety of Kaposi's sarcoma. There may be few or no initial cutaneous lesions, and death usually occurs within 2 years. In both groups of patients, high serum antibody titers to cytomegalovirus have been found (Friedman-Kien). Many of the young homosexual men with Kaposi's sarcoma also have markedly elevated serum antibody titers to the Epstein–Barr virus (Friedman-Kien) and show evidence of severe acquired immunodeficiency (Siegal et al).

Histopathology.   Two types of formations occur in the lesions of Kaposi's sarcoma: vascular formations with a predominance of endothelial cells, and spindle cell formations containing vascular slits. In addition, an inflammatory reaction may be observed in early lesions, giving some of them the appearance of granulation tissue.

In early lesions resembling *granulation tissue*, the blood vessels in the dermis are dilated and increased in number (Fig. 30-10). Their endothelial cells are large and may protrude into the lumen. There is a perivascular as well as a diffuse cellular infiltrate varying in severity. It is composed of lymphoid cells, plasma cells, and some histiocytes. There also are groups of endothelial cells attempting to form new blood vessels. Frequently, one sees small groups of extravasated erythrocytes and deposits of hemosiderin. The histologic picture in the early stage thus is not always diagnostic; however, the presence of large, protruding endothelial cells, of extravasated erythrocytes, and of hemosiderin in a granulation tissue always indicates the possibility of early Kaposi's sarcoma.

The *vascular formations* often are found intermingled with spindle cell formations within the same lesion (Fig. 30-11), but they may occur by themselves, particularly in lesions of the early patch stage of Kaposi's sarcoma.

In the early patch stage, widely dilated, anastomosing, thin-walled vascular spaces with a jagged outline may be seen in the upper half of the dermis seemingly dissecting the collagen (Gange and Wilson Jones; Ackerman). They often contain no erythrocytes in their lumina, in which case they suggest lymphatic structures (Gange and Wilson Jones). The endothelial cells lining these spaces do not appear atypical and thus differ from angiosarcoma. Small, glomeruluslike bulbs that are lined by endothelial cells and bulge into the vascular spaces are frequently observed. These connective tissue bulbs may show a small capillary lumen in their center (Schwartz et al).

In plaquelike and nodular lesions, aggregates of blood vessels may be present that show proliferation of spindle-shaped cells peripheral to the layer

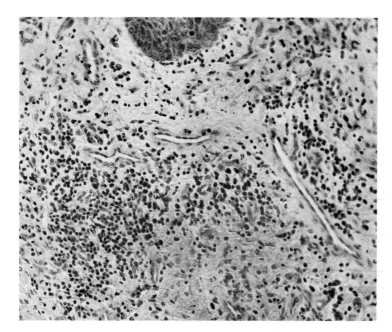

Fig. 30-10. Kaposi's sarcoma, early lesion
This early lesion resembles granulation tissue. The capillaries are dilated and increased in number, and their endothelial cells are large. A diffuse chronic inflammatory infiltrate is present. (×200)

Fig. 30-11. Kaposi's sarcoma, late lesion
On the left, spindle cell formations predominate; on the right, vascular formations are seen. (×100)

Simulants of Kaposi Histologically
Hemorrhagic Scar
Tufted angioma
Angiosiderotic Dermatofibroma

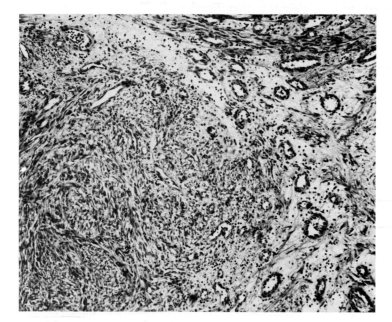

of endothelial cells (Fig. 30-12). The stroma in which the vessels are embedded usually contains extravasated erythrocytes and deposits of hemosiderin. There are also solid aggregates of endothelial cells, some of which contain elongated cells, so that it may be impossible to decide whether they are endothelial cells or spindle cells.

In addition to showing neoplastic proliferation of blood vessels, plaquelike and nodular lesions may also show neoplastic proliferations of lymph channels, resulting in formations suggestive of a lymphangioma. Considerable cystic dilatation may be seen in some of the newly formed lymphatic channels (Ronchese and Kern; Tedeschi).

In the *spindle cell formations,* one observes extensive proliferations of spindle-shaped cells lying in strands that extend irregularly in various directions (see Fig. 30-11). The elongated nuclei vary in size

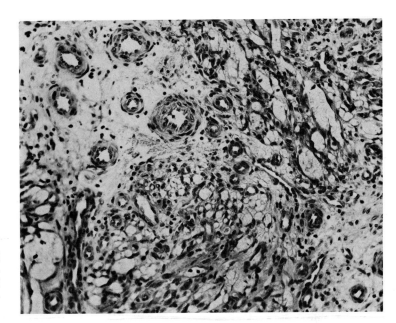

Fig. 30-12.   Kaposi's sarcoma, late lesion
There are numerous vascular lumina lined by prominent endothelial cells. Spindle-shaped cells lie peripheral to the endothelial cells. The edematous stroma contains extravasated erythrocytes. (×100)

and staining qualities, and some are atypical. Mitotic figures are present, though usually in small numbers. Thus, the histologic picture resembles that of a fibrosarcoma. One feature, however, distinguishes the spindle cell formations of Kaposi's sarcoma from fibrosarcoma: the presence among the spindle-shaped cells of narrow slits containing erythrocytes (Plate 3, facing p. 612). It is usually impossible to decide whether these slits represent newly formed capillaries with an atypical endothelial lining or whether the erythrocytes within the slits are there as a result of extravasation. Both types of formation can occur. Areas showing fairly large aggregates of erythrocytes and nearby deposits of hemosiderin can be regarded as areas of extravasation. Because of the diagnostic import of the presence of erythrocytes and hemosiderin in the tissue, staining for iron may be advisable to demonstrate deposits of hemosiderin. Granules of hemosiderin are often also seen within the spindle-shaped cells as a result of phagocytosis (Hashimoto and Lever). Although mature collagen is rarely seen within the spindle cell formations, a rather dense network of reticulum fibers is usually present (Reynolds et al).

It has not been proved that true malignant degeneration with formation of metastases ever occurs in the lesions of Kaposi's sarcoma, even though, in occasional patients with Kaposi's sarcoma, the disease has a short, fulminating course, and many of the cutaneous and visceral tumors appear anaplastic with minimal maturation toward vasoformation (Reed et al). The presence of tumor cells within pulmonary veins has been interpreted as proof of embolization and metastasis (Cox and Helwig). However, direct invasion of pulmonary veins can also produce this finding (Reynolds et al).

Histogenesis. The following three observations speak against the theory that Kaposi's sarcoma represents a true, metastasizing sarcoma and in favor of a multifocal origin of the lesions: (1) there is no primary focus that enlarges progressively; (2) some lesions regress spontaneously; and (3) histologic examination may reveal very early stages in late-appearing lesions.

The basic cell giving rise to the lesions of Kaposi's sarcoma is a vascular cell. According to this view, Kaposi's sarcoma is a multifocal angiomatosis (Becker and Thatcher; Cox and Helwig). In early electron microscopic investigations carried out around 1965, the impression was gained that two types of tumor cells were present in the lesions of Kaposi's sarcoma: proliferating endothelial cells, and proliferating pericapillary spindle cells derived from pericytes and developing into immature phagocytic fibroblasts (Hashimoto and Lever; Niemi and Mustakallio; Mottaz and Zelickson). It was noticed even then, however, that differentiation between the two types of cells was often difficult and that differences between them were in degree rather than in type. Thus, it was found that the endothelial cells lying adjacent to lumina contain only a small number of phagolysosomes with few ferritin particles, whereas the spindle cells often show several large phagolysosomes containing large aggregates of ferritin particles and, in addition, partially digested erythrocytes from which the ferritin particles are derived. On the other hand, histochemical staining for alkaline phosphatase was found to be strongly positive in the cells lying adjacent to a lumen but weak or even absent in areas of cellular proliferation (Hashimoto and Lever). In subsequent investigations, it has become apparent that the presence of a basement membrane around the proliferating cells is variable. In some instances, most of the spindle cells possess a basement membrane (Sterry et al), whereas, in others, a basement membrane surrounds spindle cell complexes as a whole but is seen only rarely around individual cells (Braun-Falco et al). It was also observed that even spindle cells may show a tendency to form capillary structures either with or without a lumen (Braun-Falco et al). Thus, it seems likely that all tumor cells are endothelial cells of different degrees of maturity or immaturity. Also, immunohistologic staining for factor-VIII-related antigen, a marker for endothelial cells, stains many cells in Kaposi's sarcoma. Although the intensity of reaction has been found to be greater in cells that line vascular channels and blood-filled clefts, many intertwining spindle cells also contain the antigen (Nadji et al).

The reason for the spindle shape of the immature endothelial cells in Kaposi's sarcoma may lie in their increased phagocytic capacity. It can be assumed that a certain number of pericytes, as well as fibroblasts, are present in the vicinity of fairly mature capillaries, but they do not participate in the neoplastic proliferation.

Differential Diagnosis.   For a discussion of differentiation of Kaposi's sarcoma from hemangiopericytoma, see p. 636; for differentiation from angiosarcoma in lymphedema, see p. 643. Pseudo-Kaposi's sarcoma, usually associated with the Klippel–Trenaunay syndrome, differs from Kaposi's sarcoma by showing no nuclear atypicality or vascular slits (see p. 624).

ANGIOSARCOMA

Angiosarcomas of the skin, also called *malignant angioendotheliomas*, are rare except for two types: (1) angiosarcoma occurring on the scalp and face of the elderly, and (2) angiosarcoma secondary to persistent chronic lymphedema, referred to as the *Stewart-Treves syndrome* (Wilson Jones, 1976). Angiosarcoma of the skin following high doses of therapeutic radiation is very rare (Maddox and Evans). A fourth type, malignant proliferating angioendotheliomatosis (see p. 645), is also very rare.

Occasional instances of fatal angiosarcoma of the skin have been described in locations other than the head, for instance, on the thigh (Girard et al), lower leg (Lambert et al), and breast (Maddox

and Evans). However, cases that have been described as low-grade angiosarcomas (Girard et al) generally are pseudoangiosarcomas. In this group are papular angioplasia (see p. 630), intravascular papillary endothelial hyperplasia (see p. 643), and angiolymphoid hyperplasia with eosinophilia (see p. 646). Even in cases of early granuloma pyogenicum, differentiation from an angiosarcoma is sometimes difficult (Girard et al).

In infants and young children, vascular tumors suggestive of angiosarcoma are invariably benign, even though they may exhibit local invasiveness and may show considerable cellularity and mitotic activity. The preferred term, therefore, is *cellular angioma of infancy* (Taxy and Gray). In some of these tumors, a histologic overlap is found with infantile hemangiopericytoma (see p. 635). So-called low-grade angiosarcomas arising in a nevus flammeus in infancy or early childhood are also clinically benign (Girard et al).

Angiosarcoma of the Scalp and Face of the Elderly

Angiosarcoma of the scalp and face of the elderly is an almost invariably fatal tumor that in many instances starts rather innocuously with erythematous or hemorrhagic macules or plaques on the scalp or, less commonly, on the face. It spreads by gradual, centrifugal infiltration, so that the greater part of the scalp and face, and often also the neck, become affected. Sooner or later, nodules and ulcerations develop. Edema of the face, especially of the eyelids, develops (Caro and Stubenrauch; Wilson Jones, 1964; Weidner and Braun-Falco). Depending on whether the tumor is predominantly a hemangiosarcoma or a lymphangiosarcoma, the involved areas show either purple blue or only slightly erythematous thickening of the skin (Bardwil et al). Metastases to the cervical lymph nodes and hematogenous metastases to the lungs, liver, and elsewhere often occur rather late, so that, in some patients, death results from the destructive ulcerations of the tumor rather than from metastases (Girard et al; Haustein). Invasion of the orbital bones (Haustein) or of the calvarium (Hori) may occur.

Histopathology.   Tumor tissue usually extends far beyond the clinically visible boundaries of the lesion (Rosai et al; Hori). A variable degree of differentiation may be seen even within the same tumor, with well-differentiated formations often present at the periphery and less differentiated areas in the heavily infiltrated, often nodular and ulcerated center (Wilson Jones, 1964; Reed et al; Bardwil et al; Girard et al; Haustein).

In well-differentiated areas, one observes irregular, often anastomosing vascular channels lined by endothelial cells that are largely single-layered and only in some places multilayered (Fig. 30-13). Such formations may easily be misdiagnosed as nonspecific granulation tissue, although, on careful study, some of the endothelial cells appear unusually large and pleomorphic, with some of them cuboidal in shape (Wilson Jones, 1964).

In less differentiated areas, the vascular spaces are lined by frankly atypical, cuboidal endothelial cells. The vascular spaces may be markedly dilated, so that they consist of tortuous sinuses into which endothelial cells proliferate as papillary projections (Figs. 30-14, 30-15) (Reed et al), or they may form several layers and completely fill the lumina (Caro and Stubenrauch).

In poorly differentiated areas, endothelial cells may be seen as invading cords between collagen bundles with only occasional small vascular lumina. In such areas, the cells may appear spindle-shaped instead of cuboidal (Caro and Stubenrauch; Wilson Jones, 1964). Elsewhere, there may be solid proliferations of more or less cuboidal endothelial cells, with poorly defined vascular spaces (Fig. 30-16) (Wilson Jones, 1976). Such solid areas of cellular proliferation may resemble malignant melanoma, in which the tumor cells often appear cuboidal (Bardwil et al).

Of considerable value in the diagnosis of angiosarcoma is the fact that the endothelial cells, even though they are variable in appearance, may be found at least in some areas as cords of cuboidal cells with rather indistinct cell boundaries between them, thus having a syncytial appearance (see Fig. 30-15) (Wilson Jones, 1964). A reticulum stain may be of definite value in identifying an angiosarcoma, because, in areas of poorly recognizable vascular lumina, a ring of reticulum outlining the basement membrane may be seen peripheral to the endothelial cells (Mach). Even solid areas of endothelial cell proliferation may show a dense network of reticulum fibers within the tumor cell complexes in some areas surrounding individual endothelial cells (Weidner and Braun-Falco; Hori).

The number of erythrocytes that are present varies. In well-differentiated areas of hemangiosarcoma, the lumina often contain numerous erythrocytes, whereas poorly differentiated areas of hemangiosarcoma, because of the immaturity of the vessels, may contain few or no erythrocytes in their lumina. However, even lymphangiosarcomas may contain some erythrocytes because of the existence of anastomoses between neoplastic lymph

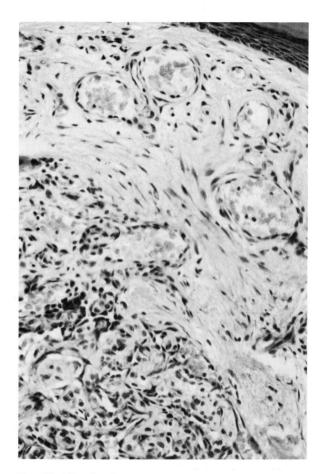

Fig. 30-13. Angiosarcoma
The tumor is fairly well differentiated in the uppermost dermis, where capillary lumina are seen. Farther down, the cells appear atypical and fill the lumina. ($\times 200$)

channels and pre-existing blood vessels secondary to blood vessel invasion (Reed et al). In addition, there are probably some tumors that are partially hemangiosarcomas and partially lymphangiosarcomas. Such a dual origin is assumed, for instance, in many cases of the Stewart–Treves syndrome (see p. 643).

Differential Diagnosis. Well-differentiated areas may at first glance suggest merely granulation tissue or a granuloma pyogenicum, but a thorough examination will reveal areas in which the endothelial cells appear atypical and are "piled up" in more than one layer. For a discussion of differentiation from hemangiopericytoma, see p. 636; for differentiation from angiolymphoid hyperplasia with eosinophilia, see p. 647. It is to be remembered that "piling up" of endothelial cells within imma-

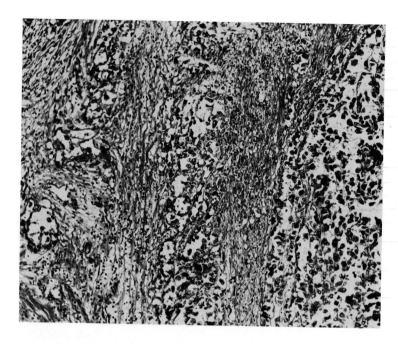

Fig. 30-14.   Angiosarcoma
Low magnification. On the left side, vascular spaces are seen infiltrating between collagen bundles. These vascular spaces, as well as a large vascular sinus on the right, are lined by atypical endothelial cells. (×100)

Fig. 30-15.   Angiosarcoma
High magnification of Figure 30-14. Cords of large, anaplastic, cuboidal endothelial cells proliferate as papillary projections within a large vascular sinus. (×400)

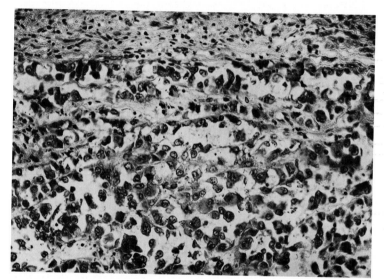

ture capillary lumina may occasionally occur in angiolymphoid hyperplasia with eosinophilia. For differentiation from intravascular papillary endothelial hyperplasia, see p. 644.

Angiosarcoma in Lymphedema (Stewart–Treves Syndrome)

The development of an angiosarcoma in an area of lymphedema was first described as postmastectomy lym-phangiosarcoma in 1948 (Stewart and Treves). It is now well recognized that cutaneous and subcutaneous nodules may develop several years after a radical mastectomy in the edematous tissue of the ipsilateral arm. The cutaneous nodules have a bluish color. They increase in number and size quite rapidly and may undergo ulceration. The clinical resemblance of the lesions to those occurring in Kaposi's sarcoma may be great. Death usually occurs within 1 to 2 years after appearance of the angiosarcoma as a result of metastases, especially to the lungs (Jessner et al; Wolff).

An angiosarcoma occasionally also arises in a chron-

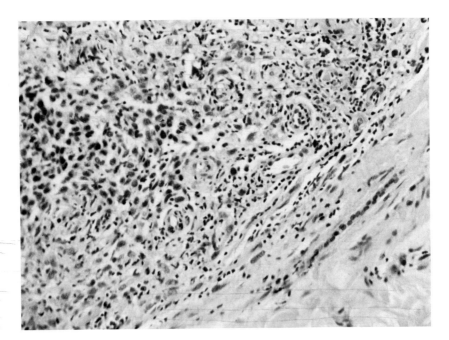

Fig. 30-16. Angiosarcoma
This poorly differentiated tumor consists largely of solid proliferations of predominantly cuboidal endothelial cells. Only a few vascular spaces are present. In the lower right corner, tumor cells are seen extending as a solid cord between collagen bundles. (×200)

ically and severely edematous extremity without a preceding tumor. Most commonly, the severe edema is congenital (Merrick et al; Laskas et al; Dubin et al). It is much less common in idiopathic lymphedema of delayed onset (Baes; Chen and Gilbert) and is rare in chronic lymphedema secondary to a filarial infection (Sordillo et al). The angiosarcoma often shows an ulcer as its first manifestation (Dubin et al), followed by the formation of nodules (Baes; Laskas et al). Although the prognosis is very poor, the best chance for long-term survival is prompt diagnosis and radical surgery (Dubin et al; Sordillo et al).

Histopathology. Angiosarcomas that develop in an edematous extremity often are particularly undifferentiated and invasive, but they generally do not differ in histologic appearance from an idiopathic angiosarcoma as seen on the scalp and face of the elderly (Wilson Jones, 1964; Reed et al; Baes). Vascular structures lined by proliferating, atypical endothelial cells are present (Jessner et al; Wolff). These angiosarcomas usually contain fewer erythrocytes than idiopathic angiosarcomas of the head, and, in some tumors developing in a chronic lymphedematous limb, no erythrocytes are seen (Dubin et al; Chen and Gilbert). Quite frequently, hyperplastic and endothelial cells are seen in clusters or infiltrating in linear strands between collagen bundles (Wolff; Laskas et al).

Histogenesis. Since the tumors arise in areas of lymphedema, it was originally thought that they were lymphangiosarcomas (Stewart and Treves). However, because of the presence of erythrocytes in some of the lumina, it is now widely thought that the tumors arise from both lymph vessels and capillaries (Jessner et al; McConnell and Haslam; Wolff; Baes). In favor of participation of blood capillaries in the formation of most tumors are also the reported presence of pericytes on electron microscopic examination (Silverberg et al) and the presence in some instances of a strongly positive reaction for alkaline phosphatase in the atypical endothelial cells (Dubin et al; Hori).

INTRAVASCULAR PAPILLARY ENDOTHELIAL HYPERPLASIA (MASSON'S PSEUDOANGIOSARCOMA)

A fairly common solitary lesion first described in 1923 (Masson), intravascular papillary endothelial hyperplasia received very little attention until 1974 (Rosai and Akerman). Since then, numerous reports have appeared. The main importance of this innocuous lesion is its histologic resemblance to and possible misinterpretation as an angiosarcoma (Salyer and Salyer).

Clinically, the lesion may or may not have the appearance of a vascular lesion. Its size can vary from 3 by 3 mm for very superficial lesions (Paslin) to 4 by 5 cm for deep-seated lesions (Kreutner et al). Most of the lesions are located in the skin or subcutaneous tissue of the head or the extremities (Kuo et al).

Histopathology. Most lesions arise within a vein, but a few have been found within a pre-existing benign vascular neoplasm, such as a venous lake (Barr et al), a granuloma pyogenicum, a cavernous hemangioma (Kuo et al), or a cavernous lymphangioma (Kuo and Gomez). In most instances, the lesion is found in association with a thrombus. Most authors therefore regard the lesion as a peculiar pattern of thrombus organization characterized by endothelialization of thrombus fragments (Salyer and Salyer; Clearkin and Enzinger; Barr et al; Kreutner et al). Occasionally, no thrombus is found, which has led some authors to believe that the lesion represents a primary endothelial proliferation with possible secondary thrombus formation (Rosai and Akerman; Kuo et al; Kuo and Gomez; Paslin). It seems most likely, however, that, in lesions without a thrombus, the endothelial hyperplasia has persisted after the thrombus has disappeared (Salyer and Salyer).

The characteristic histologic feature is the presence of irregular connective tissue stalks lined with one or, at the most, two layers of endothelial cells (Fig. 30-17). Usually, erythrocytes are seen within the irregular luminal spaces. Some of the endothelial cells may appear hyperplastic and may show hyperchromatic, somewhat pleomorphic nuclei, but there is no real nuclear atypia (Rosai and Akerman; Barr et al). In some areas, the connective tissue stalks lie widely separated and on cross sections have the appearance of irregularly shaped islands (Salyer and Salyer); in other areas, they lie closely together with so little supporting stroma that the stalks appear to be lined by multiple layers of endothelial cells (Kuo et al). In addition, endothelial cells may be found aggregated in highly cellular nodules together with small, irregular capillary lumina (Rosai and Akerman).

When such irregular endothelial proliferation is present, recognition of the intravascular location of the lesion is important for proof of the diagnosis. In some instances, all the elements of a vein wall completely surround the lesion. Quite frequently, however, only portions of the wall have remained. Identification of such remnants as the wall of a vein is best accomplished by the demonstration of fragments of the elastic lamina with the aid of an elastic tissue stain (Rosai and Akerman). Even when no vascular wall can be identified, the lesion is well circumscribed and shows no infiltrating growth (Rupec and Batzenschlager). Detection of portions of a thrombus is also helpful in the diagnosis. Even if a thrombus can no longer be found, the stalks that are lined by endothelial cells often appear fibrinous or hyalinized, suggesting that they are derived from an organized thrombus (Salyer and Salyer; Barr et al).

Differential Diagnosis. Differentiation from angiosarcoma is usually possible because of the intravascular location and the lack of significant anaplasia of the endothelial cells.

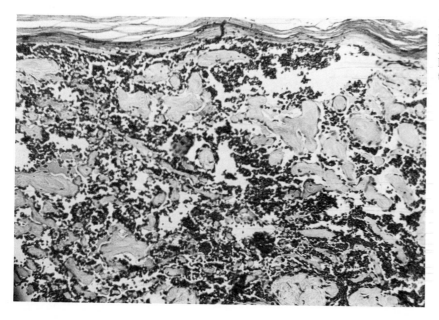

Fig. 30-17. Intravascular papillary endothelial hyperplasia Irregular connective tissue stalks are lined with a single layer of endothelial cells. (×50)

PROLIFERATING ANGIOENDOTHELIOMATOSIS

The cases that have been reported with the diagnosis of proliferating angioendotheliomatosis can be divided into a rapidly fatal neoplastic type and a benign, reactive type (Pasyk and Depowski; Martin et al; Kauh et al).

Neoplastic Proliferating Angioendotheliomatosis

Widespread erythematous or purplish patches and plaques, as well as intracutaneous and subcutaneous nodules, are present in neoplastic proliferating angioendotheliomatosis (Braverman and Lerner; Haber et al; Fievez et al; Scott et al, case 1; Kauh et al). In one patient, there were several large, ulcerating tumors as well (Midana and Ormea). Malaise, constitutional symptoms, and evidence of multisystem dysfunction exist (Martin et al). Death occurs in less than 1 year.

Histopathology. The capillaries in the cutaneous and subcutaneous lesions are dilated, and there is pronounced proliferation of the endothelial cells filling the lumina of the vessels partially or even completely (Braverman and Lerner). Many of the endothelial cells appear atypical, with hyperchromatic nuclei, often in mitosis (Fievez et al). Sub-cutaneous nodules may show a massive infiltrate of immature cells (Braverman and Lerner).

On autopsy, the blood vessels of almost every internal organ may show numerous tumor cells. Although, in some cases, the infiltrate is limited to the blood vessels (Fievez et al), in most instances extravascular extension, which may be slight, is found (Braverman and Lerner). Usually, however, an extensive extravascular neoplastic cell infiltrate composed of large, pleomorphic cells is found in many internal organs (Scott et al; Kauh et al).

Histogenesis. Electron microscopic studies have shown that the intravascular cells in the skin have the appearance of endothelial cells and, like endothelial cells, show basement membrane material on their extraluminal side (Scott et al). In view of the occurrence of extravascular lesions, however, the possibility exists that the disease represents an unusual form of lymphoma (Scott et al).

Reactive Proliferating Angioendotheliomatosis

The cutaneous lesions of the reactive type of proliferating angioendotheliomatosis resemble those of the neoplastic type, consisting of patches, plaques, and nodules (Pfleger and Tappeiner). In addition, petechiae and ecchymoses (Gottron and Nikolowski; Ruiter and Mandema; Scott et al, case 3) and small areas of necrosis are frequently observed (Gottron and Nikolowski; Pasyk and Depowski). In one case, gangrene of the lower

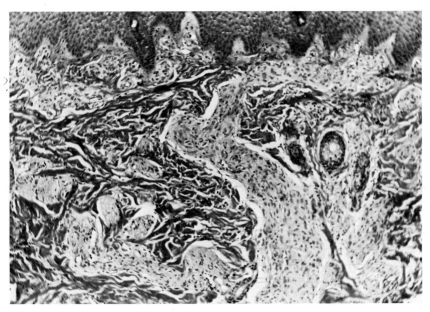

Fig. 30-18. Reactive proliferating angioendotheliomatosis
The dermal capillaries are dilated and completely filled with proliferating endothelial cells showing no atypicality. (×100) (Courtesy of Krystyna Pasyk, M.D.)

extremities developed (Abulafia et al). In some instances, the extent of the lesions is limited (Ruiter and Mandema; Pasyk and Depowski). Two patients were children (Pasyk and Depowski; Martin et al). The dermatosis usually clears within 6 to 12 months, although it may take several years (Tappeiner and Pfleger; Scott et al).

Histopathology. As in the neoplastic type, the capillaries of the dermis and subcutaneous tissue are dilated and show marked proliferation of their endothelial cells, causing occlusion of the lumen over wide areas (Fig. 30-18). In addition, fibrin thrombi may be seen. Whereas the endothelial cells show no signs of atypicality in some cases (Gottron and Nikolowski; Ruiter and Mandema; Pasyk and Depowski), they have shown a slight degree of apparent atypicality in others (Abulafia et al; Martin et al); rarely, there even is significant apparent atypicality (Pfleger and Tappeiner). Thus, on a histopathologic basis, differentiation of the reactive type from the neoplastic type is not always possible (Martin et al).

ANGIOLYMPHOID HYPERPLASIA WITH EOSINOPHILIA

Solitary or, more commonly, multiple nodules located intradermally or subcutaneously or both are seen in angiolymphoid hyperplasia usually on the head of young adults and rarely elsewhere (Mehregan and Shapiro). Whereas the dermal lesions usually measure less than 1 cm in size, the subcutaneous lesions may attain a size of 5 cm to 10 cm (Inada et al). The nodules are often quite persistent and may even gradually increase in number, but, in some instances, they ultimately resolve spontaneously (Wilson Jones and Bleehen; Reed and Terazakis; Baler). Significant eosinophilia in the peripheral blood is only occasionally present (Mehregan and Shapiro; Grimwood et al).

The subcutaneous nodules were described originally in 1948 by Kimura as eosinophilic lymphfolliculosis of the skin (Inada et al) and in 1969 as subcutaneous angiolymphoid hyperplasia with eosinophilia (Wells and Whimster). The dermal nodules were also first described in 1969 under the designation pseudogranuloma pyogenicum (Wilson Jones and Bleehen). Soon, however, it became apparent that the two represent the same disease process taking place at different tissue levels (Kandil) and that patients can have dermal and subcutaneous nodules simultaneously (Mehregan and Shapiro; Reed and Terazakis).

Histopathology. Histologically, the lesion has a vascular and a cellular component. The vascular component consists predominantly of irregularly shaped capillaries with greatly swollen, pleomorphic endothelial cells that protrude into the lumen and sometimes occlude it. The endothelial layer often appears to be two or three cells thick (Fig. 30-19) (Wilson Jones and Bleehen). One may also see cords and buds of endothelial cells, some of which show small, central lumina (Mehregan and Shapiro). In addition, there are often thick-walled vessels with a muscular coat. In some cases,

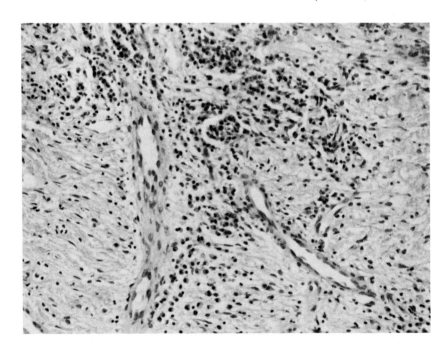

Fig. 30-19. Angiolymphoid hyperplasia with eosinophilia
The capillaries are lined by greatly swollen, pleomorphic endothelial cells that protrude into the lumen. In some areas, the endothelial cells seem to form several layers. There is a pronounced cellular infiltrate containing many eosinophils. (×200)

A.L.H.
Papular *Angioplesia*
A.L.H
P.P.G (Pseudo pyogenic gran.)
Soft. Tissue Tumor
"histiocytoid" hemangioma

these vessels have the appearance of small arteries because of the presence of an internal elastic lamina (Reed and Terazakis; Olsen and Helwig); in other cases, no internal elastic lamina is seen, indicating that they probably are venules (Vázquez and Sánchez).

The cellular component consists of an extensive cellular infiltrate of lymphocytes, histiocytes, and numerous eosinophils. Although eosinophils usually are prominent in the infiltrate, they may be few in number and can even be absent (Burrall et al). In about 40% of the cases, particularly those with subcutaneous nodules, lymphoid follicles with follicular centers can be identified (Wells and Whimster; Mehregan and Shapiro; Inada et al; Olsen and Helwig).

Histogenesis. It is likely that the proliferation of endothelial cells in angiolymphoid hyperplasia is an inflammatory reactive rather than a neoplastic process. Direct immunofluorescence has shown deposits of immunoglobulin A (IgA), IgM, and the third component of complement (C3) around many of the small vessels of the lesions, suggesting that the vascular proliferations represent an immunologic phenomenon (Grimwood et al).

Differential Diagnosis.   The proliferation of large endothelial cells and immature blood vessels may suggest the possibility of an angiosarcoma. However, the latter occurs largely on the scalp and face of elderly persons. The young age of most of the patients with angiolymphoid hyperplasia, the nodular character of the lesions, and the common presence of tissue eosinophilia help in the differentiation of angiolymphoid hyperplasia from angiosarcoma.

BIBLIOGRAPHY

Congenital Hemangiomas

BARSKY SH, ROSEN S, GEER DE et al: The nature and evolution of port wine stains. J Invest Dermatol 74:154–157, 1980

BEAN WB: Dyschondroplasia and hemangiomata (Maffucci's syndrome). Arch Intern Med 95:767–778, 1955

BEAN WB: Vascular Spiders and Related Lesions of the Skin, pp 178–185. Springfield, IL, Charles C Thomas, 1958

BLUEFARB SM: Sturge-Weber syndrome. Arch Dermatol Syph 59:531–541, 1949

BLUEFARB SM, ADAMS LA: Arteriovenous malformation with angiodermatitis. Arch Dermatol 96:176–181, 1967

BOWERS RE, GRAHAM EA, TOMLINSON KA: The natural history of the strawberry nevus. Arch Dermatol 82:667–680, 1960

DEFAUW J: Hypertension veineuse et hypertrophie des extrémités. Arch Belg Dermatol Syph 19:11–13, 1963

EARHART RN, AELING JA, NUSS DD et al: Pseudo-Kaposi Sarcoma. Arch Dermatol 110:907–910, 1974

FINLEY JL, BARSKY SH, GEER DE et al: Healing of port-wine stains from argon laser therapy. Arch Dermatol 117:486–489, 1981

FRETZIN DF, POTTER B: Blue rubber bleb nevus. Arch Intern Med 116:924–929, 1965

INCEMAN S, YUCEL T: Chronic defibrination syndrome due to a giant hemangioma associated with microangiopathic hemolytic anemia. Am J Med 46:997–1002, 1969

KASABACH HH, MERRITT KK: Capillary hemangioma with extensive purpura. Report of a case. Ann J Dis Child 59:1063–1070, 1940

KUZMA JF, KING JM: Dyschondroplasia with hemangiomatosis (Maffucci's syndrome) and teratoid tumor of the ovary. Arch Pathol 46:74–82, 1948

LANG PG, DUBIN HV: Hemangioma-thrombocytopenia syndrome. Arch Dermatol 111:105–107, 1975

LINDENAUER SM: The Klippel-Trenaunay syndrome: Varicosities, hypertrophy and hemangioma with no arteriovenous fistula. Ann Surg 162:303–314, 1965

MIESCHER G: Uber plane Angiome (Naevi hyperaemici). Dermatologica 106:176–193, 1953

MULLINS JF, LIVINGOOD CS: Maffucci's syndrome (dyschondroplasia with hemangiomas). Arch Dermatol 63:478–482, 1951

MULLINS JF, NAYLOR D, REDETZKI J: The Klippel-Trenaunay-Weber syndrome. Arch Dermatol 86:202–206, 1962

NAKAYAMA H: Clinical and histological studies of the classification and the natural course of the strawberry mark. J Dermatol (Tokyo) 8:277–291, 1981

PERSON JR, PERRY HO: Recent advances in the phacomatoses. Int J Dermatol 17:1–13, 1978

RICE JS, FISCHER DS: Blue rubber-bleb nevus syndrome. Arch Dermatol 86:503–511, 1962

ROSEN T, MARTIN S, STERN JK: Radionuclide scanning in pseudo-Kaposi's sarcoma. Arch Dermatol 115:747–748, 1979

SUKURANE HF, SUGAI T, SAITO T: The association of the blue rubber bleb nevus and Maffucci's syndrome, Arch Dermatol 95:28–36, 1968

SCHNYDER UW: Zur Klinik und Histologie der Angiome. 2. Mitteilung: Die Feuermäler (Naevi teleangiectatici). Arch Dermatol Syph (Berlin) 198:51–75, 1954

SCHNYDER UW: Zur Klinik und Histologie der Angiome. 4. Mitteilung: Die planotuberösen und tuberonodösen Angiome des Kleinkindes. Arch Klin Exp Dermatol 204:457–471, 1957

STEINWAY DM, FRETZIN DF: Acquired zosteriform cavernous hemangioma. Arch Dermatol 113:848–849, 1977

STRAUB PW, KESSLER S, SCHREIBER A et al: Chronic intravascular coagulation in Kasabach-Merritt syndrome. Arch Intern Med 129:475–478, 1972

WALSH TS JR, TOMPKINS VN: Some observations on the strawberry nevus of infancy. Cancer 9:869–904, 1956

WILKIN JK: Unilateral dermatomal cavernous hemangiomatosis. Dermatologica 161:347–354, 1980

WILSON CJ, HAGGARD ME: Giant vascular tumors and thrombocytopenia. Arch Dermatol 81:432–437, 1960

Angiokeratoma

AGGER P, OSMUNDSEN PE: Angiokeratoma of the scrotum (Fordyce). Acta Dermatol Vener (Stockh) 50:221–224, 1970

BRUCE DH: Angiokeratoma circumscriptum and angiokeratoma scroti. Arch Dermatol 81:388–393, 1960

DAMMERT K: Angiokeratosis naeviformis, a form of naevus telangiectaticus lateralis (naevus flammeus). Dermatologica 130:17–39, 1965

FISCHER H, FRIEDERICH HC: Angiokeratoma corporis circumscriptum naeviforme mit Venektasien und Osteohypertrophie. Dermatol Wochenschr 151:297–306, 1965

GOLDMAN L, GIBSON SH, RICHFIELD DF: Thrombotic angiokeratoma circumscriptum simulating melanoma. Arch Dermatol 117:138–139, 1981

HAYE KR, REBELLO DJA: Angiokeratoma of Mibelli. Acta Derm Venereol (Stockh) 41:56–60, 1961

IMPERIAL R, HELWIG EB: Angiokeratoma. Arch Dermatol 95:166–175, 1967a

IMPERIAL R, HELWIG EB: Verrucous hemangioma. Arch Dermatol 96:247–253, 1967b

JESSEN RT, THOMPSON S, SMITH EB: Cobb syndrome. Arch Dermatol 113:1587–1590, 1977

JOHNSON WC: Pathology of cutaneous vascular tumors. (Review) Int J Dermatol 15:239–270 (1976)

KNOTH W, KNOTH-BORN RC, BOERGEN G: Über das Angiokeratoma corporis circumscriptum naeviforme der Stammhaut. Hautarzt 14:452–462, 1963

LYNCH PJ, KOSANOVICH M: Angiokeratoma circumscriptum. Arch Dermatol 96:665–668, 1967

MAEKAWA Y, ARAO T: A case of angiokeratoma corporis circumscriptum neviforme. J Dermatol (Tokyo) 2:15–18, 1975

ZALA L, MUMENTHALER M: Cobb Syndrom. Dermatologica 163:417–425, 1981

Venous (Arteriovenous) Hemangioma

BIBERSTEIN HH, JESSNER M: A cirsoid aneurysm in the skin. Dermatologica 113:129–141, 1956

CARAPETO FJ, GARCIA-PEREZ A, WINKELMANN RK: Acral arteriovenous tumor. Acta Derm Venereol (Stockh) 57:155–158, 1977

GIRARD C, GRAHAM JH, JOHNSON WC: Arteriovenous hemangioma (arteriovenous shunt). J Cutan Pathol 1:73–83, 1974

WADE TR, KAMINO H, ACKERMAN AB: A histologic atlas of vascular lesions. J Dermatol Surg Oncol 4:845–850, 1978

Generalized Essential Telangiectasis

GENTELE H, LODIN A: Telangiectasia essentialis generalisata of unknown origin. Acta Derm Venereol (Stockh) 37:465–470, 1957

MCGRAE JD JR, WINKELMANN RK: Generalized essential telangiectasia. JAMA 185:909–913, 1963

Unilateral Nevoid Telangiectasia

ANDERTON RL, SMITH JG JR: Unilateral nevoid telangiectasia with gastric involvement. Arch Dermatol 111:617–621, 1975

WILKIN JK: Unilateral nevoid telangiectasia. Arch Dermatol 113:486–488, 1977

Angioma Serpiginosum

BARKER LP, SACHS PM: Angioma serpiginosum. Arch Dermatol 92:613–620, 1965

CHAVAZ P, LAUGIER P: Angiome serpigineux de Hutchinson. Ann Dermatol Venereol 108:429–436, 1981

FRAIN-BELL W: Angioma serpiginosum. Br J Dermatol 69:251–268, 1957

KUMAKIRI M, KATOH N, MIURA Y: Angioma serpiginosum. J Cutan Pathol 7:410–421, 1980

MARRIOTT PJ, MUNRO O, RYAN T: Angioma serpiginosum. Br J Dermatol 93:701–706, 1975

Hereditary Hemorrhagic Telangiectasia (Osler's Disease)

CHANDLER D: Pulmonary and cerebral arteriovenous fistula with Osler's disease. Arch Intern Med 116:277–282, 1965

DALY JJ, SCHILLER AL: The liver in hereditary hemorrhagic telangiectasia (Osler-Weber-Rendu disease). Am J Med 60:723–726, 1976

HASHIMOTO K, PRITZKER MS: Hereditary hemorrhagic telangiectasia. An electron microscopic study. Oral Surg 34:751–768, 1972

LAUGIER P: Les manifestations digestives de la maladie de Rendu-Osler. Ann Dermatol Venereol 105:1055–1058, 1978

MUGGIA FM: Osler's disease with an aortic arch aneurysm. Arch Intern Med 114:307–310, 1964

SMITH CR JR, BARTHOLOMEW LG, CAIN JC: Hereditary hemorrhagic telangiectasia and gastrointestinal hemorrhage. Gastroenterology 44:1–6, 1963

WALLER JD, GREENBERG JH, LEWIS CW: Hereditary hemorrhagic telangiectasia with cerebrovascular malformations. Arch Dermatol 112:49–52, 1976

Nevus Araneus

BEAN WB: The arterial spider and similar lesions of the skin and mucous membranes. Circulation 8:117–129, 1953

SCHUHMACHERS-BRENDLER R: Beitrag zur morphologischen Pathologie und Therapie des Naevus-araneus-Rezidivs. Dermatol Wochenschr 139:167–174, 1959

WHITING DA, KALLMEYER JC, SIMSON IW: Widespread arterial spiders in a case of latent hepatitis, with resolution after therapy. Br J Dermatol 82:32–36, 1970

Granuloma Pyogenicum

COSKEY RJ, MEHREGAN AH: Granuloma pyogenicum with multiple satellite recurrences. Arch Dermatol 96:71–73, 1967

DAVIES MG, BARTON SP, ATAI F et al: The abnormal dermis in pyogenic granuloma. J Am Acad Dermatol 2:132–142, 1980

JUHLIN L, HJERSTQUIST SO, PONTEN J et al: Disseminated granuloma pyogenicum. Acta Derm Venereol (Stockh) 50:134–136, 1970

LEYDEN JL, MASTER GH: Oral cavity pyogenic granuloma. Arch Dermatol 108:226–228, 1973

MARSCH WC: The ultrastructure of eruptive hemangioma ("pyogenic granuloma"). (Abstr) J Cutan Pathol 8:144–145, 1981

NÖDL F: Das "sogenannte" Granuloma teleangiektaticum. Z Hautkr 19:163–167, 1955

OEHLSCHLAEGEL G, MÜLLER E: Zum Granuloma pyogenicum sive teleangiektaticum als Sonderfall des capillären Hämangioms. Arch Klin Exp Dermatol 218:126–157, 1964

WARNER J, WILSON JONES E: Pyogenic granuloma recurring with multiple satellites. Br J Dermatol 80:218–227, 1968

ZAYNOUN ST, JULJULIAN HH, KURBAN AK: Pyogenic granuloma with multiple satellites. Arch Dermatol 109:689–691, 1974

Cherry Hemangioma

ŠALAMON T, LAZOVIĆ O, MILIČEĆIC M: Über einige histologische Befunde bei dem sogenannten Angioma senile. Dermatol Monatsschr 159:1021–1028, 1973

SCHNYDER UW, KELLER R: Zur Klinik und Histologie der Angiome. III. Mitteilung. Zur Histologie und Pathogenese der senilen Angiome. Arch Dermatol Syph (Berlin) 198:333–342, 1954

Papular Angioplasia

PETERSON WC JR, FUSARO RM, GOLTZ RW: Atypical pyogenic granuloma. Arch Dermatol 90:197–201, 1964

WILSON JONES E, MARKS R: Papular angioplasia. Arch Dermatol 102:422–427, 1970

WINER LH, LEVIN GH: Acquired vascular tumors of the skin in the adult. Arch Dermatol 79:17–31, 1959

Venous Lakes

BEAN WB, WALSH JR: Venous lakes. Arch Dermatol 74:459–463, 1956

Thrombosed Capillary or Vein

EPSTEIN E, NOVY FG JR, ALLINGTON HV: Capillary aneurysms of the skin. Arch Dermatol 91:335–341, 1965

HAYEN DO: Thrombosed angiokeratoma simulating malignant melanoma. Arch Dermatol 93:358–361, 1966

WEATHERS DR, FINE RM: Thrombosed varix of oral cavity. Arch Dermatol 104:427–430, 1971

WEINER MA: Capillary aneurysms of the skin. Arch Dermatol 93:670–673, 1966

Lymphangioma

BURSTEIN JH: Lymphangioma circumscriptum with congenital unilateral lymphedema. Arch Dermatol 74:689–690, 1956

FISHER I, ORKIN M: Acquired lymphangioma (lymphangiectasis). Arch Dermatol 101:230–234, 1970

FLANAGAN BP, HELWIG EB: Cutaneous lymphangioma. Arch Dermatol 113:24–30, 1977

PALMER LC, STRAUCH WG, WELTON WA: Lymphangioma circumscriptum. A case with deep lymphatic involvement. Arch Dermatol 114:394–396, 1978

PEACHEY RDG, LIM CC, WHIMSTER IW: Lymphangioma of skin. Br J Dermatol 83:519–527, 1970

PLOTNICK H, RICHFIELD, D: Tuberous lymphangiectatic varices secondary to radical mastectomy. Arch Dermatol 74:466–468, 1956

PRIOLEAU PG, SANTA CRUZ DJ: Lymphangioma circumscriptum following radical mastectomy and radiation therapy. Cancer 42:1989–1991, 1978

WHIMSTER IW: The pathology of lymphangioma circumscriptum. Br J Dermatol 94:473–486, 1976

Glomus Tumor

CHANDON JP, DE MICCO C, LEBREUIL G et al: Blue rubber bleb naevus et glomangiomatose. Unicité ou dualité? Ann Dermatol Venereol 105:123–130, 1978

FINE RM, DERBES VJ, CLARK WH JR: Blue rubber bleb nevus. Arch Dermatol 84:802–805, 1961

GOODMAN TF: Fine structure of the cells of the Suquet-Hoyer canal. J Invest Dermatol 59:363–369, 1972

GOODMAN TF, ABELE DC: Multiple glomus tumors. A clinical and electron microscopic study. Arch Dermatol 103:11–23, 1971

GORDON B, HYMAN AB: Multiple non-tender glomus tumors. Arch Dermatol 83:640–643, 1961

GUPTA RK, GILBERT EF, ENGLISH RS: Multiple painful glomus tumors of the skin. Arch Dermatol 92:670–673, 1965

ISHIBASHI Y, IKEDA S, KAWAMURA T: Multiple, schmerzhafte Glomustumoren. Jpn J Dermatol (Series B) 78:274–286, 1968

LAYMON CW, PETERSON WC JR: Glomangioma (glomus tumor). Arch Dermatol 92:509–513, 1965

LÜDERS G, SCHLOTE W, REINHARD M: Zur Ultrastruktur von Glomustumoren und Glomusorganen. Arch Klin Exp Dermatol 238:398–416, 1970

MCEVOY BF, WALDMAN PM, TYE MJ: Multiple hamartomatous glomus tumors of the skin. Arch Dermatol 104:188–191, 1971

MUKHTAR JAK, PFLEGER L: Angiomatosis cutis disseminata (Beziehungen zum Blue Rubber Bleb Nevus). Hautarzt 15:230–235, 1964

MURAD TM, VON HAAM E, MURTHY MSN: Ultrastructure of a hemangiopericytoma and a glomus tumor. Cancer 22:1239–1249, 1968

RYCROFT RJG, MENTER MA, SHARVILL DE et al: Hereditary multiple glomus tumors. Trans St John's Hosp Dermatol Soc 61:70–81, 1975

SCHNYDER UW: Über Glomustumoren. Dermatologica 131:83–88, 1965

SHUGART RR, SOULE EH, JOHNSON EW JR: Glomus tumor. Surg Gynecol Obstet 117:334–340, 1963

TARNOWSKI WM, HASHIMOTO K: Multiple glomus tumors. J Invest Dermatol 52:474–478, 1969

Hemangiopericytoma

ALTMEYER P, NÖDL F: Das Hämangioperizytom des Säuglings. Hautarzt 27:272–276, 1976

BATTIFORA H: Hemangiopericytoma. Ultrastructural study of five cases. Cancer 31:1412–1432, 1973

BIANCHI O, ABULAFIA J, MIRANDE L: Hémangiopéricytome cutané. Ann Dermatol Syph 95:269–284, 1968

COLE HN JR, REAGAN JW, LUND HZ: Hemangiopericytoma. Arch Dermatol 72:328–334, 1955

EIMOTO T: Ultrastructure of an infantile hemangiopericytoma. Cancer 40:2161–2170, 1977

ENZINGER FM, SMITH BH: Hemangiopericytoma. An analysis of 106 cases. Hum Pathol 7:61–82, 1976

FORRESTER JS, HOUSTON RA: Hemangiopericytoma with metastases. Arch Pathol 51:651–657, 1951

HAHN MJ, DAWSON R, ESTERLY JA et al: Hemangiopericytoma, an ultrastructural study. Cancer 31:255–261, 1973

HOLLMANN G, HÖPNER F, DAUM R et al: Beitrag zur Klinik des Hämangiopericytoms. Langenbecks Arch Chir 330:128–139, 1971

KUHN C III ROSAI J: Tumors arising from pericytes. Arch Pathol 88:653–663, 1969

LATTES, R: Quoted by Kuhn C III, Rosai J: Tumors arising from pericytes. Arch Pathol 88:653–663, 1969

MCMASTER MJ, SOULE EH, IVINS JC: Hemangiopericytoma. A clinicopathologic study and long-term follow-up of 60 patients. Cancer 36:2232–2244, 1975

MEADE JB, WHITWELL F, BICKFORD BJ et al: Primary hemangiopericytoma of the lung. Thorax 29:1–15, 1974

MURAD TM, VON HAAM E, MURTHY MSN: Ultrastructure of a hemangiopericytoma and a glomus tumor. Cancer 22:1239–1249, 1968

NUNNERY EW, KAHN LB, REDDICK RL et al: Hemangiopericytoma: A light microscopic and ultrastructural study. Cancer 47:906–914, 1981

O'BRIEN P, BRASFIELD RD: Hemangiopericytoma. Cancer 18:249–252, 1965

RAMSEY HJ: Fine structure of hemangiopericytoma and hemangioendothelioma. Cancer 19:2005–2018, 1966

REICH H: Das Hämangiopericytom. Arch Klin Exp Dermatol 202:390–397, 1956

REICH H: Das Hämangiopericytom. Hautarzt 24:275–285, 1973

SCHNEIDER W, UNDEUTSCH W: Seltene Blutgefässgeschwülste der Haut. Hautarzt 18:437–445, 1967

SIMS CF, KIRSCH N, MACDONALD RG: Hemangiopericytoma. Arch Dermatol Syph 58:194–205, 1948

STOUT AP: Hemangiopericytoma. Cancer 2:1047–1054, 1949

STOUT AP: Discussion in Cole HN Jr, Reagan JW, Lund HZ: Hemangiopericytoma. Arch Dermatol 72:328–334, 1955

STOUT AP, MURRAY MR: Hemangiopericytoma: A vascular tumor featuring Zimmermann's pericytes. Ann Surg 116:26–33, 1942

WEBER K, BRAUN-FALCO O: Ultrastructure of blood vessels in human granulation tissue. Arch Derm Forsch 248:29–44, 1973

Kaposi's Sarcoma

ACKERMAN AB: The patch stage of Kaposi's sarcoma. Am J Dermatopathol 1:165–172, 1979

AMAZON K, RYWLIN AM: Lymph node involvement in Kaposi's sarcoma. Am J Dermatopathol 1:173–176, 1979

ANTHONY CW, KONEMAN EW: Visceral Kaposi's sarcoma. Arch Pathol 70:740–746, 1960

BECKER SW, THATCHER HW: Multiple idiopathic hemorrhagic sarcoma of Kaposi. J Invest Dermatol 1:379–398, 1938

BRAUN-FALCO O, SCHMOECKEL C, HÜBNER G: Zur Histogenese des Sarcoma idiopathicum multiplex haemorrhagicum (Morbus Kaposi). Virchows Arch (Pathol Anat) 369:215–227, 1976

COX JW, HALPRIN K, ACKERMAN AB: Kaposi's sarcoma localized to the penis. Arch Dermatol 102:461–462, 1970

COX FH, HELWIG EB: Kaposi's sarcoma. (Review) Cancer 12:289–298, 1959

DUPERRAT B, PACOT C: Les adénopathies kaposiennes. Ann Dermatol Syph 91:241–254, 1965

ECKLUND RE, VALAITIS J: Kaposi's sarcoma of lymph nodes. Arch Pathol 74:224–229, 1962

FEUERMAN EJ, POTRUCH-EISENKRAFT S: Kaposi's sarcoma. Dermatologica 146:115–122, 1973

FRIEDMAN-KIEN AE: Disseminated Kaposi's sarcoma syndrome in young homosexual men. J Am Acad Dermatol 5:468–471, 1981

GANGE RW, WILSON JONES E: Lymphangioma-like Kaposi's sarcoma. Br J Dermatol 100:327–334, 1979

GOTTLIEB GJ, RYWLIN AM, RAGAZ A et al: A preliminary communication on extensively disseminated Kaposi's sarcoma in young homosexual men. Am J Dermatopathol 3:111–114, 1981

HARWOOD AR, OSOBA D, HOFSTADER SL et al: Kaposi's sarcoma in recipients of renal transplant. Am J Med 67:759–765, 1979

HASHIMOTO K, LEVER WF: Kaposi's sarcoma. Histochemical and electron microscopic studies. J Invest Dermatol 43:539–549, 1964

MOTTAZ JH, ZELICKSON AS: Electron microscopic observations of Kaposi's sarcoma. Acta Derm Venereol (Stockh) 46:195–200, 1966

NADJI M, MORALES AR, ZIEGLES-WEISSMAN J et al: Kaposi's sarcoma. Immunohistologic evidence for an endothelial origin. Arch Pathol 105:274–275, 1981

NIEMI M, MUSTAKALLIO KK: The fine structure of the spindle cell in Kaposi's sarcoma. Acta Pathol Microbiol Scand 63:567–575, 1965

O'BRIEN PH, BRASFIELD RD: Kaposi's sarcoma. Cancer 19:1497–1502, 1966

REED WB, KAMATH HM, WEISS L: Kaposi's sarcoma, with emphasis on the internal manifestations. Arch Dermatol 110:115–118, 1974

REYNOLDS WA, WINKELMANN RK, SOULE EH: Kaposi's sarcoma. (Review) Medicine (Baltimore) 44:419–443, 1965

RONCHESE F, KERN AB: Lymphangioma-like tumors in Kaposi's sarcoma. Arch Dermatol 75:418–428, 1957

SCHWARTZ RA, BURGESS GH, HOSHAW RA: Patch stage Kaposi's sarcoma. J Am Acad Dermatol 2:509–512, 1980

SIEGAL FP, LOPEZ C, HAMMER GS et al: Severe acquired immunodeficiency in male homosexuals, manifested by chronic perianal ulcerative herpes simplex lesions. N Engl J Med 305:1439–1444, 1981

SLAVIN G, CAMERON HM, FORBES C et al: Kaposi's sarcoma in East African children. J Pathol 100:187–199, 1970

STERRY W, STEIGLEDER GK, BODEUX E: Kaposi's sarcoma: Venous capillary haemangioblastoma. Arch Dermatol Res 266:253–267, 1979

STRAEHLEY CJ III, SANTOS JI, DOWNEY DM et al: Kaposi's sarcoma in a renal transplant recipient. Arch Pathol 99:611–613, 1975

STRIBLING J, WEITZNER S, SMITH GV: Kaposi's sarcoma in renal allograft recipients. Cancer 42:442–446, 1978

TEDESCHI CG: Some considerations concerning the nature of the so-called sarcoma of Kaposi. Arch Pathol 66:656–684, 1958

TEDESCHI CG, FOLSOM HF, CARNICELLI TJ: Visceral Kaposi's disease. Arch Pathol 43:335–357, 1947

TEMIME P, STAHL A, BERARD-BADIER M: The visceral lesions of Kaposi's disease. Br J Dermatol 73:303–309, 1961

TEMPLETON AC: Studies in Kaposi's sarcoma. Cancer 30:854–867, 1972

ULBRIGHT TM, SANTA CRUZ DJ: Kaposi's sarcoma: Relationship with hematologic, lymphoid and thymic neoplasia. Cancer 47:963–973, 1981

Angiosarcoma, Stewart–Treves Syndrome

BAES H: Angiosarcoma in a chronic lymphedematous leg. Dermatologica 134:331–336, 1967

BARDWIL JM, MOCEGA EE, BUTLER JJ et al: Angiosarcomas of the head and neck region. Am J Surg 116:548–553, 1968

CARO MR, STUBENRAUCH CH JR: Hemangioendothelioma of the skin. Arch Dermatol Syph 51:295–304, 1945

CHEN KTK, GILBERT EF: Angiosarcoma complicating generalized lymphangiectasia. Arch Pathol 103:86–88, 1979

DUBIN HV, CREEHAN EP, HEADINGTON JT: Lymphangiosarcoma and congenital lymphedema of the extremity. Arch Dermatol 110:608–614, 1974

GIRARD C, JOHNSON WC, GRAHAM JH: Cutaneous angiosarcoma. (Review) Cancer 26:868–883, 1970

JESSNER M, ZAK FG, REIN CR: Angiosarcoma in postmastectomy lymphedema (Stewart-Treves syndrome). Arch Dermatol Syph 65:123–129, 1952

HAUSTEIN UF: Angioplastisches Sarkom der Kopfhaut. Dermatol Monatsschr 160:399–408, 1974

HORI Y: Malignant hemangioendothelioma of the skin. J Dermatol Surg Oncol 7:130–136, 1981

LAMBERT D, JUSTRABO E, KNOPF JF et al: Hémangio-endothéliosarcomes cutanés. Ann Dermatol Venereol 104:549–556, 1977

LASKAS JJ JR, SHELLEY WB, WOOD MG: Lymphangiosarcoma arising in congenital lymphedema. Arch Dermatol 111:86–89, 1975

MACH K: Zur Frage des Lymphangioendothelioms. Arch Klin Exp Dermatol 226:318–326, 1966

MADDOX JC, EVANS HL: Angiosarcoma of skin and soft tissue. Cancer 48:1907–1921, 1981

MCCONNELL EM, HASLAM P: Angiolymphoid hyperplasia with eosinophilia. Br J Surg 46:322–332, 1959

MERRICK TA, ERLANDSON RA, HAJDU SJ: Lymphangiosarcoma of a congenitally lymphedematous arm. Arch Pathol 91:365–371, 1971

REED RJ, PALOMEQUE FE, HAIRSTON MA III et al: Lymphangiosarcomas of the scalp. Arch Dermatol 94:396–402, 1966

ROSAI J, SUMNER HW, KOSTIANOVSKY M et al: Angiosarcoma of the skin. Hum Pathol 7:83–109, 1976

SILVERBERG SG, KAY S, KOSS LG: Postmastectomy lymphangiosarcoma: Ultrastructural observations. Cancer 27:100–108, 1971

SORDILLO EM, SORDILLO PP, HAJDU SI et al: Lymphangiosarcoma after filarial infection. J Dermatol Surg Oncol 7:235–239, 1981

STEWART FW, TREVES N: Lymphangiosarcoma in postmastectomy lymphedema. Cancer 1:64–81, 1948

TAXY JB, GRAY SR: Cellular angiomas of infancy. Cancer 43:2322–2331, 1979

WEIDNER F, BRAUN-FALCO O: Über das angioplastische Reticulosarkom der Kopfhaut bei älteren Menschen. Hautarzt 21:60–66, 1970

WILSON JONES E: Malignant angioendothelioma of the skin. Br J Dermatol 76:21–39, 1964

WILSON JONES E: Malignant vascular tumors. (Review) Clin Exp Dermatol 1:287–312, 1976

WOLFF K: Das Stewart-Treves-Syndrom. Arch Klin Exp Dermatol 216:468–496, 1963

Intravascular Papillary Endothelial Hyperplasia (Masson's Pseudoangiosarcoma)

BARR RJ, GRAHAM JH, SHERWIN LA: Intravascular papillary endothelial hyperplasia. Arch Dermatol 114:723–726, 1978

CLEARKIN KP, ENZINGER FM: Intravascular papillary endothelial hyperplasia. Arch Pathol 100:441–444, 1976

KREUTNER A JR, SMITH RM, TREFNY FA: Intravascular papillary endothelial hyperplasia. Cancer 42:2304–2310, 1978

KUO TT, GOMEZ LG: Papillary endothelial proliferation in cystic lymphangioma. Arch Pathol 103:306–308, 1979

KUO TT, SAYERS P, ROSAI J: Masson's "vegetant intravascular hemangioendothelioma": A lesion often mistaken for angiosarcoma. Cancer 38:1227–1236, 1976

MASSON P: Hémangioendothéliome végétant intravasculaire. Bull Soc Anat 93:517–523, 1923

PASLIN DA: Localized primary cutaneous intravascular papillary endothelial hyperplasia. J Am Acad Dermatol 4:316–318, 1981

ROSAI J, AKERMAN LR: Intravascular atypical vascular proliferation. Arch Dermatol 109:714–717, 1974

RUPEC M, BATZENSCHLAGER I: Pseudoangiosarkom (Masson). Z Hautkr 56:1360–1363, 1981

SALYER WR, SALYER DC: Intravascular angiomatosis: Development and distinction from angiosarcoma. Cancer 36:995–1001, 1979

Proliferating Angioendotheliomatosis

ABULAFIA J, CIGORRAGA J, SALIVA J et al: Angioendoteliomatosis proliferante sistémica (Pfleger y Tappeiner). Dermatol Ibero Lat Am 11:23–40, 1969

BRAVERMAN IM, LERNER AB: Diffuse malignant proliferation of vascular endothelium. Arch Dermatol 84:22–30, 1961

FIEVEZ M, FIEVEZ C, HUSTIN J: Proliferating systematized angioendotheliomatosis. Arch Dermatol 104:320–324, 1971

GOTTRON HA, NIKOLOWSKI W: Extrarenale Löhlein Herdnephritis der Haut bei Endocarditis. Arch Klin Exp Dermatol 207:156–176, 1958

HABER H, HARRIS-JONES JN, WELLS AL: Intravascular endothelioma (endothelioma in situ, systemic endotheliomatosis). J Clin Pathol 17:608–611, 1964

KAUH VC, MCFARLAND JP, CARNABUCI GG et al: Malignant proliferating angioendotheliomatosis. Arch Dermatol 116:803–806, 1980

MARTIN S, PITCHER D, TSCHEN J et al: Reactive angioendotheliomatosis. J Am Acad Dermatol 2:117–123, 1980

MIDANA A, ORMEA F: A propos d'un cas d'angioendotheliomatosis proliferans systematisata (de Tappeiner et Pfleger). Ann Dermatol Syph 92:129–138, 1965

PASYK K, DEPOWSKI M: Proliferating systematized angioendotheliomatosis of a 5-month-old infant. Arch Dermatol 114:1512–1515, 1978

PFLEGER L, TAPPEINER J: Zur Kenntnis der systemisierten Endotheliomatose der cutanen Blutgefässe (Reticuloendotheliose?). Hautarzt 10:359–363, 1959

RUITER M, MANDEMA E: New cutaneous syndrome in subacute bacterial endocarditis. Arch Intern Med 113:283–290, 1964

SCOTT PWB, SILVERS DN, HELWIG EB: Proliferating angioendotheliomatosis. Arch Pathol 99:323–326, 1975

TAPPEINER J, PFLEGER L: Angioendotheliomatosis proliferans systematisata. Hautarzt 14:67–70, 1963

Angiolymphoid Hyperplasia with Eosinophilia

BALER GR: Angiolymphoid hyperplasia with eosinophilia. J Dermatol Surg Oncol 7:229–234, 1981

BURRALL BA, BARR RJ, KING DF: Cutaneous histiocytoid hemangioma. Arch Dermatol 118:166–170, 1982

GRIMWOOD R, SWINEHART JM, AELING JL: Angiolymphoid hyperplasia with eosinophilia. Arch Dermatol 115:205–207, 1979

INADA S, YAMAMOTO S, KITAURA H et al: A case of eosinophilic lymphfolliculosis of the skin (Kimura's disease). J Dermatol (Tokyo) 4:207–214, 1977

KANDIL E: Dermal angiolymphoid hyperplasia with eosinophilia versus pseudopyogenic granuloma. Br J Dermatol 83:405–408, 1970

MEHREGAN AH, SHAPIRO L: Angiolymphoid hyperplasia with eosinophilia. Arch Dermatol 103:50–57, 1971

OLSEN TG, HELWIG EB: Inflammatory angiomatous nodules. (Abstr) Arch Dermatol 115:1348, 1979

REED RJ, TERAZAKIS N: Subcutaneous angioblastic lymphoid hyperplasia with eosinophilia (Kimura's disease). Cancer 29:489–497, 1972

VÁZQUEZ MB, SÁNCHEZ JL: Angiolymphoid hyperplasia with eosinophilia: Report of a case and a review of the literature. J Dermatol Surg Oncol 4:931–936, 1978

WELLS GC, WHIMSTER IW: Subcutaneous angiolymphoid hyperplasia with eosinophilia. Br J Dermatol 81:1–15, 1969

WILSON JONES E, BLEEHEN SS: Inflammatory angiomatous nodules with abnormal blood vessels occurring about the ears and scalp (pseudo or atypical pyogenic granuloma). Br J Dermatol 81:804–816, 1969

Blood Vessel Markers

Factor 8 AG

Ulex europaeus

Lecting (other)

Alk. Phosphatase

Weibel-Palade Body

Tumors of Fatty, Muscular, and Osseous Tissue

31

NEVUS LIPOMATOSUS SUPERFICIALIS

Nevus lipomatosus superficialis is a fairly uncommon lesion showing groups of soft, flattened papules or nodules that have a smooth or wrinkled surface and are skin-colored or pale yellowish. Characteristically, the lesions are distributed on one buttock, but they may overlap onto the adjacent skin of the back or the upper thigh (Wilson Jones et al). They may be present already at birth, but they develop most commonly during the first two decades of life and occasionally later (Hönigsmann and Gschnait).

Solitary lesions have been diagnosed as nevus lipomatosus superficialis (Weitzner; Wilson Jones et al), but it seems preferable to regard them instead as solitary, baglike soft fibromas (see p. 601) (Mehregan et al). The rather common presence of fat cells within long-standing intradermal melanocytic nevi represents an involutionary phenomenon rather than an association of a nevus lipomatosus with a melanocytic nevus (see p. 684) (Maize and Foster).

Histopathology. Groups and strands of fat cells are found embedded among the collagen bundles of the dermis, often as high as the papillary dermis (Fig. 31-1) (Abel and Dougherty). The proportion of fatty tissue varies greatly, from over 50% of the dermis to less than 10% (Wilson Jones et al). In cases with only small deposits, the fat cells are apt to be situated in small foci around the subpapillary vessels. In instances with relatively large amounts of fat, the fat lobules are irregularly distributed throughout the dermis, and the boundary between the dermis and the hypoderm is ill defined or lost (Wilson Jones et al). The fat cells may all be mature (Abel and Dougherty; Hönigsmann and Gschnait), but, in some instances, an occasional small, incompletely lipidized cell may be observed (Wilson Jones et al).

The dermis may be entirely normal, but, in some instances, the density of the collagen bundles, the number of fibroblasts, and the vascularity are greater than in normal skin (Mehregan et al).

Histogenesis. It is generally agreed that nevus lipomatosus represents, as the name implies, a nevoid anomaly. The ectopic fat cells in the dermis are derived from the perivascular mesenchymal tissue (Holtz; Cramer; Wilson Jones et al).

This view has found support in *electron microscopic studies* of nevus lipomatosus superficialis, in which immature lipocytes containing numerous small lipid droplets and a centrally located nucleus have been seen in the vicinity of capillaries (Reymond et al).

Differential Diagnosis. In focal dermal hypoplasia, fat cells are also seen in the dermis, often in close approximation to the epidermis. However, this disorder differs from nevus lipomatosus by the extreme attenuation of the collagen (see p. 65).

FOLDED SKIN WITH LIPOMATOUS NEVUS

Only two instances have been reported of newborn babies showing generalized folding of the skin (Ross,

1969; Gardner et al). This appearance has given rise to the term *Michelin-tire baby*. The folding diminishes gradually during childhood (Ross, 1972).

Histopathology. The dermis appears thinned, although thick septa of dermal collagen extend into the underlying fatty tissue. An increased amount of adipose tissue extends as thick lobules into the lower dermis. The sweat glands are located within the lobules of fat (Ross, 1969; Gardner et al).

LIPOMA

Lipomas occur as single or multiple subcutaneous growths that are soft, rounded or lobulated, and movable against the overlying skin.

In three rare conditions, multiple lipomas composed of mature fat cells arise in adult life. They are (1) *adiposis dolorosa*, or Dercum's disease, in which there are tender circumscribed or diffuse fatty deposits (Szegö; Blomstrand et al); (2) *benign symmetric lipomatosis*, or Madelung's disease, characterized by large, coalescent, nontender lipomas present especially in the region of the neck in a typical "horse-collar" distribution and to a lesser degree in the occipital region, on the upper part of the trunk, and on the proximal part of the extremities (Uhlin); and (3) *familial multiple lipomatosis*, inherited as an autosomal dominant trait, with development of innumerable asymptomatic lipomas beginning in early adulthood (Rabbiosi et al; Mohar).

Histopathology. Lipomas are surrounded by a thin connective tissue capsule and are composed often entirely of normal fat cells that are indistinguishable from the fat cells in the subcutaneous tissue. In some lipomas, one finds more and in others less of a connective tissue framework than in the normal subcutaneous fat. Those containing a considerable proportion of connective tissue are called fibrolipomas.

In *adiposis dolorosa*, most authors have found the lipomas to be indistinguishable histologically from ordinary lipomas (Szegö). In some cases, however, the histologic appearance is that of an angiolipoma (Eyckmans), a tumor that is often painful (see below). In other cases, granulomas of the foreign body type have been noted within the fatty tissue (Bloomstrand et al).

In *benign symmetric lipomatosis* and *familial multiple lipomatosis*, the lipomas have the histologic appearance usually seen in ordinary lipomas (Uhlin; Rabbiosi et al; Mohar).

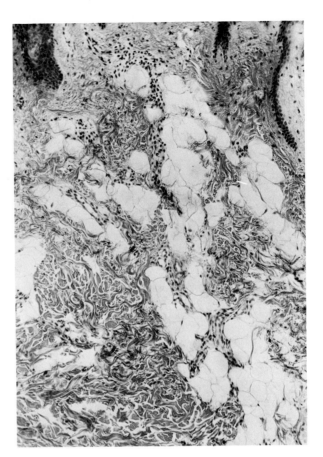

Fig. 31-1. Nevus lipomatosus superficialis
Groups and strands of mature fat cells are embedded among the collagen bundles of the dermis, extending as high as the subpapillary layer. Portions of the epidermis are seen at the top. (×100)

ANGIOLIPOMA

Angiolipomas usually occur as encapsulated subcutaneous lesions. They are found less commonly as infiltrating, yet benign, tumors that invade muscular tissue, mainly on a lower extremity (Sahl).

Encapsulated subcutaneous angiolipomas usually arise in young adults. They clinically resemble lipomas, although they have a greater tendency to be multiple. Also, they are often tender and painful (Howard and Helwig).

Histopathology. Encapsulated subcutaneous angiolipomas are composed of mature adipose tissue and varying numbers of blood vessels. The degree of vascularity is quite variable, ranging from only a few small angiomatous foci to lesions with a predominance of dense vascular and stromal tissue

(Howard and Helwig). The angiomatous foci are composed in part of well-formed, dilated capillaries engorged with erythrocytes. Other capillaries appear tortuous and have poorly formed lumina and prominent proliferation of pericytes. Nearly all angiolipomas contain fibrin thrombi within their capillaries, often to a considerable degree. These thrombi are well demonstrated by phosphotungstic acid-hematoxylin staining (Dixon et al).

BENIGN LIPOBLASTOMA

An uncommon solitary tumor originally referred to as lipoblastomatosis (Vellios et al), benign lipoblastoma arises in the subcutaneous fat between the time of birth and 7 years of age (Chung and Enzinger). The slowly growing tumor may reach considerable size. It occurs mostly in the lower extremities.

Two basic forms of benign lipoblastoma occur. One is deeply situated and poorly circumscribed and tends to grow into the surrounding tissue spaces and musculature. The other is relatively superficial and encapsulated (Chung and Enzinger).

Histopathology. Benign lipoblastoma is composed of immature, embryonic fat cells and a mucinous stroma. The size of the lipoblasts varies. Most of them contain a single vacuole that is variable in size but smaller than that found in mature fat cells. This vacuole displaces the nucleus against the cytoplasmic membrane (Vellios et al). A few small lipoblasts possess two, three, or occasionally more vacuoles (Greco et al). Only some benign lipoblastomas show also lipoblasts with finely vacuolar cytoplasm and a centrally placed nucleus resembling hibernoma cells (Chaudhuri et al). Nonvacuolated cells that are spindle-shaped or stellate are seen in the mucinous stroma.

Differential Diagnosis. The tumor must be distinguished from a myxoid liposarcoma, from which it differs by the absence of atypical lipoblasts, of mitoses, and of hyperchromatic nuclei (Chaudhuri et al). Furthermore, liposarcomas occur very rarely in infants and young children (Kauffman and Stout).

SPINDLE CELL LIPOMA

A solitary, slowly growing subcutaneous tumor, spindle cell lipoma occurs predominantly in elderly males. The back and the posterior neck are the most commonly affected areas (Enzinger and Harvey).

Histopathology. The well-circumscribed tumor contains mature fat cells and uniform, slender spindle cells within a mucinous matrix (Enzinger and Harvey). In some areas, the neoplasm consists of a pure spindle cell population, often arranged in thick bundles, without fat cells. In other areas, the spindle cells are intermingled with scattered groups of mature fat cells (Brody et al). The spindle cells, being fibroblasts, produce varying amounts of collagen. A unique feature is the presence of numerous mast cells throughout the tumor (Brody et al).

Differential Diagnosis. The diagnosis of liposarcoma or fibrosarcoma can usually be excluded without difficulty because of the uniformity of the proliferated spindle cells and the absence of lipoblasts in spindle cell lipoma (Enzinger and Harvey).

PLEOMORPHIC LIPOMA

Pleomorphic lipoma is a subcutaneous tumor that clinically resembles spindle cell lipoma (see above) in that it occurs as a solitary lesion predominantly on the back and posterior neck of elderly males (Shmookler and Enzinger).

Histopathology. The well-circumscribed tumor displays a wide morphologic spectrum. Although areas of mature fat cells are present, some of them show enlarged, hyperchromatic nuclei (Evans et al). In addition, most fat cells show marked variation in size. Also, in about half of the tumors, occasional multivacuolated cells are seen that have the appearance of lipoblasts (Shmookler and Enzinger). The mature and immature fat cells are situated singly and in groups in a mucinous stroma traversed by dense collagen bundles.

A very helpful feature in the diagnosis of pleomorphic lipoma is the presence of characteristic multinucleated giant cells, which are found in most but not all cases (Evans et al). These giant cells show within an eosinophilic cytoplasm multiple, marginally placed, and often overlapping nuclei, a peculiar arrangement not unlike that of the petals of a small flower; these giant cells are therefore referred to as *floret type giant cells* (Shmookler and Enzinger; Bryant). It is of interest that small foci of spindle cell lipoma are encountered in some pleomorphic lipomas (Evans et al; Shmookler and Enzinger).

Differential Diagnosis. Although the histologic picture may be suggestive of liposarcoma, the clinical picture does not suggest a malignancy. Liposarcomas differ from pleomorphic lipoma by their infiltrative growth, greater cellularity, more nuclear atypicality, including atypical mitoses, more numerous multivacuolated lipoblasts, and absence of thick collagen bundles. Floret type giant cells are only rarely seen in liposarcomas, and then only in small numbers (Shmookler and Enzinger).

HIBERNOMA

Hibernoma is a benign, moderately firm, solitary, subcutaneous tumor with a size generally between 3 cm (Dardick) and 12 cm (Brines and Johnson). Although usually asymptomatic, it is occasionally tender (Dardick). Hibernomas may appear in childhood and slowly increase in size (Brines and Johnson; Novy and Wilson), but, more commonly, they arise in adulthood. This rare tumor is found most commonly on the upper back, but it may occur in other locations, such as the abdomen (Dardick). Clinically, hibernomas are indistinguishable from lipomas.

Histopathology.   Histologic examination reveals that the tumor is divided into numerous lobules by well-vascularized connective tissue. The majority of cells are multivacuolated, with a granular, eosinophilic cytoplasm between the vacuoles and a centrally located nucleus (Fig. 31-2) (Brines and Johnson; Novy and Wilson). The multivacuolated cells, referred to as mulberry cells, vary considerably

in size, ranging from 20 μm to 55 μm in diameter. They also show great variability in the number and size of the vacuoles, although, within each cell, the vacuoles are equal in size. Transitional forms between multivacuolated cells and larger, univacuolated cells can be identified. The latter have peripherally located nuclei and measure up to 120 μm in size (Seemayer et al). A few lobules, particularly at the periphery of the tumor, may be composed entirely of univacuolated cells (Dardick). The vacuoles in both the multivacuolated and the univacuolated cells stain positively with Sudan black (Levine).

A third type of cell, which is lipid-free and shows an eosinophilic granular cytoplasm, can also be identified. It is smaller than the multivacuolated cell, measuring only about 12 μm in diameter. Transitional stages between this lipid-free cell and multivacuolated cells are evident (Levine).

Histogenesis. The term *hibernoma* reflects the fact that these tumors are composed of the same type of cells as found in the brown fat of hibernating animals. However, brown fat is also found in other animals as well as in human beings. In humans, brown fat is more prevalent in the newborn period than later in life. Yet remnants of brown fat persist throughout adulthood and are found in the neck, axilla, and mediastinum as well as elsewhere embedded within the common white fat (Seemayer et al).

Although the cells of both the white and the brown fat develop from a multivacuolated stage into a univac-

Fig. 31-2. Hibernoma
The tumor is composed of rounded, multivacuolated cells with centrally placed nuclei. The multivacuolated cells are referred to as *mulberry cells.* (×400) (Courtesy of Frederick J. Novy, Jr., M.D., and J. Walter Wilson, M.D.)

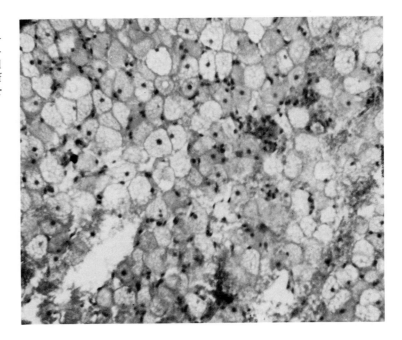

uolated stage, the two types of fat cells differ on *electron microscopic examination.* The main difference lies in the number and appearance of the mitochondria. The cells of brown fat as well as those of hibernomas contain many large mitochondria with an intricate internal structure due to the presence of numerous transverse tubular cristae, whereas the cells of white fat have only few small mitochondria with an uncomplicated internal structure (Levine; Seemayer et al; Dardick). The presence of numerous large mitochondria accounts for the granular appearance of the cytoplasm in brown fat cells (Levine).

LIPOSARCOMA

Although liposarcomas are one of the most common malignant soft tissue tumors, they only rarely arise in the subcutaneous fat. Most commonly, they originate in the intermuscular fascial planes, with a special predilection for the thighs (Enterline et al). From a fascial plane, they extend to the subcutaneous tissue. Liposarcomas arise as such and do not develop from lipomas. Even though they may occur at any age, they are rare in infants and young children (Kauffman and Stout).

Liposarcomas present themselves as a diffuse nodular infiltration of the subcutaneous tissue. Metastases are common, especially in poorly differentiated liposarcomas, the lungs and liver being the most common sites of metastasis.

Histopathology.   The degree of atypicality varies considerably among liposarcomas, making a mor-

phologic classification highly desirable. Depending on the degree of atypicality, four types of liposarcoma are generally recognized: (1) well-differentiated lipomalike, (2) well-differentiated and poorly differentiated myxoid, (3) round cell, and (4) pleomorphic liposarcoma (Enterline et al; Enzinger and Winslow). These four types can occur as pure or mixed forms.

In the well-differentiated lipomalike liposarcoma, the tumor is composed of univacuolated fat cells of varying size. The nuclei of the fat cells are slightly pleomorphic, and some of them are hyperchromatic. In addition, there are fibrous areas showing cells with large, pleomorphic, hyperchromatic nuclei. Although well-differentiated lipomalike liposarcomas do not metastasize, they can recur because of their poor demarcation. On recurring, they may dedifferentiate and become frankly atypical and then may eventually metastasize (Kindblom et al).

Myxoid liposarcomas are the most common type of liposarcoma. They have been subdivided into a well-differentiated type with little tendency to metastasize and a poorly differentiated type that commonly metastasizes (Enterline et al). A well-differentiated myxoid liposarcoma contains, in addition to lipoblasts with spindle-shaped nuclei and several lipid vacuoles, more highly differentiated fat cells, such as so-called signet ring cells, which have a single large vacuole occupying a major portion of the cytoplasm, and even mature fat cells

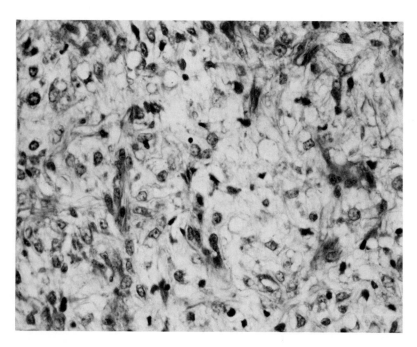

Fig. 31-3. Liposarcoma, well-differentiated myxoid type
The tumor is composed mainly of lipoblasts showing spindle-shaped nuclei and several lipid vacuoles, but it also contains more highly differentiated cells, such as univacuolated signet-ring cells and even mature fat cells. (×400)

(Fig. 31-3). The tumor cells are arranged loosely in a myxoid stroma.

In a poorly differentiated myxoid liposarcoma, the spindle-shaped lipoblasts have large, atypical nuclei and usually only small amounts of lipid droplets. Depending on the amount of myxoid stroma, there is considerable resemblance either to a myxosarcoma or to an undifferentiated fibrosarcoma, since the latter may also have a certain amount of myxoid stroma (Holtz).

Round cell liposarcomas are characterized by the presence of closely packed, rounded or oval cells with a single cytoplasmic vacuole, so-called signet ring cells, and multivacuolated lipoblasts. The nuclei are large, hyperchromatic, and atypical, with frequent mitoses (Kindblom et al).

Pleomorphic liposarcomas are composed mainly of extremely pleomorphic, huge, multivacuolated lipoblasts with one, or frequently several, irregular, hyperchromatic nuclei (Kindblom et al). The bizarre, giant lipoblasts are frequently admixed with smaller, polygonal, round or spindle-shaped lipoblasts (Saunders et al). In some instances, the presence of numerous vacuoles in the lipoblasts causes these cells to have the appearance of atypical mulberry cells, so that the tumor is suggestive of a malignant hibernoma (Fig. 31-4) (Stout; Grimmer; Kindblom et al).

Differential Diagnosis. The diagnosis of liposarcoma may be difficult in a poorly differentiated myxoid liposarcoma, which may contain very little lipid material. A lipid stain then often aids in the diagnosis. For differentiation from benign lipoblastoma, a tumor that occurs in infancy and early childhood, see p. 654.

SMOOTH MUSCLE HAMARTOMA

In smooth muscle hamartoma, a rare condition first described in 1923 (Stokes), one patch, usually several centimeters in diameter, is seen, most commonly in the lumbar region. It may be present at birth (Sourreil et al; Bonafé et al) or arise in childhood or early adulthood (Urbanek and Johnson). Usually, there are small, follicular papules throughout the patch, although the entire lesion may be slightly elevated (Sourreil et al). The patch shows hyperpigmentation and hypertrichosis in some patients (Stokes; Urbanek and Johnson; Bonafé et al) but not in others (Sourreil et al; Plewig and Schmoeckel). If hyperpigmentation and hypertrichosis are present, an association with Becker's melanosis exists (see p. 697).

Histopathology. Numerous thick, long, straight, well-defined bundles of smooth muscle fibers are seen scattered throughout the dermis and extending in various directions (Plewig and Schmoeckel). In patients with hypertrichosis, some of the smooth muscle bundles show connections with large hair follicles (Urbanek and Johnson).

Differential Diagnosis. The arrangement of the smooth muscle bundles in the dermis differs from

Fig. 31-4. Liposarcoma, pleomorphic type
The tumor is composed largely of rounded cells with multivacuolated cytoplasm and centrally placed anaplastic nuclei. The cells have the appearance of atypical mulberry cells, suggestive of a malignant hibernoma. (×200)

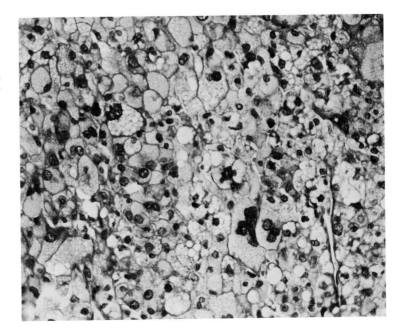

that seen in piloleiomyoma, in which the smooth muscle bundles form a large aggregate.

LEIOMYOMA

There are four types of leiomyomas of the skin: (1) multiple piloleiomyomas and (2) solitary piloleiomyoma, both arising from arrectores pilorum muscles; (3) solitary genital leiomyoma, arising from the dartoic, vulvar, or mamillary muscle; and (4) solitary angioleiomyoma, arising from the muscle of veins.

Multiple piloleiomyomas are small, firm, reddish or brownish intradermal nodules arranged in a group or in a linear fashion. Often, two or more areas are affected. Usually but not always, the lesions are tender and give rise spontaneously to occasional attacks of pain (Montgomery and Winkelmann).

Solitary piloleiomyomas are intradermal nodules that are

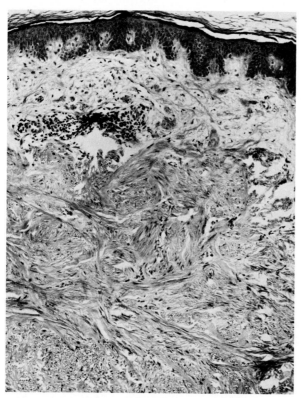

Fig. 31-5. Leiomyoma, piloleiomyoma type
The tumor is composed of interlacing bundles of smooth muscle fibers. The nuclei located in the center of the smooth muscle fibers are thin, very long, and blunt-edged. Collagen bundles are intermingled with the smooth muscle bundles. Both stain alike with hematoxylin-eosin. To differentiate them, an aniline blue stain may be used. (See Plate 4, facing p. 676.) (× 100)

usually larger than those of multiple piloleiomyomas, measuring up to 2 cm in size. Most of them are tender and also occasionally painful (Fisher and Helwig).

Solitary genital leiomyomas are located on the scrotum, the labia majora, or rarely, the nipples. Their location is intradermal. In contrast to the other leiomyomas, most genital leiomyomas are asymptomatic (Fisher and Helwig).

Solitary angioleiomyomas are usually subcutaneous and only rarely intracutaneous in location. As a rule, their size does not exceed 4 cm in diameter. The lower extremities are the most common site. Pain and tenderness are present in most, but not all, angioleiomyomas (Montgomery and Winkelmann; MacDonald and Sanderson; Bardach and Ebner).

Histopathology. *Piloleiomyomas,* whether multiple or solitary, and *genital leiomyomas* have a similar histologic appearance (Fisher and Helwig). They are poorly demarcated and are composed of interlacing bundles of smooth muscle fibers with which varying amounts of collagen bundles are intermingled (Fig. 31-5). The muscle fibers composing the smooth muscle bundles are generally straight, with little or no waviness; they contain centrally located, thin, very long, blunt-edged, "eellike" nuclei.

The muscle bundles stain pink with hematoxylin-eosin, just as collagen does, and thus are often difficult to distinguish from the collagen bundles, despite the following differences in the appearance of the nuclei and the bundles: the nuclei of the fibroblasts located in the collagen are shorter than the nuclei located in the smooth muscle fibers and show tapering at their ends; and, in contrast to the collagen bundles, the muscle bundles usually show slight vacuolization, especially in cross sections (Fisher and Helwig). A reliable differentiation between muscle and collagen bundles is possible with the aid of one of the collagen stains, such as the aniline blue stain or the Masson stain. With the aniline blue stain, muscle stains red and collagen blue (Plate 4, facing p. 676); with the Masson stain, muscle stains dark red and collagen green. Longitudinal intracytoplasmic myofibrils often can be visualized in sections stained with phosphotungstic acid-hematoxylin, where they appear as purple threads (Fields and Helwig).

Angioleiomyomas differ from the other types of leiomyoma by being encapsulated and containing numerous veins. As a rule, they contain only a small amount of collagen.

The numerous veins that are present vary in size and have muscular walls of varying thickness (Fig. 31-6). Smooth muscle bundles extend tangentially from the periphery of the veins and merge with the intervascular muscle bundles (Magner and Hill). The veins usually have a rounded or slitlike lumen, but some, because of contraction of their muscular tissue, have a stellate lumen (Saunders and Fitzpatrick). The large number and size of the veins present within angioleiomyomas are an indication that not only the muscle of veins but also the veins themselves are involved in the neoplasia (Magner and Hill). The veins possess no elastic lamina. Areas of mucinous alteration are often present, especially in large angioleiomyomas (MacDonald and Sanderson).

Histogenesis. *Electron microscopic examination* has shown that piloleiomyomas are composed of normal-appearing smooth muscle cells. These cells have a central nucleus surrounded by an area containing endoplasmic reticulum and mitochondria and, peripheral to this, numerous myofilaments arranged in bundles. Each muscle cell is surrounded by a narrow basement membrane (Mann).

In addition, electron microscopy has revealed distortion of nerve fibers and disruption of their myelin sheaths as a result of compression between adjoining muscle cells (Mann). This finding is analogous to that obtained with the Bodian stain, which has shown extension of the tumor around nerve fibers resulting in their compression (Montgomery and Winkelmann). Some authors assume that this compression of nerve fibers causes the attacks of pains (Montgomery and Winkelmann). Other authors, however, believe that the pain is a result of muscular contractions (Bardach and Ebner).

Also of interest is the observation that the smooth muscle bundles of piloleiomyomas, in contrast to normal arrector pili muscles, show a complete lack of nonspecific cholinesterase; this suggests that increased cholinergic activity causes the painfulness of piloleiomyomas (Mustakallio et al).

LEIOMYOSARCOMA

Because of their different prognosis, it is important to distinguish between cutaneous and subcutaneous leiomyosarcomas.

Cutaneous leiomyosarcomas have a good prognosis. There is usually a solitary nodule that only rarely ulcerates (Haim and Gellei). The nodule may be painful (Tappeiner and Wodniansky) or tender (Montgomery and Winkelmann), but it is often asymptomatic (Rising and Booth). In some cases, several nodules are present (Haim and Gellai; Jegasothy et al). Metastases to regional lymph nodes occur only rarely (Rising and Booth; Haim and Gellei) and are not fatal.

Subcutaneous leiomyosarcomas have a guarded prognosis. They manifest themselves as subcutaneous nodules or diffuse swellings that cause pain of either a local or a radiating nature in only a few patients (Phelan et

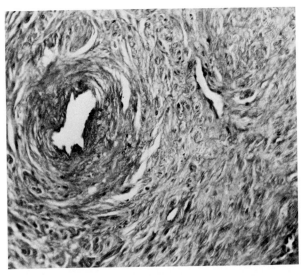

Fig. 31-6.   Leiomyoma, angioleiomyoma type
A large vein with a thick muscular wall is present. Smooth muscle bundles extend tangentially from the periphery of the vein and merge with intervascular muscle bundles. (×200)

al). They may cause hematogenous metastases, especially to the lungs, and lead to death in about one third of the patients (Phelan et al; Fields and Helwig).

Histopathology. *Cutaneous leiomyosarcomas* vary from moderately well to poorly delimited intradermal tumors that may extend into the subcutaneous tissue. In the center, the tumor shows nodular aggregates and densely packed, interlacing bundles of smooth muscle cells. At the margin of the tumor, strands of smooth muscle cells extend between collagen bundles.

Well-differentiated areas differ from leiomyomas mainly by showing a higher concentration of elongated, thin, blunt-ended nuclei. There are, however, a few plump nuclei and mitotic figures (Tappeiner and Wodniansky; Rising and Booth). Areas of lesser differentiation are present in all tumors, although to varying degrees. They show numerous irregularly shaped, anaplastic nuclei and usually also atypical giant cells with bizarre nuclei (Fig. 31-7) (Haim and Gellei; Fields and Helwig). Still, the nature of the sarcoma usually can be established even in rather anaplastic tumors, since, in some areas, one generally finds bundles of fairly well differentiated smooth muscle cells in which delicate myofibrils can be demonstrated by staining with phosphotungstic acid-hematoxylin (Haim and Gellei; Fields and Helwig). The number of mitoses

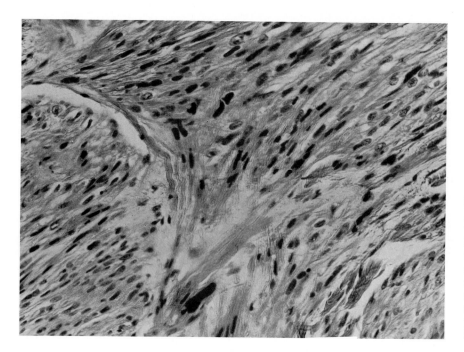

Fig. 31-7 Leiomyosarcoma Although, in some areas of this photograph, especially the lower left corner, the nuclei are thin, very long, and blunt-edged, thereby resembling those seen in a benign leiomyoma, most nuclei are irregular in shape and thus appear anaplastic. One bizarre giant cell is present. (×200)

may be high in anaplastic areas even when there are no metastases (Headington et al).

Subcutaneous leiomyosarcomas are surrounded by a compressed rim of connective tissue. Irregular aggregates of more or less atypical smooth muscle cells are seen to intertwine haphazardly without the fascicular pattern characteristic of the cutaneous leiomyosarcomas. Another way in which subcutaneous leiomyosarcomas differ from cutaneous tumors is by the presence of endothelium-lined, thin-walled blood vessels with variously shaped but often large lumina surrounded by smooth muscle cells (Field and Helwig). The presence of these blood vessels suggests that subcutaneous leiomyosarcomas are vascular in origin. No correlation seems to exist between the degree of histologic malignancy of the tumor and the occurrence of metastases (Phelan et al).

Histogenesis. *Electron microscopic examination* has shown that the tumor cells have the characteristics of smooth muscle cells even when there is marked nuclear atypicality (Headington et al). Thus, the tumor cells show bundles of myofilaments with filamentous dense bodies and attachment plaques on the cell membrane and a basement membrane surrounding individual cells (Headington et al; Seifert; Flotte et al).

Differential Diagnosis.   The presence of bizarre giant cells in leiomyosarcomas may cause a resemblance to malignant fibrous histiocytoma (Head-

ington et al). However, in some areas, one will usually find greatly elongated, thin, blunt-ended nuclei characteristic of smooth muscle cells. Also, demonstration of the presence of myofibrils by staining with phosphotungstic acid-hematoxylin will aid in the differentiation. The same holds true of subcutaneous leiomyosarcomas, in which the presence of endothelial-lined vessels may suggest a hemangiopericytoma.

CUTANEOUS OSSIFICATION

Cutaneous bone formation may be primary or secondary. If it is primary, there is no preceding cutaneous lesion; if it is secondary, bone forms through metaplasia within a pre-existing lesion. Primary cutaneous ossification can occur in Albright's hereditary osteodystrophy and as osteoma cutis.

Albright's Hereditary Osteodystrophy

In Albright's hereditary osteodystrophy, first described in 1952 (Albright et al), multiple areas of subcutaneous or intracutaneous ossification are often encountered. These areas may be present at birth or may arise later in life. No definite area of predilection seems to exist; areas of ossification have been described on the trunk (Peterson and Mandel) as well as on the extremities (Donaldson and Summerly) and the scalp (Barranco).

The areas of ossification may be so small as to be hardly perceptible or as large as 5 cm in diameter (Eyre and Reed). Those located in the skin may cause ulceration, and bony spicules may be extruded through the ulcer (Donaldson and Summerly). In addition to cutaneous and subcutaneous osteomas, bone formation may be observed in some cases along fascial planes (Eyre and Reed).

Albright's hereditary osteodystrophy includes the syndromes of pseudohypoparathyroidism and pseudopseudohypoparathyroidism. It is evident that these disorders are variants of the same disease, since both may occur in different members of the same family (Brook and Valman) and even at different times in the same patient (Spranger). Patients with pseudohypoparathyroidism have hypocalcemia with a failure to respond to parathyroid hormone, whereas patients with pseudopseudohypoparathyroidism have normal serum calcium values (Eyre and Reed). Patients with Albright's hereditary osteodystrophy have a short stature, a round facies, and multiple skeletal abnormalities, such as curvature of the radius and shortening of some of the metacarpal bones (Eyre and Reed). As a result of this shortening, several knuckles are absent when the fists are clenched, and a depression or dimple is apparent there instead. This important diagnostic sign is referred to as the Albright dimpling sign.

Additional manifestations include basal ganglia calcification and mental retardation. The mode of inheritance is dominant, possibly X-linked dominant (Eyre and Reed).

Histopathology.   Spicules of bone of varying size may be found within the dermis (Barranco) or in the subcutaneous tissue (Brook and Valman; Eyre and Reed). The bone contains fairly numerous osteocytes as well as cement lines that are best seen in polarized light (Roth et al). Haversian canals containing blood vessels and connective tissue are often present (Fig. 31-8). In addition, osteoblasts with elongated nuclei can usually be seen along the margin of the bone where new bone is being laid down. Osteoclasts are often absent but, if present, are seen as cells with multiple large nuclei resembling multinucleated foreign body giant cells. They are located within deep grooves called Howship lacunae that extend from the surface of the bone into the bone substance (Fig. 31-9).

The spicules of bone may enclose either partially or completely areas of mature fat cells (Eyre and Reed). Hematopoietic elements, however, are seen only rarely among the fat cells (Roth et al).

Histogenesis. The osteoblasts and osteocytes that form bone in primary cutaneous ossification originate from mesenchymal cells and thus form membranous rather than enchondral bone (Roth et al).

The incidence of cutaneous ossification in Albright's hereditary osteodystrophy is fairly high. It has been estimated that cutaneous ossification is found in 42% of the patients with pseudohypoparathyroidism and in 27% of those with pseudopseudohypoparathyroidism (Spranger). However, the reason for the bone formation is not clear.

Since the association of Albright's hereditary osteodystrophy with cutaneous ossification was not recog-

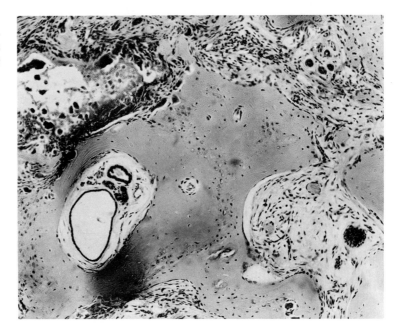

Fig. 31-8.   Osteoma cutis
Low magnification. The bone appears lamellated about several haversian canals containing blood vessels and connective tissue. (×100)

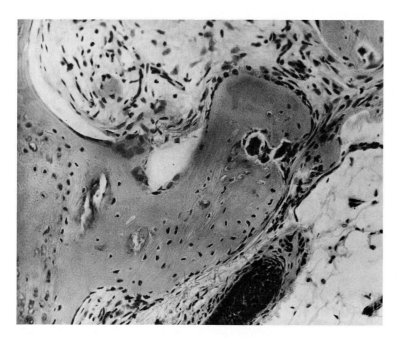

Fig. 31-9. Osteoma cutis
High magnification of Figure 31-8. The bone is lined in many areas by osteoblasts. In the center of the flield, several osteoclasts lie within a niche called Howship's lacuna. (×200)

nized until 1965 (Piesowicz), the question arises as to how many cases of primary cutaneous ossification reported before then occurred in association with Albright's hereditary osteodystrophy. In a review examining this question (Brook and Valman), several cases originally reported as primary osteoma of the skin were recognized as showing evidence of Albright's hereditary osteodystrophy (Tijdens and Ruiter; Donaldson and Summerly; Peterson and Mandel). Although the conclusion that most cases of primary osteoma cutis are associated with Albright's hereditary osteodystrophy seems somewhat exaggerated, it is nevertheless apparent that patients with extensive foci of ossification usually have Albright's hereditary osteodystrophy.

Osteoma Cutis

The term *osteoma cutis* is applied to cases of primary cutaneous ossification in which there is no evidence of Albright's hereditary osteodystrophy in either the patient or his family.

Apparently, there are four groups of patients with osteoma cutis, with the osteomas limited in extent in all but the first group. The four groups are (1) patients with *widespread osteomas* since birth or early life but without evidence of Albright's hereditary dystrophy (Vero et al; Maclean et al; O'Donnell and Geller); (2) patients with a *single, large, plaquelike osteoma* present since birth either in the skin of the scalp (Combes and Vanina; Tritsch; Franke) or in the skin or subcutaneous tissue of an extremity (Burgdorf and Nasemann; Vončina); (3) patients with a *single small osteoma* arising in later life in various locations (Burgdorf and Nasemann) and in some

instances showing transepidermal elimination of bony fragments (Duperrat and Vanbremeersch; Delacrétaz and Koenig); and (4) patients with *multiple miliary osteoma of the face,* all of them women. In some instances, the osteomas do not appear until late in life (Hopkins; Costello; Rossman and Freeman; Helm et al; Zabel). In others, they are seen in young women in association with a long-standing acne vulgaris (Leider; Jewell; Basler et al; Walter and Macknet). In the latter cases, the miliary osteomas have been interpreted as metaplastic ossification within acne scars. However, the absence of acne vulgaris among the patients in the older age group and the presence in one case of miliary osteomas also in the scalp, where acne does not occur (Helm et al), raises the possibility that the acne vulgaris is coincidental.

Histopathology. The histologic findings in osteoma cutis are the same as in primary cutaneous ossification occurring in conjunction with Albright's hereditary osteodystrophy (see p. 661). In cases with transepidermal elimination of bone, one observes fragments of bone either within a channel lined by epidermis and leading to the surface (Duperrat and Vanbremeersch) or within a break in the epidermis (Delacrétaz and Koenig).

Metaplastic Ossification

Secondary or metaplastic ossification occurs within a pre-existing lesion. It may be seen in association with cutaneous tumors, scars, or inflammatory processes (Barranco).

Histopathology. The tumor that most commonly shows metaplastic ossification is pilomatricoma, or calcifying epithelioma (see p. 532). Whereas calcification starts within the areas of shadow cells, ossification starts in the stroma of the tumor, but with the calcium-rich shadow cells acting as inducing factor. Ossification is found in 14% to 20% of pilomatricomas (Forbis and Helwig; Wiedersberg; Burgdorf and Nasemann). It also occurs on rare occasions in basal cell epitheliomas, where it takes place usually in the stroma but sometimes in degenerating areas of keratinization (Delacrétaz and Christeler). Some basal cell epitheliomas with ossification are cases of the nevoid basal cell epithelioma syndrome (Mason et al). In intradermal nevi, ossification usually is secondary to a folliculitis (Duperrat; Delacrétaz and Frenk). Finally, ossification may also occur in chondroid syringomas or mixed tumors of the skin (Roth et al). This is the only instance in which enchondral bone is formed in the skin through ossification of the chondroid cells of the tumor.

In contrast to metaplastic ossification in association with tumors, metaplastic ossification in scars (Lilga and Burns) and in inflammatory processes of the skin such as scleroderma and dermatomyositis (Roth et al) is rare.

CUTANEOUS CARTILAGINOUS TUMOR

Cutaneous cartilaginous tumor is a rare tumor that, like primary cutaneous ossification, probably arises from mesenchymal cells. It is found as an asymptomatic, firm mass moveable with the skin on a finger or toe or in the metacarpal or metatarsal region. The tumor rarely exceeds 3 cm in diameter. Metastases are not known to occur (Dahlin and Salvador).

Histopathology. The tumor is located in the dermis and extends into the subcutaneous tissue as a lobulated mass of immature-appearing hyaline cartilage with eosinophilic cytoplasm and nuclei of variable shape (Holmes and Bovenmeyer). In some instances, the nuclei are large and hyperchromatic, suggestive of malignancy, even though the tumors clinically follow a benign course (Dahlin and Salvador). Foci of calcification or ossification are seen quite commonly.

CUTANEOUS ENDOMETRIOSIS

Cutaneous endometriosis is characterized by the presence of a solitary brownish or bluish nodule measuring from 0.5 cm to 6 cm in size. The lesion, which is quite rare, is seen only in adult women. Most commonly, it occurs in a surgical scar of the abdominal or genital region, especially following a cesarean section (Steck and Helwig). However, the lesion may arise spontaneously in the umbilicus (Popoff et al) and, rarely, in the inguinal area (Steck and Helwig). Quite often, the lesion is slightly tender and painful. At the time of menstruation, these symptoms usually become more pronounced and may be associated with swelling and slight bleeding of the lesion. However, there are asymptomatic lesions, some of which are even unresponsive to menstruation (Steck and Helwig; Williams et al).

Histopathology. Irregular glandular lumina are embedded in a highly cellular and vascular stroma resembling the stroma of the functioning endometrium (Popoff et al). The lumina are lined with a single row of secretory cells that are flat in some areas and tall and columnar in others. Secretory globules are seen being extruded from the secretory cells (Steck and Helwig). Erythrocytes and hemosiderin-filled macrophages are found in the surrounding stroma, and, occasionally, erythrocytes are present also in the lumina (Popoff et al).

Histogenesis. In cases in which cutaneous endometriosis develops in surgical scars, implantation of viable endometrial cells is probably the cause. In contrast, in cases of spontaneously arising cutaneous endometriosis, it appears most likely that the endometrial tissue is transported to the area by way of lymphatic or vascular channels (Steck and Helwig).

CUTANEOUS ENDOSALPINGIOSIS

On rare occasions, multiple brownish papules averaging 5 mm in diameter develop after a salpingectomy around the umbilicus, but not necessarily within the laparotomy incision scar.

Histopathology. Each papule contains beneath an intact epidermis a unilocular cyst with papillary projections into the lumen. The lining consists of epithelium as seen in the fallopian tube, that is, of columnar cells, some of them ciliated and others secretory (Doré et al). The lining thus resembles that seen in cutaneous ciliated cysts (see p. 488) (Farmer and Helwig).

UMBILICAL OMPHALOMESENTERIC DUCT POLYP

Remnants of the omphalomesenteric duct are found on rare occasions in the skin of the umbilicus, where they

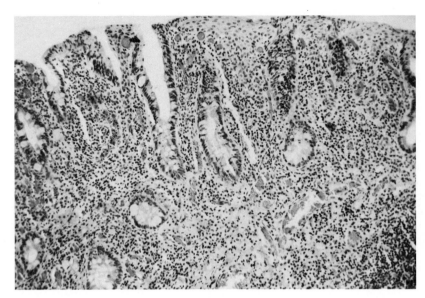

Fig. 31-10. Umbilical omphalomesenteric duct polyp
The gastrointestinal epithelium in this polyp has the appearance of the colonic mucosa, showing glandular crypts lined with goblet cells interspersed with simple columnar cells. (×100)

manifest themselves as a polyp from 2 mm to 20 mm in size. The polyp may be present at birth or appear in childhood (Hejazi). It is bright red and often has a central depression. It may be associated with an underlying sinus or cyst (Steck and Helwig).

Histopathology. Ectopic gastrointestinal epithelium is present on and near the surface of the umbilical polyp. Since the omphalomesenteric duct remnant can differentiate into epithelium of any gastrointestinal type, the gastrointestinal epithelium may have the appearance of gastric, small intestinal, or colonic mucosa (Fig. 31-10) (Steck and Helwig). The polyp also shows areas of epithelial hyperplasia often intermingled with areas of erosion, as well as proliferation of capillaries and a diffuse chronic inflammatory infiltrate (Hejazi).

Histogenesis. The omphalomesenteric duct communicates between the midgut and the yolk sac of the embryo. It usually disappears during the seventh week of embryonic life. If there is a remnant of the duct anywhere along its embryonic course from the skin to the intestine, it may give rise to the formation of polyps, sinuses, or cysts with or without connection to the intestine or the surface of the skin (Hejazi).

Differential Diagnosis. An umbilical metastasis from a carcinoma of the colon differs from an umbilical omphalomesenteric duct polyp clinically by onset late in life and histologically by the presence of nuclear atypicality (Zeligman and Schwilm).

BIBLIOGRAPHY

Nevus Lipomatosus Superficialis
ABEL R, DOUGHERTY JW: Nevus lipomatosus cutaneus superficialis (Hoffmann-Zurhelle). Arch Dermatol 85:524–526, 1962
CRAMER HJ: Zur nosologischen Stellung des Naevus lipomatodes cutaneus superficialis (Hoffmann-Zurhelle). Dermatol Wochenschr 142:1218–1222, 1960
HOLTZ KH: Beitrag zur Histologie des Naevus lipomatodes cutaneus superficialis (Hoffmann-Zurhelle). Arch Dermatol Syph (Berlin) 199:275–286, 1955
HÖNIGSMANN H, GSCHNAIT F: Naevus lipomatosus cutaneus superficialis (Hoffmann-Zurhelle). Z Hautkr 49:517–524, 1974
MAIZE JC, FOSTER G: Age-related changes in melanocytic nevi. Clin Exp Dermatol 4:49–58, 1979
MEHREGAN AH, TAVAFOGHI V, GHANDCHI A: Nevus lipomatosus cutaneus superficialis (Hoffmann-Zurhelle). J Cutan Pathol 2:307–313, 1975
REYMOND JL, STOEBNER P, AMBLARD P: Nevus lipomatosus cutaneus superficialis. An electron microscopic study of four cases. J Cutan Pathol 7:295–301, 1980
WEITZNER S: Solitary nevus lipomatosus cutaneus superficialis of scalp. Arch Dermatol 97:540–542, 1968
WILSON JONES E, MARKS R, PONGSEHIRUN D: Naevus superficialis lipomatosus. Br J Dermatol 93:121–133, 1975

Folded Skin with Lipomatous Nevus
GARDNER EW, MILLER HM, LOWNEY ED: Folded skin associated with underlying nevus lipomatosus. Arch Dermatol 115:978–979, 1979
ROSS CM: Generalized folded skin with an underlying lipomatous nevus. Arch Dermatol 100:320–323, 1969
ROSS CM: Generalized folded skin with underlying lipomatous nevus: The Michelin tyre baby. Arch Dermatol 106:766, 1972

Lipoma
BLOMSTRAND R, JUHLIN L, NORDENSTAM H et al: Adiposis dolorosa associated with defects of lipid metabolism. Acta Derm Venereol (Stockh) 51:243–250, 1971

EYCKMANS R: Adipose douloureuse de Dercum. Arch Belg Dermatol Syph 10:365–366, 1954

MOHAR N: Familial multiple lipomatosis. Acta Derm Venereol (Stockh) 60:509–513, 1980

RABBIOSI G, BORRONI G, SCUDERI N: Familial multiple lipomatosis. Acta Derm Venereol (Stockh) 57:265–267, 1977

SZEGÖ L: Gemeinsames Vorkommen der Lipomatosis dolorosa (Dercum) mit intrauteriner Amputation des linken Oberschenkels. Dermatol Wochenschr 150:641–646, 1964

UHLIN SR: Benign symmetric lipomatosis. Arch Dermatol 115:94–95, 1979

Angiolipoma

DIXON AY, MCGREGOR DH, LEE SH: Angiolipomas: An ultrastructural and clinicopathological study. Hum Pathol 12:737–747, 1981

HOWARD WR, HELWIG EB: Angiolipoma. Arch Dermatol 82:924–931, 1960

SAHL WJ JR: Mobile encapsulated lipomas. Arch Dermatol 114:1684–1686, 1978

Benign Lipoblastoma (Lipoblastomatosis)

CHAUDHURI B, RONAN SG, GHOSH L: Benign lipoblastoma. Cancer 46:611–614, 1980

CHUNG EB, ENZINGER FM: Benign lipoblastomatosis. An analysis of 35 cases. Cancer 32:483–492, 1973

GRECO MA, GARCIA RL, VULETIN JC: Benign lipomatosis. Cancer 45:511–515, 1980

KAUFFMAN SL, STOUT AP: Lipoblastic tumors of children. Cancer 12:912–925, 1959

VELLIOS F, BAEZ J, SHUMACKER HB: Lipoblastomatosis: A tumor of fetal fat different from hibernoma. Am J Pathol 34:1149–1159, 1958

Spindle Cell Lipoma

BRODY HJ, MELTZER HD, SOMEREN A: Spindle cell lipoma. Arch Dermatol 114:1065–1066, 1978

ENZINGER FM, HARVEY DA: Spindle cell lipoma. Cancer 36:1852–1859, 1975

Pleomorphic Lipoma

BRYANT J: A pleomorphic lipoma in the scalp. J Dermatol Surg Oncol 7:323–325, 1981

EVANS HL, SOULE EH, WINKELMANN RK: Atypical lipoma, atypical intramuscular lipoma, and well differentiated retroperitoneal liposarcoma. Cancer 43:574–584, 1979

SHMOOKLER BM, ENZINGER FM: Pleomorphic lipoma: A benign tumor simulating liposarcoma. Cancer 47:126–133, 1981

Hibernoma

BRINES OA, JOHNSON MH: Hibernoma, a special fatty tumor. Am J Pathol 25:467–479, 1949

DARDICK I: Hibernoma: A possible model of brown fat histogenesis. Hum Pathol 9:321–329, 1978

LEVINE GD: Hibernoma. An electron microscopic study. Hum Pathol 3:351–359, 1972

NOVY FG JR, WILSON JW: Hibernomas, brown fat tumors. Arch Dermatol 73:149–157, 1956

SEEMAYER TA, KNAACK J, WANG NS et al: On the ultrastructure of hibernoma. Cancer 36:1785–1793, 1975

Liposarcoma

ENTERLINE HT, CULBERSON JD, ROCHLIN DB et al: Liposarcoma. Cancer 13:932–950, 1960

ENZINGER FM, WINSLOW DJ: Liposarcoma. Virchows Arch (Pathol Anat) 335:367–388, 1962

GRIMMER H: Hibernoma. Z Hautkr 33:XXI–XXIV, 1962

HOLTZ F: Liposarcomas. Cancer 11:1103–1109, 1958

KAUFFMAN SL, STOUT AP: Lipoblastic tumors in children. Cancer 12:912–925, 1959

KINDBLOM LG, ANGERVALL L, JARLSTEDT J: Liposarcoma of the neck. Cancer 42:774–780, 1978

SAUNDERS JR, JAQUES DA, CASTERLINE FF et al: Liposarcomas of the head and neck. Cancer 43:162–168, 1979

STOUT AP: Liposarcoma—the malignant tumor of lipoblasts. Ann Surg 119:86–107, 1944

Smooth Muscle Hamartoma

BONAFÉ JL, GHRENASSIA-CANAL S, VANCINA S: Naevus musculaire lisse. Ann Dermatol Venereol 107:929–931, 1980

PLEWIG, G, SCHMOECKEL C: Naevus musculi arrector pili. Hautarzt 30:503–505, 1979

SOURREIL P, BEYLOT C, DELFOUR MM: Hamartome par hyperplasie des muscles arrecteurs des poils chez un nourrisson d'un mois. Bull Soc Fr Dermatol Syph 76:602, 1969

STOKES JH: Nevus pilaris with hyperplasia of nonstriated muscle. Arch Dermatol Syph 7:479–481, 1923

URBANEK RW, JOHNSON WC: Smooth muscle hamartoma associated with Becker's nevus. Arch Dermatol 114:104–106, 1978

Leiomyoma

BARDACH H, EBNER H: Das Angioleiomyom der Haut. Hautarzt 26:638–642, 1975

FIELDS JP, HELWIG EB: Leiomyosarcoma of the skin and subcutaneous tissue. Cancer 47:156–169, 1981

FISHER WC, HELWIG EB: Leiomyomas of the skin. Arch Dermatol 88:510–520, 1963

MACDONALD DM, SANDERSON KV: Angioleiomyoma of the skin. Br J Dermatol 91:161–168, 1974

MAGNER D, HILL DP: Encapsulated angiomyoma of the skin and subcutaneous tissue. Am J Clin Pathol 35:137–141, 1961

MANN PR: Leiomyoma cutis: An electron microscope study. Br J Dermatol 82:463–469, 1970

MONTGOMERY H, WINKELMANN RK: Smooth-muscle tumors of the skin. Arch Dermatol 79:32–41, 1959

MUSTAKALLIO KK, LEVONEN E, NIEMI M: Histochemical studies on cutaneous leiomyomatosis. Br J Dermatol 75:60–70, 1963

SAUNDERS TS, FITZPATRICK TB: Cutaneous leiomyoma. Arch Dermatol 74:389–392, 1956

Leiomyosarcoma

FIELDS JP, HELWIG EB: Leiomyosarcoma of the skin and subcutaneous tissue. Cancer 47:156–169, 1981

FLOTTE TJ, BELL DA, SIDHU GS et al: Leiomyosarcoma of the dartos muscle. J Cutan Pathol 8:69–74, 1981

HAIM S, GELLEI B: Leiomyosarcoma of the skin. Dermatologica 140:30–35, 1970

HEADINGTON JT, BEALS TF, NIEDERHUBER JE: Primary leiomyosarcoma of skin: A report and critical appraisal. J Cutan Pathol 4:308–317, 1977

JEGASOTHY BV, GILGOR RS, HULL DM: Leiomyosarcoma of the skin and subcutaneous tissue. Arch Dermatol 117:478–481, 1981

MONTGOMERY H, WINKELMANN RK: Smooth-muscle tumors of the skin. Arch Dermatol 79:32–41, 1959

PHELAN JT, SHERER W, MESA P: Malignant smooth-muscle tumors (leiomyosarcomas) of soft-tissue origin. N Engl J Med 266:1027–1030, 1962

RISING JA, BOOTH E: Primary leiomyosarcoma of the skin with lymphatic spread. Arch Pathol 81:94–96, 1966

SEIFERT HW: Elektronenmikroskopische Untersuchung am cutanen Leiomyosarkom. Arch Dermatol Res 263:159–169, 1978

TAPPEINER J, WODNIANSKY P: Solitäres Leiomyom-Leiomyosarkom. Hautarzt 12:160–163, 1961

Cutaneous Ossification

ALBRIGHT F, FORBES AP, HENNEMAN PH: Pseudopseudohypoparathyroidism. Trans Assoc Am Phys 65:337–350, 1952

BARRANCO VP: Cutaneous ossification in pseudohypoparathyroidism. Arch Dermatol 104:643–647, 1971

BASLER RSW, TAYLOR WB, PEACOR DR: Postacne osteoma cutis. Arch Dermatol 110:113–114, 1974

BROOK CGD, VALMAN HG: Osteoma cutis and Albright's hereditary osteodystrophy. Br J Dermatol 85:471–475, 1971

BURGDORF W, NASEMANN T: Cutaneous osteomas: A clinical and histopathologic review. Arch Dermatol Res 260:121–135, 1977

COMBES FC, VANINA R: Osteosis cutis. Arch Dermatol Syph 69:613–615, 1954

COSTELLO MJ: Metaplasia of bone. Arch Dermatol Syph 56:536–537, 1947

DELACRÉTAZ J, CHRISTELER A: Les phénomènes d'ossification dans les épithéliomas cutanés. Dermatologica 134:305–311, 1967

DELACRÉTAZ J, FRENK E: Zur Pathogenese des Osteo-Naevus Nanta. Hautarzt 15:487–489, 1964

DELACRÉTAZ J, KOENIG R: Osteoma perforant. Dermatologica 156:251–254, 1978

DONALDSON EM, SUMMERLY R: Primary osteoma cutis and diaphyseal aclasis. Arch Dermatol 85:261–265, 1962

DUPERRAT B: Ostéomes cutanés. Ann Dermatol Syph 88:11–31, 1961

DUPERRAT B, VANBREMEERSCH F: Ostéome perforant verruciforme post-traumatique. Ann Dermatol Syph 90:37–39, 1963

EYRE WG, REED WB: Albright's hereditary osteodystrophy with cutaneous bone formation. Arch Dermatol 104:636–642, 1971

FORBIS R JR, HELWIG EB: Pilomatrixoma (calcifying epithelioma). Arch Dermatol 83:606–618, 1961

FRANKE H: Beitrag zum Krankheitsbild der Osteosis cutis circumscripta. Hautarzt 7:270–272, 1956

HELM F, DE LA PAVA S, KLEIN E: Multiple miliary osteomas of the skin. Arch Dermatol 96:681–682, 1967

HOPKINS JG: Multiple miliary osteomas of the skin. Arch Dermatol Syph 18:706–715, 1928

JEWELL EW: Osteoma cutis. Arch Dermatol 103:533–555, 1971

LEIDER M: Osteoma cutis as a result of severe acne vulgaris of long duration. Arch Dermatol Syph 62:405–407, 1950

LILGA HV, BURNS DC: Osteomatosis cutis. Arch Dermatol Syph 46:872–874, 1942

MACLEAN GD, MAIN RA, ANDERSON TE et al: Connective tissue ossification presenting in the skin. Arch Dermatol 94:168–174, 1966

MASON JK, HELWIG EB, GRAHAM JH: Pathology of the nevoid basal cell carcinoma syndrome. Arch Pathol 79:401–408, 1965

O'DONNELL TF JF, GELLER SA: Primary osteoma cutis. Arch Dermatol 104:325–326, 1971

PETERSON WC JR, MANDEL SL: Primary osteomas of skin. Arch Dermatol 87:626–632, 1963

PIESOWICZ AT: Pseudohypoparathyroidism with osteoma cutis. Proc Roy Soc Med 58:126–218, 1965

ROSSMAN RE, FREEMAN RG: Osteoma cutis, a stage of preosseous calcification. Arch Dermatol 89:68–73, 1964

ROTH SI, STOWELL RE, HELWIG EB: Cutaneous ossification. Arch Pathol 76:44–54, 1963

SPRANGER J: Skeletal dysplasia: Albright's hereditary osteodystrophy. In Birth Defects: The First Conference, p. 122. White Plains, NY, National Foundation March of Dimes, 1968

TIJDENS EF, RUITER M: Über "Osteosis kutis." Acta Derm Venereol (Stockh) 29:140–153, 1949

TRITSCH H: Osteome der Kopfhaut. Arch Klin Exp Dermatol 221:336–347, 1965

VERO R, MACHACEK GF, BARTLETT FH: Disseminated congenital osteoma of the skin with subsequent development of myositis ossificans. JAMA 129:728–734, 1945

VONČINA D: Osteoma cutis. Dermatologica 148:257–261, 1974

WALTER JF, MACKNET KD: Pigmentation of osteoma cutis caused by tetracycline. Arch Dermatol 115:1087–1088, 1979

WIEDERSBERG H: Das Epithelioma calcificans Malherbe. Dermatol Monatsschr 157:867–883, 1971

ZABEL R: Osteosis cutis multiplex faciei. Dermatol Montsschr 156:798–801, 1970

Cutaneous Cartilaginous Tumor

DAHLIN DC, SALVADOR AH: Cartilaginous tumors of the soft tissues of the hands and feet. Mayo Clin Proc 49:721–726, 1974

HOLMES HS, BOVENMEYER DA: Cutaneous cartilaginous tumor. Arch Dermatol 112:839–840, 1976

Cutaneous Endometriosis

POPOFF L, RAITCHEV R, ANDREEV VC: Endometriosis of the skin. Arch Dermatol 85:186–189, 1962

STECK WD, HELWIG EB: Cutaneous endometriosis. JAMA 191:167–170, 1965

WILLIAMS HE, BARSKY S, STORINO W: Umbilical endometrioma (silent type). Arch Dematol 112:1435–1436, 1976

Cutaneous Endosalpingiosis

DORÉ N, LANDRY M, CADOTTE M et al: Cutaneous endosalpingiosis. Arch Dermatol 116:909–912, 1980

FARMER ER, HELWIG EB: Cutaneous ciliated cysts. Arch Dermatol 114:70–73, 1978

Umbilical Omphalomesenteric Duct Polyp

HEJAZI N: Umbilical polyp: A report of two cases. Dermatologica 150:111–115, 1975

STECK WD, HELWIG EB: Cutaneous remnants of the omphalomesenteric duct. Arch Dermatol 90:463–470, 1964

ZELIGMAN I, SCHWILM A: Umbilical metastasis from carcinoma of the colon. Arch Dermatol 110:911–912, 1974

Tumors of Neural Tissue

32

Three major types of benign nerve sheath tumors occur in the skin: (1) neurofibromas, (2) neurilemmomas, and (3) neuromas. In neurofibromas, the characteristic finding is a proliferation of both Schwann cells and endoneurial fibroblasts embedded in a considerable amount of endoneurial collagen. In neurilemmomas, the tumor consists of Schwann cells that possess numerous cytoplasmic processes forming so-called Verocay bodies. In neuromas, there is a proliferation of nerve fascicles that often are surrounded by a conspicuous perineurium.

NEUROFIBROMATOSIS

Neurofibromas may occur as solitary cutaneous lesions, in which case one finds no café-au-lait spots and no family history of the disease (Winkelmann and Johnson; Knight et al). When multiple cutaneous lesions are present, the disorder is referred to as neurofibromatosis, or von Recklinghausen's disease. It can arise as an autosomal dominant condition, but, in nearly half of the patients, it arises by spontaneous mutation (Crowe et al). About 90% of the patients have at least one café-au-lait spot, and multiple café-au-lait spots are usually present (Crowe and Schull). Whereas solitary neurofibromas generally arise in adulthood, the multiple cutaneous tumors of neurofibromatosis in most instances first appear in late childhood or in adolescence and gradually increase in size and number. There also is a localized or segmental form of neurofibromatosis with only a few cutaneous neurofibromas and a negative family history. Café-au-lait spots are present in some of these cases (Miller and Sparks) but absent in others (Winkelmann and Johnson).

Both solitary and multiple neurofibromas have a soft consistency. They usually are flesh-colored but occasionally have a violaceous color. They are either semiglobular or pedunculated.

The multiple neurofibromas of neurofibromatosis vary considerably in number and size. In some cases, subcutaneous tumors are also present. They usually consist of firm, discrete nodules attached to a nerve. In rare instances, large, pendulous, flabby masses are encountered in which numerous thickened, tortuous nerves can be felt. They are referred to as plexiform neuromas.

Café-au-lait spots are usually present at birth, but they may take months, and perhaps up to 1 year, to appear. They continue to increase in number and size during the first decade of life, especially in the first 2 years (Riccardi). They usually precede the cutaneous tumors. Although a few café-au-lait spots are occasionally seen in patients without neurofibromatosis, the presence of more than six spots exceeding 1.5 cm in diameter is indicative of neurofibromatosis (Crowe and Schull). Frecklelike pigmentation of the axilla is a highly characteristic feature of neurofibromatosis (Crowe).

Histopathology. Histologic examination of cutaneous neurofibromas shows the same findings in solitary neurofibromas and in neurofibromatosis. Although usually well circumscribed, they are not encapsulated (Reed). Occasionally, they are not sharply separated from the surrounding dermis but infiltrate the dermal connective tissue (Winkelmann and Johnson). Large tumors often extend into the subcutaneous fat. In typical areas, neu-

667

rofibromas are composed of faintly eosinophilic, thin, wavy fibers lying in loosely textured strands that extend in various directions (Fig. 32-1). Embedded among the wavy fibers, one finds a fairly large number of nuclei that are oval to spindle-shaped and quite uniform in size. Occasionally, the nuclei lie in parallel rows, but well-developed Verocay bodies, as in neurilemmomas, are uncommon. A Giemsa stain reveals a considerable number of mast cells in most neurofibromas. Nuclei of mast cells constitute, on the average, 5% of all nuclei present in neurofibromas (Jurecka et al). Elastic fibers are absent in the tumors. Staining with special nerve stains, such as Bodian's stain, reveals scattered, long, thin nerve fibers in most but not all tumors (McNairy and Montgomery). The presence of nerve fibers in neurofibromas has also been confirmed by the staining of thick sections with methylene blue (Shelley and Arthur). Staining for reticulum fibers reveals that many of the thin, loosely textured, wavy fibers are reticulum fibers (McNairy and Montgomery).

Occasionally, mucoid degeneration of the stroma is observed in parts of a tumor or in an entire tumor. In such areas, the nuclei are embedded in a homogeneous, pale blue ground substance (Fig. 32-2). This ground substance consists of acid mucopolysaccharides that are digested by hyaluronidase (Nürnberger and Korting). One must be familiar with this type of mucoid degeneration, because it results in a histologic picture that is quite different from that usually associated with neurofibroma.

Subcutaneous neurofibromas show diffuse involvement of the nerve or origin. In contrast to cutaneous tumors, they are encapsulated, with the perineurium of the involved nerve forming the capsule of the tumor (Reed).

The café-au-lait spots show in sections stained with silver, in comparison with the surrounding skin, (1) an increase in the total amount of melanin in both melanocytes and keratinocytes and (2) scattered giant melanin granules measuring up to 5 μm in diameter in both melanocytes and basal cells (Benedict et al). In addition, the dopa reaction, when applied to skin sections, indicates (3) an increase in the activity of melanocytes, and, when applied to epidermal sheets, (4) an increased concentration of melanocytes per square millimeter (Benedict et al; Johnson and Charneco).

In regard to the presence of giant melanin granules, they are occasionally absent in the café-au-lait spots of adult patients with neurofibromatosis (Johnson and Charneco), and they seem to be regularly absent in the café-au-lait spots of children with neurofibromatosis (Silvers et al). Furthermore, giant melanin granules are not specific for the café-au-lait spots of neurofibromatosis but are also found occasionally in the café-au-lait spots of persons without neurofibromatosis (Eady and Cowen) as well as in various other pigmentary conditions, including the melanotic macules of

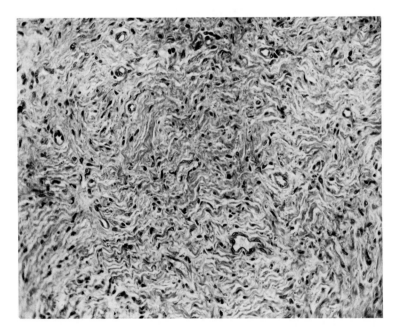

Fig. 32-1. Neurofibromatosis (von Recklinghausen's disease)
Thin, wavy fibers lie in loosely textured strands extending in various directions. Most nuclei appear elongated. (×200)

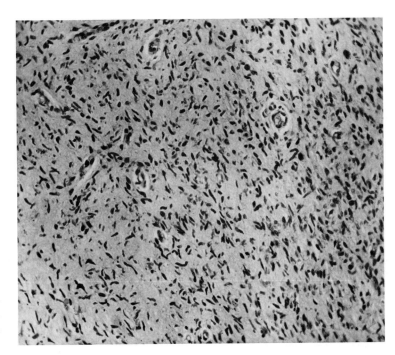

Fig. 32-2. Neurofibromatosis (von Recklinghausen's disease)
In this tumor, mucoid degeneration of the stroma has taken place, so that the nuclei are embedded in a homogeneous ground substance. (×200)

Albright's syndrome, melanocytic nevi, speckled lentiginous nevus (or nevus spilus), and the multiple lentiginosis syndrome (Ortonne and Perrot). They have been observed even in normal human epidermis (Konrad and Hönigsmann). (For a further discussion of giant melanin granules, see p. 695.)

Histogenesis. In 1882, von Recklinghausen postulated that neurofibromas are mainly fibrous tumors arising from the connective tissue of nerve sheaths. In 1910, having observed nerve fibers in the tumors, Verocay asserted that the cells of the tumors are Schwann cells and that the tumors are neuroectodermal in origin. He suggested that they be called *neurinomas.* Subsequently, some authors (Penfield) supported von Recklinghausen's view, and others (Masson) inclined to Verocay's, whereas still others expressed the opinion that probably both ectodermal Schwann cells and connective tissue cells participate in the formation of the tumors (Foot; McNairy and Montgomery).

The demonstration of nonspecific cholinesterase activity in neurofibromas has provided evidence that the tumors contain neuroectodermal tissue (Winkelmann and Johnson). However, the localization of the nonspecific cholinesterase activity in neurofibromas is uneven and patchy, indicating that neurofibromas also contain mesodermal tissue.

On *electron microscopic examination,* neurofibromas appear as a complex aggregate of Schwann cells (neurilemmal cells), endoneurium, and perineurium in which axons are sporadically present (Reed). Schwann cells predominate.

Schwann cells (EM 44) are characterized by the presence of a basement membrane 50 nm to 70 nm wide peripheral to the plasma membrane. Some of the Schwann cells contain axons within invaginations of their cytoplasm, each axon being surrounded by a basement membrane (EM 44, inset). In contrast to normal Schwann cells, in which the axons are found largely in the central cytoplasm, the Schwann cells present in neurofibromas have their axons almost entirely at their periphery within long cellular processes (Weber and Braun-Falco).

The endoneurium is represented by endoneurial fibroblasts that produce collagen fibrils of a smaller caliber than dermal fibroblasts. Thus, the average diameter of these collagen fibrils lies well below that of dermal collagen fibrils, which is about 100 nm. The Schwann cells in many areas are widely separated from one another by considerable numbers of collagen fibrils generally aggregated into collagen fibers but only rarely into collagen bundles (Waggener).

Perineurial cells are present in significant numbers only at the site at which the cutaneous nerve enters the neurofibroma. There, they may still be recognized as a multilayered perineurium, but they split up farther into the tumor and then are seen in only small numbers, recognizable by their elongated nuclei, multiple cell processes, and discontinuous basement membrane (Lassmann et al).

Electron microscopic examination of the giant melanin granules that are found in most café-au-lait spots of neurofibromatosis within both melanocytes and keratinocytes reveals that they are rounded and measure from 2 μm to 5 μm in diameter (Jimbow et al; Bhawan et al). This is in contrast to normal melanosomes, which are ellipsoidal and on the average measure 0.7 μm by 0.3 μm in diameter (Jimbow et al). The giant melanin granules have a variable appearance in different cases. They may be membrane-bound (Jimbow et al; Hirone and Eryu) or may have no limiting membrane (Bhawan et al; Ortonne and Perrot). In some instances, they have an electron-dense, homogeneous structure (Ortonne and Perrot), whereas, in others, they contain numerous electron-lucid microvesicles (Jimbow et al; Bhawan et al; Hirone and Eryu). They have been regarded as macro-melanosomes by some (Jimbow et al; Konrad et al) and as melanosome-filled phagolysosomes by others (Bhawan et al; Hirone and Eryu; Ortonne and Perrot). (For a discussion of this problem, see p. 695.)

Systemic Lesions. Extracutaneous neurofibromas may occur in deep peripheral nerves and nerve roots and in or on viscera and blood vessels innervated by the autonomic nervous system. Such neurofibromas may be nodular or diffuse (Riccardi). Spinal root tumors may cause compression of the spinal cord (Crowe et al). Tumors of the central nervous system occur in 5% to 10% of the patients with neurofibromatosis; they include optic gliomas and other astrocytomas, acoustic neuromas, neurilemmomas, meningiomas, and neurofibromas (Riccardi). Involvement of the bones may consist either of intraosseous neurofibromas or of erosive defects caused by the pressure of adjacent neurofibromas on bone. In addition, nonspecific bone lesions, such as kyphoscoliosis or an increase in the length of long bones, may occur (Levene). Of interest is the relatively common association of neurofibromatosis with pheochromocytoma (Healey and Mekelatos).

Malignant Changes. Neurofibrosarcomas, also referred to as malignant schwannomas, may arise in patients with neurofibromatosis, but this is not common. Thus, in a series of 678 patients, a malignant schwannoma was observed in only 21, or 3.1% of the patients (D'Agostino et al). Formation of a malignant schwannoma is particularly rare in cutaneous neurofibromas; it occurred in only 2 of the 678 patients. Neurofibrosarcomas usually arise contiguous with a subcutaneous neurofibroma or within a large nerve trunk, such as a femoral, tibial, or intercostal nerve (Undeutsch), but, in some instances, no such connections are apparent (Taxy et al).

On histologic examination, various degrees of malignant changes are seen. In malignant neurofibrosarcomas of low malignancy, the appearance of the tumor may be nearly indistinguishable from that of a benign neurofibroma except for a mild to moderate increase in cellularity and the presence of mitoses (Storm et al). Since mitoses are exceedingly rare in neurofibromas, the identification of even a single mitosis is cause for concern, necessitating careful scrutiny of the neoplasm for additional mitotic figures. However, the absence of mitoses does not preclude the existence of malignancy (Trojanowski et al). In tumors of somewhat greater malignancy, the nuclei are enlarged and closely packed and show moderate variation in size and shape. Collagen production is reduced, and mitotic figures are present (Fig. 32-3). Highly malignant tumors show dense cellularity, minimal collagen production, bizarre nuclei, and a lack of any wavy pattern. Differentiation from a fibrosarcoma may then be impossible without evidence of associated neurofibromatosis (Storm et al). In some malignant neurofibrosarcomas, mast cells can be identified with the aid of a Giemsa stain (Sordillo et al).

The prognosis of neurofibrosarcomas is very serious, even in tumors with fairly good differentiation. Extensive spread along the involved nerve requires aggressive surgical treatment (Sordillo et al).

Differential Diagnosis. A histologic differentiation of a neural nevus from a solitary neurofibroma is impossible in routinely stained sections if, as seen occasionally, the neural nevus shows no nevus cell nests in its upper portion (Becker). Staining for nerve fibers is of no value in this differentiation, since intradermal melanocytic nevi contain more nerve fibers than are seen in most neurofibromas (Shelley and Arthur). On staining for nonspecific cholinesterase, neural nevi show diffuse staining (Winkelmann), whereas neurofibromas show uneven and patchy staining (Winkelmann and Johnson). However, distinction is possible by electron microscopy, since the melanocytes of neural nevi contain melanosomes, whereas the Schwann cells of neurofibromas contain axons, and by an immunohistochemical technic showing the absence of myelin basic protein in neural nevi (see pp. 684 and 686).

Storiform Neurofibroma

Storiform neurofibroma is a rare solitary intradermal tumor first described in 1957 (Bednář). It grows slowly and usually measures 5 cm to 6 cm in diameter. It is well circumscribed, has a firm consistency, and is found most commonly on the trunk (Nishio and Koda).

Histopathology. The tumor is composed of two types of cells, spindle-shaped Schwann cells and

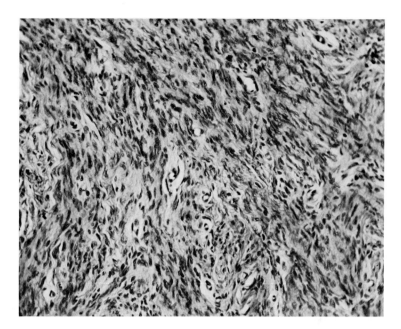

Fig. 32-3. Neurofibrosarcoma arising in von Recklinghausen's disease
The wavy pattern characteristic of neurofibromatosis is preserved, but the nuclei are increased in number and atypical. (×200)

dendritic melanocytes. It is well circumscribed but not encapsulated. It may extend from the dermis into the subcutaneous tissue.

The spindle-shaped Schwann cells constitute the majority of cells. They are arranged in intertwining bundles resulting in a matlike (storiform) pattern (Santa Cruz and Yates). In some areas, the tumor cells show a cartwheellike arrangement (Nishio and Koda) and may even undergo sudden rotations of about 90° (Bednář, 1970). Scattered throughout the tumor are deeply pigmented dendritic melanocytes (Santa Cruz and Yates).

Differential Diagnosis.   The relationship of storiform neurofibroma to cellular blue nevus (see p. 701) is not clear. As long as no electron microscopic studies of storiform neurofibromas are available, it seems quite possible that this tumor is identical to cellular blue nevus (Nishio and Koda).

NEURILEMMOMA

Neurilemmomas occur almost invariably as solitary tumors along the course of peripheral or cranial nerves. Their usual size is between 2 cm and 4 cm. They are most commonly found in a subcutaneous location on the head or extremities and only rarely on the trunk. They have also been reported as occurring on the tongue (Kuske and Soltermann; Mercantini and Mopper). In addition, they may occur in internal organs, particularly the stomach (Stout), and in bones (Fawcett and Dahlin).

Neurilemmomas may be asymptomatic, but they are not infrequently associated with pain, which may be localized to the tumor or radiate along the nerve from which the neurilemmoma arises (Izumi et al). Occasionally, neurilemmomas are encountered in persons who also have neurofibromatosis (Das Guptas et al; Izumi et al).

Malignant degeneration of neurilemmomas is a rare event, and only a few cases have been reported (Carstens and Schrodt).

Histopathology.   Neurilemmomas are well encapsulated. They are composed of two types of tissue, referred to as Antoni types A and B.

Antoni type A tissue is composed of cells whose nuclei are elongated and tightly packed. In most areas, the nuclei are arranged in a wavy pattern or in whorls. A highly characteristic feature is the arrangement of the nuclei in two parallel rows enclosing between them a space of nearly homogeneous anucleate material. Such formations are called Verocay bodies (Fig. 32-4). In some instances, the Verocay bodies consist of an entire circle of palisading nuclei surrounding the homogeneous anucleate material (Izumi et al). Only few collagen fibers are found in Antoni type A tissue.

Antoni type B tissue consists of an edematous stroma containing relatively few haphazardly arranged cells with nuclei of variable shape. In some instances, the edema leads to the formation of microcysts, which, by coalescence, may form large, fluid-filled cystic spaces (Stout). In other cases, the

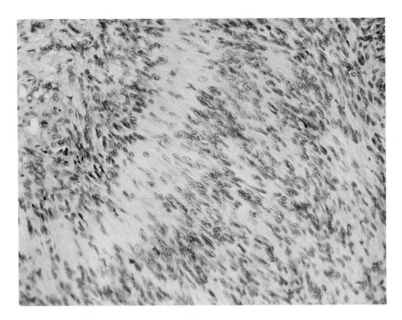

Fig. 32-4. Neurilemmoma
Numerous elongated nuclei are arranged in a streaming fashion. In the center of the field lies a so-called Verocay body formed by a double palisade of nuclei enclosing between them a space of homogeneous material that is nearly devoid of nuclei. (×200)

stroma shows mucoid changes, or there may be hemorrhage and necrosis. Between the type A and the type B tissue, there is often an intermediate zone in which the tightly packed cells as seen in type A tissue are separated by intercellular fluid (Sian and Ryan).

Staining for nerves with the Bodian stain reveals, in contrast with neurofibromas, very few or no nerve fibers (Reed et al). However, like neurofibromas, neurilemmomas show fairly numerous mast cells (Das Guptas et al).

Histogenesis. The presence of nonspecific cholinesterase in neurilemmoma is consistent with the presence of Schwann cells in this tumor (Winkelmann and Johnson).

Electron microscopy reveals that the Verocay bodies in Antoni type A tissue are composed of Schwann cells whose nuclei are largely arranged in palisading rows. The homogeneous material between two rows of nuclei consists of numerous thin, greatly elongated cytoplasmic processes that extend from the Schwann cells and are oriented in a parallel alignment (Fischer and Vuzevski). The interstitial tissue in Antoni type A areas is scantier than in neurofibromas but also consists of collagen fibrils and occasional fibroblasts (Waggener).

Antoni type B tissue results from degenerative changes occurring in type A tissue. On electron microscopy, the cells are seen to be widely separated by an electron-lucid homogeneous matrix containing strands of fibrin and detached segments of basement membrane. The cells show varying degrees of degeneration. Autophagic lysosomes, some of them containing myelin figures, are seen in many cells. Also, the cells show extensive loss of their basement membrane, disruption of their cell

membrane, and degenerative changes in their nuclei (Sian and Ryan).

NEUROMA

Neuromas can be divided into three types: (1) traumatic neuromas, (2) idiopathic solitary or multiple neuromas, and (3) multiple mucosal neuromas occurring in multiple endocrine neoplasia, type 2b.

The *traumatic neuromas* include the amputation neuromas and the so-called rudimentary supernumerary digits. The latter are smooth or verrucous papules that are found at the same site as true supernumerary digits, that is, at the base of the ulnar side of the fifth finger. They arise as a result of either postnatal destruction of a supernumerary digit or its autoamputation in utero (Shapiro et al). Whereas amputation neuromas are very sensitive to pressure, the rudimentary supernumerary digits usually are asymptomatic.

Idiopathic cutaneous neuromas are quite rare. As solitary neuromas, they may arise either in early childhood (Altmeyer, 1979a) or in adulthood (Dupré et al). Multiple neuromas arise in adulthood. They may be limited to the skin (Holm et al) or involve both the skin and oral mucosa (Altmeyer and Merkel), but they show no evidence of multiple endocrine neoplasia. Both the solitary and the multiple cutaneous neuromas are asymptomatic.

The *multiple mucosal neuromas* are part of the syndrome of multiple endocrine neoplasia, type 2b, first described in 1968 (Gorlin et al). It is the only one of the three types of multiple endocrine neoplasia, referred to as types 1, 2, and 2b, to show mucosal and cutaneous neuromas. The disorder may be inherited as an autosomal dominant trait (Khairi et al; Bazex et al). The mucosal neuromas are often the earliest manifestation of the type 2b syndrome, since they may begin to appear in early childhood. They are seen as small nodules, often in large numbers, on the mucosa of the lips, tongue, and oral mucosa (Jacobi and Kleine-Natrop; Hurwitz; Khairi et al; Bazex et al). Conjunctival and scleral neuromas may also be present (Thies). In addition, some patients show small, nodular neuromas on the skin of the face, usually only in small numbers (Khairi et al) but occasionally in large numbers on and around the nose and on the eyelids (Thies). Quite frequently, the lips are thick, fleshy, and protruding (Jacobi and Kleine-Natrop; Hurwitz). Marfanoid features and skeletal abnormalities may be present (Ayala et al). The recognition of this syndrome is of great importance because of its frequent association, beginning at an early age, with medullary thyroid carcinoma, which is diagnosable through elevated urinary calcitonin levels, and with pheochromocytoma, which causes elevated urinary catecholamine excretion (Khairi et al). Many patients also have diffuse alimentary tract ganglioneuromatosis (Carney et al).

Histopathology. In all three types of neuroma, large bundles of peripheral nerves extend in various directions and are sharply demarcated from the dermal connective tissue. Whereas the bundles of nerves show no capsule in some instances (Khairi et al), a capsule composed of perineurial cells and collagen can be found in most instances (Fig. 32-5) (Thies; Jacobi and Kleine-Natrop; Holm et al; Altmeyer and Merkel). Nerve bundles located close to the epidermis may resemble Meissner's corpuscles (Shapiro et al). Nerve stains, such as the Bodian stain, reveal numerous axons scattered throughout the nerve bundles (Thies; Jacobi and Kleine-Natrop; Holm et al). Staining for myelin with Luxol fast blue (Holm et al) or with osmium zinc iodide (Thies) reveals the presence of a myelin sheath around some of the nerves.

Histogenesis. *Electron microscopy* in both traumatic neuromas (Waggener) and spontaneously arising neuromas (Altmeyer and Merkel) shows multiple nerve fascicles composed of myelinated and nonmyelinated axons and Schwann cells. The fascicles are ensheathed by multiple lamina of perineurial cells. Intermingled with the perineurial cells lie dense bundles of collagen (Waggener).

Pacinian Neurofibroma

Pacinian neurofibroma is a rare tumor that usually occurs as a solitary lesion, most commonly on the hands and feet. Quite often, it is tender (Prose et al; Bennin et al). In most instances, it arises in adulthood, but it may be present at birth (Altmeyer, 1979b). In one reported

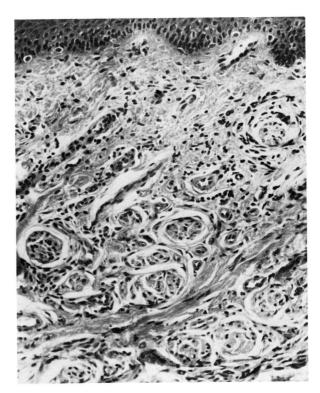

Fig. 32-5. Neuroma
Large bundles of peripheral nerves are present. They are surrounded by a capsule formed by perineurial cells and collagen. (×200)

instance, multiple tumors were observed on one finger (Levi and Curri).

Histopathology. The tumor is well demarcated and often encapsulated (MacDonald and Wilson Jones). It contains numerous round or ovoid lobules, each showing a central homogeneous, acellular, eosinophilic core surrounded by as many as 30 pale-staining concentric collagenous lamellae. These formations greatly resemble pacinian corpuscles (Bennin et al). In some tumors, there are areas in which the tissue surrounding the lobules is quite cellular and contains poorly formed nerve bundles of various diameters (Prose et al). In such areas, the lobules contain numerous elliptic or spindle-shaped nuclei both in the central core and in the surrounding lamellae (King and Barr); however, with increasing maturity, the number of nuclei decreases greatly (Levi and Curri). In some instances, the stroma of the lobules shows mucinous alterations (King and Barr).

Histogenesis. Several authors at first regarded the lobules as maturing and mature pacinian corpuscles

(Prose et al; Bennin et al; MacDonald and Wilson Jones; Levi and Curri). *Electron microscopic examination,* however, has indicated that the concentric lamellae are a result of the proliferation of perineurial cells (Weiser). Thus, the tumor may be regarded as a neuroma in which the central axons are still present in early neural formations but are gradually destroyed by a neoplastic proliferation of the perineurium (Altmeyer, 1979b).

GRANULAR CELL TUMOR

Granular cell tumors were originally described in 1926 (Abrikossoff) as granular cell myoblastomas. They usually occur as solitary tumors but are multiple in about 10% of the cases (White et al). As many as 64 tumors have been observed in a single patient (Apisarnthanarax). They occur most commonly on the tongue, where 40% of them are located, on the skin, and in the subcutaneous tissue. However, they may also occur in many other areas, such as the esophagus, stomach, appendix, larynx, bronchus, pituitary gland, uvea, and skeletal muscle (Aparicio and Lumsden).

Intradermal granular cell tumors consist of a well-circumscribed, raised, firm nodule usually from 0.5 cm to 3 cm in diameter. The tumor is in some instances tender or pruritic and occasionally has a verrucous surface (Apisarnthanarax).

Histopathology.   On histologic examination, the cells of the tumor appear large and often elongated. Most cells measure from 30 μm to 60 μm in diameter, but some are even larger. They have a

distinct cellular membrane and a pale cytoplasm filled with faintly eosinophilic, coarse granules (Fig. 32-6). The nuclei are small, round to oval, and centrally located. A few of the cells may possess more than one nucleus. Mitoses are seen only rarely. A characteristic feature of tumors located in the skin is the arrangement of the tumor cells in clusters and strands that are surrounded by a periodic acid-Schiff (PAS)-positive, diastase-resistant membrane, strands of collagen fibers, and occasional flattened fibroblasts referred to as *satellite fibroblasts* (Aparicio and Lumsden). Similarly, in tumors of the tongue, a PAS-positive, diastase-resistant membrane and slender, striated muscle fibers may surround groups of tumor cells (Fig. 32-7).

The characteristic faint granules within the tumor cells are PAS-positive and diastase-resistant. In some instances, the cytoplasmic granules are slightly sudanophilic, especially on staining with Sudan black, indicating that they contain a phospholipid rather than neutral fat (Fisher and Wechsler; Haisken and Langer). In other instances, the granules stain entirely negative for lipid (Aparicio and Lumsden).

The overlying epidermis is usually hyperplastic and not infrequently shows downward proliferation, often with horn-pearl formation (Fig. 32-8) It is important that this pseudocarcinomatous hyperplasia not be mistaken for squamous cell carcinoma (Bloom and Ginzler).

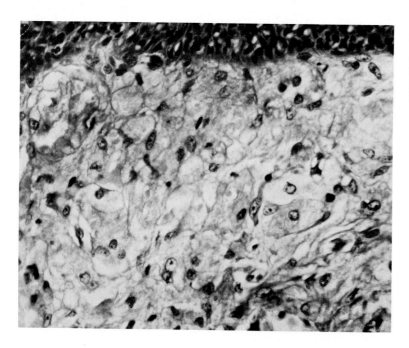

Fig. 32-6.   Granular cell tumor
The tumor is composed of large cells with a pale cytoplasm filled with numerous fine granules. Wedged in among the tumor cells are scattered flattened fibroblasts. (× 400)

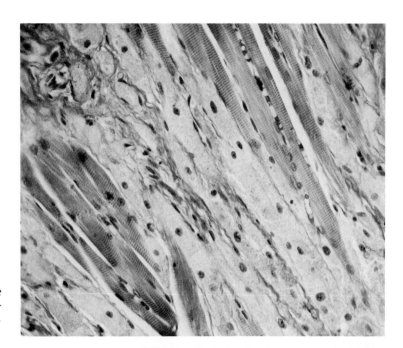

Fig. 32-7. Granular cell tumor of the tongue
The granular cells are infiltrating into the striated muscle. Thus, striated muscle fibers are seen among rows of tumor cells. (×400)

Histogenesis. For many years after its original description in 1926 (Abrikossoff), this tumor was thought to be composed of immature striated muscle cells, or myoblasts, and it was therefore named granular cell myoblastoma. This view arose because of the frequent close association between tumor cells and striated muscle fibers of the tongue, suggesting transitions between them (see Fig. 32-7).

Although histochemical and electron microscopic studies have eliminated myoblasts as the source of the tumor cells (Alkek et al), there is no agreement as to the nature of the tumor cells. It is agreed that the cytoplasmic granules are largely phagolysosomes (EM 45); it is possible, however, that some granules are derived from mitochondria (Tamaki et al). Most granules contain lysosomal enzymes, such as acid phosphatase (Sobel et al, 1971). On *electron microscopy*, they appear as membrane-bound vacuoles measuring 200 nm to 900 nm in diameter. Some appear almost empty, whereas others contain fine filamentous or electron-dense amorphous material (Chrestian et al; Tamaki et al). Also, some of the cytoplasmic granules have the appearance of residual bodies or myelin figures (Garancis et al; Sobel et al, 1971). The myelin figures, which represent the end stage of lysosomes, are probably responsible for the presence of phospholipid in some of the granules.

Concerning the nature of the tumor cells, most authors believe that they are Schwann cells. The following arguments have been offered in favor of this assumption: (1) granular cells may be seen inside of nerve sheaths both within and in the vicinity of the tumor, by light microscopy as well as by electron microscopy (Ashburn and Rodger; Tamaki et al; White et al); (2) on electron microscopy, many tumor cells, like Schwann cells, are surrounded by a basement membrane (Garancis et al);

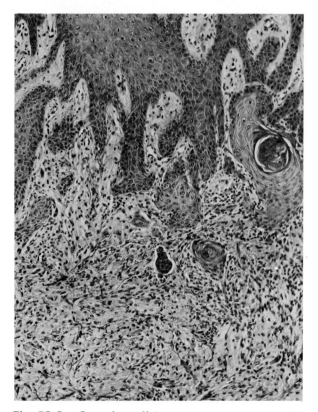

Fig. 32-8. Granular cell tumor
The epidermis exhibits pseudocarcinomatous hyperplasia. The dermis contains many large, pale tumor cells. In many areas, thin strands of collagen surround groups of tumor cells. (×200)

(3) some tumor cells show axons in their cytoplasm (Fisher and Wechsler); (4) the flattened satellite cells surrounding the clusters of tumor cells often show a partial basement membrane and thus may represent perineurial cells (Tamaki et al); (5) numerous lysosomal granules can be found in Schwann cells undergoing wallerian degeneration (Fisher and Wechsler; Weiser and Propst); and (6) myelin basic protein, a substance found in neural structures, has been demonstrated in granular cell tumors by use of a monoclonal antibody generated against myelin basic protein and an immunoperoxidase method (Penneys et al).

In contrast, several authors doubt that the tumor cells are Schwann cells for the following reasons: (1) most investigators have found no axons in the tumor cells (Moscovic and Azar), and the illustrations of Fisher and Wechsler purporting to show axons in granular cells are unconvincing (Sobel et al, 1973); (2) no fully acceptable transitions of Schwann cells to granular cells have been demonstrated in electron microscopic studies (Sobel et al, 1973; Chrestian et al); and (3) the presence of a basement membrane around each tumor cell nest with extensions into the cell nests and along the satellite fibroblasts represents a rather nonspecific process (Chrestian et al). Thus, although some of these authors favor an origin from undifferentiated mesenchymal cells (Moscovic and Azar; Sobel et al, 1973), it has also been stated that the ultrastructural data do not provide definitive proof of any histogenetic hypothesis (Chrestian et al).

Differential Diagnosis.   On cursory examination, the large, pale cells of the tumor resemble the foam cells of xanthoma. However, the cells of the granular cell tumor contain a granular rather than a foamy cytoplasm. The granules are strongly PAS-positive and take fat stains only faintly, if at all. The tumor cells in granular cell tumors, in contrast to xanthoma cells, are often surrounded by fine strands of collagen. Furthermore, the overlying epidermis tends to be hyperplastic in granular cell tumors, rather than atrophic as in xanthoma.

Care must be taken not to regard the pseudo-carcinomatous hyperplasia overlying many granular cell tumors as carcinoma. This danger exists especially in biopsy specimens from the tongue and the upper respiratory or digestive tract, if excision of the biopsy specimen is so superficial that the few granular cells present are overlooked.

MALIGNANT GRANULAR CELL TUMOR

Malignant granular cell tumor, originally called malignant granular cell myoblastoma, is a rare tumor. Most of the reported cases have occurred on the skin or in the subcutaneous tissue, but, as in benign granular cell tumors, a few cases have been reported from other areas, such as the bladder (Ravich et al) and the larynx (Busanni-Caspari and Hammar).

In the skin and subcutaneous tissue, the tumor manifests itself as a quite rapidly growing, poorly defined nodule or mass that may reach considerable size. Extensive visceral metastases occur either in association with regional lymph node metastases (Ross et al) or without them (Svejda and Horn). Widespread metastases to the skin and skeletal musculature have also been observed (Haustein).

Histopathology.   Histologically, two types of malignant granular cell tumors have been recognized (Gamboa). In one type, in spite of the clinically malignant course, the histologic appearance of the primary lesion and even of the metastases is benign, except for mild pleomorphism of the cells manifesting itself by the presence of slightly larger and darker nuclei than seen in benign granular cell tumors, and occasional mitotic figures (Ravich et al; Crawford and DeBakey; Gamboa; Svejda and Horn; Usui et al). In the other type, the primary lesion and the metastases appear histologically malignant inasmuch as they show transitions from typical granular cells through pleomorphic granular cells to pleomorphic nongranular spindle and giant cells with numerous mitotic figures (Fig. 32-9) (Ross et al; Krieg; Al-Sarraf et al; Haustein; Gartmann).

In an evaluation of the malignant potential of granular cell tumors with a benign histologic appearance, it should be kept in mind that clinical data such as the large size of the tumor, its rapid growth, and invasion into adjacent tissue are of greater diagnostic value than the histologic features (Strong et al). The average diameter of the "histologically benign, clinically malignant" granular cell tumors has been found to be 9 cm, as compared with 1.85 cm for the benign variety (Gamboa; Strong et al).

Differential Diagnosis.   The presence of granules in the cytoplasm of tumor cells has been observed on rare occasions in squamous cell carcinoma and in basal cell epithelioma. The granules in squamous cell carcinoma, in contrast to those of benign and malignant granular cell tumors, are PAS-negative, and desmosomes are seen on electron microscopy (Gilliet et al). In granular cell basal cell epithelioma, as in granular cell tumors, the granules are PAS-positive. However, typical palisading basalioma cells are located at the periphery of the tumor lobules showing a gradual transition into granular

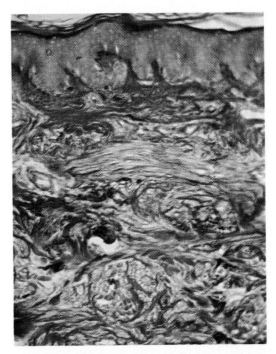

Leiomyoma. Aniline blue stain. This stain serves to differentiate collagen from smooth muscle. With hematoxylin-eosin, both stain red, but with aniline blue, collagen stains blue, and muscle red. (See p. 658.) (×150)

Blue nevus. Greatly elongated, deeply pigmented melanocytes with long dendritic processes are located in the lower dermis. (See p. 701.) (×150)

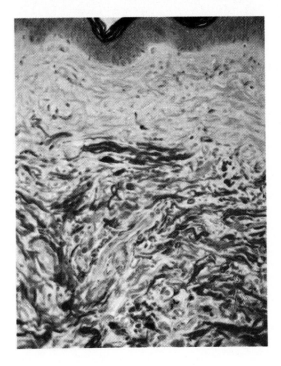

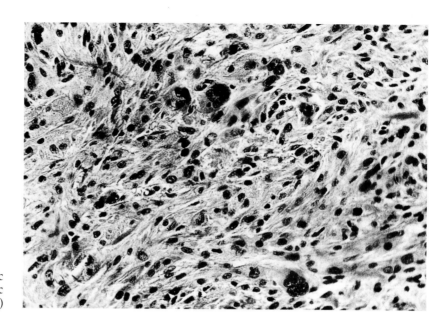

Fig. 32-9.   Malignant granular cell tumor
The tumor shows pleomorphic granular cells with hyperchromatic nuclei and bizarre giant cells. (× 400)

cells. In the latter cells, the nuclei lie in an eccentric position and are not centrally located as in granular cell tumors (Barr and Graham).

NASAL GLIOMA

Nasal glioma represents an intrauterine herniation of brain tissue. It is found most commonly on the skin near the root of the nose. It consists of a firm, smooth, red to purple protrusion that is quite large, measuring 2 cm to 3 cm in diameter, and resembles a hemangioma. Gliomas may also be located intranasally, or they may be both extranasal and intranasal, in which case they are connected through a defect in the nasal bone (Baran et al).

Nasal gliomas and encephaloceles have the same clinical and histologic appearance but differ in that encephaloceles are connected to the subarachnoid space by a sinus tract, whereas nasal gliomas lose this connection prior to birth. Their clinical similarities makes an ordinary biopsy inadvisable, since a septic encephalitis may ensue in the case of an encephalocele. Thus, radiography and neurosurgical consultation should precede any operative intervention (Kopf and Bart).

Histopathology.   The lesion shows interweaving strands of neural and fibrous tissue beneath a flattened epidermis (Kopf and Bart). In addition, there may be dilated blood vessels. The neural tissue consists of glial cells, or astrocytes, and loosely textured intercellular glial substance (Fig. 32-10) (Christianson). The astrocytes possess fairly light-staining, oval nuclei. Neurons may be absent; in some nasal gliomas, however, they are focally prominent and are recognizable by their triangular shape, eccentric nucleus, and ample cytoplasm, which often contains Nissl's granules. On staining with silver, neurites are seen protruding from the neurons (Mirra et al). Scattered foci of calcification are encountered in some lesions (Mirra et al).

CUTANEOUS MENINGIOMA

Meningiomas are tumors arising from the meninges of the brain or spinal cord, specifically from the arachnoid villi, which are normally found as inclusions within the dura mater (Waterson and Shapiro). Cutaneous meningiomas may develop in the scalp secondary to an intracranial meningioma either by means of erosion of the skull (Laymon and Becker) or by extension through an operative defect of the skull (Waterson and Shapiro). Such secondary cutaneous meningiomas may attain considerable size. Extracranial metastases are rare, but they have been found, for instance, in the cervical lymph nodes (Laymon and Becker).

In addition, primary cutaneous meningiomas of the scalp have been described in very rare instances as small solitary nodules that may be present at birth or appear later in life (Bain and Shnitka). They are benign and do not increase in size. The existence of primary cutaneous meningiomas is open to question; they may merely represent intradermal nevi containing psammoma bodies (see Histogenesis).

Histopathology.   Secondary cutaneous meningiomas of the scalp show sharply circumscribed

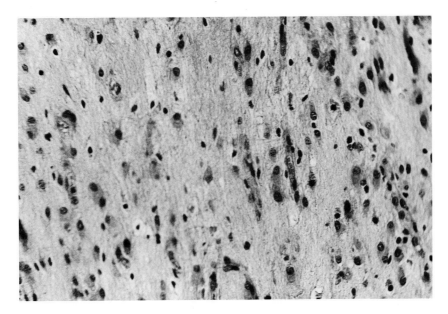

Fig. 32-10. Nasal glioma
The lesion shows loosely textured glial tissue containing two types of cells: glial cells, or astrocytes, and neurons. The latter show an eccentric nucleus and ample cytoplasm. (×400)

islands of cells in a dense, hyalinized stroma. The cells have oval, vesicular nuclei and moderately abundant, pale-staining cytoplasm (Waterson and Shapiro). Psammoma bodies are usually absent (Laymon and Becker).

Primary cutaneous meningiomas have been described as showing small groups or strands of cells embedded in a loose, fibrous stroma. The cells possess large, oval, vesicular nuclei and abundant cytoplasm. As a characteristic feature, one observes large and small, concentrically laminated, hyaline psammoma bodies showing varying degrees of calcification. The hyaline material forming the psammoma bodies originates in the cytoplasm of the tumor cells (Bain and Shnitka).

Histogenesis. The traditional view has been that primary cutaneous meningiomas develop from ectopic arachnoidal cells and thus represent true meningiomas. However, there is great histologic resemblance between the cells of primary cutaneous meningioma and those of intradermal melanocytic nevi, the only difference being the presence of psammoma bodies in primary cutaneous meningioma (Bain and Shnitka). Since psammoma bodies have also been noted in intradermal melanocytic nevi (Weitzner), it appears likely that primary cutaneous meningiomas are merely intradermal melanocytic nevi in which psammoma bodies have formed as a result of degeneration of some of the nevus cells.

BIBLIOGRAPHY

Neurofibromatosis
BECKER SW: Diagnosis and treatment of pigmented nevi. Arch Dermatol Syph 60:44–65, 1949

BEDNÁŘ B: Storiform neurofibromas of the skin, pigmented and nonpigmented. Cancer 10:368–376, 1957

BEDNÁŘ B: Storiform neurofibroma in the core of naevocellular naevi. J Pathol 101:199–201, 1970

BENEDICT PH, SZABO G, FITZPATRICK TB et al: Melanotic macules in Albright's syndrome and in neurofibromatosis. JAMA 205:618–626, 1968

BHAWAN J, PURTILO DT, RIORDAN JA et al: Giant and "granular melanosomes" in Leopard syndrome. J Cutan Pathol 3:207–216, 1976

CROWE FW: Axillary freckling as a diagnostic aid in neurofibromatosis. Ann Intern Med 61:1142–1143, 1964

CROWE FW, SCHULL WJ: Diagnostic importance of café-au-lait spot in neurofibromatosis. Arch Intern Med 91:758–766, 1953

CROWE FW, SCHULL WJ, NEEL JV: (eds) Clinical, Pathological, and Genetic Study of Multiple Neurofibromatosis. Springfield, IL, Charles C Thomas, 1956

D'AGOSTINO AN, SOULE EH, MILLER RH: Sarcomas of the peripheral nerves and somatic soft tissues associated with multiple neurofibromatosis (von Recklinghausen's disease). Cancer 16:1015–1027, 1963

EADY RAJ, COWEN TC: Naevus spilus. Br J Dermatol 93, Suppl 11:16, 1975

FOOT NC: Histology of tumors of the peripheral nerves. Arch Pathol 30:772–808, 1940

HEALEY FH, MEKELATOS CJ: Pheochromocytoma and neurofibromatosis. N Engl J Med 258:540–543, 1958

HIRONE T, ERYU Y: Ultrastructure of giant pigment granules in lentigo simplex. Acta Derm Venereol (Stockh) 58:223–229, 1978

JIMBOW K, SZABO G, FITZPATRICK TB: Ultrastructure of giant pigment granules (macromelanosomes) in the cutaneous pigmented macules of neurofibromatosis. J Invest Dermatol 61:300–309, 1973

JOHNSON BL, CHARNECO DR: Café-au-lait spot in neurofibromatosis and in normal individuals. Arch Dermatol 102:442–446, 1970

JURECKA W, LASSMANN H, GEBHART W et al: Classification of peripheral nerve sheath tumors. (Abstr) Arch Dermatol Res 258:100, 1977

KNIGHT WA III, MURPHY WK, GOTTLIEB JA: Neurofibromatosis

associated with malignant neurofibromas. Arch Dermatol 107:747–750, 1973

KONRAD K, HÖNIGSMANN H: Riesenmelanosomen in Naevuszellnaevi und in normaler menschlicher Epidermis. Wien Klin Wochenschr 87:173–177, 1975

KONRAD K, HÖNIGSMANN H, WOLFF K: The giant melanosome: A model of deranged melanosome morphogenesis. J Ultrastruct Res 48:102–123, 1974

LASSMANN H, JURECKA W, GEBHART W: Some electron microscopic and autoradiographic results concerning cutaneous neurofibromas in von Recklinhausen's disease. Arch Dermatol Res 255:69–81, 1976

LEVENE LJ: Bone changes in neurofibromatosis. Arch Intern Med 103:570–580, 1959

MASSON P: Experimental and spontaneous schwannomas (peripheral gliomas). Am J Pathol 8:367–415, 1932

MCNAIRY DJ, MONTGOMERY H: Cutaneous tumors of von Recklinghausen's disease (neurofibromatosis). Arch Dermatol Syph 51:384–390, 1945

MILLER RM, SPARKS RS: Segmental neurofibromatosis. Arch Dermatol 113:837–838, 1977

NISHIO K, KODA H: A case of storiform neurofibroma. J Dermatol (Tokyo) 2:143–148, 1975

NÜRNBERGER F, KORTING GW: Zum Vorkommen saurer Mucopolysaccharide in Neurofibromen und Neurofibrosarkomen. Arch Klin Exp Dermatol 235:97–114, 1969

ORTONNE JP, PERROT H: Giant melanin granules in vitiliginous achromia with malignant melanoma. Acta Derm Venereol (Stockh) 58:475–480, 1978

PENFIELD W: Tumors of the sheaths of the nervous system. Arch Neurol Psychiatr 27:1298–1309, 1932

REED RJ: Cutaneous manifestations of neural crest disorders (neurocristopathies). (Review) Int J Dermatol 16:807–826, 1977

RICCARDI VM: Von Recklinghausen neurofibromatosis. (Review) N Engl J Med 305:1617–1627, 1981

SANTA CRUZ DJ, YATES AJ: Pigmented storiform neurofibroma. J Cutan Pathol 4:9–13, 1977

SHELLEY WB, ARTHUR RP: Nerve fibers, a neglected component of intradermal cellular nevi. J Invest Dermatol 34:59–65, 1960

SILVERS DN, GREENWOOD RS, HELWIG EB: Café au lait spots without giant pigment granules. Arch Dermatol 110:87–88, 1974

SORDILLO PP, HELSON L, HAJDU SI et al: Malignant schwannoma: Clinical characteristics, survival, and response to therapy. Cancer 47:2503–2509, 1981

STORM FK, EILBER FR, MIRRA J et al: Neurofibrosarcoma. Cancer 45:126–129, 1980

TAXY JB, BATTIFORA H, TRUJILLO Y et al: Electron microscopy in the diagnosis of malignant schwannoma. Cancer 48:1381–3191, 1981

TROJANOWSKI JQ, KLEINMAN GM, PROPPE KH: Malignant tumors of nerve sheath origin. Cancer 46:1202–1212, 1980

UNDEUTSCH W: Zum Problem der malignen Entartung der Neurofibromatosis Recklinghausen. Dermatol Wochenschr 136:1145–1153, 1957

VEROCAY J: Zur Kenntnis der Neurofibrome. Beitr Pathol Anat Allg Pathol 48:1–69, 1910

VON RECKLINGHAUSEN FD: Über die multiplen Fibrome der Haut und ihre Beziehung zu den multiplen Neuromen. Berlin, A Hirschwald, 1882

WAGGENER JD: Ultrastructure of benign peripheral nerve sheath tumors. Cancer 19:699–709, 1966

WEBER K, BRAUN-FALCO O: Zur Ultrastruktur der Neurofibromatose. Hautarzt 23:116–122, 1972

WINKELMANN RK: Cholinesterase nevus: Cholinesterase in pigmented tumors of the skin. Arch Dermatol 82:17–23, 1960

WINKELMANN RK, JOHNSON LA: Cholinesterases in neurofibromas. Arch Dermatol 85:106–114, 1962

Neurilemmoma

CARSTENS PHB, SCHRODT GR: Malignant transformation of a benign encapsulated neurilemmoma. Am J Clin Pathol 51:144–149, 1969

DAS GUPTAS TK, BRASFIELD RD, STRONG EW et al: Benign solitary schwannoma (neurilemmoma). Cancer 24:355–366, 1969

FAWCETT KJ, DAHLIN DC: Neurilemmoma of bone. Am J Clin Pathol 47: 759–766, 1967

FISCHER ER, VUZEVSKI VD: Cytogenesis of schwannoma (neurilemmoma), neurofibroma, dermatofibroma, and dermatofibrosarcoma as revealed by electron microscopy. Am J Clin Pathol 49:141–154, 1967

IZUMI AK, ROSATO FE, WOOD MG: Von Recklinghausen's disease assoicated with multiple neurilemmomas. Arch Dermatol 104:172–176, 1971

KUSKE H, SOLTERMANN W: Neurinom der Zunge nach Zungenbiss. Dermatologica 116:386–387, 1958

MERCANTINI ES, MOPPER C: Neurilemmoma of the tongue. Arch Dermatol 79:542–544, 1959

REED RJ, FINE RM, MELTZER HD: Palisaded, encapsulated neuromas of the skin. Arch Dermatol 106:865–870, 1972

SIAN CS, RYAN SF: The ultrastructure of neurilemoma with emphasis on Antoni B tissue. Hum Pathol 12:145–160, 1981

STOUT AP: The peripheral manifestations of the specific nerve sheath tumor (neurolemoma). Am J Cancer 24:751–796, 1935

WAGGENER JD: Ultrastructure of benign peripheral nerve sheath tumors. Cancer 19:699–709, 1966

WINKELMANN RK, JOHNSON LA: Cholinesterases in neurofibromas. Arch Dermatol 85:106–114, 1962

Neuroma, Pacinian Neurofibroma

ALTMEYER P: Zur Histologie des pigmentierten granulären Rankenneuroms. Arch Dermatol Res 264:161–168, 1979a

ALTMEYER P: Histologie eines Rankenneuroms mit Vater-Pacini-Lamellenkörper-ähnlichen Strukturen. Hautarzt 30:248–252, 1979b

ALTMEYER P, MERKEL KH: Multiple systematisierte Neurome der Haut und Schleimhaut. Hautarzt 32:240–244, 1981

AYALA F, DEROSA G, SCIPPA L et al: Multiple endocrine neoplasia, type IIb. Dermatologica 162:292–299, 1981

BAZEX A, BOULARD C, DELSOL G et al: Syndrome de Sipple héréditaire. Ann Dermatol Venereol 104:103–114, 1977

BENNIN B, BARSKY S, SALGIA K: Pacinian neurofibroma. Arch Dermatol 112:1558, 1976

CARNEY JA, GO VLW, SIZEMORE GW et al: Alimentary-tract ganglioneuromatosis. A major component of the syndrome of multiple endocrine neoplasia, type 2b. N Engl J Med 295:1287–1291, 1976

DUPRÉ A, CHRISTOL B, BONAFÉ JL et al: Neurome cutané à tumeur unique avec importantes altérations des cellules schwanniennes. Ann Dermatol Syph 101:271–276, 1974

GORLIN RJ, SEDANO HO, VICKERS RA et al: Multiple mucosal neuromas, pheochromocytoma and medullary carcinoma of the thyroid. A syndrome. Cancer 22:293–299, 1968

HOLM TW, PRAWER SE, SAHL WJ JR et al: Multiple cutaneous neuromas. Arch Dermatol 107:608–610, 1973

HURWITZ S: Sipple syndrome. Arch Dermatol 110:139–140, 1974

JACOBI H, KLEINE-NATROP HE: Beitrag zum "Syndrom der angeborenen fibrillären Neurome." Dermatol Monatsschr 156:644–652, 1970

KHAIRI MRA, DEXTER RN, BURZYNSKI NJ et al: Mucosal neuroma, pheochromocytoma and medullary thyroid carcinoma: Multiple endocrine neoplasia type 3. (Review) Medicine (Baltimore) 54:89–112, 1975

KING DT, BARR RJ: Bizarre cutaneous neurofibromas. J Cutan Pathol 7:21–31, 1980

LEVI L, CURRI SB: Multiple pacinian neurofibroma. Br J Dermatol 102:345–349, 1980

MACDONALD DM, WILSON JONES E: Pacinian neurofibroma. Histopathology 1:247–255, 1977

PROSE PH, GHERARDI GJ, COBLENZ A: Pacinian neurofibroma. Arch Dermatol 76:65–69, 1957

SHAPIRO L, JUHLIN EA, BROWNSTEIN HM: Rudimentary polydactyly. Arch Dermatol 108:223–225, 1973

THIES W: Multiple echte fibrilläre Neurome (Rankenneurome) der Haut und Schleimhaut. Arch Klin Exp Dermatol 218:561–573, 1964

WAGGENER JD: Ultrastructure of benign peripheral nerve sheath tumors. Cancer 19:699–709, 1966

WEISER G: An electron microscope study of "Pacinian neurofibroma." Virchows Arch (Pathol Anat) 366:331–340, 1975

Granular Cell Tumor

ABRIKOSSOFF A: Über Myome, ausgehend von der quergestreiften, willkürlichen Muskultur. Virchows Arch (Pathol Anat) 260:215–233, 1926

ALKEK DS, JOHNSON WC, GRAHAM JH: Granular cell myoblastoma. Arch Dermatol 98:543–547, 1968

APARICIO SR, LUMSDEN CE: Light and electron microscopic studies on the granular cell myoblastoma of the tongue. J Pathol 97:339–355, 1969

APISARNTHANARAX P: Granular cell tumor. (Review) J Am Acad Dermatol 5:171–182, 1981

ASHBURN LL, RODGER RC: Myoblastomas, neural origin. Am J Clin Pathol 22:440–448, 1952

BLOOM D, GINZLER AM: Myoblastoma. Arch Dermatol Syph 56:648–658, 1947

CHRESTIAN MA, GAMBARELLI D, HASSOUN J et al: Granular cell myoblastoma. J Cutan Pathol 4: 80–89, 1977

FISHER ER, WECHSLER H: Granular cell myoblastoma, a misnomer. Cancer 15:936–954, 1962

GARANCIS JC, KOMOROWSKI RA, KUZMA JF: Granular cell myoblastoma. Cancer 25:542–550, 1970

HAISKEN W, LANGER E: Die submikroskopische Struktur des sogenannten Myoblastenmyoms (Lipidfibrom, granuläres Neurom). Frankfurt Z Pathol 71:600–616, 1962

MOSCOVIC EA, AZAR HA: Multiple granular cell tumors ("myoblastomas"). Cancer 20:2032–2047, 1967

PENNEYS NS, ADACHI K, ZIEGELS-WEISMAN J et al: Granular cell tumors of the skin contain myelin basic protein. Arch Pathol, in press

SOBEL HJ, MARQUET E, AVRIN E et al: Granular cell myoblastoma. Am J Pathol 65:59–78, 1971

SOBEL HJ, MARQUET E, SCHWARZ R: Is schwannoma related to granular cell myoblastoma? Arch Pathol 95:396–401, 1973

TAMAKI K, ISHIBASHI Y, KUKITA A: A granular cell tumor. J Dermatol (Tokyo) 5:127–133, 1978

WEISER G, PROPST A: Elektronenoptische Untersuchung zur Histogenese des granulären Neuroms. Virchows Arch (Pathol Anat) 358:193–204, 1973

WHITE SW, GALLAGER RL, RODMAN OG: Multiple granular-cell tumors. J Dermatol Surg Oncol 6:57–61, 1980

Malignant Granular Cell Tumor

AL-SARRAF M, LOUD AV, VAITKEVICIUS VK: Malignant granular cell tumor. Histochemical and electron microscopic study. Arch Pathol 91:550–558, 1971

BARR RJ, GRAHAM JH: Granular cell basal cell carcinoma. Arch Dermatol 115:1064–1067, 1979

BUSANNI-CASPARI W, HAMMAR CH: Zur Malignität der sogenannten Myoblastenmyome. Zentralbl Allg Pathol 98:401–406, 1958

CRAWFORD ES, DE BAKEY ME: Granular-cell myoblastoma: Two unusual cases. Cancer 6:786–789, 1953

GAMBOA LG: Malignant granular-cell myoblastoma. Arch Pathol 60:663–668, 1955

GARTMANN H: Malignant granular cell tumor. Hautarzt 28:40–44, 1977

GILLIET F, MACGEE W, STOIAN M et al: Zur Histogenese granuliertzelliger Tumoren. Hautarzt 24:52–57, 1973

HAUSTEIN UF: Malignes metastasierendes Granularzellmyoblastom Abrikosow mit symptomatischer Dermatomyositis. Dermatol Monatsschr 160:318–328, 1974

KRIEG AF: Malignant granular cell myoblastoma. Arch Pathol 74:251–256, 1962

RAVICH A, STOUT AP, RAVICH RA: Malignant granular cell myoblastoma involving the urinary bladder. Ann Surg 121:361–372, 1945

ROSS RC, MILLER TR, FOOTE FW: Malignant granular-cell myoblastoma. Cancer 5:112–121, 1952

STRONG EW, MCDIVITT RW, BRASFIELD RD: Granular cell myoblastoma. Cancer 25:415–422, 1970

SVEJDA J, HORN V: Disseminated granular-cell pseudotumour: So-called metastasizing granular-cell myoblastoma. J Pathol Bacteriol 76:343–348, 1958

USUI M, ISHII S, YAMAWAKI S et al: Malignant granular cell tumor of the radial nerve. Cancer 39:1547–1555, 1977

Nasal Glioma

BARAN R, KOPF A, SCHNITZLER L: Le gliome nasal. Ann Dermatol Syph 100:395–407, 1973

CHRISTIANSON HB: Nasal glioma. Arch Dermatol 93:68–76, 1966

KOPF AW, BART RS: Nasal glioma. J Dermatol Surg Oncol 4:128–130, 1978

MIRRA SS, PEARL GS, HOFFMAN JC et al: Nasal "glioma" with prominent neuronal component. Arch Pathol 105:540–541, 1981

Cutaneous Meningioma

BAIN GO, SHNITKA TK: Cutaneous meningioma (psammoma). Arch Dermatol 74:590–594, 1956

LAYMON CW, BECKER FT: Massive metastasizing meningioma involving the scalp. Arch Dermatol Syph 59:626–635, 1949

WATERSON KW JR, SHAPIRO L: Meningioma cutis: Report of a case. Int J Dermatol 9:125–129, 1970

WEITZNER S: Intradermal nevus with psammoma body formation. Arch Dermatol 98:287–289, 1968

Melanocytic Nevi and Malignant Melanoma

33

Melanocytic tumors are composed of one of the following three types of cells: nevus cells, epidermal melanocytes, or dermal melanocytes.

Benign tumors composed of nevus cells are called melanocytic nevi. They can be divided into junctional nevi, compound nevi, and intradermal nevi. Special variants of melanocytic nevi are (1) the balloon cell nevus, (2) the halo nevus, (3) the Spitz nevus, and (4) the congenital melanocytic nevus.

Benign tumors composed of epidermal melanocytes include (1) lentigo simplex, (2) freckles, (3) the melanotic macules of Albright's syndrome, (4) Becker's melanosis, and (5) lentigo senilis. (The café-au-lait patches of neurofibromatosis have been described on p. 668.)

Benign tumors derived from dermal melanocytes include the Mongolian spot, the nevi of Ota and of Ito, and the blue nevus.

Malignant melanoma either is located in situ or is invasive. Malignant melanoma in situ can be divided into (1) lentigo maligna, (2) superficial spreading malignant melanoma in situ, and (3) acral lentiginous malignant melanoma in situ. Invasive malignant melanoma has the following five types: (1) lentigo maligna melanoma, (2) superficial spreading malignant melanoma, (3) acral lentiginous malignant melanoma, (4) nodular malignant melanoma, and (5) melanoma arising within the dermis either from a congenital melanocytic nevus or, rarely, from an intradermal nevus. Finally, there is the rare malignant blue nevus.

MELANOCYTIC NEVUS

Melanocytic nevi vary considerably in their clinical appearance. Aside from the four special variants of melanocytic nevi mentioned above, which will be discussed separately, five clinical types of melanocytic nevi may be recognized: (1) flat lesions, (2) slightly elevated lesions, (3) papillomatous lesions, (4) dome-shaped lesions, and (5) pedunculated lesions. The first three types are always pigmented; the latter two may or may not be pigmented. Dome-shaped lesions often show several coarse hairs. Although exceptions occur, one can predict to a certain degree from the clinical appearance of a melanocytic nevus whether on histologic examination it will prove to be a junctional nevus, a compound nevus, or an intradermal nevus. Most flat lesions represent either a junctional nevus or a lentigo simplex; most slightly elevated lesions and some papillomatous lesions represent a compound nevus; and most papillomatous lesions and nearly all dome-shaped and pedunculated lesions represent an intradermal nevus (Shaffer).

Melanocytic nevi are only rarely present at birth (see Congenital Melanocytic Nevus). Most nevi appear in adolescence and early adulthood (see Histogenesis). In this age period, they may occur in crops and, rarely, as widespread eruptive nevi (Eady et al).

Histopathology. Melanocytic nevi are composed of nevus cells, which, even though they are basically identical with melanocytes, differ from melanocytes by being arranged in clusters, or "nests," and by not showing dendritic processes, as best demonstrated by staining with silver. (For details, see Histogenesis.)

681

Although a histologic subdivision of melanocytic nevi into junctional, compound, and intradermal nevi is very useful and is generally accepted, it should be realized that lesions in an intermediate state between junctional and compound nevus and between compound and intradermal nevus are frequently encountered. Such intermediate states can be interpreted as transitional stages in the "life cycle" of melanocytic nevi, which start out as junctional nevi and, after having become intradermal nevi, undergo involution (see Histogenesis).

Nevus cells show considerable variation in their appearance, so that they are often recognizable as nevus cells largely by their arrangement in clusters or nests rather than by their cellular characteristics. As the result of a shrinkage artifact, nevus cell nests often appear partially separated from their surrounding stroma. In the lower epidermis and upper dermis, nevus cells commonly resemble epithelioid cells, since they usually are cuboidal or oval in shape and possess a distinctly outlined homogenous cytoplasm and a large, round or oval nucleus. Frequently, they contain melanin. Nevus cells in the middermis usually are smaller than those in the upper dermis and may resemble lymphoid cells; they rarely contain melanin. Nevus cells in the lower dermis resemble fibroblasts, or Schwann cells, since they are usually elongated and possess a spindle-shaped nucleus. They often lie in strands and hardly ever contain melanin. Some authors refer to the nevus cells in the upper, middle, and lower dermis as *types A, B,* and *C,* respectively (Miescher and von Albertini; Mishima).

Junctional Nevus.   In a junctional nevus, or junction nevus, nevus cells lie in well-circumscribed nests either entirely within the lower epidermis (Fig. 33-1) or bulging downward into the dermis but still in contact with the epidermis, thus being in the stage of "dropping off." The nevus cells constituting these nests generally have a regular, cuboidal appearance, although they are occasionally spindle-shaped. In addition, varying numbers of diffusely arranged nevus cells are seen in the lowermost epidermis, especially in the basal cell layer. Varying amounts of melanin granules are seen in the nevus cells. Some of the well-pigmented spindle-shaped nevus cells within the nests and, often, the diffusely arranged nevus cells, on staining with silver, show dendritic processes, making them indistinguishable from melanocytes.

The upper epidermis usually appears normal, since nevus cells only occasionally penetrate into the upper layers of the epidermis. However, in deeply pigmented junctional nevi, aggregates of melanin granules may be seen in the stratum corneum. Not infrequently, the upper dermis contains an infiltrate of melanophages and mononuclear cells.

Lesions in which there is a significant degree of diffuse arrangement of nevus cells and a pronounced inflammatory infiltrate may be difficult to differentiate from a malignant melanoma in situ

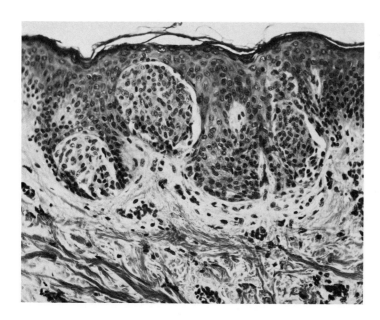

Fig. 33-1. Junctional nevus
Well-circumscribed nevus cell nests are present in the lower epidermis. (×200)

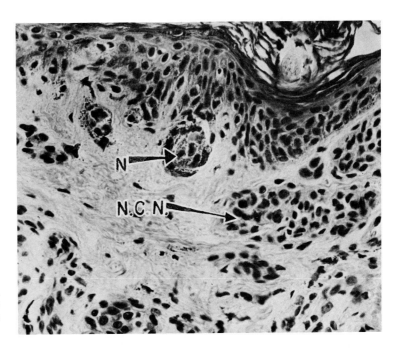

Fig. 33-2. Compound nevus, mature type
Nevus cell nests are seen within the epidermis and in the dermis. One nevus cell nest (*N*) is in the state of "dropping off." Typical nevus cell nests (*N.C.N.*) also lie free in the dermis. Considerable amounts of melanin are present in the nevus cell nests in the upper dermis, whereas no melanin is seen in the nevus cell nests further down. (×200)

(see p. 702). The most important points of differentiation are the lack of nuclear atypicality and the fairly sharp lateral demarcation in junctional nevi.

Compound Nevus.   A compound nevus possesses features of both a junctional and an intradermal nevus. Nevus cell nests may be seen in the epidermis, as well as "dropping off" from the epidermis into the dermis and in the dermis (Fig. 33-2). Usually, the nevus cells in the upper dermis are cuboidal and show abundant cytoplasm containing varying amounts of melanin granules. They represent type A cells (see p. 682). Melanophages are often seen in the surrounding stroma. The cells in the middermis usually are type B cells; they are distinctly smaller than the type A cells, display less cytoplasm and less melanin, and generally lie in well-defined aggregates. This decrease in size and good nesting is often referred to as maturation and is regarded as evidence of benignity, since the size of the cells in a malignant melanoma usually does not decrease with depth.

Compound nevi with a significant degree of junctional activity, referred to as early compound nevi, show no type B or C cells but only type A cells. Not infrequently, such early compound nevi show some pleomorphism of their type A melanocytes in the upper dermis, so that some of them appear spindle-shaped rather than cuboidal or oval, or they contain abundant cytoplasm with fine, dusty melanin granules. Also, there may be

an inflammatory infiltrate intermingled with melanophages. Distinction from an incipient malignant melanoma (see p. 708) and particularly from a dysplastic nevus (see p. 716 and Fig. 33-28) requires careful weighing of all histologic as well as clinical data.

In contrast to early compound nevi, "mature" compound nevi show few areas of junctional activity and usually display significant amounts of type B and C cells. They are then easily recognized as benign. (For a description of type C cells, see Intradermal Nevus below.)

Intradermal Nevus.   Intradermal nevi show usually only very slight and occasionally no junctional activity. The upper dermis shows nests and cords of nevus cells (Fig. 33-3). Not infrequently, one encounters within the nests and cords multinucleated nevus cells in which small nuclei lie either in a rosettelike arrangement or close together in the center of the cell. These giant cells occur only in well-matured nevi and therefore can be taken as evidence of the benign nature of the nevus in which they occur. They differ significantly in appearance from the irregularly and even bizarrely shaped giant cells that are seen frequently in the Spitz nevus and occasionally also in malignant melanoma. As a result of shrinkage during tissue processing, clefts may form between some nests of nevus cells and the surrounding stroma, leaving a space that simulates a lymphatic space. This may

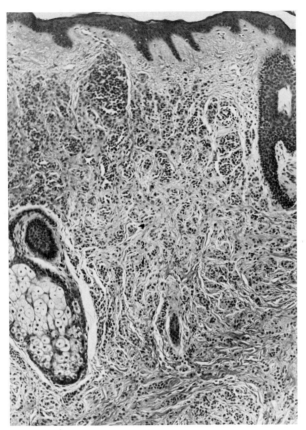

Fig. 33-3.   Intradermal nevus
In the upper dermis, the nevus cells lie in nests and
cords. In the lower dermis, the nevus cells appear
spindle-shaped and are embedded in collagenous fibers.
($\times 100$)

give the impression that a group of nevus cells is
located within a lymphatic space, simulating lymphatic invasion (Sagebiel).

Whereas the nevus cell nests located in the
upper dermis often contain a moderate amount of
melanin, the nevus cells in the midportion and the
lower dermis rarely contain melanin. Instead, these
nevus cells, referred to as type C cells, appear
spindle-shaped, are arranged in bundles, and are
embedded in collagenous fibers having a loose,
pale, wavy appearance similar to that of the fibers
in a neurofibroma. Such formations have been
referred to as neuroid tubes. In other areas, the
nevus cells lie within concentrically arranged, loosely
layered filamentous tissue, forming so-called nevic
corpuscles that resemble Meissner's tactile bodies
and are referred to as lames foliacées (Masson).
Occasionally, small aggregates of type A cells
containing abundant amounts of melanin and sur-

rounded by melanophages are observed in the
lower portion of an intradermal nevus, where they
are surrounded by type B or type C cells.

An occasional intradermal nevus is devoid of
nevus cell nests in the upper dermis and contains
only spindle-shaped nevus cells embedded in
abundant, loosely arranged collagenous tissue
(Fig. 33-4). Such nevi are referred to as neural nevi.
Their differentiation from a solitary neurofibroma
may be impossible in routinely stained sections
(Becker). Staining for nerves is also of no help in
this differentiation, since both neural nevi and
neurofibromas contain numerous nerves (Shelley
and Arthur). Both also show nonspecific cholinesterase activity, which is diffuse in neural nevi,
whereas, in neurofibromas, it shows irregular patchy
and fibrillar distribution (Winkelmann; Winkelmann and Johnson). A distinction is possible only
with the ultrastructural dopa technic, and with an
immunohistochemical technic employing myelin
basic protein (see Histogenesis and p. 670).

Some intradermal and, less commonly, compound nevi show hyperkeratosis and papillomatosis, which may be associated with a lacelike,
downward growth of epidermal strands and with
horn cysts (Fig. 33-5). Such nevi show a resemblance to seborrheic keratoses in their epidermal
architecture (Bentley-Phillips and Marks). In other
instances, large hair follicles are observed. Rupture
of a large hair follicle may manifest itself clinically
in an increase in the size of the nevus associated
with an inflammatory reaction, leading to suspicion
of a malignant melanoma. Histologic examination
in such instances shows a partially destroyed epidermal follicular lining with a pronounced inflammatory infiltrate containing foreign body giant cells
as a reaction to the presence of keratin in the
dermis (Freeman and Knox).

Occasionally, intradermal nevi contain scattered, large fat cells within the aggregates of nevus
cells (Fig. 33-6). Since this fatty infiltration is seen
largely in nevi removed from persons over 50 years
of age, it can be regarded as a regressive phenomenon in which fat cells replace involuting nevus
cells, rather than as a combination of a nevus
lipomatosus and a melanocytic nevus (Stegmaier;
Maize and Foster). The infrequent presence of
spicules of bone in intradermal nevi is regarded as
metaplastic ossification secondary to an inflammatory reaction (see p. 663) (Delacrétaz and Frenk;
Roth et al). In rare instances, psammoma bodies,
that is, hyaline bodies with slight calcification, are
observed within intradermal nevi (see p. 678)
(Weitzner).

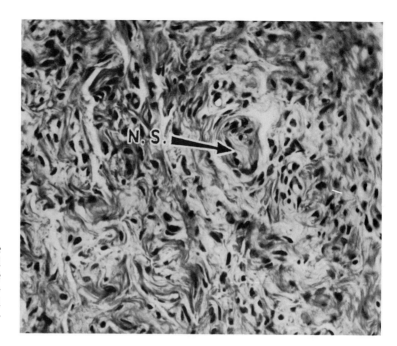

Fig. 33-4.   Neural nevus
The nevus cells are spindle-shaped and are embedded in abundant, loosely arranged collagenous tissue, which has the same loose, wavy, pale appearance as in neurofibroma. In the center, one sees a neuroid structure (*N.S.*) or nevic corpuscle resembling a Meissner tactile body. (×200)

Fig. 33-5.   Papillomatous intradermal nevus
One observes hyperkeratosis and papillomatous as well as lacelike downward growth of epidermal strands and horn cysts. The nevus contains numerous multinucleated nevus cells in which the nuclei lie either in a rosettelike arrangement or close together in the center of the cell. (×50)

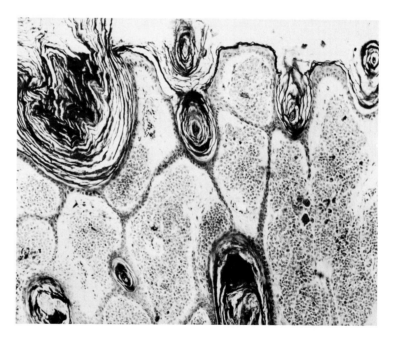

The term *fibrous papule of the nose* was given in 1965 to a usually solitary, flesh-colored, dome-shaped lesion of the nose (Graham et al). The lesion was then regarded as an involuting melanocytic nevus, and this view has since been shared by several subsequent observers. Other authors, however, have interpreted some of the lesions with this clinical appearance as either a solitary angiofibroma or a solitary perifollicular fibroma. (For a detailed discussion of fibrous papule of the nose, see p. 602.)

Histogenesis. For many years, Masson's theory of the dual origin of nevus cells was widely accepted. As stated

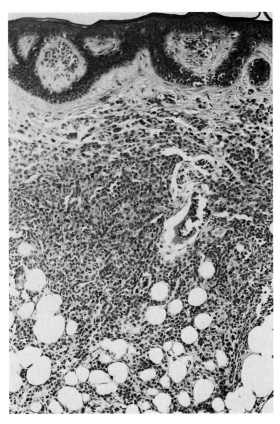

Fig. 33-6. Intradermal nevus containing scattered large fat cells
This fatty infiltration represents a regressive phenomenon in which involuting nevus cells are replaced by fat cells. (×100)

by Masson in 1951, he believed that the nevus cells in the upper dermis developed from epidermal melanocytes, whereas the nevus cells in the lower dermis developed from Schwann cells. The Schwann cell origin of the nevus cells in the lower dermis was suggested to Masson by the frequent presence of nervelike structures, such as neuroid tubes and nevic corpuscles, in the deep portions of compound and intradermal nevi (see p. 684). The fact that both epidermal melanocytes and Schwann cells are derived from the neural crest and thus are related to one another seemed to support Masson's view. Also in favor of a relationship between the nevus cells in the deep dermis and Schwann cells were the presence of a strongly positive nonspecific cholinesterase reaction in both types of cells and the absence of melanin and of a positive dopa-oxidase reaction in the nevus cells in the deep dermis (Winkelmann).

The first ultrastructural investigation of the dopa reaction by Mishima seemed to confirm that the nevus cells in the deep dermis, referred to as C type nevus cells, are dopa-negative. However, Mishima also found

that cholinesterase activity was present in all nevus cells, although the reaction was more pronounced in the B and C types of nevus cells than in the A type.

An important clarification was achieved in 1971 by Thorne et al, who used a more sensitive method for the ultrastructural dopa reaction than Mishima had used. They demonstrated the presence of melanosomes with dopa-oxidase activity even in nevus cells deep in the dermis that had a neuroid appearance on light microscopy. For the demonstration of the electron microscopic dopa reaction, Thorne et al used glutaraldehyde as fixative in place of formalin that had been used by Mishima. In addition, after incubating the ultrathin sections in dopa solution, they postfixed them in osmium tetroxide. An electron microscopic examination of nevic corpuscles (Niizuma) revealed that, even though these corpuscles resemble Meissner corpuscles by light microscopy, they contain no Schwann cells but are instead composed exclusively of nevus cells. These nevus cells were found to contain premelanosome-like dense bodies in their perikaryon, whereas axons were absent. Furthermore, with use of an immunoperoxidase method, myelin basic protein has been found to be regularly present in Schwann cells and absent in all types of melanocytic nevi (Penneys et al).

Another important point in favor of a single origin of the nevus cell is to be found in the life cycle of melanocytic nevi. Although there are exceptions, most nevi appear in childhood, adolescence, and early adulthood, and, with advancing age, there is a progressive decrease in the number of melanocytic nevi (Stegmaier). The evolution and regression of melanocytic nevi correlate with their histologic appearance. Junctional proliferation of nevus cells is present in almost every melanocytic nevus in children, in about half of the nevi in young adults, and only in 10% to 20% of nevi in adults more than 50 years of age (Stegmaier; Maize and Foster). Intradermal nevi, by contrast, are most unusual in the first decade of life, and their proportion increases progressively with age (Lund and Stobbe; Maize and Foster). The incidence of fibrosis, fatty infiltration, and neuroid changes increases with age (Maize and Foster). Thus, the formation of cylindrical neuroid structures represents the end stage of differentiation and not a source of origin of intradermal nevi (Lund and Stobbe).

Concerning the relationship between epidermal melanocytes and nevus cells, some authors believe that these two types of cells have a different embryologic genesis, the nevus cell originating from a neural crest precursor cell referred to as nevoblast (Mishima; Lupulescu et al). Most authors, however, regard the two cell types as identical (Clark and Mihm; Gottlieb et al; Maize and Foster). It would seem that all morphologic features by which nevus cells differ from melanocytes, such as the absence of dendrites as seen by light microscopy, their arrangement in cell nests, and their larger size, are secondary adjustments of the cells. Electron microscopy has shown that the fine structure of nevus cells is comparable to that of epidermal melanocytes

(EM 46, 47). Thus, the mitochondria, Golgi complexes, and, in particular, melanosomes are identical in the two types of cells. In addition, nevus cells possess pseudopodic cytoplasmic processes that, even though they are shorter, are similar to the dendritic processes of melanocytes (Gottlieb et al). In conclusion, it seems established that nevus cells differ from Schwann cells but are identical to melanocytes.

Pseudomelanomatous Changes in Melanocytic Nevi

A traumatized nevus as well as a nevus recurring after incomplete removal may show a histologic picture that can be misinterpreted as malignant.

Histopathology. A *traumatized* melanocytic nevus, in addition to demonstrating a diffuse inflammatory infiltrate and crusting, may show intraepidermal proliferation and hyperplasia of melanocytes with apparent nuclear atypicality (Connors and Ackerman). The focal nature of the changes, the presence of neutrophils in the infiltrate, and the normal appearance of the tumor cells in areas devoid of inflammation aids in differentiation from a malignant melanoma.

The recurrent lesion that forms after the *incomplete removal* of a melanocytic nevus may show a considerable number of nevus cells, both singly and in nests, mainly along the epidermal-dermal junction and in the epidermis but occasionally also in the upper dermis (Fig. 33-7). These cells may appear atypical by showing large hyperchromatic and pleomorphic nuclei. Usually, they contain considerable amounts of melanin. A chronic inflammatory infiltrate containing melanophages may be seen in the upper dermis (Kornberg and Ackerman). Distinction from a superficial spreading malignant melanoma may be difficult without a pertinent history. However, the presence of fibrosis in the upper dermis and often also of remnants of a melanocytic nevus beneath the zone of fibrosis, as well as the sharp lateral demarcation, usually make a correct diagnosis possible.

Histogenesis. The nevus cells in the recurrent lesion originate from residual nevus calls located either at the periphery of the lesion or along the outer root sheath of hairs (Schoenfeld and Pinkus).

Melanonychia Striata

Melanonychia striata refers to a pigmented band extending in the long axis of the nail. Such bands are common in blacks and Orientals and therefore regarded as normal (Kouskoukis et al). However, the sudden appearance of melanonychia striata in whites is cause for concern, requiring a punch biopsy of the nail matrix after avulsion of the nail plate and retraction of the proximal nail fold subsequent to lateral incisions into the nail fold (Scher). An exception is the melanonychia striata seen in the Laugier–Hunziker syndrome in association with pigmented macules of the lips or the buccal mucosa, since this type of melanonychia is always benign (Baran). Some authors prefer an excision of the pigmented nail

Fig. 33-7.
Pseudomelanomatous changes in a recurrent melanocytic nevus Melanocytes with atypical-appearing nuclei extend along the epidermal-dermal border lying singly and in nests. On the right, a nest is seen in the upper dermis.

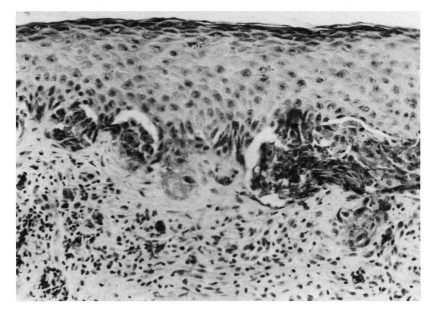

matrix lesion to a punch biopsy (Strempel and Horn; Kopf and Waldo).

Histopathology. Histologic examination in some instances shows merely hyperpigmentation without an obvious increase in the number of melanocytes (Kouskoukis et al). In others, a junctional nevus, a compound nevus, or an acral lentiginous melanoma, either in situ or invasive, is found (Kopf and Waldo).

Differential Diagnosis. Differentiation of a junctional nevus from an acral lentiginous melanoma in situ may be very difficult (see p. 706) (Bart and Kopf). For this reason, an excision may be preferable to a punch biopsy.

BALLOON CELL NEVUS

Balloon cell nevi possess no clinical features through which they can be differentiated from other melanocytic

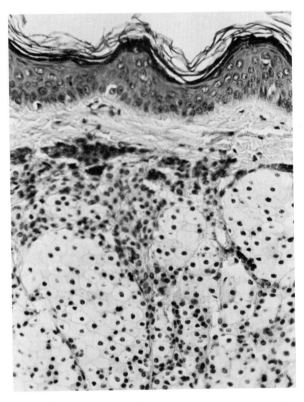

Fig. 33-8. Balloon cell nevus
Ballooned melanocytes lie in the dermis aggregated into lobules. Above the lobules of balloon cells are small groups of nonballooned, moderately pigmented melanocytes. Two solitary balloon cells are seen in the basal cell layer of the overlying epidermis. (×200)

nevi. They are quite rare. As a rule, they occur as solitary, slightly elevated, soft lesions of light brown color. They rarely exceed a size of 5 mm (Schrader and Helwig) and have no specific site of predilection. Although more common during the first three decades of life, they may also be found in elderly persons.

Histopathology. The presence of a few solitary or focally aggregated balloon cells in the dermis or epidermis of melanocytic nevi is not very uncommon; nearly 2% of melanocytic nevi show this phenomenon (Gartmann). However, the designation *balloon cell nevus* should be used only when balloon cells form the majority of cells in a nevus (Schrader and Helwig). On the basis of this criterion, only 31 cases of balloon cell nevus were reported up to 1978, and only 5 of them were composed entirely of balloon cells (Goette and Doty).

Balloon cell nevi may show balloon cells in direct contact with the overlying epidermis (Hornstein), but, in some instances, no connection with the epidermis is seen (Fig. 33-8). In either case, balloon cells may be seen within the epidermis singly or in groups. In the dermis, the balloon cells lie arranged in lobules of varying size. The lobules are separated by thin strands of connective tissue. In balloon cell nevi with an admixture of nevus cells, the latter are found mainly at the periphery of the lesion (Wilson Jones and Sanderson), although, in some cases, the two cell types appear intermingled (Schrader and Helwig). Transitions between nevus cells and balloon cells are seen in some instances (Wilson Jones and Sanderson).

The balloon cells are considerably larger than ordinary nevus cells, usually measuring 20 μm to 40 μm in diameter (Hornstein). Their nucleus is small, round, and usually centrally placed (Goette and Doty). Multinucleated balloon cells that resemble the rosette type of giant cells seen in intradermal nevi are commonly present and may be numerous (Wilson Jones and Sanderson). The cytoplasm of balloon cells appears either empty or finely granular. A few small melanin granules are commonly seen in subepidermally located balloon cells, especially with the Fontana–Masson stain (Hornstein), and coarse clumps of melanin granules are occasionally present (Goette and Doty). Stains for lipids, glycogen, and acid or neutral mucopolysaccharides are negative in the balloon cells.

Histogenesis. *Electron microscopic examination* reveals in balloon cells numerous large vacuoles that have formed by progressive enlargement, degeneration, and coalescence of melanosomes (Hashimoto and Bale). Because of the vacuolar degeneration of the melanosomes, melanization of the lamellar matrix of melanosomes usually does not take place. Vacuoles similar to those seen in the balloon cells of the dermis can also be found within balloon cells located in the epidermis, as well as within some keratinocytes as a result of transfer of altered melanosomes from balloon cells to keratinocytes (Okun et al).

The significance of the ballooning transformation is not clear. It is thought to represent a self-destructive process (Hashimoto and Bale). However, the presence of ribonucleic acid in the balloon cells indicates that they are metabolically active (Schrader and Helwig).

Differential Diagnosis.   Balloon cell nevus must be differentiated from balloon cell melanoma (for a description of balloon cell melanoma, see p. 712). The large fat cells that are present in some intradermal nevi as a result of a regressive fatty infiltration (see p. 684) differ from balloon cells by having a flattened nucleus that is located at the periphery of the cell and by showing a positive fat stain.

HALO NEVUS

A halo nevus represents a pigmented melanocytic nevus surrounded by a depigmented zone, or halo. In the common type of halo nevus, which is characterized histologically by an inflammatory infiltrate and is therefore referred to as *inflammatory halo nevus*, the central nevus only rarely shows erythema or crusting (Frank and Cohen); however, it undergoes involution in most instances, a process that extends over a period of several months. The area of depigmentation shows no clinical signs of inflammation and, even though it may persist for many months and even years, ultimately disappears in most cases. However, there are well-documented examples in which a halo nevus fails to involute, even though an inflammatory infiltrate is present, and repigmentation of the halo takes place (Berman). Most persons with halo nevi are young adults, and the back is the most common site. Not infrequently, halo nevi are multiple, occurring either simultaneously or successively.

Multiple halo nevi have been noted to develop following the excision of a malignant melanoma (Epstein et al). In rare instances, a halo of depigmentation forms around a congenital nevus, a Spitz nevus, a blue nevus, a malignant melanoma, or metastases of a malignant melanoma (Kopf et al; Shapiro and Kopf).

Besides the more common inflammatory halo nevus, there also are cases of *noninflammatory halo nevi* in which histologic examination shows no inflammatory infiltrate (Brownstein et al; King and King; Brownstein). In such instances, the nevus does not involute. Multiple halos without histologic inflammation and without involution

have been observed on rare occasions also around neurofibromas (Smith and Moseley).

In addition, there is the so-called *halo nevus phenomenon* (Brownstein), also referred to as *halo nevus without halo* (Happle et al). In such instances, there may be a nevus clinically showing signs of inflammation but no halo and histologically showing the characteristic inflammatory infiltrate (Happle et al). In other cases, a diagnosis of halo nevus is made solely on histologic grounds on a nevus that clinically has shown neither inflammation nor a halo (Brownstein).

Histopathology.   An inflammatory halo nevus in its early stage shows, embedded in a dense inflammatory infiltrate, numerous nests of nevus cells in the upper dermis and, in the case of a compound nevus, also at the epidermal-dermal junction. Later, a greater number of scattered nevus cells than of nests are seen. Even when melanin is still present in the nevus cells, these cells often show evidence of damage to their nucleus and cytoplasm. Most of the cells in the dense inflammatory infiltrate in the dermis have the appearance of lymphoid cells (Fig. 33-9). However, some of them are macrophages, in which varying amounts of melanin are seen. As the infiltrate invades the nevus cell nests, it often is impossible to distinguish between the lymphoid cells of the infiltrate and the type B nevus cells in the middermis, since they, too, have the appearance of lymphoid cells (see p. 682) (Kopf et al; Swanson et al). The infiltrate extends upward into the lower portion of the epidermis. In most instances, the infiltrate is characterized by dense cellular packing without vasodilatation or intercellular edema and by sharp demarcation along its lower border (Findlay).

At a later stage, only a few, and finally no distinct nevus cells can be identified (Findlay; Frank and Cohen). Gradually, after all nevus cells have disappeared, the inflammatory infiltrate subsides.

In both the inflammatory and the noninflammatory halo nevus, the epidermis of the halo at first shows a reduction in the amount of melanin on staining with silver and fewer dopa-positive melanocytes than are seen in the normal epidermis (Stegmaier et al). Ultimately, there is complete absence of melanin and also a negative dopa reaction (Stegmaier et al). The melanin in the epidermis overlying the nevus persists longer than that in the halo, but it ultimately also disappears after the involution of the nevus.

Histogenesis. Patients with an involuting halo nevus show circulating antibodies against the cytoplasm of malignant melanoma cells. These antibodies disappear

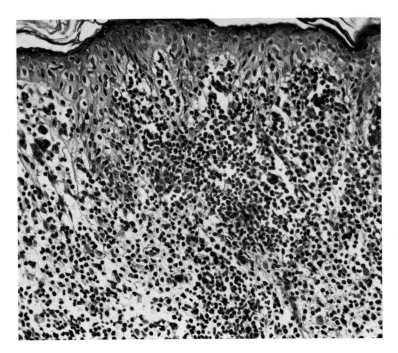

Fig. 33-9.   Halo nevus
In the upper dermis are scattered nevus cells, some of which contain melanin granules. Intermingled with the nevus cells and extending more deeply into the dermis is a dense infiltrate of cells. Most of them have the appearance of lymphoid cells, but some may be either nevus cells or melanophages. (×200)

from the blood stream once resolution of the nevus is complete (Copeman et al). Also, on direct immunofluorescence testing, halo nevus cells in frozen sections react with sera from patients with a halo nevus or a malignant melanoma (Bennett and Copeman). These findings imply that the entire population of melanocytic cells in the halo nevus has undergone mutation, because melanocytes elsewhere in the skin do not react.

Electron microscopic study reveals that, under the influence of the lymphocytic infiltrate, all nevus cells and melanocytes within reach of the infiltrate at first are damaged and ultimately disappear. In the nevus, many nevus cells appear vacuolated and contain only few melanosomes, while large aggregates of melanosomes are seen within macrophages. Some of the lymphocytes are in a transitional stage to plasma cells. It thus seems that the halo nevus cells produce an antigen and that the lymphocytes in the infiltrate carry antibodies against these nevus cells that destroy them (Stegmaier et al). Also, the presence of endoplasmic reticulum in the lymphocytes of the infiltrate suggests that they are antigenically stimulated (Swanson et al).

In the depigmenting halo, the melanocytes show various kinds of degeneration, such as vacuolization and coagulation of the cytoplasm and autophagocytosis of melanosomes. The melanocytes are seen partially in the upper layers of the epidermis and are apparently shed from the epidermis (Hashimoto). As long as damaged melanocytes are still present in the epidermis, one may observe in the Langerhans cells melanosome complexes enclosed within lysosomes (Ebner and Niebauer). Ultimately, all melanocytes disappear and only Langerhans cells remain; these cells are then seen also in the basal cell layer immediately above the basement membrane (Ebner and Niebauer). It is of interest that, both in halo

nevi and in vitiligo, the depigmentation takes place through disappearance of the melanocytes. However, the association of vitiligo and halo nevus is not sufficiently common for halo nevus to be regarded as a form of vitiligo.

Differential Diagnosis.   It can be difficult to differentiate early lesions of inflammatory halo nevus from a malignant melanoma; both types of lesions may have a dense cellular infiltrate in the dermis, and, in halo nevi, the nevus cell nests, as a result of having been invaded by the cellular infiltrate, may appear as if they were atypical. The danger of misinterpretation is greatest in halo nevi without a halo, the so-called halo nevus phenomenon. However, the inflammatory infiltrate in inflammatory halo nevi is more pronounced than in malignant melanoma and extends diffusely through the lesion, rather than being present largely at the periphery as in malignant melanoma.

If no identifiable nevus cells are present, the diagnosis of halo nevus is suggested by the presence of melanophages in the dense cellular infiltrate and by the absence of melanin in the epidermis on staining with silver.

SPITZ NEVUS

The Spitz nevus, now generally named after the author who first described it in 1948 (Spitz), is known also as *benign juvenile melanoma* and as *spindle and epithelioid cell nevus*. The lesion was originally thought to occur largely in children (Allen), but it is now recognized that more than half of the patients with a Spitz nevus are older than 14 (Paniago-Pereira et al), and about one fourth over 30 years of age (Barr et al, 1978). The lesion usually is solitary and is encountered most commonly on the face and extremities. In most instances, it consists of a dome-shaped, hairless, small nodule that in three quarters of the cases measures 6 mm or less. In 95% of the patients, the size of the tumor is below 1 cm (Weedon and Little). Its color is usually pink because of the sparsity of melanin, and it is then often diagnosed clinically as granuloma pyogenicum. However, it may be tan in color and, in some cases, brown and even black. Ulceration is seen only rarely (Paniago-Pereira et al).

In rare instances, multiple tumors are encountered either agminated in one area (Weimar and Zuehlke; Burket) or widely disseminated (Capetanakis; Burket).

Histopathology. The Spitz nevus in most instances has the architecture of a compound nevus, but it can have the appearance of an intradermal nevus and in some instances that of a junctional nevus. Because of the pleomorphism of the cells and the frequent presence of an inflammatory infiltrate, the histologic picture often closely resembles that of a nodular malignant melanoma, and there is no doubt that, prior to its recognition as an entity in 1948, many cases were misdiagnosed as malignant melanoma. Even today, differentiation from a malignant melanoma can occasionally be very difficult and even impossible (Okun).

Two types of cells may be found in Spitz nevi, spindle cells and epithelioid cells. In about half of the cases, spindle cells predominate (Fig. 33-10), in about 20%, epithelioid cells predominate (Fig. 33-11), and in the rest, the two types of cells are intermingled (Paniago-Pereira et al; Rupec et al). The cells in Spitz nevi are large. This feature, more than any other, sets the Spitz nevus apart from the common melanocytic nevus (McWhorter and Woolner).

The nevus cells in the Spitz nevus are arranged mostly in fairly well circumscribed nests. In Spitz nevi with junctional activity, one observes in nearly half of the cases artifactual clefts above the nests of nevus cells at the epidermal-dermal junction. Since this is rarely seen in malignant melanoma, it may be a useful diagnostic feature (Weedon and Little). Although there may be diffuse junctional activity, permeation of the epidermis by tumor cells is relatively slight. If present, it usually consists of single nevus cells or small groups of cells and is generally limited to the lower part of the epidermis (Paniago-Pereira et al). The epidermis is often hyperplastic and may show elongated rete ridges. However, it may be thinned and even ulcerated (Saksela and Rintala; Weedon and Little). Although found in fewer than half of the patients, diffuse edema and telangiectasia in the papillary dermis, if present, are of diagnostic importance. The edema may cause a loose arrangement of the nevus cell nests.

Fig. 33-10. Spitz nevus, with spindle cells predominating
Like most Spitz nevi, this is a compound nevus with edema in the subepidermal region and little or no melanin. Artifactual clefts are seen above the nests of nevus cells and the epidermis. (× 100)

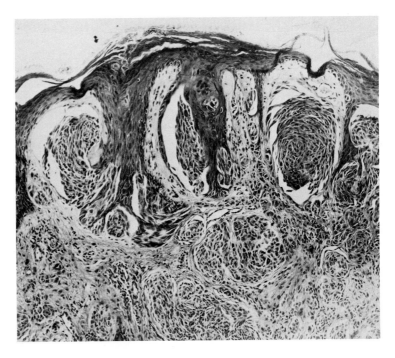

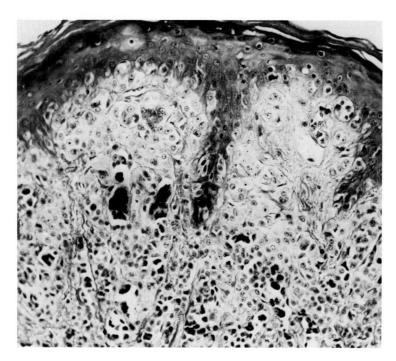

Fig. 33-11. Spitz nevus, with epithelioid cells predominating
The tumor cells vary in size and shape. Several rather large, irregularly shaped, bizarre giant cells are present. Other features are junctional activity, edema in the subepidermal region, and little or no melanin. (×200)

An important feature quite frequently present and helpful in the distinction of a Spitz nevus from malignant melanoma is maturation of the cells with increasing depth, so that they become smaller and look more like the cells of a common melanocytic nevus (Weedon and Little). In contrast, the sharp lateral demarcation of the junctional nests is of limited value, since lack of horizontal spread is also seen in nodular malignant melanoma.

Whereas spindle-shaped cells are characteristically arranged in whorls and only rarely show multinucleated giant cells, frequently, some of the epithelioid cells are multinucleated. The epithelioid cells are large, polygonal, and sharply demarcated, and they often have an eosinophilic cytoplasm. The nuclei of multinucleated epithelioid cells often appear bizarre, being large and hyperchromatic and having an irregular outline (Allen). The multinucleated epithelioid cells tend to stand out clearly, because they are often surrounded by edema.

Melanin is in many instances completely or nearly completely absent in Spitz nevi. Nevertheless, in about 10% of the cases, moderate amounts of melanin are found, and, in about 5%, melanin is heavily deposited (Paniago-Pereira et al). Mitoses are found in about half of the cases (Weedon and Little; Rupec et al). Usually, there are only a few, but occasionally, they are quite numerous. However, atypical mitoses are uncommon, and, if they

are found, the lesion should be interpreted with great caution (Weedon and Little).

An inflammatory infiltrate is found in many Spitz nevi and may be quite heavy. Its distribution can be bandlike, mainly at the base, as in malignant melanoma (Allen; Weedon and Little). Often, however, the infiltrate has a patchy distribution around blood vessels and is seen throughout the lesion (Paniago-Perreira et al). In some instances, diffuse fibrosis is present (Barr et al, 1980). Such desmoplastic Spitz nevi generally show no junctional activity, nesting, or pigmentation. The nevus cells are predominantly spindle-shaped and compressed by a desmoplastic stroma. However, they differ from a dermatofibroma by the presence of epithelioid and multinucleated cells.

A recent observation is the presence within the epidermis of reddish globules resembling colloid bodies in about 60% of Spitz nevi. Similar-appearing eosinophilic globules have been noted in the epidermis in only 2% of malignant melanomas and 0.9% of ordinary melanocytic nevi, and they are periodic acid-Schiff (PAS)-negative, whereas those seen in Spitz nevi are PAS-positive and diastase-resistant. Thus, the presence of eosinophilic globules appears to be an important diagnostic feature (Kamino et al).

On comparing Spitz nevi occurring in adults with those of children, it appears that pure epithelioid cell nevi are rare in adults. Also, lesions in adults often are more pigmented than in children (Echevarria and Ackerman). Furthermore, desmoplastic Spitz nevi occur predominantly in adults (Paniago-Pereira et al; Rupec et al).

Histogenesis. In Spitz nevi, in contrast to malignant melanoma, no circulating antibodies against the cytoplasm of malignant melanoma cells are found, indicating that the Spitz nevus is a biologically benign lesion (Copeman et al).

On *electron microscopic examination*, Spitz nevi show in their upper portion melanocytes with numerous melanosomes, whereas, in their lower portion, the number of melanosomes in the melanocytes decreases. Melanization is incomplete in most melanosomes. In addition, there is considerable lysosomal degradation of melanosome complexes within the tumor cells, even though the melanosomes are poorly melanized (Schreiner and Wolff). The almost complete absence of melanin in most Spitz nevi is thus explained.

Differential Diagnosis.   Differentiation of a Spitz nevus from a nodular malignant melanoma can be difficult and even impossible in some cases, since all of the changes seen in the Spitz nevus may also be observed in malignant melanoma (Helwig). Thus, there are cases on record that were diagnosed as instances of Spitz nevus but later proved to be malignant melanoma (Okun). The diagnosis of a Spitz nevus depends on an assessment of multiple morphological features, including clinical data such as size: whereas 95% of Spitz nevi measure less than 1 cm, 63% of malignant melanomas are larger than 1 cm (Weedon and Little). In borderline cases, histologic features that favor a diagnosis of malignant melanoma rather than Spitz nevus are (1) the presence of atypical mitoses; (2) prominent upward epidermal spread of tumor cells; (3) lack of nevus cell maturity at the base of the lesion; and (4) nuclear hyperchromasia in mononuclear tumor cells (Weedon and Little). Deep invasion, intense melanization, especially when it is deep, and arrangement of epithelioid cells in large, contiguous aggregates are additional possible signs of malignancy in borderline lesions, particularly when they are encountered in persons at or beyond puberty (Okun). Because of the difficulty of making an absolutely certain differentiation from malignant melanoma, it is advisable as a precautionary measure that all lesions diagnosed as Spitz nevi be excised in persons at or beyond puberty, particularly since such lesions are usually small in size. Also, one should never be biased by the age of the patient, because a malignant melanoma may arise in children, although this is rare (see p. 707).

CONGENITAL MELANOCYTIC NEVUS

Congenital melanocytic nevi are found in about 1% of newborn infants (Walton et al). In most instances, congenital melanocytic nevi are larger than acquired nevi, measuring more than 1.5 cm in diameter (Mark et al). Although generally they measure only a few centimeters in diameter, some are of considerable size. Those measuring more than 20 cm in greatest diameter are referred to as giant congenital melanocytic nevi (Kopf et al).

Nongiant congenital melanocytic nevi are usually slightly raised and often pigmented, and they may show a moderate growth of hair. Special forms are the *cerebriform congenital nevus,* which is found on the scalp as a skin-colored, convoluted mass (Gross and Carter; Orkin et al); the *spotted grouped pigmented nevi,* showing closely set brown to black papules that are either eccrine-centered (Mishima) or follicle-centered (Morishima et al); and the *congenital acral melanocytic nevus,* which consists of a bluish black patch on the sole or the distal portion of a finger clinically resembling an acral lentiginous melanoma (Botet et al).

Giant congenital melanocytic nevi often have the distribution of a garment and may follow the outline of a bathing trunk, a cap, a shoulder stole, a coat sleeve, or a stocking. They usually are deeply pigmented and are covered with a moderate growth of hair. Often, there are many scattered satellite lesions of a similar appearance (Slaughter et al). Leptomeningeal melanocytosis is found especially in cases in which the giant congenital melanocytic nevus involves the neck and scalp. There may be not only epilepsy and mental retardation but also a primary leptomeningeal malignant melanoma (Touraine; Reed et al; Slaughter et al).

Incidence of Cutaneous Malignant Melanoma. The incidence of a malignant melanoma arising either in a giant melanocytic nevus or, as seen occasionally, in one of the many smaller satellite nevi is high, averaging 12% (Kopf et al). The malignant melanoma may be present at birth, or it may arise in infancy or any time later in life. The mortality of such malignant melanomas is very high (Reed et al). It is therefore generally agreed that they should be excised as soon as possible, if this is feasible. The incidence of malignant melanoma in nongiant congenital melanocytic nevi, that is, in those less than 20 cm in greatest diameter, is at least 1% (Solomon), whereas the predicted percentage of malignant melanoma in the general population is 0.4%. The incidence of malignant melanoma is higher in the larger nongiant congenital melanocytic nevi, such as cerebriform nevi (Gross and Carter). The excision of all nongiant congenital melanocytic nevi is advised by many (Solomon; Rhodes et al) though not by all authors (Kopf et al). As an argument in favor of removal of all congenital melanocytic nevi, it has been pointed out that one or more histologic features of congenital nevi can be detected in 8% of melanoma specimens (Rhodes et al).

Histopathology. The histologic appearance of congenital melanocytic nevi generally differs from that of acquired nevi. Also, the appearance in neonates differs from that in patients older than 3 months, and it may differ in nongiant and giant congenital melanocytic nevi.

Nongiant congenital melanocytic nevi in neonates, that is, during the first 3 months of life, show nests of melanocytes as well as individual melanocytes scattered through the epidermis and within pilosebaceous and eccrine sweat units. Some of these melanocytes appear quite atypical and in some instances simulate the atypical melanocytic hyperplasia seen in the epidermis of superficial spreading malignant melanoma (Silvers and Helwig). The nevus cells within the dermis show a striking predilection either to originate from or to lie in close proximity to adnexal structures (Silvers and Helwig).

In children and adults, nongiant congenital melanocytic nevi are either compound or intradermal nevi. They differ from acquired nevi by the following features: (1) deeper extension of the nevus cells into the lower two thirds of the reticular dermis in nearly all, and into the subcutis in more than half of the cases; (2) extension of nevus cells between collagen bundles singly or in double rows; (3) distribution of nevus cells largely in the vicinity of the cutaneous appendages; and (4) presence of nevus cells within hair follicles, in sweat ducts and glands, in sebaceous glands, in vessel walls, and in the perineurium of nerves (Mark et al). Neuroid structures may be present in the lower portion of the nevus.

Among the special forms of nongiant congenital melanocytic nevi, the *cerebriform congenital nevus* usually presents as an intradermal nevus with neuroid changes simulating those seen in neurofibroma (Orkin et al). The *spotted grouped pigmented nevi* also are intradermal nevi. When they are eccrine-centered, each eccrine sweat duct is tightly enveloped by nevus cells, whereas hair follicles are involved only slightly (Mishima). When they are follicle-centered, nevus cell nests are found mainly around the hair follicles (Morishima et al). In the *acral melanocytic nevus,* a compound melanocytic nevus is seen with considerable pigmentation in the upper dermis, and aggregates of nonpigmented nevus cells are seen around blood vessels and eccrine glands deep in the dermis (Botet et al).

Giant congenital melanocytic nevi often are more complex than nongiant congenital nevi. Three patterns may be found within them: a compound or intradermal nevus, a "neural nevus," and a blue nevus (Reed et al). In some instances, the compound or intradermal nevus component predominates, whereas, in others, the "neural nevus" component predominates. In the latter case, formations such as neuroid tubes and nevic corpuscles are present (see p. 684). Such areas may show a great similarity to a neurofibroma (Santa Cruz and Bashiti). A component resembling a blue nevus is found in only some of the giant pigmented nevi and then usually only as a minor component (Reed et al). In rare instances, however, the entire congenital scalp lesion consists of a giant blue nevus, which, in one patient, was reported to extend to the dura (Menter et al) and in another infiltrated the brain (Silverberg et al).

If a malignant melanoma arises in a congenital melanocytic nevus, it usually originates at the epidermal-dermal junction. Occasionally, however, the malignant melanoma in a giant congenital melanocytic nevus, in contrast with nearly all other cutaneous malignant melanomas, arises deep in the dermis (Reed et al; Penman and Stringer). In such cases, it consists largely of undifferentiated cells resembling lymphoblasts and containing little or no melanin (Reed et al). In rare instances, the malignant melanoma arises from an area of blue nevus and thus represents a malignant blue nevus (Pack and Davis; Grouls et al).

In cases of leptomeningeal melanocytosis, one finds a diffuse infiltration of the leptomeninges with pigmented melanocytes. Also, the blood vessels entering the brain and spinal cord may be surrounded by melanocytes, and there may be areas of infiltration of the brain or spinal cord with melanocytes. Leptomeningeal malignant melanoma can infiltrate the leptomeninx and form multiple nodules in the brain (Touraine; Slaughter et al; Williams).

LENTIGO SIMPLEX

Three types of lentigo are recognized: lentigo simplex, lentigo senilis, and lentigo maligna. Lentigo simplex most frequently arises in childhood, but it may appear at any age (Gartmann). Usually in lentigo simplex, there are only a few scattered lesions without predilection to areas of sun exposure. They are evenly pigmented but vary individually from brown to black. They are not infiltrated and usually measure only a few millimeters in diameter. Clinically lentigo simplex is indistinguishable from a junctional nevus.

Special forms of lentigo simplex are lentiginosis profusa, the multiple lentigines syndrome or leopard syndrome, and speckled lentiginous nevus, referred to also as nevus spilus.

Lentiginosis profusa shows innumerable small, pigmented macules either from birth on (Kaufmann et al) or starting in childhood or early adulthood (Eady et al) without any other abnormalities. The mucous membranes are spared. There is no family history.

The *multiple lentigines syndrome*, like lentiginosis profusa, is characterized by the presence of thousands of flat, dark brown macules on the skin but not on the mucous surfaces. The lentigines begin to appear in infancy and gradually increase in number (Capute et al). The syndrome is inherited as a dominant trait. Although most macules vary from pinpoint dots to 5 mm in size, occasional dark spots are much larger, up to 5 cm in diameter (Selmanowitz). Features of this rare syndrome known also by the mnemonic *leopard syndrome*, may be, besides the lentigines (L), electrocardiographic conduction defects (E), ocular hypertelorism (O), pulmonary stenosis (P), and abnormalities of the genitalia (A) consisting of gonadal or ovarian hypoplasia, retardation of growth (R), and neural deafness (D) (Gorlin et al; Capute et al). Not all of these manifestations are present in every case (Voron et al; Weiss and Zelickson).

The *speckled lentiginous nevus*, or *nevus spilus*, consists of a light brown patch or band present from the time of birth that in childhood becomes dotted with small, dark brown macules (Cohen et al; Stewart et al; van der Horst and Dirksen).

Histopathology.   Lentigo simplex shows a slight to moderate elongation of the rete ridges, an increase in the concentration of melanocytes in the basal layer, an increase in the amount of melanin in both the melanocytes and the basal keratinocytes, and the presence of melanophages in the upper dermis. In some instances, melanin is also seen in the upper layers of the epidermis, including the stratum corneum. A mild inflammatory infiltrate may be found intermingled with the melanophages (Gartmann). Occasionally, small nests of nevus cells are seen at the epidermal-dermal junction, especially at the lowest pole of rete ridges. Such lesions then combine features of a lentigo simplex and a junctional nevus (Stewart et al; Gartmann).

In *lentiginosis profusa* and the *multiple lentiginosis syndrome*, as a rule, the lesions are "pure" lentigines without the formation of nevus cell nests (Eady et al; Gorlin et al; Capute et al). In large spots, however, there may be junctional nevus cell nests, and there may even be nevus cell nests in the upper dermis (Selmanowitz).

In *speckled lentiginous nevus*, or nevus spilus, the light brown patch or band shows the histologic features of lentigo simplex. The speckled areas show not only junctional nests of nevus cells at the lowest pole of some of the rete ridges but also diffuse junctional activity and dermal aggregates of nevus cells (Cohen et al; Stewart et al).

Histogenesis. The presence of occasional giant melanin granules has been described in several cases of lentigo simplex (Hirone and Eryu), lentiginosis profusa (Eady et al), multiple lentigines syndrome (Weiss and Zelickson; Bhawan et al), and speckled lentiginous nevus or nevus spilus (Konrad et al, 1974a). However, they also occur in several other conditions associated with hyperpigmentation, particularly in the café-au-lait spots of neurofibromatosis (Jimbow et al) (see p. 668) and, less commonly, in café-au-lait spots without neurofibromatosis, in the melanotic macules of Albright's syndrome (Benedict et al), in Becker's melanosis (Bhawan and Chang), in melanocytic nevi (Konrad et al, 1974b), and, on occasion, even in normal skin of healthy persons (Konrad and Hönigsmann).

Giant melanin granules vary in size from 1 µm to 6 µm. Because of their size and heavy melanization, the larger granules are readily recognized by light microscopy. Although seen largely within melanocytes, they also occur in keratinocytes and melanophages to which they have been transferred (Weiss and Zelickson).

On *electron microscopy*, giant melanin granules usually are found to be spheric. When fully melanized, they are uniformly electron-dense and are surrounded by a trilaminar membrane. However, in not fully melanized giant granules, one observes mainly at the periphery numerous densely set microvesicles 30 nm to 40 nm in diameter (Jimbow et al; Konrad et al, 1974b). Most authors regard these microvesicles as the basic component and the giant granule as a macromelanosome, rather than as a compound melanophagosome (Jimbow et al; Konrad et al, 1974b; Weiss and Zelickson; Bhawan et al). In favor of this view is the complete absence of melanofilaments, which are present in normal melanosomes and in the giant melanophagosomes of Chédiak–Higashi disease (see p. 442). Furthermore, the lysosomal enzyme acid phosphatase is absent (Konrad et al, 1974b). Nevertheless, some authors regard the giant melanin granules as completely degraded melanophagosomes (Hirone and Eryu; Ortonne and Perrot). Their main argument is the presence of still fairly small macromelanosomes within compound melanophagosomes. However, there is no reason why fairly small macromelanosomes should not occasionally be phagocytized (Bhawan et al), but this observation does not imply that, in a melanophagosome containing an early, still fairly small macromelanosome, all melanosomes will undergo this type of transformation and change the melanophagosome into a macromelanophagosome.

Peutz–Jeghers Syndrome

The Peutz–Jeghers syndrome shows dark brown macules clinically resembling lentigines in the perioral region.

Similar macules are seen on the vermilion border and the oral mucosa. Often, the dorsa of the fingers are also involved. Although a few cases of this dominantly inherited disorder have shown only the pigmentary anomaly (Bologa et al), there are usually multiple polyps in the gastrointestinal tract, mainly in the small intestine (Jeghers et al). The polyps often cause repeated episodes of intussusception and intestinal bleeding, but they rarely become malignant. In only 2% to 3% of the cases of Peutz–Jeghers syndrome does an adenocarcinoma develop in one of the polyps in the gastrointestinal tract (Reid), most commonly in the stomach (Achord and Proctor) or in the duodenum (Case Records, Massachusetts General Hospital).

Histopathology.   The basal cell layer shows marked hyperpigmentation. Although some authors have stated that the number of melanocytes is increased (Bologa et al; Blank et al), no increase has been found in dopa-stained sections (Yamada et al).

Histogenesis. *Electron microscopic examination* has led to different results on the pigmented macules located on the lips and those located on the fingers. On the lips, large, singly dispersed, deeply pigmented melanosomes, as seen in Negroid skin, are found largely within keratinocytes, rather than in melanocytes (Blank et al; Yamada et al). In contrast, the pigment macules on the fingers show a conspicuous pigment blockade, so that many melanosomes are located within dendrites of melanocytes and few melanosomes lie within keratinocytes (Yamada et al). No giant melanosomes have been observed in Peutz–Jeghers syndrome (Blank et al; Yamada et al).

It is evident that the intestinal polyps are hamartomas, since the glandular elements are intermingled with bundles of smooth muscle (Case Records, Massachusetts General Hospital).

FRECKLES

Freckles, or ephelides, are small, brown, macules scattered over skin exposed to the sun. Exposure to the sun deepens the pigmentation of freckles, in contrast to lentigo simplex.

Histopathology.   Freckles show hyperpigmentation of the basal cell layer, but, in contrast to lentigo simplex, show no elongation of the rete ridges and, in particular, no increase in the concentration of melanocytes. In fact, in epidermal spreads of freckled skin, the number of dopa-positive melanocytes within the freckles appears decreased on comparison with the adjacent epidermis. However, the melanocytes that are present are more strongly dopa-positive and larger, and they show more

numerous and longer dendritic processes than the melanocytes of the surrounding epidermis (Breathnach).

Histogenesis. On *electron microscopy*, the melanocytes within freckles are found to be essentially similar to those of dark-skinned persons. Melanocytes of the surrounding epidermis, by contrast, show markedly fewer and minimally melanized melanosomes, many of which are rounded rather than elongated and thus resemble the melanosomes encountered in red hair (Breathnach and Wyllie).

MELANOTIC MACULES OF ALBRIGHT'S SYNDROME

Albright's syndrome is characterized by usually unilateral polyostotic fibrous dysplasia, precocious puberty in females, and melanotic patches. The patches usually are large in size and few in number, are located on only one side of the midline, often on the same side as the bone lesions, and have a jagged, irregular border, like the "coast of Maine," in contrast to the smooth "coast of California" type of border of the café-au-lait patches of neurofibromatosis.

Histopathology.   Except for hyperpigmentation of the basal layer, there is no abnormality, and both the number and the size of the melanocytes are normal (Benedict et al).

Histogenesis. *Electron microscopic examination* reveals that many melanosomes are enlarged, measuring from 600 nm to 800 nm in length, that is, about twice the normal length (Frenk). Because of their enlarged size, most melanosomes within keratinocytes lie dispersed rather than in melanosome complexes. The rarity of melanosome complexes thus is similar to that observed in Negroid skin as opposed to Caucasoid skin (see p. 18). The increased melanization can thus be explained on the basis of a reduced degradation of melanin.

Differential Diagnosis.   The melanotic macules of Albright's syndrome only rarely show the "giant" melanin granules that are commonly seen in some of the melanocytes and keratinocytes within the café-au-lait patches of neurofibromatosis (see p. 668) (Benedict et al).

BECKER'S MELANOSIS

Becker's melanosis, also called Becker's pigmented hairy nevus, was first described in 1949 (Becker). It occurs most commonly as a large, unilateral patch showing hyperpigmentation and hypertrichosis on the shoulder or chest of a man. Usually, the patch is sharply but irregularly demarcated, but, occasionally, one observes netlike coalescing macules instead of a patch (Gartmann et al). The lesion commonly appears during the second decade of life. In some instances, Becker's melanosis affects areas other than the shoulder and chest (Tymen et al). Also, it may be multiple and bilateral and may be found in women (Copeman and Wilson Jones; Gartmann et al).

The hairiness always appears after the pigmentation, and, quite frequently, no hypertrichosis is seen (Gartmann et al; Tymen et al). It is therefore possible that cases described as progressive cribiform and zosteriform hyperpigmentation represent a variant of Becker's melanosis without hypertrichosis (Rower et al).

Of interest is the association of a smooth muscle hamartoma with Becker's melanosis, first reported in 1978 (see p. 657) (Urbanek and Johnson). Although a smooth muscle hamartoma may occur without Becker's melanosis (Plewig and Schmoeckel) and may be present from birth on together with pigmentation and hairiness (Bonafé et al), the association of a smooth muscle hamartoma with Becker's melanosis does not seem to be uncommon (Haneke). In such cases, the area of Becker's melanosis may show slight perifollicular papular elevations or slight induration (Urbanek and Johnson).

Histopathology. The epidermis shows slight acanthosis and regular elongation of the rete ridges. There is hyperpigmentation of the basal layer, and melanophages are seen in the upper dermis (Becker; Copeman and Wilson Jones; Frenk and Delacrétaz). The number of melanocytes is increased (Gebhart et al). This increase is particularly evident when melanocytes are stained for dopa-oxidase activity in both involved and uninvolved skin nearby (Tate et al). The hair structures appear normal.

In cases with an associated smooth muscle hamartoma, irregularly arranged, thick bundles of smooth muscle are present in the dermis (Urbanek and Johnson; Haneke). (For details, see p. 657.)

Histogenesis. *Electron microscopic examination* reveals an increased number of melanosomes within the melanocytes. The number and size of the melanosome complexes within the keratinocytes are increased, with many of the complexes containing more than ten melanosomes, rather than the usual average of three melanosomes (Frenk and Delacrétaz; Gebhart et al). Pronounced activity of the melanocytes and marked complexing of melanosomes similar to that found in Becker's melanosis also occur in the hyperpigmentation following exposure to sunlight.

LENTIGO SENILIS

Lentigo senilis commonly occurs as multiple lesions in areas exposed to the sun and is therefore also referred to as solar lentigo (Montagna et al). The lesions rarely occur before the fourth or fifth decade of life and slowly increase in size and number. They are found in more than 90% of Caucasoids over 70 years of age, most commonly on the dorsa of the hands (Hodgson). They are not infiltrated, possess a uniform dark brown color, and have an irregular outline. They vary in size from minute to more than 1 cm and may coalesce (Cawley and Curtis). Malignant degeneration does not occur (Braun-Falco and Schoefinius).

Senile lentigines and seborrheic keratoses may resemble each other in clinical appearance, and both are commonly referred to as liver spots. Seborrheic keratoses in general show more hyperkeratosis clinically. However, there exists a close relationship between lentigo senilis and the reticulated type of seborrheic keratosis, and it is believed by some that lentigo senilis can develop into a reticulated seborrheic keratosis (Mehregan) (see below). In contrast, lentigo maligna differs from lentigo senilis in clinical appearance by its irregular distribution of pigment (see p. 703).

Histopathology. The rete ridges are significantly elongated (Fig. 33-12). They either appear club-shaped or are tortuous and show small, budlike extensions (Cawley and Curtis). Between the elongated rete ridges, the epidermis may appear atrophic (Braun-Falco and Schoefinius). The elongated rete ridges are composed, especially in their lower portion, of deeply pigmented basaloid cells intermingled with melanocytes. The melanocytes appear significantly increased in number in some cases (Montagna et al) but only slightly increased (Hodgson) or not at all increased in others (Mehregan). They possess an increased capacity for melanin production, as shown by the fact that, on staining with dopa, they show more numerous as well as longer and thicker dendritic processes than the melanocytes of control skin (Hodgson). No junctional activity is observed. The upper dermis often contains melanophages and sometimes a mild, perivascular lymphoid infiltrate.

In some lesions, the rete ridges are elongated to such an extent that strands of basaloid cells form anastomosing branches, resulting in a reticulated pattern closely resembling that seen in the reticulated pigmented type of seborrheic keratosis (Mehregan).

Histogenesis. On *electron microscopy,* the basal layer of keratinocytes is seen to contain increased amounts of melanosomes and melanosome complexes (Braun-Falco and Schoefinius). Also, the melanosome complexes inside the keratinocytes appear larger than those found in uninvolved skin (Montagna et al). Even in the upper layers of the epidermis, including the horny layer,

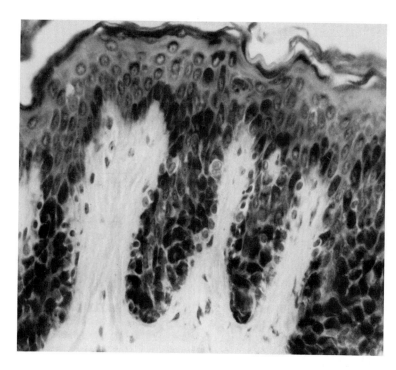

Fig. 33-12. Lentigo senilis
The rete ridges are significantly elongated. They show considerable hyperpigmentation of the basal keratinocytes and a moderate increase in the concentration of melanocytes. However, there is no nesting of the melanocytes or junctional activity. (×400)

numerous melanosomes are present largely in a dispersed state rather than as complexes. Thus, it seems that, in addition to increased melanin synthesis in the melanocytes, there is also a delay in the lysosomal destruction of melanosomes (Braun-Falco and Schoefinius).

Differential Diagnosis.   In lentigo simplex, there is much less elongation of the rete ridges than in lentigo senilis, the elongations are not tortuous or budlike, and junctional nevus cell nests are occasionally present. Lentigo maligna shows flattening or even absence of the rete ridges together with anaplasia of its melanocytes, and it usually possesses a more pronounced dermal infiltrate than lentigo simplex.

MONGOLIAN SPOT

The typical Mongolian spot occurs in the sacrococcygeal region as a uniformly bluish discoloration resembling a bruise. It consists of a noninfiltrated, round or ovoid, rather ill defined patch of varying size. It is found very frequently in Mongoloid and Negroid infants, but it also occurs occasionally in Caucasoid infants. It is present at birth and usually disappears spontaneously within 3 to 4 years. However, among Japanese, it is still found to be present in about 4% of young adults (Hidano) and in about 3% of middle-aged persons (Kikuchi and Inoue).

Occasionally, Mongolian spots occur outside the lumbosacral region as aberrant Mongolian spots, such as on the middle or upper part of the back; they may then be multiple and bilateral and persist (Cole et al). Extensive and persistent Mongolian spots are commonly seen in patients with bilateral nevus of Ota (Hidano et al).

Histopathology.   In the Mongolian spot, the dermis shows in its lower half or two thirds greatly elongated, slender, often slightly wavy dendritic cells containing melanin granules. These cells are present in a low concentration and lie widely scattered between the collagen bundles, and, like the collagen bundles, generally lie parallel to the skin surface. They are bipolar and from 5 µm to 10 µm wide and from 25 µm to 75 µm long. They often show several branching dendritic processes at either pole (Cole et al). Even though they are melanocytes, these cells show little or no increase in their pigment content on incubation with dopa compared with unincubated sections (Inoue; Konrad et al; Mevorah et al). No melanophages are seen (Konrad et al).

Histogenesis. The Mongolian spot is a result of the delayed disappearance of dermal melanocytes. Melanocytes are found in the dermis of Negroid embryos beginning with the 10th week. Between the 11th and 14th weeks, they start migrating into the epidermis. They gradually disappear from the dermis after the 20th week, and, at birth, dermal melanocytes are found in only a few areas, especially in the sacral region (Zimmermann and Becker).

The blue color depends upon the phenomenon that light passing through a turbid medium, such as the skin, is scattered as it strikes dark particles, such as melanin. Owing to the Tyndall effect, the colors of light that have a longer wavelength, such as red, orange, and yellow, tend to be less scattered and therefore continue to travel in a forward direction, whereas the colors of shorter wavelength, such as blue, indigo, and violet, are scattered to the side and backward to the skin surface (Kopf and Weidman).

On *electron microscopy*, the dermal melanocytes are seen to contain numerous fully melanized melanosomes (Inoue). Only a few melanocytes show premelanosomes as evidence of melanoneogenesis. The adjoining connective tissue cells contain very little phagocytized melanin (Konrad et al). The rather weak or even negative dopa reaction in the dermal melanocytes is due to the fact that most or all enzyme activity has been used up in the process of forming melanin.

NEVUS OF OTA AND OF ITO, DERMAL MELANOCYTE HAMARTOMA

Nevi of Ota and Ito and dermal melanocyte hamartoma are types of dermal melanocytosis that differ from the Mongolian spot by usually having a speckled rather than a uniform bluish appearance and by showing a greater concentration of dermal melanocytes, with location in the upper rather than in the lower portion of the dermis (Burkhart and Gohara).

The *nevus of Ota* represents a usually unilateral discoloration of the face composed of bluish and brownish, partially confluent macular lesions. The periorbital region, temple, forehead, malar area, and nose are apt to be involved. Because of this usual distribution, Ota has called the lesion nevus fuscocaeruleus ophthalmomaxillaris. There is frequently also a patchy bluish discoloration of the sclera of the ipsilateral eye and occasionally also of the conjunctiva, cornea, and retina (Kopf and Weidman). In some instances, the oral and nasal mucosa is similarly affected (Mishima and Mevorah). In about 10% of the cases, the lesions are bilateral rather than unilateral (Hidano et al, 1967). The lesions of the nevus of Ota may be present at birth; they may also appear during the first year of life or during adolescence but only rarely in childhood (Hidano et al, 1967). They have a tendency toward gradual extension. Malignant change in the cutaneous lesions of a nevus of Ota is extremely rare. So far, only two such cases have been reported, with death from metastases in one (Dorsey and Montgomery). In several instances, a primary malignant melanoma of the choroid, iris, orbit, or brain has developed in patients with a nevus of Ota involving an eye (Enriquz et al).

In the nevus of Ota, the involved areas of the skin show a brown to slate-blue mottled discoloration, usually without any infiltration. Occasionally, however, some areas are slightly raised. Also, in some patients, discrete nodules varying in size from a few millimeters to a few centimeters and having the appearance of blue nevi are found within the areas of discoloration (Kopf and Weidman).

The *nevus of Ito* differs from the nevus of Ota by its location in the supraclavicular, scapular, and deltoid regions. It may occur alone or in association with an ipsilateral or bilateral nevus of Ota (Mishima and Mevorah; Hidano et al, 1965). Like the nevus of Ota, it has a mottled, macular appearance.

In the *dermal melanocyte hamartoma,* there may be a single, very extensive area of gray-blue pigmentation present from the time of birth (Burkhart and Gohara). In other instances, there are several coalescing bluish macules that have gradually extended within a circumscribed area from the time of childhood (Mevorah et al), or widely scattered bluish patches that have gradually developed during childhood (Carleton and Biggs).

Histopathology. The noninfiltrated areas of the nevus of Ota, as well as the nevus of Ito and the dermal melanocyte hamartoma, show, similar to the Mongolian spot, elongated, dendritic melanocytes scattered among the collagen bundles. However, in these three forms of dermal melanocytosis, the melanocytes generally are more numerous and more superficially located than in the Mongolian spot (Mishima and Mevorah; Burkhart and Gohara). Although most of the fusiform melanocytes lie in the upper third of the reticular dermis, one can observe melanocytes also in the papillary layer in some lesions and extending as far down as the subcutaneous tissue in others (Mishima and Mevorah). Melanophages are seen in only few lesions (Mevorah et al). The dopa reaction is variable, even within the same lesion, since melanocytes that are scantily pigmented show a positive reaction, whereas heavily pigmented melanocytes react either weakly or not at all (Carleton and Biggs; Mishima and Mevorah). A negative dopa reaction is due to all melanogenic enzyme having been consumed in heavily pigmented melanocytes.

Slightly raised and infiltrated areas show a larger number of elongated, dendritic melanocytes than do noninfiltrated areas, thus approaching the histologic picture of a blue nevus, and nodular areas are indistinguishable histologically from a blue nevus (Dorsey and Montgomery).

In the two cases of nevus of Ota in which malignant changes occurred in the skin, the histologic appearance of the tumors was that of a malignant blue nevus arising within an area of cellular blue nevus (see p. 718) (Dorsey and Montgomery).

Histogenesis. Since the concentration of melanocytes in the nevi of Ota and Ito and in the dermal melanocyte hamartoma is larger than in the Mongolian spot, it is evident that these melanocytes do not merely represent residual dermal melanocytes, as in the Mongolian spot, but rather a hamartoma or nevoid lesion, analogous to the blue nevus (Dorsey and Montgomery; Burkhart and Gohara).

BLUE NEVUS

Blue nevi generally occur on the skin, although, in rare instances, they have been observed elsewhere, such as in the oral mucosa (Bogomoletz), the vagina (Rodriguez and Ackerman), the uterine cervix (Qizilibash), and the prostate gland (Jao et al).

On the skin, three types of blue nevi are recognized: the common blue nevus, the cellular blue nevus, and the combined nevus.

The *common blue nevus* occurs as a small, well-circumscribed, dome-shaped nodule of slate-blue or bluish black color. The lesion rarely exceeds 1 cm in diameter. About half of all common blue nevi are found on or near the dorsa of the hands and feet (Dorsey and Montgomery). Usually, there is only one lesion, but there may be several. A rare manifestation is the plaque type of blue nevus, which shows within a circumscribed area numerous macules and papules. This type of lesion may be present at birth (Pittman and Fisher) or appear in childhood (Hendricks). Malignant degeneration does not occur in the common blue nevus.

The *cellular blue nevus* consists of a bluish nodule that is usually larger than the common blue nevus. It generally measures 1 cm to 3 cm in diameter, but it may be larger (Dorsey and Montgomery). It shows either a smooth or an irregular surface (Kersting and Caro; Gartmann, 1965). About half of all cellular blue nevi have been found located over the buttocks or in the sacrococcygeal region (Rodriguez and Ackerman). Although rare, malignant degeneration of cellular blue nevi can occur (see Malignant Blue Nevus, p. 718). (For a discussion of congenital giant blue nevus, see Congenital Melanocytic Nevus, p. 694.)

The term *combined nevus* is applied to the association of a blue nevus with an overlying melanocytic nevus (Leopold and Richards). This association is found on histologic examination in about 1% of all nevi (Gartmann and Müller). Clinically, combined nevi are usually deeply pigmented.

Histopathology. In the *common type* of blue nevus, the melanocytes have the same appearance as those seen in the Mongolian spot and in the nevus of Ota, but their number is much greater. Greatly elongated, slender, often slightly wavy melanocytes with long, occasionally branching dendritic processes lie grouped in irregular bundles in the dermis (Fig. 33-13). The bundles of cells may extend into the subcutaneous tissue or lie close to

the epidermis. However, the epidermis is normal, except in the combined nevus (see below). The greatly elongated melanocytes lie predominantly with their long axis parallel to the epidermis (Plate 4, facing p. 676). Most of them are filled with numerous fine granules of melanin, often so completely that their nuclei cannot be visualized. The melanin granules may also fill the long, often wavy, occasionally branching dendritic processes (Fig. 33-14). Thus, on impregnation with silver, they resemble nerve fibers, inasmuch as both nerve fibers and melanin appear impregnated (Gartmann, 1965). Melanophages are frequently seen near the bundles of melanocytes. The melanophages differ from the melanocytes by being shorter and thicker, by showing no dendritic processes, and by containing larger granules (Dorsey and Montgomery). In contrast to the melanocytes, the melanophages are dopa-negative. The number of fibroblasts and the amount of collagen are often also increased, resulting in disruption of the normal architecture of the connective tissue.

In the *cellular type* of blue nevus, one observes, usually in addition to areas of deeply pigmented dendritic melanocytes, as seen also in the common type of blue nevus, cellular islands composed of closely aggregated, rather large spindle-shaped cells with ovoid nuclei and abundant pale cytoplasm often containing little or no melanin (Fig. 33-15). Melanophages with abundant melanin may surround the islands (Gartmann, 1961). Also, the spindle-shaped cells are occasionally pigmented, at least in some areas. The diagnosis of cellular blue nevus is generally easy in "biphasic" lesions with both dendritic and spindle-shaped cells, but it can be difficult in occasional lesions without dendritic cells and without melanin, which, however, often becomes apparent when a silver stain is used.

Larger islands composed of spindle-shaped cells may consist of many intersecting bundles of cells extending in various directions and resembling the storiform pattern seen in a neurofibroma (Santa Cruz and Yates). In some of the intersecting bundles, the spindle-shaped cells appear rounded as a result of cross sectioning (Fig. 33-16). Not infrequently, the cellular islands penetrate into the subcutaneous fat. If, in addition, the nuclei show pleomorphism, and if bizarre, atypical-appearing cells, including multinucleated giant cells, are present together with a surrounding inflammatory infiltrate, differentiation from a malignant blue nevus or a malignant melanoma can be difficult (Gartmann, 1961; Avidor and Kessler). The absence

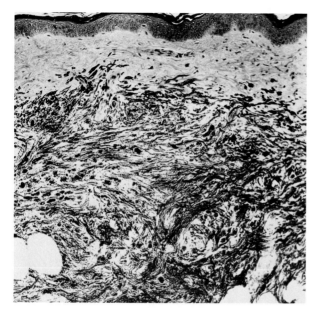

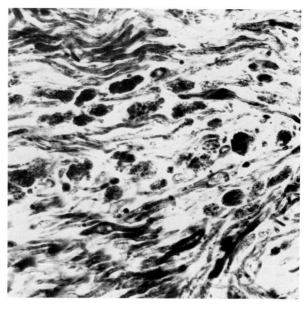

Fig. 33-13.   Blue nevus, common type
Low magnification. Numerous greatly elongated, slender, often slightly wavy melanocytes show dendritic processes and are filled with melanin. They lie grouped in irregular bundles in the lower dermis and in the subcutaneous fat. (×50)

Fig. 33-14.   Blue nevus, common type
High magnification of Figure 33-13. The greatly elongated melanocytes and their long dendritic processes are filled with fine melanin granules. In addition, melanophages filled with coarse melanin granules and showing no dendritic processes are present. (×400)

Fig. 33-15.   Blue nevus, cellular type
Low magnification. A large island of cells is seen extending into the subcutaneous fat. The cells are spindle-shaped, but where cross-sectioned, they appear rounded. They possess abundant pale cytoplasm without melanin. (×100)

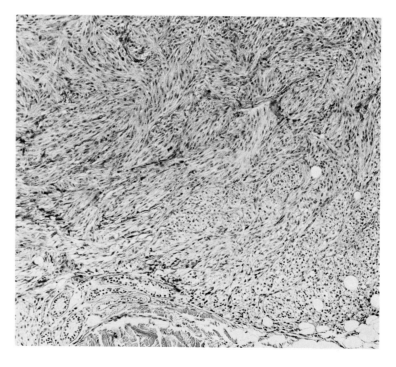

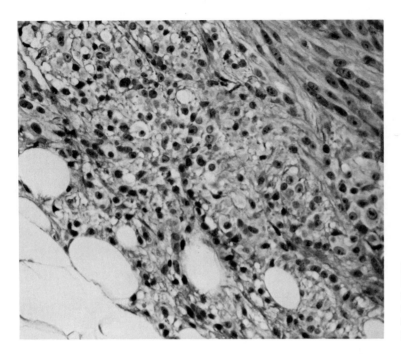

Fig. 33-16.   Blue nevus, cellular type
High magnification of Figure 33-15. The cells appear spindle-shaped or rounded, depending on the angle at which they are sectioned. No melanin is apparent in them. (×400)

or sparsity of mitotic figures and the absence of areas of necrosis are evidence against a diagnosis of malignant blue nevus, and the presence of areas of dendritic cells elsewhere in the tumor speaks against a diagnosis of malignant melanoma.

Occasionally in cellular blue nevi, small groups of well-differentiated nevus cells are found in the marginal sinuses of the regional lymph nodes. It can be assumed that these cells do not represent true metastases but were passively transported to the lymph nodes and lodged there as inert deposits (Rodriguez and Ackerman).

In the *combined type* of nevus, the blue nevus may be either a common or a cellular blue nevus, and the overlying melanocytic nevus may be a junctional, compound, intradermal or, rarely, a Spitz nevus (Gartmann and Müller).

Histogenesis. Whereas there is general agreement that the cells of the common blue nevus are melanocytes, some differences of opinion exists about the derivation of the spindle-shaped cells in cellular blue nevi, which often are free of of melanin.

As long as only light microscopic examination was available and silver impregnation was the usual method for demonstrating nerve fibers, a clear distinction between nerve fibers and melanin-filled dendritic processes was often impossible. It was thus understandable that some observers recognized numerous nerve fibers within cellular blue nevi and regarded these tumors as neural in origin (Dupont and Bourlond; Cramer). Since the

spindle-shaped cells are often arranged in intertwining bundles resembling Schwann cells, the cellular blue nevus was regarded as related to a neurinoma or neurofibroma, and, for cellular blue nevi containing melanin in the spindle-shaped cells, the term *pigmented storiform neurofibroma* was proposed (see p. 670) (Bird and Willis; Santa Cruz and Yates).

On *electron microscopic examination,* it becomes apparent that melanosomes are present both in the tumor cells of the common blue nevus (EM 48) and in the Schwann-like cells of the cellular blue cells. Even though the melanosomes in the spindle-shaped cells of the cellular blue nevus may show only little melanization, the electron microscopic dopa reaction indicates that they have considerable melanogenic potential (Mishima).

Even on electron microscopic examination, a neural origin of the cellular blue nevus has been regarded as likely by some authors either because of the enclosure of unmyelinated nerve fibers within the cytoplasm of the tumor cells (Merkow et al) or because of the invasion of the endoneurium by cellular blue nevus cells (Bhawan and Edelstein). However, these observations have not been confirmed by others (Hernandez; Bourlond).

Since transitions between dendritic and spindle-shaped cells can be seen, it may be concluded that the spindle-shaped cells are not Schwann cells but melanocytes, like the dendritic cells (Mishima; Hernandez).

MALIGNANT MELANOMA IN SITU

It is generally agreed that, aside from malignant blue nevus, there are four types of malignant melanoma.

Three types have an early *horizontal growth phase* within the confines of the epidermis, also referred to as in situ growth. This is followed after varying lengths of time by the *vertical growth phase*, or dermal invasion. The three types of malignant melanoma with a preceding in situ phase are (1) lentigo maligna melanoma, preceded by lentigo maligna; (2) superficial spreading melanoma, preceded by superficial spreading melanoma in situ; and (3) acral lentiginous melanoma, preceded by acral lentiginous melanoma in situ. The fourth type of malignant melanoma, nodular melanoma, arises as such (Clark et al, 1969; McGovern, 1970; Lopansri and Mihm).

In most instances, a histologic distinction between a malignant melanoma arising from a lentigo maligna and one arising from a superficial spreading or an acral lentiginous melanoma in situ can be made without difficulty through study of the adjacent intraepidermal component of the tumor. Nevertheless, there are instances in which the adjacent in situ portion cannot be classified with certainty either as lentigo maligna, or as superficial spreading or acral lentiginous melanoma in situ. Clinical data as to site and duration are then often of great value, but there are instances in which, even with this information, a decision as to whether a malignant melanoma has arisen within a lentigo maligna or a superficial spreading melanoma in situ is impossible (Flegel). A designation such as "malignant melanoma with adjacent intraepidermal component unclassifiable" is then advisable (McGovern et al, 1973).

The fact that categorization of an individual case is occasionally difficult does not mean that classification of malignant melanoma is unnecessary, aside from location and depth of penetration (Ackerman). Even when thickness is considered, the prognosis of lentigo maligna melanoma is better than that of other melanomas (McGovern et al, 1980).

The reason for a discussion of malignant melanoma in situ separate from that of invasive malignant melanoma is the same as that for the discussion of squamous cell carcinoma in situ, that is, solar keratosis, precancerous leukoplakia, and Bowen's disease, separate from that of squamous cell carcinoma in Chapter 26. Malignant melanoma in situ, like squamous cell carcinoma in situ, is a lesion that is still biologically benign, even though it is morphologically already malignant.

Lentigo Maligna

Lentigo maligna, also referred to as melanosis circumscripta preblastomatosa of Dubreuilh and as melanotic freckle of Hutchinson, occurs on the exposed cutaneous surfaces of the elderly, most commonly on the face, and only rarely on the forearms or the lower legs (Pitman et al). The lesion evolves slowly over many years. It starts as an unevenly pigmented macule that gradually extends peripherally and may thus attain a diameter of several centimeters. The lesion has an irregular border and, as long as it remains a malignant melanoma in situ, shows no induration. While extending in some areas, it may show spontaneous regression in others. The color of the lesion shows shadings from light brown to brown with minute dark brown to black flecks. In addition, there may be depigmented areas at sites of spontaneous regression (Clark and Mihm). In rare instances only, a primary lesion (Cramer; Paver et al) or a recurrent lesion (Su and Bradley) of lentigo maligna lacks melanin pigmentation. The clinical appearance then resembles that of a solar keratosis or of Bowen's disease.

Progression into an invasive lentigo maligna melanoma occurs in about one third of all lesions. Usually, invasion does not take place until the lentigo maligna has been in existence for 10 to 15 years and has reached a size of 4 cm to 6 cm (McGovern et al, 1973). Occasionally, however, invasive melanoma occurs in quite small lesions of 1 cm to 2 cm in diameter (McGovern, 1976). (For a clinical and histologic description of lentigo maligna melanoma, see Malignant Melanoma.)

Histopathology.   In its earliest stage, lentigo maligna may show merely hyperpigmentation, mainly of the basal cell layer, although, in some areas, the hyperpigmentation may extend to the higher layers of the epidermis, even to the stratum corneum. Usually, however, one also observes, at least in some areas, an increase in the concentration of basal melanocytes and some irregularity in their arrangement. The upper dermis at this stage may or may not contain some melanophages and a mild inflammatory infiltrate (Anton-Lamprecht et al). The epidermis is frequently flattened.

In more advanced lesions of lentigo maligna, the basal melanocytes in the epidermis show a marked increase in concentration, so that their number in some areas exceeds that of the basal keratinocytes (Clark and Mihm). The melanocytes in many areas are haphazardly arranged along the epidermal-dermal junction, and many of them are elongated and spindle-shaped. Their nuclei appear atypical, being enlarged, hyperchromatic, and pleomorphic (Fig. 33-17). The cytoplasm of some of the melanocytes appears vacuolated (Mishima). Frequently, atypical melanocytes extend along the basal cell layer of hair follicles, often for a considerable distance. Usually, the proliferating melanocytes contain a considerable amount of melanin. There is often some upward extension of atypical melanocytes, but it may be difficult to differentiate them from melanin-filled keratinocytes. Some nesting of melanocytes in the basal layer may be seen, but this is not pronounced until invasion of the lentigo maligna into the dermis is developing (McGovern, 1970, 1976; Cramer and Kiehn). The atypical melanocytes within the nests usually retain

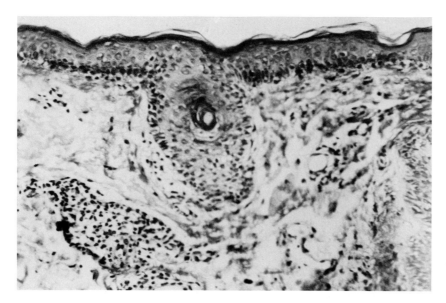

Fig. 33-17. Lentigo maligna, early stage
The basal melanocytes show a marked increase in concentration, appear pleomorphic, and contain a considerable amount of melanin. Atypical melanocytes extend along the basal cell layer of hair follicles. (×100)

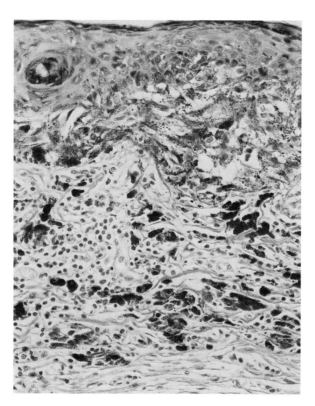

Fig. 33-18. Lentigo maligna, late stage
Spindle-shaped melanocytes with atypical nuclei and vacuolated cytoplasm are arranged along the epidermal-dermal border. Some nesting of melanocytes is apparent. The upper dermis contains a bandlike inflammatory infiltrate intermingled with melanophages. (×200)

their spindled shape, and they often lie with their long axis oriented in a horizontal direction (Fig. 33-18). Except in areas of nesting, the melanocytes retain their dendritic processes. If the melanocytes are heavily melanized, some dendrites may be visible even in sections stained with hematoxylin-eosin; otherwise, staining with silver demonstrates the dendrites well.

The upper dermis, in addition to showing solar degeneration, contains numerous melanophages and a rather pronounced, often bandlike, inflammatory infiltrate. The bandlike dermal infiltrate may extend for a considerable distance beyond the obviously altered epidermis. Careful scrutiny of the apparently normal epidermis overlying the dermal infiltrate, however, reveals in it an increased number of melanocytes and, among them, some atypical melanocytes (Clark et al, 1969).

Since transformation of a lentigo maligna into a lentigo maligna melanoma is a gradual process, dermal invasion by the atypical melanocytes may be present in some areas but not in others. It is therefore advisable to cut step sections throughout the block of tissue in order not to miss such areas (Ollstein et al).

Histogenesis. Lentigo maligna, on the average, requires a much longer time to become an invasive malignant melanoma than the superficial spreading malignant melanoma in situ; and, even after it has become invasive, the lentigo maligna melanoma shows a distinctly slower rate of growth and less of a tendency to give rise to metastases than the superficial spreading melanoma. As explanation for the relatively benign behavior of lentigo maligna, the theory has been offered that lentigo maligna is derived from spindle-shaped junctional melanocytes and thus represents a melanocytic malignant melanoma in situ, whereas the superficial spreading melanoma in situ is derived from rounded junctional nevus cells and can be regarded as a nevocytic malignant melanoma in situ (Mishima and Matsunaka).

Against the validity of this theory is the lack of evidence that the melanocyte and the nevus cell are two different types of cells. The fine structure of nevus cells is seen by electron microscopy to be very similar to that of melanocytes (see p. 686) (Gottlieb et al). The presence of large dendrites on melanocytes and their absence on nevus cells results from the solitary arrangement of melanocytes, which through their dendrites, supply the cells surrounding them with melanin, whereas nevus cells, being arranged in nests, do not supply surrounding cells with melanin.

It seems that, from its onset, lentigo maligna is a slowly growing tumor, thus allowing the tumor cells to exist for a long time as individual melanocytes with dendrites (Paul and Illig). Only when dermal invasion is about to take place do the tumor cells start to grow in nests in a manner similar to nevus cells and malignant melanoma cells. The fact that lentigo maligna and lentigo maligna melanoma usually arise in the exposed skin of elderly persons, which has been modified by many years of exposure to the sun, probably also contributes to the relatively benign biologic behavior of these lesions. A similar benign clinical course is seen in solar keratosis and in squamous cell carcinoma arising from a solar keratosis (see p. 490). Although solar keratosis, like lentigo maligna, contains anaplastic cells, the rate of metastasis of a squamous cell carcinoma arising from it is extremely low, amounting to only about 0.5% (see p. 499) (Lund).

Electron microscopy has shown no specific changes in the melanocytes of lentigo maligna. They are large, synthetically active cells with many dendrites. The melanosomes are essentially normal, except that they appear somewhat more elongated than those present in normal melanocytes (Anton-Lamprecht and Tilgen). This is in contrast to superficial spreading malignant melanoma in situ, in which the melanosomes show considerable abnormalities (see p. 706).

Superficial Spreading Melanoma in Situ

The superficial spreading melanoma in situ, also referred to as pagetoid melanoma in situ (McGovern, 1970) may occur on exposed skin but is also found quite commonly on unexposed skin. The most frequently involved sites are the upper back, especially in men, and the lower legs, especially in women. Superficial spreading melanoma in situ is usually a smaller lesion than lentigo maligna, rarely measuring more than 2.5 cm in diameter (McGovern, 1970). In contrast to lentigo maligna, it may be slightly or definitely elevated. It has an irregular, partly arciform outline. The lesion may show a variation in color that is even greater than that of lentigo maligna, since it includes not only tan, brown, and black, but also pink, blue, and grey. White areas may be seen, as in lentigo maligna, at sites of spontaneous regression (Clark and Mihm). Invasion of the dermis occurs much sooner than in lentigo maligna, often within a year, and is indicated by the development of nodularity and sometimes also ulceration. Frequently, in its early stage of development, superficial spreading melanoma in situ is misdiagnosed clinically as a melanocytic nevus.

Histopathology. Rather uniformly rounded, large melanocytes are scattered in a pagetoid pattern throughout the epidermis (Fig. 33-19). The large cells lie predominantly in nests in the lower epidermis and singly in the upper epidermis (McGovern, 1970). They have atypical, hyperchromatic nuclei and abundant cytoplasm containing varying amounts of melanin. The tumor cells are almost

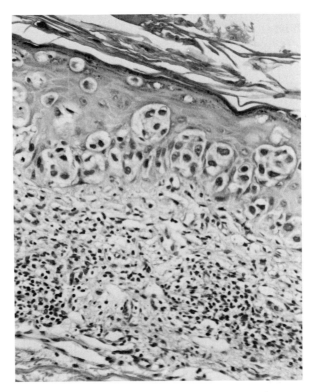

Fig. 33-19. Superficial spreading melanoma in situ
Rounded, large melanocytes with atypical, hyperchromatic nuclei are seen. They lie predominantly in nests in the lower epidermis and singly in the upper epidermis, where they are scattered in a pagetoid pattern. (× 400)

entirely devoid of dendrites. The probable reason for this is that they lie in nests in the lower epidermis and that those lying singly in the upper epidermis were carried to this level passively from the nests in the lower epidermis. The epidermis generally lacks the flattening seen in lentigo maligna and often is acanthotic. Dermal melanophages and a dermal infiltrate are regularly present and, as in lentigo maligna, may extend beyond the obviously altered epidermis under an apparently normal epidermis. Careful examination of such apparently normal epidermis, however, reveals the presence of atypical melanocytes (Clark et al, 1969).

Histogenesis. Melanosomes are present in great numbers in the large pagetoid tumor cells. Their shape is largely spheroid, rather than ellipsoid as in normal melanocytes and in the tumor cells of lentigo maligna (Mishima and Matsunaka). They often also show other abnormalities, such as absence of cross linkages of the filaments within the melanosomes (Clark et al, 1975). Melanization within the melanosomes is variable but often incomplete.

Differential Diagnosis.   A junctional nevus differs from superficial spreading melanoma in situ by a lack of atypicality in the tumor cells, particularly in their nuclei, by a lack of pagetoid upward extension of tumor cells, by the absence of a significant inflammatory infiltrate in the upper dermis, and by a sharper lateral demarcation (see p. 682). (For a discussion of the potentially premalignant "B-K-mole," see p. 716. For differentiation from Paget's disease, see p. 511.)

A clear-cut decision as to whether a malignant melanoma in situ is a lentigo maligna or a superficial spreading melanoma in situ is possible in most but not in all instances (McGovern et al, 1973; Flegel). A distinction between the two types is of no clinical importance in lesions that are found on step sections to be still completely located in situ, since the prognosis is excellent in either case if the tumor is completely excised, but the distinction is very important in those tumors that show invasion into the dermis. (For differentiation between lentigo maligna melanoma and superficial spreading malignant melanoma, see p. 716.)

Acral Lentiginous Melanoma in Situ

Acral lentiginous melanoma in situ has only recently been recognized as a histologic entity (Clark et al, 1975). It occurs on the hairless skin of the palms and soles and in the ungual and periungual regions. It is characterized not only by its specific location but also by its usually short period of in situ growth before invasive growth occurs. Thus, a contradiction exists between the tumor's aggressive behavior in most cases and the usually conspicuous presence of dendritic spindle cells, which, as a rule, are indicative of a relatively benign course.

Clinically, acral lentiginous melanoma in situ shows uneven pigmentation with an irregular, often indefinite border (Lupulescu et al). The soles of the feet are most commonly involved (Coleman et al). If the tumor is situated in the nail matrix, the nail and nail bed may show a longitudinal pigmented band (see p. 687).

Histopathology.   Early in situ lesions may show a deceptively benign histologic picture consisting of an increase in basal melanocytes and hyperpigmentation with only focal atypia of the melanocytes (Silvers). Even in more advanced in situ lesions, all tumor cells occasionally appear spindle-shaped, but some of them are located in the upper layers of the epidermis. The histologic picture is then similar to that of lentigo maligna (Lupulescu et al; Seiji and Takahashi), except for the presence of irregular acanthosis. In most instances, however, both spindle-shaped and rounded, pagetoid tumor cells are seen, and, in some cases, pagetoid cells are the preponderant cell type (Fig. 33-20) (Lopansri and Mihm). Pigmentation is often pronounced, resulting in the presence of melanophages in the upper dermis and of large aggregates of melanin in the broad stratum corneum (Lopansri and Mihm).

MALIGNANT MELANOMA

There are four major types of cutaneous malignant melanoma. They differ in mode of onset, course, prognosis, and incidence. The two most common types are the superficial spreading melanoma and the nodular melanoma, which amount to 70% and 15%, respectively, of all cutaneous malignant melanomas; acral lentiginous melanoma account for only 8%, lentigo maligna melanoma for 5%, and unclassifiable malignant melanomas for 2% (Lopansri and Mihm). If there is no clinical evidence of metastases, one speaks of *stage I;* in the presence of only regional lymph node metastases, of *stage II;* and in the presence of disseminate metastases, of *stage III.* The various types of malignant melanoma are discussed in the same sequence as in malignant melanoma in situ (see p. 702).

Lentigo maligna melanoma develops from a lentigo maligna (see p. 703). Development into an invasive malignant melanoma is often indicated clinically by the development of induration or of one or several intradermal nodules that have a bluish black color. Because of this tumor's slow rate of growth, the lateness of metastases, and the tendency for metastases to be limited at first to

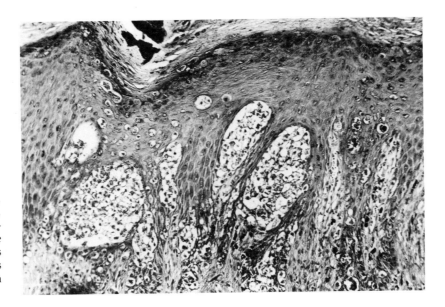

Fig. 33-20.   Acral lentiginous melanoma in situ
Although some of the melanocytes, especially in the lower epidermis, are spindle-shaped, others, especially in the upper epidermis, are rounded and pagetoid. There is acanthosis. Considerable amounts of melanin are seen in the stratum corneum. (×200)

the regional lymph nodes, the survival rate is high, lying between 90% and 94% (Clark and Mihm; van der Esch et al).

Superficial spreading melanoma develops from a superficial spreading melanoma in situ (see p. 705). It is referred to also as pagetoid melanoma. Development into an invasive malignant melanoma is usually indicated by the appearance of papules and nodules or by diffuse induration. Ulceration, if it occurs, is a late feature. The prognosis depends on the stage of the disease and the depth of penetration, and less so on other factors (see Prognosis, p. 712). The 5-year survival rate of patients in stage I averages about 70% (McGovern, 1970).

Nodular melanoma from the beginning shows both horizontal and vertical spread and, because of a more rapid invasion, has a poorer prognosis than superficial spreading melanoma. It starts as an elevated, usually deeply pigmented nodule that increases in size quite rapidly and often undergoes ulceration. When nodular melanoma is treated in stage I, the 5-year survival rate lies between 50% and 60% (Clark; McGovern, 1970; Huvos et al).

Acral lentiginous melanoma occurs on the palms and soles and in the ungual and periungual regions, the soles being the most common site. Even though it accounts for only 8% of all malignant melanomas, it is the most common type in black patients. Tumefaction and ulceration, as well as metastases, often occur within a short time, resulting in very low survival rates of only 11% to 15% (Coleman et al; Fleming et al).

Multiple Primary Melanomas. All patients who have had a cutaneous malignant melanoma are at risk of developing additional malignant melanomas, with an incidence varying from 3.4% to 5.3% (Bellet et al; Moseley et al). It is important to differentiate an additional malignant melanoma from a metastatic melanoma, especially from an epidermotropic metastasis (see p. 714).

Malignant Melanoma in Children. The incidence of prepubertal malignant melanoma is very low. In a few instances, it has occurred as multiple metastases resulting from transplacental transmission (Skov-Jensen et al). Occasionally, a malignant melanoma arises already in infancy or childhood in a giant congenital melanocytic nevus (see p. 693). In addition, two types of primary malignant melanoma can occur in children (Helwig). In most instances, the melanoma shows a histologic picture similar to that seen in adults and follows an aggressive, fatal course. In a few instances, however, the histologic picture is reminiscent of that seen in Spitz nevi, metastases are limited to the regional lymph nodes, and the child survives after adequate treatment (Skov-Jensen et al; Lerman et al; Helwig).

Frequency of a Pre-existing Melanocytic Nevus. It is well known that malignant melanomas can develop in congenital melanocytic nevi (see p. 693) and in the dysplastic nevus syndrome (see p. 716) but both are rather rare types of nevi. The frequency with which a malignant melanoma develops from a pre-existing ordinary nevus cannot be determined on a clinical basis, because the pre-existing lesion, although it may have looked clinically like a melanocytic nevus, may have been the earliest manifestation of the malignant melanoma. However, histologically, remnants of a benign melanocytic nevus are found in about 35% of malignant melanomas (see p. 708) (Lopansri and Mihm).

Juxtacutaneous Malignant Melanoma. Next to the skin and eyes, malignant melanoma is most apt to arise in the juxtacutaneous mucous membranes, such as the oral mucosa (Trodahl and Sprague), upper respiratory tract (Mesara and Burton), vagina (Norris and Taylor), and anorectal mucosa (Wanebo et al, 1981). Mucosal melanomas are analogous to the acral lentiginous melanoma in histologic appearance and aggressiveness.

Histopathology.   The question of whether an *incisional biopsy* is permissible in a lesion that is highly suspected of being a malignant melanoma has been widely discussed. Several authors, especially from Europe, have opposed the performance of an incisional biopsy, because they believe it may cause metastatic spread (Miescher). In two series in which two groups of patients were compared, one group of patients had first a punch biopsy and then an excision, whereas the other group of patients had an immediate excision. It was thought that performance of an incisional biopsy caused a reduction in the 5-year survival rate, from 70% to 53% in one series (Ironside et al) and from 75% to 62% in the other (Rampen et al). In contrast, in two similar comparative series from the United States, no deleterious effect of a preceding punch biopsy was noted (Epstein et al; Bagley et al). Since a correct diagnosis is more likely to be made when the entire tumor can be studied, an excisional biopsy is advisable whenever feasible, and only in large lesions is an incisional biopsy indicated (Harris and Gumport). A shave biopsy or curetting is contraindicated, because it may result in inadequate material for diagnosis; it may also make impossible a determination of the depth of penetration of the tumor, which is very

important for prognosis and for planning of the extent of surgical procedures, including regional lymph node dissection (see Prognosis).

In *all four major types of malignant melanoma,* lentigo maligna melanoma, superficial spreading melanoma, nodular melanoma, and acral lentiginous melanoma, the tumor originates at the epidermal-dermal junction. This also applies to cases of malignant melanoma that have not arisen de novo but have arisen in a junctional or compound nevus. Not infrequently, one may observe beneath an early malignant melanoma, as evidence that it has arisen in a compound nevus, nests of mature nevus cells in the dermis (Fig. 33-21). An exception to the general rule of malignant melanoma arising at the epidermal-dermal border is observed occasionally in congenital melanocytic nevi, in which a malignant melanoma may arise deep in the dermis (Herzberg, 1963; Reed et al). Also, in very rare instances, a malignant melanoma may develop within or beneath an intradermal nevus, resulting in a large nodular growth (Okun and Bauman; Okun et al; Benisch et al). In two of the four cases reported, fatal metastases developed.

In a typical malignant melanoma, one observes considerable irregular junctional activity with downward streaming from the epidermis into the dermis of tumor cells possessing anaplastic nuclei (Fig. 33-22). In conjunction with the downward streaming of the atypical tumor cells, the epidermis may show considerable irregular downward proliferation of its rete ridges. The rete ridges may

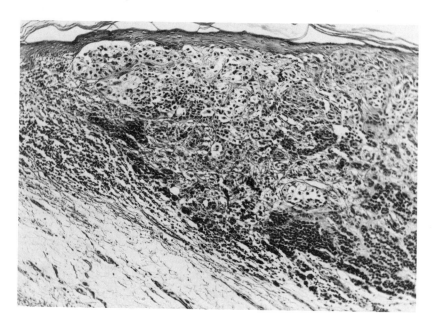

Fig. 33-21.   Malignant melanoma with underlying melanocytic nevus

It can be assumed that the malignant melanoma has developed along the epidermal-dermal border in a melanocytic nevus. (× 100)

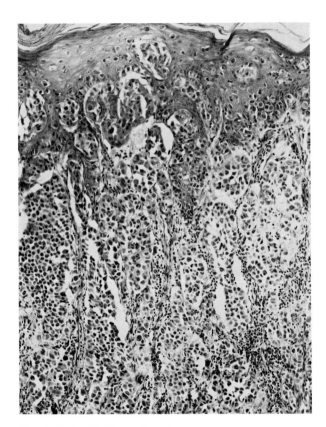

Fig. 33-22.   Malignant melanoma
Low magnification. There is considerable junctional activity with downward streaming from the epidermis into the dermis of tumor cells possessing atypical nuclei. In addition, there is upward extension of tumor cells into the epidermis. The tumor cells are largely of the epithelioid type and lie in alveolar formations. (×100)

appear as if drawn down by the downward migration of the tumor cells. A very common phenomenon is the upward extension of tumor cells into the epidermis overlying the malignant melanoma. This may lead to disintegration of the epidermis and ulceration. Whereas, in nodular malignant melanoma, permeation of the epidermis with tumor cells is limited to that portion overlying the dermal tumor, lateral intraepidermal extension of melanoma cells beyond the confines of the dermal tumor is seen in lentigo maligna melanoma, superficial spreading melanoma, and acral lentiginous melanoma. This phenomenon greatly aids in histologic recognition of the latter three types of tumors.

The *tumor cells* in the dermis show great variation in size and shape. Nevertheless, two major types of cells can be recognized; an epithelioid and a spindle-shaped cell type (Clark et al, 1969). Most tumors show both types of cells, but, as a rule, one type predominates. On the average, cells of the epithelioid type are seen much more commonly than spindle-shaped cells, since only the two relatively rare forms of malignant melanoma, the lentigo maligna melanoma and the acral lentiginous melanoma, tend to show a predominance of spindle-shaped cells, whereas the two common forms of malignant melanoma, the superficial spreading and the nodular melanoma, are composed largely of an epithelioid type of cells (Clark et al, 1969). The epithelioid type of cells tends to lie in alveolar formations (Fig. 33-23), and the spindle-shaped type of cells in irregularly branching formations (Fig. 33-24). The alveolar formations of the epithelioid cells are surrounded by thin fibers of collagen containing a few fibroblasts. In the case of small,

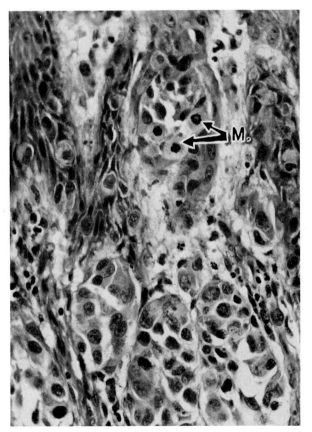

Fig. 33-23.   Malignant melanoma
High magnification of Figure 33-22. The field shows the epidermal-dermal junction. The majority of cells are epithelioid, but some are spindle-shaped. There are several mitotic figures in the tumor cells (*M.*). (×400)

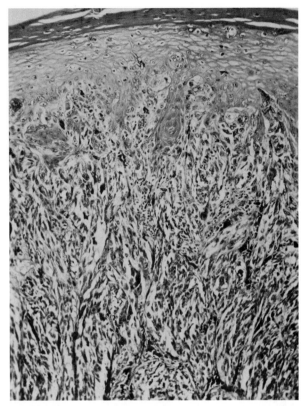

Fig. 33-24. Malignant melanoma
The tumor cells are spindle-shaped and lie in irregularly branching formations. Only small amounts of melanin are present. (×100)

outlying alveolar formations, it is important not to mistake the fibroblasts for endothelial cells and to regard the tumor cells as lying within lymphatics or capillaries, although this is seen occasionally. Tumors in which fusiform cells predominate resemble fibrosarcomas but differ from them by the presence of junctional activity. (For a discussion of desmoplastic melanoma, which is in most instances a variant of spindle cell malignant melanoma, i.e., of lentigo maligna melanoma or acral lentiginous melanoma, see below.)

Mitotic figures are generally present in malignant melanoma, but usually only in small numbers (see Fig. 33-23). Although they are absent in ordinary melanocytic nevi, they are not infrequently seen in Spitz nevi (see p. 692). Similarly, bizarre giant cells may be seen in both malignant melanoma and Spitz nevi, the difference being that, in the latter, they are often surrounded by a clear space caused by edema.

The *amount of melanin* present varies greatly in malignant melanomas. In some tumors, considerable amounts of melanin are found not only within the tumor cells but also within melanophages located in the stroma. In others, there may be no evidence of melanin in hematoxylin-eosin stains. However, staining with ammoniated silver nitrate, that is, the Fontana–Masson stain, then reveals in many amelanotic-appearing malignant melanomas, although not in all, at least a few cells containing melanin (Azar et al). If fresh tissue is available, the dopa reaction can be carried out, invariably showing a positive reaction in at least part of the tumor.

The amount of *inflammatory infiltrate* in malignant melanomas varies. As a rule, early invasive malignant melanoma shows a bandlike inflammatory infiltrate, often intermingled with melanophages, at the base of the tumor. This corresponds to the band of inflammatory cells seen beneath malignant melanoma in situ. In a malignant melanoma in situ that has invaded the dermis, the bandlike inflammatory infiltrate often extends beyond the invasive and the in situ portions of the tumor along the normal-appearing epidermis (Fig. 33-25). Careful examination of this normal-appearing epidermis, however, reveals the presence of atypical melanocytes in it (Clark et al, 1969). In tumors that extend deep into the dermis, the inflammatory infiltrate is quite variable, but it is often only slight to moderate rather than pronounced (Wanebo et al, 1975).

Three rare histologic variants of malignant melanoma deserve a brief description: desmoplastic, pedunculated, and balloon cell melanoma.

Desmoplastic malignant melanoma may occur as a primary lesion (Frolow et al) but often occurs in a recurrent malignant melanoma (Conley et al). Desmoplasia is a common feature of the vertical growth phase of acral lentiginous melanoma (Arrington et al) and can occur also in lentigo maligna melanoma (Labrecque et al; Valensi). However, desmoplastic changes are not observed exclusively in tumors with predominantly spindle-shaped melanoma cells; they can also be seen occasionally in tumors with rounded or completely undifferentiated melanoma cells (Frolow et al; Gartmann).

Histologic examination of desmoplastic malignant melanoma reveals melanoma cells that are usually elongated and amelanotic and are embedded in a markedly fibrotic stroma, so that it is often difficult to decide which are fibroblasts and which are melanoma cells (Fig. 33-26). If there is a lack of melanin and the Fontana–Masson stain

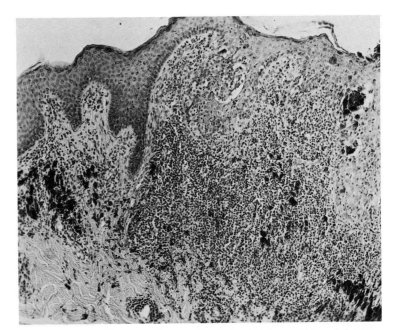

Fig. 33-25. Margin of a superficial spreading melanoma
On the right side, invasive melanoma is seen. In the center, the melanoma is still in situ. The dermis beneath the tumor shows a dense, bandlike inflammatory infiltrate intermingled with numerous melanophages. The infiltrate extends on the left beyond the margin of the tumor underneath the normal-appearing epidermis, which, however, on careful scrutiny shows several atypical melanocytes. (×100)

Fig. 33-26. Desmoplastic lentigo maligna melanoma
Elongated and largely amelanotic cells are embedded in a fibrotic stroma, so that it is difficult to decide which are fibroblasts and which are melanoma cells. (×200)

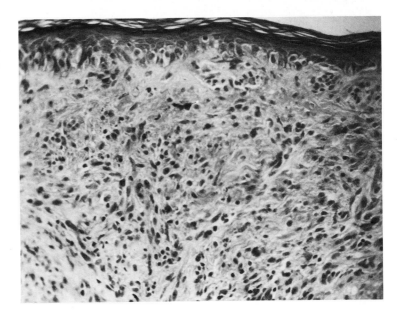

is negative, differentiation from a fibrosarcoma may be very difficult (Conley et al). Because of the great depth of the tumor, the prognosis is very poor, even in cases arising in a lentigo maligna melanoma (Labrecque et al; Valensi).

Pedunculated malignant melanoma, referred to also as polypoidal melanoma, designates a malignant melanoma that is confined, at least at first, to a nodule connected to the underlying skin by a pedicle or stalk. The surface of the nodule often

shows erosion or ulceration (Niven and Lubin; Rosenberg et al). In spite of its superficial location, the prognosis of this tumor is often poor (Beardmore).

On histologic examination, the protruding nodule is found to be filled with melanoma cells, whereas the underlying stalk or pedicle is free of tumor cells at first (Rosenberg et al). Later, the tumor may infiltrate the pedicle and the dermis adjacent to the pedicle (Shafir et al). The reticular dermis, however, is only rarely invaded (Rosenberg et al). The depth of the tumor cannot be accurately measured, and the tumor is "nonstageable" in regard to its level (Beardmore) (see below for a discussion of level). Regional lymph node metastases are often present even in tumors still confined to the area above the pedicle (Niven and Lubin).

Balloon cell melanoma shows, in addition to melanoma cells of the epithelioid type, aggregates of balloon cells (Fig. 33-27). These balloon cells may show relatively little nuclear atypicality and thus may greatly resemble those seen in a balloon cell nevus (see p. 688), so that the danger exists of the lesion being diagnosed as such. It is only through a study of the cells of the epithelioid type that one is able to recognize the tumor as a malignant melanoma, since these cells show the nuclear anaplasia that is associated with a malignant melanoma. Transitions from the melanoma cells to balloon cells are usually seen (Gardner and Vazquez). In some instances, the metastases of a balloon cell melanoma are composed largely of balloon cells (Gardner and Vazquez; Ranchod), whereas, in other cases, the metastases show the usual pattern of a malignant melanoma (Hula).

Prognosis. Of the two less common types of malignant melanoma, lentigo maligna melanoma in stage I has a survival rate of 90% to 94% (see p. 706), and acral lentiginous melanoma has a mortality rate of 85% to 89% within 3 to 4 years (see p. 707). These are therefore usually excluded from any statistics on prognosis, and only the superficial spreading and the nodular melanomas, which together account for over 85% of all malignant melanomas, are included (Lopansri and Mihm). The numerous reviews assessing prognosis generally include only patients in clinical stage I, that is, without palpable regional lymph node swelling, since, in stage II, the chances for survival are quite poor (see below).

THICKNESS OF THE TUMOR. Tumor thickness is the single most important factor in predicting survival for stage I patients (Balch). Originally, the depth of invasion was determined by the five levels suggested by Clark (Clark et al, 1969). They are as follows:

Level I: confinement of the malignant melanoma cells to the epidermis and its appendages

Level II: extension into the papillary dermis, with at most only a few melanoma cells extending to the interface between papillary and reticular dermis

Level III: extension of the tumor cells throughout the papillary dermis, filling it and impinging upon the reticular dermis without, however, invading it

Level IV: invasion of the reticular dermis

Level V: invasion of the subcutaneous fat

Clark et al (1969) showed that the 5-year mortality increased with each level, from 8% in level II to 35% in level III, 46% in level IV, and 52% in level V. However, after 10 years, the mortality rate was found to be the same for levels III and IV (McGovern, 1976; Elias et al).

Breslow, in 1970, first measured tumor thickness

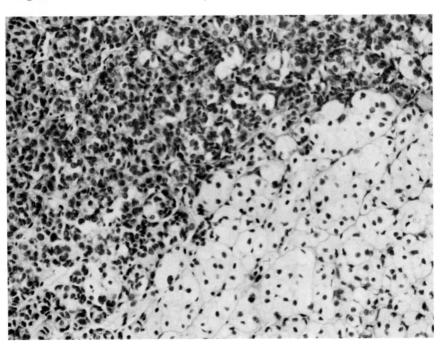

Fig. 33-27. Balloon cell malignant melanoma
In the upper left portion, a malignant melanoma is seen composed largely of atypical cells of the epithelioid type. In the lower right portion, balloon cells constitute the tumor. These cells resemble the balloon cells seen in the balloon cell nevus shown in Figure 33-8.

objectively with a micrometer placed in the ocular of the microscope. He recommended that the depth of invasion be measured from the top of the granular layer to the deepest extension of the tumor; in ulcerated lesions, he recommended that measurement be carried out from the ulcer base overlying the deepest point of invasion, rather than from the top of the granular layer. Breslow stated that malignant melanomas less than 0.76 mm thick did not metastasize and therefore required no regional lymph node dissection, whereas, in melanomas greater than 1.5 mm thick, prophylactic lymph node dissection doubled the rate of survival. The figures for melanomas from 0.76 mm to 1.5 mm thick were inconclusive with respect to the value of lymph node dissection. Breslow (1975) also pointed out that, in 17% of patients with level II melanoma, the tumor was thicker than 0.76 mm and, in 25% of patients with level III melanomas, it was less than 0.76 mm thick, so that measurement with a micrometer gave more reliable prognostic information than Clark's levels. Breslow (1979) furthermore stated that it is often difficult to identify the junction between the papillary and the reticular dermis and that, in such cases, separation of level III and level IV melanomas is quite subjective.*

Various attempts have been made to combine the Clark and Breslow methods of measurement. A good combination is the following, using the thickness of the melanoma as the governing parameter and its level as a modifier (Bagley et al), thus dividing stage I melanomas into three risk groups:

Low-risk: melanomas less than 0.76 mm thick and level II or III

Moderate-risk:

(a) melanomas less than 0.76 mm thick and level IV

(b) melanomas between 0.76 mm and 1.5 mm thick

(c) melanomas more than 1.5 mm thick and level III

High-risk: melanomas more than 1.5 mm thick and level IV or V

Bagley et al found the mortality rates for these three risk groups to be 0%, 23%, and 37%, respectively.

OTHER PROGNOSTIC FACTORS. Various factors in addition to thickness of the tumor have been cited as influencing the prognosis of clinical stage I malignant melanoma but many of them are directly related to

---

* In determining the depth of penetration, whether by level or by measurement, the following rules apply. (1) Melanocytes in junctional nests are not considered invasive, even though they may extend deep into the papillary dermis. (2) If deep nests of melanoma cells arise from the epithelium of cutaneous appendages, they are not used in measurement. (3) If one finds a column of melanocytes extending from the lower border of the lesion into the deep dermis at nearly a right angle, it is not measured, since it is likely that the column arises from an appendage; this supposition can usually be verified by serial sections (Breslow, 1979).

the growth rate of the tumor and thus to the depth of penetration. Among the *clinical factors* that have a favorable effect is location of the tumor on the hair-bearing portions of the extremities, in contrast to an axial location on the trunk, neck, or head (Balch). Also, women have a better prognosis than men, owing largely, although not entirely, to the higher incidence in women of lesions on the extremities (Shaw et al). Clinical factors that are closely related to an increased rate of growth and thus have an adverse prognostic effect are age of the patient (Balch), diameter of the lesion (Huvos et al), and ulceration. The presence of ulceration reduces the 5-year survival rate from 80% to 55% (Balch et al, 1980).

Among the *histologic factors*, the type of tumor, that is, whether nodular or superficial spreading, has an effect on the prognosis (see p. 708). This is due to the fact that nodular melanoma usually has a more rapid rate of growth than superficial spreading melanoma. However, at similar depths, the two types of tumor have similar mortality rates (Larsen and Grude; Rampen et al). A high mitotic index (Schmoeckel and Braun-Falco), the presence of vascular or lymphatic invasion (Elias et al), and the sparsity or absence of melanin in the tumor cells, indicative of poor differentiation (Bhawan), affect the prognosis adversely, but they do so largely because they correlate with tumor thickness (Balch). In contrast, the presence of a lymphocytic infiltrate around the tumor, especially at its base, is regarded as a favorable prognostic sign (Huvos et al; Day et al, 1981), but this is so largely because maximum lymphocyte infiltration is seen in superficially located melanomas, and lymphocytosis decreases with the depth of penetration and is apt to be absent in deeply invasive tumors (Wanebo et al, 1975). Some authors, however, have found the degree of inflammatory reaction of no prognostic significance (van der Esch et al).

LYMPH NODE INVOLVEMENT AND ELECTIVE LYMPH NODE DISSECTION. The incidence of regional lymph node involvement increases with the thickness of the tumor. As first stated by Breslow in 1970 (see p. 712) and confirmed by many subsequent observers, involvement of the regional lymph nodes is extremely rare in melanomas with a thickness of less than 0.76 mm. It is therefore generally agreed that regional lymph node dissection is not indicated.

With regard to tumors 0.76 mm thick or thicker, there are three schools of thought. (1) Elective node dissection in stage I results in no improvement in survival over therapeutic node dissection in stage II (Veronesi et al in a WHO study; Elias et al; Sim et al; Bagley et al). It has even been stated that the regional lymph nodes are an important immunologic defense mechanism (Sim et al). However, the WHO study has been criticized, because 80% of the study population consisted of women, and "women seem to survive stage I melanoma better than men"; furthermore, the study actually shows that men do better with elective node dissection than without it— 65% versus 56% survival at 5 years (Krementz). (2)

Elective node dissection is indicated in patients with a tumor depth range from 1.5 mm to 4 mm. In these patients, the 5-year survival rate has been significantly increased by lymph node dissection, as much as from 37% to 83% (Balch et al, 1979). However, in the depth range from 0.76 mm to 1.5 mm, elective lymph node dissection has not resulted in any increased survival rate, largely because the percentage of patients with positive lymph nodes is small (Breslow, 1975; Rampen et al). (3) All patients with tumor thickness between 0.76 mm and 4 mm should undergo a prophylactic node dissection in order to improve their survival rate (Wanebo et al, 1975; Day et al, 1981) and those with greater tumor thickness should have it as a staging procedure (Balch). The number of involved lymph nodes as well as the depth of the tumor are important factors in the prognosis of patients with clinical stage I melanoma, since patients who have metastases in less than 20% of their resected regional lymph nodes and a tumor thickness of less than 3.5 mm have a 5-year disease-free survival rate of 80%, as compared to only 18% for those patients who have a tumor thickness greater than 3.5 mm and/or metastases in 20% or more of their resected lymph nodes (Day et al, 1981).

Stage II melanoma patients with palpable lymph nodes are at a high risk of having distant metastases from which they will ultimately die. Only patients with involvement of few lymph nodes have a reasonable chance for cure. Involvement of one, two to four, and more than four lymph nodes resulted in one study in 5-year survival rates of 45%, 28%, and 9%, respectively (Balch).

Therapy. The margin of resection of the primary tumor is regarded by most authors as optimal at about 5 cm beyond the perimeter of the lesion (Rampen et al). However, a narrower margin has been recommended recently for some tumors. Thus, a margin of 2 cm has been regarded as adequate for melanomas less than 0.76 mm thick, whereas thicker lesions may be excised using a 3-cm to 5-cm skin margin (Balch et al, 1979). It has also been recommended that the margin be made twice the diameter of the lesion (Bagley et al). More intricate suggestions for resection margins distinguish between melanomas of the BANS region (upper *b*ack, posteriolateral *a*rm, posterior and lateral *n*eck, and posterior *s*calp) and other superficial spreading and nodular melanomas, since melanomas of the BANS region may metastasize even when only 0.85 mm to 1.69 mm thick. A margin of 1.5 cm is recommended for all melanomas less than 0.85 mm thick located anywhere and for non-BANS melanomas 0.85 mm to 1.69 mm thick. All other melanomas should be excised with a 3-cm margin (Day et al, 1982).

Metastases. Metastatic spread is very common in malignant melanoma, particularly in tumors thicker than 1.5 mm, with extension taking place at first to the regional lymph nodes (see Prognosis).

Spread through the blood stream generally occurs later, and, when it occurs, metastases are apt to be widespread.

On autopsy, the following organs have been found to be involved in more than half of the cases: lungs (88%), brain, dura, or spinal cords (75%), gastrointestinal tract (73%), heart (70%), liver (63%), peritoneum (58%), and adrenal glands (53%) (Amer et al). Metastases to the skin and subcutaneous tissue are present on autopsy in 54% to 75% of the patients (Einhorn et al; Das Gupta and Brasfield).

In about 4% of the patients with metastases of malignant melanoma, no primary tumor can be found (Das Gupta et al; Baab and McBride). Although the primary tumor may in some instances be in an internal organ, it can be assumed that it was in most instances located in the skin and regressed spontaneously. In some instances, there is a history of a spontaneously resolving pigmented lesion, and one may see at that site either a hypopigmented area (Das Gupta et al; Smith and Stehlin) or an irregular, flat, pigmented lesion (Pellegrini).

Histopathology. The histologic appearance of melanoma *metastases in the skin* usually differs from that of the primary melanoma by the absence of an inflammatory infiltrate and of junctional activity. However, neither of these two criteria is reliable. In the first place, primary tumors of malignant melanoma may also not show an inflammatory infiltrate, particularly when they are deeply invasive (see p. 710); and secondly, even metastases can contact the overlying epidermis in a way that is suggestive of junctional activity (Klostermann). It has been stated that the dopa reaction in such cases may show that no true junctional activity exists, since a sharp line of demarcation exists between the strongly dopa-positive tumor islands and the single line of dopa-positive basal melanocytes in the overlying epidermis (Herzberg, 1964). However, there are truly epidermotropic melanoma metastases in which, in addition to dermal aggregates of atypical melanocytes, aggregates of atypical melanocytes are seen either within the epidermis (Kornberg et al) or in a truly junctional position (Warner et al). Distinction from a primary malignant melanoma in such cases is very difficult, although the diagnosis of epidermotropic metastasis is suggested by (1) thinning of the epidermis by aggregates of atypical melanocytes within the dermis, (2) inward turning of the rete ridges at the periphery of the lesion, and (3) no lateral extension of atypical melanocytes within the epidermis beyond the concentration of the metastasis in the dermis (Kornberg et al).

In cases of metastatic malignant melanoma with nearly complete *regression of the primary tumor,* histologic examination shows in the case of depigmented lesions telangiectasia and some pigmented macrophages deep in the dermis (Das Gupta et al) and in the case of still pigmented lesions a band of melanophages and inflammatory cells in the upper part of the dermis (Pellegrini). In some cases, a few melanoma cells are still present either in the dermis or in the subcutaneous tissue (Smith and Stehlin).

Histogenesis. On *electron microscopic examination,* lentigo maligna melanoma shows most melanosomes to be ellipsoidal and of normal appearance (EM 49). In superficial spreading and nodular melanoma, most melanosomes are spheroidal and show a reduction in the cross linkage of their melanofilaments. In addition, some melanosomes are grossly abnormal, having a granular, lamellar, or vacuolar appearance (Hunter et al). The diagnostic value of electron microscopy in borderline melanocytic lesions is greatly limited by the fact that benign melanocytic lesions may also show abnormal melanosome formations (Mintzis and Silvers).

The *lymphocytic infiltrate* that is often found around early invasive malignant melanomas (see p. 710) represents a delayed hypersensitivity reaction. This can be concluded from the fact that the large majority of the cells in the infiltrate are T lymphocytes (Edelson). Also, a great number of the cells in the infiltrate can be labeled with tritiated thymidine, indicating that they are stimulated cells synthesizing deoxyribonucleic acid (DNA) (Pullmann and Steigleder). This finding is in line with the observation that blood lymphocytes of patients with malignant melanoma are cytotoxic to cultured autologous tumor cells (DeVries et al).

In addition to cellular antibodies in circulating lymphocytes, humoral antibodies against the cytoplasm of malignant melanoma cells are also present in the plasma of patients with malignant melanoma prior to the development of metastases. These antibodies disappear when metastases develop (Copeman et al). (For a discussion of the presence of these antibodies in halo nevus, see p. 689).

Differential Diagnosis.   Great difficulty may be encountered in the differentiation of malignant melanoma from a junctional or compound nevus. The actual incidence of a wrong diagnosis is not inconsiderable, judging from the frequency with which pathologists or dermatopathologists disagree in their opinions. Also, in a retrospective analysis, it became apparent that, in at least 7% of the cases diagnosed as malignant melanoma, the subsequent course proved this diagnosis to be incorrect (Truax et al). Still, in a disease with such a serious prognosis, it seems better to "overdiagnose" than to "underdiagnose" and thus to err

on the safe side. Also, since a junctional or compound nevus may develop into a malignant melanoma, a phenomenon well exemplified by the dysplastic nevus syndrome (see p. 716), and since this development may proceed slowly, an intermediate stage may be encountered in which no clear-cut decision is possible.

Several features are generally regarded as being suggestive of malignant melanoma, but there is actually only one absolute sign of malignancy, and that is often difficult to decide upon: nuclear anaplasia or atypicality associated with pleomorphism. The indications for anaplasia are the same as in other malignant tumors and include large size, irregular shape and hyperchromasia of the nuclei, and presence of atypical mitoses. The presence of large amounts of irregularly distributed melanin may give benign cells a "wild," anaplastic appearance. It is advisable to judge such cells as if they contained no melanin and, if necessary, to bleach the melanin in them with potassium permanganate. Although melanocytes with abundant, pale-staining cytoplasm and fine, dusty melanin particles are quite typical of malignant melanoma, especially the superficial spreading type, nests of such cells lacking nuclear atypicality may be seen along the epidermal-dermal junction in compound nevi.

Features suggestive but not indicative of malignancy are the following:

1. Presence of melanocytes within the upper portion of the epidermis singly or in groups.
2. Irregular scattering of the melanocytes in the basal cell layer, in addition to their arrangement in nests.
3. Poor lateral circumscription of the intraepidermal or basal layer melanocytic component due to lateral spread (Price et al). The phenomenon of lateral spread is commonly seen in lentigo maligna melanoma, superficial spreading melanoma, and acral lentiginous melanoma but is absent in nodular melanoma.
4. Failure of the melanocytes in the deeper layers of the dermis to decrease in size (absence of "maturation"). This must not be confused, however, with the presence of an intradermal nevus beneath a malignant melanoma, a fairly common feature (see p. 708).
5. Presence of mitotic figures. They are found in nearly all melanomas (McGovern, 1976; Schmoeckel and Braun-Falco; Price et al). By contrast, mitotic figures are rarely seen in benign melanocytic nevi other than Spitz nevi (Lund and Stobbe).

The presence of an inflammatory infiltrate and the distribution of melanin have little diagnostic significance (Price et al).

An inflammatory infiltrate, often intermingled with melanophages, is found more commonly in malignant melanoma than in melanocytic nevi. However, it may be mild or absent in malignant melanoma and may be quite pronounced in melanocytic nevi, not only in Spitz nevi and halo nevi but also in junctional nevi and early compound nevi. In addition, trauma, infection, or rupture of a hair follicle may cause inflammation.

Melanin in malignant melanoma is usually found throughout the tumor, whereas melanin is generally seen only in the upper portion of melanocytic nevi. However, many melanomas show little or no melanin, and nevi may show melanin in their deeper as well as their upper portions, so that the distribution of melanin has very little diagnostic value.

It is important to decide in malignant melanoma with an adjacent intraepidermal component whether this component is of the lentigo maligna type or of the superficial spreading type, since lentigo maligna melanoma has a much better prognosis. Although this decision is possible in most cases, it cannot be made in all. Cases in which a decision is impossible are referred to as "invasive malignant melanoma with adjacent intraepidermal component unclassifiable" (McGovern et al). The following similarities may exist between the intraepidermal components of lentigo maligna melanoma and superficial spreading melanoma, thus occasionally making their distinction difficult. (1) Both may show formation of nests at the epidermal-dermal junction, although the nests in lentigo maligna melanoma are usually composed of spindle-shaped rather than of rounded cells (see p. 709 and Fig. 33-26) (Clark; McGovern, 1970). (2) Both may show upward extension of atypical melanocytes in the epidermis. (3) Although, in typical cases, the epidermis is flattened in lentigo maligna melanoma and acanthotic in superficial spreading melanoma, exceptions occur. Also, clinical location is an important factor, since lentigo maligna melanoma occurs only in sun-exposed areas, particularly the face. However, superficial spreading melanoma can also occur in these locations.

For differentiation of a Spitz nevus from malignant melanoma, which may be very difficult, see p. 693.

So far, the differentiation of malignant melanoma from other melanocytic tumors has been discussed. However, in some instances, it may be difficult to recognize a *highly undifferentiated malignant melanoma* as such. Generally, these tumors are amelanotic and, although some of them show at least in some cells a positive Fontana–Masson silver stain, others do not (Azar et al). Unfortunately, the dopa reaction requires fresh tissue, and electron microscopy requires especially fixed tissues, and these procedures thus cannot always be carried out. The dopa reaction is always positive in at least part of the tumor, and electron microscopy shows occasional melanosomes and premelanosomes in most but not in all cases (Azar et al). The two tumors from which an undifferentiated melanoma must usually be differentiated are anaplastic squamous cell carcinoma and large cell lymphoma. Since many antigens survive the processes of formalin fixation and paraffin embedding, peroxidase–antiperoxidase reactions can be carried out on previously fixed tissues, with rabbit antihuman keratin antiserum reacting with the cells of squamous cell carcinoma, and with rabbit antisera against human immunoglobulin heavy chains and/or kappa and lambda light chains reacting with B-cell lymphoma (Azar et al).

Dysplastic Nevus Syndrome

The occasional occurrence of a malignant melanoma in more than one member of a family has long been known (Cawley; Anderson et al). However, the association of familial malignant melanoma, often occurring in multiple lesions, with "dysplastic" nevi in both the melanoma patients and many of their relatives has been described only recently under the designation of *B-K mole syndrome* (Clark et al, 1978). The dysplastic nevi usually are larger than ordinary melanocytic nevi, measuring from 5 mm to 15 mm in size. They have an irregular border and show a haphazard mixture of tan, brown, black, and pink. There is often a small, palpable central component. The nevi are located on exposed and unexposed skin and form throughout adult life. Since a dysplastic nevus may transform itself into a malignant melanoma, its recognition is important.

In addition to its familial occurrence, the dysplastic nevus syndrome can be observed as a sporadic phenomenon in patients with a primary malignant melanoma (Elder et al) or in patients without a melanoma but at a high risk of developing one (Rahbari and Mehregan).

Histopathology. Dysplastic nevi have the histologic appearance of a compound nevus in which some individual melanocytes and nests of melanocytes appear atypical. Individual atypical melanocytes are usually located in the basal cell layer, whereas the nests of atypical melanocytes extend downward into the upper dermis, where the long axis of the nests tends to lie parallel to the epidermal-dermal interface. The atypical-appearing melanocytes in the junctional nests are frequently spindle-shaped, but they may be large and epithelioid and show abundant cytoplasm and fine, dusty melanin granules (Clark et al, 1978). Some nests lying free in the upper part of the papillary dermis may also show atypical melanocytes, but most nests have melanocytes with a uniform appearance as seen in a compound nevus. The nests are generally limited to the papillary dermis, and neuroid structures are absent (Rahbari and Mehregan). An inflammatory infiltrate intermingled with melanophages is commonly present in the dermis beneath areas of junctional activity (Fig. 33-28). Mitotic figures are infrequent (Elder et al).

Extension of atypical-appearing melanocytes into the upper layers of the epidermis can be seen, but without intraepidermal lateral, pagetoid spread (Elder et al). If pagetoid spread is apparent, transformation into a superficial spreading melanoma in situ has occurred (Rahbari and Mehregan). Borderline lesions occur in which a decision is difficult as to whether the lesion is a dysplastic nevus or an early superficial spreading melanoma that is either still in situ or early invasive.

It should be emphasized that some lesions in the dysplastic nevus syndrome are unremarkable compound nevi (Elder et al). Furthermore, not all malignant melanomas in patients with the dysplastic nevus syndrome arise within a pre-existing dysplastic nevus but may arise de novo (Clark et al, 1978).

By no means every "borderline" melanocytic lesion represents the dysplastic nevus syndrome, which is actually quite rare; however, when seeing histologic changes analogous to those seen in the dysplastic nevus syndrome, the dermatopathologist can alert the clinician to the possible presence of this syndrome (Rahbari and Mehregan).

Generalized Melanosis in Metastatic Melanoma

Generalized melanosis in metastatic melanoma is associated with widespread melanoma metastases and with melanuria. It is characterized by diffuse slate-blue discoloration of the entire skin, the conjunctivae, and the oral and pharyngeal mucous membranes (Fitzpatrick et al; Holcomb et al). Autopsy reveals a similar discoloration in the intima of the large arteries and of many visceral organs (Konrad and Wolff).

Histopathology. Numerous melanin granules are seen located within macrophages throughout the dermis, especially around capillaries (Fitzpatrick et al). They stain with the Fontana–Masson stain and are dopa-positive (Adrian et al). In addition, some dermal vessels are focally plugged with dark, amorphous dopa-positive material (Adrian et al). In most instances, only melanophages have been found (Silberberg et al; Holcomb et al; Bork et al; Rowden et al); however, in a few cases, two types of pigmented cells have been identified in the dermis, particularly in semithin sections: melanophages, and individually scattered melanoma cells

Fig. 33-28.   Dysplastic compound nevus
The nests of melanocytes at the epidermal-dermal junction are irregularly shaped and extend with their long axis parallel to the epidermal surface. These junctional nests are composed of spindle-shaped cells. Individual, atypical melanocytes are seen scattered not only along the basal cell layer but also within the epidermis. The melanocytes of the nests in the papillary dermis appear much more uniform than the melanocytes of the nests at the epidermal-dermal junction. An inflammatory infiltrate intermingled with melanophages is present in areas of junctional activity. (×100)

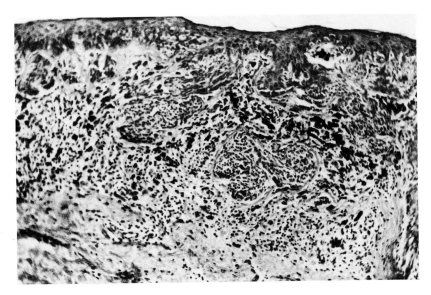

appearing larger and less pigmented than the melanophages (Konrad and Wolff; Schuler et al).

On autopsy, melanin phagocytosis is seen in many organs, especially in the Kupffer cells of the liver and the cells lining the sinusoids of the lymph nodes, spleen, and adrenal glands (Sohn et al).

Histogenesis. On *electron microscopic examination,* most authors have found in the dermis only macrophages and no scattered melanoma cells (Silberberg et al; Bork et al; Rowden et al; Adrian et al). The macrophages contain membrane-bound vacuoles that are filled with numerous electron-dense granules measuring approximately 50 nm in diameter. These granules differ from melanosomes by the absence of any internal substructure and by their small size. (Melanosomes usually measure more than 300 nm in diameter; see p. 17.) The granules have been interpreted as particulate melanin aggregates within phagolysosomes (Adrian et al). The finding of dopa-positive, amorphous plugs within vessel lumina suggests diffusion of precursor substances from blood vessels into the perivascular tissue and subsequent accumulation of these substances within macrophages, where they are nonenzymatically oxidized to form visible melanin granules (Adrian et al). In some cases, the dermal melanophages contain not only melanin granules but also melanosomes. It is assumed that the melanosomes are produced by distant primary and metastatic melanoma cells, from which they are released and then carried by the blood stream to the skin, where they are deposited within dermal melanophages (Silberberg et al). In still other cases, electron microscopy has shown in the dermis both melanophages and scattered individual melanoma cells. The major source of the melanin in the dermis in such cases is myriads of individual melanoma cells continuously dispersed by the blood to the skin and other organs, the production of melanosomes within these cells, and the phagocytosis of released melanosomes by macrophages in the dermis as well as elsewhere (Konrad and Wolff; Schuler et al). The scattered dermal melanocytes differ from the dermal melanophages by containing largely singly dispersed melanosomes in all stages of melanization and only few vacuoles with aggregated melanosomes (Schuler et al).

MALIGNANT BLUE NEVUS

Malignant blue nevus is a rare tumor. It may arise in a blue nevus (Kwittken and Negri; Merkow et al) or in a nevus of Ota (Dorsey and Montgomery), or it may be malignant from the start (Gartmann and Lischka; Hernandez). Malignant blue nevi may show ulceration if they are superficially located (Herzberg and Klein), but they may merely show an increase in size without ulceration if they are deeply located (Gartmann and Lischka; Hernandez). With regard to the prognosis, two forms of malignant blue nevus are recognized. In one form, the metastases are limited to the regional lymph nodes, and the patient survives after removal of the tumor and the involved lymph nodes (Merkow et al; Gartmann and Lischka). In the other form, however, death occurs as the result of widespread metastases (Kwittken and Negri; Mishima; Hernandez).

Histopathology.   Recognition of the lesion as a malignant blue nevus is based on the absence of junctional activity and the presence of at least some bipolar tumor cells with branching dendritic processes containing melanin granules (Fig. 33-29) (Herzberg and Klein; Mishima; Hernandez). This

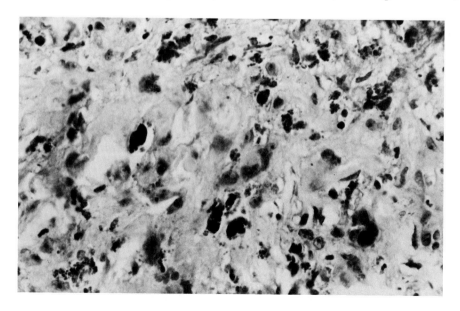

Fig. 33-29. Malignant blue nevus
The tumor contains many anaplastic nuclei, some of which are elongated. Melanin is present in many tumor cells and, in some, lies within branching dendritic processes. (×400)

may require staining with ammoniated silver nitrate, since melanin is often scanty owing to the fact that most malignant blue nevi arise from areas of cellular blue nevus and are composed of cells of this type. However, considerable amounts of melanin are seen in some malignant blue nevi (Gartmann and Lischka; Hernandez).

In addition to showing the standard features of malignancy, such as invasiveness of the tumor, atypicality and pleomorphism of the nuclei, and presence of atypical mitoses, malignant blue nevi often show areas of necrosis as evidence of their malignant nature (Herzberg and Klein; Merkow et al; Hernandez).

Histogenesis. Although some authors have regarded the tumor cells as being related to Schwann cells (Merkow et al), *electron microscopic studies* have shown a lack of cytoplasmic enclosures of unmyelinated axons, which would be seen if the tumor cells were Schwann cells, and the presence of melanosomes in all cells. Although the melanosomes in many cells are devoid of melanin (Hernandez), incubation with dopa has shown that such melanosomes are strongly dopa-positive (Mishima). Thus, it is evident that all tumor cells are melanocytes.

Differential Diagnosis. Malignant blue nevus differs from primary malignant melanoma by the absence of junctional activity. However, distinction of a malignant blue nevus from a metastatic malignant malignant melanoma can be difficult, since metastatic malignant melanoma is occasionally found without a demonstrable primary malignant melanoma. The primary malignant melanoma either may have involuted or may be located at an obscure internal site (see p. 714). The presence of dendritic cells is then the most reliable criterion favoring a diagnosis of malignant blue nevus over that of a metastatic malignant melanoma.

BIBLIOGRAPHY

Melanocytic Nevus

BARAN R: Longitudinal melanotic streaks as a clue to Laugier-Hunziker syndrome. Arch Dermatol 115:1448–1449, 1979

BART RS, KOPF AW: A darkly pigmented lesion of a great toe (acral lentiginous melanoma). J Dermatol Surg Oncol 3:158–159, 1977

BECKER SW: Diagnosis and treatment of pigmented nevi. Arch Dermatol Syph 60:44–65, 1949

BENTLEY-PHILLIPS CB, MARKS R: The epidermal component of melanocytic nevi. J Cutan Pathol 3:190–194, 1976

CLARK WH JR, MIHM MC JR: Lentigo maligna and lentigo-maligna melanoma. Am J Pathol 55:39–67, 1969

CONNORS RC, ACKERMAN AB: Histologic pseudomalignancies of the skin. Arch Dermatol 112:1767–1780, 1976

DELACRÉTAZ J, FRENK E: Zur Pathogenese des Osteo-Naevus Nanta. Hautarzt 15:487–489, 1964

EADY RAJ, GILKES JJH, WILSON JONES E: Eruptive naevi: Report of two cases. Br J Dermatol 97:267–278, 1977

FREEMAN RG, KNOX JM: Epidermal cysts associated with pigmented nevi. Arch Dermatol 85:590–594, 1962

GOTTLIEB B, BROWN AL JR, WINKELMANN RK: Fine structure of the nevus cell. Arch Dermatol 92:81–87, 1965

GRAHAM JH, SANDERS JB, JOHNSON WC: Fibrous papule of the nose. J Invest Dermatol 45:194–203, 1965

KOPF AW, WALDO E: Melanonchyia stratia. Aust J Dermatol 21:59–70, 1980

KORNBERG R, ACKERMAN AB: Pseudomelanoma. Recurrent melanocytic nevus following partial surgical removal. Arch Dermatol 111:1588–1590, 1975

KOUSKOUKIS CE, SCHER RK, HATCHER VA: Melanonychia striata longitudinalis. J Dermatol Surg Oncol 8:284–286, 1982

LUND HZ, STOBBE GD: The natural history of the pigmented nevus: Factors of age and anatomic location. Am J Pathol 25:1117–1147, 1949

LUPULESCU A, PINKUS H, BIRMINGHAM DJ et al: Lentigo maligna of the fingertip. Arch Dermatol 107:717–722, 1973

MAIZE JC, FOSTER G: Age-related changes in melanocytic naevi. Clin Exp Dermatol 4:49–58, 1979

MASSON P: My conception of cellular nevi. Cancer 4:9–38, 1951

MIESCHER G, VON ALBERTINI A: Histologie de 100 cas de naevi pigmentaires d'après les méthodes de Masson. Bull Soc Fr Dermatol Syph 42:1265–1273, 1935

MISHIMA Y: Macromolecular changes in pigmentary disorders. Arch Dermatol 91:519–557, 1965

NIIZUMA K: Electron microscopic study of nevic corpuscle. Acta Derm Venereol (Stockh) 55:283–289, 1975

PENNEYS NS, MOGOLLON R, KOWALCZYK A: A survey of cutaneous neural lesions for the presence of myelin basic protein. Arch Dermatol, in press

ROTH SI, STOWELL RE, HELWIG EB: Cutaneous ossification. Arch Pathol 76:44–54, 1963

SAGEBIEL RW: Histologic artifacts of benign pigmented nevi. Arch Dermatol 106:691–693, 1972

SCHER RK: Biopsy of the matrix of a nail. J Dermatol Surg Oncol 6:19–21, 1980

SCHOENFELD RJ, PINKUS H: The recurrence of nevi after incomplete removal. Arch Dermatol 78:30–35, 1958

SHAFFER B: Pigmented nevi. Arch Dermatol 72:120–132, 1955

SHELLEY WB, ARTHUR RP: Nerve fibers, a neglected component of intradermal cellular nevi. J Invest Dermatol 34:59–65, 1960

STEGMAIER OC: Natural regression of the melanocytic nevus. J Invest Dermatol 32:413–419, 1959

STREMPEL H, HORN W: Melanosis striata longitudinalis ungium. Z Hautkr 54:861–865, 1979

THORNE EG, MOTTAZ JH, ZELICKSON AS: Tyrosinase activity in dermal nevus cells. Arch Dermatol 104:619–624, 1971

WEITZNER S: Intradermal nevus with psammoma body formation. Arch Dermatol 98:287–289, 1968

WINKELMANN RK: Cholinesterase nevus: Cholinesterases in pigmented tumors of the skin. Arch Dermatol 82:17–23, 1960

WINKELMANN RK, JOHNSON LA: Cholinesterase in neurofibromas. Arch Dermatol 85:106–114, 1962

Balloon Cell Nevus

GARTMANN H: Über blasige Zellen im Naevuszellnaevus. Z Hautkr 28:148–159, 1960

GOETTE DK, DOTY RD: Balloon cell nevus. Arch Dermatol 114:109–111, 1978

HASHIMOTO K, BALE GF: An electron microscopic study of balloon cell nevus. Cancer 30:530–540, 1972

HORNSTEIN O: Zur Kenntnis des sogenannten Blasenzellnaevus. Arch Klin Exp Dermatol 226:97–110, 1966

OKUN MR, DONNELLAN B, EDELSTEIN L: An ultrastructural study of balloon cell nevus. Cancer 34:615–625, 1974

SCHRADER WA, HELWIG EB: Balloon cell nevi. Cancer 20:1502–1514, 1967

WILSON JONES E, SANDERSON KV: Cellular nevi with peculiar foam cells. Br J Dermatol 75:47–54, 1963

Halo Nevus

BENNETT C, COPEMAN PWM: Melanocyte mutation in halo nevus and malignant melanoma. Br J Dermatol 100:423–426, 1979

BERMAN A: Halo nevus with exceptional clinical features. Arch Dermatol 114:1081–1082, 1978

BROWNSTEIN MH: Halo nevi without dermal infiltrate. Arch Dermatol 114:1718, 1978

BROWNSTEIN MH, KAZAN BB, HASHIMOTO K: Halo congenital nevus. Arch Dermatol 113:1572–1575, 1977

COPEMAN PWM, LEWIS MG, PHILLIPS TM et al: Immunological associations of the halo nevus with cutaneous malignant melanoma. Br J Dermatol 88:127–137, 1973

EBNER H, NIEBAUER G: Elektronenoptische Befunde zum Pigmentverlust beim Naevus Sutton. Dermatologica 137:345–357, 1968

EPSTEIN WL, SAGEBIEL R, SPITLER L et al: Halo nevi and melanoma. JAMA 225:373–377, 1973

FINDLAY GH: The histology of Sutton's nevus. Br J Dermatol 69:389–394, 1957

FRANK SB, COHEN HJ: The halo nevus. Arch Dermatol 89:367–373, 1964

HAPPLE R, ECHTERNACHT K, SCHOTOLA I: Halonaevus ohne Halo. Hautarzt 26:44–46, 1975

HASHIMOTO K: A case of halo nevus with effete melanocytes. Acta Derm Venereol (Stockh) 55:87–95, 1975

KING LA, KING DT: Halo congenital nevus without histological inflammation. Arch Dermatol 114:1242, 1978

KOPF AW, MORRILL SD, SILBERBERG I: Broad spectrum of leukoderma acquisitum centrifugum. Arch Dermatol 92:14–35, 1965

SHAPIRO L, KOPF AW: Leukoderma acquisitum centrifugum. Arch Dermatol 92:64–68, 1965

SMITH WE, MOSELEY JC: Multiple halo neurofibromas. Arch Dermatol 112:987–990, 1976

STEGMAIER OC, BECKER SW JR, MEDENICA M: Multiple halo nevi. Arch Dermatol 99:180–189, 1969

SWANSON JL, WAYTE DM, HELWIG EB: Ultrastructure of halo nevi. J Invest Dermatol 50:434–437, 1968

Spitz Nevus

ALLEN AC: Juvenile melanomas of children and adults and melanocarcinomas of children. Arch Dermatol 82:325–335, 1960

BARR RJ, MORALES V, GRAHAM JH: Spindle cell and epithelioid cell nevi. (Abstr) Arch Dermatol 114:1833, 1978

BARR RJ, MORALES RV, GRAHAM JH: Desmoplastic nevus. A distinct variant of mixed spindle cell and epithelioid cell nevus. Cancer 46:557–564, 1980

BURKET JM: Multiple benign juvenile melanoma. Arch Dermatol 115:229, 1979

CAPETANAKIS J: Juvenile melanoma disseminatum. Br J Dermatol 92:207–211, 1975

COPEMAN PWM, LEWIS MG, PHILLIPS TM et al: Immunological associations of the halo nevus with cutaneous malignant melanoma. Br J Dermatol 88:127–137, 1973

ECHEVARRIA R, ACKERMAN LV: Spindle and epithelioid cell nevi in the adult. Cancer 20:175–189, 1967

HELWIG EB: Malignant melanoma in children. In Freitag SB, Culhane DL, Demec JC (eds): Neoplasms of the Skin and Malignant Melanoma, pp 11–26. Chicago, Year Book Medical Publishers, 1976

KAMINO H, MISHELOFF E, ACKERMAN AB et al: Eosinophilic globules in Spitz's nevi. New findings and a diagnostic sign. Am J Dermatopathol 1:319–324, 1979

MCWHORTER HE, WOOLNER LB: Pigmented nevi, juvenile melanomas and malignant melanomas in children. JAMA 156:695–698, 1954

OKUN MR: Melanoma resembling spindle and epithelioid cell nevus. Arch Dermatol 115:1416–1420, 1979

PANIAGO-PEREIRA C, MAIZE JC, ACKERMAN AB: Nevus of large spindle and/or epithelioid cells (Spitz's nevus). Arch Dermatol 114:1811–1923, 1978

RUPEC M, KINT A, HORN W: Das juvenile Melanom. Hautarzt 30:581–585, 1979

SAKSELA E, RINTALA A: Misdiagnosis of prepubertal malignant melanoma. Cancer 22:1308–1314, 1968

SCHREINER E, WOLFF K: Die Ultrastruktur des benignen juvenilen Melanoms. Arch Klin Exp Dermatol 237:749–768, 1970

SPITZ S: Melanomas of childhood. Am J Pathol 24:591–609, 1948

WEEDON D, LITTLE JH: Spindle and epithelioid cell nevi in children and adults. A review of 211 cases of the Spitz nevus. Cancer 40:217–225, 1977

WEIMAR VM, ZUEHLKE RL: Multiple agminate spindle and epithelioid cell nevi in an adult. Arch Dermatol 114:1383–1384, 1978

Congenital Melanocytic Nevus

BOTET MV, CARO FR, SÁNCHEZ JL: Congenital acral melanocytic nevi clinically resembling acral lentiginous melanoma. J Am Acad Dermatol 5:406–410, 1981

GROSS PR, CARTER DM: Malignant melanoma arising in a giant cerebriform nevus. Arch Dermatol 96:536–539, 1967

GROULS V, HELPAP B, CRNIC A: Kombination eines malignen blauen Naevus mit einem congenitalen Tierfellnaevus. Z Hautkr 56:943–946, 1981

KOPF AW, BART RS, HENNESSEY P: Congenital nevocytic nevi and malignant melanomas. J Am Acad Dermatol 1:123–130, 1979

MARK GJ, MIHM MC, LITEPLO MG et al: Congenital melanocytic nevi of the small and garment type. Hum Pathol 4:395–418, 1973

MENTER MA, GRIESSEL PJC, DE KLERK DJ: Giant blue naevus of the scalp with underlying scalp defect. Br J Dermatol 85, Suppl 7:73–75, 1971

MISHIMA Y: Eccrine-centered nevus. Arch Dermatol 107:59–61, 1973

MORISHIMA T, ENDO M, IMAGAWA I et al: Clinical and histopathological studies on spotted grouped pigmented nevi with special reference to eccrine-centered nevus. Acta Derm Venereol (Stockh) 56:345–351, 1976

ORKIN M, FRICHOT BC III, ZELICKSON AS: Cerebriform intradermal nevus. Arch Dermatol 110:575–582, 1974

PACK GT, DAVIS J: Nevus giganticus pigmentosus with malignant transformation. Surgery 49:347–354, 1961

PENMAN HG, STRINGER HCW: Malignant transformation in giant congenital pigmented nevus. Arch Dermatol 103:428–432, 1971

REED WB, BECKER WS JR, BECKER WS SR et al: Giant pigmented nevi, melanoma, and leptomeningeal melanocytosis. Arch Dermatol 91:100–199, 1965

RHODES AR, SOBER AJ, DAY CL et al: The malignant potential of small congenital nevocellular nevi. J Am Acad Dermatol 6:230–241, 1982

SANTA CRUZ DJ, BASHITI H: Bathing trunk nevus with extensive vascular involvement. J Cutan Pathol 6:513–516, 1979

SILVERBERG GD, KADIN ME, DORFMAN RF et al: Invasion of the brain by a cellular blue nevus of the scalp. Cancer 27:349–354, 1971

SILVERS DN, HELWIG EB: Melanocytic nevi in neonates. J Am Acad Dermatol 4:166–175, 1981

SLAUGHTER JC, HARDMAN JM, KEMPE LG et al: Neurocutaneous melanosis and leptomeningeal melanomatosis in children. Arch Pathol 88:298–304, 1969

SOLOMON LM: The management of congenital melanocytic nevi. Arch Dermatol 116:1017, 1980

TOURAINE A: Les mélanoses neuro-cutanées. Ann Dermatol Syph VIII, 9:489–524, 1949

WALTON RG, JACOBS AH, COX AJ: Pigmented lesions in newborn infants. Br J Dermatol 95:389–396, 1976

WILLIAMS HI: Primary malignant meningeal melanoma associated with benign hairy nevi. J Pathol 99:171–172, 1969

Lentigo Simplex, Peutz–Jeghers Syndrome

ACHORD JL, PROCTOR HD: Malignant degeneration and metastasis in Peutz-Jeghers syndrome. Arch Intern Med 111:498–502, 1963

BENEDICT PH, SZABO G, FITZPATRICK TB et al: Melanotic macules in Albright's syndrome and in neurofibromatosis. JAMA 205:618–626, 1968

BHAWAN J, CHANG WH: Becker's melanosis. Dermatologica 159:221–230, 1979

BHAWAN J, PURTILO DT, RIORDAN JE et al: Giant and "granular melanosomes" in leopard syndrome. J Cutan Pathol 3:207–216, 1976

BLANK AA, SCHNEIDER BV, PANIZZON R: Pigmentfleckenpolypose (Peutz-Jeghers-Syndrom). Hautarzt 32:296–300, 1981

BOLOGA EI, BENE M, PASZTOR P: Considérations sur la lentiginose éruptive de la face. Ann Dermatol Syph 92:277–286, 1965

CAPUTE AJ, RIMOIN DL, KONIGSMARK BW et al: Congenital deafness and multiple lentigines. Arch Dermatol 100:207–213, 1969

Case Records of the Massachusetts General Hospital, Case 24–1976. Peutz-Jeghers syndrome. N Engl J Med 292:1340–1345, 1975

COHEN HJ, MINKIN W, FRANK SB: Nevus spilus. Arch Dermatol 102:433–437, 1970

EADY RAJ, GILKES JJH, WILSON JONES E: Eruptive naevi, report of two cases. Br J Dermatol 97:267–278, 1977

GARTMANN H: Zur Dignität der naevoiden Lentigo. Z Hautkr 53:91–100, 1978

GORLIN RJ, ANDERSEN RC, BLAW M: Multiple lentigines syndrome. Am J Dis Child 117:652–662, 1969

HIRONE T, ERYU Y: Ultrastructure of giant pigment granules in lentigo simplex. Acta Derm Venereol (Stockh) 58:223–229, 1978

JEGHERS H, MCKUSICK BA, KATZ KH: Generalized intestinal polyposis and melanin spots of the oral mucosa, lips and digits. N Engl J Med 241:993–1005, 1031, 1036, 1949

JIMBOW K, SZABO G, FITZPATRICK TB: Ultrastructure of giant pigment granules (macromelanosomes) in the cutaneous pigmented macules of neurofibromatosis. J Invest Dermatol 61:330–309, 1973

KAUFMANN J, EICHMANN A, NEVES C et al: Lentiginosis profusa. Dermatologica 153:116, 1976

KONRAD K, HÖNIGSMANN H: Riesenmelanosomen in Naevuszellnaevi und in normaler menschlicher Epidermis. Wien Klin Wochenschr 87:173–177, 1975

KONRAD K, HÖNIGSMANN H, WOLFF K: Naevus spilus: Ein Pigmentnaevus mit Riesenmelanosomen. Hautarzt 25:585–593, 1974a

KONRAD K, WOLFF K, HÖNIGSMANN H: The giant melanosome: A model of deranged melanosome-morphogenesis. J Ultrastruct Res 48:102–123, 1974b

ORTONNE JP, PERROT H: Giant melanin granules in vitiliginous achromia with malignant melanoma. Acta Derm Venereol (Stockh) 58:475–480, 1978

REID JD: Intestinal carcinoma in the Peutz-Jeghers syndrome. JAMA 229:833–834, 1974

SELMANOWITZ VJ: Lentiginosis profusa syndrome (multiple lentigines syndrome). Acta Derm Venereol (Stockh) 51:387–393, 1971

STEWART DM, ALTMAN J, MEHREGAN AH: Speckled lentiginous nevus. Arch Dermatol 114:895–896, 1978

VAN DER HORST JC, DIRKSEN HJ: Zosteriform lentiginous nevus. Br J Dermatol 104:104, 1981

VORON DA, HATFIELD HH, KALKHOFF RK: Multiple lentigines syndrome. Am J Med 60:447–456, 1976

WEISS LW, ZELICKSON AS: Giant melanosomes in multiple lentigines syndrome. Arch Dermatol 113:491–494, 1977

YAMADA K, MATSUKAWA A, HORI Y et al: Ultrastructural studies on pigmented macules of Peutz-Jeghers syndrome. J Dermatol (Tokyo) 8:367–377, 1981

Freckles

BREATHNACH AS: Melanocyte distribution in forearm epidermis of freckled human subjects. J Invest Dermatol 29:253–261, 1957

BREATHNACH AS, WYLLIE LM: Electron microscopy of melanocytes and melanosomes in freckled human epidermis. J Invest Dermatol 42:389–394, 1964

Melanotic Macules of Albright's Syndrome

BENEDICT PH, SZABO G, FITZPATRICK TB: Melanotic macules in Albright's syndrome and in neurofibromatosis. JAMA 205:618–626, 1968

FRENK E: Étude ultrastructurale des taches pigmentaires du syndrome d'Albright. Dermatologica 143:12–20, 1971

Becker's Melanosis

BECKER SW: Concurrent melanosis and hypertrichosis in distribution of nevus unius lateris. Arch Dermatol Syph 60:155–160, 1949

BONAFÉ JL, GHRENASSIA-CANAL S, VANCINA S: Naevus musculaire lisse. Ann Dermatol Venereol 107:929–301, 1980

COPEMAN PWM, WILSON JONES E: Pigmented hairy epidermal nevus (Becker). Arch Dermatol 92:249–251, 1965

FRENK E, DELACRÉTAZ J: Zur Ultrastruktur der Beckerschen Melanose. Hautarzt 21:397–400, 1970

GARTMANN H, NEUHAUS D, TRITSCH H: Melanosis naeviformis. Z Hautkr 43:973–984, 1968

GEBHART W, KIDD RL, NIEBAUER G: Beckersche Melanosis. Arch Dermatol Forsch 241:166–178, 1971

HANEKE E: The dermal component in melanosis naeviformis Becker. J Cutan Pathol 6:53–58, 1979

PLEWIG G, SCHMOECKEL C: Naevus musculi arrector pili. Hautarzt 30:503–505, 1979

ROWER JM, CARR RD, LOWNEY ED: Progressive cribiform and zosteriform hyperpigmentation. Arch Dermatol 114:98–99, 1978

TATE PR, HODGE SJ, OWEN LG: A quantitative study of melanocytes in Becker's nevus. J Cutan Pathol 7:404–409, 1980

TYMEN R, FORESTIER JF, BOUTET B et al: Naevus tardif de Becker. Ann Dermatol Venereol 108:41–46, 1981

URBANEK RW, JOHNSON WC: Smooth muscle hamartoma associated with Becker's nevus. Arch Dermatol 114:98–99, 1978

Lantigo Senilis

BRAUN-FALCO O, SCHOEFINIUS HH: Lentigo senilis. Hautarzt 22:277–283, 1971

CAWLEY EP, CURTIS AC: Lentigo senilis. Arch Dermatol Syph 62:635–641, 1950

HODGSON C: Lentigo senilis. Arch Dermatol 87:197–207, 1963

MEHREGAN AH: Lentigo senilis and its evolution. J Invest Dermatol 65:429–433, 1975

MONTAGNA W, HU F, CARLISLE K: A reinvestigation of solar lentigines. Arch Dermatol 116:1151–1154, 1980

Mongolian Spot

COLE HR JR, HUBLER WR, LUND HZ: Persistent, aberrant Mongolian spots. Arch Dermatol Syph 61:244–260, 1950

HIDANO A: Persistent Mongolian spot in the adult. Arch Dermatol 103:680–681, 1971

HIDANO A, KAJIMA H, IKEDA S et al: Natural history of nevus of Ota. Arch Dermatol 95:187–195, 1967

INOUE S: Studies on nevus of Ota. Jpn J Dermatol (Series B) 77:130–138, 1967

KIKUCHI I, INOUE S: Natural history of the Mongolian spot. J Dermatol 7:449–450, 1980

KONRAD K, HÖNIGSMANN H, WOLFF K: Bindegewebsmelanocyten beim Menschen. Arch Dermatol Forsch 244:273–275, 1972

KOPF AW, WEIDMAN A: Nevus of Ota. Arch Dermatol 85:195–208, 1962

MEVORAH B, FRENK E DELACRÉTAZ J: Dermal melanocytosis. Dermatologica 154:107–114, 1977

ZIMMERMANN AA, BECKER SW JR: Precursors of epidermal melanocytes in the Negro fetus. In Gordon M (ed): Pigment Cell Biology, pp 159–170. New York, Academic Press, 1959

Nevus of Ota and of Ito, Dermal Melanocyte Hamartoma

BURKHART CG, GOHARA A: Dermal melanocyte hamartoma. Arch Dermatol 117:102–104, 1981

CARLETON A, BIGGS R: Diffuse mesodermal pigmentation with congenital cranial abnormality. Br J Dermatol 60:10–13, 1948

DORSEY CS, MONTGOMERY H: Blue nevus and its distinction from Mongolian spot and the nevus of Ota. J Invest Dermatol 22:225–236, 1954

ENRIQUEZ R, EGBERT B, BULLOCK J: Primary malignant melanoma of central nervous system. Arch Pathol 95:392–395, 1973

HIDANO A, KAJIMA H, ENDO Y: Bilateral nevus Ota associated with nevus Ito. Arch Dermatol 91:357–359, 1965

HIDANO A, KAJIMA H, IKEDA S et al: Natural history of nevus of Ota. Arch Dermatol 95:187–195, 1967

KOPF AW, WEIDMAN AI: Nevus of Ota. Arch Dermatol 85:195–208, 1962

MEVORAH B, FRENK E, DELACRÉTAZ J: Dermal melanocytosis. Dermatologica 154:107–114, 1977

MISHIMA Y, MEVORAH B: Nevus Ota and Nevus Ito in American Negroes. J Invest Dermatol 36:133–154, 1961

Blue Nevus

AVIDOR I, KESSLER E: "Atypical" blue nevus, a benign variety of cellular blue nevus. Dermatologica 154:39–44, 1977

BHAWAN J, EDELSTEIN LM: Bands in cellular blue nevus. Arch Dermatol 113:1130, 1977

BIRD CC, WILLIS RA: The histogenesis of pigmented neurofibromas. J Pathol 97:631–637, 19698

BOGOMOLETZ W: Blue naevus of oral mucosa. Br J Dermatol 80:611–613, 1968

BOURLOND A: Bands in cellular blue nevus. Arch Dermatol 113:1129–1130, 1977

CRAMER HJ: Über den "Neuro-nevus blue" (Masson). Hautarzt 17:16–21, 1966

DORSEY CS, MONTGOMERY H: Blue nevus and its distinction from Mongolian spot and the nevus of Ota. J Invest Dermatol 22:225–236, 1954

DUPONT A, BOURLOND A: Les naevi bleus. Ann Dermatol Syph 89:261–269, 1962

GARTMANN H: Über den zellreichen blauen Naevus. Dermatol Wochenschr 143:297–307, 1961

GARTMANN H: Neuronaevus bleu Masson—Cellular blue nevus Allen. Arch Klin Exp Dermatol 221:109–121, 1965

GARTMANN H, MÜLLER HD: Über das gemeinsame Vorkommen von blauem Naevus und Naevuszellnaevus. Z Hautkr 52:389–398, 1977

HENDRICKS WM: Eruptive blue nevi. J Am Acad Dermatol 4:50–53, 1981

HERNANDEZ FJ: Malignant blue nevus. Arch Dermatol 107:741–744, 1973

JAO W, FRETZIN DF, CHRIST ML et al: Blue nevus of the prostate gland. Arch Pathol 91:187–191, 1971

KERSTING DW, CARO MR: Cellular blue nevus of Ota followed for 22 years. Arch Dermatol 74:59–62, 1956

LEOPOLD JG, RICHARDS DB: The interrelationship of blue and common nevi. J Pathol 95:37–43, 1968

MERKOW LP, BURT RC, HAYESLIP DW et al: A cellular and malignant blue nevus. Cancer 24:886–896, 1969

MISHIMA Y: Cellular blue nevus. Melanogenic activity and malignant transformation. Arch Dermatol 101:104–110, 1970

PITTMAN JL, FISHER BK: Plaque-type of blue nevus. Arch Dermatol 112:1127–1128, 1976

QIZILIBASH AH: Blue nevus of the uterine cervix. Am J Clin Pathol 59:803–806, 1973

RODRIGUEZ HA, ACKERMAN LV: Cellular blue nevus. Cancer 21:393–405, 1968

SANTA CRUZ DJ, YATES AJ: Pigmented storiform neurofibroma. J Cutan Pathol 4:9–13, 1977

Malignant Melanoma in Situ

ACKERMAN AB: Malignant melanoma. A unifying concept. Am J Dermatopathol 2:309–313, 1980

ANTON-LAMPRECHT J, SCHNYDER UW, TILGEN W: Das "Stade éphélide" der melanotischen Präcancerose. Arch Dermatol Forsch 240:61–78, 1971

ANTON-LAMPRECHT I, TILGEN W: Zur Ultrastruktur der melanotischen Präcancerose. Arch Dermatol Forsch 244:264–269, 1972

CLARK WH JR: A classification of malignant melanoma in man correlated with histogenesis and biologic behavior. In Advances in Biology of the Skin, Vol 8: The Pigmentary System, pp 621–647. Oxford, Pergamon Press, 1967

CLARK WH JR, AINSWORTH AM, BERNARDINO EA et al: The developmental biology of malignant melanomas. Sem Oncol 2:83–103, 1975

CLARK WH JR, FROM L, BERNARDINO EA et al: Histogenesis and biologic behavior of primary human malignant melanoma of the skin. Cancer Res 29:705–727, 1969

CLARK WH JR, MIHM MC JR: Lentigo maligna and lentigo-maligna melanoma. Am J Pathol 55:39–67, 1969

COLEMAN WP III, LORIA PR, REED RJ et al: Acral lentiginous melanoma. Arch Dermatol 116:773–776, 1980

CRAMER HJ: Unpigmentierte Melanosis praeblastomatosa. Hautarzt 18:203–206, 1967

CRAMER SF, KIEHN CL: Sequential histologic study of evolving lentigo maligna melanoma. Arch Pathol 106:121–125, 1982

FLEGEL H: Melanotische Problastomatosen. Dermatol Monatsschr 167:517–522, 1981

GOTTLIEB B, BROWN L, WINKELMANN RK: Fine structure of the nevus cell. Arch Dermatol 92:81–87, 1965

LOPANSRI S, MIHM MC JR: Clinical and pathological correlation of malignant melanoma. J Cutan Pathol 6:180–194, 1979

LUND HZ: How often does squamous cell carcinoma of the skin metastasize? Arch Dermatol 92:635–637, 1965

LUPULESCU A, PINKUS H, BIRMINGHAM DJ et al: Lentigo maligna of the fingertip. Arch Dermatol 107:717–722, 1973

MCGOVERN VJ: The classification of melanoma and its relationship with prognosis. Pathology 2:85–98, 1970

MCGOVERN VJ: Malignant Melanoma: Clinical and Histological Diagnosis. New York, John Wiley & Sons, 1976

MCGOVERN VJ, MIHM MC JR, BAILLY C et al: The classification of malignant melanoma and its histologic reporting. Cancer 32:1446–1457, 1973

MCGOVERN VJ, SHAW HM, MILTON GW et al: Is malignant melanoma arising in Hutchinson's melanotic freckle a separate disease entity? Histopathology 4:235–242, 1980

MISHIMA Y: Melanocytic and nevocytic malignant melanoma. Cancer 20:632–649, 1967

MISHIMA Y, MATSUNAKA M: Pagetoid premalignant melanosis and melanoma: Differentiation from Hutchinson's melanotic freckle. J Invest Dermatol 65:434–440, 1975

OLLSTEIN RN, KAPLAN HS, CRIKELAIR GF et al: Is there a malignant freckle. Cancer 19:767–775, 1966

PAUL E, ILLIG L: Melanin-producing dendritic cells and histogenesis of malignant melanoma. Arch Dermatol Res 257:163–177, 1976

PAVER K, STEWART M, KOSSARD S et al: Amelanotic lentigo maligna. Aust J Dermatol 22:106–108, 1981

PITMAN GH, KOPF AW, BART RS et al: Treatment of lentigo maligna and lentigo maligna melanoma. J Dermatol Surg Oncol 5:727–737, 1979

SEIJI M, TAKAHASHI M: Plantar malignant melanoma. J Dermatol (Tokyo) 2:163–170, 1975

SILVERS DN: Focus on melanoma. J Dermatol Surg Oncol 2:108–110, 1976

SU WPD, BRADLEY RR: Amelanotic lentigo maligna. Arch Dermatol 116:82–83, 1980

Malignant Melanoma

ADRIAN RM, MURPHY GF, SATO S et al: Diffuse melanosis secondary to metastatic malignant melanoma. J Am Acad Dermatol 5:308–318, 1981

AMER MH, AL-SARRAF M, BAKER LH et al: Malignant melanoma and central nervous system metastases. Cancer 42:660–668, 1978

ANDERSON DE, SMITH JL, MCBRIDE CM: Hereditary aspects of malignant melanoma. JAMA 200:81–86, 1967

ARRINGTON JR III, REED, RJ, ICHINOSE H et al: Plantar lentiginous melanoma. Am J Surg Pathol 1:131–143, 1977

AZAR HA, ESPINOZA CG, RICHMAN AV et al: "Undifferentiated" large cell malignancies: An ultrastructural and immunocytochemical study. Hum Pathol 13:323–333, 1982

BAAB GH, MCBRIDE CM: Malignant melanoma. The patient with an unknown site of primary origin. Arch Surg 110:896–900, 1975

BAGLEY FH, CADY B, LEE A et al: Changes in clinical presentation and management of malignant melanoma. Cancer 47:2126–2134, 1981

BALCH CM: Surgical management of regional lymph nodes in cutaneous melanoma. J Am Acad Dermatol 3:511–524, 1980

BALCH CM, MURAD TM, SOONG SJ et al: Tumor thickness as a guide to surgical management of clinical stage I melanoma patients. Cancer 43:883–888, 1979

BALCH CM, WILKERSON JA, MURAD TM et al: The prognostic significance of ulceration of cutaneous melanoma. Cancer 45:3012–3017, 1980

BEARDMORE GL: Primary cutaneous polypoidal non-stageable melanomas in Queensland. Aust J Dermatol 18:73–76, 1977

BELLET RE, VAISMAN J, MASTRANGELO MJ et al: Multiple primary malignancies in patients with cutaneous melanoma. Cancer 40:1974–1981, 1977

BENISCH B, PEISON B, KANNERSTEIN M et al: Malignant melanoma originating from intradermal nevi. Arch Dermatol 116:696–698, 1980

BHAWAN J: Amelanotic melanoma or poorly differentiated melanoma. J Cutan Pathol 7:55–56, 1980

BORK K, KORTING GW, RUMPELT HJ: Diffuse Melanose bei malignem Melanom. Hautarzt 28:463–468, 1977

BRESLOW A: Thickness, cross-sectional areas and depth of invasion in the prognosis of cutaneous melanoma. Ann Surg 172:902–908, 1970

BRESLOW A: Tumor thickness, level of invasion and node dissection in stage I cutaneous melanoma. Ann Surg 182:572–575, 1975

BRESLOW A: Prognostic factors in the treatment of cutaneous melanoma. J Cutan Pathol 6:208–212, 1979

CAWLEY EP: Genetic aspects of malignant melanoma. Arch Dermatol 65:440–450, 1952

CLARK WH JR: A classification of malignant melanoma in man correlated with histogenesis and biologic behavior. In Montagna W, Hu F (eds): Advances in Biology of Skin, Vol 8, The Pigmentary System, pp 621–647. New York, Pergamon Press, 1966

CLARK WH JR, FROM L, BERNARDINO EH et al: Histogenesis and biologic behavior of primary human malignant melanoma of the skin. Cancer Res 29:705–727, 1969

CLARK WH JR, MIHM MC JR: Lentigo maligna and lentigo-maligna melanoma. Am J Pathol 55:39–67, 1969

CLARK WH JR, REIMER RR, GREENE M et al: Origin of familial malignant melanomas from heritable melanocytic lesions. Arch Dermatol 114:732–738, 1978

COLEMAN WP III, LORIA PR, REED RJ et al: Acral lentiginous melanoma. Arch Dermatol 116:773–776, 1980

CONLEY J, LATTES R, ORR W: Desmoplastic malignant melanoma. Cancer 28:914–936, 1971

COPEMAN PWM, LEWIS MG, PHILLIPS TM et al: Immunological associations of the halo nevus with cutaneous malignant melanoma. Br J Dermatol 88:127–137, 1973

DAS GUPTA T, BOWDEN L, BERG JW: Malignant melanoma of unknown primary origin. Surg Gynecol Obstet 117:341–345, 1963

DAS GUPTA T, BRASFIELD R: Metastatic melanoma. Cancer 17:1323–1339, 1964

DAY CL JR, MIHM MC JR, SOBER AJ et al: Narrower margins for clinical stage I malignant melanoma. N Engl J Med 306:479–482, 1982

DAY CL JR, SOBER AJ, LEW RA et al: Malignant melanoma patients with positive nodes and relatively good prognosis. Cancer 47:955–962, 1981

DE VRIES JR, RÜMKE P, BERNSTEIN JL: Cytotoxic lymphocytes in melanoma patients. Int J Cancer 9:567–576, 1972

EDELSON RL: Membrane markers of lymphocytes in lymphomas, melanoma and lupus erythematosus. Int J Dermatol 15:577–586, 1976

EINHORN LH, BURGESS MA, VALLEJOS C et al: Prognostic correlations and response to treatment in advanced metastatic malignant melanoma. Cancer Res 34:1955–2004, 1974

ELDER DE, GOLDMAN LI, GOLDMAN SC et al: Dysplastic nevus syndrome. Cancer 46:1787–1794, 1980

ELIAS EG, DIDOLKAR MS, GOEL IP et al: A clinicopathologic study of prognostic factors in cutaneous malignant melanoma. Surg Gynecol Obstet 144:327–334, 1977

EPSTEIN E, BRAGG K, LINDEN G: Biopsy and prognosis of malignant melanoma. JAMA 208:1369–1371, 1969

FITZPATRICK TB, MONTGOMERY H, LERNER AB: Pathogenesis of generalized dermal pigmentation secondary to malignant melanoma and melanuria. J Invest Dermatol 22:163–172, 1954

FLEMING ID, BARNAWELL JR, BURLISON PE et al: Skin cancer in black patients. Cancer 35:600–605, 1975

FROLOW GR, SHAPIRO L, BROWNSTEIN MH: Desmoplastic malignant melanoma. Arch Dermatol 111:753–754, 1975

GARDNER WA JR, VAZQUEZ MD: Balloon cell melanoma. Arch Pathol 89:470–472, 1970

GARTMANN H: Desmoplastisches malignes Melanom. Z Hautkr 54:107–114, 1979

HARRIS MN, GUMPORT SL: Biopsy technique for malignant melanoma. J Dermatol Surg Oncol 1:24–27, 1975

HELWIG EB: Malignant melanoma in children. In McBride CM, Smith JL (eds): Neoplasms of the Skin and Malignant Melanoma, pp 11–26. Chicago, Year Book Medical Publishers, 1976

HERZBERG JJ: Naevus und Melanom. Hautarzt 14:111–114, 1963

HERZBERG JJ: Tyrosinasenachweis bei Metastasen des malignen Melanoms. Arch Klin Exp Dermatol 220:480–485, 1964

HOLCOMB BW, THIGPEN JT, PUCKETT JF et al: Generalized melanosis complicating disseminated malignant melanoma in pregnancy. Cancer 35:1459–1464, 1975

HULA M: Clear cell melanoblastoma. Dermatologica 146:86–89, 1973

HUNTER JAA, ZAYNOON S, PATERSON WD et al: Cellular fine structure in the invasive nodules of different histogenetic types of malignant melanoma. Br J Dermatol 98:255–272, 1978

HUVOS AG, SHAH JP, MIKÉ V: Prognostic factors in cutaneous malignant melanoma. Hum Pathol 5:347–357, 1974

IRONSIDE P, PITT TTE, RANK BK: Malignant melanoma: Some aspects of pathology and prognosis. Aust NZ J Surg 47:70–75, 1977

KLOSTERMANN GF: Zur Frage der multizentrischen Entstehung beim malignen Melanom. Arch Klin Exp Dermatol 215:379–388, 1962

KONRAD K, WOLFF K: Pathogenesis of diffuse melanosis secondary to malignant melanoma. Br J Dermatol 91:635–655, 1974

KORNBERG R, HARRIS M, ACKERMAN AB: Epidermotropically metastatic malignant melanoma. Arch Dermatol 114:67–69, 1978

KREMENTZ ET: Node dissection for extremity melanoma? N Engl J Med 297:664–665, 1977

LABRECQUE PG, HU CH, WINKELMANN RK: On the nature of desmoplastic melanoma. Cancer 38:1205–1213, 1976

LARSEN TE, GRUDE TH: A retrospective histological study of 669 cases of primary cutaneous malignant melanoma in clinical stage I. Acta Pathol Microbiol Scand (A) 87:131–138, 1979

LERMAN RJ, MURRAY D, O'HARA JM et al: Malignant melanoma in childhood. Cancer 25:436–449, 1970

LOPANSRI S, MIHM MC JR: Clinical and pathological correlation of malignant melanoma. J Cutan Pathol 6:180–194, 1979

LUND HZ, STOBBE GD: The natural history of the pigmented nevus. Am J Pathol 25:1117–1155, 1959

MCGOVERN VJ: The classification of melanoma and its relationship with prognosis. Pathology 2:85–98, 1970

MCGOVERN VJ: Malignant Melanoma: Clinical and Histological Diagnosis, p 125. New York, John Wiley & Sons, 1976

MCGOVERN VJ, MIHM MC JR, BAILLY C et al: The classification of malignant melanoma and its histologic reporting. Cancer 32:1446–1457, 1973

MESARA BW, BURTON WD: Primary malignant melanoma of the upper respiratory tract. Cancer 21:217–225, 1968

MIESCHER G: Uber Klinik und Therapie der Melanome. Arch Dermatol Syph (Berlin) 200:215–251, 1955

MINTZIS MM, SILVERS DN: Ultrastructural study of superficial spreading melanoma and benign simulants. Cancer 42:502–511, 1978

MOSELEY HS, GIULIANO AE, STORM FK III et al: Multiple primary melanoma. Cancer 43:939–944, 1979

NIVEN J, LUBIN J: Pedunculated malignant melanoma. Arch Dermatol 111:755–756, 1975

NORRIS HJ, TAYLOR HB: Melanomas of the vagina. Am J Clin Pathol 46:420–426, 1966

OKUN MR, BAUMAN L: Malignant melanoma arising from an intradermal nevus. Arch Dermatol 92:69–72, 1965

OKUN MR, DI MATTIA A, THOMPSON J et al: Malignant melanoma developing from intradermal nevi. Arch Dermatol 110:599–601, 1974

PELLEGRINI AE: Regressed primary malignant melanoma with regional metastases. Arch Dermatol 116:585–586, 1980

PRICE NM, RYWLIN AM, ACKERMAN AB: Histologic criteria for the diagnosis of superficial spreading malignant melanoma. Cancer 38:2434–2441, 1976

PULLMANN H, STEIGLEDER GK: A study of cellular inflammatory reaction in human malignant melanoma, using in vitro labelling techniques with H^3-thymidine. Arch Dermatol Forsch 249:285–289, 1974

RAHBARI H, MEHREGAN AH: Sporadic atypical mole syndrome. Arch Dermatol 117:329–331, 1981

RAMPEN F: Changing concepts in melanoma management. Br J Dermatol 104:341–348, 1981

RAMPEN FHJ, VAN HOUTEN WA, HOP WCJ: Incisional procedures and prognosis in malignant melanoma. Clin Exp Dermatol 5:313–320, 1980

RANCHOD M: Metastatic melanoma with balloon cell changes. Cancer 30:1006–1013, 1972

REED WB, BECKER SW SR, BECKER SW JR et al: Giant pigmented nevi, melanoma, and leptomeningeal melanocytosis. Arch Dermatol 91:100–119, 1965

ROSENBERG L, GOLDSTEIN J, BEN-YAKAR Y et al: The pedunculated malignant melanoma. J Dermatol Surg Oncol 7:123–126, 1981

ROWDEN G, SULICA VI, BUTLER TP et al: Malignant melanoma with melanosis. J Cutan Pathol 7:125–139, 1980

SCHMOECKEL C, BRAUN-FALCO O: The prognostic index in malignant melanoma. Arch Dermatol 114:871–873, 1978

SCHULER G, HÖNIGSMANN H, WOLFF K: Diffuse melanosis in metastatic melanoma. J Am Acad Dermatol 3:363–369, 1980

SHAFIR R, DAVID R, SLUTZKI S: Pedunculated malignant melanoma. Arch Dermatol 114:626–627, 1978

SHAW HM, MCGOVERN VJ, MILTON GW et al: Malignant melanoma: Influence of site of lesion and age of patient in the female superiority in survival. Cancer 46:2731–2735, 1980

SILBERBERG I, KOPF AW, GUMPORT SL: Diffuse melanosis in malignant melanoma. Arch Dermatol 97:671–677, 1968

SIM FH, TAYLOR WF, IVINS JC ET AL: A prospective randomized study of the efficacy of routine elective lymphadenectomy in management of malignant melanoma. Preliminary results. Cancer 41:948–956, 1978

SKOV-JENSEN T, HASTRUP J, LAMBRETHSEN E: Malignant melanoma in children. Cancer 19:620–626, 1966

SMITH JL, STEHLIN JS JR: Spontaneous regression of primary malignant melanomas with regional metastases. Cancer 18:1399–1415, 1965

SOHN N, GANG H, GUMPORT SL et al: Generalized melanosis secondary to malignant melanoma. Cancer 24:897–903, 1969

TRODAHL JN, SPRAGUE WG: Benign and malignant melanocytic lesions of the oral mucosa. Cancer 25:812–823, 1970

TRUAX H, BARNETT RN, HUKILL PB et al: Effect of inaccurate diagnosis on survival statistics for melanoma. Cancer 19:1543–1547, 1966

VALENSI QJ: Desmoplastic malignant melanoma. Cancer 39:286–292, 1977

VAN DER ESCH EP, CASCINELLI N, PREDA F et al: Stage I melanoma of the skin. Cancer 48:1668–1673, 1981

VERONESI U, ADAMUS J, BANDIERA DC et al: Inefficacy of immediate node dissection in stage I melanoma of the limbs. N Engl J Med 297:627–630, 1977

WANEBO HJ, WOODRUFF JM, FARR GH et al: Anorectal melanoma. Cancer 47:1891–1900, 1981

WANEBO HJ, WOODRUFF J, FORTNER JG: Malignant melanoma of the extremities: A clinicopathological study using levels of invasion (microstage). Cancer 35:666–676, 1975

WARNER TFCS, GILBERT EF, RAMIREZ G: Epidermotropism in melanoma. J Cutan Pathol 7:55–56, 1980

Malignant Blue Nevus

DORSEY CS, MONTGOMERY H: Blue nevus and its distinction from Mongolian spot and the nevus of Ota. J Invest Dermatol 22:225–235, 1954

GARTMANN H, LISCHKA G: Maligner blauer Naevus (Malignes dermales Melanozytom). Hautarzt 23:175–178, 1972

HERNANDEZ FJ: Malignant blue nevus. Arch Dermatol 107:741–744, 1973

HERZBERG JJ, KLEIN UE: Blauer Naevus mit Solitär-Metastasen in Lunge und Nebennieren. Arch Klin Exp Dermatol 212:158–172, 1961

KWITTKEN J, NEGRI L: Malignant blue nevus. Arch Dermatol 94:64–69, 1966

MERKOW LP, BURT RC, HAYESLIP DW et al: A cellular and malignant blue nevus. Cancer 24:888–896, 1969

MISHIMA Y: Cellular blue nevus. Melanogenic activity and malignant transformation. Arch Dermatol 101:104–110, 1970

34 Lymphoma and Leukemia

Lymphoma designates a group of malignant neoplasias derived either from B or T lymphocytes or from histiocytes (macrophages). The lymphomas are subdivided into (1) Hodgkin's disease, probably derived from macrophages; (2) the "non-Hodgkin's" or monomorphous lymphomas, largely derived from B lymphocytes; and (3) mycosis fungoides with its variant, the Sézary syndrome, derived from T lymphocytes. Malignant histiocytosis consists of actively phagocytic histiocytes. Leukemia and multiple myeloma represent neoplastic diseases of the hematopoietic system, with primary plasmacytoma of the skin representing a variant of multiple myeloma. Waldenström's macroglobulinemia, like multiple myeloma a plasma cell dyscrasia, only rarely shows specific cutaneous lesions. Finally, the pseudolymphomas of the skin, particularly lymphocytoma cutis, are discussed.

HODGKIN'S DISEASE

In about 90% of the cases, Hodgkin's disease is initially limited to the lymph nodes, with superficial lymph nodes, particularly the cervical lymph nodes, more commonly the first site of involvement than visceral lymph nodes. In most instances, Hodgkin's disease originates in a single lymph node region (Rosenberg and Kaplan). Whether it starts in a lymph node or in an extralymphatic location, subsequent spreading tends to take place through lymphatic vessels to contiguous groups of lymph nodes. Ultimately, vascular invasion within lymph nodes may lead to hematogenous spread to distant lymph nodes or to extranodal sites, resulting in widespread disease (Strum et al). Less widespread disease may occur as a result of retrograde lymphatic spread from obstructed lymph nodes to organs such as the skin, liver, or lung (Benninghoff et al).

The usually orderly extension of Hodgkin's disease in its early stages has led to the widely accepted "staging" of the disease by lymphangiography and exploratory laparotomy consisting of splenectomy, liver biopsy, and biopsy of iliac and para-aortic lymph nodes in order to determine the extent of the disease and, based upon this, the type of treatment (Prosnitz et al). In some cases, exploratory thoracotomy is indicated (Kaplan and Rosenberg). Although bone marrow involvement is rare, bone marrow biopsy may also be done. In the Ann Arbor Staging Classification, four stages are recognized (Carbone et al):

Stage I: Involvement of a single lymph node region (I) or of a single extralymphatic organ or site (I_E)

Stage II: Involvement of two or more lymph node regions on the same side of the diaphragm (II) or localized involvement of an extralymphatic organ or site and of one or more lymph node regions on the same side of the diaphragm (II_E)

Stage III: Involvement of lymph node regions on both sides of the diaphragm (III), which may be accompanied by involvement of the spleen (III_S) or by localized involvement of an extralymphatic organ or site (III_E) or both III_{SE})

Stage IV: Diffuse or disseminated involvement of one or more extralymphatic organs or tissues, with or without associated lymph node involvement

Whether general symptoms, such as fever and weight loss, are present or absent is denoted by the suffix letters B and A, respectively. Biopsy-proved lesions of the liver

726

or bone marrow are invariably defined as stage IV disease, whereas lesions of other extralymphatic tissues, such as the lung, pleura, or bone, may be either E lesions, if localized, or stage IV disease, if multiple or disseminated, and thus call for individualized judgment (Kaplan and Rosenberg).

Involvement of the skin in Hodgkin's disease may consist of nonspecific or specific lesions. The former most commonly consist of excoriations, erythema, and lichenification secondary to generalized pruritus, or ichthyosis vulgaris. Herpes zoster is a fairly common nonspecific cutaneous reaction caused by a decrease in cell-mediated immune responses (see Histogenesis, p. 729) (Reboul et al).

Specific cutaneous lesions are rare. They occur in about 0.5% of the cases (Smith and Butler). They usually consist of papules, nodules, or plaques that may undergo ulceration as they increase in size (Senear and Caro; Benninghoff et al; Smith and Butler). In most instances, the cutaneous lesions are caused by retrograde lymphatic spread from involved lymph nodes (Benninghoff et al; Smith and Butler). In other cases, they are caused by hematogenous spread (Ultmann and Moran). Because most patients die within a few months following the development of the skin lesions, such lesions may be considered an indication of stage IV disease (Smith and Butler).

Occasionally, the skin may be infiltrated by contiguity from underlying cervical, axillary, or inguinal nodes (Saxe et al; Bardach and Kühböck). In such a situation, a diagnosis of stage IV disease appears unwarranted (Ultmann and Moran).

There is no convincing evidence that cutaneous lesions occur as the only manifestation of Hodgkin's disease. Such cases, although reported (Dupont; Szur et al), in reality represent instances of lymphomatoid papuloses (see p. 173) (Smith and Butler). Similarly, cases of Hodgkin's disease in stage IIA with a largely papular eruption (Rubins; Gordon et al) probably do not represent examples of cutaneous Hodgkin's disease, but rather of lymphomatoid papulosis in coincidental association with Hodgkin's disease.

Histopathology. The so-called Rye histopathologic classification (Lukes et al) is now generally used. It has evolved out of the following considerations: (1) an inverse relationship exists between the abundance of lymphocytes and that of giant cells; (2) two distinctively different types of connective tissue reactions may be observed: nodular sclerosis, characterized by interconnecting bands of collagen surrounding nodules of lymphoid tissue, and diffuse fibrosis, a disorderly, finely fibrillar deposit of collagen; (3) there is an association between the occurrence of diffuse fibrosis and depletion of lymphocytes; and (4) in addition to classic Reed–Sternberg cells and mononuclear Hodgkin's cells, a distinctive type of giant cell designated *lacunar cell* is found in the nodular sclerosis type of Hodgkin's disease (Kaplan). These considerations have yielded the four types of the Rye classification. The first two types, called *lymphocytic predominance* and *nodular sclerosis*, since they spread slowly, are often diagnosed while still in stage I or II and then show a good response to adequate treatment; the latter two, called *mixed cellularity* and *lymphocytic depletion,* carry a poor prognosis. The histologic type remains constant in over 90% of the cases with the nodular sclerosis type, in contrast with only about 40% of the cases with lymphocytic predominance and about 70% of those with mixed cellularity. In cases requiring reclassification, the change is toward a histologically more malignant form of Hodgkin's disease (Strum and Rappaport).

In *lymphocytic predominance*, cellular proliferation is composed largely of lymphocytes, with or without benign histiocytes. The lymph nodal architecture may be only partially effaced. Only few immature or atypical mononuclear cells and few Reed–Sternberg giant cells are present, so that examination of multiple sections may be necessary for identification of diagnostic Reed–Sternberg cells. Eosinophils, plasma cells, and neutrophils are usually few or absent, and necrosis and fibrosis are not seen. The majority of patients are clinically in stage I or II and asymptomatic, and the prognosis is very favorable (Mann et al).

In *nodular sclerosis*, interconnecting, thick bands of collagenous tissue subdivide the lymphoid tissue into circumscribed nodules. Although classic Reed–Sternberg giant cells are few, a large, pale variant, referred to as lacunar cell, may be prominent (see below). Lymphocytes, eosinophils, neutrophils, plasma cells, fibroblasts, and histiocytes as well as immature, atypical mononuclear cells are present in varying amounts. Necrosis is occasionally seen. The majority of patients are clinically in stage II at presentation. Patients with nodular sclerosis, particularly those in stage I or II, have an excellent prognosis (Mann et al).

The *mixed cellularity* type occupies an intermediate position between lymphocytic predominance and lymphocytic depletion with respect to both proportion of neoplastic cells and prognosis. Reed–Sternberg cells and their mononuclear precursors are easily found. In addition, lymphocytes, eosinophils, neutrophils, plasma cells, and histiocytes are present. Mild focal necrosis and disorderly, fine, diffuse or focal fibrosis are seen. However, there are no thick bands of collagen (Franssila et al). This type is often associated with systemic symptoms and occurs in all clinical stages. The prognosis is intermediate between that of lymphocytic predominance and that of lymphocytic depletion (Mann et al).

In *lymphocytic depletion*, lymphocytes are scarce. There are many classic Reed–Sternberg giant cells, foci of necrosis, and extensive diffuse fibrosis without collagen band formation. The majority of patients are symptomatic, and the disease is usually disseminated, that is, in stage III or IV, at the time of diagnosis. This is the most aggressive form of Hodgkin's disease; it has a median survival of 25 months, and only 21% of the patients survive 4 years or longer (Bearman et al).

The presence of Reed–Sternberg cells is essential for the histologic diagnosis of Hodgkin's disease. Typical Reed–Sternberg giant cells have the following characteristics. They are large cells measuring from 15 μm to 45 μm in diameter. They contain either several nuclei or one multilobular nucleus.

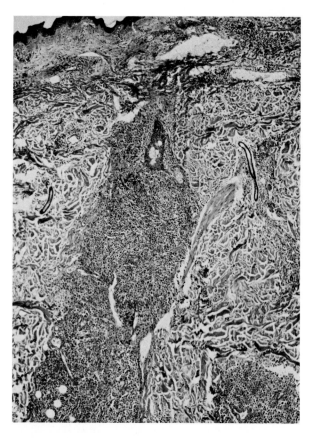

Fig. 34-1. Hodgkin's disease
Low magnification. There are two large masses of neoplastic cells. In addition, numerous small aggregates of cells are present throughout the dermis. (×50)

Often, one sees either two nuclei or a bilobed nucleus that has a "mirror-image" appearance. The nucleoli are large, stain either eosinophilic or amphophilic, and are surrounded by a chromatin-free, clear halo (Franssila et al). If the cells are multinucleated, the nuclei may be either peripherally or centrally located. The so-called lacunar cell, a particular variant of the Reed–Sternberg cell found in the nodular sclerosis category, has abundant pale-staining eosinophilic cytoplasm with a well-defined border, a multilobated nucleus, and multiple small nucleoli. In formalin-fixed tissue, the cytoplasm of these cells artifactually retracts, so that the cells lie within clear spaces or "lacunae" (Mann et al). The mononuclear precursor cell to the Reed–Sternberg giant cells, referred to as Hodgkin's cell, shows a large, atypical nucleus with a conspicuous nucleolus.

The *cutaneous lesions* occurring in Hodgin's disease, if nonspecific, merely show a chronic inflammatory infiltrate. The specific nodules and plaques show large masses of cells often extending into the subcutaneous tissue (Fig. 34-1) (Senear and Caro). The histologic findings are rarely as typical as in the lymph nodes, and assignment to one of the four histologic types is more difficult than in the lymph nodes and often impossible. It may even happen that the changes in the skin suggest a different histologic type than those seen in the lymph nodes of the same patient (Smith and Butler). The number of Reed–Sternberg giant cells, on the presence of which the diagnosis depends, is often small. In some sections, only large, atypical mononuclear cells are observed in association with a chronic inflammatory infiltrate (Smith and Butler). Since the atypical mononuclear cells resemble mycosis cells, the histologic changes may suggest mycosis fungoides. A finding in favor of Hodgkin's disease is the presence of large nucleoli within these cells (Fig. 34-2). Also, a thorough examination of multiple biopsy specimens by means of step sections often shows a few multilobular and multinucleated giant cells, although these cells may not necessarily show the characteristic large, eosinophilic nucleolus with surrounding halo (EM 50).

Histogenesis. On incubation with tritiated thymidine, the Reed–Sternberg cell shows no labeling, indicating that it is incapable of cell division (Azar). It is formed through nuclear division without cellular division from its precursor cell, the Hodgkin's cell, a mononuclear cell with an atypical-appearing nucleus and a prominent nucleolus. This tumor cell replicates readily and is the active malignant cell, with the Reed–Sternberg cell representing its end stage (Azar).

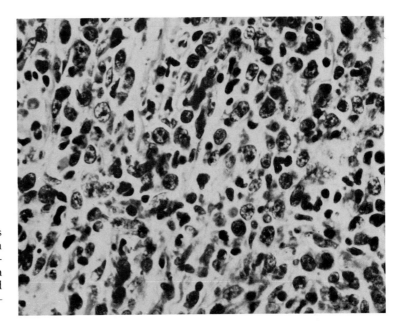

Fig. 34-2. Hodgkin's disease
High magnification of Figure 34-1. There is a dense, polymorphous infiltrate, as seen in the "mixed cellularity" type. The infiltrate contains many mononuclear cells with atypical nuclei and large nucleoli, so-called Hodgkin's cells. A few multinucleated Reed–Sternberg cells are present. (×400)

The derivation of the Hodgkin's and Reed–Sternberg cells has not been determined satisfactorily. However, it seems that, even though the Hodgkin's and Reed–Sternberg cells share some *morphological* features with lymphocytes, their *functional* characteristics are analogous to those of macrophages. From the *morphological* point of view, it has been found that Hodgkin's and Reed–Sternberg cells, similar to transformed lymphocytes, possess large nuclei with dispersed chromatin, large nucleoli, and great numbers of dispersed cytoplasmic polyribosomes and lack lysosomal granules (Glick et al). Also, a developmental sequence has been observed from lymphocyte to transformed lymphocyte to the abnormal mononuclear Hodgkin's cell to the Reed–Sternberg cell (Anagnostou et al). From the *functional* point of view, however, the following findings speak in favor of a derivation of the Hodgkin's and Reed–Sternberg cells from macrophages. (1) Polyclonal immunoglobulins (Ig) and immune complexes are found within viable Reed–Sternberg cells as a result of phagocytosis (Kadin et al). (2) Long-term cultures of lymph nodes from Hodgkin's disease have shown that the Hodgkin's cell is strongly phagocytic and has a number of cytochemical properties typical of macrophages (Roberts et al). (3) Like the macrophage, the Hodgkin's cell has receptors for both complement and the Fc portion of IgG (Kaplan and Gartner). (4) The adherence of T lymphocytes to the surface of isolated Hodgkin's cells is a well-documented phenomenon. It does not represent a cytotoxic attack, however, as was originally thought. Rather, it represents an interaction analogous to that between lymphocytes and macrophages, thus supporting the theory of the macrophage origin of Hodgkin's cells (Payne et al).

A decrease in delayed hypersensitivity reactions, caused by a deficiency in T-cell function, is already evident early in Hodgkin's disease and becomes more pronounced in the course of the disease. In an evaluation of the cell-mediated immune response in Hodgkin's disease, it must be kept in mind that radiation therapy and chemotherapy can also decrease the delayed hypersensitivity reactions (Han and Sokal). When protein synthesis by lymphocytes of untreated patients with Hodgkin's disease is measured after in vitro stimulation of the lymphocytes with varying concentrations of phytohemagglutinin, a phytohemagglutinin dose-dependent defect in lymphocyte stimulation is apparent, even in patients with limited disease (stages I and II). The defect is more pronounced in patients with more extensive disease (stages III and IV) (Levy and Kaplan). Additional defects in delayed hypersensitivity reactions may or may not be present at the same time, but, if absent, they often develop later in the course of the disease. Among the defects may be failure to develop contact sensitivity to dinitrochlorobenzene; unresponsiveness to skin testing with tuberculin, mumps antigen, and various fungal antigens (Schein and Vickers); and an increase in the incidence and severity of viral and fungal infections, particularly herpes zoster and varicella (Sell; Reboul et al). The defect in delayed hypersensitivity responses may reach the state of total anergy in the late stage of the disease, especially in patients with lymphocytic depletion (Young et al). In contrast to the T lymphocytes, the B lymphocytes are not affected in Hodgkin's disease, except perhaps in the terminal stage, so that, as a rule, immunoglobulin values in the serum are normal.

Differential Diagnosis. The dermal infiltrate in lymphomatoid papulosis, even though this is a benign disorder, may be indistinguishable from that occurring in Hodgkin's disease. Even giant cells resembling Reed–Sternberg giant cells may be found (Dupont; Macaulay; Szur et al). Thus, only the clinical features of lymphomatoid papulosis, in which the lesions are predominantly papular rather than nodular and furthermore come and go spontaneously, make a differentiation from Hodgkin's disease possible. For a discussion of differentiation of the tumor stage of mycosis fungoides from Hodgkin's disease, see Mycosis Fungoides (p. 742).

NON-HODGKIN'S LYMPHOMA

Classification.   The great majority of non-Hodgkin's lymphomas originate in the germinal centers, or follicles, of lymph nodes and are monoclonal neoplasms of the cells that are formed in these reaction centers, even in tumors arising in extralymphatic locations. The cells forming the follicles are B lymphocytes. The small B lymphocytes present in the perifollicular mantle of cells, referred to as well-differentiated lymphocytes (Rappaport et al; Rappaport), are transformed within the follicles or germinal centers over an intermediate stage of "poorly differentiated lymphocytes" (Rappaport), "cleaved follicular center cells" (Lukes and Collins), or "centrocytes" (Lennert et al) into large cells referred to as "histiocytes" (Rappaport), "large noncleaved follicular center cells" (Lukes and Collins), or "centroblasts" (Lennert et al). In normal lymph nodes, these transformed lymphocytes move through the lymphocytic mantle into the interfollicular tissue. In this location, either they continue to proliferate as immunoblasts and give rise to plasma cells, or they revert to a dormant state as small lymphocytes as the stimulus subsides (Lukes and Collins; Rywlin).

The different designations given to the germinal center lymphocytes have resulted in apparently different classifications. In the United States, the old classification of Rappaport (1966) still is regarded as the most useful (Rosenberg; Nathwani). This is because of the ease of its histologic application and the prognostic significance inherent in the separation of non-Hodgkin's lymphomas into nodular and diffuse types. It should be realized, however, that the term *nodular* actually signifies "follicular" and that the term *histiocyte* indicates "immunoblast." Generally, in non-Hodgkin's lymphoma, a nodular or follicular pattern can be clearly recognized only in the lymph nodes and spleen, where there are pre-existing follicles. In the Rap-

paport Classification, the non-Hodgkin's lymphomas are divided into the following categories:

1. Well-differentiated lymphocytic lymphoma
2. Poorly differentiated lymphocytic lymphoma
3. Mixed lymphocytic–histiocytic lymphoma
4. Histiocytic lymphoma (large cell lymphoma)
5. Undifferentiated lymphoma (Burkitt's lymphoma)

The histologic architecture may be either nodular or diffuse in the poorly differentiated, mixed, and histiocytic types of lymphoma, since these three types are composed of follicular center cells that may aggregate into follicular or nodular formations. The well-differentiated lymphocytic lymphomas and the undifferentiated lymphomas are always diffuse and never nodular or follicular. This is the case because the former type is derived from lymphocytes that are located at the periphery of the follicles and the latter type is composed of highly undifferentiated cells.

Since nodular configuration indicates a differentiation toward lymph follicles, non-Hodgkin's lymphomas with a nodular pattern have a significantly better prognosis than their diffuse counterparts. Although the pattern, whether nodular or diffuse, is prognostically more important than the cell type, patients with smaller, "more differentiated" cell types have a survival advantage over those with larger, "more immature" cell types. One may thus divide the non-Hodgkin's lymphomas into those with a favorable outlook, which include all nodular lymphomas as well as the diffuse, well-differentiated lymphocytic lymphoma, and into aggressive lymphomas, which include all others with a diffuse pattern (Ezdinli et al). Naturally, other factors besides the pattern and the size of the cells are important to both prognosis and management. They include (1) the extent of the disease or stage of the patient; (2) the site, or sites, of involvement; (3) the size or mass of the tumor in various sites; (4) the symptoms of the patient, both local and systemic; (5) bone marrow function; (6) the age of the patient; and (7) the speed of the patient's tumor progression (Rosenberg).

Clinical Manifestations. Non-Hodgkin's lymphoma differs from Hodgkin's disease in its clinical manifestations in several respects: (1) localized nodal disease, which is common in the early stage of Hodgkin's disease, is less common in the early stage of non-Hodgkin's lymphoma, occurring in only about 11% of the patients (Hellman et al); (2) primary extranodal disease is much more frequently encountered in patients with non-Hodgkin's lymphoma than in patients with Hodgkin's disease; (3) secondary spread in non-Hodgkin's lymphoma occurs predominantly to distant sites, whereas spreading in Hodgkin's disease tends to take place to contiguous groups of lymph nodes; and (4) whereas bone marrow involvement occurs in less than 1% of the patients with Hodgkin's disease, marrow infiltration with lymphomatous cells occurs in at least 10% of the patients with non-Hodgkin's lymphoma (Carbone). Paradoxically, bone marrow involvement is found frequently in patients in the well-differentiated lymphocytic group, who have a good prognosis, and infrequently in the histiocytic group (Rosenberg).

Staging of the disease is done, as in Hodgkin's disease, according to the Ann Arbor Staging Classification (Carbone et al) (see p. 726). It should include, in addition to routine laboratory tests, bone marrow evaluation, lower extremity lymphograms for the detection of periaortic and iliac nodal disease, and computerized tomographic scanning. Diagnostic laparotomy is used less frequently in non-Hodgkin's than in Hodgkin's disease and is indicated primarily for patients who, after all other testing, seem to be in stage I or II. The purpose of laparotomy in these patients is to rule out stage III or IV disease, because radiation therapy is not recommended in stage III or IV, whereas it is in localized disease (Rosenberg). Even though 80% of the patients with localized disease (stage I or II) survive for 5 years, as opposed to only 45% with disseminated disease (stage III or IV), the high relapse rate in stages I and II indicates that few patients who present with localized disease can actually be cured (Qazi et al).

Involvement of the skin with specific lesions is more common in non-Hodgkin's lymphoma than in Hodgkin's disease. In Hodgkin's disease, only about 0.5% of the patients have specific skin lesions, and these lesions are not present at the beginning of the disease or as the only manifestation (see p. 727). In contrast, in non-Hodgkin's lymphoma, around 17% of the patients have specific cutaneous lesions, and, in about 5%, these lesions are the initial manifestation of the disease (Rosenberg et al). The skin lesions may precede all other manifestations by as much as 1 year (Fisher et al) or even by several years (Long et al). In the latter series, the interval ranged from 6 months to 5 years, averaging 21 months (Long et al). The initial cutaneous lesions may consist of a single cutaneous nodule, especially on the scalp, face, or neck (Long et al) or of multiple nodules or plaques that are either localized or diffuse in their distribution (Saxe et al; Evans et al). Purely subcutaneous nodules may occur (Long et al), although extension of large cutaneous nodules into the subcutaneous fat is more common.

The question is unresolved as to whether non-Hodgkin's lymphoma can consist solely of cutaneous lesions. Some authors do not label as lymphoma but rather as lymphoid hyperplasia cases with cutaneous lesions that are clinically suspected of being lymphoma and are histologically indistinguishable from lymphoma when there has been no evidence of extracutaneous lymphoma for a minimum of 4 years (Caro and Helwig; Fisher et al; Evans et al). Other authors, however, recognize the existence of non-Hodgkin's lymphoma only with cutaneous lesions (Long et al; Burke et al). (See also Histiocytic Lymphoma, which on rare occasions has caused death with extensive cutaneous lesions but without lymph nodal or visceral lesions being found on autopsy, p. 735.)

Histopathology. In the *lymph nodes*, the diagnosis of non-Hodgkin's lymphoma requires two determinations: whether the pattern is nodular or diffuse, and which cell type predominates.

The *nodular pattern* imitates the follicles or germinal centers in which normally small, round, "well-differentiated" B lymphocytes located at the periphery of the follicles are transformed into large immunoblasts. This transformation takes place with a "cleaved" cell as an intermediate stage. Thus, the neoplastic nodules or follicles of non-Hodgkin's lymphoma in the lymph nodes consist either predominantly of cleaved cells or predominantly of immunoblasts, or of a mixture of these two cell types. (For a description of cleaved cells and of immunoblasts, see below under Skin.) The neoplastic follicles are larger and much more numerous than the follicles in normal lymph nodes. Usually, the abnormal follicles appear lighter than the surrounding tissue, but they may appear darker (Hurst and Meyer). Whether they are lighter or darker depends on whether the lymphocytes in the abnormal follicles are predominantly large immunoblasts with pale nuclei or cleaved lymphocytes with dark nuclei. A perifollicular mantle of small lymphocytes, as seen around normal lymph follicles, may be present or absent around the follicles of nodular lymphoma. In most instances of nodular lymphoma, the follicles assume an irregular shape and coalesce as the lymphoma progresses, and, finally, the follicular pattern disappears and diffuse lymphoma emerges. In some cases, however, the pattern is still nodular even at autopsy (Wright).

In the *skin* and *subcutaneous tissue*, a diagnosis of lymphoma is often more difficult to make than in the lymph nodes, except in cases with obviously anaplastic large lymphoma cells. There are two reasons for this: first, a nodular pattern is only rarely found in the skin, and, secondly, variation in the size of the nuclei and fairly numerous mitotic figures can also be found in so-called pseudolymphomas.

A *nodular pattern* in the skin has been described by only a few authors. It has been stated that this pattern is most readily recognizable in tissue sections stained with a reticulin stain (Long et al; Burke et al). Still, it is not entirely clear whether this does not just represent a patchy distribution of the infiltrate, which is common in lymphomatous infiltrates of the skin. Other authors regard as "follicular" a pattern in which large atypical immunoblasts are surrounded by small lymphocytes (Kwittken and Goldberg), but this in reality indicates a mixed lymphocytic–histiocytic lymphoma. Thus, there is justification for doubting the existence of a truly nodular pattern in lymphoma of the skin (Evans et al). On the contrary, the presence of germinal centers in a cutaneous infiltrate is a well-established indicator of benignity, since it is often seen in pseudolymphomas such as lymphocytoma cutis (see p. 753) (Caro and Helwig; Fisher et al; Evans et al).

Indeed, it is hazardous, except in cases with obviously anaplastic cells, to base the diagnosis of lymphoma of the skin merely on histologic findings in the skin (Clark et al). Therefore, before a diagnosis of lymphoma of the skin is made, multiple specimens of the skin should be taken for biopsy if more than one lesion is present. In addition, staging procedures should be carried out, such as chest x-ray examination, bone marrow biopsy, gallium scan or computerized tomography, and, in cases with enlarged lymph nodes, lymph node biopsy.

The following histologic features speak in favor of a diagnosis of lymphoma rather than of an inflammatory infiltrate or of pseudolymphoma. (1) There are large masses or small scattered patches of cells that may show atypical nuclei and atypical mitoses. The large masses of cells that clinically appear as cutaneous tumors usually spare the papillary dermis and the epidermis. If, however, the infiltrate extends to the epidermis, ulceration rather than permeation of the epidermis with tumor cells is apt to occur (Long et al). Frequently, one observes extension of the large masses of tumor cells from the reticular dermis deep into the subcutaneous tissue. The small patches of lymphoma cells are distributed haphazardly throughout the dermis and the subcutaneous tissue. Occasionally, patches of lymphoma cells are found in the subcutaneous tissue even in areas of normal-appearing skin, suggesting that the subcutaneous fat can be the primary site of involvement (Trubowitz and Sims; Long et al). (2) The cells within the masses and patches are often so tightly packed that their nuclei may coalesce, whereas, in an inflammatory infiltrate, the cells are generally separated by edema. (3) The masses and patches of cells are quite sharply demarcated at their borders. (4) Frequently, single rows of lymphoma cells not only extend from the otherwise sharply demarcated masses and patches of cells but often lie independent of the masses and patches of cells within the spaces between intact bundles of collagen, like "Indians in a file" (Saxe et al). This phenomenon of single-row invasion also occurs in metastatic carcinoma of the skin, especially in cancer en cuirasse of the breast, and, to a lesser degree, in granuloma annulare (see pp. 591 and 235). For further points of differentiation of lymphoma from inflammatory infiltrates, see pp. 449 and 733; for differentiation from pseudolymphoma, particularly from lymphocytoma, see p. 755.

Well-Differentiated Lymphocytic Lymphoma

Histopathology.   In well-differentiated lymphocytic lymphoma of the skin, one observes either large masses of cells (Fig. 34-3) or scattered patches of cells (Fig. 34-4). In either case, the predominating cell is indistinguishable from a normal lymphocyte. As such, it shows a small, round nucleus with coarsely clumped chromatin and hardly any visible cytoplasm. In some instances, there is an admixture of lymphocytes that have the appearance of "poorly differentiated" lymphocytes with cleaved nuclei. (For their description, see below.) Mitotic figures are sparse. At the periphery of the large masses or scattered patches of cells, one may see single rows of tumor cells extending between and even around intact collagen bundles. In contrast to most inflammatory infiltrates, no edema separates the cells within the patchy or massive aggregates, and, in some areas, one may see coalescence of the nuclei. This feature, occasionally seen in the skin in all types of lymphoma but hardly ever in inflammatory infiltrates, is most commonly observed in well-differentiated lymphocytic lymphoma, because the tumor cells not only lie closely aggregated, as in most cases of lymphoma, but also possess very little cytoplasm.

Although any form of non-Hodgkin's lymphoma may be occasionally associated with leukemia, well-differentiated lymphocytic lymphoma is frequently associated with chronic lymphocytic leukemia. In most instances, leukemic conversion occurs relatively early in the course of the disease;

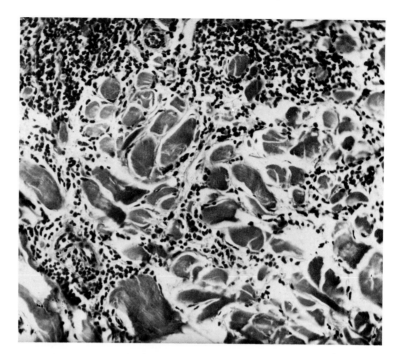

Fig. 34-3. Well-differentiated lymphocytic lymphoma

In the upper third of the photograph, one sees the periphery of a large mass of cells. Rows of tumor cells extend from the mass into the spaces between intact collagen bundles like "Indians in a file." The cells are indistinguishable from normal lymphocytes. (×200)

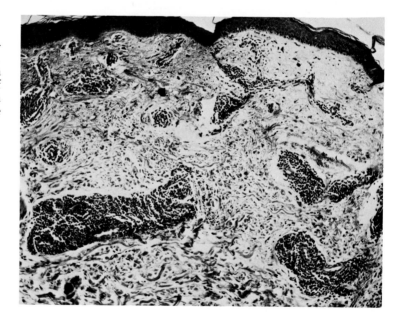

Fig. 34-4. Well-differentiated lymphocytic lymphoma

Sharply demarcated patches of lymphocytes are distributed through the dermis. Because of the small amount of cytoplasm and the absence of edema, the nuclei of the lymphocytes lie closely aggregated. In the patch near the lower left corner, one sees coalescence of the nuclei. (×100)

however, it occasionally develops late during the disease (Pangalis et al).

Differential Diagnosis. Lymphocytic lymphoma with scattered patches of cells, especially without immature cells and mitotic figures, must be differentiated from four diseases that also show a patchy infiltrate. They together form the five patchy dis-

eases beginning with an **L**, which comprise, aside from well-differentiated lymphocytic Lymphoma, chronic discoid Lupus erythematosus, the patchy type of polymorphous Light eruption, Lymphocytic infiltration of the skin of Jessner, and Lymphocytoma cutis.

Chronic discoid lupus erythematosus differs from well-differentiated lymphocytic lymphoma by usually showing characteristic epidermal changes (see p. 447). In addition, the patchy infiltrate of chronic discoid lupus erythematosus appears less sharply demarcated than the infiltrate of lymphocytic lymphoma, and the cells within it are less tightly packed. Also, since it is an inflammatory infiltrate, the cells are more loosely arranged, and there may be a slight admixture of plasma cells and histiocytes. Furthermore, the cellular infiltrate shows no single-row invasion between the collagen bundles, but it often shows a tendency toward arrangement in the vicinity of the cutaneous appendages and may even invade them. Nevertheless, the appearance and composition of the dermal infiltrate in chronic discoid lupus erythematosus may not differ sufficiently from that of lymphocytic lymphoma to permit a clear differentiation on a histologic basis.

Polymorphous light eruption of the plaque type (see p. 211) and lymphocytic infiltration of the skin of Jessner (see p. 456), both of which are probably related to chronic discoid lupus erythematosus, nevertheless lack the epidermal changes that are seen in chronic discoid lupus erythematosus. The dermal infiltrate in these disorders, like that in chronic discoid lupus erythematosus, often does not differ sufficiently from that seen in lymphocytic lymphoma to allow reasonably certain differentiation. Thus, clinical data and possibly a therapeutic test with hydroxychloroquine sulfate (Plaquenil) may be required in order to differentiate chronic discoid lupus erythematosus, polymorphous light eruption of the plaque type, and Jessner's lymphocytic infiltration of the skin from well-differentiated lymphocytic lymphoma.

In lymphocytoma, the infiltrate often differs from that seen in lymphocytic lymphoma by showing two types of cells, mature small lymphocytes and mature follicle center cells, often in a germinal center arrangement. Differentiation then is easy. In other cases, however, lymphocytoma shows a monomorphous lymphocytic infiltrate just like that seen in well-differentiated lymphocytic lymphoma, and a distinction between these two entities can be impossible (see p. 755) (Fisher et al).

Poorly Differentiated Lymphocytic Lymphoma

Histopathology. In poorly differentiated lymphocytic lymphoma of the skin, the infiltrate is composed of cells that vary in nuclear configuration (Fig. 34-5). Many of the cells have cleaved, indented nuclei (Long et al). The nuclei are larger and, because of dispersion of their chromatin, stain lighter than the nuclei of well-differentiated lymphocytic lymphoma cells. Because of the small amount of cytoplasm, the nuclei lie close together (Fig. 34-6). These cells are referred to as cleaved follicular center cells (Lukes and Collins) or centrocytes (Lennert et al). They are intermediate between the small, well-differentiated lymphocytes and the larger immunoblasts in both size and nuclear structure.

Mixed Lymphocytic–Histiocytic Lymphoma

Histopathology. The cutaneous infiltrate in the mixed lymphocytic–histiocytic type of lymphoma contains in varying proportions both partially transformed, cleaved, poorly differentiated lymphocytes and fully transformed large lymphocytes formerly thought to be histiocytes (Fig. 34-7). The latter type of cells, referred to also as immunoblasts (Lukes and Collins) and centroblasts (Lennert et al), has a large, pale-staining, irregularly shaped,

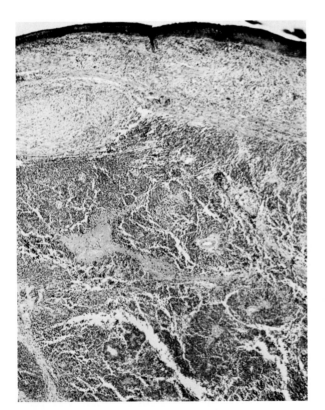

Fig. 34-5. Poorly differentiated lymphocytic lymphoma
Low magnification. Masses of densely packed tumor cells are present in the lower dermis. (× 50)

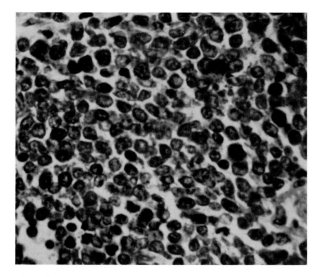

Fig. 34-6. Poorly differentiated lymphocytic lymphoma
High magnification of Figure 34-5. Many of the cells have cleaved, indented large nuclei. The cells possess only a small amount of cytoplasm and therefore lie close together. (×400)

atypical nucleus. (For a detailed description of the "histiocytes," see Histiocytic Lymphoma below.)

Differential Diagnosis. Two types of cells are found in the dermal infiltrate not only in mixed lymphocytic–histiocytic lymphoma but also in some

cases of lymphocytoma. The latter differs from mixed lymphocytic–histiocytic lymphoma by usually not showing atypical nuclei (see p. 755).

Histiocytic Lymphoma (Large Cell Lymphoma)

Histiocytic lymphoma, also referred to as large cell lymphoma (Evans et al; Rywlin; Warnke et al), immunoblastic lymphoma (Lukes and Collins), and centroblastic lymphoma (Lennert et al), was formerly called reticulum cell sarcoma. Large cell lymphoma may present as a solitary tumor that remains localized for a long period, and some patients are cured by local treatment alone (Warnke et al). Occasionally, the first lesion or group of lesions occurs in the skin as nodules or plaques (Kim et al, 1963). In rare instances, innumerable large nodules, some of them ulcerated, are widely distributed over the skin, causing the patient's death, while autopsy reveals no lymph nodal or visceral lesions (Kalkoff; Winkler; Sonck). Clinically, the nodules seen in histiocytic lymphoma may resemble those of the tumor stage of mycosis fungoides (see p. 739). Leukemic transformation is seen only rarely (Rosenberg et al).

Histopathology. The cells present in the lesions, even though still often referred to as histiocytes, represent fully transformed, malignant lymphocytes referred to as immunoblasts (Lukes and Collins) or centroblasts (Lennert et al). These cells usually are present as large masses (Fig. 34-8).

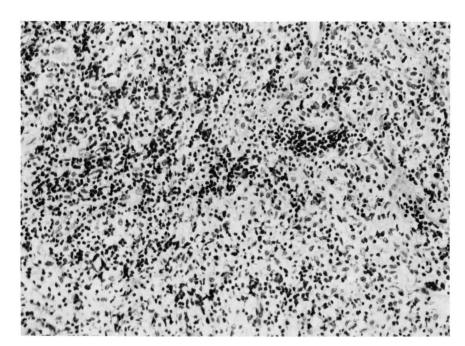

Fig. 34-7. Mixed lymphocytic–histiocytic lymphoma
The infiltrate contains two types of cells. One cell type shows a fairly small and dark nucleus; it represents a poorly differentiated lymphocyte. The other cell type possesses a large, pale-staining, irregularly shaped nucleus; it represents a centroblast or immunoblast, formerly regarded as a histiocyte. (×200)

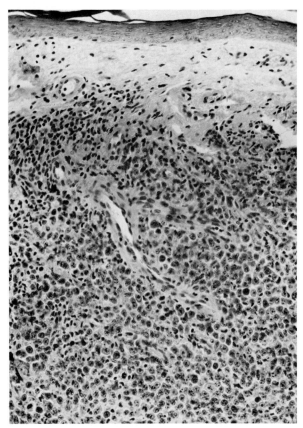

Fig. 34-8. Histiocytic or large cell lymphoma
Low magnification. A mass of cells with large, pale, pleomorphic nuclei is present in the dermis. (×100)

They have a large vesicular nucleus two or three times the diameter of a small lymphocyte with a well-defined nuclear membrane, only few chromatin particles, and one or two distinct nucleoli. The nuclei may be round to oval, but many have an irregular outline and thus an anaplastic appearance (Fig. 34-9). The cytoplasm is ample but stains poorly with hematoxylin-eosin, so that its outline is ill defined. With the Giemsa stain, however, the cytoplasm stains moderately basophilic and thereby becomes clearly visible (Stein et al). Mitotic figures usually are numerous among the immunoblasts, some of them atypical in appearance. Scattered throughout the tumor, one may find varying numbers of lymphocytes with cleaved nuclei and often also macrophages.

Differential Diagnosis.   The large masses of tumor cells seen in immunoblastic (histiocytic) lymphoma must be differentiated from those seen in the tumor stage of mycosis fungoides (see p. 741).

This may be difficult, since the infiltrate in both conditions may consist of tumor cells with large, pale, irregularly shaped nuclei. However, as a rule, the infiltrate in the tumor stage of mycosis fungoides appears more pleomorphic by containing a significant admixture of mycosis cells with dark-staining, cerebriform nuclei and occasionally also multinucleated giant cells resembling Reed–Sternberg cells (Cyr et al). Although ulceration may occur in both conditions, the epidermis next to ulcerations is generally not invaded by the infiltrate in immunoblastic lymphoma. In contrast, one may observe epidermotropism and even scattered Pautrier microabscesses within the epidermis overlying the tumors of mycosis fungoides (Petrozzi et al). Immunologic studies may also be of value, since immunoblastic lymphoma is usually a B-lymphocyte tumor (see p. 730) and mycosis fungoides a T-lymphocyte tumor (see p. 744).

Burkitt's Lymphoma

Burkitt's lymphoma is seen predominantly in Central Africa, although it occasionally occurs elsewhere, including the United States (Ziegler). It is a disorder seen largely but not exclusively among children. It is often multifocal. Whereas most tumors in African patients are extranodal, occurring particularly in the maxillae and the mandible, in nonendemic areas, intra-abdominal tumors originating from mesenteric lymph nodes are common. The skin is only rarely affected but may show multiple infiltrated plaques (Rogge; Evans et al).

Histopathology.   The dermal infiltrate appears monomorphous, being composed of moderately large lymphocytes with predominantly rounded nuclei, rather finely distributed chromatin, and numerous mitotic figures (Evans et al). Scattered among the lymphocytes are usually macrophages with abundant light-staining cytoplasm, resulting in small, clear spaces referred to as a starry sky pattern (Ziegler et al). This phenomenon, however, may be absent in the cutaneous lesions (Rogge).

Lennert's Lymphoma

Lennert's lymphoma, a diffuse type of lymphoma of lymph nodes first described in 1968 (Lennert and Mestdagh), regularly affects the cervical lymph nodes. In some instances, multiple cutaneous nodules are present (Saxe et al; Kim et al, 1978; Roundtree et al).

Histopathology.   Both the lymph nodes and the cutaneous lesions show a diffuse infiltrate of preponderantly small, atypical lymphocytes intermin-

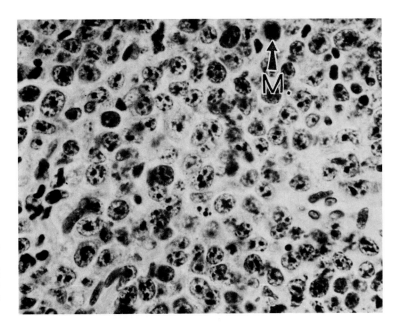

Fig. 34-9.   Histiocytic or large cell lymphoma
High magnification of Figure 34-8. The cells possess abundant cytoplasm and large, pleomorphic nuclei. Because of clumping of the chromatin, most nuclei appear quite pale-staining. A mitotic figure (*M.*) is present in the upper right corner. (× 400)

gled with clusters of epithelioid cells and scattered giant cells. Large, atypical lymphocytes (immunoblasts) are also present in some cases, but only in small numbers (Roundtree et al). Whereas the giant cells in the lymph nodes may resemble Reed–Sternberg giant cells (Kim et al, 1978), those seen in the skin either have the appearance of Langhans type giant cells (Saxe et al) or appear wreath-shaped (Roundtree et al).

Histogenesis. It is evident that the epithelioid cells are not neoplastic cells but reactive, since they are not consistently present in all lesions of Lennert's lymphoma (Roundtree et al). Furthermore, an admixture of epithelioid cells can be found in skin lesions of other types of lymphoma and thus is not specific for Lennert's lymphoma (Saxe et al).

Lymphoma in Angioimmunoblastic Lymphadenopathy

Angioimmunoblastic lymphadenopathy shows cutaneous lesions in about 40% of the cases (see p. 190). However, even though angioimmunoblastic lymphadenopathy progresses into immunoblastic lymphoma in about one third of the cases, the skin shows evidence of lymphoma only rarely (Nathwani et al, 1978b).

Histopathology.   The dermis shows cellular infiltrates around the vessels and appendages composed predominantly of large, fully transformed lymphocytes, that is, immunoblasts, together with

a scattering of plasma cells and small lymphocytes. The small vessels show proliferation within these areas (Nathwani et al, 1978b).

Histogenesis of Non-Hodgkin's Lymphoma. It is generally assumed that the non-Hodgkin's lymphomas are true neoplasms. The tumor cells, as in Hodgkin's disease, are thought to be antigenically altered, possibly by a virus. However, the only human type of lymphoma in which a causal relationship with a virus has been established is the endemic form of Burkitt's lymphoma (see below).

Whereas the tumor cells in Hodgkin's disease are derived from macrophages (see p. 729) and in mycosis fungoides from T lymphocytes (see p. 744), most non-Hodgkin's lymphomas are composed of B lymphocytes. This fact has been well established for all nodular lymphomas and for diffuse lymphomas derived from nodular types of lymphomas, as well as for Burkitt's lymphoma. A certain percentage of diffuse and large cell lymphomas, however, are not B-cell lymphomas. It has been estimated that 50% to 60% of large cell lymphomas have characteristics of B lymphocytes, 5% to 15% have T-cell markers, 5% have features consistent with monocytes or true histiocytes, and approximately one third of the cases have no specific markers, their cells being termed null cells (Mann et al). Among the diffuse large cell lymphomas recognized as predominantly T-cell lymphomas are the lymphoblastic lymphoma (Nathwani et al, 1976), Lennert's lymphoma (Nathwani), and some of the "reticulum cell sarcomas" (large cell lymphomas) arising in the skin (Burg et al; Edelson).

It should be emphasized, however, that an overall subdivision of non-Hodgkin's lymphomas into the immunologic subgroups of T, B, undefined, and true histiocytic has little clinical significance, since each of these subgroups is too heterogeneous (Nathwani). A morphologic classification that clearly defines homogeneous groups, like that proposed by Rappaport, is therefore preferable, even though its terminology may be outdated (Nathwani et al, 1978a).

From the immunologic point of view, however, recognition of the fact that all nodular lymphomas are B-lymphocyte lymphomas is of considerable importance. Since the germinal centers, or follicles, in lymph nodes and the spleen are composed largely of B lymphocytes, and since the nodular lymphomas and all diffuse lymphomas developing from nodular lymphomas are B-lymphocyte lymphomas, it has been concluded that such lymphomas are derived from follicles (Lukes and Collins; Lennert et al).

The commonly used methods for identifying T lymphocytes, B lymphocytes, and histiocytes employ the induction of rosette formation. Whereas testing for identification of B lymphocytes or histiocytes can be carried out either with cell suspensions or with frozen sections, rosette testing for T lymphocytes requires living cells and thus can be done only with cell suspensions. T lymphocytes are identified by their spontaneous rosette formation with neuraminidase-treated sheep erythrocytes (Edelson et al). In addition, testing for T cells can be carried out either on cell suspensions or on frozen sections with antisera against human T cells in combination with the peroxidase–antiperoxidase technic (Burg et al). Also, T lymphocytes show granular staining with acid nonspecific alpha-naphthyl acetate esterase (A-EST) (Sterry et al). Furthermore, the recently developed OKT series of hybridoma monoclonal antibodies reacts with human T cells and T-cell malignancies (see also p. 744). (Knowles and Halper).

B lymphocytes as well as histiocytes have receptors for the activated third component of complement (C3), identifiable by their rosette formation with erythrocytes coated with IgM antibody and complement (IgM EAC). However, only histiocytes have receptors for cytophilic antibodies and thus bind erythrocytes coated with IgG antibody (IgG EA) (Edelson et al; Jaffe et al). In addition, histiocytes show diffuse staining with the nonspecific esterases A-EST (alpha-naphthyl acetate esterase) and B-EST (alpha-naphthyl butyrate esterase) (Mann et al).

IMMUNE DEFECT. In nodular or follicular lymphoma, the lymphomatous cells within the follicles are defective. There is a block in their development, and they proliferate within the follicles without moving into the interfollicular tissue, where they would normally become plasma cells. Antibody production is therefore deficient. In comparison with nodular or follicular lymphoma, diffuse lymphoma has an even more severe immune defect. It shows a tremendous accumulation of defective B lymphocytes, which are unable to function and fail to form lymphoid follicles in the lymph nodes and spleen (Lukes and Collins). Analogous to the finding of a proliferation of defective B lymphocytes, the amount of circulating immunoglobulins in B-cell lymphomas is often reduced; however, delayed hypersensitivity is not impaired in non-Hodgkin's lymphoma, in contrast to Hodgkin's disease (Miller).

DEVELOPMENT OF LEUKEMIA. The transformation of a non-Hodgkin's lymphoma to leukemia of the same cell line indicates that these two processes are related and represent merely different stages in the evolution of the process. Whereas non-Hodgkin's lymphoma is a more or less localized process, leukemia is characterized by diffuse bone marrow involvement associated with diffuse involvement of spleen, liver, and lymph nodes (Rubin).

BURKITT'S LYMPHOMA. The Epstein–Barr virus (EBV) is associated with nearly all cases of African Burkitt's lymphoma, as indicated by significantly elevated antibody titers to EBV in patients with this kind of lymphoma. Between 80% and 90% of Burkitt's tumors contain EBV deoxyribonucleic acid (DNA) (Ziegler). It is assumed that the EBV transforms B lymphocytes into malignant cells and that viral DNA then persists in these cells. In contrast to patients with African Burkitt's lymphoma, patients with American Burkitt's lymphoma, on the average, have only slightly higher EBV antibody titers than the general population, and no EBV DNA has been found in the tumor tissue (Pagano et al).

MYCOSIS FUNGOIDES

Mycosis fungoides affects the skin primarily, but, ultimately, lymph nodes and visceral organs are frequently involved (Clendenning et al; Cyr et al; Epstein et al).

Clinically as well as histologically, mycosis fungoides in typical cases can be divided into three stages: erythematous, plaque, and tumor. The three stages overlap, so that lesions of all three stages may be present simultaneously.

In the *erythematous stage,* one observes a patchy eruption. The patches are usually flat and not atrophic, but, in some patients, they appear atrophic. The flat, non-atrophic patches often show scaling and then resemble psoriasis or some form of dermatitis. The atrophic patches appear shiny and show easy wrinkling, loss of normal skin markings, telangiectases, and hypo- and hyperpigmentation (Sanchez and Ackerman). Clinically, they have the appearance either of the large plaque type of parapsoriasis en plaques* (see p. 148) or of parapsoriasis variegata (see p. 149). Whereas the flat, *non-atrophic* patches are generally followed by infiltrated plaques within several months to several years, and later on usually also by visceral lesions, the flat, *atrophic* patches undergo clinical transition into aggressive mycosis fungoides in only about 12% of the cases, while persisting in the remainder without significant change (see p. 150) (Samman).

---

* It must be kept in mind that, in French, the term *plaque* refers to a flat patch, whereas, in English, it refers to an indurated lesion.

In the *plaque stage,* irregularly shaped, well-demarcated, slightly indurated plaques occur. They may show central clearing, resulting in serpiginous lesions.

In the *tumor stage,* one observes round or irregularly shaped, raised tumors of a brownish red color. They often undergo ulceration. The tumors that occur in the tumor stage of mycosis fungoides have the same clinical appearance as the tumors that are seen in other forms of lymphoma. Once the tumor stage has begun in a patient with mycosis fungoides, death usually occurs within a few years, with 50% of the patients dying within 2½ years (Epstein et al).

In some patients, the erythematous stage of mycosis fungoides becomes generalized. This *erythrodermic form* of mycosis fungoides has the appearance of a generalized exfoliative dermatitis or generalized erythroderma (Clendenning et al; Epstein et al). In most of these cases Sézary cells are present in the blood (see p. 746). Such cases represent the Sézary syndrome. A close relationship exists between the Sézary syndrome and mycosis fungoides, as shown by the fact that both are T-cell lymphomas caused by the same infiltrating cell referred to as either mycosis cell or Sézary cell (see Histogenesis). In addition, circulating Sézary cells can occasionally be seen in mycosis fungoides (Clendenning et al), and plaques and tumors may occur in the Sézary syndrome (Schein et al). Both diseases show progressive involvement of lymph nodes and visceral organs.

In the rare *d'emblée form* of mycosis fungoides, tumors of the skin develop without the previous presence of erythematous or plaque lesions (Lapière; Epstein et al; Blasik et al). The diagnosis of mycosis fungoides d'emblée of course requires that, on histologic examination, the tumors show an infiltrate that is compatible with the histologic diagnosis of mycosis fungoides.

Histopathology. The division of mycosis fungoides into three stages as described for the clinical picture pertains also to the histologic picture.

In the *erythematous stage,* the histologic picture varies, depending on whether the lesions are flat, nonatrophic patches or flat, atrophic patches. Although it is generally agreed that mycosis fungoides starts as such in every case and does not develop from another dermatosis, it may be difficult in the early phase of the disease to establish the diagnosis with certainty, particularly in the flat, nonatrophic patches. It is therefore recommended that multiple specimens be taken for biopsy (Chu et al, 1982a).

In *flat, nonatrophic patches,* the dermis at first often shows merely a banal inflammatory infiltrate in the papillary and subpapillary portions of the dermis. The infiltrate is composed mainly of lymphocytes but also contains varying numbers of histiocytes. Several repeat biopsies may be required before the diagnosis of mycosis fungoides can be confirmed (Chu et al, 1982b). However even at a very early stage of the disease, one frequently observes epidermotropism, a feature that is highly suggestive of mycosis fungoides (Sanchez and Ackerman). *Epidermotropism* refers to the presence in the epidermis of mononuclear cells and differs from the common phenomenon of exocytosis, seen for instance in the various forms of dermatitis (see p. 96), by showing usually very little or no spongiosis. In epidermotropism, one observes scattered through the epidermis mononuclear cells that usually lie singly and are separated from the surrounding keratinocytes by a clear space or halo (Fig. 34-10). Occasionally, one may see several mononuclear cells lying close together and surrounded by a halolike clear space suggestive of a small Pautrier microabscess (see below). Cells with hyperchromatic and irregularly shaped nuclei, analogous to mycosis cells, are usually absent. Even if they are present in small numbers in the cellular infiltrate, their presence cannot be regarded as evidence of mycosis fungoides, since a few cells with this appearance are also occasionally present in the dermal infiltrate of various inflammatory dermatosis (see p. 744) (Flaxman et al).

In *flat, atrophic patches,* the histologic picture resembles that of poikiloderma atrophicans vasculare by showing flattening of the epidermis with vacuolization of the basal cell layer and a bandlike mononuclear infiltrate lying in close apposition to the epidermis and invading the epidermis in some areas. In addition, there may be telangiectases, small extravasations of red cells, and pigmentary incontinence. The infiltrate in early poikilodermatous lesions of mycosis fungoides may be nonspecific, but it is more pronounced than in poikiloderma atrophicans vasculare associated with dermatomyositis or systemic lupus erythematosus (see p. 460) (Janis and Winkelmann). In more advanced lesions, cells with hyperchromatic, convoluted nuclei may be seen within the dermal infiltrate and within the epidermis. In the epidermis, they lie mostly singly as "haloed cells" but also in small collections (Sanchez and Ackerman). Only occasionally does one observe pronounced epidermotropism, that is, permeation of the epidermis by numerous cells with hyperchromatic nuclei (see p. 741) (Haneke et al).

In the indurated *plaque stage,* the histologic picture is diagnostic in most instances. The following three changes are generally present: (1) a fairly high percentage of so-called mycosis cells with hyperchromatic and irregularly shaped nuclei, giving the mycosis cells a pleomorphic appearance;

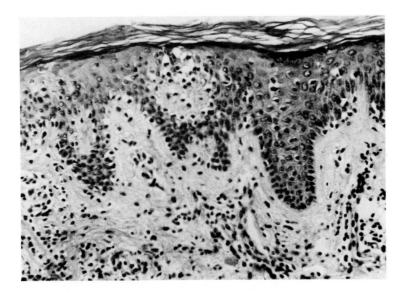

Fig. 34-10.   Mycosis fungoides, flat, nonatrophic patch
The epidermis shows epidermotropism without spongiosis. Mononuclear cells surrounded by a halo are scattered through the epidermis. The dermal infiltrate is nonspecific. No mycosis cells are seen. (×100)

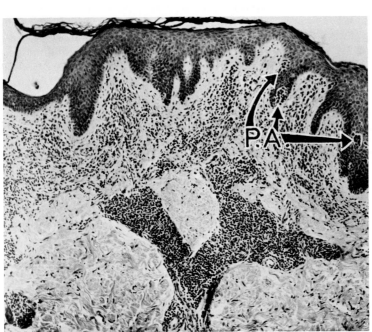

Fig. 34-11.   Mycosis fungoides, plaque
Low magnification. The infiltrate in the upper dermis is diffuse, while in the lower dermis it consists of sharply demarcated patches of various sizes. The epidermis contains several Pautrier microabscesses (*P.A.*). (×100)

(2) arrangement of the dermal infiltrate in a band-like and patchy pattern in the dermis; and (3) presence of epidermotropism and often also of Pautrier microabscesses in the epidermis.

The presence of *mycosis cells*, which represent T lymphocytes with hyperchromatic, irregularly shaped nuclei, is diagnostic of the plaque stage of mycosis fungoides, provided that the mycosis cells form a fairly high percentage of the cells in the dermal infiltrate. The size of their nuclei is not significantly greater than the size of other nuclei in the infiltrate of the plaques, so that they stand out more by virtue of their hyperchromasia than their size. Mitoses of such nuclei can be found, but their number is usually not large. It is only during the late plaque stage that the nuclei of some of the mycosis cells become significantly larger than the other nuclei in the infiltrate. Such cells have been referred to as true mycosis cells (Rappaport and Thomas).

The *arrangement of the cellular infiltrate* in the plaque stage of mycosis fungoides is often patchy. In addition to a diffuse or bandlike infiltrate in the upper dermis, as seen also in a nonspecific chronic inflammation, one frequently finds patches of cellular infiltration in the lower dermis (Fig. 34-11). If the patches are fairly large and show a rather sharp demarcation, they are strong evidence in favor of a diagnosis of mycosis fungoides. Aside from showing the presence of lymphocytes, histiocytes, and varying numbers of mycosis cells, the dermal infiltrate in some instances shows an admixture of eosinophils and plasma cells.

A very helpful diagnostic feature is the presence of *epidermotropism* and of *Pautrier microabscesses* in the epidermis, found in the majority of cases in the plaque stage, particularly if several biopsy specimens are examined. Epidermotropism is characterized by the presence within the epidermis of scattered single mononuclear cells often surrounded by a halolike clear space. Pautrier microabscesses consist of small intraepidermal groups of often tightly aggregated mononuclear cells located within a vacuole (Fig. 34-12). In contrast to the erythematous stage, in which the epidermotropic cells and the cells within Pautrier microabscesses usually have the appearance of ordinary lymphocytes, some of the intraepidermal mononuclear cells in the plaque stage have the appearance of mycosis cells. Not only the epidermis but also the epithelium of adnexa, especially hair follicles, may be invaded by scattered mononuclear cells (Altmeyer and Nödl; Sanchez and Ackerman). The epidermis in the plaque stage usually shows acanthosis with elongation of the rete ridges and thus may have an appearance similar to that of psoriasis. Spongiosis and microvesiculation, as seen in dermatitis, are generally absent in mycosis fungoides but it can nevertheless be very difficult in some instances to distinguish the intraepidermal aggregates of cells that have formed as a result of vesiculation in cases of dermatitis from the aggregates seen in the Pautrier microabscesses of mycosis fungoides (see Differential Diagnosis, p. 745). Occasionally, epidermotropism with or without Pautrier microabscesses is pronounced, with mononuclear cells diffusely infiltrating the epidermis, so that one may speak of an epidermotropic form of mycosis fungoides (Castermans-Elias; Smoes-Charles and Dupont; Degreef et al). (For a discussion of the Woringer–Kolopp form of mycosis fungoides which is characterized by a single lesion or a localized area of cutaneous involvement showing marked epidermotropism, see p. 747.)

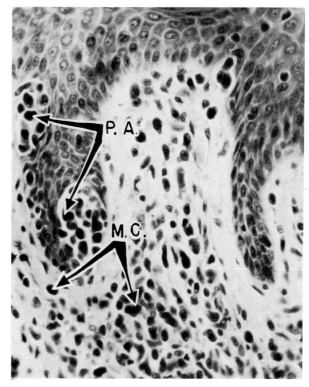

Fig. 34-12.   Mycosis fungoides, plaque
High magnification of Figure 34-11. The dermal infiltrate contains several cells with hyperchromatic, irregularly shaped nuclei, so-called mycosis cells (*M.C.*). There are several Pautrier microabscesses in the epidermis (*P.A.*). (×400)

In rare instances, plaque lesions of mycosis fungoides show accumulations of acid mucopolysaccharides within hair follicles and sebaceous glands at the site of degenerating epithelial cells, resulting in a histologic picture identical to that seen in alopecia mucinosa (see p. 205) (Emmerson). The mucinous degeneration in such cases is secondary to the invasion of the pilosebaceous structures by mononuclear cells (Altmeyer and Nödl).

In the *tumor stage,* the infiltrate consists of large masses of cells occupying extensive areas of the dermis and often penetrating into the subcutaneous tissue. The infiltrate may compress and destroy the epidermis, so that ulceration results. In most cases, the infiltrate consists mainly of mycosis cells with pleomorphic, hyperchromatic nuclei showing considerable variation in size (Fig. 34-13) (Vonderheid et al). In some cases, however, the infiltrate shows many cells that appear to have undergone blastic transformation and possess large, vesicular nuclei causing resemblance

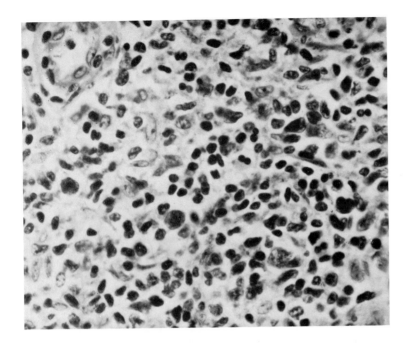

Fig. 34-13. Mycosis fungoides, tumor
The infiltrate consists mainly of mycosis cells with pleomorphic, hyperchromatic nuclei showing considerable variation in size. (×400)

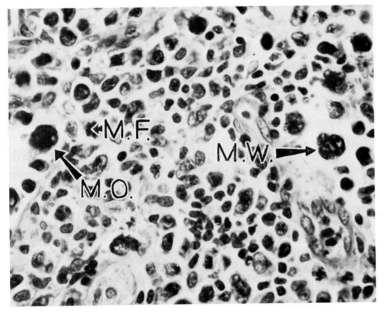

Fig. 34-14. Mycosis fungoides, tumor
Many cells appear to have undergone blastic transformation and possess large nuclei as seen in "histiocytic" lymphoma. Several mycosis cells are multilobular (*M.O.*) or multinucleated (*M.W.*). Mitotic figures (*M.F.*) are present. (×400)

to a histiocytic lymphoma (Camisa and Goldstein; Schmoeckel et al). Mitotic figures are common among these cells. Occasionally, the blastic cells are pleomorphic and appear as mono- and multinucleated giant cells (Cyr et al; Brehmer-Andersson). They may then resemble the Reed–Sternberg cells of Hodgkin's disease, from which they differ, however, by greater hyperchromasia of their nuclei and by the absence of large, eosinophilic nucleoli

(Fig. 34-14). The difficulty of recognizing such tumors as representing mycosis fungoides is increased by the fact that epidermotropism is often absent in the tumors, although it may still be found in coexisting plaque-type lesions (Edelson).

Staging and Involvement of Peripheral Lymph Nodes in Vivo. Staging procedures are important in all patients with mycosis fungoides with the exception of those with a limited erythematous eruption or with plaques covering less than 10% of the skin surface (T-1). In patients in the T-1 stage, only radiographic examination of the chest and repeated examination of smears of peripheral blood for Sézary cells are indicated. All patients with plaques covering more than 10% of the skin (T-2), with tumors (T-3), with generalized erythroderma (T-4, Sézary syndrome), or with more than 4% of Sézary cells in their differential white blood cell count, even without palpable lymph nodes, should have a "blind" biopsy of a lymph node draining an involved skin area (Lamberg and Bunn). All patients with palpable lymph nodes (stage II) should have a biopsy of one or several enlarged lymph nodes, as well as liver and bone marrow biopsies (Lamberg and Bunn).

Bipedal lymphangiograms contribute little to the evaluation of mycosis fungoides, in contrast with Hodgkin's disease, because of poor correlation (Hamminga et al). Similarly, liver and spleen scans frequently give false-negative or false-positive results. Even with computed tomography, false-negative results may be obtained, since there may be histologic involvement of visceral lymph nodes or of the spleen without sufficient organ enlargement to be considered abnormal (Doyle and Winkelmann, 1981a). Thus, staging laparotomy is the most accurate method of staging, and, in patients with positive findings, it may lead to more aggressive therapy and thus to improved long-term survival (Fuks et al; Variakojis et al; Griem et al; Doyle and Winkelmann, 1981b).

The presence of palpably enlarged *lymph nodes* in patients with mycosis fungoides has an unfavorable effect on the prognosis. Even when dermatopathic lymphadenopathy is the only apparent histologic change, survival is affected adversely. In one study, the median length of survival was found to be 34 months in patients in whom the biopsy of palpable lymph nodes revealed dermatopathic lymphadenopathy and only 18 months if the histologic examination revealed lymphoma (Levi and Wiernik). Although other authors have also found a longer survival period in patients with palpable lymph nodes diagnosed as having dermatopathic lymphadenopathy than in patients diagnosed as having lymphoma (Rappaport and Thomas; Scheffer et al), some studies have shown no significant difference in survival among the various grades of lymph node involvement ranging from dermatopathic lymphadenopathy to diffuse involvement by mycosis fungoides (Colby et al). This finding, as well as the frequently observed progression of dermatopathic lymphadenopathy into mycosis fungoides on a subsequent lymph node biopsy (Block et al; Fuks et al; Scheffer et al; Colby et al), suggests that many cases of mycosis fungoides diagnosed as dermatopathic lymphadenopathy on histologic grounds are in reality instances of early lymph node involvement with mycosis fungoides.

Histopathology of Lymph Nodes. The statement has been made that mycosis fungoides of lymph nodes can be reliably diagnosed only when there are clusters or sheets of cells with hyperchromatic, irregularly shaped nuclei (Rappaport and Thomas). However, it has been pointed out that large numbers of cells with hyperchromatic, convoluted nuclei analogous to mycosis cells can be found in dermatopathic lymphadenopathy associated with nonneoplastic conditions (Colby et al). It is thus apparent that a definite diagnosis of mycosis fungoides in the early phase of the disease is even more difficult in the lymph nodes than it is in the skin. In the late stage, when clearly malignant lymphocytes have largely replaced the nodal architecture, the diagnosis of mycosis fungoides is easy. In the lymph nodes, as in the skin, there may be blast cells and giant cells resembling Reed–Sternberg cells (Colby et al).

Visceral Lesions. Clinically apparent visceral lesions are relatively rare, in spite of their often widespread presence on autopsy. However, occasional instances are encountered of multiple osteolytic lesions (Greer et al) or of fatal involvement of the brain (Pariser), lungs (Wolfe et al), or gastrointestinal tract (Camisa and Goldstein).

The *mortality rate* among patients with mycosis fungoides from the disease itself is estimated to be about 80%, with about one half of the patients dying of infection, largely pneumonia or sepsis, and one half dying of the consequences of disseminated lymphoma (Epstein et al). Since many patients with mycosis fungoides are elderly and the erythematous and plaque stages can extend over many years, about 20% of the patients die of causes unrelated to mycosis fungoides.

On *autopsy*, 72% of the patients who have died with mycosis fungoides show extracutaneous involvement, as revealed by a compilation of 13 series reported between 1940 and 1974 (Carney and Bunn). This frequency is significantly higher than expected from clinical symptoms prior to death. The involvement is often widespread. The lymph nodes, affected in 61% of the cases, are the most common site of visceral involvement (Carney and Bunn). However, almost any organ may be affected. The lungs, liver, and spleen are involved in 43% to 52% of the cases, and the bone marrow, gastrointestinal tract, kidneys, heart, and central nervous sytem in 18% to 32% (Carney and Bunn). The number of organs with lymphomatous infiltrate may vary from 1 to 25, with an average of 6.3 per patient (Epstein et al).

Histopathology of Internal Organs. Involvement of internal organs may consist of diffuse interstitial infiltration that can be detected only on microscopic examination. This is especially true of the liver, spleen, and kidneys. There may be a striking degree of epitheliotropism, analogous to that seen in the skin, with invasion of epithelial tissues by lymphomatous cells, for instance, in the renal tubules and thyroid tissue (Rappaport and Thomas; Blasik et al). Some visceral lesions, like cutaneous lesions in the tumor stage, consist largely of mycosis cells with large, hyperchromatic nuclei or of blastic cells with either large, vesicular nuclei or pleomorphic mono- and multinucleated giant nuclei. The infiltrate may then resemble other forms of lymphoma, such as non-Hodgkin's lymphoma or Hodgkin's disease. At one time, therefore, some authors assumed that transitions could occur from mycosis fungoides to "reticulum cell sarcoma" or to Hodgkin's disease (Cyr et al). If, however, previous sections of such cases are reviewed and sections of various organs obtained at autopsy are compared with one another, it becomes apparent that transitions exist between mycosis cells and such blastic cells. These cells are thus a manifestation of the tumor stage of mycosis fungoides (Epstein et al).

It is of interest that, whereas involvement of the bone marrow in vivo is rare, autopsy studies have shown involvement in 32% of patients, suggesting that bone marrow infiltration represents a common terminal event (Carney and Bunn).

Histogenesis. It is generally accepted that mycosis fungoides in its plaque stage and especially in its tumor stage represents a neoplastic disease, a malignant lymphoma in which the mycosis cell, a T lymphocyte, represents the neoplastic cell. However, it is still an open question whether the mycosis cell in the initial phase of the disease is a tumor cell arising from a malignant clone or whether it is the product of chronic immunologic stimulation (Claudy).

The view has been widely held that mycosis fungoides is a malignant process from its beginning (Lapière; Degos et al; Epstein et al; Fuks et al; Rappaport and Thomas; Edelson et al; Wilson Jones). The fact that the number of mycosis cells is small in the beginning is thought to be due to a pronounced inflammatory defense reaction of the tissue against the presence of lymphoma cells, as first suggested in 1925 (Fraser). As the disease advances and the number and atypicality of the lymphoma cells increases, the host reaction slackens until, in the tumor stage, lymphoma cells predominate (Rosas-Uribe et al). This theory is supported by the observation that, in other malignant diseases, such as squamous cell carcinoma, malignant melanoma, and Hodgkin's disease, an inflammatory host reaction is also often present in the early stage but disappears as the malignancy of the tumor cells increases. Also, the presence of chromosomal abnormalities in the cells even of early skin infiltrates (Erkman-Balis and Rappaport) and of abnormal contents of DNA (Prunieras) has been thought to indicate that mycosis fungoides is a neoplastic disorder from the beginning.

The other view, that mycosis fungoides starts as an immunologic disorder and only later develops into a lymphoma, has received increasing support in recent years. The possibility of such a development has been convincingly demonstrated by the rather frequent progression of angioimmunoblastic lymphadenopathy into an immunoblastic lymphoma (see p. 737) (Nathwani et al). The following observations speak in favor of an immunologic origin of mycosis fungoides. First, incubation of normal human lymphocytes with pokeweed mitogen or phytohemagglutinin results in the presence of 5% to 11% of cells with the light microscopic and ultrastructural appearance of mycosis or Sézary cells, indicating that they are a product of stimulated lymphocytes (Yeckley et al). The finding that mycosis cells are stimulated or transformed lymphocytes explains their presence on electron microscopic examination in the dermal infiltrate of a variety of randomly selected inflammatory infiltrates, such as lupus erythematosus, lichen planus, and solar keratosis (Flaxman et al). Second, epidermotropism and the formation of Pautrier microabscesses in mycosis fungoides represent an immunologic phenomenon in which Langerhans cells present antigens to T lymphocytes, resulting, as in contact dermatitis, in an apposition of T lymphocytes to Langerhans cells. Interaction with Langerhans cells acts as the focus for the development of Pautrier microabscesses (Rowden et al; Schmitt and Thivolet). The fact that this process, in contrast with contact dermatitis, is chronic suggests a defect in antigen processing that results in the persistence of an as yet unidentified antigen (Tan et al, 1974). Malignant transformation is assumed to take place as a result of the chronicity of this reactive process (Schuppli).

The mycosis cells, as well as the circulating Sézary cells, are T lymphocytes. The T-cell identity of a majority of cells in the cellular infiltrate of mycosis fungoides was at first established by the preparation of cell suspensions from lesions of mycosis fungoides and determination of the percentage of cells forming sheep erythrocyte rosettes, as T cells do. It was found that the skin infiltrate of mycosis fungoides contains from 66% to 86% T lymphocytes (Tan et al, 1975). More recently, in situ identification of lymphocytes became possible with a specific antihuman T-lymphocyte antiserum and an indirect peroxidase staining technic. It was thus shown that, in mycosis fungoides, the dermal and epidermal infiltrates consist predominantly of cells bearing the specific human T-lymphocyte antigen (HTLA), and, in Pautrier microabscesses, all cells show positive T-lymphocyte labeling (Chu and MacDonald, 1979). The presence also in large plaque (atrophic) parapsoriasis of a high percentage of HTLA-positive cells in the dermal and epidermal infiltrates supports the theory of a relationship between this condition and mycosis fungoides (McMillan et al).

Quite recently, a series of mouse monoclonal antibodies has been developed against various T-cell antigens. These antigens are identifiable by labeling of the antibody with either fluorescein or peroxidase. All peripheral T cells react with the OKT3 antibody. Within this population, cells with inducer (helper) function react with the OKT4 antibody, whereas T cells with cytotoxic and suppressor function react with the OKT8 antibody. In the dermal infiltrate of mycosis fungoides, the great majority of T cells, usually 80% to 90%, express the inducer (helper) phenotype, and only 10% to 20% are of the suppressor/cytotoxic type (Thomas et al).

During the early, "premalignant" phase of mycosis fungoides, most of the inducer (helper) type of cells are in contact with Langerhans cells exhibiting large amounts of immune-response associated (Ia) antigen. This contact is indicative of a close functional relationship (Thomas et al). In the later stages of the disease, the T-cell populations become self-sustained and more independent of Ia-antigen-positive cells. At this stage, mycosis fungoides is a malignant monoclonal proliferation of inducer T cells (Thomas et al).

On *electron microscopic examination*, the mycosis cell shows only scant cytoplasm but a relatively large nucleus with numerous infoldings of the nuclear membrane resulting in fingerlike projections of the nucleoplasm. Thus, in three-dimensional reconstructions, the nucleus appears to be cerebriform (Lutzner et al). Dense aggregates of chromatin particles are concentrated at the nuclear membrane and are scattered throughout the nucleus (Brownlee and Murad; Lutzner et al; Rosas-Uribe et al). A great resemblance exists in electron microscopic appearance among the mycosis cell, the Sézary cell (Lutzner et al), and the cells in the dermal and epidermal infiltrates of large plaque parapsoriasis (McMillan et al).

Attempts have been made to use electron microscopic measurement of lymphocyte nuclear contours in skin biopsies for diagnostic purposes. In one investigation, significant differences were found between the group mean nuclear contour index for early mycosis fungoides and that for benign inflammatory dermatoses, so that patients could be classified correctly with a probability of over 95% (Meijer et al). However, there is overlapping in controversial cases (McNutt and Crain). Lymphocytes with a high nuclear contour index of 16 or more appear specific for mycosis fungoides but are not found in all cases of the disease (McNutt and Crain).

Study of the *Langerhans cells* and their interaction with the mycosis cells by electron microscopy has shown the presence of Langerhans cells, recognizable by their characteristic granules (see p. 18), throughout the epidermis. There, they are always present in Pautrier microabscesses and are often seen in direct apposition to lymphoid cells. Langerhans cells are also present in the dermal infiltrate in all stages of mycosis fungoides in close apposition to lymphoid cells, whereas Langerhans cells are normally seen only rarely in the dermis (Jimbow et al).

Since Langerhans cells are OKT6-reactive, use of either fluorescein-labeled or peroxidase-labeled OKT6 has shown in mycosis fungoides an increased number of labeled cells in the epidermis and, in addition, labeled cells in the dermis (MacKie). In the dermal infiltrate, OKT6-reactive cells account for up to 5% of the cells (Chu et al, 1982a).

Immunologic evaluation of patients with mycosis fungoides has revealed in the early stage of the disease normal T- and B-lymphocyte populations, as well as a normal mitogen blastogenic response, normal antibody production, and normal skin test reactivity (Blaylock et al). Some patients show a decreased mitogen blastogenic response in the plaque stage (Cooperrider and Roenigk), but only in the tumor stage do many patients show a defect in their cell-mediated immune responses, including prolonged skin graft survival and decreased dinitrochlorobenzene (DNCB) sensitization (Clendenning and Van Scott), as well as a significant decrease in the mitogen blastogenic response (Langner et al).

Hematologic examination has revealed the presence of circulating Sézary cells in mycosis fungoides in from 12% to 20% of the patients (Winkelmann and Hoagland; Clendenning et al). However, their concentration is usually less than 15%, the minimum level required for the diagnosis of the Sézary syndrome (Winkelmann and Hoagland). Also, circulating Sézary cells at low concentrations are not a specific finding; they are often found intermittently in various inflammatory dermatoses, generally at levels below 10% or 1000 per mm³ (Duncan and Winkelmann). It is very rare for mycosis fungoides to terminate in a T-cell leukemia without the development of erythroderma (Harrington and Slater).

Differential Diagnosis.   The diagnosis of mycosis fungoides in its early stage can be very difficult, so that, often, only a presumptive diagnosis of mycosis fungoides can be made, and additional biopsies and correlation with the clinical findings are necessary. The reason for the difficulty in the histologic diagnosis of the early stage of mycosis fungoides lies in the fact that occasional cells with hyperchromatic, irregularly shaped nuclei corresponding to "early" mycosis cells and representing transformed lymphocytes can be seen in many nonspecific chronic inflammatory infiltrates (see p. 739) (Flaxman et al). The presence of epidermotropism and/or of Pautrier microabscesses containing mononuclear cells can then be of great value, especially if a fairly high percentage of the mononuclear cells have the appearance of mycosis cells or at least appear haloed. Otherwise, it can be very difficult to distinguish between epidermotropism and exocytosis. The latter is commonly seen in the various forms of dermatitis and shows within the epidermis scattered mononuclear cells in association with spongiosis. Even Pautrier microabscesses containing mononuclear cells cannot always be differentiated from intraepidermal aggregates of mononuclear cells that have formed as a result of exocytosis in cases of dermatitis (Ackerman et al). Such "spongiotic simulants of Pautrier microabscesses" usually show spongiosis in their vicinity, whereas spongiosis is rare in mycosis fungoides. Even in the spongiotic simulants of Pautrier microabscesses, as seen in dermatitis, some of the mononuclear cells may possess hyperchromatic, irregularly shaped nuclei (Ackerman et al).

Sézary Syndrome

The Sézary syndrome, first described in 1938 (Sézary and Bouvrain), is characterized by generalized erythroderma with intense itching, peripheral lymphadenopathy, and the presence of Sézary cells in the cellular infiltrate of the skin and in the peripheral blood. The Sézary cell, as present in the skin, is indistinguishable from the mycosis cell by both light and electron microscopy (Lutzner and Jordan).

Clinically, the entire skin shows erythema and, in addition, edema and lichenification. The general health of the patient remains good for several years. Death occurs as a result of either an intercurrent disease or the involvement of peripheral as well as visceral lymph nodes and of various viscera (Fleischmajer and Eisenberg; Edelson et al; Weber et al; Kienitz et al). In some patients, one observes, in addition to generalized erythroderma, plaques or tumors indistinguishable from those seen in mycosis fungoides (Schein et al; Kienitz et al).

There is a group of patients with a "pre-Sézary erythroderma syndrome" who have intractable erythroderma but show no specific histologic findings in the skin and have benign dermatopathic lymphadenopathy, no lymphocytosis, and only a few Sézary cells in their differential count not exceeding 6%. In some of these patients, the condition evolves into the Sézary syndrome (Winkelmann et al).

Histopathology. The skin in the Sézary syndrome shows in the upper dermis a dense infiltrate composed of lymphocytes, histiocytes, and varying numbers of Sézary cells. The Sézary cell in the dermis is indistinguishable from the mycosis cell seen in the plaque stage of mycosis fungoides and shows a hyperchromatic, irregularly shaped nucleus. In addition, Pautrier microabscesses are often present in the epidermis, as in mycosis fungoides, containing Sézary cells and other cells of the dermal infiltrate (Sézary; Fleischmajer and Eisenberg; Weber et al).

The circulating blood reveals a moderate leukocytosis, showing commonly between 10,000 and 30,000 but occasionally as many as 60,000 leukocytes (Taswell and Winkelmann) or even more

than 200,000 (Edelson et al) per cubic millimeter of blood. Atypical mononuclear cells, or Sézary cells, usually account for 15% to 30% of the white blood cells. It is well recognized that the percentage of Sézary cells can fluctuate considerably (Miller et al). The Sézary cell is characterized in blood smears as having a large, grooved nucleus occupying at least four fifths of the cell. The cytoplasm appears as a narrow rim around the nucleus. There are two types of Sézary cells: the large, typical cell, 12 μm to 14 μm in diameter, and the small cell variant, of the same size as a normal lymphocyte, 8 μm to 11 μm in diameter, but differing from it by the grooved pattern of its nucleus (Flandrin and Brouet). In addition to the presence of Sézary cells, the blood shows a rather high percentage of normal lymphocytes. In the bone marrow, however, less than 50% of the nucleated cells are lymphocytes, and the other marrow-derived cell lines are well preserved, indicating extramedullary production of some of the lymphocytes and of the Sézary cells (Edelson et al).

The enlarged peripheral lymph nodes may show only nonspecific dermatopathic lymphadenopathy (Fleischmajer and Eisenberg). In some instances, however, the normal nodal architecture is completely replaced by a diffuse proliferation of Sézary cells (Tedeschi and Lansinger; Edelson et al). The visceral infiltrates are indistinguishable from those seen in mycosis fungoides (Schein et al).

Histogenesis. By *electron microscopy,* the Sézary cell that is present in the skin and in the circulating blood shows, like the mycosis cell, a nucleus that is characterized by numerous infoldings of the nuclear membrane, resulting in fingerlike projections of the nucleoplasm (Brownlee and Murad; Lutzner and Jordan; Lutzner et al). The Sézary cell has been identified by immunologic studies as a thymus-derived lymphocyte, since it can be stimulated by phytohemagglutinin in vitro to synthesize DNA (Crossen et al), forms sheep erythrocyte rosettes, and is killed by a specific rabbit antihuman T-cell antiserum (Flandrin and Brouet). Like the mycosis cell, the Sézary cell has been identified as a malignant proliferation of helper T cells (Broder et al).

The Sézary syndrome is now generally regarded as an erythrodermic, leukemic variant of mycosis fungoides (Edelson et al; Schein et al). The Sézary syndrome differs from other forms of leukemia in that usually the Sézary cells do not originate in the bone marrow, which is normal in appearance (Edelson et al). Only in patients with large numbers of Sézary cells in the blood has bone marrow infiltration been noted (Flandrin and Brouet; Büchner). It has not been clarified where the Sézary cells present in the circulating blood originate. Since Sézary cells in the circulating blood have the same appearance as those in the skin, some authors believe that they originate in the skin (Main et al; Taswell and Winkelmann). Others assume that they arise from lymph nodes (Crossen et al). Radioisotopic scanning has suggested that the Sézary cell migrates from the blood to the skin, a finding that makes lymph nodes the most likely site for its origin (Miller et al).

Differential Diagnosis. There is no doubt that cases of the Sézary syndrome have in the past been mistaken for chronic lymphocytic leukemia with erythroderma. However, chronic lymphocytic leukemia represents an overproduction of B lymphocytes in the bone marrow, which is usually not involved in the Sézary syndrome. The bone marrow in chronic lymphocytic leukemia hardly ever shows, as it does in the Sézary syndrome, more than 50% of the nucleated cells to be nonlymphocytic cells. As a rule, 80% or more of the nucleated cells in the bone marrow are lymphocytes in chronic lymphocytic leukemia (Edelson et al).

Woringer–Kolopp Disease

Woringer–Kolopp disease is a rare, benign disorder that was first described in 1939 (Woringer and Kolopp). Referred to also as pagetoid reticulosis (Braun-Falco et al, 1973), it most likely represents a localized form of mycosis fungoides with prominent epidermotropism (Lever). It usually shows only a single, slowly enlarging skin lesion, but, occasionally, there are several closely aggregated lesions (Braun-Falco et al, 1973, 1979). The sites of predilection are the extremities, mainly the lower ex-

tremities (Mandojana and Helwig). The lesion or lesions consist of asymptomatic, erythematous, scaly, sometimes hyperkeratotic plaques with a slightly raised, circinate border and a tendency toward central healing.

Histopathology. The epidermis, particularly its lower portion, is infiltrated by numerous mononuclear cells. Their nuclei are rather large, hyperchromatic, and irregular in shape and thus appear atypical (Fig. 34-15) (Lever). The infiltrating cells have very little cytoplasm and, as a rule, are surrounded by a halolike clear space. Quite frequently, two or more nuclei are arranged in nests and have a nonstaining halo at their periphery, thus greatly resembling Pautrier microabscesses (Medenica and Lorincz). The dermis contains only a mild nonspecific inflammatory infiltrate (Mandojana and Helwig).

Histogenesis. On *electron microscopic examination*, the cells infiltrating the epidermis are seen to lack desmosomes and tonofilaments. They possess convoluted nuclei with numerous infoldings. They are thus indistinguishable from mycosis cells (Braun-Falco et al, 1973; Medenica and Lorincz; Toribio et al; Mandojana and Helwig). Also, as in mycosis fungoides (see p. 745), the lymphoid cells with convoluted, cerebriform nuclei are often seen in close apposition to Langerhans cells or indeterminate cells, suggesting a functional interaction between them (Geerts et al). In addition, the lymphoid cells bear T-cell markers, inasmuch as they form rosettes with sheep erythrocytes and have receptors for anti-T-cell globulin (Burg et al). Thus, it appears likely that Woringer–Kolopp disease is a T-cell lymphoma and a

Fig. 34-15. Woringer–Kolopp disease
The nuclei in the epidermal infiltrate are hyperchromatic, irregular in shape, and variable in size. Many cells in the epidermal infiltrate are surrounded by a halolike clear space. (×200)

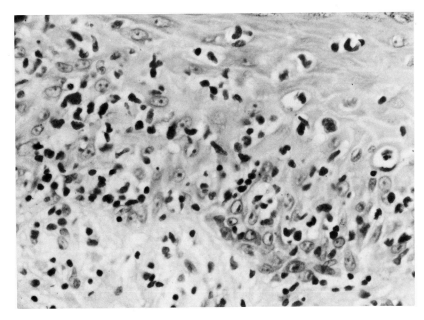

special form of mycosis fungoides (Burg et al). Also in favor of a relationship with mycosis fungoides is the fact that a similar pronounced epidermotropism may be seen in some cases of disseminated, fatal mycosis fungoides, so that they have even been regarded as disseminated Woringer–Kolopp disease (Castermans-Elias; Degreef et al; Bourlond et al). However, it seems preferable to classify such cases as disseminated epidermotropic mycosis fungoides (see p. 741) and to limit the diagnosis Woringer–Kolopp disease to the localized cases (Medenica and Lorincz; Wood et al).

MALIGNANT HISTIOCYTOSIS

Malignant histiocytosis, originally described in 1939 as histiocytic medullary reticulosis (Scott and Robb-Smith), is a rare histiocytic proliferative disorder that often shows an acute onset with severe malaise and used to progress to death within a few months. Recently, however, complete remissions were observed in 9 of 13 patients who underwent an intensive combination chemotherapy regimen (Zucker et al). The disease occurs in children as well as in adults. It is characterized by fever, lymphadenopathy, and hepatosplenomegaly. Later on, pancytopenia, jaundice, and purpura develop.

Involvement of the skin or of the subcutaneous tissue with specific lesions has been estimated to occur in about 10% of the cases (Abele and Griffin). In children, however, the incidence seems to be higher, since, in one series, 18 of 22 children had such lesions (Zucker et al). The cutaneous or subcutaneous lesions may consist of papules, nodules, or plaques that often undergo ulceration (Abele and Griffin; Robinowitz et al; Nishio et al). They may be an early manifestation of the disease (Warnke et al).

Histopathology.   The cutaneous infiltrate is usually located in the middle to lower portion of the dermis and in the subcutaneous fat. It consists of masses of normal and atypical histiocytes with focal areas of necrosis and acute and chronic inflammation. The atypical histiocytes display large, pleomorphic, vesicular nuclei (Robinowitz et al). Some of the histiocytes contain in their cytoplasm phagocytized erythrocytes, nuclear debris, and fragments of leukocytes (Engstrom et al).

Histogenesis. The phagocytic activity of the histiocytes present in all involved organs, including the bone marrow, causes the pancytopenia, as well as the jaundice and the purpura. The histiocytic nature of the infiltrate can be proved by the presence of acid phosphatase and of naphthol AS acetate esterase activity. This activity is more pronounced in well-differentiated than in poorly differentiated histiocytes (Huhn and Meister). On electron microscopy, no Langerhans granules are seen in the histiocytes (Piñol-Aguadé et al; Huhn and Meister).

Differential Diagnosis. Distinction from lymphoma and Letterer–Siwe disease is usually possible by the pronounced erythrophagia of the histiocytes in malignant histiocytosis, often best seen in the lymph nodes (Zucker et al). Also, the infiltrate in Letterer–Siwe disease is located in the upper rather than in the lower layers of the dermis (see p. 393). Erythrophagia of histiocytes is also seen in cytophagic histiocytic panniculitis, in which, however, the histiocytes appear benign with normal nuclei (see p. 194).

LEUKEMIA

The leukemias represent malignant neoplasias of white blood cells. They are characterized by a diffuse infiltration of the bone marrow with immature leukocytes and by the presence of these leukocytes in the blood stream, often in abnormal numbers. In addition, there is usually widespread infiltration of liver, spleen, and lymph nodes, and often also of other organs, including the skin.

Leukemia usually arises as a primary systemic disorder without developing from a lymphoma. As already stated in the description of the non-Hodgkin's lymphomas, the development of a leukemia in the course of a lymphoma is rather rare (see p. 731), with the exception of well-differentiated lymphocytic lymphoma (see p. 732). Four major groups of leukemia are recognized: (1) chronic lymphocytic leukemia, (2) acute lymphocytic leukemia, (3) chronic granulocytic leukemia, and (4) acute granulocytic leukemia (Saarni and Linman).

Chronic Lymphocytic Leukemia

Chronic lymphocytic leukemia is the most common cause for specific leukemic infiltrates in the skin, which usually consist of nodules or plaques (Kerl et al).

Histopathology.   The infiltrates are composed of small, mature lymphocytes with only occasional mitoses. Larger, irregularly shaped nuclei are seen only in some cases.

Differential Diagnosis.   Histologic differentiation from well-differentiated lymphocytic lymphoma is not possible on histologic grounds (see p. 732). In both instances, the tumor cells are B lymphocytes.

Acute Lymphocytic Leukemia

Specific cutaneous infiltrates are seen in only about 3% of the cases of acute lymphocytic leukemia (Boggs et al). In addition to cutaneous and subcutaneous nodules, purpuric lesions are commonly seen (Bernengo et al, 1976). The cutaneous lesions in some cases precede the appearance of leukemic cells in the peripheral blood (Cochrane and Milne; Yoder and Schuen).

Histopathology. Diffuse dermal and subcutaneous infiltrates of cells with large, irregular nuclei are seen (Yoder and Schuen). There may be extensive areas of hemorrhage within or near the infiltrates (Cochrane and Milne).

Histogenesis. The cells of acute lymphocytic leukemia are T lymphocytes in 26%, B lymphocytes in 4%, and null cells in 70% of the cases (Kerl and Kresbach).

Differential Diagnosis. The rarity of B-cell markers may aid in the differentiation of the infiltrate from non-Hodgkin's lymphoma.

Chronic Granulocytic Leukemia

Specific cutaneous manifestations are quite rare in chronic granulocytic leukemia. If they occur, it is usually during the terminal phase of the disease, although, in exceptional cases, leukemic infiltration of the skin can be demonstrated before characteristic changes are found in the bone marrow and in the peripheral blood (Conrad et al). Terminally, there may be a transformation into acute granulocytic leukemia. This may be preceded by a few months or may be accompanied by the appearance of one or several lesions of granulocytic sarcoma (Neiman et al) (see Acute Granulocytic Leukemia below).

Clinically, the specific cutaneous lesions of chronic granulocytic leukemia consist of papules and nodules of varying size that may coalesce into plaques. They rarely ulcerate. They may have a hemorrhagic appearance. In addition, purpuric lesions and hemorrhagic bullae may be seen (Costello et al).

Eosinophilic leukemia, a rare variant of chronic granulocytic leukemia, occasionally has cutaneous manifestations consisting of widespread nodules (Deme; Carmel et al). Eosinophilic leukemia has also been described as occurring in the hypereosinophilic syndrome in association with cardiac dysfunction (see p. 192) (Kazmierowski et al). The skin eruption in such cases is pruritic and polymorphous. However, since the eosinophils are mature, the pronounced eosinophila may not be truly neoplastic but reactive, as in Löffler's syndrome (Hardy and Anderson).

Histopathology. Histologic examination of the specific cutaneous lesions in chronic granulocytic leukemia shows the presence of dense cellular infiltrates in the dermis, often extending into the subcutaneous tissue (Costello et al). In addition to large areas of infiltration, small groups of cells may be found. The cells are in part mature neutrophils with a lobated nucleus, but, in addition, there are cells that are larger than neutrophils and have round, oval, or indented nuclei without recognizable granules. These cells represent myelocytes and myeloblasts and are indistinguishable from the immature cells seen in lymphoma (Costello et al). In addition, there often are mature eosinophils and eosinophilic myelocytes (Conrad et al). The latter cells possess an irregularly shaped nucleus and abundant cytoplasm containing eosinophilic granules (Kerl and Kresbach).

Of great value in confirming the granulocytic nature of the tumor cells are two cytochemical stains that can be carried out on formalin-fixed, paraffin-embedded tissue: the chloroacetate esterase and the antilysozyme immunoperoxidase stains, both of which are negative in lymphocytes and thus exclude lymphocytic leukemia and lymphoma. The chloroacetate esterase (naphthol AS-D chloroacetate esterase) stain is positive in myelocytes but negative in myeloblasts and eosinophilic myeloid cells. In contrast, the antilysozyme immunoperoxidase technic is positive not only in myelocytes but also in leukemic myeloblasts and eosinophilic myeloid cells (Neiman et al).

In *eosinophilic leukemia,* the cellular infiltrate in the dermis and subcutis contains, in addition to immature, mononuclear cells, some eosinophilic myelocytes (Carmel et al) or even mature eosinophils (Deme).

Acute Granulocytic Leukemia

In addition to a pure form of acute granulocytic leukemia in which myeloblasts and young myelocytes predominate, there are two variants: myelomonocytic leukemia, with a proliferation of immature granulocytes and monocytes, and erythroleukemia, in which immature erythrocytes are found in association with immature granulocytes. In all three forms, fever, malaise, anemia, purpura, and hepatosplenomegaly are found, and death usually occurs within a few months.

Acute granulocytic leukemia shows specific cutaneous lesions relatively rarely, although vegetating, necrotic tumor masses may form in the course of the disease (Bernengo et al, 1975). The most common specific cutaneous manifestation, however, is the appearance of one or several tumors referred to as granulocytic sarcomas. Such tumors were formerly called chloromas because, as a result of the presence of myeloperoxidase, they often display a greenish color that fades on exposure to air (Neiman et al). They also occur at sites other than the skin, especially in bones and lymph nodes. They either arise in chronic granulocytic leukemia shortly before its change into the acute form (Neiman et al) or occur as a very early manifestation of acute granulocytic leukemia, often at a time when there are not yet any immature granulocytes in the peripheral blood (Wiernik and Serpick; Long and Mihm; Sun and Ellis). Their size varies from 1 cm to 3 cm, and they may be either soft and tender (Long and Mihm) or firm and nontender (Sun and Ellis). They have no tendency to ulcerate.

Two dermatoses that occasionally precede or accompany acute granulocytic or myelomonocytic leukemia are pyoderma gangrenosum, showing bullae and superficial ulcers (Perry and Winkelmann; Pye and Choudhury), and febrile neutrophilic dermatosis (Raimer and Duncan; Behm et al).

Myelomonocytic leukemia, or the Naegeli type of leukemia, is the most common type of acute leukemia (Saarni and Linman). Granulocytic as well as monocytic cells are present in various proportions not only in the bone marrow but also in the peripheral blood and in the various infiltrates owing to the fact that both originate from a common stem cell (Shaw). Most cases of acute monocytic leukemia, or the Schilling type of leukemia, will at some time also show granulocytic cells, making recognition of this type of leukemia as a separate entity unnecessary (Wohlenberg et al).

Both myelomonocytic and monocytic leukemia not infrequently show skin lesions ranging from papules (Berger et al) to plaques (Hubler and Netherton) and nodules (Brynes et al; Burg et al). In nearly half of the cases, ulcers of the mouth and hypertrophy of the gums are observed and are regarded as characteristic of myelomonocytic leukemia (Hubler and Netherton; Shaw).

Erythroleukemia, often referred to as DiGuglielmo's disease, is initially characterized by a proliferation of both megaloblasts and myeloblasts. In the beginning, the proliferation of immature, nucleated erythrocytes may predominate, and immature granulocytes are relatively inapparent. In patients surviving long enough, the disease usually terminates as acute granulocytic leukemia (Scott et al). The skin, in addition to demonstrating purpuric lesions, occasionally shows macules, nodules, plaques, and ulcers (Belisario et al; Shaklai et al).

Histopathology. The diagnosis of acute granulocytic leukemia is usually made by a correlation of the histologic findings in the skin with those in the peripheral blood and in the bone marrow. However, the cutaneous lesions may precede the appearance of leukemic cells in the blood both in acute granulocytic leukemia (Wiernik and Serpick; Long and Mihm; Sun and Ellis) and in myelomonocytic leukemia (Burg et al). The cutaneous infiltrate in acute leukemia consists largely of undifferentiated cells, so that, in the absence of abnormal hematologic findings, acute leukemia may be misinterpreted as non-Hodgkin's lymphoma, leading to omission of a bone marrow examination (Long and Mihm). Distinction from non-Hodgkin's lymphoma, however, is readily made by cytochemical tests that can be carried out on formalin-fixed, paraffin-embedded tissue (see below) (Long and Mihm).

Acute granulocytic leukemia shows in the specific infiltrates of the skin and subcutis, including the granulocytic sarcomas, a pleomorphic infiltrate of cells varying in size and nuclear configuration. Larger cells show a vesicular nucleus, and smaller cells a folded or cleaved nucleus. In some cases, mature eosinophils admixed with eosinophilic myelocytes can be readily detected in hematoxylin-eosin-stained sections, whereas, in other cases, examination of Giemsa and periodic acid-Schiff (PAS)-stained sections is necessary for identification of the eosinophilic granules in eosinophilic myelocytes (Long and Mihm). Still, in occasional instances, no eosinophilic granules can be found, and only cytochemical staining will identify the granulocytic nature of the infiltrate.

In most lesions, some of the tumor cells are sufficiently mature to show chloroacetate esterase activity, indicated by red staining of granules in the cell cytoplasm (Long and Mihm). Some tumors, however, are very immature and contain only myeloblasts, which show no chloroacetate esterase activity but do show brown granules on staining with the antilysozyme immunoperoxidase technic (Sun and Ellis; Neiman et al).

Myelomonocytic leukemia shows an infiltrate of atypical monocytes and myelocytes that are often difficult to distinguish from one another on light microscopy. However, they can be distinguished by the double esterase stain, in which the myelocytes stain red for naphthol AS-D chloroacetate esterase and the monocytes stain blue for alpha-naphthol acetate esterase, also referred to as nonspecific esterase (Long and Mihm; Shaw; Sun and Ellis; Neiman et al).

In *erythroleukemia,* the infiltrate contains erythroid as well as myeloid cells, with occasional nucleated red cells among them (Belisario et al).

Cutaneous Extramedullary Hematopoiesis

Extramedullary hematopoiesis occurs in patients with myelofibrosis. The myelofibrosis is either primary or secondary to polycythemia vera. It shows proliferation of connective tissue cells in the bone marrow and proliferation of bone marrow elements in various organs, particularly the spleen, liver, and lymph nodes, resulting in splenomegaly. The skin only rarely participates in the hematopoiesis. If it does, it may show one nodule only (Kuo et al) or numerous papules and subcutaneous nodules (Tagami et al).

Histopathology. Within a myxoid, vascular stroma, one observes a polymorphic cellular infiltration consisting of myeloid cells and nucleated red blood cells (Kuo et al). In some cases, a few megakaryocytes are also seen (Tagami et al).

MULTIPLE MYELOMA

Multiple myeloma, or myelomatosis, shows (1) multiple areas of bone rarefaction; (2) plasma cell infiltration of varying degrees in a random sample of aspirated bone marrow, with at least some of the plasma cells appearing atypical; and (3) the presence of a monoclonal immunoglobulin or light chain in the serum and/or urine. At least two of these three criteria must be met for a diagnosis of multiple myeloma to be made (Wiltshaw). The disease usually begins with bone pain. The osteolytic lesions often lead to pathologic fractures. The disease is almost always fatal. The median survival period has been found to be 20 months, and the most common causes of death are infection as a result of lowered resistance and renal insufficiency (Kyle). Although, on autopsy, about 70% of the patients show metastatic spread, organ involvement usually is diffuse, so that grossly visible tumor nodules are found in only 10% of the cases (Hayes et al). Only 1% to 3% of patients with IgA- or IgG-producing myelomatosis show evidence of extraosseous involvement during life, in contrast to 10% of patients with myeloma producing only Bence Jones light chains, and 63% of patients with the rare type of IgD myeloma (Gomez et al).

Staging procedures in patients suspected of having multiple myeloma include bone marrow aspiration and biopsy, full skeletal roentgenograms, and serum and urine protein electrophoresis and immunoelectrophoresis (Alberts and Lynch).

The cutaneous manifestations of multiple myeloma can be divided into specific and nonspecific lesions. The nonspecific lesions may consist of amyloid deposits in the skin occurring, in association with visceral deposits, in primary systemic amyloidosis (see p. 407), or of monoclonal cryoglobulinemic purpura (see p. 170) or diffuse normolipemic plane xanthoma (see p. 397).

Specific involvement of the skin with metastases is quite rare. A review of the literature has revealed cutaneous lesions in only 4 of 182 cases of multiple myeloma with extramedullary lesions (Hayes et al). Individual series have shown cutaneous involvement in 1 of 38 cases of multiple myeloma (Hayes et al), in 2 of 78 cases (Edwards and Zawadzki), and in 2 of 57 cases (Wuepper and MacKenzie). This contrasts with one series in which cutaneous lesions were found in 9 of 88 cases of multiple myeloma (Bluefarb). The cutaneous lesions consist of violaceous nodules, often several centimeters in size. There are usually many nodules (Walzer and Shapiro; Wuepper and MacKenzie) and rarely only one or two nodules (Bluefarb; River and Schorr). Ulceration is rare (Bluefarb; Wuepper and MacKenzie). Also, subcutaneous masses may be present, either in association with cutaneous nodules (Walzer and Shapiro; Gomez et al) or without them (Tschen et al). Very rarely, cutaneous metastases precede the clinical, radiologic, and laboratory evidence of multiple myeloma by several months (Stankler and Davidson). In other cases without clinical and radiologic evidence, at least laboratory evidence of multiple myeloma existed (Wuepper and MacKenzie, case 1; Bork and Weigand). No specific association of cutaneous plasmacytomas with any particular class of myeloma protein exists (Wuepper and MacKenzie).

Histopathology. The specific cutaneous lesions of multiple myeloma show a dense infiltrate of plasma cells (Fig. 34-16). Most of the plasma cells appear atypical and show variation in the size, shape, and staining intensity of their nuclei as well as atypical mitotic figures. Also, multinucleated plasma cells may be present (Walzer and Shapiro). Because of their immaturity, the plasma cells are often difficult to identify as such. They may resemble atypical lymphocytes and thus suggest the presence of lymphoma (River and Schorr; Wuepper and MacKenzie). However, methyl green pyronin stains the cytoplasm of the cells dark red (Wuepper and MacKenzie).

Histogenesis. On *electron microscopy,* the plasma cells are readily recognizable as such, particularly through the presence of numerous cisternae lined by rough endoplasmic reticulum (see p. 51) (Klein and Grishman; Swanson et al). Also, immunoperoxidase staining on formalin-fixed, paraffin-embedded tissue shows selective staining of the plasma cells by samples of antiserum to the immunoglobulin and/or light chain type secreted by them (Tschen et al). In contrast, demonstration of immunoglobulins in cutaneous plasmacytomas by direct immunofluorescence has been unsuccessful (Wuepper and MacKenzie; Jorizzo et al).

Extramedullary Plasmacytoma

Extramedullary plasmacytoma differs from multiple myeloma in that the primary lesion, which is usually solitary, arises outside the bone marrow. The primary lesion is most commonly located in the upper air passages but occurs occasionally in the skin. Although the primary

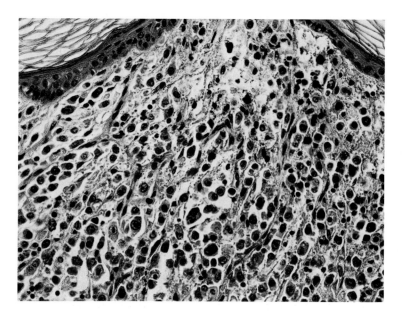

Fig. 34-16.   Multiple myeloma metastatic to the skin
Beneath a flattened epidermis is a dense infiltrate of plasma cells, most of which appear atypical. (×200) (Courtesy of Lewis Shapiro, M.D.)

lesion in some cases remains localized and then is curable, there are extensive metastases in other cases, particularly to the soft tissues and lymph nodes. Spread to bone occurs frequently, causing one or several osteolytic lesions without bone marrow involvement at first. Only few patients in whom the disease is widespread show plasma cell infiltration of the bone marrow similar to that seen in multiple myeloma (Wiltshaw). Patients with localized disease often show no measurable amount of myeloma protein (Wiltshaw; Klein and Grishman). However, patients with large primary tumors or with metastases usually show increased amounts of a monoclonal immunoglobulin in the serum (Swanson et al) and/or Bence Jones protein in the urine (Parra et al).

Involvement of the skin is rare in extramedullary plasmacytoma, but it can occur either as a solitary primary lesion or as multiple metastatic lesions. *Solitary primary cutaneous lesions* may remain limited to the skin and be cured by excision (La Perriere et al) or by radiation (Klein and Grishman), or they may cause a regional lymph node metastasis (Mikhail et al). In some cases, death has occurred with widespread metastases but without bone marrow involvement (Johnson and Taylor; Canlas et al).

Multiple metastatic cutaneous lesions may arise from a primary plasmacytoma in the upper air passages (Parra et al; Alberts and Lynch), from a retroperitoneal mass (Swanson et al), or from a solitary cutaneous lesion (Canlas et al). The disease may be very chronic (Parra et al), or it may be fatal (Alberts and Lynch; Canlas et al).

Histopathology.   Both primary and metastatic extramedullary plasmacytomas of the skin, irrespective of whether the course is favorable or not, show sheets of plasma cells with evidence of atypicality and occasional mitotic figures (La Perriere et al). Binucleated and multinucleated plasma cells may be seen (Mikhail et al; Klein and Grishman). Atypicality is most pronounced in metastatic cutaneous lesions, which may show resemblance to a non-Hodgkin's lymphoma, but the presence of cytoplasmic pyrinophilia establishes that the tumor cells are plasma cells (Swanson et al).

Differential Diagnosis.   Primary extramedullary plasmacytoma must be differentiated from other plasma cell aggregates, as seen, for instance, in the vicinity of a syringocystadenoma (Agarwal). Such aggregates, in contrast to the cutaneous lesions of extramedullary plasmacytoma, show no nuclear atypicality.

MACROGLOBULINEMIA OF WALDENSTRÖM

Waldenström's macroglobulinemia, first described in 1944 (Waldenström), represents a monoclonal gammopathy involving cells that deal with the synthesis of IgM globulin. There may be lymphadenopathy, hepatosplenomegaly, and/or purpura, but the diagnosis generally requires laboratory studies (see Histogenesis). In spite of chemotherapy, patients succumb to the disease, usually within a few years.

Specific cutaneous lesions occur infrequently. There are two types, but, so far, they have not been described as occurring together. The more common type consists of large infiltrative diffuse plaques or nodules of a red or violaceous color. The other type consists of multiple translucent papules only a few millimeters in diameter.

Histopathology. The large plaques or nodules show an infiltrate identical to that seen also in the bone marrow, liver, spleen, lymph nodes, and elsewhere. One observes in the reticular dermis, and occasionally also in the subcutaneous tissue, a dense, diffuse infiltrate of atypical lymphoid cells, some of which show partial differentiation toward plasma cells (Orfanos and Steigleder; Bureau et al; Dupré et al). In some instances, one observes in a few cells intranuclear, PAS-positive inclusions (Gottron et al) that represent small deposits of IgM (Mascaro et al). In some cases, the cells of the infiltrate appear embedded in an amorphous, PAS-positive gel; this gel contains IgM (Bureau et al).

The translucent papules, referred to as *storage papules*, contain eosinophilic, homogeneous material occupying the papillary and upper reticular dermis (Tichenor et al; Hanke et al). The material may show parallel cleft artifacts similar to those seen in amyloid and colloid (Mascaro et al). It contains stored IgM and is strongly PAS-positive.

Histogenesis. Large amounts of IgM are present in the blood serum. They are produced by the lymphoplasmacytoid cells present in the bone marrow and elsewhere. This IgM production results in an increase in total serum protein, an increase in serum viscosity, and an elevated gamma-globulin peak on serum protein electrophoresis. Agar immunoelectrophoresis with specific IgM antiserum shows an aberrant IgM band (Tichenor et al).

Direct immunofluorescence studies with IgM antiserum reveals in the large plaques or nodules strongly fluorescent material between the cells of the infiltrate (Mascaro et al). Similarly, the homogeneous material in the storage papules fluoresces strongly with IgM antiserum (Hanke et al).

LYMPHOCYTOMA (PSEUDOLYMPHOMA OF SPIEGLER–FENDT)

The term *pseudolymphoma* is applied to a group of benign dermatoses with histologic features that often make a distinction from lymphoma very difficult, if not impossible. Among these dermatoses are (1) lymphomatoid papulosis (see p. 172), (2) actinic reticulosis (see p. 213), (3) Jessner's lymphocytic infiltration (see p. 456), (4) angioimmunoblastic lymphadenopathy (see p. 190), (5) arthropod bites and stings (see p. 216), and persistent nodules of scabies (see p. 219), (6) phenytoin-induced drug eruption (see p. 268), and (7) lymphocytoma.

Lymphocytoma is known also under a variety of other designations, such as pseudolymphoma of Spiegler–Fendt, Spiegler–Fendt sarcoid, lymphadenosis benigna cutis (Bäfverstedt), cutaneous lymphoid hyperplasia (Caro and Helwig), and cutaneous lymphoplasia (Mach and Wilgram). In two thirds of the cases, it shows a solitary nodule that is most commonly located on the face (Caro and Helwig). In other cases, there are several grouped lesions or numerous widespread lesions. The lesions may vary from a small nodule measuring only a few millimeters to large plaques several centimeters in diameter. The lesions usually are asymptomatic, have a firm consistency, and may be skin-colored, red, or violaceous. Clinical differentiation from non-Hodgkin's lymphoma is generally impossible, since both may start as a solitary cutaneous nodule (Caro and Helwig; Long et al). The clinical resemblance to lymphoma is greatest in patients with multiple large nodules or plaques (Evans et al). In contrast with lymphoma, the lesions heal spontaneously, even though they may persist for months or years and there may be recurrences (Caro and Helwig). Thus, in retrospective studies, a diagnosis of lymphoma has been excluded only when, after a minimum of 4 to 5 years, no lesions in the lymph nodes or the viscera have become evident (Caro and Helwig; Fisher et al; Evans et al).

Although lymphocytoma is generally benign, any persistent lesion, even though histologically benign at first, may ultimately prove to be a malignant lymphoma. Histologically benign lesions may even coexist with such a malignant lesion (Pegum and Landells; Shelley et al).

Histopathology. A heavy infiltrate is present in the dermis, usually separated from the epidermis by a narrow grenz zone of normal collagen. The infiltrate in larger lesions often extends into the subcutaneous tissue. In most cases, the infiltrate consists of two types of cells, generally referred to as lymphocytes and histiocytes (see Histogenesis). The two types of cells lie either intermingled with one another or in a follicular arrangement. In the latter type of arrangement, one sees lymphocytes surrounding aggregates of histiocytes, resulting in structures that resemble the follicles of lymph nodes (Fig. 34-17) (Caro and Helwig; Fisher et al). The lymphocytes and histiocytes are easily differentiated. The lymphocytes have small, round or occasionally folded or cleaved nuclei that lie closely packed, because lymphocytes possess little cytoplasm. The histiocytes have large, irregularly shaped, pale-staining or vesicular nuclei lying in a loose arrangement, because these cells possess ample amounts of cytoplasm, to separate the nuclei from one another (Fig. 34-18). Not infrequently, nuclear fragments can be seen within or near histiocytes (Caro and Helwig; Bernstein et al).

Frequently, there are variations of the histologic picture just described. In some instances, only few histiocytes are seen, and the infiltrate consists

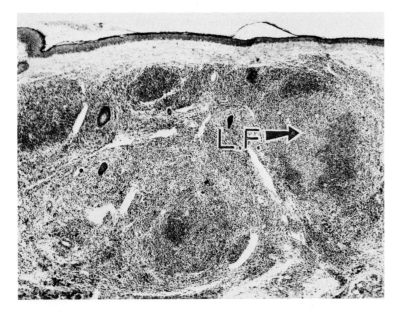

Fig. 34-17. Lymphocytoma
Low magnification. The infiltrate is composed of two types of cells: lymphocytes, which lie in the dark-staining areas, and histiocytes, which lie in the light-staining areas. On the right, the arrangement of the two types of cells resembles that encountered in a lymph follicle (*L.F.*). (×50)

Fig. 34-18. Lymphocytoma
High magnification of Figure 34-17. Lymphocytes are seen in the upper left portion of the illustration and histiocytes in the lower right portion. (×200)

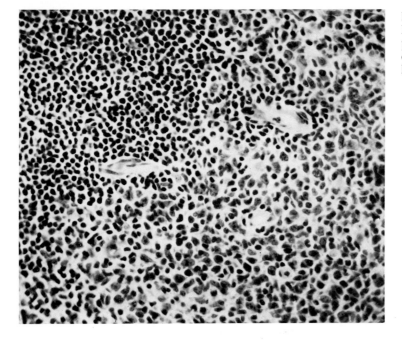

almost entirely of a monomorphous, mature lymphocytic infiltrate (Fisher et al). In other instances, some of the pale, histiocytic cells have large, atypical-appearing nuclei (Kawada et al). Also, there may be fairly numerous mitoses (Clark et al), and, as in lymphoma, one may observe at the periphery of the infiltrate single rows of lymphocytes extending between and around intact collagen bundles like "Indians in a file" (Fig. 34-19)

(Caro and Helwig). An admixture of plasma cells or eosinophils is seen in some cases, and their presence speaks against a diagnosis of lymphoma (Connors and Ackerman).

A special variant described as large cell lymphocytoma shows a distinctive histologic picture suggestive of lymphoma but with a benign course (Duncan et al). One observes nodular infiltrates of large cells with pleomorphic, pale-staining

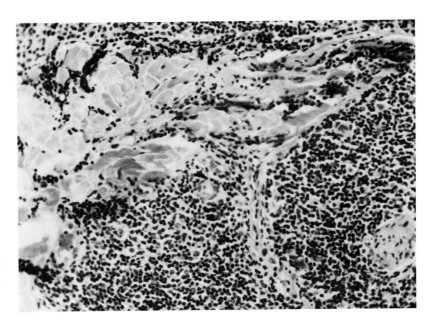

Fig. 34-19. Lymphocytoma
Nearly all cells have the appearance of lymphocytes. In several areas, single rows of lymphocytes extend between collagen bundles like "Indians in a file," as seen also in lymphoma. (×100)

nuclei and frequent mitoses suggestive of histiocytic lymphoma. As a characteristic feature, dense clusters of small lymphocytes surround or infiltrate the aggregates of large cells, whereas medium-sized lymphocytes are few or absent.

Histogenesis. It is generally agreed that lymphocytoma represents a reactive hyperplasia (Caro and Helwig; Clark et al).

In lesions with follicular formations, the large, pale cells in the center represent follicular center B lymphocytes, as shown by the fact that, in cryostat sections, they do not stain with acid phosphatase or nonspecific esterase, as histiocytes would, but react on incubation with IgM EAC (see p. 738) (Burg and Braun-Falco) and fluoresce with antihuman B-cell serum (Jimbow et al). Outside of the follicles, however, the scattered large, pale cells stain with acid phosphatase and nonspecific esterase and thus represent histiocytes (Burg and Braun-Falco). The proportions of B and T cells among the lymphocytes apparently depends on the presence or absence of follicular structures. In the presence of such structures, B cells predominate (Braun-Falco and Burg), whereas, in their absence, T cells form the majority of lymphocytes (David et al).

Electron microscopic studies have confirmed the presence of both lymphocytes and phagocytic histiocytes. Some of the lymphocytes have a cleaved nucleus corresponding to centrocytes and a few have a lightly stained and larger nucleus corresponding to centroblasts (Schmoeckel et al).

In preliminary studies, an immunoperoxidase technic has been used on paraffin-embedded tissue for the staining of cytoplasmic immunoglobulins contained in B lymphocytes. These studies have shown that, whereas a lesion of lymphoma showed monoclonal staining with IgG-lambda only, a lesion of reactive lymphoid hyperplasia showed polyclonal IgG-lambda and kappa staining (Barr et al).

Differential Diagnosis. Identification of lymphocytoma and differentiation from lymphoma generally is easy in lesions with a distinct follicular arrangement in at least some areas (Caro and Helwig; Clark et al). A true follicular pattern is not seen in the skin lesions of lymphoma, not even in nodular or follicular lymphoma (Evans et al).

If the two types of cells lie intermingled, the diagnosis of lymphocytoma can be made with certainty only if the histiocytes show no atypicality. Even though it is generally accepted that lymphocytoma in some instances shows a significant admixture of histiocytes with large, atypical-appearing nuclei, great caution is indicated in making an outright diagnosis of lymphocytoma in such cases, because mixed lymphocytic–histiocytic lymphoma also shows two types of cells that lie intermingled. However, in lymphocytic–histiocytic lymphoma, in contrast to lymphocytoma, both types of cells appear atypical, since most lymphocytes are cleaved and larger than small, round, well-differentiated lymphocytes and represent poorly differentiated lymphocytes (see p. 734).

Caution in diagnosing lymphocytoma is also indicated in cases that show a monomorphous infiltrate of small, round, well-differentiated lymphocytes, because this type of infiltrate is seen also in well-differentiated lymphocytic lymphoma (see

p. 732), as well as in lymphocytic leukemia (see p. 748) and Jessner's lymphocytic infiltration (see p. 456). It has therefore been suggested that all monomorphous, mature lymphocytic infiltrates be designated "unclassified lymphocytic infiltrates" that require investigation into the possibility of lymphoma (Fisher et al).

BIBLIOGRAPHY

Hodgkin's Disease

ANAGNOSTOU D, PARKER JW, TAYLOR CR et al; Lacunar cells of nodular sclerosing Hodgkin's disease. Cancer 39:1032–1043, 1977

AZAR HA: Significance of the Reed-Sternberg cell. Hum Pathol 6:479–484, 1975

BARDACH H, KÜHBÖCK J: Lokalisierte Poikilodermia vascularis atrophicans als Frühmanifestation eines Morbus Hodgkin vom nodulär-sklerosierenden Typ. Hautarzt 32:126–129, 1981

BEARMAN RM, PANGALIS GA, RAPPAPORT H: Hodgkin's disease, lymphocyte depletion type. Cancer 41:293–302, 1978

BENNINGHOFF DL, MEDINA A, ALEXANDER L et al: The mode of spread of Hodgkin's lymphoma. Cancer 26:1135–1140, 1970

CARBONE PP, KAPLAN HS, MUSSHOFF K et al: Report of the committee on Hodgkin's disease staging classification. Cancer Res 31:1860–1861, 1971

DUPONT A: Langsam verlaufende und klinisch gutartige Reticulopathie mit höchst maligner histologischer Struktur. Hautarzt 16:284–286, 1965

FRANSSILA KO, KALIMA TV, VOUTILAINEN A: Histologic classification of Hodgkin's disease. Cancer 20:1594–1601, 1967

GLICK AD, LEECH JH, FLEXNER JM et al: Ultrastructural study of Reed-Sternberg cells. Am J Pathol 85:195–208, 1976

GORDON RA, LOOKINGBILL DP, ABT AB: Skin infiltration in Hodgkin's disease. Arch Dermatol 116:1038–1040, 1980

HAN T, SOKAL JE: Lymphocyte response to phytohemagglutinin in Hodgkin's disease. Am J Med 48:728–734, 1970

KADIN ME, STITES DP, LEVY R et al: Exogenous immunoglobulin and the macrophage origin of Reed-Sternberg cells in Hodgkin's disease. N Engl J Med 299:1208–1214, 1978

KAPLAN HS: Hodgkin's disease: Unfolding concepts concerning its nature, management and prognosis. (Review) Cancer 45:2439–2474, 1980

KAPLAN HS, GARTNER S: "Sternberg-Reed" giant cells of Hodgkin's disease: Cultivation in vitro, heterotransplantation, and characterization as neoplastic macrophages. Int J Cancer 19:511–525, 1977

KAPLAN HS, ROSENBERG SA: The management of Hodgkin's disease. Cancer 36:796–803, 1975

LEVY R, KAPLAN HS: Impaired lymphocyte function in untreated Hodgkin's disease. N Engl J Med 290:181–186, 1974

LUKES RJ, BUTLER JJ, HICKS EB: Natural history of Hodgkin's disease as related to its pathologic picture. Cancer 19:317–344, 1966

MACAULAY WL: Lymphomatoid papulosis. Arch Dermatol 97:23–30, 1968

MANN RB, JAFFE ES, BERARD CW: Malignant lymphoma: A conceptual understanding of morphologic diversity. A review. Am J Pathol 94:105–192, 1979

PAYNE SV, NEWELL DC, JONES DB et al: The Reed-Sternberg/lymphocyte interaction. Am J Pathol 100:7–24, 1980

PROSNITZ LR, NULAND SB, KLIGERMAN MM: Role of laparotomy and splenectomy in the management of Hodgkin's disease. Cancer 29:44–50, 1972

REBOUL F, DONALDSON SH, KAPLAN SH: Herpes zoster and varicella infection in children with Hodgkin's disease. Cancer 41:95–99, 1978

ROBERTS AN, SMITH KL, DOWELL BL et al: Cultural, morphological, cell membrane, enzymatic, and neoplastic properties of cell lines derived from a Hodgkin's disease lymph node. Cancer Res 38:3033–3043, 1978

ROSENBERG SA, KAPLAN HS: Evidence for an orderly progression in the spread of Hodgkin's disease. Cancer Res 26:1225–1231, 1966

RUBINS J: Cutaneous Hodgkin's disease. Cancer 42:1219–1221, 1978

SAXE N, KAHN LB, KING H: Lymphoma of the skin. J Cutan Pathol 4:111–122, 1977

SCHEIN PS, VICKERS HR: Lupus vulgaris and Hodgkin's disease. Arch Dermatol 105:244–246, 1972

SELL S: Immunological deficiency diseases. Arch Pathol 86:95–107, 1968

SENEAR FE, CARO MR: Ulcerative Hodgkin's disease of the skin. Arch Dermatol Syph 35:114–128, 1937

SMITH JL JR, BUTLER JJ: Skin involvement in Hodgkin's disease. Cancer 45:354–361, 1980

STRUM SB, ALLEN LW, RAPPAPORT H: Vascular invasion in Hodgkin's disease: Its relationship to involvement of the spleen and other extranodal sites. Cancer 28:1329–1334, 1971

SZUR L, HARRISON CV, LEVENE GM et al: Primary cutaneous Hodgkin's disease. Lancet 1:1016–1020, 1970

ULTMANN JE, MORAN EM: Clinical course and complications in Hodgkin's disease. Arch Intern Med 131:332–353, 1973

YOUNG RC, CORDER MP, HAYNES HA et al: Delayed hypersensitivity in Hodgkin's disease. Am J Med 52:63–72, 1972

Non-Hodgkin's Lymphoma

BURG G, BRAUN-FALCO O, HOFFMANN-FEZER G et al: Patterns of cutaneous lymphomas. Dermatologica 157:282–291, 1978

BURKE JS, HOPPE RT, CIBULL ML et al: Cutaneous malignant lymphoma. Cancer 47:300–310, 1981

CARBONE PP: Management of patients with non-Hodgkin's lymphoma. Arch Intern Med 131:455–459, 1973

CARBONE PP, KAPLAN HS, MUSSHOFF K et al: Report of the committee on Hodgkin's disease staging classification. Cancer Res 31:1860–1861, 1971

CARO WA, HELWIG EB: Cutaneous lymphoid hyperplasia. Cancer 24:487–502, 1969

CLARK WH, MIHM MC JR, REED RJ et al: The lymphocytic infiltrates of the skin. Hum Pathol 5:25–43, 1974

CYR DP, GEOKAS MC, WORSLEY GH: Mycosis fungoides. Arch Dermatol 94:558–573, 1966

EDELSON RL: Membrane markers of lymphocytes in lymphomas, melanoma and lupus erythematosus. Int J Dermatol 15:577–586, 1976

EDELSON RL, SMITH RW, FRANK MM et al: Identification of subpopulations of mononuclear cells in cutaneous infiltrates. J Invest Dermatol 61:82–89, 1973

EVANS HL, WINKELMANN RK, BANKS PM: Differential diagnosis of malignant and benign cutaneous lymphoid infiltrates. Cancer 44:699–717, 1979

EZDINLI EZ, COSTELLO W, WASSER LP et al: Eastern Cooperative Oncology Group experience with the Rappaport classification on non-Hodgkin's lymphoma. Cancer 43:544–550, 1979

FISHER ER, PARK EJ, WECHSLER HL: Histologic identification of malignant lymphoma cutis. Am J Clin Pathol 65:149–158, 1976

HELLMAN S, ROSENTHAL DS, MOLONEY WC et al: The treatment of non-Hodgkin's lymphoma. Cancer 36:804–808, 1975

HURST DW, MEYER OO: Giant follicular lymphoblastoma. Cancer 14:753–778, 1961

JAFFE ES, SHEVACH EM, FRANK MM et al: Nodular lymphoma—Evidence for origin from follicular B lymphocytes. N Engl J Med 290:813–819, 1974

KALKOFF KW: Über eine primäre isolierte Reticulumzellensarkomatose der Haut. Z Hautkr 14:3–8, 1953

KIM H, JACOBS C, WARNKE RA et al: Malignant lymphoma with a high content of epithelioid histiocytes. Cancer 41:620–635, 1978

KIM R, WINKELMANN RK, DOCKERTY M: Reticulum cell sarcoma of the skin. Cancer 16:646–655, 1963

KNOWLES DM II, HALPER JP: Human T-cell malignancies. Am J Pathol 106:187–203, 1982

KWITTKEN J, GOLDBERG AF: Follicular lymphoma of the skin. Arch Dermatol 93:177–183, 1966

LENNERT K, MESTDAGH J: Lymphogranulomatosen mit konstant hohem Epitheloid-zellgehalt. Virchows Arch (Pathol Anat) 344:1–20, 1969

LENNERT K, MOHRI N, STEIN H et al: The histopathology of malignant lymphoma. Br J Haematol 31 (Suppl): 193–203, 1975

LONG JC, MIHM MC, QAZI R: Malignant lymphoma of the skin. Cancer 38:1282–1296, 1976

LUKES RJ, COLLINS RD: Immunologic characterization of human malignant lymphomas. Cancer 34:1488–1503, 1974

MANN RB, JAFFE ES, BERARD CW: Malignant lymphoma, a conceptual understanding of morphologic diversity. A review. Am J Pathol 94:105–175, 1979

MILLER DG: Immunological deficiency and malignant lymphoma. Cancer 20:579–588, 1967

NATHWANI BN: A critical analysis of the classifications of non-Hodgkin's lymphomas. Cancer 44:347–384, 1979

NATHWANI BN, KIM H, RAPPAPORT H: Malignant lymphoma, lymphoblastic. Cancer 38:964–983, 1976

NATHWANI BN, KIM H, RAPPAPORT H et al: Non-Hodgkin's lymphomas. A clinicopathologic study comparing two classifications. Cancer 41:303–325, 1978a

NATHWANI BN, RAPPAPORT H, MORAN EM et al: Malignant lymphoma arising in angioimmunoblastic lymphadenopathy. Cancer 41:578–606, 1978b

PAGANO JS, HUANG CH, LEVINE P: Absence of Epstein-Barr viral DNA in American Burkitt's lymphoma. N Engl J Med 289:1395–1399, 1973

PANGALIS GA, NATHWANI BN, RAPPAPORT H: Malignant lymphoma, well differentiated lymphocytic. Cancer 39:999–1010, 1977

PETROZZI JW, RAQUE CJ, GOLDSCHMIDT H: Malignant lymphoma, reticulum cell type. Ultrastructural and cytologic demonstration of Lutzner cells. Arch Dermatol 104:38–44, 1971

QAZI R, AISENBERG AC, LONG JC: The natural history of nodular lymphoma. Cancer 37:1923–1927, 1976

RAPPAPORT H: Tumors of the hematopoietic system. In Atlas of Tumor Pathology, Sect 3, Fascicle 8. Washington DC, Armed Forces Institute of Pathology, 1966

RAPPAPORT H, WINTER WJ, HICKS EB: Follicular lymphoma. Cancer 9:792–831, 1956

ROGGE T: Ein Burkitt-Lymphoma mit Hautinfiltraten. Hautarzt 26:379–382, 1975

ROSENBERG SA: Current concepts in cancer. Non-Hodgkin's lymphoma. N Engl J Med 301:924–928, 1979

ROSENBERG SA, DIAMOND HD, JASLOWITZ B et al: Lymphosarcoma: A review of 1269 cases. Medicine (Baltimore) 40:31–84, 1961

ROUNDTREE JM, BURGDORF W, HARKEY MR: Cutaneous involvement in Lennert's lymphoma. Arch Dermatol 116:1291–1294, 1980

RUBIN P: Comment: The non-Hodgkin's lymphomas. JAMA 223:175–178, 1973

RYWLIN AM: Non-Hodgkin's malignant lymphomas. Brief historical review and simple unifying classification. Am J Dermatopathol 2:17–25, 1980

SAXE N, KAHN LB, KING H: Lymphoma of the skin. J Cutan Pathol 4:111–122, 1977

SONCK CE: Primäre Reticulumzellsarcomatose der Haut. Acta Derm Venereol (Stockh) 37:129–139, 1957

STEIN H, KAISERLING E, LENNERT K: Evidence for B-cell origin of reticulum cell sarcoma. Virchows Arch (Pathol Anat) 364:51–67, 1974

STERRY W, STEIGLEDER GM, PULLMANN H: In situ identification and enumeration of T lymphocytes in cutaneous T-cell lymphomas by demonstration of granular activity of acid nonspecific esterase. Br J Dermatol 103:67–72, 1980

TRUBOWITZ S, SIMS CF: Subcutaneous fat in leukemia and lymphoma. Arch Dermatol 86:520–524, 1962

WARNKE R, MILLER R, GROGAN T et al: Immunologic phenotype in 30 patients with diffuse large-cell lymphoma. N Engl J Med 303:293–300, 1980

WINKLER K: Neoplastische Wucherungen des RES der Haut. Z Hautkr 20:9–14, 1956

WRIGHT CJE: Macrofollicular lymphoma. Am J Pathol 32:201–233, 1956

ZIEGLER JL: Burkitt's lymphoma. N Engl J Med 305:735–745, 1981

Mycosis Fungoides, Sézary Syndrome, Woringer–Kolopp Disease

ACKERMAN AB, BREZA TS, CAPLAND L: Spongiotic simulants of mycosis fungoides. Arch Dermatol 109:218–220, 1974

ALTMEYER P, NÖDL P: Die "besonderen" Beziehungen maligner Lymphome der Haut zu der Epidermis und den ektodermalen Adnexen. Arch Dermatol Res 262:113–123, 1978

BLASIK LG, NEWKIRK RE, DIMOND RL et al: Mycosis fungoides d'emblée. Cancer 49:742–747, 1982

BLAYLOCK WK, CLENDENNING WE, CARBONE P: Normal immunologic reactions in patients with the lymphoma mycosis fungoides. Cancer 19:233–236, 1966

BLOCK JB, EDGCOMB J, EISEN A et al: Mycosis fungoides. Natural history and aspects of its relationship to other malignant lymphomas. Am J Med 34:228–235, 1963

BOURLOND A, DELBROUCK-POOT F, PHILIPPART JL et al: Lymphome épidermotrope type Woringer-Kolopp. Dermatologica 159:101–114, 1979

BRAUN-FALCO O, MARGHESCU S, WOLFF HH: Pagetoide Reticulose. Morbus Woringer-Kolopp. Hautarzt 24:11–21, 1973

BRAUN-FALCO, SCHMOECKEL C, BURG G et al: Pagetoid reticulosis. Acta Derm Venereol (Stockh) Suppl 85:11–21, 1979

BREHMER-ANDERSSON E: Mycosis fungoides. Acta Derm Venereol (Stockh) 56, Suppl 75, 1976

BRODER S, EDELSON RL, LUTZNER MA et al: The Sézary syndrome: A malignant proliferation of helper T cells. J Clin Invest 58:1297–1306, 1976

BROWNLEE TR, MURAD TM: Ultrastructure of mycosis fungoides. Cancer 26:686–698, 1970

BÜCHNER SA: Sézary syndrome after successful treatment of Hodgkin's disease. Arch Dermatol 117:50–54, 1981

BURG G, WOLFF HH, BRAUN-FALCO O et al: Pagetoid reticulosis, a cutaneous T cell lymphoma. (Abstr) J Invest Dermatol 68:249, 1977

CAMISA C, GOLDSTEIN A: Mycosis fungoides. Small-bowel involvement complicated by perforation and peritonitis. Arch Dermatol 117:234–237, 1981

CARNEY DN, BUNN PA JR: Manifestations of cutaneous T-cell lymphoma. J Dermatol Surg Oncol 6:369–377, 1980

CASTERMANS-ELIAS S: Reticulose épidermotrope (maladie de Woringer-Kolopp). Arch Belg Dermatol Syph 30:187–194, 1974

CHU A, BERGER CL, KUNG P et al: In situ identification of Langerhans cells in the dermal infiltrate of cutaneous T cell lymphoma. J Am Acad Dermatol 6:350–354, 1982a

CHU AC, MACDONALD DM: Identification in situ of T lymphocytes in the dermal and epidermal infiltrates of mycosis fungoides. Br J Dermatol 100:177–182, 1979

CHU AC, MORGAN WE, MACDONALD EM: An ultrastructural study of the mononuclear cell infiltrate of mycosis fungoides and poikiloderma atrophicans vasculare. Clin Exp Dermatol 7:11–19, 1982b

CLAUDY AL: The immunological identification of the Sézary cell. Br J Dermatol 91:597–600, 1974

CLENDENNING WE, BRECKER G, VAN SCOTT EJ: Mycosis fungoides. Arch Dermatol 87:785–792, 1964

CLENDENNING WE, VAN SCOTT EJ: Skin allografts and homografts in patients with the lymphoma mycosis fungoides. Cancer Res 25:1844–1853, 1965

COLBY TV, BURKE JS, HOPPE RT: Lymph node biopsy in mycosis fungoides. Cancer 47:351–359, 1981

COOPERRIDER PA, ROENIGK HH JR: Selective immunological evaluation of mycosis fungoides. Arch Dermatol 114:207–212, 1978

CROSSEN PE, MELLOR JEL, FINLEY AG et al: The Sézary syndrome. Am J Med 50:25–34, 1971

CYR DP, GEOKAS MC, WORSLEY GH: Mycosis fungoides. Arch Dermatol 94:558–573, 1966

DEGOS R, CIVATTE J, TOURAINE R et al: Confrontation anatomo-clinique de 129 hémoréticulopathies malignes cutanées. Ann Dermatol Syph 92:121–127, 1965

DEGREEF H, HOLVOET C, VAN VLOTEN WA et al: Woringer-Kolopp disease. An epidermotropic variant of mycosis fungoides. Cancer 38:2154–2165, 1976

DOYLE JA, WINKELMANN RK: Staging laparotomy in cutaneous T-cell disease. Arch Dermatol 117:543–546, 1981a

DOYLE JA, WINKELMANN RK: Staging procedures in cutaneous T-cell disease. Aust J Dermatol 22:64–67, 1981b

DUNCAN SC, WINKELMANN RK: Circulating Sézary cells in hospitalized dermatology patients. Br J Dermatol 99:171–178, 1978

EDELSON RL: Cutaneous T-cell lymphoma. J Am Acad Dermatol 2:89–106, 1980

EDELSON RL, KIRKPATRICK CH, SHEVACH EM et al: Preferential cutaneous infiltration by neoplastic thymus-derived lymphocytes. Ann Intern Med 80:685–692, 1974

EMMERSON RW: Follicular mucinosis. Br J Dermatol 81:395–413, 1969

EPSTEIN EH, LEVIN DL, CROFT JO JR et al: Mycosis fungoides. Medicine (Baltimore) 51:61–72, 1972

ERKMAN-BALIS B, RAPPAPORT H: Cytogenetic studies in mycosis fungoides. Cancer 34:626–633, 1974

FLANDRIN G, BROUET JC: The Sézary cell: Cytology, cytochemical and immunological studies. Mayo Clin Proc 49:575–583, 1974

FLAXMAN BA, ZELAZNY G, VAN SCOTT EJ: Nonspecificity of characteristic cells in mycosis fungoides. Arch Dermatol 104:141–147, 1971

FLEISCHMAJER R, EISENBERG S: Sézary's reticulosis. Arch Dermatol 89:9–19, 1964

FRASER JF: Mycosis fungoides. Arch Dermatol Syph 12:814–828, 1925

FUKS ZY, BAGSHAW MA, FARBER EM: Prognostic signs and the management of mycosis fungoides. Cancer 32:1385–1395, 1973

GEERTS ML, KAISERLING E, KINT A: Microenvironment of Woringer-Kolopp's disease. Dermatologica 164:15–29, 1982

GREER KE, LEGUM LL, HESS CE: Multiple osteolytic lesions in a patient with mycosis fungoides. Arch Dermatol 113:1242–1244, 1977

GRIEM ML, MORAN EM, FERGUSON DJ et al: Staging procedures in mycosis fungoides. Br J Cancer 31, Suppl 2:362–367, 1975

HAMMINGA L, MULDER JD, EVANS C et al: Staging lymphography with respect to lymph node histology, treatment, and follow-up in patients with mycosis fungoides. Cancer 47:692–697, 1981

HANEKE E, TULUSAN AH, WEIDNER F: Histological features of "pagetoid reticulosis" (Woringer-Kolopp) in pre-mycosis fungoides. Arch Dermatol Res 258:265–273, 1972

HARRINGTON CI, SLATER DN: Mycosis fungoides with blast cell transformation. Arch Dermatol 114:611–612, 1978

JANIS JF, WINKELMANN RK: Histopathology of the skin in dermatomyositis. Arch Dermatol 97:640–650, 1968

JIMBOW K, CHIBA M, HORIKOSHI T: Electron microscopic identification of Langerhans cells in the dermal infiltrates of mycosis fungoides. J Invest Dermatol 78:102–107, 1982

KIENITZ T, BURG G, SCHMOECKEL C et al: High-grade malignant lymphoma arising fromn Sézary syndrome. Dermatologica 158:126–139, 1979

LAMBERG SI, BUNN PA JR: Cutaneous T-cell lymphoma. Summary of the Mycosis Fungoides Cooperative Group and National Cancer Institute Workshop. Arch Dermatol 115:1103–1105, 1979

LANGNER A, GLINSKI W, PAWINSKA M et al: Lymphocyte transformation in mycosis fungoides. Arch Dermatol Forsch 251:249–257, 1975

LAPIÈRE S: The realm and frontiers of mycosis fungoides. J. Invest Dermatol 42:101–103, 1964

LEVER WF: Localized mycosis fungoides with prominent epidermotropism. Woringer-Kolopp disease. Arch Dermatol 113:1254–1256, 1977

LEVI JA, WIERNIK PH: Management of mycosis fungoides: Current status and future prospects. Medicine (Baltimore) 54:73–88, 1975

LUTZNER MA, HOBBS JW, HORVATH P: Ultrastructure of abnormal cells in Sézary syndrome, mycosis fungoides, and parapsoriasis en plaques. Arch Dermatol 103:375–386, 1971

LUTZNER MA, JORDAN HW: The ultrastructure of an abnormal cell in Sézary's syndrome. Blood 31:719–726, 1968

MACKIE RM: A monoclonal antibody technique to demonstrate an increase in Langerhans cells in cutaneous lesions of mycosis fungoides. Clin Exp Dermatol 7:43–47, 1982

MAIN RA, GOODALL HB, SWANSON WC: Sézary's syndrome. Br J Dermatol 71:335–343, 1959

MANDOJANA RM, HELWIG EB: Woringer-Kolopp disease. (Abstr) Arch Dermatol 116:1392, 1980

MCMILLAN EM, WASIK R, MARTIN D et al: T cell nature of exocytic and dermal lymphoid cells in atrophic parapsoriasis. J Cutan Pathol 8:355–360, 385–391, 1981

MCNUTT NS, CRAIN WR: Quantitative electron microscopic comparison of lymphocyte nuclear contours in mycosis fungoides and in benign infiltrates in skin. Cancer 47:698–709, 1981

MEDENICA M, LORINCZ AL: Pagetoid reticulosis (Woringer-Kolopp disease). Arch Dermatol 114:262–268, 1978

MEIJER CJLM, VAN DER LOO EM, VAN VLOTEN et al: Early diagnosis of mycosis fungoides and Sézary's syndrome by morphometric analysis of lymphoid cells in the skin. Cancer 45:2864–2871, 1980

MILLER RA, COLEMAN CN, FAWCETT HD et al: Sézary syndrome: A model for migration of T lymphocytes to skin. N Engl J Med 303:89–92, 1980

NATHWANI BN, RAPPAPORT H, MORAN EM et al: Malignant

lymphoma arising in angioimmunoblastic lymphadenopathy. Cancer 41:578–606, 1978

PARISER DM: Mycosis fungoides involving the brain and optic nerves. Arch Dermatol 114:397–399, 1978

PRUNIERAS M: DNA content and cytogenetics of the Sézary cell. Mayo Clin Proc 49:548–552, 1974

RAPPAPORT H, THOMAS LB: Mycosis fungoides. The pathology of extracutaneous involvement. Cancer 34:1198–1229, 1974

ROSAS-URIBE A, VARIAKOJIS D, MOLNAR Z et al: Mycosis fungoides: An ultrastructural study. Cancer 34:634–645, 1974

ROWDEN G, PHILLIPS TM, LEWIS MG et al: Target role of Langerhans cells in mycosis fungoides: Transmission and immuno-electron microscopic studies. J Cutan Pathol 6:364–382, 1979

SAMMAN PD: The natural history of parapsoriasis en plaques (chronic superficial dermatitis) and prereticulotic poikiloderma. Br J Dermatol 87:405–411, 1972

SANCHEZ JL, ACKERMAN AB: The patch stage of mycosis fungoides. Am J Dermatophol 1:5–26, 1979

SCHEFFER E, MEIJER CJLM, VAN VLOTEN WA: Dermatopathic lymphadenopathy and lymph node involvement in mycosis fungoides. Cancer 45:137–148, 1980

SCHEIN PS, MACDONALD JS, EDELSON R: Cutaneous T-cell lymphoma. Cancer 38:1859–1861, 1976

SCHMITT D, THIVOLET J: Lymphocyte-epidermis interactions in malignant epidermotropic lymphomas. I. Ultrastructural aspects. Acta Derm Venereol (Stockh) 60:1–11, 1980

SCHMOECKEL C, BURG G, BRAUN-FALCO O et al: Mycosis fungoide à forte malignité avec transformation cytologique. Ann Dermatol Venereol 108:231–241, 1981

SCHUPPLI R: Is mycosis fungoides an "immunoma"? Dermatologica 153:1–6, 1976

SÉZARY A: Une nouvelle réticulose cutanée. Ann Dermatol Syph VIII, 9:5–26, 1949

SÉZARY A, BOUVRAIN Y: Erythrodermie avec présence de cellules monstreuses dans derme et sang circulant. Bull Soc Fr Dermatol Syph 45:254–260, 1938

SMOES-CHARLES J, DUPONT A: A propos d'une forme particulière generalisée de réticulose épidermotrope. Arch Belg Dermatol Syph 29:205–211, 1973

TAN RSH, BUTTERWORTH CM, MCLAUGHLIN H et al: Mycosis fungoides, a disease of antigen persistence. Br J Dermatol 91:607–616, 1974

TAN RSH, BYROM NA, HAYES JP: A method of liberating living cells from the dermal infiltrate. Br J Dermatol 93:271–276, 1975

TASWELL HF, WINKELMANN RK: Sézary syndrome, a malignant reticulemic erythroderma. JAMA 177:465–472, 1971

TEDESCHI LG, LANSINGER DT: Sézary syndrome. Arch Dermatol 92:272–262, 1965

THOMAS JA, JANOSSY G, GRAHAM-BROWN RAC et al: The relationship between T lymphocyte subsets and Ia-like antigen positive nonlymphoid cells in early stages of cutaneous T cell lymphoma. J Invest Dermatol 78:169–176, 1982

TORIBIO J, QUIÑONES PA, VIGIL TR: Woringer-Kolopp disease, pagetoid reticulosis. Dermatologica 156:283–291, 1978

VARIAKOJIS D, ROSAS-URIBE A, RAPPAPORT H: Mycosis fungoides: Pathologic findings in staging laparotomies. Cancer 32:18–30, 1973

VONDERHEID EC, TAM DW, JOHNSON WC et al: Prognostic significance of cytomorphology in the cutaneous T-cell lymphomas. Cancer 47:119–125, 1981

WEBER K, BURG G, WOLFF HH et al: Sézary-Syndrom. Ein Bericht anhand eines Falles. Hautarzt 26:255–259, 1975

WILSON JONES E: Prospectives in mycosis fungoides in relation to other lymphomas. Trans St John's Hosp Dermatol Soc 61:16–30, 1975

WINKELMANN RK, HOAGLAND HC: The Sézary cell in the blood of patients with mycosis fungoides. Dermatologica 160:73–79, 1980

WINKELMANN RK, PERRY HO, MULLER SA et al: The pre-Sézary erythroderma syndrome. Mayo Clin Proc 49:588–589, 1974

WOLFE JD, TREVOR ED, KJELDSBERG CR: Pulmonary manifestations of mycosis fungoides. Cancer 46:2648–2653, 1980

WOOD WS, KILLBY VAA, STEWART WD: Pagetoid reticulosis (Woringer-Kolopp disease). J Cutan Pathol 6:113–123, 1979

WORINGER F, KOLOPP P: Lésion érythémato-squameuse polycyclique de l'avant-bras évoluant depuis 6 ans chez un garçonnet de 13 ans. Ann Dermatol Syph VII, 10:945–958, 1939

YECKLEY JA, WESTON WL, THORNE C et al: Production of Sézary-like cells from normal human lymphocytes. Arch Dermatol 111:29–32, 1976

Malignant Histiocytosis

ABELE DC, GRIFFIN TB: Histiocytic medullary reticulosis. Arch Dermatol 106:319–329, 1972

ENGSTROM PF, AELING JL, SURINGA DWR: Histiocytic medullary reticulosis with cutaneous lesions. Arch Dermatol 106:369–371, 1972

HUHN D, MEISTER P: Malignant histiocytosis. Cancer 42:1341–1349, 1978

NISHIO K, KODA H, URABE H: Über einen Fall von Histiocytic Medullary Reticulosis. Arch Dermatol Forsch 251:259–269, 1975

PIÑOL-AGUADÉ J, FERRANDO J, TOMÁS JM et al: Necropsy and ultrastructural findings in histiocytic medullary reticulosis. Br J Dermatol 95:35–44, 1976

ROBINOWITZ BN, NOGUCHI S, BERGFELD WF: Tumor cell characterization of histiocytic medullary reticulosis. Arch Dermatol 113:927–929, 1977

SCOTT RB, ROBB-SMITH AHT: Histiocytic medullary reticulosis. Lancet 2:194–198, 1939

WARNKE RA, KIM H, DORFMAN RF: Malignant histiocytosis (histiocytic medullary reticulosis). Cancer 35:215–230, 1975

ZUCKER JM, CAILLEAUX JM, VANEL D et al: Malignant histiocytosis in childhood. Cancer 45:2821–2829, 1980

Leukemia

BEHM FG, KAY S, APORTELA R: Febrile neutrophilic dermatosis associated with acute leukemia. Am J Clin Pathol 76:344–347, 1981

BELISARIO JC, MCGOVERN VJ, DAWSON IE: Erythraemic myelosis (di Guglielmo's disease). Aust J Dermatol 4:191–198, 1958

BERGER BJ, GROSS PR, DANIELS RB et al: Leukemia cutis masquerading as guttate psoriasis. Arch Dermatol 108:416–418, 1973

BERNENGO MG, LEIGHEB G, ZINA G: A case of acute promyelocytic leukemia with bullous, haemorrhagic and necrotic skin lesions. Dermatologica 151:184–190, 1975

BERNENGO MG, ZINA A, ZINA G: Leucosis and skin: Acute lymphoid immunoblastic leukaemia. Br J Dermatol 95:45–49, 1976

BOGGS DP, WINTROBE MM, CARTWRIGHT GE: The acute leukemias: Analysis of 322 cases and review of the literature. Medicine (Baltimore) 41:163–225, 1962

BRYNES RK, GOLOMB HM, DESSER RK et al: Acute monocytic leukemia. Am J Clin Pathol 65:471–482, 1976

BURG G, SCHMOECKEL C, BRAUN-FALCO O et al: Monocytic leukemia. Arch Dermatol 114:418–420, 1978

CARMEL WJ, MINNO AM, COOK WL: Eosinophilic leukemia with report of a case. Arch Intern Med 87:280–286, 1951

COCHRANE T, MILNE JA: A leukaemic acute lymphoblastic leukaemia presenting with cutaneous lesions. Br J Dermatol 91:587–589, 1974

CONRAD ME, RAPPAPORT H, CROSBY WH: Chronic granulocytic leukemia in the aged. Arch Intern Med 116:765–775, 1965

COSTELLO MJ, CANIZARES O, MONTAGUE M et al: Cutaneous manifestations of myelogenous leukemia. Arch Dermatol 71:605–614, 1955

DEME I: Eosinophile Leukämie mit Hautsymptomen. Dermatologica 98:150–157, 1949

HARDY WR, ANDERSON RE: The hypereosinophilic syndromes. Ann Intern Med 68:1120–1228, 1968

HUBLER WR, NETHERTON EW: Cutaneous manifestations of monocytic leukemia. Arch Dermatol 56:70–89, 1947

KAZMIEROWSKI JA, CHUSID MJ, PARILLO JE et al: Dermatologic manifestations of the hypereosinophilic syndrome. Arch Dermatol 114:531–535, 1978

KERL H, KRESBACH H, HÖDEL S: Klinische und histologische Kriterien zur Diagnose und Klassifikation der Leukämien der Haut. Hautarzt 29, Suppl 3:97–101, 1978

KUO T, UHLEMANN J, REINHARD EH: Cutaneous extramedullary hematopoiesis. Arch Dermatol 112:1302–1303, 1976

LONG JC, MIHM MC: Multiple granulocytic tumors of the skin. Cancer 39:2004–2016, 1977

NEIMAN RS, BARCOS M, BERARD C et al: Granulocytic sarcoma. Cancer 48:1426–1437, 1981

PERRY HO, WINKELMANN RK: Bullous pyoderma gangrenosum and leukemia. Arch Dermatol 106:901–905, 1972

PYE RJ, CHOUDHURY C: Bullous pyoderma as a presentation of acute leukemia. Clin Exp Dermatol 2:33–38, 1977

RAIMER SS, DUNCAN WC: Febrile neutrophilic dermatosis in acute myelogeneous leukemia. Arch Dermatol 114:413–414, 1978

SAARNI MI, LINMAN JW: Myelomonocytic leukemia: Disorderly proliferation of all marrow cells. Cancer 27:1221–1230, 1971

SCOTT RB, ELLISON RR, LEY AB: A clinical study of 20 cases of erythroleukemia (di Guglielmo's syndrome). Am J Med 37:162–171, 1964

SHAKLAI M, NIR M, FEUERMAN E: Cutaneous involvement in erythroleukemia. Dermatologica 149:385–387, 1974

SHAW MT: Monocytic leukemias. Hum Pathol 11:215–227, 1980

SUN NCJ, ELLIS R: Granulocytic sarcoma of the skin. Arch Dermatol 116:800–802, 1980

TAGAMI H, TASHIMA M, UEHARA N: Myelofibrosis with skin lesions. Br J Dermatol 102:109–112, 1980

WIERNIK PH, SERPICK AA: Granulocytic sarcoma (chloroma). Blood 35:361–369, 1970

WOHLENBERG H, GRISS P, GOOS M et al: Zur Zytochemie von Hautinfiltraten myelomonocytärer Leukämien. Dtsch Med Wochenschr 95:1439–1443, 1970

YODER FW, SCHUEN RL: Aleukemic leukemia cutis. Arch Dermatol 112:367–369, 1976

Multiple Myeloma, Extramedullary Plasmacytoma

AGARWAL SC: Extramedullary plasmacytoma: Report of a case. Arch Dermatol 74:679–680, 1956

ALBERTS DS, LYNCH P: Cutaneous plasmacytomas in myeloma. Arch Dermatol 114:1784–1787, 1978

BLUEFARB SM: Cutaneous manifestations of multiple myeloma. Arch Dermatol 72:506–523, 1955

BORK K, WEIGAND V: Multiple Plasmacytome der Haut mit IgA-Vermehrung im Serum ohne Knochenmarkbeteiligung. Arch Dermatol Res 254:245–252, 1975

CANLAS MS, DILLON ML, LOUGHRIN JJ: Primary cutaneous plasmacytoma. Arch Dermatol 115:722–724, 1979

EDWARDS GA, ZAWADZKI ZA: Extraosseous lesions in plasma cell myeloma. Am J Med 43:194–205, 1967

GOMEZ EC, MARGULIES M, RYWLIN A et al: Cutaneous involvement by IgD myeloma. Arch Dermatol 114:1700–1703, 1978

HAYES DW, BENNETT WA, HECK FJ: Extramedullary lesions in multiple myeloma. Arch Pathol 53:262–272, 1952

JOHNSON WH JR, TAYLOR BG: Solitary extramedullary plasmacytoma of the skin. Cancer 26:65–68, 1970

JORIZZO JL, GAMMON WR, BRIGGAMAN RA: Cutaneous plasmacytomas. J Am Acad Dermatol 1:59–66, 1979

KLEIN M, GRISHMAN E: Single cutaneous plasmacytoma with crystalloid inclusions. Arch Dermatol 113:64–68, 1977

KYLE RA: Multiple myeloma. Review of 869 cases. Mayo Clin Proc 50:29–40, 1975

LA PERRIERE RJ, WOLF JE, GELLIN GA: Primary cutaneous plasmacytoma. Arch Dermatol 107:99–100, 1973

MIKHAIL GR, SPINDLER AC, KELLY AP: Malignant plasmacytoma cutis. Arch Dermatol 101:59–62, 1970

PARRA CA, RIVERO I, MONCUNILL ALM: Mucocutaneous gamma G polyclonical plasmacytoma with two Bence Jones proteins (BJK and BJL). Arch Dermatol Forsch 242:353–360, 1972

RIVER GL, SCHORR WF: Malignant skin tumors in multiple myeloma. Arch Dermatol 93:432–438, 1966

STANKLER L, DAVIDSON JF: Multiple extramedullary plasmacytomas of the skin. Br J Dermatol 90:217–221, 1974

SWANSON NA, KEREN DF, HEADINGTON JT: Extramedullary IgM plasmacytoma presenting in skin. Am J Dermatopathol 3:79–83, 1981

TSCHEN JA, MIGLIORE PJ, MCGAVRAN MH: Multiple myeloma with cutaneous involvement. Arch Dermatol 116:1394, 1980

WALZER RA, SHAPIRO L: Multiple myeloma with cutaneous metastases. Dermatologica 134:449–454, 1967

WILTSHAW E: The natural history of extramedullary plasmacytoma and its relation to solitary myeloma of bone and myelomatosis. Medicine (Baltimore) 55:217–238, 1976

WUEPPER KD, MACKENZIE MR: Cutaneous extramedullary plasmacytomas. Arch Dermatol 100:155–164, 1969

Macroglobulinemia of Waldenström

BUREAU Y, BARRIÈRE H, BUREAU B et al: Les localisations cutanées de la macroglobulinémie de Waldenström. Ann Dermatol Syph 95:125–137, 1968

DUPRÉ A, BONAFÉ JL, FONTAN B et al: Nodules cutanés d'une macroglobulinémie de Waldenström. Ann Dermatol Venereol 108:961–967, 1981

GOTTRON HA, KORTING GW, NIKOLOWSKI W: Die makroglobulinämische retikuläre Hyperplasie der Haut. Arch Klin Exp Dermatol 210:176–201, 1960

HANKE CW, STEEK WD, BERGFELD WF et al: Cutaneous macroglobulinosis. Arch Dermatol 116:575–577, 1980

MASCARO JM, MONTSERRAT E, ESTRACH T et al: Specific cutaneous manifestations of Waldenström's macroglobulinemia. Br J Dermatol 106:217–222, 1982

ORFANOS C, STEIGLEDER GK: Die tumorbildende kutane Form des Morbus Waldenström. Dtsch Med Wochenschr 92:1449–1454, 1475–1477, 1967

TICHENOR RE, RAU JM, MANTZ FA: Macroglobulinemia cutis. Arch Dermatol 114:280–281, 1978

WALDENSTRÖM J: Incipient myelomatosis or "essential" hyperglobulinemia with fibrinogenopenia: A new syndrome? Acta Med Scand 117:216–247, 1944

Lymphocytoma (Pseudolymphoma of Spiegler-Fendt)

BÄFVERSTEDT B: Lymphadenosis benigna cutis. Acta Derm Venereol (Stockh) 48:1–6, 1968

BARR RJ, SUN NCJ, KING DF: Immunoperoxidase staining of cytoplasmic immunoglobulins. J Am Acad Dermatol 3:58–62, 1980

BERNSTEIN H, SHUPACK J, ACKERMAN AB: Cutaneous pseudolymphoma resulting from antigen injections. Arch Dermatol 110:756–757, 1974

BRAUN-FALCO O, BURG G: Lymphoretikuläre Proliferationen der Haut. Hautarzt 26:124–132, 1975

BURG G, BRAUN-FALCO O: Cutaneous non-Hodgkin's lymphoma: Reevaluation of histology using enzyme-cytochemical and immunologic studies. Int J Dermatol 17:496–505, 1978

CARO WA, HELWIG EB: Cutaneous lymphoid hyperplasia. Cancer 24:487–502, 1969

CLARK WH, MIHM MC JR, REED RJ et al: The lymphocytic infiltrates of the skin. Hum Pathol 5:25–43, 1974

CONNORS RC, ACKERMAN AB: Histologic pseudomalignancies of the skin. Arch Dermatol 112:1767–1780, 1976

DAVID M, SHOHAT B, HAZAZ B et al: Identification of T and B lymphocytes on skin sections from patients with lymphoproliferative disorders of the skin. J Invest Dermatol 75:491–494, 1980

DUNCAN SC, EVANS HL, WINKELMANN RK: Large cell lymphocytoma. Arch Dermatol 116:1142–1146, 1980

EVANS HL, WINKELMANN RK, BANKS PM: Differential diagnosis of malignant and benign cutaneous infiltrates. Cancer 44:699–717, 1979

FISHER ER, PARK EJ, WECHSLER HL: Histologic identification of malignant lymphoma cutis. Am J Clin Pathol 65:149–158, 1976

JIMBOW K, KATOH M, NISHIO C et al: Characterization of surface markers and cytoplasmic organelles in benign and malignant lymphoid lesions of skin. J Cutan Pathol 8:283–298, 1981

KAWADA A, MORI S, HAYASHI T: Lymphadenosis benigna cutis: Pseudomalignant form and its imprint smear cytology. Dermatologica 141:339–347, 1970

LONG JC, MIHM MC, QAZI R: Malignant lymphoma of skin. Cancer 38:1282–1296, 1976

MACH KW, WILGRAM GF: Characteristic histopathology of cutaneous lymphoplasia (lymphocytoma). Arch Dermatol 94:26–32, 1966

PEGUM JS, LANDELLS JW: Lymphosarcoma supervening on lymphocytoma. Trans St John's Hosp Dermatol Soc 56:149–155, 1970

SCHMOECKEL C, BURG G, WOLFF HH et al: The ultrastructure of lymphadenosis benigna cutis (pseudolymphoma cutis). Arch Dermatol Res 258:161–167, 1977

SHELLEY WB, WOOD MG, WILSON JF et al: Premalignant lymphoid hyperplasia. Arch Dermatol 117:500–503, 1981

Glossary

NOTE: Many terms not defined in this Glossary are listed in the Index, with the main reference indicated in bold numerals.

The measurements in size are expressed in centimeters (cm)

millimeters (mm; 1000 mm = 1 m)

micrometers (μm; 1000 μm = 1 mm)

nanometers (nm; 1000 nm = 1 μm)

The term *Angstrom* (10 A = 1 nm) has been avoided.

Acantholysis: Loss of coherence between epidermal or epithelial cells. This process may be primary or secondary. *Primary acantholysis* occurs among unaltered cells as a result of dissolution of the intercellular substance. It is seen in pemphigus vulgaris, pemphigus foliaceus, benign familial pemphigus, Darier's disease, transient acantholytic dermatosis, warty dyskeratoma, and incidental focal acantholytic dyskeratosis. *Secondary acantholysis* occurs among altered or damaged cells. It may occur in viral vesicles, impetigo, subcorneal pustular dermatosis, solar keratosis, and adenoid dyskeratotic squamous cell carcinoma.

Acanthosis: Increase in the thickness of the stratum malpighii.

Anaplasia: Atypical appearance of the nuclei found in malignant neoplasia. Anaplastic nuclei are usually large, irregularly shaped, and hyperchromatic. Atypical mitotic figures may be present.

Apoptosis: Dropping off of colloid bodies (see *Colloid bodies*) from the epidermis into the dermis. It is seen in many dermatoses in which damage to basal cells occurs, such as lichen planus, benign lichenoid keratosis, and lupus erythematosus. The amyloid in macular and lichenoid amyloidosis and the colloid in juvenile colloid milium are also formed by degenerating basal cells dropping off into the dermis.

Argentaffin: Ability to reduce silver salts to metallic silver. Melanin possesses phenolic groups capable of reducing the silver salts that are present in ammoniated silver nitrate to free black silver. (The Fontana–Masson stain contains ammoniated silver nitrate.) (See p. 16.)

Argyrophilic: Substances like melanin, nerves, and reticulum fibers that can be impregnated with silver nitrate solutions and that, by reducing the silver nitrate with hydroquinone to metallic silver, stain black (see p. 16).

Atypia: Identical to anaplasia (see *Anaplasia*).

Ballooning degeneration of epidermis: A type of degeneration of epidermal cells causing marked swelling of the cells with loss of the intercellular bridges. Acantholysis results, and a bulla forms. Ballooning degeneration occurs in viral vesicles and is diagnostic of them. See also under *Reticular degeneration*.

Basal lamina: Identical to basement membrane (see *Basement membrane*).

Basement membrane: A homogeneous band composed of filaments extending along the undersurface of the epidermal basal cells. Measuring only 35 nm to 45 nm in thickness, it is a submicroscopic structure visible only by electron microscopy (see p. 13).

Basement membrane zone: Visible by light microscopy with the PAS reaction. Located beneath the basal cell layer, it measures between 0.5 µm and 1 µm in thickness and thus, on the average, is 20 times thicker than the basement membrane. The basement membrane zone is not homogeneous; it consists not only of the basement membrane but also of the lamina lucida, anchoring fibrils, and reticulum fibers (see p. 9).

Birefringence: On microscopic examination with polarized light, birefringent or doubly refracticle substances are visible as bright white bodies in a dark field (see p. 44).

Bulla: A cavity forming either within or beneath the epidermis and filled with tissue fluid, blood plasma, and, often, inflammatory and/or epidermal cells. A bulla smaller than 5 mm in diameter generally is called a *vesicle,* and a small, slitlike, intraepidermal bulla, as seen in Darier's disease and solar keratosis, is referred to as a *lacuna.*

Cartwheel pattern: Occurs in various fibrous tumors when the elongated cells radiate from a central hub of fibrous tissue in a whorllike fashion. This pattern is often associated with a storiform pattern (see *Storiform pattern*).

Caseation necrosis: Originally described as a type of tissue death characteristic of tuberculosis, syphilis, and some other infections, it is now regarded as identical to coagulation necrosis and ischemic necrosis and thus is the prototype of tissue necrosis. The affected tissue has lost its structural outline and consists of pale eosinophilic, amorphous, finely granular material. Unless the necrosis is far advanced, some shrunken (pyknotic) nuclei or fragments of nuclei (nuclear dust) are still present.

Civatte bodies: See *Colloid bodies.*

Colliquative necrosis: Necrosis associated with the formation of pus (invasion of neutrophils).

Colloid: Homogeneous eosinophilic material of variable composition. The colloid in juvenile colloid milium is of epidermal derivation, whereas the colloid in adult colloid milium is synthesized by fibroblasts. For colloid in colloid bodies, see below.

Colloid bodies: Also referred to as *Civatte bodies.* They are round to ovoid, have an eosinophilic, homogeneous appearance, and measure ap-

proximately 10 µm in diameter. They are seen in the lower epidermis or upper dermis. Although not specific for any disease, they occur most commonly in lichen planus and lupus erythematosus. They form through degeneration of epidermal cells and are extruded into the dermis, a process referred to as *apoptosis* (see *Apoptosis*).

Corps ronds: See *Dyskeratosis.*

Crust: Coagulated tissue fluid and blood plasma intermingled with degenerated inflammatory and epithelial cells.

Degeneration, ballooning, of epidermis: See under *Ballooning.*

Degeneration, fibrinoid, of connective tissue: See under *Fibrinoid.*

Degeneration, granular, of epidermis: See under *Granular.*

Degeneration, hydropic, of basal cell layer: See under *Hydropic.*

Degeneration, liquefaction, of basal cell layer: See under *Liquefaction.*

Degeneration, reticular, of epidermis: See under *Reticular.*

Dyskeratosis: Faulty and premature keratinization of individual keratinocytes. Two types of dyskeratosis are recognized, one occurring in certain acantholytic diseases and the other in certain epidermal neoplasias. *Acantholytic dyskeratosis* occurs as corps ronds, which consist of a central, homogeneous, basophilic, pyknotic nucleus surrounded by a clear halo. Peripheral to the halo lies a shell of basophilic, dyskeratotic material. Corps ronds are seen in Darier's disease, warty dyskeratoma, focal acantholytic dyskeratoma, occasionally in transient acantholytic dermatosis, and rarely in familial benign pemphigus. *Neoplastic dyskeratosis,* referred to also as individual cell keratinization, manifests itself as homogeneous, eosinophilic bodies about 10 µm in diameter that occasionally still show remnants of their nucleus. They may be seen in Bowen's disease, solar keratosis, and squamous cell carcinoma, especially its pseudoglandular or adenoid variant, but also in keratoacanthoma and trichilemmal tumor of the scalp. The occurrence of neoplastic dyskeratosis in the latter two conditions indicates that it is not necessarily an indication of malignancy.

Epidermolytic hyperkeratosis: Also referred to as granular degeneration. One observes the following: (1) perinuclear clear spaces in the upper stratum malpighii; (2) peripheral to the clear spaces, indistinct cellular boundaries formed either by lightly staining material or by keratohyaline granules; (3) a markedly thickened granular layer containing an increased number of keratohyaline granules; and (4) hyperkeratosis. It occurs regularly in epidermolytic hyperkeratosis, also referred to as dominant congenital ichthyosiform erythroderma (see p. 58), in epidermolytic keratosis palmaris et plantaris (see p. 61), in solitary and disseminated epidermolytic acanthoma (see p. 474), and in incidental epidermolytic hyperkeratosis (see p. 475). It is also found occasionally in linear epidermal nevus, usually the systematized type (see p. 473).

Epidermotropism: Presence of mononuclear cells in the epidermis without spongiosis occurring in mycosis fungoides. The cells lie either singly, surrounded by a clear halo, or aggregated as in a Pautrier microabscess (see p. 739). Epidermotropism must be differentiated from exocytosis (see *Exocytosis*).

Erosion: Area in which the epidermis is absent but the dermis is intact, so that, in contrast with an ulcer, healing takes place without scarring.

Exocytosis: Presence of mononuclear cells in the epidermis with spongiosis and often also with microvesiculation occurring in various inflammatory dermatoses, especially subacute dermatitis. Exocytosis must be differentiated from epidermotropism (see *Epidermotropism*).

Fibrinoid degeneration of connective tissue: Permeation of collagen with fibrin giving the involved area a brightly eosinophilic, homogeneous appearance. Often, there are additional degenerative changes. For instance, in allergic vasculitis, the fibrin deposits within and around the vascular walls are associated with vascular damage and often with extravasation of erythrocytes (see p. 168). In rheumatoid nodules, the area of fibrinoid permeation of the collagen appears anuclear (see p. 240). In lupus erythematosus, the fibrinoid deposits in the subepidermal region, around vessels, and on the surface as well as within collagen bundles cause these areas to appear homogeneous and thickened (see p. 450).

Granular degeneration of epidermis: See *Epidermolytic hyperkeratosis*.

Granulation tissue: Newly formed edematous collagenous tissue arising in healing wounds and ulcers and in chronic inflammatory processes. It shows numerous fibroblasts, newly formed capillaries, and a rather dense cellular infiltrate consisting of lymphoid cells, macrophages, and plasma cells.

Granuloma: A chronic proliferative lesion containing, besides mononuclear cells (lymphocytes, monocytes, macrophages), either epithelioid cells or multinucleated giant cells or both. Granulomas arise either as a foreign body reaction or as an allergic granuloma. *Foreign body granulomas* can form as a response either to substances introduced into the skin from the outside, such as various oils or starch powder, or to substances formed endogenously, such as urates or keratin (see p. 221). Foreign body granulomas usually show macrophages and multinucleated giant cells but few or no epithelioid cells. *Allergic granulomas* arise in persons in whom a delayed type of hypersensitivity has already developed to the foreign body material or to the type of microorganism that is being phagocytized. Among the foreign substances capable of producing allergic granulomas are zirconium, beryllium, and various dyes used for tattoos (see p. 223); among the microorganisms are *Mycobacterium tuberculosis, M. Leprae, Treponema pallidum,* and the various fungi causing "deep" fungus infections. In addition, there are idiopathic allergic granulomas, such as those seen in sarcoidosis and allergic granulomatosis. Allergic granulomas are characterized by the presence of epithelioid cells; they often also contain multinucleated giant cells. The multinucleated giant cells in allergic granulomas, often referred to as Langhans giant cells, usually but not always are smaller than the giant cells in foreign body granulomas and often show a peripheral arrangement of their nuclei in a horseshoe pattern, rather than in an irregular arrangement. Still, there is considerable overlapping between Langhans and foreign body giant cells.

Grenz zone: The narrow space that may be found between the epidermis and a dermal lesion, as often seen in granuloma faciale, lepromatous leprosy, and lymphocytoma.

Histiocyte: See *Macrophage*.

Hyalin: Homogeneous eosinophilic material that is PAS-positive and diastase-resistant and has glycoprotein as a major component. Hyalin is present in the lesions of hyalinosis cutis et mucosae (see p. 414), as well as in the lesions of porphyria (see p. 418) and cylindroma (see p. 548). On electron microscopy, a major component of hyalin is seen to be an excessive amount of basement membrane material related to the basement membranes of capillaries in hyalinosis cutis et mucosae and porphyria and to subepithelial basement membranes in cylindroma.

Hydropic degeneration of basal cells: A type of degeneration causing vacuolization of the basal cells, it is referred to also as liquefaction degeneration. It occurs in lupus erythematosus, dermatomyositis, poikiloderma atrophicans vasculare, erythema dyschromicum perstans, and lichen sclerosus et atrophicus. It may also be seen in early lesions of lichen planus, in which, however, it usually progresses to disappearance of the basal cell layer. Hydropic degeneration of the basal cells may cause incontinence of pigment (see below). In lupus erythematosus, lichen sclerosus et atrophicus, and lichen planus, the damage to the basal cells may be severe enough to cause formation of subepidermal bullae (see Classification of Bullae at the beginning of Chapter 7, p. 93).

Hypersensitivity reactions: Four types are recognized:

Type I is the immediate hypersensitivity reaction, or anaphylactic reaction. It is IgE-mediated and results from an antigen reacting with specifically sensitized IgE that is fixed to mast cells and basophils. This results in degranulation of these cells and the release of mediators, which cause vasodilatation. This reaction occurs in anaphylactic shock and in urticaria.

Type II, the cytotoxic reaction, does not occur in the skin.

Type III is the immune complex reaction. In this reaction, the antigen reacts with specific circulating antibodies produced by plasma cells. The resulting antigen–antibody complexes fix complement. The resultant immune reaction attracts neutrophils and/or eosinophils, which participate in the inflammatory response. This represents the Arthus phenomenon. This reaction occurs, for instance, in allergic vasculitis and bullous pemphigoid.

Type IV is the delayed hypersensitivity reaction, or cell-mediated reaction. It is mediated by specifically sensitized T lymphocytes. Lymphokines are released from sensitized lymphocytes at the site of the antigen and produce tissue damage. This reaction occurs, for instance, in allergic contact dermatitis.

Incontinence of pigment: Loss of melanin from the cells of the basal layer due to damage to these cells, with accumulation of the melanin in the upper dermis within melanophages. It occurs particularly in incontinentia pigmenti, lichen planus, lupus erythematosus, poikiloderma atrophicans vasculare, erythema dyschromicum perstans, and fixed drug eruption.

Indian filing of cells: Extension of single rows of cells between and around collagen bundles. It is seen commonly in non-Hodgkin's lymphoma and metastatic scirrhous carcinoma and occasionally in lymphocytoma (pseudolymphoma of Spiegler–Fendt) and granuloma annulare.

Intercellular edema of epidermis: See *Spongiosis*.

Intracellular edema of epidermis: See *Reticular degeneration of epidermis*.

Karyorrhexis: Fragmentation of nuclei resulting in nuclear dust.

Keratin: Two forms of keratin exist: "soft" keratin, found in the stratum corneum of the epidermis, and "hard" keratin, found in the hair cortex and nails. In the sudden keratinization process that takes place in the epidermis, the tonofibrils contain no disulfide bonds and thus remain soft, with keratohyalin providing strength and stability to the tonofibrils (see *Keratohyalin*). In the slow keratinization of the hair cortex, the tonofibrils form disulfide bonds from sulfhydryl groups and become hard keratin, and keratohyalin does not participate.

Keratinocyte: Designation for all epidermal cells with the exception of the dendritic cells (*i.e.,* melanocytes and Langerhans cells). The potential of these epidermal cells is to form keratin.

Keratohyalin: Deeply basophilic, irregularly shaped granules present in the cells of the granular layer of the epidermis. Keratohyaline granules form two structures: the interfibrillary matrix, which cements the keratin fibrils, or tonofibrils, together, and the marginal band of the horny cells. Keratohyalin contains many disulfide bonds and thus provides strength and stability to the tonofibrils, which contain no disulfide bonds and thus remain soft and flexible (see p. 13).

Lacuna: See *Bulla*.

Langerhans cell: A dendritic cell present in the upper layers of the stratum malpighii. Seen in routinely prepared light microscopic sections as "high-level clear cells." Langerhans cells stain well with adenosine triphosphatase. They play an important role in contact dermatitis (see p. 97) and mycosis fungoides (see p. 744).

Langhans giant cell: See *Granuloma.*

Leukocytoclasis: Disintegration of leukocytes, occurring especially in allergic vasculitis, and resulting in nuclear dust.

Liquefaction degeneration of basal cells: See *Hydropic degeneration of basal cells.*

Lymphoid cells: Cells having the histologic appearance of lymphocytes. The term is often used in place of the term lymphocyte, since, in routinely processed and stained histologic sections, lymphocytes and monocytes are indistinguishable, both cells showing a small, round, deeply basophilic nucleus and hardly any cytoplasm. For details about monocytes, see *Macrophage.*

Lysosome: Primary lysosomes are small, membrane-bound organelles containing a variety of hydrolytic enzymes. Because of their small size, primary lysosomes can be seen only by electron microscopy. However, their content of enzymes can be demonstrated in the light microscope by histochemical staining for acid phosphatase, aryl sulfatase, or beta-galactosidase, among others. The lysosomal enzymes are capable of digesting a variety of endogenous or exogenous material. The material to be digested is engulfed by membrane-bound phagosomes. Primary lysosomes then discharge their enzymes into such phagosomes, which thus become phagolysosomes. Phagolysosomes containing exogenous material that the cell has phagocytized by means of endocytosis are called heterophagolysosomes. After completion of the digestion, the phagolysosomes are present as residual bodies, referred to also as myelin bodies because of their resemblance to myelin and their content of phospholipids. (See also pp. 48 and 53.)

Macrophage: The precursors of macrophages are present in the bone marrow and the circulating blood as monocytes. Monocytes that accumulate in the dermis after leaving the blood stream are indistinguishable from lymphocytes in routinely processed and stained histologic sections (see *Lymphoid cells*). They can be distinguished from lymphocytes histochemically by their content of lysosomal enzymes (see *Lysosome*). As monocytes change into actively phagocytizing macrophages, referred to also as histiocytes, their light microscopic appearance changes: the nucleus, instead of being small, round, and deeply basophilic, as in a lymphocyte, becomes larger, elongated, and lightly staining, with a clearly visible nuclear membrane. The nucleus of a macrophage or histiocyte thus is often indistinguishable from that of a fibroblast or an endothelial cell. After completion of their phagocytosis, macrophages may fuse into multinucleated giant cells (see p. 52). Epithelioid cells form from macrophages, usually in foreign body reactions and infections that have provoked a delayed hypersensitivity reaction. Epithelioid cells may also fuse into multinucleated giant cells (see *Granuloma*).

Melanocyte: A dendritic cell normally present in the basal cell layer of the epidermis and of the hair matrix. It is seen in routinely prepared light microscopic sections as a "basal layer clear cell." Melanocytes possess the ability to form melanin through the enzymatic oxidation of tyrosine (see p. 16).

Melanophage: A phagocytizing macrophage, or histiocyte, that has ingested melanin granules, or melanosomes.

Metachromasia: The phenomenon of reacting with a different color from that of the dye used for the staining. Metachromasia can be observed in the presence of acid mucopolysaccharides or of amyloid. Acid mucopolysaccharides, also referred to as glycosaminoglycans, may be sulfated or sulfur-free. Sulfated acid mucopolysaccharides consisting largely of dermatan sulfate are present in the granules of mast cells and in the hair papilla of anagen hair. They stain metachromatically, that is, purple, with methylene blue, toluidine blue, and the Giemsa stain at both pH 3.0 and pH 1.5. Sulfur-free acid mucopolysaccharides consisting largely of hyaluronic acid are present in the dermal mucin of the mucinoses (see p. 424). They stain metachromatically at pH 3.0 but not at pH 1.5. Amyloid shows reddish metachromasia with crystal violet (see p. 407). The exact nature of the substance responsible for the metachromasia of amyloid is not known. The same metachromasia occurs occasionally also in colloid milium (see p. 413).

Metaplasia: Change of one type of tissue into another. It occurs, for instance, as metaplastic ossification within cutaneous tumors, such as pilomatricoma and intradermal nevi (see p. 663).

Microabscesses: Small accumulations of cells in the epidermis or the subepidermal papillae. Three types of microabscesses occur: the Munro microabscess, composed of disintegrated neutrophils in the parakeratotic horny layer in psoriasis (see p. 141); the Pautrier microabscess, composed of mononuclear cells and mycosis cells in the stratum malpighii in mycosis fungoides (see p. 741); and the papillary microabscess, composed predominantly of neutrophils in dermatitis herpetiformis (see p. 119) and of eosinophils in the inflammatory lesions of bullous pemphigoid (see p. 114).

Mucin: There are two types of mucin: dermal and epithelial. *Dermal mucin* forms the ground substance and consists of acid mucopolysaccharides, largely hyaluronic acid. It (1) is PAS-negative, (2) stains with alcian blue at *p*H 2.5 but not at *p*H 0.4, (3) stains metachromatically with methylene blue and toluidine blue at *p*H 3.0 but not at *p*H 1.5, and (4) is hyaluronidase-labile (see p. 424). *Epithelial mucin,* referred to as sialomucin, contains both neutral and acid mucopolysaccharides. It is present in the skin in the granules of the dark, mucoid secretory cells of eccrine glands (see p. 21), in some of the granules of apocrine secretory cells (see p. 23), within oral mucous cysts and the cells lining them (see p. 617), in the cells of cutaneous metastases of gastrointestinal carcinoma (see p. 593), and in the cells of only some cases of mammary and extramammary Paget's disease but regularly in the cells of "secondary" extramammary Paget's disease extending from a mucus-secreting adenocarcinoma (see p. 513). Epithelial mucin (1) is PAS-positive and diastase-resistant, (2) stains with alcian blue at *p*H 2.5 but not at *p*H 0.4, (3) does not stain metachromatically with methylene blue or toluidine blue, and (4) is hyaluronidase-resistant (see p. 21).

Munro's microabscess: See *Microabscesses* and under *Spongiform pustule.*

Myoepithelial cells: Cells forming the peripheral cell row in the secretory segment of eccrine and apocrine glands. They contain contractile myofibrils just like those present in glomus cells and in the smooth muscle cells of blood vessels and arrector pili muscles, from which they differ, however, by their epithelial derivation.

Necrosis: See *Caseation necrosis, Colliquative necrosis,* and under *Fibrinoid degeneration.*

Nevus: For a definition of this term, see p. 524.

Nuclear dust: See *Karyorrhexis* and *Leukocytoclasis.*

Papilla: A pine-cone-shaped elongation of the dermis protruding into the epidermis as subepidermal papillae surrounded by rete ridges and into the bulb-shaped hair matrix as hair papillae.

Papilloma: A tumor or tumorlike proliferation of the skin characterized by papillomatosis (see below) and hyperkeratosis. Five lesions show this type of proliferation: linear epidermal nevus, solar keratosis, seborrheic keratosis, verruca vulgaris, and acanthosis nigricans. In typical instances, histologic differentiation of these five lesions is easy, but, occasionally, a diagnosis no more specific than papilloma can be made. For a discussion of histologic differentiation, see p. 474.

Papillomatosis: Upward proliferation of subepidermal papillae causing the surface of the epidermis to show irregular undulation.

Parakeratosis: Incomplete keratinization characterized by retention of nuclei in the horny layer and associated with a marked underdevelopment or absence of the granular layer. It is seen especially in psoriasis. Parakeratosis at one time was interpreted as being the result of a too rapid cell proliferation interfering with cellular maturation. However, it has since been shown that a defect in cellular differentiation is the primary event. (See p. 144 for details.)

Pautrier microabscess: See *Microabscesses.*

Phagosome: See *Lysosome.*

Pigmentary incontinence: See *Incontinence of pigment.*

Plaque: As used in English, the term refers to a circumscribed thickened or indurated area, as in the plaque stage of mycosis fungoides. In French, however, it means a patch without thickening or induration, as in parapsoriasis en plaques.

Pleomorphism: Variation in the appearance of the nuclei of the same cell type. If pleomorphism is pronounced, it is associated with the presence of large, irregularly shaped, hyperchromatic nuclei referred to as anaplastic or atypical nuclei. Anaplasia is often an indication of malignant neoplasia (see *Anaplasia*).

Polymorphism: Variation in types of cells. This phenomenon is commonly seen in a variety of inflammatory diseases and thus is not an indication of malignancy.

Pustule: A vesicle or bulla containing numerous neutrophils or, in some instances, eosinophils, as in pemphigus vegetans and in erythema toxicum neonatorum. For a definition of *spongiform pustule,* see below.

Pyknosis: Shrinking of nuclei.

Reticular degeneration of epidermis: A process in which severe intracellular edema causes bursting of epidermal cells and formation of a multilocular bulla. The septa inside the bulla are formed by resisting cell walls. Reticular degeneration is found in the blisters of acute dermatitis, usually in association with spongiosis (see *Spongiosis*) and, in viral blisters, usually in association with ballooning degeneration (see under *Ballooning degeneration*).

Reticuloses: This term is rarely used and should be avoided because of its vagueness. The term *malignant reticulosis* as a designation for lymphoma is a misnomer, since it has been shown that mycosis fungoides is a T-lymphocyte lymphoma and that nearly all non-Hodgkin's lymphomas, including reticulum cell sarcomas or histiocytic lymphomas, are composed of altered B or T lymphocytes.

Sialomucin: See *Mucin*.

Spongiform pustule of Kogoj: A multilocular pustule located in the upper stratum malpighii and characterized by the intercellular presence of neutrophils within a spongelike network that is composed of flattened, degenerated keratinocytes (see p. 141). This type of pustule is typical of all variants of pustular psoriasis, including Reiter's disease (see p. 148). Ordinary psoriasis shows small spongiform pustules only if the lesions are in an early and acute stage. As the spongiform pustules move with the proliferating epidermis into the horny layer, they manifest themselves as Munro microabscesses. Although spongiform pustules are highly suggestive and usually diagnostic of psoriasis and its pustular variants, they have also been observed in the lesions of geographic tongue (see p. 476) and, in rare instances, in the cutaneous pustules of candidiasis (see p. 332).

Spongiosis: A process in which intercellular edema between the squamous cells of the epidermis causes an increase in the width of the spaces between the cells. It occurs frequently in inflammatory processes of the skin. In acute and subacute dermatitis, spongiosis in the epidermis is the essential factor in producing the spongiotic blister that is characteristic of dermatitis (see p. 94). Severe spongiosis may be accompanied by intracellular edema resulting in reticular degeneration of the epidermis (see under *Reticular degeneration*).

Storiform pattern: Occurs in various fibrous tumors when the elongated cells intersect or intertwine at various angles so as to resemble the weaving of a doormat (Latin: *storia*). This pattern is often associated with a cartwheel pattern (see *Cartwheel pattern*).

Stratum malpighii: Term applied to the nucleated, viable portion of the epidermis consisting of the basal, squamous, and granular layers.

Trichohyalin: In contrast with the hard keratin of the hair cortex, which consists of tonofibrils rich in disulfide bonds and contains no keratohyalin, the three components of the inner root sheath, that is, the inner root sheath cuticle, the Huxley layer, and the Henle layer, keratinize by means of trichohyaline granules (see p. 27). Although trichohyaline granules stain eosinophilic, in contrast to the basophilic staining of the keratohyaline granules in the epidermis, these two types of granules have similar functions.

Touton giant cell: A giant cell showing a wreath of nuclei around a central area of nonfoamy cytoplasm and a peripheral area of foamy, lipidized cytoplasm. These cells are seen in various types of xanthoma and in juvenile xanthogranuloma.

Ulcer: An area in which, besides the epidermis, part of the dermis is also absent. Thus, in contrast with an erosion, healing takes place with scarring.

Vesicle: A small bulla generally less than 5 mm in diameter. (See *Bulla*.)

Villi: Elongated and often tortuous papillae that as a rule are covered with only a single layer of epidermal cells and that extend into a bulla, vesicle, or lacuna that has formed as a result of suprabasal acantholysis. Villi are observed in pemphigus vulgaris, particularly in its variant pemphigus vegetans, familial benign pemphigus, Darier's disease, warty dyskeratoma, and transient acantholytic dermatosis.

Appendix

Electron Micrographs

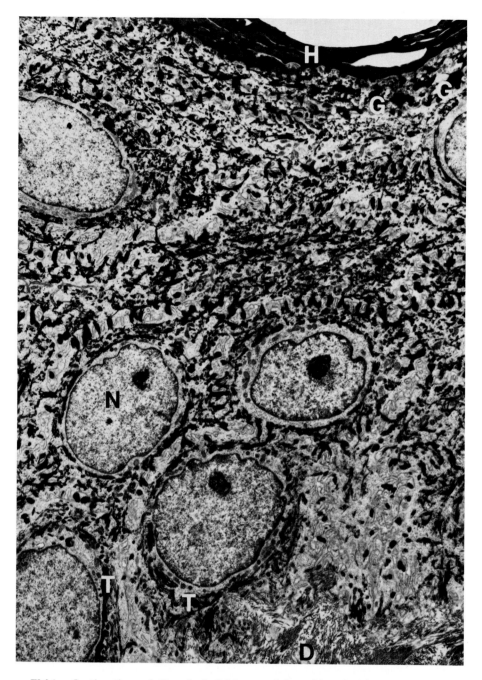

EM 1.   **Section through the whole thickness of the epidermis.** The stratum corneum is at the top and the dermis at the bottom of the micrograph. *H,* horny cells; *G,* keratohyaline granules in granular cells; *N,* nucleus of squamous cells; *T,* tonofilaments in basal cells; *D,* dermis. (×7500) (See p. 12.)

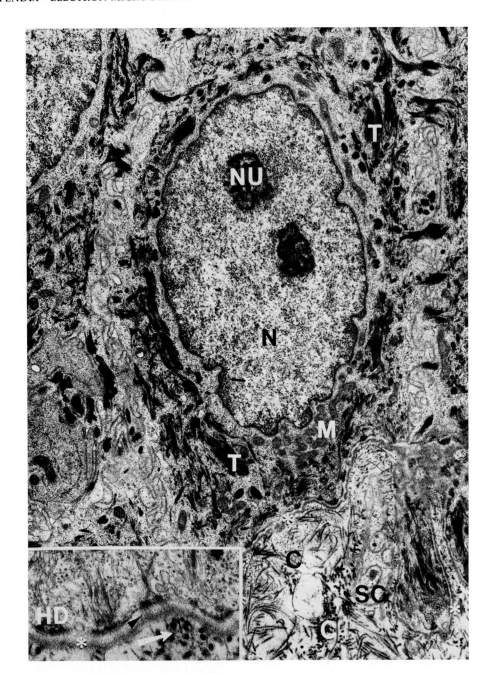

EM 2.   **Basal cell.** *Inset:* **Dermal-epidermal junction.** *N,* nucleus; *NU,* nucleolus; *T,* tonofilaments; *M,* mitochondria; *asterisk,* basement membrane; *SC,* Schwann cell in the dermis; *C,* collagen. (×12,500) (See p. 12.) **Inset:** *Asterisk,* basement membrane; *HD,* half-desmosome with sub-basal cell dense plaque beneath; *pointer,* anchoring filaments; *arrow,* anchoring fibrils in the dermis. (×25,000) (See p. 13.)

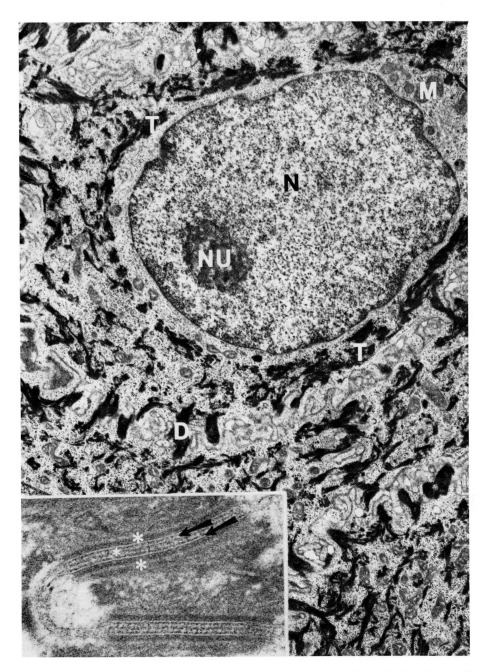

EM 3. **Squamous cell.** *Inset:* **Desmosomes.** *N,* nucleus; *NU,* nucleolus; *T,* tonofilaments; *D,* desmosome; *M,* mitochondria. (×12,500). (See p. 12.) **Inset:** Desmosomes
at higher magnification. A desmosome connecting two adjoining keratinocytes consists
of nine lines—five electron-dense lines and four electron-lucid lines. The two peripheral
dense, thick lines (*large asterisks*) are the attachment plaques. The single electron-dense
line in the center of the desmosome (*small asterisk*) is the intercellular contact layer.
The two electron-dense lines between the intercellular contact layer and the two
attachment plaques represent the cell surface coat together with the outer leaflet of the
trilaminar plasma membrane of each keratinocyte (*arrows*). The two inner electron-
lucid lines adjacent to the intercellular contact layer represent intercellular cement. The
two outer electron-lucid lines are the central lamina of the trilaminar plasma membrane.
(×100,000) (See p. 12.)

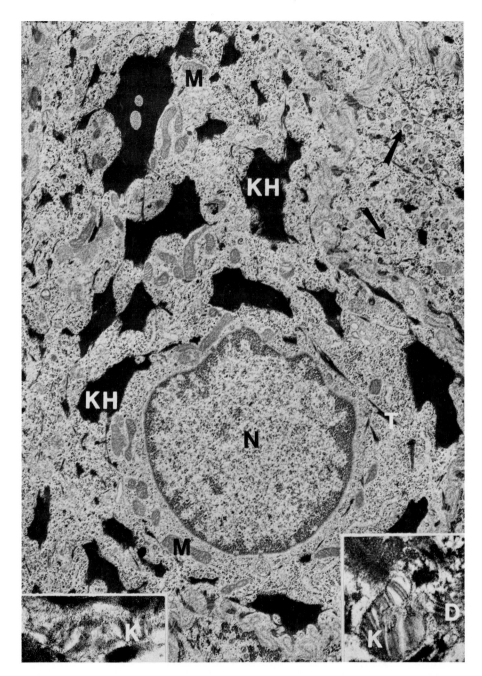

EM 4. **Granular cell.** *Inset:* **Keratinosomes** or **Odland bodies.** *N,* nucleus of granular cell; *KH,* keratohyaline granules; *M,* mitochondria; *arrows,* keratinosomes; *T,* tonofilaments. (×12,500) (See p. 13.) **Left inset:** *K,* intracellular keratinosome. (×50,000) (See p. 14.) **Right inset:** *K,* keratinosome in intercellular space; *D,* desmosome. (×50,000) (See p. 14.)

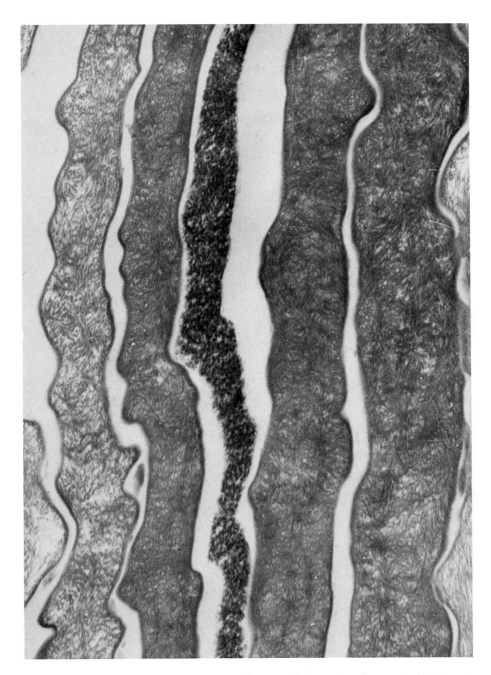

EM 5.   **Horny cells.** The cytoplasm of horny cells contains electron-lucid filaments and an electron-dense amorphous substance. The filaments are believed to derive from tonofilaments, the amorphous substance from keratohyaline granules. (×50,000) (See p. 13.)

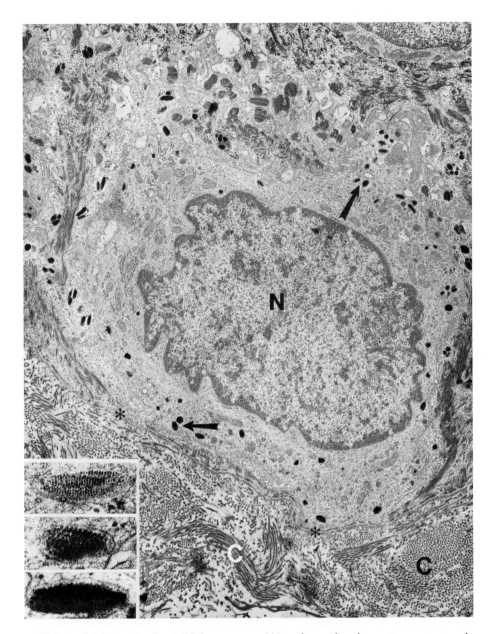

EM 6. **Melanocyte.** *Inset:* **Melanosomes.** *N,* nucleus of melanocyte; *arrows,* melanosomes; *C,* collagen in the dermis; *asterisk,* basal lamina. (×10,000) (See p. 17.) **Insets:**
Melanosomes in different stages of development: Stage II (*upper inset*), Stage III (*middle
inset*), and Stage IV (*lower inset*). (×75,000) (See p. 17.)

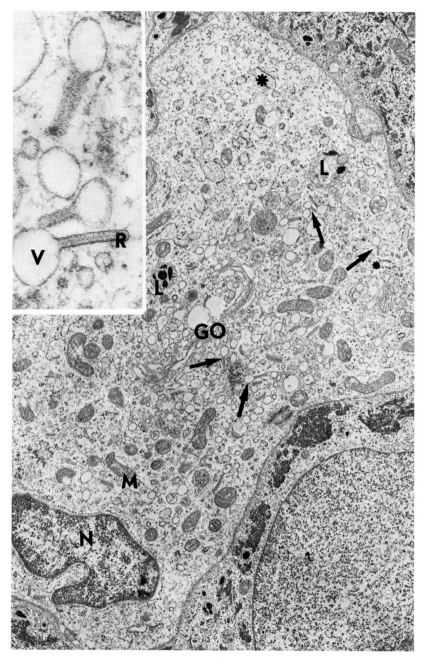

EM 7. **Langerhans cell.** *Inset:* **Langerhans granules.** *N,* nucleus of Langerhans cell; *L,* lysosomes containing melanosomes; *GO,* Golgi complex; *M,* mitochondrium; *asterisk,* rough endoplasmic reticulum; *arrows,* Langerhans granules. (×12,500) (See p. 18.) **Inset:** Langerhans granules at higher magnification consisting of a vesicle (*V*) and a rod (*R*), both giving the appearance of a tennis racquet. (×75,000) (See p. 18.)

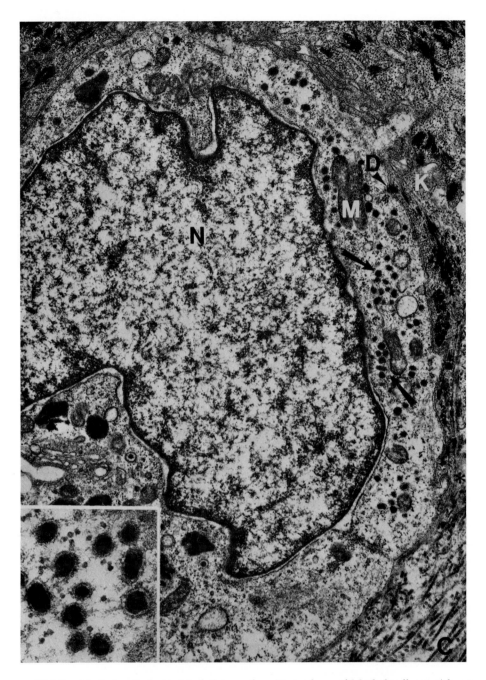

EM 8.   **Merkel cell.** *Inset:* **Merkel granules.** *N,* nucleus of Merkel cell; *asterisk,* on basal lamina; *M,* mitochondria; *arrows,* specific granules of the Merkel cell; *D with pointer,* desmosome between Merkel cell and keratinocyte (*K*); *C,* collagen with cross striation. (×20,000) (See p. 20.) **Inset:** Specific membrane-bound granules at higher magnification. (×75,000) (See p. 20.)

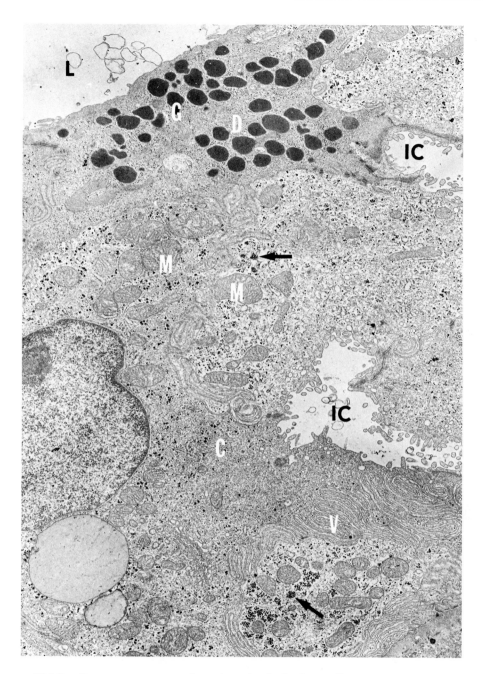

EM 9. **Secretory segment of eccrine gland.** *C,* clear cells; *arrows,* aggregates of glycogen granules; *V,* villous folds between clear cells; *M,* mitochondria; *IC,* intercellular canaliculi; *D,* dark cell with large mucoid granules (*G*); *L,* lumen of the eccrine gland. (×12,500) (See p. 21.)

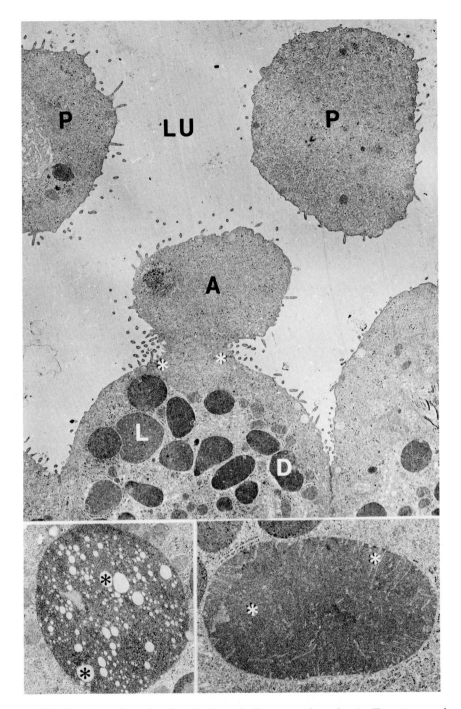

EM 10.   **Apocrine gland with decapitation secretion.** *Insets:* **Two types of granules.** *P*, pinched-off parts of secretory cells; *A*, apical portion of apocrine cell, which is partly decapitated; *asterisks*, membranes that extend from each side of the cell toward the middle of the cell. When they fuse in the middle, the apical portion of the cell has become detached (''decapitated''). *D*, dark granule; *L*, light granule; *LU*, lumen of gland. (×5000) (See p. 24.) **Left inset:** Dark granule with lipid droplets (*asterisk*). (×10,000) (See p. 24.) **Right inset:** Light granule with cristae (*asterisk*). (×12,500) (See p. 24.)

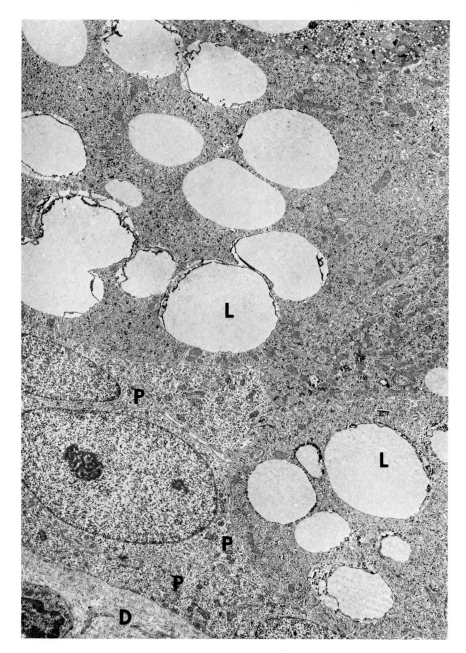

EM 11.   **Sebaceous gland.** *P,* cells of peripheral cell layer without lipid droplets; *D,* dermis; *L,* lipid droplets. (×6000) (See p. 25.)

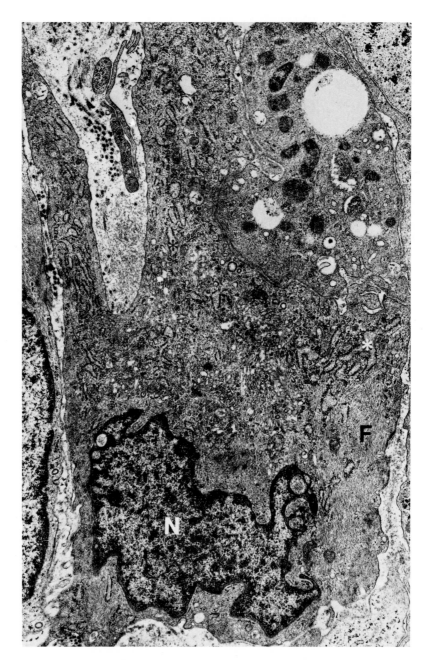

EM 12.   **Fibroblast that actively synthesized collagen.** *Asterisks,* cisternae of rough endoplasmic reticulum filled with amorphous material; *F,* intracytoplasmic filaments; *N,* nucleus. (Courtesy of B. Mihatsch-Konz, M.D.) (×15,000) (See p. 31.)

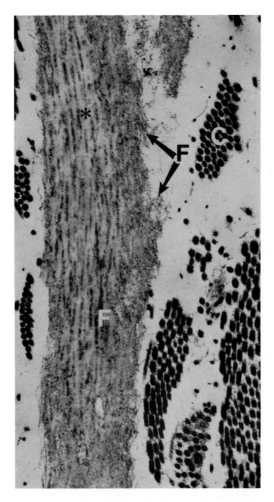

EM 13.   **Elastic fiber.** Within the amorphous part of the elastic fiber (*asterisk*), skeins of microfibrils (*F*) are visible. They are also visible at the periphery of the elastic fiber (*arrows*). C, collagen. (×25,000) (See p. 31.)

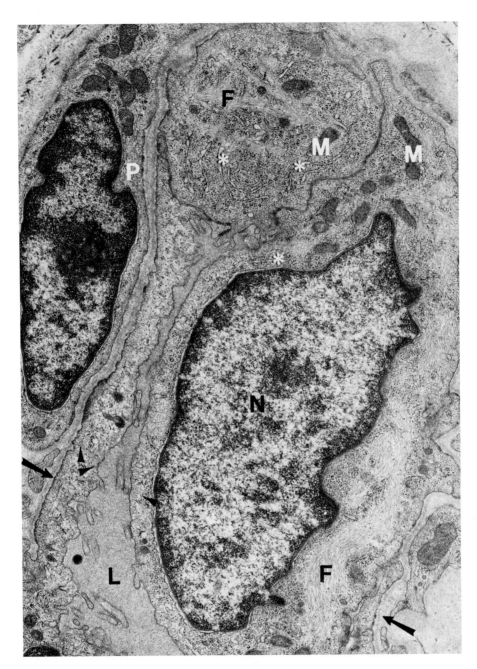

EM 14.   **Capillary.** *N,* nucleus of endothelial cell; *asterisks,* well-developed endoplasmic reticulum; *F,* cytoplasmic filaments in endothelial cells; *pointers,* pinocytotic
vesicles; *M,* mitochondria; *arrows,* basal lamina; *L,* capillary lumen; *P,* pericyte.
(×17,000) (See p. 35.)

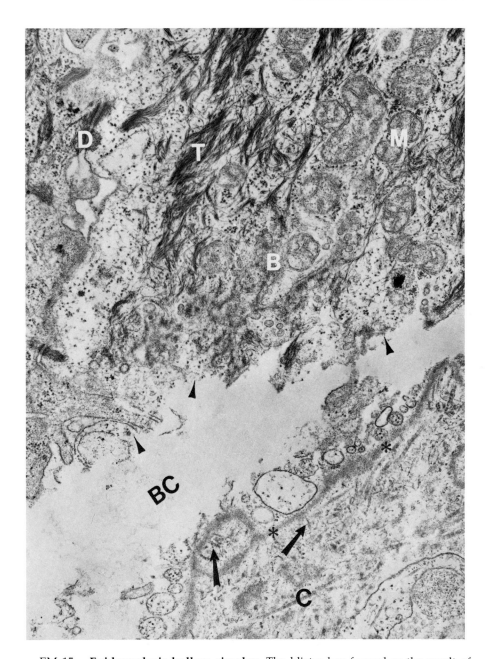

EM 15. **Epidermolysis bullosa simplex.** The blister has formed as the result of degenerative, cytolytic changes in the basal cells (*B*). The bulla cavity (*BC*) is situated above the basement membrane (*asterisk*). The basal cells are severely damaged, lacking a plasma membrane (*pointers*). *T*, tonofilaments; *M*, mitochondria; *D*, desmosome. (×25,000) (See p. 69.)

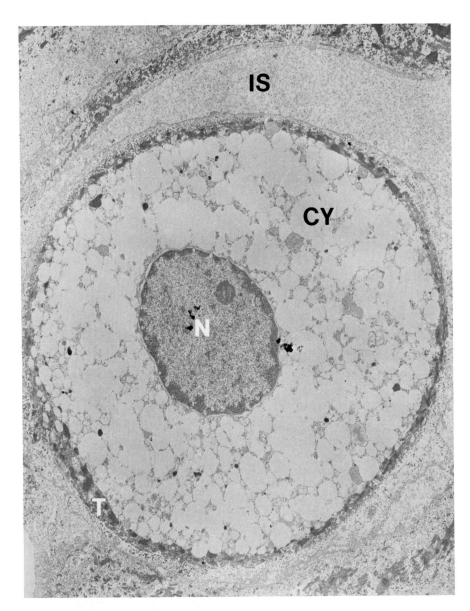

EM 16.   **Darier's disease: corps rond.** A corps rond consists of a pyknotic nucleus (*N*), an autolyzed electron-lucid cytoplasm (*CY*), and a shell of homogenized tonofilaments (*T*). *IS*, widened intercellular space due to disappearance of desmosomes. (×10,000) (See p. 72.)

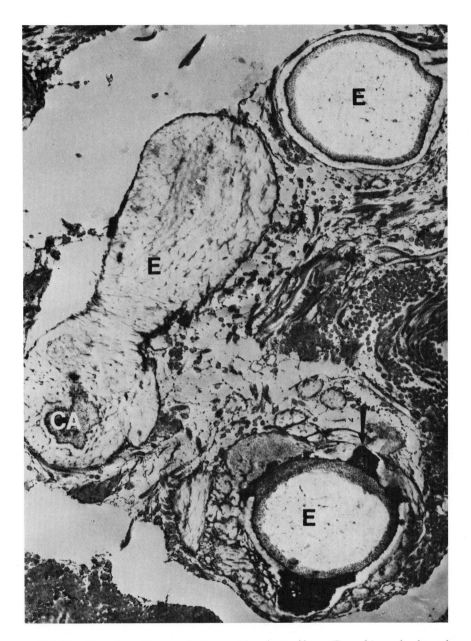

EM 17.   **Pseudoxanthoma elasticum.** The elastic fibers (*E*) are bizarrely shaped. Calcium (*CA; arrows*) is deposited on or around elastic fibers. (×12,500) (See p. 76.)

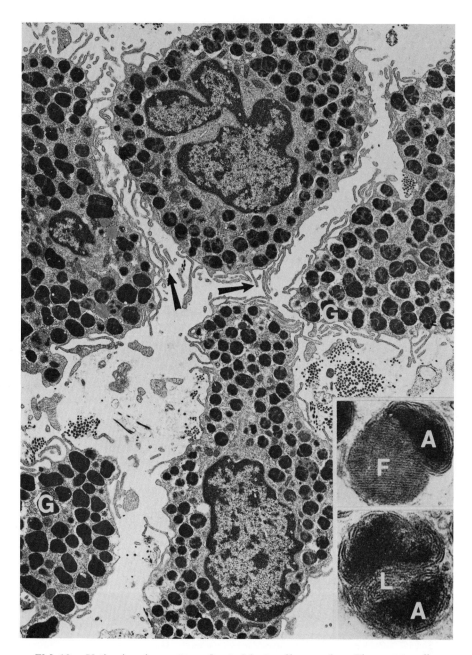

EM 18. **Urticaria pigmentosa.** *Inset:* **Mast cell granules.** The mast cells are increased above normal in number. They do not differ from normal mast cells. Mast cells have numerous long villous projections (*arrows*) and contain characteristic granules (G). (×6000) (See p. 83.) **Insets:** Mast cell granules at higher magnification. *Upper inset:* This granule shows dense filaments in parallel arrangement (F). *Lower inset:* This granule shows curved parallel lamellae (L) reminding one of fingerprints. In addition, both granules show amorphous, dense material (A). (×75,000) (See p. 54.)

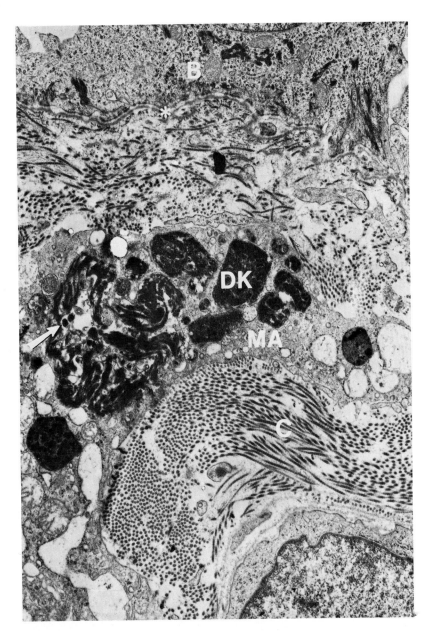

EM 19.   **Incontinentia pigmenti.** In this disease, dyskeratotic cells are found in the epidermis. Macrophages migrate into the epidermis, phagocytize these dyskeratotic cells as well as melanosomes, and subsequently return to the dermis. *MA,* macrophage containing dyskeratotic material (*DK*) and melanosomes (*arrow*); *B,* basal cell; *asterisk,* basal lamina; *C,* collagen. (×12,500) (See p. 84.)

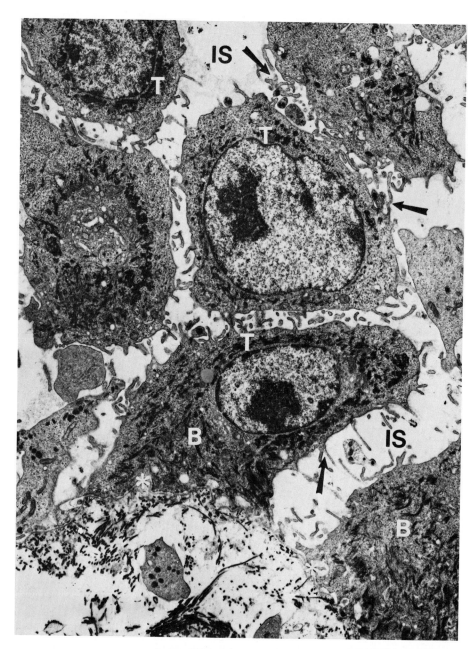

EM 20. **Pemphigus vulgaris—beginning acantholysis.** The dissolution of the intercellular cement substance and the disappearance of desmosomes lead to widening of the intercellular space (*IS*). Keratinocytes form microvilli (*arrows*). Tonofilaments (*T*) retract to the perinuclear area. The basal cells (*B*) remain attached to the basement membrane (*asterisks*). (×8000) (See p. 107.)

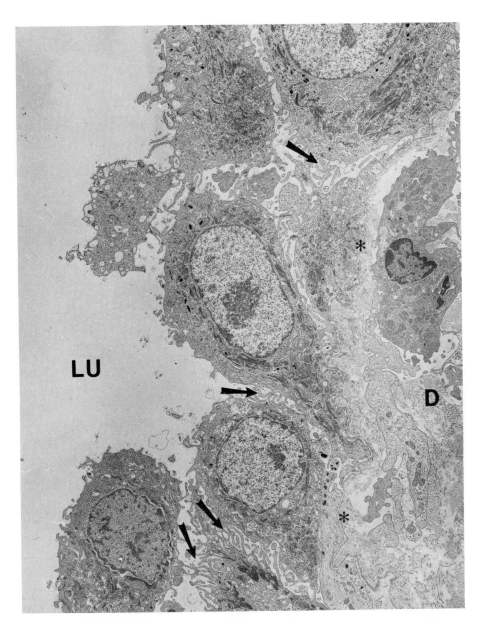

EM 21. **Pemphigus vulgaris—tombstone row.** The dissolution of the intercellular cement has led to the formation of a blister. At the base of the blister, one or two rows of keratinocytes are left. The cohesion of the basal cells with the dermis is well preserved. *LU*, blister lumen; *asterisks*, basement membrane; *arrows*, microvilli of keratinocytes; *D*, dermis. (×5000) (See p. 108.)

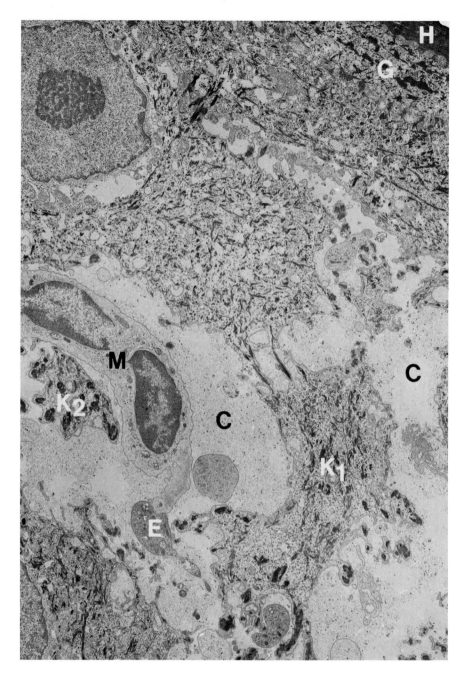

EM 22. **Pemphigus foliaceus.** The upper portion of the epidermis, in which the acantholysis is most pronounced, is shown. *K1,* partly acantholytic cell in the upper stratum spinosum; *K2,* completely acantholytic cell; *C,* cleft in the upper epidermis; *M,* macrophage; *E,* eosinophil; *G,* granular cell; *H,* horny cells. (×6000) (See p. 112.)

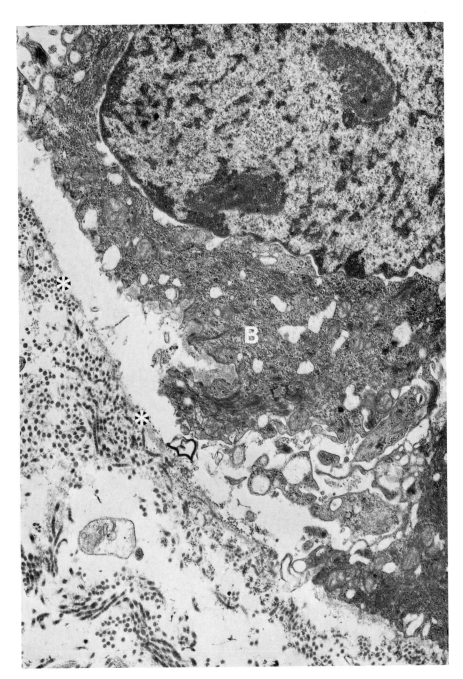

EM 23. **Bullous pemphigoid—noninflamed type.** In this type of bullous pemphigoid, the blister forms between the basal cell (*B*) and the basement membrane (*asterisks*). (×15,000) (See p. 115.)

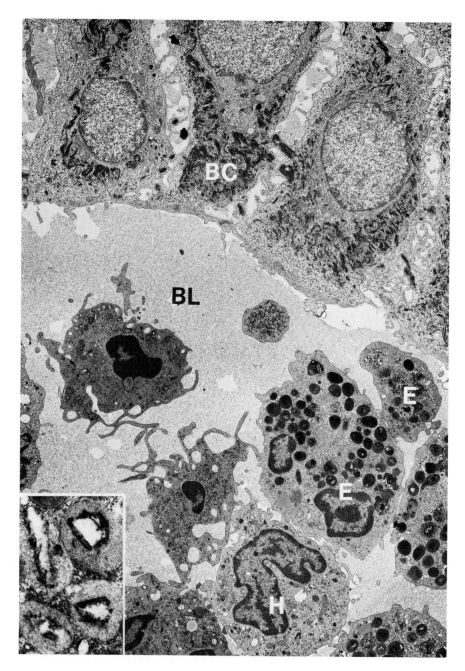

EM 24.   **Bullous pemphigoid—inflamed type.** *Inset:* **Granules of eosinophils.**
The blister (*BL*) contains several histiocytes (*H*) and eosinophils (*E*). The basement
membrane has disappeared. The basal cells (*BC*) at the top of the blister are well
preserved. (×5000) (See p. 115.) **Inset:** Eosinophilic granules at higher magnification
show a ''crystal'' at their center. (×25,000) (See p. 48.)

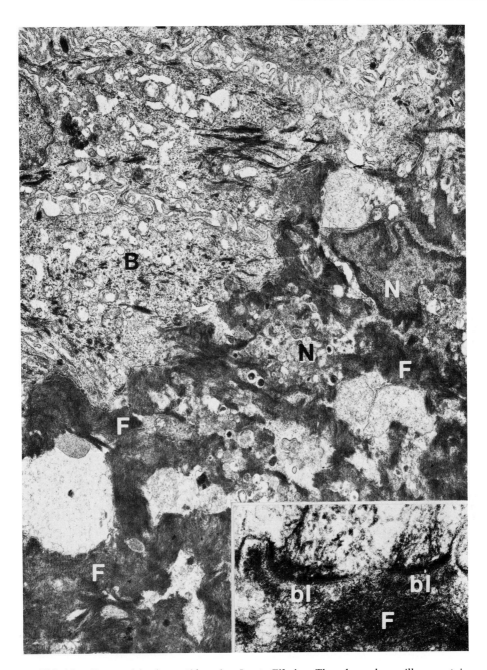

EM 25. **Dermatitis herpetiformis.** *Inset:* **Fibrin.** The dermal papillae contain abundant amounts of fibrin (*F*). Between the meshes of fibrin, fragments of neutrophilic leukocytes (*N*) can be seen. *B,* basal cell. (×12,500) (See p. 120.) **Inset:** The fibrin (*F*) is attached to the dermal side of the basement membrane or basal lamina (*bl*). The basement membrane shows discontinuities. (×60,000) (See p. 120.)

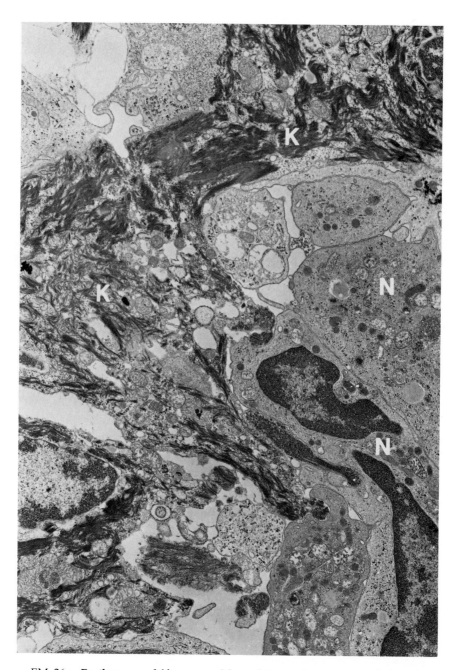

EM 26. **Erythema multiforme—epidermal type.** Among necrotic keratinocytes (*K*) with abundant tonofilaments, neutrophils (*N*) are found. (×10,000) (See
p. 124.)

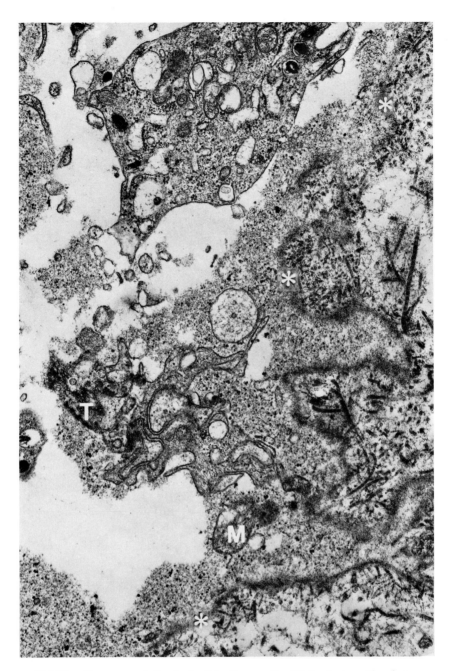

EM 27. **Herpes gestationis.** In this disease, the blister forms either between basal cells and basement membrane or, subsequent to dissolution of basal cells, between squamous cells and basement membrane. A disintegrated basal cell containing tonofilaments (*T*) and mitochondria (*M*) and the basement membrane (*asterisks*) form the floor of the blister. *D,* dermis. (×25,000) (See p. 118.)

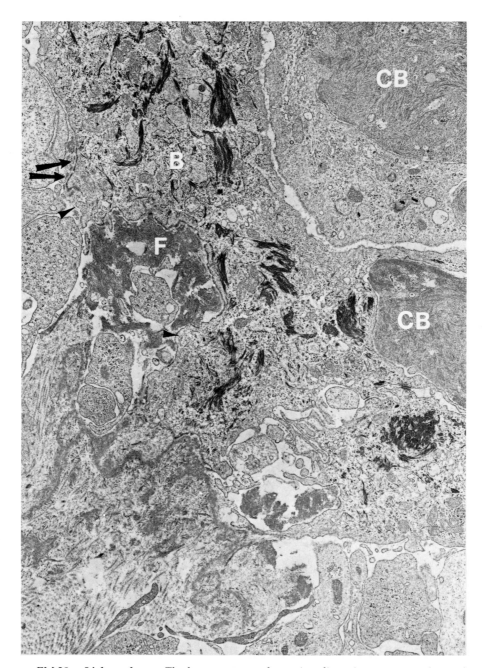

EM 28. **Lichen planus.** The basement membrane is split up in some areas (*arrows*) and has disappeared in others (*pointers*). The lower epidermis contains colloid bodies (*CB*) consisting of numerous filaments and remnants of organelles. *F,* fibrin beneath the basal cell (*B*). (×10,000) (See p. 155.)

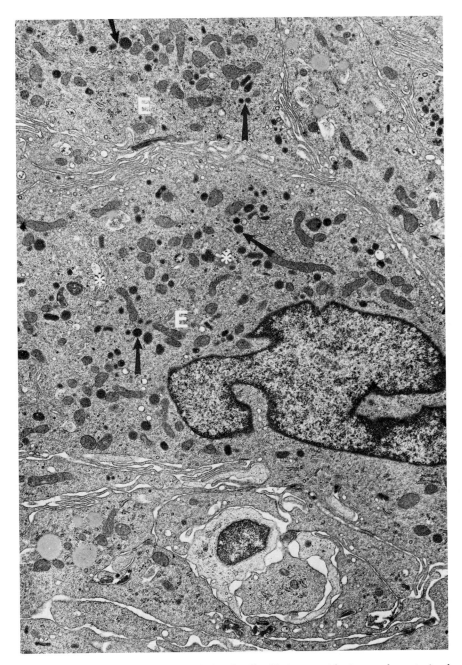

EM 29.   **Sarcoidosis.** The epithelioid cells (*E*) in sarcoidosis are characterized by the presence of many primary lysosomes (*arrows*) and a few autophagic vacuoles (*asterisks*). (×17,500) (See p. 232.)

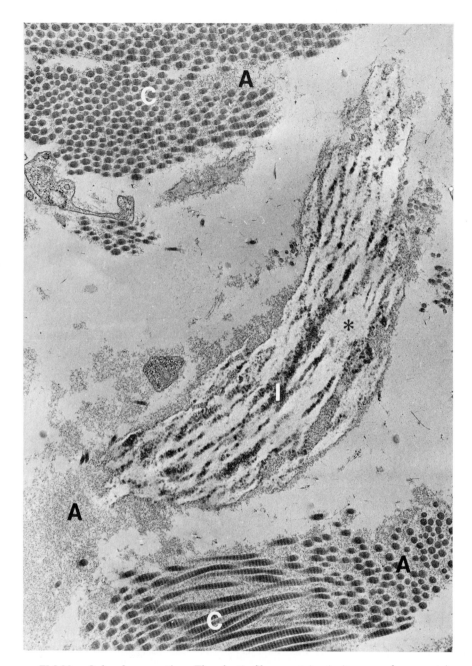

EM 30.   **Solar degeneration.** The elastic fiber contains in its amorphous matrix (*asterisk*) numerous electron-dense inclusions (*I*). Extensive amorphous material (*A*) can be seen around the elastotic fiber and among the collagen fibrils (*C*). (×20,000) (See p. 271.)

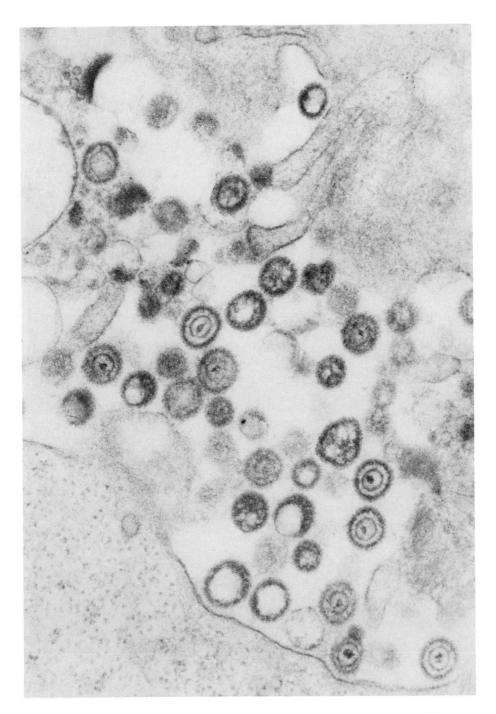

EM 31. **Varicella-zoster virus.** Numerous mature virus particles or virions are located extracellularly between two keratinocytes. Many virus particles show in their center a small, electron-dense, round to oval nucleoid or core that is surrounded by the capsid. Having replicated in the nucleus, the virus particles possess an outer coat derived from the nuclear membrane. (Courtesy of C. M. Orfanos, M.D.) (×57,000) (See p. 367.)

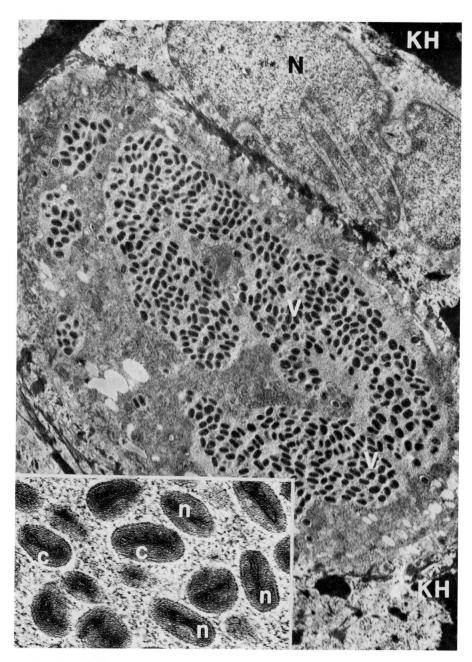

EM 32. **Molluscum contagiosum.** *Inset:* **High magnification of viruses.** The granular cell contains an inclusion body consisting of numerous molluscum contagiosum viruses (*V*). The nucleus (*N*) of the cell has been displaced to the periphery of the cell. *KH*, keratohyaline granules. (×12,500) (See p. 370.) **Inset:** The virus consists of the dumbbell-shaped nucleoid (*n*) surrounded by the capsid (*c*). (×75,000) (See p. 371.)

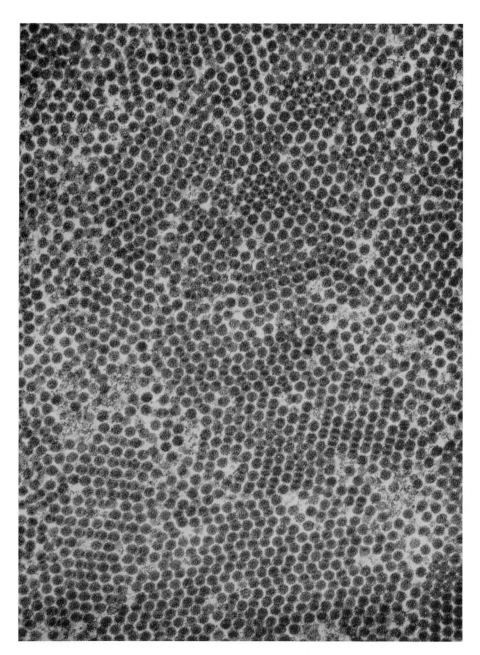

EM 33.   **Deep palmoplantar wart (myrmecia).** The wart viruses form aggregates in a semicrystalloid arrangement within the nucleus of parakeratotic cells. The viruses appear round and stippled. ($\times$80,000) (See p. 374.)

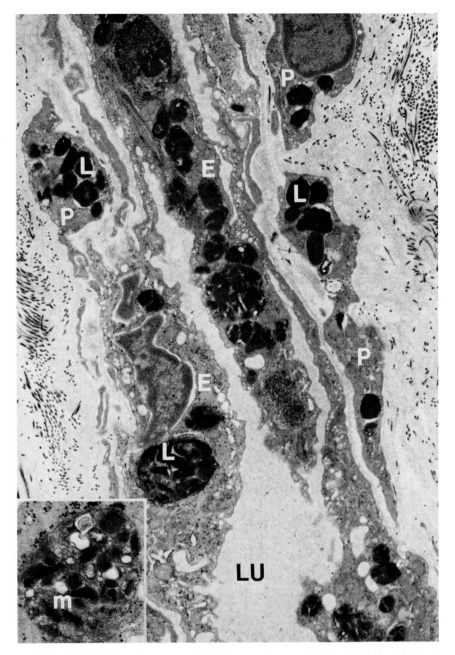

EM 34. **Angiokeratoma corporis diffusum (Fabry's disease).** *Inset:* **Lysosomal residual body.** Endothelial cells (*E*) and pericytes (*P*) contain lipid deposits (*L*) within greatly enlarged lysosomes. *LU,* lumen of capillary. (×12,500) (See p. 391.) **Inset:** A large matured lysosome as a residual body shows laminated myelin figures (*m*). (×25,000) (See p. 391.)

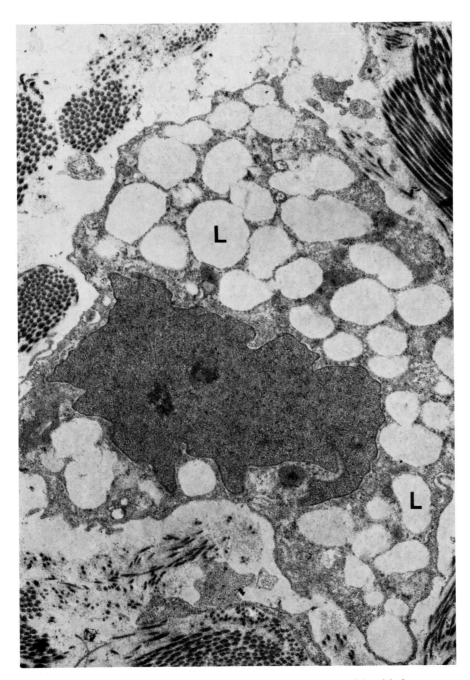

EM 35. **Juvenile xanthogranuloma.** The lesion consists of lipid-laden macro-phages. The lipid material (*L*) is not bound by a membrane. (×12,500) (See p. 398.)

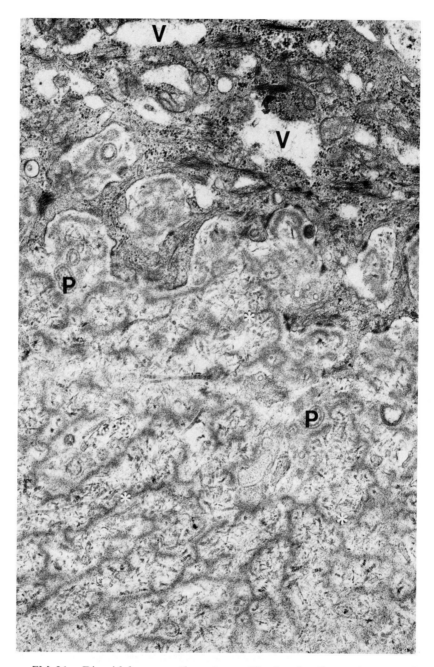

EM 36. **Discoid lupus erythematosus.** The basal cell contains several vacuoles (*V*), which ultimately may cause disintegration of the cell. Many cross-sectioned projections (*P*) of the basal cell into the dermis can be seen, as can a greatly increased amount of basal lamina material (*asterisks*). (×25,000) (See p. 455.)

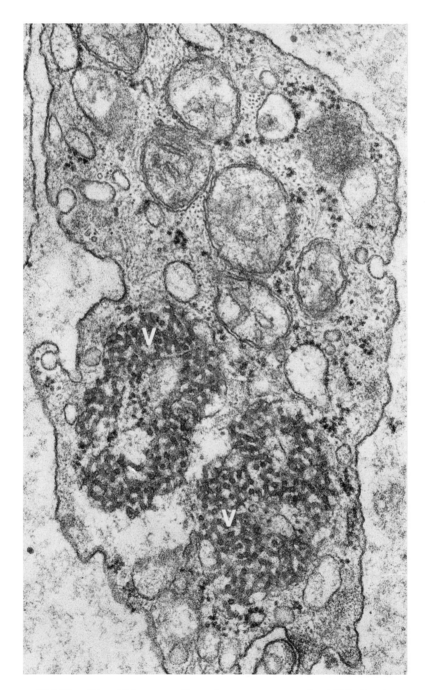

EM 37.   **Discoid lupus erythematosus: paramyxovirus.** Tubular structures of paramyxovirus (*V*) can be seen within a fibroblast. (×60,000) (See p. 455.)

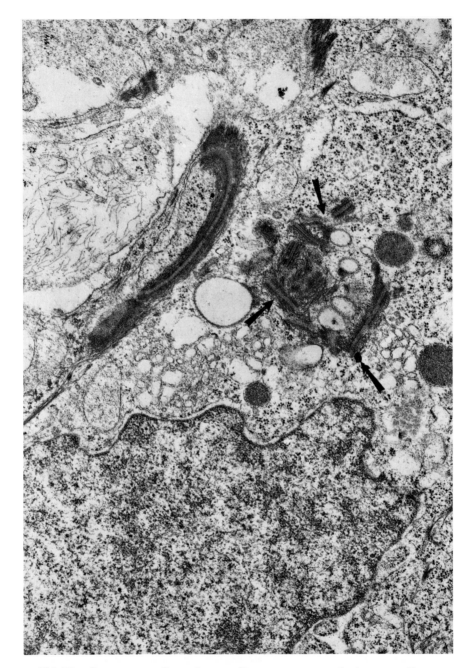

EM 38. **Squamous cell carcinoma.** Desmosomes attached to tonofilaments (*arrows*) can be seen within the cytoplasm of the tumor cells. (×25,000) (See p. 502.)

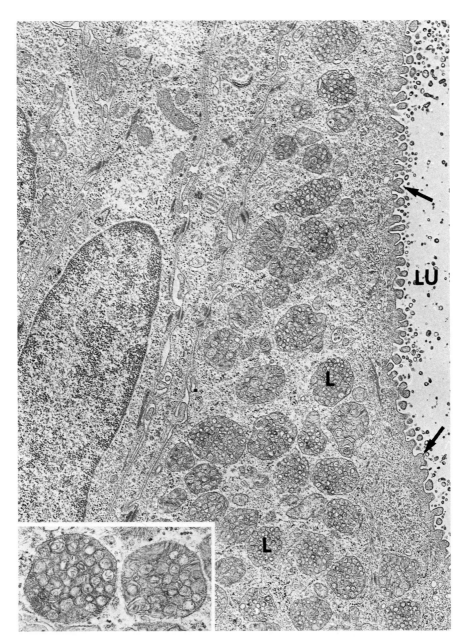

EM 39. **Syringoma.** *Inset:* **Lysosomes.** The lumen (*LU*) of a duct is lined by ductal cells showing numerous microvilli (*arrows*) and many lysosomes (*L*). (×15,000) (See p. 552.) **Inset:** Two lysosomes at higher magnification. (×37,500) (See p. 53.)

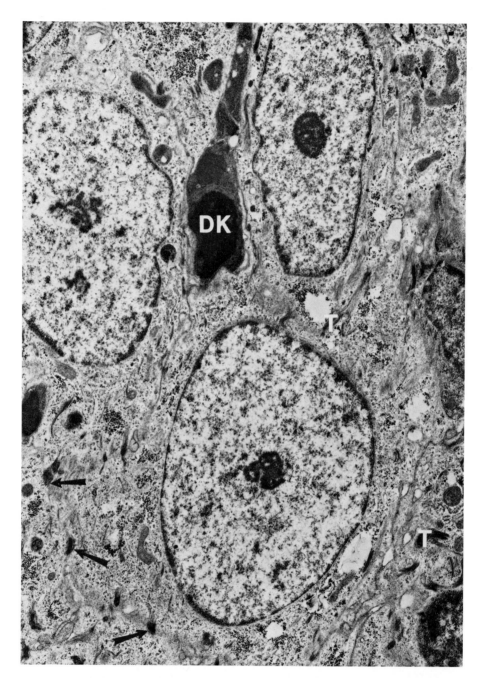

EM 40. **Basal cell epithelioma.** The cells show evidence of keratinization. In addition to tonofilaments (*T*) and desmosomes (*arrows*), some dyskeratotic material (*DK*) is present. (×10,000) (See p. 574.)

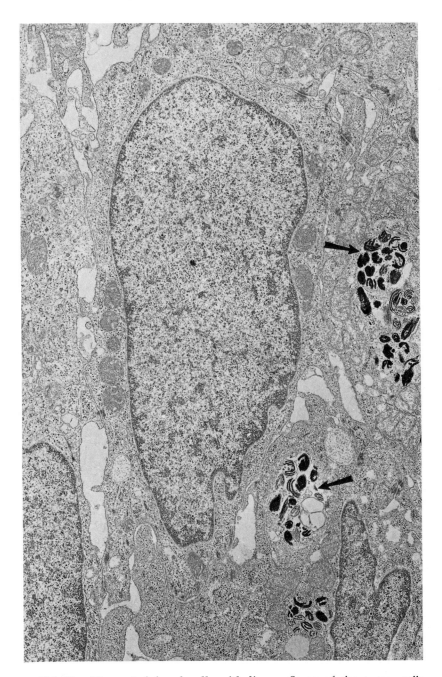

EM 41. **Pigmented basal cell epithelioma.** Some of the tumor cells contain melanosome complexes located within lysosomes (*arrows*). (× 12,500) (See p. 574.)

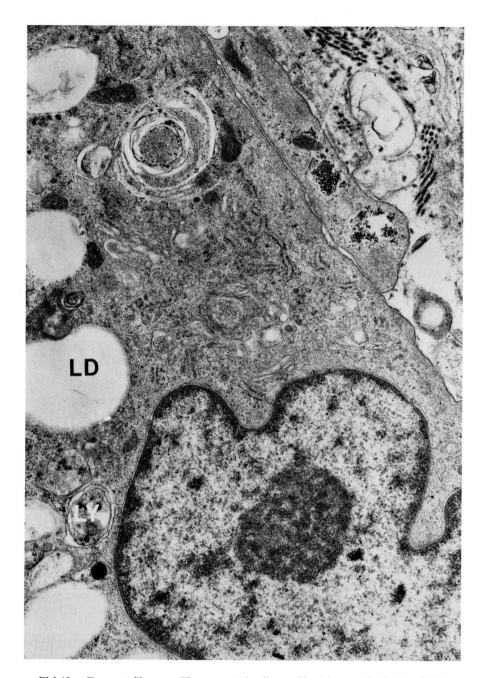

EM 42.   **Dermatofibroma.** The essential cells are fibroblasts, which, in addition to producing collagen, are engaged in phagocytosis and storage of lipid. *LY*, lysosome; *LD*, lipid droplets. (Courtesy of B. Mihatsch-Konz, M.D.) (×20,000) (See p. 600.)

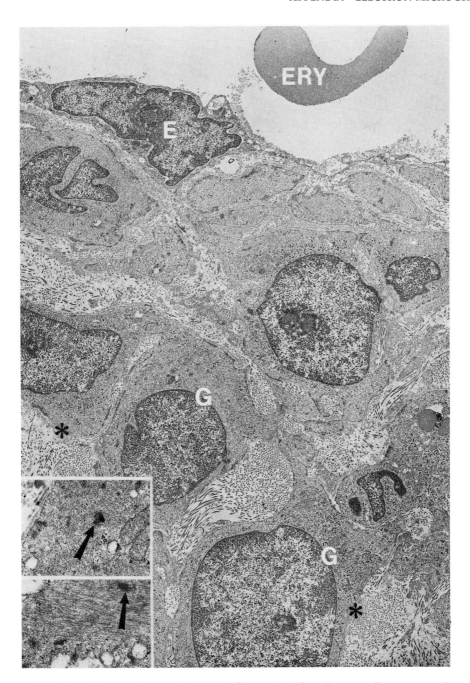

EM 43. **Glomus tumor.** *Inset:* **Myofilaments.** The glomus cells are smooth muscle cells. Each glomus cell is surrounded by a basal lamina (*asterisk*). *E*, endothelial cell of capillary; *G*, glomus cell; *ERY*, erythrocyte within capillary lumen. (×7500) (See p. 634.) **Insets:** The *upper* inset shows the myofilaments in cross section, the *lower* inset in longitudinal section. *Arrows* point to so-called dense bodies. (×30,000) (See p. 35.)

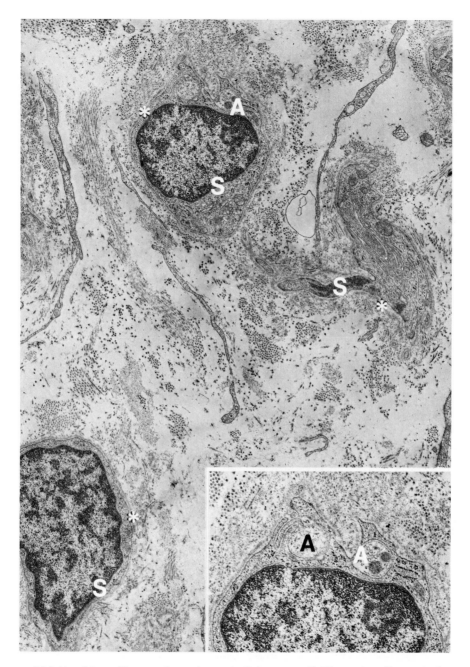

EM 44.   **Neurofibroma.** *Inset:* **Axons in Schwann cell.** The main cell type is the Schwann cell (*S*). Each cell is surrounded by a basal lamina (*asterisks*). Schwann cells contain axons (*A*) in their cytoplasm. (×10,000) (See p. 634.) **Inset:** Two axons (*A*) of the upper Schwann cell are shown at higher magnification. (×20,000) (See p. 634.)

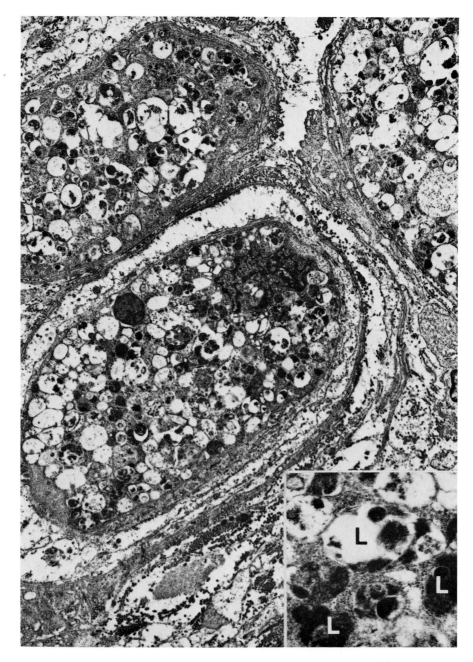

EM 45. **Granular cell tumor.** *Inset:* **Cytoplasmic granules.** The cells contain numerous cytoplasmic granules, which are lysosomes. (×8250) (See p. 675.) **Inset:** The lysosomes (*L*) are shown at higher magnification. (×25,000) (See p. 53.)

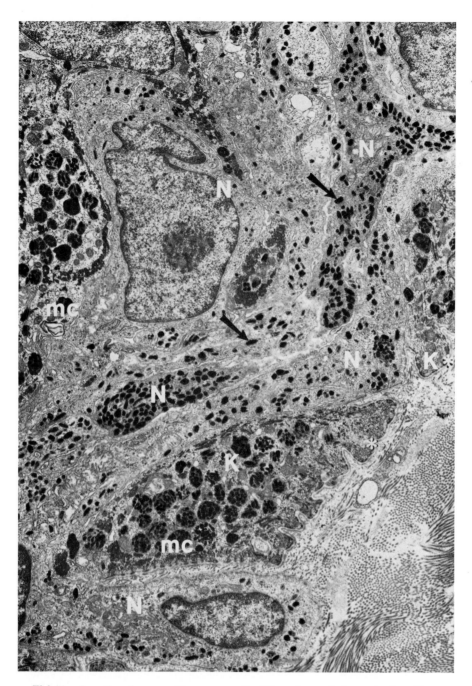

EM 46. **Junctional nevus.** The nevus cells (*N*) are located above the basal lamina (*asterisks*) and contain an abundance of melanosomes (*arrows*). Adjacent keratinocytes (*K*) contain numerous melanosome complexes (*mc*). (×7500) (See p. 686.)

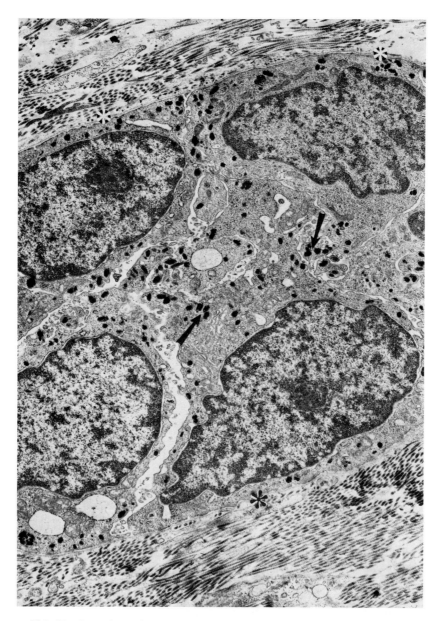

EM 47. **Intradermal nevus cell nest.** The nevus cell nest is surrounded by a basal lamina (*asterisk*). There are no desmosomes between adjacent nevus cells. The nevus cells contain numerous melanosomes (*arrows*). (×10,000) (See p. 687.)

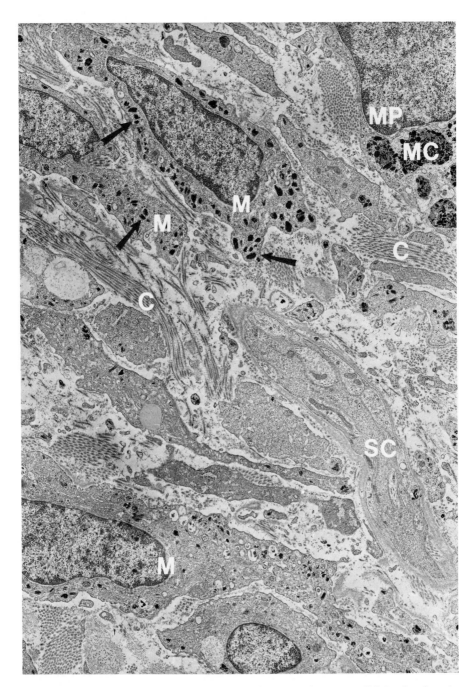

EM 48.   **Blue nevus.** The predominant cells are melanocytes (*M*) in the dermis. In addition, melanophages (*MP*) containing melanosome complexes (*MC*) are found. *Arrows*, melanosomes in melanocytes; *SC*, Schwann cell; *C*, collagen. (×8000) (See p. 702.)

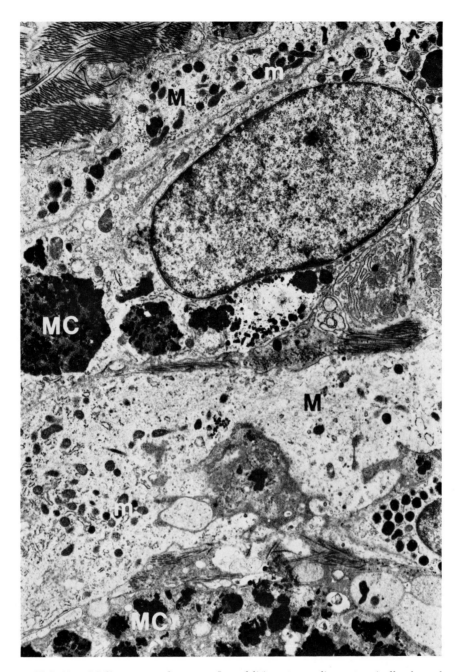

EM 49. **Malignant melanoma.** In addition to malignant spindle-shaped melanocytes (*M*) containing an abundance of melanosomes (*m*), melanophages with melanosome complexes (*MC*) are found. (×8000) (See p. 715.)

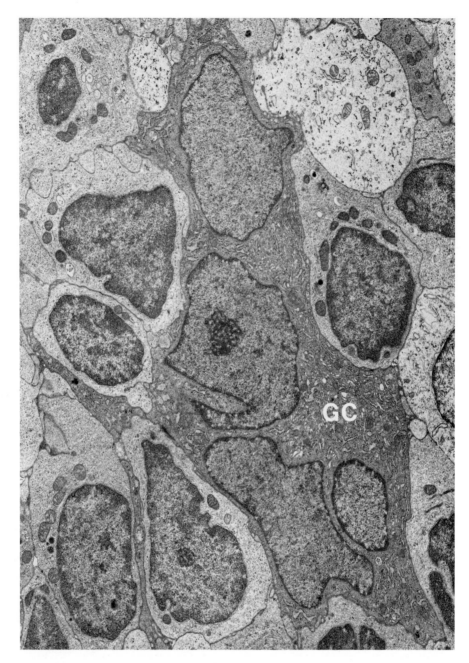

EM 50. **Hodgkin's disease: Sternberg–Reed giant cell.** This giant cell (*GC*) either is multinucleated or has a multilobular nucleus. (×8000) (See p. 728.)

Index

Index

The principal discussion of each subject is indicated by **boldface** type. Page numbers in *italics* indicate illustrative or tabular material. The letter "n" indicates a footnote.